Pharmacology

Drug Therapy and Nursing Considerations

Fourth Edition

Pharmacology

Drug Therapy and Nursing Considerations

Roger T. Malseed, PhD
Adjunct Associate Professor of Pharmacology
The University of Pennsylvania School of Nursing
Philadelphia College of Pharmacy and Science
Philadelphia, Pennsylvania

Frederick J. Goldstein, PhD, FCP
Professor of Pharmacology
Department of Physiology and Pharmacology
Philadelphia College of Osteopathic Medicine
and
Clinical Research Associate
Department of Anesthesia
City Avenue Hospital, Graduate Health System
Philadelphia, Pennsylvania

Nancy Balkon, MS, RN, CS, ANP
Clinical Assistant Professor
Adult Health Nursing
State University of New York at Stony Brook
Stony Brook, New York

Fourth Edition

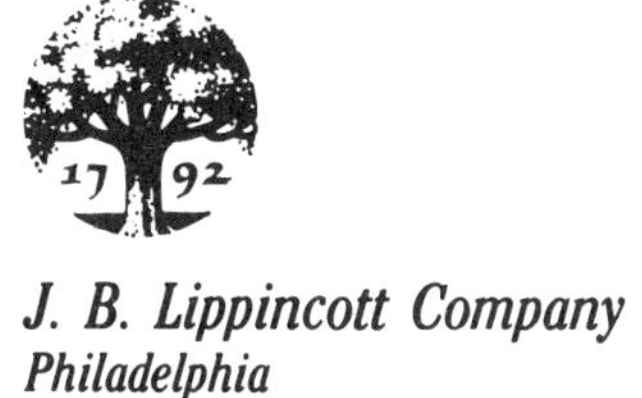

J. B. Lippincott Company
Philadelphia

Sponsoring Editor: Margaret Belcher
Coordinating Editorial Assistant: Emily Cotlier
Project Editor: Susan Deitch
Indexer: Alexandra Nickerson
Design Coordinator: Melissa Olson
Interior Designer: Anne O'Donnell
Cover Designer: Larry Pezzatto
Production Manager: Helen Ewan
Production Coordinator: Robert Randall
Compositor: Circle Graphics
Printer/Binder: Courier Book Company/Kendallville
Cover Printer: Lehigh Press Lithographers

Fourth Edition

6 5 4 3 2 1

Library of Congress Cataloging-in-Publication Data

Malseed, Roger T. (Roger Thomas)
Pharmacology, drug therapy and nursing considerations / Roger T. Malseed, Frederick J. Goldstein, and Nancy Balkon. — 4th ed.
p. cm.
Includes bibliographical references and index.
ISBN 0-397-55061-8
I. Goldstein, Frederick J. II. Balkon, Nancy. III. Title.
[DNLM: 1. Pharmacology—nurses' instruction. 2. Drug Therapy—nurses' instruction. QV 4 M259p 1995]
RM300.M183 1995
615.5'8'024613—dc20
DNLM/DLC
for Library of Congress 94-23363
CIP

Any procedure or practice described in this book should be applied by the health-care practitioner under appropriate supervision in accordance with professional standards of care used with regard to the unique circumstances that apply in each practice situation. Care has been taken to confirm the accuracy of information presented and to describe generally accepted practices. However, the authors, editors, and publisher cannot accept any responsibility for errors or omissions or for any consequences from application of the information in this book and make no warranty express or implied, with respect to the contents of the book.

Every effort has been made to ensure drug selections and dosages are in accordance with current recommendations and practice. Because of ongoing research, changes in government regulations and the constant flow of information on drug therapy, reactions and interactions, the reader is cautioned to check the package insert for each drug for indications, dosages, warnings and precautions, particularly if the drug is new or infrequently used.

To my children, Mark and Natalie, for their continued commitment to excellence in their own educational endeavors.

Roger T. Malseed

To my children, Marty, Eric, and Aliza, for their probing questions, which keep my cerebral cortical neurons operating at a high level, and to my wife, Malkeh, for providing liberal doses of understanding and patience throughout this project.

Fred Goldstein

To my husband, Joe, who always remained optimistic and graciously gave much encouragement, expertise, and time.
To my children, Bryan and Craig, who were always tolerant of deadlines, non-home-cooked meals, and my mood.
To Susan Shapiro, RN, whose enthusiasm and support will never be forgotten.
To my friends, Donna, Kathy, Elayne, and Maryanne, who are *always there*.

Nancy Balkon

Contributors

Joseph Balkon, PhD, DABFT
Professor of Pharmaceutical Sciences
College of Pharmacology & Allied Health Professions
St. John's University
Jamaica, NY

Ara derMarderosian, PhD
Professor of Pharmacognosy and Medicinal Chemistry
Philadelphia College of Pharmacology
Adjunct Professor of Pharmacology and Toxicology
College of Veterinary Medicine, University of Pennsylvania
Adjunct Professor of Pharmacology
Pennsylvania College of Podiatric Medicine
Philadelphia, PA

Henry Hitner, PhD
Department of Physiology & Pharmacology
Philadelphia College of Osteopathic Medicine
Philadelphia, PA

Bruce Livengood, PharmD
Associate Professor
Duquesne University
Pittsburgh, PA

Zoriana Kawka Malseed, PhD
Associate Professor
University of Pennsylvania School of Nursing
Philadelphia, PA

Preface

The provision of adequate health care is the responsibility of numerous members of a therapeutic team. Increasingly, the nurse's role in the delivery and maintenance of safe and efficient drug treatment of disease is expanding, and with such expansion comes the necessity for a broadened base of knowledge relating to the administration and monitoring of drug therapy. Responsible and appropriate intervention on the part of the nurse represents a primary determinant of the overall success of drug treatment. With an increasing number of therapeutic agents available for treatment of disease states, the need for nurses to have access to a current comprehensive source of drugs—one that provides not only detailed pharmacologic information but also topical relative nursing considerations—is acute.

The completely revised and updated fourth edition of *Pharmacology: Drug Therapy and Nursing Considerations* offers just such a source for both the nursing student as well as the practitioner. While the easy-to-use format found in the first three editions of the book has been retained in this new edition, many changes have been introduced in both content and style in order to provide readers with a detailed information base from which they may quickly extract the information needed to administer and monitor drug therapy in the safest and most efficient manner. Most importantly, two additional authors have been employed to bring their expertise and experience to bear in the shaping of the pharmacologic and nursing content. In addition, several other contributors have been recruited to update and expand those sections of the book that relate to their areas of specialty. The result of these additional contributions is evident in the expanded and updated content of many chapters as well as the extensive and relevant nursing content that has been reconceptualized and re-refined.

Among the salient pedagogical features of the fourth edition are:

- Five new chapters dealing with the nurse's role in management of drug therapy, therapeutic drug monitoring, new macrolide antibiotics, dermatologic drugs, and immunomodulatory agents, including a concise review of the functioning of the immune system
- The addition of over 100 new drugs, with both pharmacologic and nursing considerations
- A current bibliographic list following each chapter, encompassing both pharmacologic and nursing-oriented references from recent literature sources
- Revised physiologic review chapters, providing new terminology, including discussions of G-proteins, new second messengers, regulatory digestive peptides, and the role of inflammatory processes in bronchial asthma
- Updated information on anti-infective drugs of choice for treating common infections, including new treatment regimens for tuberculosis and AIDS

In addition, the nursing content has been completely revised and reorganized for the fourth edition, recognizing the prominent position that the nursing profession is assuming in health care. Regardless of educational background, specialty credentials, or practice setting, nurses plan and implement care regimens within the context of a patient's actual and/or potential health problems. Patient advocacy, principles of patient education, and the recognition that each patient is a unique individual and member of a social unit are themes that are central to this process. Within this spirit, the nursing alerts, nursing considerations, and nursing care plans appearing in previous editions have been replaced with guidelines for the nursing management of drug therapy. Specifically, attention is focused on assessment (pretherapy) and the nursing interventions of medication administration, surveillance during therapy, and patient teaching.

The book is divided into 13 sections. Section I presents general principles of pharmacology, including drug administration, pharmacokinetics, sites and mechanisms of drug action, adverse drug effects, interactions, and a new chapter on therapeutic drug monitoring. In addition, revised chapters devoted to pediatric and geriatric aspects of drug therapy present important information regarding proper monitoring procedures in these patient populations. Finally, the legal aspects of drug usage, particularly as they relate to the nurse, are considered as well.

Sections II through XI feature the principal classes of drugs in clinical use today, arranged according to organ system (ie, drugs acting on the nervous system, the cardiovascular system, the renal system, and so forth). Most sections begin with a chapter discussing the physiology of the organ system involved, followed by chapters detailing the individual classes of drugs that affect that particular system. The drugs to be discussed in each chapter are listed at the beginning of the chapter. Aspects of each drug or drug class considered include *Mechanism*, *Uses*, *Dosage*, *Fate*, *Common Side Effects*, *Significant Adverse Reactions*, *Contraindications (including Cautions)*, *Interactions*, and *Nursing Management*. Tables are used frequently throughout the text to group similar drugs, thus facilitating comparisons.

Section XII of the text addresses the problem of drug abuse and dependence. Many different drugs that have the potential for abuse are discussed, and guidelines for recognition and treatment are offered. An extensive listing of "street names" for drugs favored by abusers also is provided.

The Appendices, Section XIII, contain listings of common abbreviations, laboratory values, pregnancy categories, and an IV drug compatibility guide. A general bibliography also is included.

Today, nurses and other health care providers must administer and monitor an enormous array of drug products and are faced with the challenging task of maintaining their knowledge base regarding these drugs as current and accurate as possible.

The fourth edition of *Pharmacology: Drug Therapy and Nursing Considerations* represents a joint effort by several health care professionals and academicians to provide a comprehensive, relevant, and up-to-date source from which nurses and other health care providers may quickly obtain the requisite information to dispense and monitor drugs in a safe and efficient manner.

Acknowledgments

The authors would like to acknowledge the following individuals for their contributions to the book:

Margaret Belcher, Senior Editor, J.B. Lippincott Co.

Susan Deitch, Project Editor, J.B. Lippincott Co.

Joseph Balkon, PhD, DABFT, Contributing Author

Ara derMarderosian, PhD, Contributing Author

Henry Hitner, PhD, Contributing Author

Bruce Livengood, PharmD, Contributing Author

Zoriana Malseed, PhD, Contributing Author

Contents

I

General Principles of Pharmacology

1

The Nurse's Role in the Management of Drug Therapy

From a historical perspective, the past 50 years have been a time of change within nursing. Nurses are defining the profession in terms of its uniqueness, addressing practice issues, and moving the profession into a prominent position within healthcare.

Nurses are educated to recognize and respect the uniqueness of the individual and the effects of this uniqueness on maintenance of health, recovery from illness, the progression of chronic illness, and attainment of peaceful death. They claim to be holistic in their practice, emphasizing a collaborative nurse–patient relationship that recognizes the whole person (biologic, psychological, social, and spiritual) framed within the context of his or her environment.

Regardless of educational background, specialty credentials, or practice setting, nurses are united by the definition of professional nursing, which empowers them to "diagnose and treat human responses to actual and potential health problems" (American Nurses Association, 1980, p. 9), within the context of health promotion (Neuman, 1989; Rogers, 1970). This is true for nurses in staff positions as well as for those nurses who are specially educated and credentialed for advanced practice to diagnose and prescribe.

The nurse's role in the management of drug therapy is intentionally positioned against this backdrop. Medication administration should not be viewed simply as a task-oriented function, emphasizing the five rights of medication administration (right drug, right dose, right time, right route, right patient). Instead, it is an opportunity to combine these basic principles with the nursing process (assessment, diagnosis, planning, implementation, evaluation) to develop safe, appropriate, and effective nursing interventions to 1) prepare and administer drugs, 2) evaluate responses to therapy, 3) teach the patient/family, 4) seek consultation, and 5) make appropriate referrals.

Pretherapy Assessment

An ongoing, accurate, and detailed nursing assessment of the client's physical, psychosocial, and functional characteristics is perhaps the most essential component of the nursing process as it relates to the nursing management of drug therapy. Diagnosis (North American Nursing Diagnosis Association nursing diagnoses), planning (goal setting), implementation (intervention), and evaluation all depend on skilled assessment. Assessment provides the data base from which all planning and intervention are derived. The evaluation of outcomes also depends on an accurate, unbiased assessment.

The assessment process begins before the initiation of drug therapy and continues on an ongoing basis throughout therapy. The nurse should obtain, record, or review important baseline data that will assist in making nursing judgments and in the early detection of expected and undesirable adverse effects. The type of data to review varies from drug to drug, but usually includes nursing assessment data (subjective and objective), baseline vital signs, height and weight, and laboratory work and diagnostic studies. In addition, medical history should be reviewed to determine the presence of conditions that may contraindicate the use of a drug or suggest that it be administered with caution. Such conditions include current physical status, history of chronic illness, patient age, allergy to drug or drug family, and pregnancy or lactation (Table 1-1).

Specific interventions related to the pretherapy assessment are as follows:

- Assess and record important baseline data necessary for detection of adverse effects (perform a detailed, individualized nursing assessment).
- Review past medical history and documents for evidence of existing or previous medical history related to conditions that require cautious administration of a prescribed drug.
- Review past medical history and documents for evidence of existing or previous medical history related to conditions that contraindicate use of a drug.

Assessing and Recording Baseline Data

The purpose of the use of a therapeutic medication is to provide a beneficial effect. The decision to use pharmacologic therapy is fundamentally based on the assessment of the benefit-to-risk ratio. The more difficult component of this assessment often is the determination of risk, the potential for a detrimental outcome in the patient as a result of the use of the drug. Sometimes, this is not realized until the patient actually has received the medication, is experiencing its therapeutic effect, and begins to experience an adverse or toxic effect as well. The adverse effects of drugs appear in many forms and may present in subtle ways, often indistinguishable from "normal" aberrations in physiologic function. In addition, adverse effects, like therapeutic responses, may develop slowly. An accurate baseline assessment focused on those physiologic functions where the typical adverse effects of the drug are expressed is crucial for the detection of incipient changes due to the drug. Some baseline parameters are target organ focused (cardiovascular [blood pressure, heart rate, electrocardiogram] or central nervous system [orientation, bilateral grip strength]), whereas others are derived from laboratory data (liver function tests, hematologic parameters).

From a practical perspective, it is not unusual for the nurse to suspect that a patient is beginning to experience an adverse response to therapy and to report his or her perception to the practitioner–prescriber. Often the detection of an adverse effect is contingent on the observation of a *change* in the patient's condition or physiologic and biochemical parameters.

Table 1-1. Nursing Management of Drug Therapy

Pretherapy Assessment

- Assess and record important baseline data necessary for detection of adverse effects (perform a detailed, individualized nursing assessment).
- Review past medical history and documents for evidence of existing or previous medical history related to conditions that
  a. require cautious administration of a prescribed drug: pregnancy; lactation; patient age; patient medical history.
  b. contraindicate use of a drug: allergy to prescribed drug or drug family; pregnancy; lactation; patient age; patient medical history.

Nursing Interventions

Medication Administration

- Administer drugs to maximize their intended effects and minimize their adverse effects. For example, administer diuretics in the morning to reduce the need to void at night.
- Plan and implement individualized nursing interventions that
  a. inform the patient about the expected actions and adverse effects of a prescribed drug.
  b. identify the early onset of (expected or undesirable) adverse effects and intervene appropriately.
  c. minimize the symptoms produced by the expected adverse effects of the prescribed drug.
  d. identify the safety needs of the patient and intervene appropriately to minimize environmental hazards or risk of injury.

Surveillance During Therapy

- Always monitor the drug dose being administered. Rationale: to ensure that it is within acceptable limits for the diagnosis and patient being treated.
- Compare current status with previous status to detect improvements or deterioration in the patient's condition.
- Monitor patient for therapeutic drug effect.
- Monitor for adverse effects, toxicity, and interactions.
- Monitor for signs of hypersensitivity, which may require discontinuation of drug.
- Facilitate acquisition of diagnostic tests ordered for ongoing assessment of drug response.
- Monitor diagnostic test results obtained over the course of therapy.
- Interpret results of diagnostic tests and contact practitioner–prescriber as appropriate.
- Monitor for possible drug–laboratory test interactions.
- Monitor for possible drug–drug and drug–nutrient interactions.

Patient Teaching

- Instruct patient about expected actions and possible adverse effects of prescribed drug.
- Instruct patient about appropriate action to take if adverse effects occur:
  a. how to manage symptoms related to expected adverse effects of prescribed drugs.
  b. when to notify practitioner–prescriber.
  c. under which conditions to discontinue administration of prescribed drug before notification of practitioner–prescriber.
  d. under which conditions to seek immediate medical attention if adverse side effects develop.
- Instruct patient about the importance of completing the full course of therapy as prescribed, that is, not to discontinue the drug once signs and symptoms have subsided.
- Inform patient of the consequences of not taking or abruptly discontinuing a prescribed drug.
- Instruct patient that a prescribed drug is to be taken only in the manner and for the condition for which it is prescribed.
- Instruct patient to keep all medications out of the reach of children.

Medication History

A medication history should be obtained during the pretherapy assessment. This includes a listing of all prescribed drugs and over-the-counter (OTC) drugs, as well as alcohol (ethanol), caffeine, nicotine, and illegal drugs. The medication history is used to identify drugs the patient is currently taking as well as those that the patient may have taken in the past.

The *profile of current medications* provides the necessary data (type of medication, route of administration, frequency of administration) required to determine the 1) adequacy/efficacy of the current therapeutic drug regimen, 2) the degree of patient compliance with therapy, and 3) the presence of expected and/or unanticipated and adverse effects.

A *profile of drugs previously taken* often is elicited while obtaining the past medical history. Such information provides valuable insight into the progression of disease, the patient's responsiveness to treatment, the effectiveness of teaching, compliance with therapy, and drug hypersensitivity or adverse reactions.

Over-the-Counter Drugs

A careful history of OTC drugs also is warranted. Because OTC drugs are available without prescription and may be taken at will, the identification of their use in the patient's medical record often is overlooked. Although OTC medications generally are considered "weaker" drugs, which have a wider margin of safety in their use, the interaction of OTC pharmaceuticals with legend (prescribed) pharmaceuticals remains a significant problem.

It is not unusual to find that OTC products are being used by the patient, without the knowledge of the prescriber, to mask or symptomatically deal with side effects produced by prescription medications the patient is currently using—for example, the use of nasal decongestants to offset the side effects of antihypertensive agents, or the use of laxatives or antacids to ameliorate gastrointestinal side effects. The patient may not even be aware that the symptoms the OTC product is being used to treat are a side effect of a prescribed drug, but a careful assessment of potential OTC drug use can uncover such use and the patient's reasons for it.

Alcohol

Alcohol (ethanol) is the most frequently used drug in today's society. Obtaining an accurate history of past and current alcohol consumption provides information necessary for patient teaching regarding alcohol consumption in relation to the medication about to be prescribed. Many medications cannot be used with patients who ingest alcohol because the drug effect can be additive or diminutive in the presence of alcohol. In addition, an accurate history regarding alcohol usage may provide insights into possible contraindications or cautions to the use of the prescribed medication in view of possible diminished hepatic or renal function.

Nicotine

A careful history of current and past use of nicotine-containing products also is important before drug administration. Nicotine-containing products include tobacco that is smoked (cigarettes, cigars, pipe tobacco) as well as tobacco that is chewed or self-administered buccally. Nicotine has powerful effects on the body, including the liver, where it may enhance or retard metabolic capacity. There are numerous examples of the impact of nicotine (tobacco use) on drug metabolism, which may alter the dose of the medication that the patient requires.

For the smoker, the extent of tobacco use is commonly characterized in the form of "pack-years" of use; represented by the number of packs of cigarettes smoked per day multiplied by the number of years of smoking. For example, a person who has smoked one pack of cigarettes per day for the last 20 years would be described as having smoked 20 pack-years. For those who smoke cigars or use a pipe, there is no comparable characterization; however, it is important to ascertain in these people the degree to which inhalation of the smoke from these sources occurs. For those who use tobacco products orally, careful documentation of the frequency of use is often important.

Illegal Drugs

The use of an illegal drug while being treated with a prescribed medication can result in life-threatening outcomes. Typical illegal drugs that are commonly abused today include marijuana, cocaine, opioids, amphetamines, central nervous system depressants, and volatile inhalants, such as butane and nitrous oxide. It also is important to remember that a *prescription medication* used by a person without a prescription is an *illegal use* of a drug.

It often is difficult to get a patient to reveal illegal drug use, because identification of such carries strong social connotations. It is very important, however, to identify such use because of the potential impact of these agents on responses to prescribed medications, and because of the impact of this information on patient teaching.

Reviewing Conditions That Require Cautious Administration of a Prescribed Drug

All prescribed medications have associated with their use situations or conditions in which the benefit-to-risk ratio is diminished compared to the "average" patient. Typical considerations include impaired liver and/or renal function that may impede the elimination of the drug from the body; altered cardiovascular function, which may alter the manner in which the drug is distributed in the body; altered central nervous system responsiveness, which may affect the way the person behaves in response to the drug; and preexisting hematologic, gastrointestinal, pulmonary, and other system disorders that place the patient at greater risk for adverse effects.

An important area of concern that requires caution in drug administration relates to the impact of maternal drug usage on the fetus (use of a medication in pregnancy) and on the neonate (use of a medication in the nursing mother).

Fetal Risk

The framework for the consideration of use of a medication in the pregnant patient *or* the patient who intends or desires pregnancy has been codified by the Food and Drug Administration (FDA) in the form of Pregnancy Categories. Almost all prescription medications are characterized by a Pregnancy Category. The following summarizes the FDA risk factor categories for drugs used in the pregnant patient:

Pregnancy Category A: controlled studies in women fail to demonstrate a risk to the fetus in the first trimester (the most sensitive teratogenic period) and no evidence exists for risk in later trimesters; therefore the possibility of fetal harm related to the use of the drug by the mother appears remote.

Pregnancy Category B: no controlled studies have been performed in pregnant women, but animal studies have not demonstrated a fetal risk related to maternal drug use, *or* adverse effects seen in animal reproductive studies have not been confirmed in controlled studies with women pregnant in the first trimester. In addition, there is no evidence of risk to the fetus in later trimesters.

Pregnancy Category C: Either animal studies have revealed teratogenic, embryotoxic, or other adverse effects on the fetus (and no controlled studies have been performed on pregnant women), *or* no studies of the drug have been performed on animals or women. The risk to the human fetus is unknown. The drug should be administered in pregnancy only if the potential benefit justifies the potential risk to the fetus.

Pregnancy Category D: Positive evidence of adverse risk to the human fetus has been obtained; however, the benefits of use in the pregnant woman may outweigh the risk to the fetus (ie, use of a drug in a life-threatening situation, or for a serious disorder for which safer drugs are not available or are ineffective). A careful assessment of the benefit-to-risk ratio is a requirement for Category D drugs before they can be used in the pregnant woman.

Pregnancy Category X: Fetal abnormalities have been demonstrated in animals or women, and there is evidence of significant fetal risk based on human experience. The risk of fetal hazard as a result of the use of the drug in the pregnant woman clearly outweighs any possible benefit. Here the drug is *contraindicated* in women who are or *may become* pregnant.

Pregnancy Category NR: The drug has not been rated by the FDA for a pregnancy risk factor category.

Neonatal Risk

An equally important concern is that of neonatal exposure to a drug as a result of administration of that drug to the mother, where the neonatal exposure occurs as a result of breast-feeding. Most drugs administered to the mother appear in breast milk. The evaluation of the possible effect of this occurrence on the neonate often is complicated by the absence of information on many drugs, or the lack of complete information relating drug concentrations in breast milk to dose and dose timing. In addition, some information on drugs in breast milk is derived solely from animal studies, and in some cases, reports of toxic effects in the neonate do not include the information on the quantity of the drug in breast milk or the quantity of breast milk ingested. These are necessary for the estimation of the neonatal dose.

Because of these uncertainties, the recommendations regarding the use of a medication in the nursing mother may fall within three broad categories:

No reported effects: either the drug is not secreted in breast milk *or* the concentrations of the drug in breast milk are far below those consistent with the production of a pharmacologic or toxicologic effect in the neonate.

Use with caution: concentrations of the medication are known to be present in breast milk and are possibly sufficient to produce a pharmacologic effect; however, such an effect is considered to be of minimal significance or hazard to the neonate.

Use is contraindicated: The drug is secreted in breast milk in concentrations sufficient to produce an undesired response in the neonate; therefore the drug should not be administered to the nursing mother, *or* the mother should discontinue nursing the infant while on the medication. Examples of drugs known to be contraindicated during the breast-feeding period include cimetidine, cyclophosphamide, cyclosporine, doxorubicin, ergotamine, gold salts, methimazole, methotrexate, and lithium.

Reviewing Conditions That Contraindicate Use of a Drug

Contraindication

A contraindication is basically an absolute warning that, in certain conditions or situations, a particular drug must never be used or the patient almost certainly will be severely harmed. A careful consideration of any preexisting conditions in relation to known contraindications (as published by the manufacturer and appearing in the medication's package insert) is an important safety measure for the protection of the patient. If a contraindicating condition is identified, the drug normally would not be appropriate for use; the benefit-to-risk ratio would be strongly shifted in the risk direction. A common contraindication for all drugs is that of hypersensitivity or allergy to that particular drug or drug group.

Allergy

Drug allergy can occur in four different ways:

1. *Immediate reactivity* (*Type I*) may result in life-threatening anaphylaxis.
2. *Drug-induced autoimmune disorders* (*Type II*) typically are reflected in disturbances of hematologic function.
3. *Tissue reactions* (*Type III*) are evidenced by skin eruptions, painful joints, and drug fever.
4. *Reexposure episodes* (*Type IV*) (dermatologic) usually are exhibited in the form of contact dermatitis.

Once sensitization has occurred, the allergic reaction produced by a drug may vary in intensity from an immediate, life-threatening anaphylactic reaction to a delayed reaction in the form of contact dermatitis.

Other common contraindicating conditions to use of many drugs include hepatic and renal disorders, cardiovascular disease, psychiatric disorders, and disturbances of endocrine function.

Nursing Interventions

Three nursing interventions are central to the nursing management of drug therapy: *Medication Administration*, *Surveillance During Therapy*, and *Patient Teaching*. They serve as broad categories within which other interventions are included as appropriate for each drug and clinical situation.

Medication Administration

Medication administration, as an intervention, focuses on methods for 1) giving medications, 2) evaluating response to drug therapy (surveillance during therapy), 3) patient/family teaching, and 4) providing for patient safety. It is expected that these interventions will be specific for each drug and reflect the requirements of each patient as a unique individual (see Table 1-1).

Surveillance During Therapy

The assessment process continues throughout drug therapy and includes the periodic comparison of baseline data with current data to identify actual and potential problems and assess outcomes of nursing interventions, patient responses to drug therapy (evaluation), the need for patient/family teaching, and the need for consultation and referral. If necessary, the nursing process is updated; that is, diagnoses, plans (goals), and interventions are modified and made current to correspond with changes noted (see Table 1-1).

Typical ongoing assessment considerations include the following:

Monitoring the drug dose being administered.

It is important to ensure that the dose is within acceptable limits for the diagnosis and patient being treated. This is particularly important in situations in which the drug is being used to treat a chronic disorder. Chronic disorders exhibit a variety of disease severity profiles that have one common feature: The severity of the disease state is in a continual state of change. The implication of this observation is that the dose of a therapeutic medication used in the treatment of a chronic disorder would be expected to change.

Comparing current status with previous status to detect improvements or deterioration in the patient's condition.

Comparative evaluation of the patient's condition often provides the best reflection of the effectiveness or lack thereof of the therapeutic regimen.

Monitoring patient for therapeutic drug effect.

Therapeutic effects of a drug during the early phases of therapy may be present only during a portion of the dosage interval. Once steady-state concentrations have been attained, the response of the patient to the drug would be expected to exhibit a sustained pattern. The absence of a sustained response over the dosage interval may be an indication for dose adjustment. Monitoring the response of the patient to the medication can identify whether the patient's disorder is responsive to the pharmacotherapeutic regimen. Monitoring pharmacotherapeutic response also can identify changes in the patient's ability to respond, secondary to factors such as the development of drug tolerance or an increased rate of drug metabolism. In the case of antibiotic therapy, changes in the patient's status may point to the development of superinfection induced by the antibiotic therapy.

Monitoring for adverse effects, toxicity, and interactions.
In the care of a patient, there is one constant factor that provides for continuity in the clinical setting: the continuing presence of the patient's nurse! The nurse is in the optimum position to identify changes in the patient's status reflecting the onset of adverse effects, drug toxicity, or interaction between therapeutic modalities.

Monitoring for signs of hypersensitivity, which may require discontinuation of drug.
The typical presentations of drug allergy have been discussed. It is important that the nurse be aware of the symptoms of drug hypersensitivity, so that if a patient manifests a drug allergy, it will be recognized, and the drug regimen discontinued before the development of possible life-threatening anaphylactoid symptoms.

Facilitating and monitoring diagnostic test results obtained over the course of therapy.
As stated, adverse drug responses occur in many forms. Often, adverse responses to drug regimens initially are indicated by changes in laboratory parameters, ranging from changes in serum electrolytes or serum enzymes to changes in hematologic parameters. Significant changes often are recognized first by the nurse. The nurse needs to be aware of the potential for drug-induced changes in laboratory parameters.

Monitoring for possible drug–laboratory test interactions.
In addition to observing for adverse drug effects as reflected in changes in the patient's laboratory findings, the nurse also needs to be aware of the potential of some drugs to alter the results of laboratory measurements. This can make accurate interpretation of laboratory findings difficult.

Monitoring for possible drug–drug and drug–nutrient interactions.
The necessity for recognizing potential drug–drug and drug–nutrient interactions continues throughout the patient's therapeutic course as new medications are added to the therapeutic regimen. The nurse should be continually vigilant of the possibilities for drug–drug and drug–nutrient interactions that are harmful to the patient.

Patient Teaching

Patient teaching is central to the nursing management of drug therapy, because it begins with the pretherapy nursing assessment and continues for the duration of therapy. Patient teaching may be informal and incidental, as, for example, when a patient is taught the proper method of drug administration or what to expect in terms of drug response during an emergency situation. Patient teaching also is formal, such as teaching a newly diagnosed type I diabetic about insulin, its administration, and how to obtain and monitor blood glucose by fingerstick. To teach, the nurse must assess the learner (readiness to learn, mental and physical abilities) and devise a teaching plan that is tailored to the individual. Formal teaching should be planned and initiated well enough in advance so that modifications can be made as needed, and ample time is allowed for return demonstration and evaluation of "student" achievement. Family should be taught along with the patient, especially if they will be copartners in care (see Plan of Nursing Care 1-1).

Compliance With Drug Therapy

Compliance with drug therapy or the potential for poor compliance or noncompliance lie within the framework of nursing management of drug therapy because they are directly linked to the accurate evaluation of patient responses to drug therapy (therapeutic outcomes) and outcomes of nursing interventions.

Compliance, to do what is asked with regard to drug therapy, is a desired patient outcome. Poor compliance or noncompliance are labels commonly used when an unsuccessful therapeutic regimen can be linked to patient behavior. These labels easily shift responsibility away from the health professionals, suggesting that the patient or family has done something wrong. Instead, one might consider poor compliance or noncompliance with pharmacologic therapy as a "symptom" indicating failure of the healthcare system adequately to assess and anticipate a patient or family's needs, and plan appropriate interventions and follow-up.

Poor compliance may result in inadequate therapy, prolongation of treatment, recurrence of illness, unnecessary hospitalization, adverse effects and toxicity, and added financial expense. Several factors typically impair compliance with drug therapy, and should be assessed. They include the patient's: 1) attitude toward his or her illness (especially in the presence of long-term therapy or chronic disease); 2) health beliefs; 3) knowledge of the disease process and its management; 4) mental–cognitive functioning; 5) physical ability (presence of physical disability, vision impairment, decreased manual dexterity); 6) social and emotional support systems; 7) access to care; and 8) financial status and health insurance coverage (because drugs are expensive and may not be reimbursed by a health plan). The nurse also must be aware that certain prescriptive practices such as prescribing dosage forms that are inappropriate for the patient or difficult to use, prescribing multiple drugs (polypharmacy), use of frequent dosing schedules, and using multiple prescribers increase the risk of poor compliance (see Plan of Nursing Care 1-2).

Summary

Certain behaviors, if observed by the nurse, indicate the need for immediate reassessment of a drug regimen because patient safety is at risk. They include: 1) the inability of a patient to give an adequate current drug history (drug, indication for use, dosing, and so forth); 2) acute changes in physical status, behavior, or mental–cognitive function; 3) evidence (or reports) of injury or falls; 4) intense symptoms of expected or undesirable adverse drug effects; 5) requests for changes in drug therapy; 6) frequent requests for prescription refills or long periods between prescription refills; 7) excessive or inappropriate use of OTC drugs; and 8) saving previously prescribed drugs when no longer indicated for use.

Nursing assessment before and during drug therapy assists the practitioner–prescriber in uncovering issues related to compliance and facilitates the initiation of timely interventions on the patient's behalf, such as the reevaluation of therapy; adjusting the dosing regimen, route of administration, or method of administration; or patient education.

Plan of Nursing Care 1-1

Patients Whose Knowledge of Drug Regimen is Deficient

Nursing Diagnosis: *Knowledge Deficit Regarding Drug Therapy Related to: (cite etiology specific to each patient situation)*

Goal: *Patient will possess knowledge and skills needed to implement drug regimen and related actions.*

Intervention	Rationale
Assess patient's readiness to learn, current level of understanding, and factors likely to influence learning.	Learning can be impeded by physical, emotional, or social factors such as pain, extreme anxiety, and cultural background. To help ensure success, teaching should begin at current level of understanding.
Initiate planning when patient is ready to learn.	Motivation significantly affects learning.
Explain the need for and the benefits of learning.	Learning is enhanced when information is presented in response to expressed need.
Determine whether patient is likely to benefit more from individual or group sessions, formal or incidental teaching.	Drug instruction may be provided to individuals or groups. In formal teaching, instruction is the primary activity. Incidental teaching occurs in conjunction with other activities.
Establish goals and teaching plan with patient.	Identification of objectives, responsibilities, approaches, tools, and sequence of instruction improves teaching/learning efficiency. Patient involvement promotes cooperation and success.
Involve different senses and include active learning experiences.	Involvement of multiple senses and active learning experiences enhances learning and improves retention.
Sequence learning from simple to complex.	Learning is easier if content progresses from simple to complex.
Arrange for significant others to attend teaching sessions.	Significant others can support and reinforce desired behavior and can administer drug if patient is unable to do so.
Select quiet, private times and environments for teaching.	Distraction and other environmental obstacles impede learning.
Use terminology patient understands and relate content to patient's own experiences.	The patient may be too embarrassed to acknowledge lack of familiarity with complex terminology. Content that relates to the patient's own experiences is more meaningful and easier to grasp.
Pace sessions to correspond to patient's attention span and ability to retain information.	Frequent, short teaching sessions may be more effective than a few lengthy ones.
Teach the following information related to the prescribed drug:	
1. Name of drug and availability of generic preparations	Where generic prescribing exists, the patient needs to know that generic substitutes are available in order to take advantage of them.
2. Drug action, purpose, response expected, length of time it takes to become effective	Compliance improves when the patient's expectations of results are realistic and the patient accepts susceptibility to or diagnosis of the condition being prevented or treated.
3. Dosage, route, and schedule of administration (including whether an oral drug is to be taken before or during meals, how much water or other fluid to take with it, and at what intervals it is to be taken)	Prescription labels may not clearly specify all requirements. Absorption of some drugs, for example, is greatly affected by food.
4. Importance of adhering to prescribed regimen and impact of deviation on drug effects and the condition being prevented or treated	Rigid adherence to the prescribed dosage schedule often is necessary to maintain stable, effective blood levels and minimize adverse reactions. The patient may believe, for example, that if one dose helps, two may be twice as good, possibly paving the way for adverse reactions.

(continued)

Plan of Nursing Care 1-1 (Continued)
Patients Whose Knowledge of Drug Regimen is Deficient

Intervention	Rationale
5. Technique for administration (see Chapter 2 for specific information regarding techniques for particular routes of administration)	Unfamiliar routes of administration may require special explanations (eg, sublingual tablets and troches). Injections usually require multiple demonstration and practice sessions.
6. Length of time drug is to be taken, risks entailed in premature discontinuation	For some drugs, such as antibiotics, effective use may depend on administration over a period of time, even though the patient may feel better before the entire course has been taken. Serious reactions may ensue from sudden cessation of certain drugs, such as some antihypertensives.
7. Usual side effects and how to manage them	Some side effects may be quite alarming if the patient is unaware of their cause, such as black stools from iron tablets or urine discoloration from other drugs. Also, the patient is less likely to discontinue medication when side effects appear if he or she expects them and knows what to do about them.
8. Signs of adverse reactions that should be immediately reported and person to whom they should be reported	The patient needs to be evaluated quickly if signs of serious adverse reactions appear. Symptoms of adverse reactions to some drugs may seem relatively innocuous to the uninformed patient (eg, sore throat, mild fever, itching).
9. Potential interactions with other prescription drugs, OTC drugs, food, and laboratory tests	Serious interactions and toxic effects can occur when medications are combined, even OTC preparations. This can happen if the patient visits more than one healthcare provider, each of whom may be unaware of drugs prescribed by others. Furthermore, the patient may not consider OTC preparations to be drugs, may take drugs prescribed for someone else, and may be unaware of interactions with food and laboratory tests.
10. Techniques for monitoring drug effects and the importance of these	To ensure safe and effective use, some drugs require periodic laboratory tests, such as blood counts or prothrombin times. With certain drugs, such as cardiac glycosides and beta blockers, the patient may need to monitor his or her pulse. The patient receiving hypoglycemics may need to test his or her urine or blood for glucose.
11. Storage requirements	Some drugs need special handling such as refrigeration or storage in light-resistant containers.
12. When and where to get prescription filled and obtain other supplies or services	
13. Safety measures to prevent injury or poisoning	
Encourage patient to ask questions and verbalize understanding of what is taught.	An atmosphere of trust and rapport facilitates the learning process.
Provide positive feedback regarding learning progress.	Learning is enhanced when the patient is aware of progress. Rewarded behaviors tend to be repeated.
Repeat information in various ways.	Repetition improves retention.
Provide written material to supplement content taught in other ways.	Written material serves as memory aid and reference source.
Refer patient to appropriate community healthcare agencies for follow-up or further instruction as needed.	The elderly or chronically ill patient or one with few support systems may need additional evaluation or instruction in the home setting.

OTC, over-the-counter.

Plan of Nursing Care 1-2

Patient Compliance With a Prescribed Drug Regimen

Nursing Diagnosis: *Potential Noncompliance With Drug Therapy Related to: (cite etiology specific to each patient situation)*

Goal: *Patient will follow prescribed drug regimen.*

Intervention	**Rationale**
Assess patient's attitude towards drug therapy; if problematic, devise strategies to resolve.	Numerous complex factors affect compliance with drug therapy, including attitudes about drug therapy and the nature of the condition being prevented or treated. Compliance tends to be better when evidence that drugs control symptoms or disease is apparent to the patient, which is more often the case in short-term, acute conditions.
Assess patient's level of knowledge and skills related to drug therapy: if inadequate, see **Plan of Nursing Care 1-1 (Knowledge Deficit).**	The patient cannot comply without the knowledge or skills needed to implement the drug regimen.
Ascertain ability to pay for drugs; if problematic, refer patient to appropriate resources.	The elderly and the poor are most likely to need prescription drugs and least able to pay for them.
Assess ability to remember to take drugs at prescribed times; if problematic, devise individualized, mutually agreeable, and realistic strategies to encourage and facilitate compliance, such as the use of home-made or purchased memory aids.	The elderly, in whom memory may be failing, are most likely to require pharmacologic therapy.
Assess ability to prepare drugs for administration: if childproof caps are too difficult to manage, inform patient that a regular cap may be requested. If vision is impaired, select an appropriate visual aid, teach a significant other to prepare the drug, or refer patient to a home healthcare agency, which may be able to prepare multiple doses during a home visit (eg, a week's supply of daily insulin injections drawn up in syringes).	The patient may have handicaps, such as arthritis or visual impairments, that interfere with appropriate drug use.
Determine ability to obtain medications; if problematic, explore options for acquired prescriptions and delivery of drugs to patient's home that are appropriate for each given situation.	Difficulty going up and down steps to get outdoors; weather that is too hot or too cold; lack of safe, affordable, convenient public transportation; inability to drive a car; and other factors may impede patient visits to either the drug practitioner–prescriber or the drugstore.
Assess support systems; if inadequate, suggest to healthcare provider that patient be followed more closely or refer patient for home help.	Support systems affect motivation and ability to use drugs (obtain, remember to take, administer). If inadequate, closer follow-up is indicated (eg, frequent, short telephone calls from care providers improve compliance, as do short waiting periods for visits to care providers).
Collaborate with patient, significant others, and practitioner–prescriber to ensure that the following are as few, as simple, and as convenient as possible:	The simpler the drug regimen and the more conveniently it fits into daily living patterns, the more likely the patient is to comply with it.
1. Numbers of dosage forms (eg, one-half, one, two)	Most drugs are available in several dosages. Sometimes one preparation can be substituted for two that contain half the dose. Many oral preparations combine two or more drugs in one product (eg, many antihypertensive drug combinations), reducing the number of different formulations that need to be taken.

(continued)

Plan of Nursing Care 1-2 (Continued)
Patient Compliance With a Prescribed Drug Regimen

Intervention	Rationale
2. Types of dosage forms (eg, tablet, capsule, solution)	Many patients find it easier to swallow capsules than tablets, easier to swallow liquids than capsules. The dosage form should suit individual needs and preferences to the extent possible.
3. Numbers of times a day drugs are taken	For a drug with a long half-life, it may be possible to increase the dosage and reduce the number of times a day it is taken; or, a timed-release (sustained-action) preparation, if available, might be used.
4. Routes of administration	Certain routes of administration tend to be more objectionable than others (eg, rectal, parenteral) and more difficult to fit into certain lifestyles.
Assist patient to plan a daily dosing schedule for all medications being used.	Many patients take numerous drugs and have difficulty figuring out an appropriate daily dosing schedule.
Promote patient's faith and trust in the drug prescriber.	Faith and trust in the person prescribing the drug tends to improve compliance.

Nursing Bibliography

American Nurses Association: Nursing: A Social Policy Statement. Kansas City, MO, American Nurses Association, 1980

Kilroy R, Iafrate R: Provision of pharmaceutical care in the I.C.U. Critical Care Nursing Clinics of North America 5(2):221–226, 1993

McCloskey JC, Bulechek GM (eds). Nursing Interventions Classification (NIC). St. Louis, Mosby Year Book, 1992

Neuman B. The Neuman Systems Model. Norwalk, CT, Appleton and Lange, 1989

Sommer C, Kravitz M: Analysis of a pharmacology test. Journal Staff Development 5(2):274–277, 1992

2

Methods of Drug Administration

Selection of the route by which a drug will be administered depends on several major considerations: how fast the pharmacologic actions of the drug are needed by the patient, the extent of hepatic metabolism (biotransformation) of the drug, and the ability of the patient to take medications by mouth. For some drugs, the route of administration has a very significant influence on their pharmacologic activity. For example, diazoxide is a potent, rapidly acting hypotensive agent when given by intravenous (IV) injection, but has minimal effects on blood pressure when given orally. Magnesium sulfate is a laxative when taken by mouth, reduces swelling of joints when applied as a concentrated solution, and exerts powerful anticonvulsant effects when given by IV or intramuscular (IM) injection.

Although some drugs can be used both locally and systemically, many agents are given by a single mode of administration (ie, topically, orally, or parenterally). The different methods of drug administration—and the dosage forms most commonly used with each route of administration—are presented in this chapter.

Nursing Management: General Principles of Medication Administration

Assess and record important baseline data necessary for:
- a. detection of adverse effects of prescribed drug.
- b. selection of appropriate route of administration.
- c. selection of appropriate drug administration method.

Review past medical history and documents for evidence of existing or previous medical history related to conditions that:
- a. require caution with administration of prescribed drug.
- b. contraindicate use of a drug: allergy to prescribed drug or drug family; age/physiologic development; medical history; pregnancy; lactation.

Nursing Interventions

Medication Administration

Plan the most convenient and individualized drug regimen (route of administration, dosage form, dosing schedule) that takes into account the individualized needs of the patient or family.

Plan and implement individualized nursing interventions that:
- a. inform the patient or family about the expected actions and adverse effects of a prescribed drug.
- b. identify the early onset of (expected or unexpected) adverse effects and intervene appropriately.
- c. minimize the symptoms produced by the expected adverse effects of the prescribed drug.
- d. identify the safety needs of the patient and intervene appropriately to minimize environmental hazards and risk of injury.

Recognize the patient's concerns and fears.

Answer questions honestly, providing information that is clear, accurate, developmentally appropriate, and specific to the question asked.

Encourage family and significant others to assist in medication administration regimen (especially pertinent for home care).

Surveillance During Therapy

Perform ongoing assessment of method of drug administration related to achieving desired outcomes and ensuring patient safety.

Perform ongoing physical assessment (inspection, palpation) of drug administration site for evidence of findings that may alter the rate and extent of drug absorption and distribution. Examples: pruritus, edema, inflammation, infection, eschar, sterile abscess from repeated injections into same site, lipoatrophy, lipodystrophy, IV catheter or needle obstruction.

Monitor for therapeutic drug effect.

Monitor for adverse effects, toxicity, and interactions.

Monitor for signs of hypersensitivity that may require discontinuation of drug.

Patient Teaching

Instruct patient or family about medication administration (dose, dose frequency, administration technique, and equipment) to ensure safety.

Instruct patient or family that a prescribed drug is to be taken only in the manner and for the condition for which it is prescribed.

Instruct patient or family about expected actions and possible adverse effects related to administration of prescribed drug.

Instruct patient or family about appropriate action to take if adverse effects related to drug administration occur:
- a. how to manage symptoms related to expected adverse effects of prescribed drug.
- b. when to notify practitioner or prescriber.
- c. under which conditions to discontinue administration of prescribed drug before notification of practitioner or prescriber.
- d. under which conditions to seek immediate medical attention if adverse effects develop.

Instruct patient or family regarding the importance of completing the full course of therapy as prescribed, that is, not to discontinue the drug once signs and symptoms have subsided.

Inform patient or family of the consequences of not taking or abruptly discontinuing a prescribed drug.

Instruct patient or family to keep all medications out of the reach of children.

Topical Application

Most topically applied drugs are indicated for their local effects and are applied to the surface of the skin or mucous membranes (oral, nasal, vaginal, urethral, rectal, or as otic, optic, or inhaled forms).

Dermatologic Application

Medications are applied to the skin in several forms: lotions, creams, ointments, sprays, and liquids (wet dressings, baths, soaks). Systemic absorption is limited by the keratinized structure of the skin, which prevents passage of significant amounts of most drugs. Absorption may be enhanced when drugs are applied to damaged skin (wounds, burns). Incorporation of the drug in a fatty ointment or using a keratolytic agent such as salicylic acid to break down the keratin layer also will increase absorption.

Major uses for dermatologically applied drugs are the following:

1. Antiseptic–anti-infective (antibiotics, antifungal agents, alcohol, hexachlorophene)
2. Anti-inflammatory (corticosteroids)
3. Astringent (aluminum acetate, zinc oxide)
4. Antipruritic (local anesthetics, antihistamines)
5. Emollient (vitamins A, D, and E, glycerin, lanolin, mineral oil)
6. Keratolytic (salicylic acid, resorcinol)
7. Vasodilator (nitroglycerin, clonidine)
8. Anti–motion sickness (scopolamine)
9. Pain control (fentanyl)
10. Antismoking (nicotine)
11. Hormone replacement (estrogen, testosterone)

Dermatologically applied drugs may also be used as protectives, absorbents, or counterirritants, and as corrosives to aid in sloughing off or removing damaged tissue. Diseases and conditions commonly treated by local application of drugs to the skin surface include burns, decubitus ulcers, acne, psoriasis, allergic dermatoses, skin cancers, infestations of lice, and topical bacterial and fungal infections. In addition, certain systemic conditions such as angina or hypertension are amenable to treatment by locally applied drugs that are sufficiently absorbed through the intact skin from specialized dosage vehicles (eg, transdermal patches).

Mucous Membrane Application

Absorption of drugs from mucous membranes is generally good, primarily because of the thinness and vascularity of the membrane. In addition to all the forms used for dermatologic application, drugs may be applied to mucous membranes in the form of suppositories (rectal, vaginal), powders (nasal), lozenges (oral), and tablets (buccal, sublingual). Because absorption is good, especially from aqueous solution, many drugs exert significant **systemic** actions after application to mucous membranes. Therefore, because the toxic effects of drugs may be increased by systemic absorption, mucous membrane application must be undertaken more cautiously than dermatologic administration.

Major uses of drugs applied to various mucous membranes are the following:

Local Effects

1. Antiseptic (oral lozenges, sprays, mouthwashes)
2. Antibacterial and antifungal (vaginal creams, suppositories)
3. Decongestant (nasal sprays, drops)
4. Antihemorrhoidal (rectal astringents, local anesthetics, emollients)
5. Contraceptive (vaginal foams, tablets, lotions)
6. Ocular examinations (drops)

Systemic Effects

1. Antianginal (sublingual vasodilators)
2. Laxative (rectal suppositories, retention enemas)
3. Migraine relief (sublingual ergotamine)

The rectal route (suppository, retention enema) also may be used with antiemetics (prochlorperazine), bronchodilators (aminophylline), analgesics (morphine, acetaminophen, aspirin), sedatives (phenobarbital), and many other drugs that cannot be administered orally because the patient is unconscious or uncooperative, or is vomiting. Rectal absorption is unpredictable, and a small, cleansing enema before drug administration may improve absorption.

Nursing Management: General Principles of Topical Application

Refer to "General Principles of Medication Administration."

Prepare and administer topicals recognizing the indications for use and methods of administration for the various:

a. dosage forms: troches, lotions, creams, ointments, powders, gels, liquids (soaks, wet dressings, irrigation, enema, retention enema), suppository, aerosols (topical, inhalation), occlusive dressings, transdermal patches.
b. routes of administration: dermal, optic, otic, inhalation, mucous membrane (oral, vaginal, rectal).

Differentiate between sterile and nonsterile administration sites to choose appropriate technique for medication administration.

Dermatologic Application

Remove desired quantity of topical medication dispensed in a multidose container with a sterile tongue depressor or applicator stick. Rationale: avoid contaminating remaining contents.

Use aseptic technique when cleansing site, applying topical medication, and applying dressings if skin is broken or abraded.

Apply most ointments and creams in a thin layer, covering site thoroughly using firm but gentle pressure.

Use protective coverings (dressings, plastic film) as indicated or if medication has the potential to stain clothing and linens.

Use caution if applying adhesive tape near a wound or an abraded area.

Seek clarification if local corticosteroids are prescribed for an existing topical infection without concurrent antibiotic therapy. Rationale: this may cause the infection to spread.

When interacting with patient, use appropriate communication (verbal, nonverbal) techniques:

a. Recognize that patient may experience low self-esteem and social isolation related to alteration in body image.
b. Avoid showing signs of aversion or rejection.
c. Provide emotional support and encourage expression of feelings.

Application to Mucous Membranes

Oral Mucosa

Teach patient proper technique for administration of locally and systemically acting oral topical medications.

Administer medications to treat disorders of mucous membranes of the mouth, pharynx, and esophagus after meals, other oral medications, and appropriate oral hygiene. Rationale: ensure maximum contact of drug with mucous membrane.

Do not administer buccal or sublingual dosage forms (used to produce systemic effects) with food or water.

Nasal Mucosa

Assess upper airway condition and intervene appropriately before administration. Rationale: for maximum effect, drug must come in contact with nasal mucosa.

Teach patient proper technique for administration of locally and systemically acting topical medications.

Instruct patient to limit use of drops and sprays containing nasal decongestants (vasoconstrictors) to a period of 3 to 5 days. Rationale: avoid the development of tolerance.

CAUTION

Tolerance lessens the drug effect and often produces *rebound congestion* of nasal membranes (inflammation, edema).

Teach patient with hypertension or other cardiovascular disorders that systemic absorption of nasal sprays containing vasoconstrictors may elevate blood pressure.

Teach patient that repeated, excessive use of any nasal preparation may result in significant systemic absorption, especially if substantial amounts of the drug are swallowed rather than inhaled.

Vaginal Mucosa

Teach patient proper technique for administration of locally acting topical medications (all dosage forms).

Before self-administration, assess patient's understanding of procedure, assist patient if appropriate, and ensure privacy.

Emphasize the importance of taking the prescribed medication for the prescribed length of time. Rationale: many vaginal infections are difficult to treat and can be very resistant to drugs.

If preparation causes stains, suggest wearing a sanitary napkin to prevent staining of clothing or bed linen.

Discuss potential harm of excessive douching. If patient douches, provide instructions for mixing, administration, and prevention of excessive force of flow.

If contraceptive foams and jellies are used, ensure that patient understands package instructions regarding timing and method of application. Discuss limitations of effectiveness.

Rectal Mucosa

Encourage bowel evacuation before administration of drug per rectum. Rationale: to ensure maximum contact of drug with rectal mucosa.

Ophthalmic Application

Drugs intended for use in the eye may be administered as drops, ointments, or washes. In addition, a special type of preparation intended for use in glaucoma is available in the form of sterile insertion units called Ocuserts. All ophthalmic medications are packaged sterile; thus, aseptic technique is essential when handling these drugs.

Major indications for local administration of drugs in the eye are the following:

1. Glaucoma (miotics, decongestants)
2. Inflammation (corticosteroids)
3. Infection (antibiotics)

Ophthalmic drugs also may be used to facilitate eye examinations. Mydriatics produce pupillary dilation, cycloplegics paralyze accommodation, and local anesthetics permit manipulative procedures such as tonometry. Artificial "tears" can be used to provide lubrication.

Nursing Management

Use aseptic technique in handling ophthalmic drugs. Wash hands before administering; do not allow tip of dropper or ointment tube to come into contact with eyelid; discard any unused portion of each dose.

Check solution, suspension, or ointment for expiration date, and make sure solution is clear and free from discoloration.

Hold bottle or applicator parallel to the eye, rather than perpendicular, to prevent injury should the patient move or jerk.

Have patient look up during administration; place medication in the conjunctival sac, not directly on the cornea; wipe area near the eyes gently with a cotton ball; and instruct patient to lie or sit with head tilted backward.

When using ophthalmic ointment, place *small* ribbon of medication into everted lower eyelid and tell patient to close eye. Body heat will cause dispersion of drug over eye surface.

Ensure that the patient with glaucoma understands that the drug regimen must be maintained regularly to prevent deterioration of eyesight.

Otic Application

Drugs intended for use in the ear usually are administered as drops, although irrigation of the external auditory canal can also be performed. When the tympanic membrane is intact, sterile technique is not essential.

Principal conditions for which drugs are instilled into the ear are the following:

1. Infections (antibiotics)
2. Inflammation (corticosteroids)
3. Pain (local anesthetics)
4. Obstruction with wax (hydrogen peroxide)

Self-medication should be reserved for those minor conditions (eg, impacted wax) that can be treated safely. Most patients with ear disorders require professional diagnosis and treatment.

Nursing Management

Warm ear drops to body temperature before instilling in ear canal.

Place patient on his or her side with affected ear uppermost; instruct patient to remain in that position for several minutes after drugs have been administered to allow sufficient time for medication to reach affected area.

Use the proper method for instilling drops:

a. *Adults and children 3 years and older*: Pull pinna up and back to straighten external auditory canal.

b. *Children (age 3 years and under)*: Pull pinna down and back.

If cotton is to be inserted into ear after drug administration, insert *loosely*.

For irrigation, place tip of special irrigating syringe inside auditory meatus, and pull pinna up and back while directing a slow, gentle stream of warmed solution toward the roof of the auditory canal. The patient may sit or lie with head tilted toward the side of the affected ear. Allow fluid to escape freely, and collect it in a basin placed below the ear and against the face. Stop irrigation if pain or dizziness occurs.

After irrigation, place patient with affected ear downward and allow ear to drain.

Inhalation Application

Inhaled drugs are generally intended for their local effects on the respiratory system. Many drugs, however, are rapidly absorbed by the alveoli of the lungs because of the large surface area and high permeability of the alveolar epithelium; because of this and the extensive vascularity of this area, a drug given for its local effects in the lungs can easily be absorbed systemically. Such absorption can produce undesirable side effects in other areas of the body; this possibility must be understood (certain drugs, however, such as general anesthetics, are given *via* the respiratory tract for the exact purpose of producing systemic effects). The most important factor in determining the depth of penetration into the bronchial tree, and hence the extent of systemic absorption, is the particle size of the administered drug.

Major indications for inhaled drugs are the following:

1. Anesthesia (general anesthetics)
2. Obstructive pulmonary diseases, such as asthma and emphysema (corticosteroids, bronchodilators, mucolytics, antibiotics)
3. Respiratory aid (oxygen)

Inhalation of drugs is accomplished most easily by use of a metered-dose nebulizer or atomizer, available in prepackaged form, although patients require careful instruction for effective use of this product. Alternatively, an intermittent positive-pressure breathing apparatus may be used, most often in a hospital setting. This method provides greater depth and more extensive distribution of the drug in the bronchial tree. Certain powdered drugs (eg, cromolyn) may be delivered by insufflation, a method in which the powder is blown into the respiratory passages by a pressurized container.

Nursing Management

Teach patient correct procedure for using metered-dose inhaler or hand-held nebulizer, such as when to inhale and exhale, and how long breath should be held.

Teach patient proper technique for administration of medication by inhalation such as:

a. Sit in an upright position.
b. Close lips tightly around mouthpiece.
c. Breathe *only* through mouth.

Clean nebulizer or atomizer carefully after each use to prevent obstruction and contamination. Discard unused medication left in nebulizer.

Oral Administration

The oral (per os; p.o.) route of administration is the simplest, most convenient, most economic, and generally the safest way to give a drug.

Commonly used oral dosage forms are tablets, capsules, and liquids. Most drugs are well absorbed from the gastrointestinal (GI) tract, and absorption usually is enhanced if the drug is in liquid form or is administered with water. Some drugs, such as anti-inflammatory drugs, may irritate the GI mucosa and are best given with food, whereas other agents (eg, some penicillins) may be inactivated by the presence of food-induced digestive enzymes and are best given between meals.

After oral administration of a drug, the onset of action is slower—and the duration of effect more prolonged—than after sublingual and most forms of parenteral administration. This is of little importance in most cases, but becomes significant in emergencies (eg, acute pain, cardiac arrest, acute asthmatic attacks).

Important disadvantages of the oral route of administration are the following:

1. Some drugs are rapidly inactivated in the GI tract (eg, insulin) or are not absorbed (eg, tubocurarine).
2. Some drugs undergo extensive first-pass hepatic metabolism (ie, are largely inactivated in the liver after absorption into the portal circulation). Thus, a large fraction of the dose never reaches the systemic circulation. Differences in the rate and extent of hepatic metabolism among patients can lead to significant variations in steady-state plasma levels, and hence to widely differing dosage requirements. Sublingual drug administration avoids first-pass hepatic metabolism and generally results in higher plasma levels for those drugs extensively metabolized in the liver.
3. Some drugs have an objectionable odor or taste (eg, liquid potassium).

4. Some drugs (such as large doses of aspirin) may produce local stomach irritation and cause nausea and vomiting. Drugs that may irritate the stomach can be given in the form of enteric-coated tablets, which dissolve only in the intestine where the environment is more alkaline.
5. Some drugs (such as liquid iron or gastric acids) may stain or destroy the tooth enamel.

In addition, unconscious, uncooperative, or vomiting patients or those without a gag reflex should not be given drugs by the oral route.

Nursing Management

Refer to "General Principles of Medication Administration."

Know whether or not prescribed drug may be administered with meals or other drugs. Rationale: may affect bioavailability.

Determine the patient's ability to swallow a solid dosage form.

Instruct patient to take oral medications with a full glass of water.

Do not attempt to break unscored tablets, divide capsules, or crush coated tablets. Rationale: may affect bioavailability.

Note expiration date and discard if outdated.

Keep preparations requiring refrigeration cold and discard unused portion on expiration date.

Do not mix liquids together unless so instructed. Rationale: drug–drug incompatibilities may result.

Advise patient to avoid indiscriminate use of over-the-counter (OTC) drugs when taking prescribed oral medications. Rationale: many OTC products produce drug–drug interactions.

Administration of Parenteral Medications

Although the term *parenteral* literally means any route *other* than enteral (GI tract), it is usually used to refer to the different methods of *injection* of drugs. Parenteral administration requires aseptically prepared drugs and sterile techniques, critical regulation of dosage, careful selection of site and rate of injection, and more technical skill than that required for other routes.

There often are significant differences in onset of drug action, extent of drug effects, dosage of drug required, skill in administration, and potential hazards depending on the specific parenteral route of administration selected.

Intravenous

Intravenous administration is accomplished by either rapid (*bolus*) or slow (*infusion*) injection of drug directly into the bloodstream. Bolus IV injection is often used in emergency situations because it provides an extremely rapid onset of action. Also, some drugs (eg, diazoxide) require bolus injection to achieve their desired effect. Because the drug is injected directly into the bloodstream, however, IV injection is also a very hazardous method; *extreme care* must be taken to ensure that the proper preparation and accurate dose have been selected. Antidotal therapy must be *immediately* available in case an overdose occurs. IV injections are most commonly made into the median cubital (antecubital) or basilic vein near the bend of the elbow (Fig. 2-1), although any accessible vein may be used in an emergency.

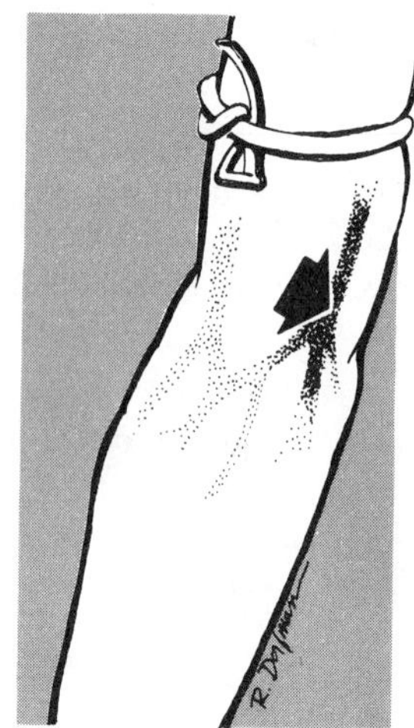

Figure 2-1 The most common bolus IV injection site is into the median cubital (antecubital) or basilic vein near the bend of the elbow (*arrow*).

Irritating substances that cannot be given by other parenteral routes of injection because they produce tissue damage can sometimes be administered by slow IV injection diluted in 100 to 200 mL of suitable liquid (eg, sterile water for injection). The lining of the blood vessels is quite resistant to the irritative effects of many drugs, and the buffering capacity of the blood may reduce local necrosis. This procedure requires selection of a large vein and assurance that the injection is properly placed into the flowing bloodstream.

Slow IV infusions are used most commonly to replace depleted blood volume, to supply nutrients and electrolytes, to prevent or relieve tissue dehydration, and to administer drugs. The veins of the dorsal venous plexus or the cephalic vein (Fig. 2-2) are commonly used for these purposes. Very large volumes of fluids can be given by IV infusion, although care must be taken to avoid overloading the patient's circulatory capacity. A controlled rate of flow is maintained and may vary depending on the nature of the drug and the patient's age, weight, and condition. Drugs are either contained in the infusion system itself or added to the flowing infusion.

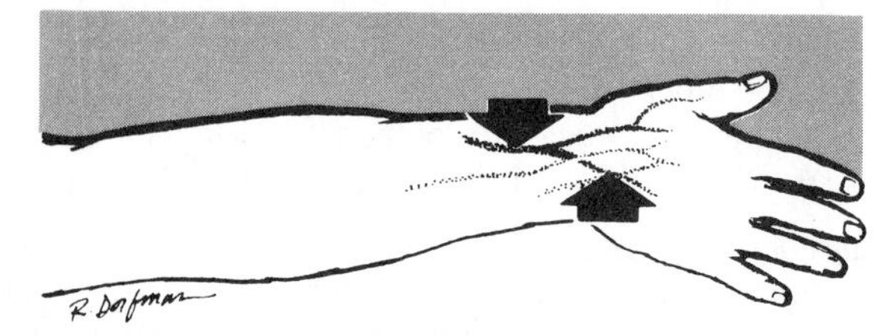

Figure 2-2 The veins of the dorsal venous plexus or the cephalic vein can be used for IV infusions.

Advantages

Major advantages of the IV route of administration are the following:

1. Effect is immediate.
2. Dosage can be adjusted (titrated) to response.
3. Fairly constant blood levels can be maintained by a proper rate of infusion.
4. Irritating drugs (such as antineoplastic agents) often can be given with minimal trauma because of the buffering capacity of the blood.
5. Administration can be performed easily in the patient who is unconscious or unable to swallow

Disadvantages

Several disadvantages to IV administration also exist:

1. Termination—or reduction—of pharmacologic effect of drug is difficult owing to its rapid action (drug is essentially irretrievable once it has been injected).
2. Toxic effects may develop quickly and may be exacerbated by an injection made too rapidly.
3. Many incompatibilities exist among drugs and IV solutions because of such variables as pH, temperature of solution, and salt content.
4. Intravenous administration is technically more difficult than most other methods, often causes pain, and may result in infection.

Intra-arterial

Injection of a drug directly into an artery is an infrequently used method of administration, the purpose of which is to perfuse a specific area or organ of the body to achieve a high local concentration of the drug.

Types of drugs most frequently given by the intra-arterial route are the following:

1. Diagnostic agents (radiographic contrast media)
2. Antineoplastic drugs
3. Vasodilators

Subcutaneous

Subcutaneous (SC) injections are given beneath the skin into the fat and connective tissue underlying the dermis. The most common sites of SC injections are the upper lateral aspect of the arm, the anterior portion of the thigh, and the abdomen (Fig. 2-3). Absorption from these sites through the capillary network is generally rapid (although slower than with IM injection), but can be reduced by local cooling of the area or by the addition of vasoconstrictors to the injection solution. The maximum volume that can be given comfortably by this route is about 2 mL, and the drugs used must be highly soluble and nonirritating to tissues.

In a special form of SC injection termed *hypodermoclysis*, large volumes of fluid are given *very slowly* into the loose connective tissue on the upper surface of the thigh or the outer side of the upper body surface. This procedure can be used to administer an isotonic sodium chloride solution, glucose, or other parenteral fluids that cannot be given IV for some reason. Hyaluronidase, an enzyme that breaks down the connective tissue matrix, is sometimes added to the mixture to facilitate the spread and absorption of the large volume of injection. It may also reduce the discomfort associated with the injection of such a large volume (500–>1000 mL) of fluid. Absorption from SC sites can also be prolonged by suspending the drug in a protein colloid or gelatin solution.

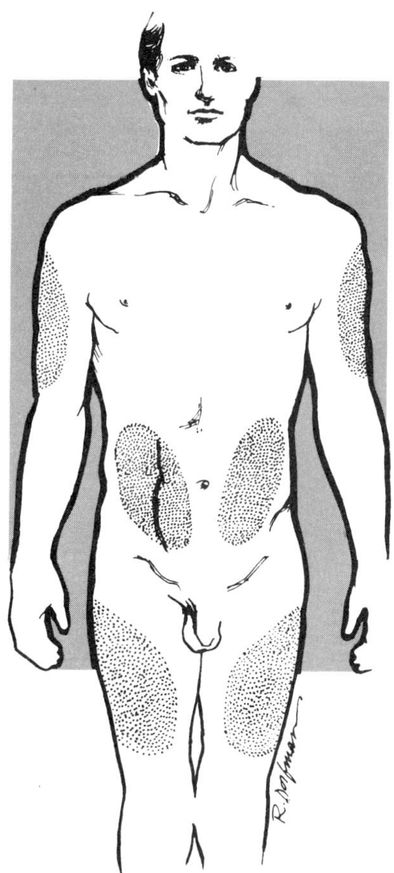

Figure 2-3 The shaded areas show the most common sites for SC injections.

Flexible capsules can be implanted subcutaneously to provide a "depot" form of a drug, which is continuously and evenly absorbed systemically over a long time. This procedure requires a small incision, and sterility is essential. The Norplant System consists of six such capsules, each of which contains a drug (levonorgestrel) that is gradually released—and will prevent conception—for up to 5 years.

Intramuscular

Drug injections can be made into several of the larger muscle masses. Sites most commonly used are the deltoid muscle (Fig. 2-4*A*), the gluteal muscles (dorsogluteal and ventrogluteal sites; see Fig. 2-4*B*), and the vastus lateralis (especially in infants; see Fig. 2-4*C*). Injections usually are made with a longer, thicker needle than that used in SC injections; larger volumes can be given IM (up to 5 mL per site) than SC. Absorption usually is rapid because of the vascularity of muscle and the large absorbing surface. The deltoid has perhaps the greatest blood flow of any muscle routinely used for IM injection.

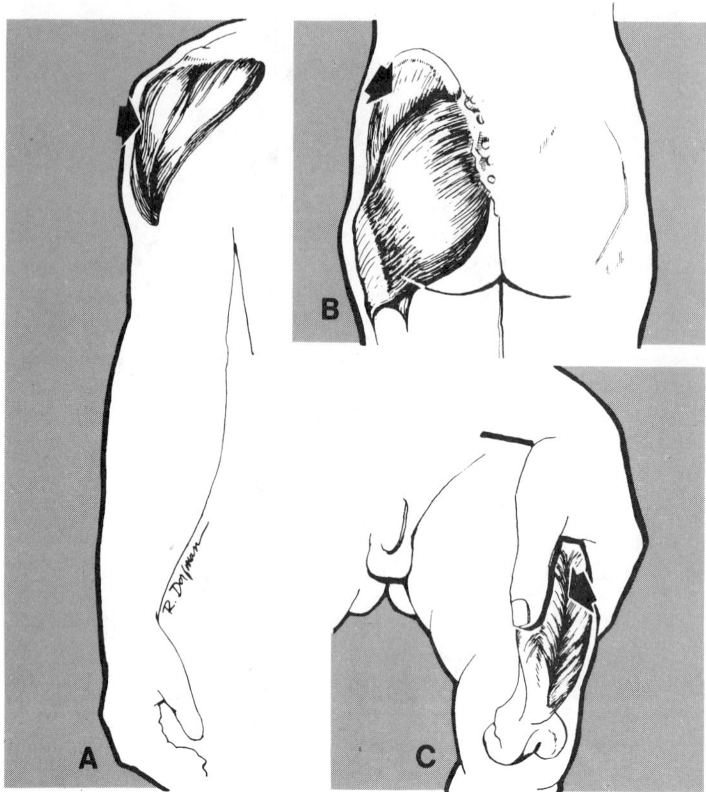

Figure 2-4 Sites most commonly used for drug injections into the larger muscle masses. (**A**) The deltoid muscle. (**B**) The gluteal muscles. (**C**) The vastus lateralis, especially in infants. With gluteal injections, *always* use bony prominences to identify correct injection site (see Nursing Management [General Principles of Parenteral Administration]).

The danger of inadvertent IV administration is increased with an IM injection because of the large number of blood vessels in muscle. Therefore, aspiration of the syringe for blood before injecting is essential to ensure proper needle placement. There is also an increased likelihood of nerve damage if the injection is performed incorrectly.

Drugs may be given IM as solutions or suspensions in either water or oil. Aqueous solutions are rapidly absorbed, whereas suspensions or solutions of different drugs (eg, hormones) in oil provide a depot form from which drug is slowly absorbed for a long-lasting effect. Caution must be exercised when injecting oil-based preparations; some patients may have allergic reactions to the oil, and in some cases the oil may not be absorbed, requiring excision and drainage.

Depth of needle insertion is very important. It depends mainly on the site and volume of injection and on the condition of the patient (age, weight, extent of body fat).

In small children, IM injections are associated with special difficulties, primarily because of the limited muscle mass. Generally, the vastus lateralis (see Fig. 2-4*C*) on the anterolateral aspect of the thigh is used. Needle lengths should be shorter than with adults, and the child should be restrained to minimize the risk of sudden movement during needle insertion and injection.

Three basic techniques are used when giving an IM injection: stretching, pinching, and the "Z" method. In *stretching*, the skin is pressed down and stretched between the thumb and fingers. This method is used often for obese patients to reduce the thickness of subcutaneous fat that must be pierced to reach the muscle. *Pinching* is accomplished by gathering the tissue between the thumb and fingers. This tends to raise the underlying muscle tissue and is helpful with emaciated adults and infants. Finally, the "Z" method (sometimes called the Z-track method) is used with medications that might discolor the skin (eg, iron preparations) or cause subcutaneous irritation should they leak from the underlying muscle. It involves pulling the overlying skin to one side of the injection site, inserting the needle at a right angle to the skin, injecting, and withdrawing the needle quickly while releasing the pulled-back skin at the same time. This maneuver "seals off" the puncture tract.

Other Parenteral Routes

Intradermal

Drugs may be injected superficially into the outer layers of the skin in very small amounts. Local anesthetics can be given intradermally to facilitate deeper injections, but this method is used primarily for diagnostic purposes, as in skin testing for allergies or in tuberculin testing. The injection sites commonly used are the medial forearm area and the surface of the back. Injections are best performed with a small needle (26 gauge) and syringe, and the injection volume is usually 0.5 mL or less. Systemic absorption of intradermally injected agents is very limited, so the method is applicable only to those drugs used locally.

Intra-articular

This method of injection, directly into a joint, is used primarily for administration of corticosteroids in the treatment of acute local inflammatory conditions. The major advantage is attainment of high local concentrations of steroid in the affected area with minimal systemic absorption, thus reducing toxicity. The procedure requires skill and is painful to the patient.

Intrathecal

Intrathecal injections (into the spinal subarachnoid space) are used most often with local anesthetics, antibiotics, and radiographic contrast media. This technically difficult procedure usually is performed by a physician. It is used frequently to induce localized anesthesia during labor and delivery, although epidural administration (*outside* of the subarachnoid space) of local anesthetics is often preferred because of a lower frequency of toxic reactions and less danger of postanesthetic complications.

Several other methods of parenteral administration of drugs are available, but are used only infrequently. These are briefly summarized as follows:

Intraperitoneal. Injection of drugs directly into the peritoneal cavity of the abdomen; absorption is rapid but this route is not used in humans because of the danger of infection and adhesions. Peritoneal dialysis is performed in cases of renal failure, intractable edema, hepatic coma, azotemia, and uremia, and in therapy for peritonitis.

Intracardiac. Direct injection into the heart; occasionally used with epinephrine and isoproterenol for emergency treatment of cardiac arrest.

Intrapleural. Administration of drugs between the lungs and chest wall (pleural cavity). Antibiotics occasionally are given this way.

Intra-amniotic. Instillation of drugs into the amniotic sac surrounding the fetus.

Nursing Management: General Principles of Parenteral Administration

Refer to "General Principles of Medication Administration."

Use appropriate technique for the administration and management of medications given parenterally (SC, intradermal, IM, IV, intraperitoneal, intra-articular, intrathecal, epidural, intra-arterial, and so forth).

Ensure provision of patient safety with SC, intradermal, and IM administration:

a. Use aseptic technique at all times.
b. Rotate injection sites.
c. Consider dosage form and patient characteristics when selecting volume of medication per injection, needle size, needle length, and injection site.
d. Assess injection sites (inspect, palpate) for evidence of sterile abscess formation, inflammation, local edema, lipodystrophy, lipoatrophy, and the like, and initiate appropriate interventions to prevent or alleviate symptoms.

Ensure provision of patient safety during infusions:

a. Use aseptic technique at all times.
b. Check that tubing is not occluded, all connections are tight, and that proper drug, dose, and route are ordered.
c. Inspect area immediately around IV injection or infusion site for evidence of local infiltration, inflammation, or extravasation.
d. Initiate appropriate nursing interventions if IV infiltration, inflammation, or extravasation occurs.
e. Frequently monitor parenteral infusion rate. Use nursing judgment or protocol to determine if use of infusion controller or pump is indicated.
f. Frequently monitor patient response to parenteral infusion and be familiar with procedure to follow in the event of development of undesirable response to the prescribed medication.

After an intra-articular injection, instruct patient not to overuse the affected joint when pain is relieved, because further damage to the joint may occur.

Caution patient that pain may intensify for several hours after an intra-articular injection before relief is obtained.

Inform patient that headache may follow intrathecal injection.

Selected Bibliography

Cramer JA: Feedback on medication dosing enhances patient compliance. Chest 104(2):333, 1993

Draine J, Solomon P: Explaining attitudes toward medication compliance among a seriously mentally ill population. J Nerv Ment Dis 182:50, 1994

Gregoriadis G, Florence AT: Liposomes in drug delivery: Clinical, diagnostic and ophthalmic potential. Drugs 45(1):15, 1993

Harris D, Robinson JR: Drug delivery via the mucous membranes of the oral cavity. J Pharm Sci 81(1):1, 1992

Kauffman RE, Banner W, Berlin CM, et al.: The transfer of drugs and other chemicals into human milk. Pediatrics 93(1):137, 1994

Labrecque GL, Belanger PM: Biological rhythms in the absorption, distribution, metabolism and excretion of drugs. Pharmacol Ther 52:95, 1991

Nahata MC: Intravenous infusion conditions: Implications for pharmacokinetic monitoring. Clin Pharmacokinet 24(3):221, 1993

VanBree JBMM, DeBoer AG, Danhof M, Breimer DD: Drug transport across the blood–brain barrier. III. Mechanisms and methods to improve drug delivery to the central nervous system. Pharmacy World & Science 15:2, 1993

Nursing Bibliography

Crane R: Intermittent subcutaneous infusion of opioids in hospice home care: An effective economical manageable option. The American Journal of Hospice and Palliative Care 11(1):8-12, 1994

Dross J: What you need to know about insulin injections. Nursing '92 22(11):40–43, 1993

Falls P, Kinney ML: The abdomen, thigh and arm as sites for subcutaneous sodium heparin injections Nursing Research 40(4): 204-207, 1991

Goode C, Titler M, Rakel B: A meta analysis of effects of heparin flush and saline flush—quality and cost implications. Nursing Research 40(6):324–330, 1991

Gullo S: Implanted ports: Technological advances and nursing care issues. Nursing Clinics of North America 28(4):859–872, 1993

Haddad A, Keefer R, Stein J: Teamwork in home infusion therapy: The relationship between nursing and pharmacy. Home Health Care Nurse 11(1):40-47, 1993

Hahn K, Wietor G: Helpful tools for medication screening. Geriatric Nursing 13(3):160–166, 1992

Keegan-Wells D, Stewart J: The use of venous access devices in pediatric oncology nursing practice. Journal of Pediatric Oncology Nursing 9(4):159–169, 1992

Lazzara D: Patient controlled analgesia in the I.C.U. Critical Care Nursing Quarterly 16(1):26-36, 1993

Luberow T, Ivankovich A: Patient controlled analgesia for postoperative pain. Critical Care Nursing Clinics of North America 3(1):35-42, 1991

McAllister C, Lenaghan P, Tosone N: Changing from heparin to saline flush solutions: A research utilizatioin model for implementation. Journal of Emergency Nursing 19(4):306–312, 1993

Rogers A, Rosas J, O'Hanlan-Nichols T: How to inject a subcutaneous abdominal implant. Nursing '94, 24(N):63-64, 1994

Weakland B: Administering insulin through an indwelling catheter. Nursing '93, 23(11):58-61, 1993

3

Interaction of Drugs With Body Tissues: Pharmacokinetics

A drug must reach the target tissue to produce its pharmacologic actions. Many factors control the **quantity** of drug that reaches the site of action and the **rate** of its entrance.

The most important of these factors are the following:

Absorption: those processes involved in transferring a drug across one or more biologic membranes to the target tissue. In the case of systemic administration, a drug will enter the bloodstream.

Distribution: the means by which drugs are transported by blood or other body fluids to their intended sites of action, biotransformation, storage, or elimination.

Biotransformation: the enzymatic processes by which a drug is converted to a **metabolite** that—most often—is less active and more readily eliminated than the parent drug.

Elimination: the mechanisms that remove a drug and its metabolite(s) from the body.

Each of these processes depends on many variables and can be modified in several ways. It is important to understand these processes and how they can be altered. An outline of the major factors that influence the concentration of a drug at its site of action is shown in Figure 3-1.

To travel from the site of administration to its target tissue, a drug usually must pass across several biologic membranes. A typical membrane is composed of phospholipid and protein molecules. The phospholipid molecules are arranged in two parallel rows (ie, a *lipid bilayer*). The protein molecules appear to occur randomly, some near the inner or outer surfaces of the membrane and others penetrating the membrane to varying degrees. This arrangement is dynamic; that is, the phospholipid and protein molecules possess the ability to move. This concept, termed the *fluid mosaic hypothesis*, may explain how drugs attach to specific receptor areas on the cell membrane. There are openings (eg, pores, channels) at various intervals along the surface of the membrane.

Because cell membranes are composed largely of lipids (fats), the lipid-soluble form of a drug is the one that most readily crosses these membranes; this occurs by *passive diffusion*. Drugs either carry an electrical charge (ie, are **ionized**) or have no charge (ie, are electrically neutral or **nonionized**). *Ionized* drugs are very water soluble; this form does not easily penetrate biologic membranes and, therefore, is more readily removed from the body. In contrast, *nonionized* drugs are very lipid soluble; this type will easily cross membranes, is readily stored in fat (adipose) tissues, and is easily eliminated.

Depending on their chemical structure, most drugs are either *weak acids* or *weak bases*. When dissolved in fluids (biologic or other), they will exist in both the ionized *and* nonionized forms. The amount of each form (ie, nonionized and ionized) that is present depends on the pH of the fluid in which the drug is placed. The pK_a (ionization constant) is the pH at which a drug is 50% nonionized and 50% ionized. At a pH *below* its pK_a, acidic drugs will be largely (>50%) nonionized; basic drugs will be largely ionized. In contrast, if the pH of the fluid is *greater* than the pK_a, acidic drugs will be largely (>50%) ionized; basic drugs will be largely nonionized.

For example, an acidic drug such as aspirin (pK_a 3.5) exists largely in the nonionized state in the stomach (pH 1.0–3.0), and therefore is well absorbed there. Basic drugs, such as morphine (pK_a 7.9), however, exist predominantly in the ionized state at this site, and are not well absorbed. As the drugs travel through the intestinal tract, the pH increases and acidic drugs become more ionized, whereas basic drugs are converted more to the nonionized state. Therefore, absorption of basic drugs is more extensive in the upper intestinal tract.

Absorption

Gastrointestinal Tract

Drugs may be absorbed from several regions of the gastrointestinal (GI) tract, but most absorption occurs throughout the upper region of the small intestine. The main reasons for this are: 1) the presence of many small folds, or *villi*, which greatly increase the absorbing surface area; and 2) the highly permeable nature of the intestinal epithelium. Other factors that make the small intestine the primary site for absorption of most drugs include the presence of special transport systems (for absorption of sugars, amino acids, nutrients, and other substances), fairly rapid emptying of many drugs from the stomach (delivers unabsorbed drug to the upper intestine), and an extensive capillary network within intestinal villi.

In general, absorption of most drugs from the GI tract is best explained by diffusion of the lipid-soluble (nonionized) form of the drug across the mucosal barrier. Some absorption, especially of low–molecular-weight drugs, also occurs by way of diffusion through aqueous pores in the membrane. With some substances, absorption involves active (energy-requiring) transport mechanisms in which a carrier moves a drug molecule *against* a concentration gradient. For example, iodide is absorbed by the thyroid and glucose is reabsorbed by the renal tubules in this manner. Facilitated diffusion also is a carrier-mediated process, but unlike active transport, it does not require energy and moves *down* the concentration gradient. It is used to move less lipid-soluble drugs across the membrane.

Absorption of drugs from the GI tract is influenced by several factors, including the following:

Nature of the Drug

1. Lipid solubility of the nonionized form (it is this form that more readily crosses GI membranes)

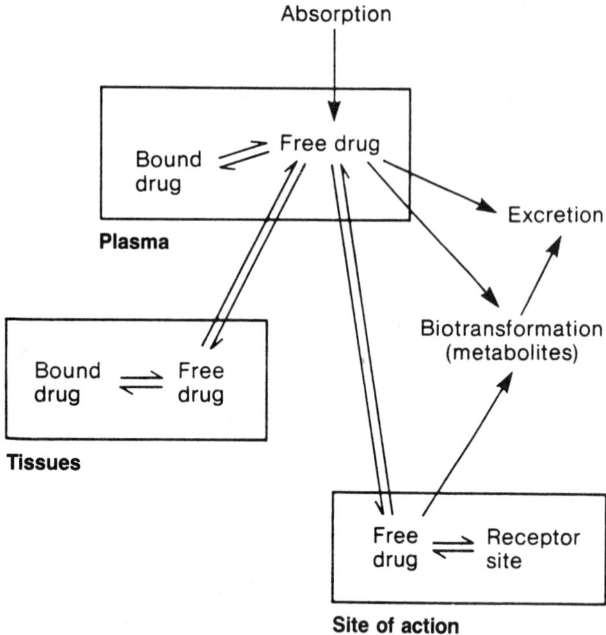

Figure 3-1 Factors influencing concentration of a drug at its site of action.

2. Stability of the drug in GI fluid
3. Molecular weight and configuration of the drug molecule, which may influence its passage through the membrane pores (smaller molecules have a better chance of "squeezing" through the pores)

Nature of the Dosage Form

1. Concentration of the drug if administered in solution
2. Dissolution rate of a solid dosage form of the drug
3. Presence of special (enteric) coatings on the drug molecules that resist breakdown and hence prevent absorption in the stomach

Nature of the Absorbing Barrier (Biologic Membrane)

1. Permeability of the mucosal epithelium
2. Blood flow in the absorbing area
3. pH of the region, which determines the ratio of the nonionized to ionized forms of the drug present
4. Amount of absorbing surface exposed, which is a function of the total surface area present (the length of the absorbing segment, and the presence of surface modifications such as villi)

Other Factors

1. Length of time the drug is in contact with the absorbing surface (depends on peristaltic activity, which influences gastric emptying time, eg, an increase in GI motility increases gastric emptying and reduces the time that a drug will spend in the GI tract)
2. Presence of food (reduces the rate of absorption of most drugs but can increase bioavailability of some drugs, presumably by reducing first-pass hepatic metabolism [see below])
3. Presence of other drugs or substances that can retard absorption by binding free drug molecules (eg, cholestyramine) or alter GI motility (eg, laxatives, anticholinergics); "bound" drugs usually cannot be absorbed efficiently

Absorption From Parenteral Sites

In general, most parenteral sites provide for a more rapid and predictable rate of absorption than the intestinal tract; the drug will not be subjected to the "first-pass" effect. Absorption after subcutaneous (SC) or intramuscular (IM) injection depends primarily on two factors:

1. Solubility of the drug in the interstitial fluid
2. Area of the absorbing capillary membrane

Drugs in aqueous solution are absorbed more rapidly than drugs in suspension. Often, however, drugs are suspended in certain fluids to slow their rate of absorption and to provide a prolonged action. Examples of this are some penicillins (benzathine and procaine penicillin G) and long-acting hormones and steroidal agents. Certain types of insulin, such as NPH, are combined with proteins or zinc to delay their rate of absorption.

Absorption of drugs from IM sites is usually more rapid than from SC areas because of the more extensive blood vessel network in muscle tissue compared with subcutaneous tissue. The decreased peripheral blood flow present during circulatory failure (as in cases of shock or secondary local edema, cellulitis, sterile abscesses, and multiple injections) may significantly reduce the rate of absorption of drugs injected from IM and SC sites, and can greatly reduce their therapeutic effects. Blood flow to these areas can be increased—and absorption enhanced—by application of heat, local vasodilators, or massage; conversely, decreased blood flow and delayed absorption can result from use of cold packs, a tourniquet, or vasoconstrictors. All these factors can exert a profound influence on the onset and extent of a drug's action.

Intravenous (IV) administration, of course, provides the most rapid drug action because the drug enters the bloodstream directly without crossing any membranes. The advantages as well as the hazards of this method were discussed in Chapter 2.

Absorption From Skin and Mucous Membranes

Absorption of most drugs through the intact skin is very poor, primarily because of the keratinized structure of the epidermis. The underlying dermis, however, is quite permeable, and significant drug absorption can occur if the overlying skin is abraded or denuded. In general, drug absorption occurs to a greater extent through mucous membranes, which present a much thinner and more permeable absorbing surface than the skin. Enhanced absorption of topically applied drugs can be obtained by dissolving the drug in an oily base, by vigorously massaging it into the area of application, or by simultaneously applying a keratin-softening agent such as salicylic acid.

Increasingly, drugs intended for systemic action are being formulated in specialized topical dosage forms, such as transdermal patches, to take advantage of their ability to be absorbed consistently through the skin. Examples of such drugs are nitroglycerin, scopolamine, clonidine, fentanyl, nicotine, and estrogen.

Drugs absorbed from a sublingual site are very rapidly absorbed, owing to the extremely thin epithelial membrane and extensive capillary network in the area of administration.

Absorption of inhaled medication depends to a large extent on the particle size of the drug, which determines the extent of penetration into the alveoli of the lungs. Patient compliance and administration technique are also important parameters. This is the primary site of systemic absorption of inhaled medications because of the close proximity of capillaries to the alveolar membrane. Although most inhaled drugs are intended for their local effects, systemic absorption may be large, leading to unwanted adverse effects.

Distribution

After a drug is absorbed, it is distributed throughout the body by the circulatory system. To produce a significant pharmacologic effect, a drug must reach adequate levels in tissues on which it exerts its principal actions. Because the distribution of a drug depends ultimately on its ability to cross body membranes, the principles governing membrane transport of a drug, discussed earlier in the chapter, apply here as well. In general, the initial distribution of a drug depends on cardiac output and blood flow to local tissue. In addition, several other factors addressed in the following sections can determine the amount of active drug that ultimately reaches the intended site of action.

Binding of the Drug

Drugs may bind either to plasma proteins (eg, albumin, α_1-acid glycoprotein) or to specific areas of cells (eg, nucleoproteins). Binding to plasma proteins slows the disappearance of the drug from the plasma, limits the rate of accumulation in tissues, and prolongs the time that the drug remains in the body. A protein-bound drug usually is inactive because it is only the free drug that is capable of diffusing across membranes to reach its site of action in the tissues. A dynamic equilibrium, however, usually exists between the bound and free forms of a drug (see Fig. 3-1), and some drug will be present in either state. Plasma protein binding may provide a reservoir of drug that gradually dissociates from the binding sites to replace the free drug that has been inactivated.

The binding capacity of plasma proteins is limited, and saturation of these binding sites may occur. Once protein-binding sites are completely occupied, further administration of the drug may increase its effects or produce toxic reactions because of the presence of large amounts of free (non–protein-bound) drug. The same type of problem can occur when two drugs, each protein bound to a large degree, are given *simultaneously*; competition for the binding sites on these plasma proteins occurs, with displacement. The drug that is bound more strongly will displace the drug with weaker binding, increasing the pharmacologic and toxicologic effects of the drug that is more weakly bound. This type of drug interaction is discussed more fully in Chapter 6.

Lipid Solubility of the Drug

Because most membranes are lipid in nature, drug distribution across these membranes, and ultimately to the site of action, depends to an extent on the lipid solubility of the drug. Moreover, highly lipid-soluble drugs tend to localize in adipose (fat) tissue, where they may be stored for extended periods because blood flow in these regions is usually sparse. In the case of some drugs, slow release of active drug from these storage sites can result in prolonged subtherapeutic effects (eg, continued drowsiness after use of a central nervous system depressant that is highly lipid soluble, such as flurazepam).

Blood–Brain Barrier

It is well established that some drugs enter the central nervous system (CNS) with relative ease, whereas others do not enter at all. The is due, in part, to the existence of the blood–brain barrier, composed of very tightly joined endothelial cells, which lack pores, and are surrounded by poorly permeable cells (*glial* cells). This barrier prevents many water-soluble drugs from entering the CNS while permitting some highly lipid-soluble drugs to pass. For a drug to pass the blood–brain barrier more easily, it should possess the following properties:

1. Low ionization at plasma pH
2. High lipid solubility of the nonionized form of the drug
3. Minimal plasma protein binding

Placental Barrier

Although some form of a barrier probably exists between the bloodstream and the placenta, it is very nonselective. Most drugs (except for strongly charged and high–molecular-weight molecules) are capable of readily entering the placental circulation. During the first trimester of pregnancy, many drugs have a potentially damaging effect on the developing fetus, even though they may not be harmful to the mother. Other drugs, such as alcohol, barbiturates, and narcotics, have adverse effects on both the mother and the fetus. No drug should be taken during pregnancy without consulting the prescriber, and drugs should be used during pregnancy *only* when the advantages are *much greater* than the potential for toxicity.

Biotransformation

Most drugs entering the body are converted into metabolites that usually are more water soluble and less active than the parent drug. These metabolic changes usually occur in the liver by way of hepatic microsomal enzyme systems, but other enzyme systems found in the lungs, plasma, intestines, kidneys, and nerve endings also can biotransform drugs.

Biotransformation does not always lead to formation of *less active* compounds. The metabolic changes occurring with some drugs (eg, fluoxetine) result in formation of active metabolites, whereas other drugs are transformed into *more toxic* metabolites (eg, ethanol → acetaldehyde, meperidine → normeperidine).

Some drugs are administered in the form of an inactive *prodrug*, which is then converted to an active metabolite. An example of such a drug is dipivefrin, an eye drop that is converted to epinephrine, the active component, in the eye. Dipivefrin is better absorbed than epinephrine, and hence less drug is required. Another example of a prodrug is the antineoplastic agent cyclophosphamide.

Biotransformation of drugs usually occurs in two phases. The initial phase involves reactions that produce a chemical change in the drug molecule, such as *oxidation*, *reduction*, and *hydrolysis*. The second phase involves the coupling of the drug or its metabolic product formed in phase one to another chemical group (eg, sulfate, acetate) or substrate (eg, carbohydrate, amino acid). This coupling, or *conjugation*, results in the formation of a more water-soluble and hence more readily excretable product.

There often is considerable variation in the rate at which different people metabolize drugs. Several factors are important in determining the capacity of a patient to inactivate a drug, including:

1. Diseases that alter liver function (eg, hepatic disease can reduce biotransformation)
2. Age (immature liver in the infant and impaired hepatic function in the geriatric patient)
3. Presence of other drugs, such as (a) barbiturates, or phenytoin, which can increase liver enzyme function and *enhance* metabolism of many other drugs, or (b) drugs such as allopurinol and cimetidine that inhibit drug-metabolizing enzymes and therefore reduce metabolism of many other drugs. See Chapter 6 for further discussion of drug interactions based on alterations in liver enzyme function.
4. Genetically determined differences in metabolic activity (which may explain hypersensitivity, resistance, or tolerance to drugs)

A significant factor in determining the efficacy of many orally administered drugs is *hepatic first-pass metabolism*. After absorption from the stomach or intestines, drugs enter the portal circulation and are immediately transported to the liver, where they may be taken up by hepatic cells and metabolized. In some cases, the metabolism of the drug is extensive on first pass, and drugs such as morphine and nitroglycerin, which undergo extensive first-pass metabolism, must be given in higher doses when used orally than when given by other routes of administration that avoid first-pass metabolism, such as SC or sublingually. Some drugs, such as propranolol, also undergo extensive first-pass metabolism, but are converted in part to an active intermediate. Other drugs cleared to a considerable extent by first-pass inactivation include desipramine, reserpine, and verapamil.

Elimination

Excretion of a drug and its metabolites from the body occurs by several routes, including the kidneys, lungs, intestines, and, to a lesser extent, the sweat, salivary, and mammary glands. Of these, the most important for most drugs is the kidneys.

Kidneys

Renal excretion of drugs involves the interaction of three processes: glomerular filtration, active tubular secretion, and tubular reabsorption. The first two of these processes remove drugs from the plasma, whereas tubular reabsorption promotes retention of the drug in the body by returning it to the plasma. The net *excretion* of a drug substance therefore depends on the sum total of these three processes.

Glomerular Filtration

Glomerular filtration is the process whereby drug molecules diffuse out of the blood perfusing the glomeruli of the nephron and pass into the tubules of the kidney. The drug may then either be reabsorbed into the bloodstream at different segments of the tubule or excreted in the urine. Several factors can influence renal excretion by glomerular filtration:

Molecular size: The amount of drug filtered by the glomerulus depends on its molecular size; smaller molecules are more easily filtered.

Plasma protein binding: Because only free drug can be filtered by the kidney, binding to plasma proteins reduces renal excretion.

Blood level of the drug: The greater the drug concentration in the plasma, the more readily the drug can be filtered and ultimately excreted.

Tubular Secretion

The proximal renal tubule can actively secrete certain drugs, transporting them from the bloodstream directly into the tubular fluid. This process is not significantly affected by protein binding if the binding is reversible. Many drugs that are secreted are also filtered by the glomeruli and thus have a very short period of action; an example is penicillin. The tubular secretion process for one drug can be inhibited by another drug. For example, probenecid competes with penicillin for a saturable transport system, and is often given with penicillin to inhibit its active tubular secretion; the duration of action of penicillin in the body is therefore prolonged.

Tubular Reabsorption

Throughout much of the length of the renal tubules, drugs are reabsorbed back into the surrounding capillary network. Renal tubular reabsorption is in many respects similar to absorption from the GI tract; that is, drug molecules are *passively* transported through the tubular epithelial cells. Thus, a drug existing in the nonionized (lipid-soluble) form in tubular fluid will be more rapidly and more completely reabsorbed than a drug that is highly ionized (water soluble) in tubular fluid. Altering the pH of the urine can markedly affect excretion of a drug. Weak acids such as salicylates, barbiturates, and sulfonamides are excreted more readily as the pH of tubular fluid increases because weak acids ionize more as the urine becomes more basic. Conversely, weak bases like amphetamines, ephedrine, and meperidine are excreted more efficiently in an acidic urine because they are largely ionized at a low pH. The techniques of acidification or alkalinization of the urine with drugs such as ascorbic acid and sodium bicarbonate, respectively, can be used to hasten excretion of certain drugs taken in overdosage. For example, barbiturate intoxication may be managed in part by administration of sodium bicarbonate to raise the urinary pH, thus promoting ionization of the drug molecules in the tubular fluid and reducing tubular reabsorption.

Intestine

Drugs that are not absorbed from the GI tract—or drugs and metabolites that are **secreted into** the GI tract by the bile, salivary glands, and digestive glands—can be excreted in the feces. Because many drugs are metabolized in the liver, their metabolites often are secreted into the bile, which passes into the intestine. The metabolite may then be excreted in the feces, but most often it is *reabsorbed* from the intestine into the bloodstream and ultimately excreted in the urine. Thus, biliary and fecal excretion are important mainly for those drugs (eg, penicillin, colchicine) that cannot be reabsorbed from the intestine because ionization occurs at the intestinal pH.

Lungs

The lungs are a relatively minor route of elimination. This route is important primarily in the case of the gaseous and volatile liquid general anesthetics, which exit the bloodstream, travel across the alveolar membrane, and enter air, which is then expired. Many other volatile substances (including alcohol) that are mainly biotransformed in the liver and excreted by the kidneys do appear in the expired air in limited amounts. Enough alcohol can be eliminated unchanged by the lungs to be detected and measured, and this procedure (breathometer) often is used to determine the degree of intoxication.

Mammary Glands

Many drugs enter breast milk and are transferred to the nursing infant. Although the amount is only approximately 1% of the dose taken by the mother, it can be sufficient for some drugs to exert a pharmacologic effect on the infant; for example, after ingestion by the mother, diazepam can sedate the infant to the point of reducing the ability to suckle. Other drugs, however, such as anticoagulants, barbiturates, corticosteroids, penicillins, and sulfonamides, may be transferred to the infant in breast milk in significant amounts. Use of any drugs during lactation should be restricted as much as possible.

Blood Level Ranges

When a drug enters the blood, its final level (concentration) depends on many factors; the dose, of course, is of primary importance. If the blood level is below that necessary to exert a therapeutic response, the drug will be in the *subtherapeutic* range; however, there may be enough drug present to produce some pharmacologic effects. The next higher range is that level at which the drug will produce the desired therapeutic effect; this is the *therapeutic* range. Finally, when the dose is too high, the blood level of the drug will rise to the point where the patient exhibits toxic effects—the *toxic* range.

The ranges for any drug are **not** absolute, however; that is, a patient may experience serious toxic effects even though the blood level of the drug being taken is in the therapeutic range.

In addition, a patient who is taking a daily dose of a drug that is in the therapeutic range could experience an increase in the blood level—possibly into the toxic range—by the addition of a second drug added to therapy. This is an important type of drug interaction (see Chapter 6 for more information).

Although the therapeutic blood level has not been established for every drug, there are many medications for which the effective range is known. For example, a patient who has epilepsy and is taking phenytoin (eg, Dilantin) will be less likely to experience seizures if the blood level is kept in the therapeutic range of 10 to 20 mg/L.

Monitoring blood levels of drug is a very important procedure to help the patient on prolonged (maintenance) therapy receive the maximum benefit. Drugs for which blood level monitoring is extremely important include lithium and digoxin. This expanding area of pharmacology is considered in greater detail in Chapter 7.

Steady-State Blood Levels

After a *single* dose of a drug, the blood level will decline (due primarily to biotransformation and elimination processes) at a fairly predictable rate. The term *elimination (biologic) half-life* ($T_{1/2}$) is the **time** required for the blood level of a drug to decrease by 50%. The variation in drug half-lives ranges from short (eg, morphine: $T_{1/2}$ = 2–4 hours) to long (eg, alprazolam [Xanax]: $T_{1/2}$ = 12–15 hours) to extremely long (eg, fluoxetine [Prozac]: $T_{1/2}$ = 2–3 days).

During chronic administration, the desired goal is to achieve a fairly constant—or *steady-state*—blood level of the drug. This is accomplished by giving the drug at a rate approximately equal to the rate at which it is eliminated from the blood, that is, administering the dose at an interval that is the same as its $T_{1/2}$. After a period of time equal to **five** biologic half-lives, the steady-state condition will have been achieved. This does **not** mean that the drug is in the *therapeutic* range; it means only that the amount of drug *entering* the blood is approximately equal to the amount of drug *exiting* the blood. It is important to understand that steady-state levels could occur in either the **subtherapeutic** or **toxic** ranges.

As an example, assume morphine has a $T_{1/2}$ of approximately 4 hours. To reach steady-state conditions, the selected dose of morphine should be given once every 4 hours. After about 20 hours (5 × 4 hours [$T_{1/2}$]), there should be a fairly constant blood level of morphine; if the dose was the correct one, the blood level will be in the therapeutic range and the patient will receive a good degree of analgesia.

If the interval between doses is *shorter* than the $T_{1/2}$, the blood level will continually increase, that is, steady-state conditions will **not** be achieved, and the drug concentration will eventually reach the toxic range. This method is used, however, under certain *limited* conditions in which it is necessary to get a drug into the therapeutic range as quickly as possible; this is called a *loading dose*. For example, in the emergency treatment of cardiac arrhythmias, lidocaine, an antiarrhythmic drug, is given by an IV bolus; dosing is then continued by IV infusion. A loading dose also can be used with oral administration of drugs. An example is the initiation of antibiotic therapy; the patient may be instructed to take two capsules for the first and second doses to increase the blood level more rapidly; dosing then continues following the usual pattern for maintenance therapy, that is, giving the drug—one antibiotic capsule in this case—at intervals equal to its $T_{1/2}$. A common example of the use of a loading dose approach is that of *digitalization* (see Chapter 31), used to achieve rapid therapeutic concentrations of digoxin in the patient with acute-onset congestive heart failure.

Selected Bibliography

Edgar B, Bailey R, Bergstrand R, et al.: Acute effects of drinking grapefruit juice on the pharmacokinetics and dynamics on felodipine—and its potential clinical relevance. Eur J Clin Pharmacol 42:31, 1992

Greenblatt DJ: Presystemic extraction: Mechanisms and consequences. J Clin Pharmacol 33:650, 1993

Guengerich FP: Cytochrome P450 enzymes. Am Scientist 81:440, 1993

Montella KR, Powrie R: Critical illness in pregnancy 4. Pharmacological considerations. Emerg Med 26(1):99, 1994

Murray M: P450 enzymes: Inhibition mechanisms, genetic regulations and effects of liver disease. Clin Pharmacokinet 23(2):132, 1992

Somberg J, Shroff G, Khosla S, Ehrenpreis S: The clinical implications of first-pass metabolism: Treatment strategies for the 1990s. J Clin Pharmacol 33:670, 1993

Vesell ES, DeAngelo TM, Katz IR: Reproducibility of antipyrine half-lives in elderly subjects. Clin Pharmacol Ther 54:150, 1993

4

Basic Sites and Mechanisms of Drug Action: Pharmacodynamics

Pharmacologic effects produced by drugs are the result of complex biochemical and/or physical interactions with cells. Although more research is required to obtain further information about the molecular basis of drug activity, sufficient data are available to identify for many drugs *where* they act (sites of action) and *how* they produce their pharmacologic effects (mechanisms of action).

Drugs are classified as either *pharmacodynamic* or *chemotherapeutic* agents. The effect of a pharmacodynamic agent is strictly quantitative; that is, it can increase or decrease the rate of existing physiologic functions (eg, reduction in blood pressure, slowing of heart rate, increased urine output) but it cannot change the type of function. In contrast, a chemotherapeutic agent (eg, antibiotic, antineoplastic) reduces or eliminates invading organisms (eg, bacteria, viruses) or growths (eg, tumors). Most drugs are in the former category.

Virtually all body tissues are exposed to systemically administered drugs, but certain tissues appear to be affected much more than others. Most drugs exert their *primary* actions at specific sites in the body, although they may affect several tissues or organs, depending on their distribution.

Many drugs produce their effects by combining with specific parts of a cell, altering the function of the target cell and ultimately the target tissue. This combination is, for many drugs, due to the formation of some type of chemical bond with reactive sites that have an affinity for the drug; these sites are termed *receptors*. Although the precise structure of most receptors is still uncertain, several concepts relating to drug–receptor interactions can be stated:

- Drugs exert a *quantitative*, not a qualitative, effect at receptor sites; that is, drugs alter the *rate* of ongoing physiologic processes but cannot create new functions.
- Receptors have specific shapes; drug molecules with similar shapes can then fit into the receptor ("lock" [receptor] and "key" [drug] theory).
- Forces must be present to attract and hold a drug in contact with a receptor so that the drug may exert its effect.
- Drugs "fitting" the receptor may either activate the receptor (*agonists*) or inhibit it (*antagonists*).
- Not all receptors on a particular cell need to be occupied for a drug effect to occur; potent drugs may be effective at very low concentrations, occupying only a fraction of the available receptors.

In considering drug–receptor interactions, it is important to understand several basic concepts. Drugs capable of binding to receptor sites and eliciting a pharmacologic effect are termed *agonists*. Depending on the maximal effect that ensues when all receptors are occupied by a particular drug, agonists may be divided into *full agonists* and *partial agonists*. Partial agonists produce a lesser response at full receptor occupancy than full agonists.

Drugs that have affinity for a receptor site but lack intrinsic activity at that site are termed *antagonists*. They prevent agonists from binding with and activating that particular receptor.

Potency Versus Efficacy

Two terms relating to drug action that often are confused are *potency* and *efficacy*. A drug is said to be *potent* when it possesses a high degree of pharmacologic activity at low doses. Knowledge of a drug's potency is important for selection of the appropriate dose to be administered, but is relatively unimportant in deciding which of two drugs—both exhibiting the same maximal effect—should be used. It makes little difference if the dose of drug A is 5 mg and that of drug B is 500 mg as long as the dosage of each is easy to administer. The major concern then becomes which of the two drugs is the safest (ie, has the lowest toxicity).

Efficacy refers to the maximal effect produced by a drug, and is very important in deciding which drug to use. For example, oral administration of 4 mg of hydromorphone (Dilaudid) results in much greater pain relief than 65 mg of propoxyphene (Darvon). Therefore, hydromorphone is more effective *and* more potent than propoxyphene.

Therapeutic Index

The therapeutic index (TI) for a given drug is a measure of its safety margin and is defined as the TD_{50}/ED_{50}, where the TD_{50} is the dose causing toxic reactions in 50% of patients, and the ED_{50} is the dose producing the desired therapeutic effect in 50% of patients. The larger the TI, the greater the safety (ie, a large TI = a wide range of safe doses). It is important to recognize, however, that the TI is simply one measure of a drug's safety; the TI cannot be used to evaluate the efficacy of a drug. Further, the TI must be viewed in general terms because some patients display an extreme sensitivity to certain drugs, and therefore have a very low TI for that particular drug. As an example, aspirin is a very safe drug in normal doses in for most people; however, severe hypersensitivity reactions to small doses of aspirin have occurred in some patients. Therefore, although the TI for aspirin is quite high in the general population, certain patients are extremely sensitive to very low doses of aspirin.

Malseed, RT; Goldstein, FJ; and Balkon, N: PHARMACOLOGY: DRUG THERAPY AND NURSING CONSIDERATIONS, Fourth Edition.

Non–Receptor-Mediated Drug Effects

Some drugs produce their respective therapeutic effects without acting on any receptors. For example, *osmotic diuretics* (eg, mannitol) reduce body fluid by increasing the osmolarity of plasma and promoting an increase in urine output, and *metal-chelating agents* such as EDTA (ethylenediaminetetraacetic acid) form a chemical complex with heavy metals to prevent poisoning by these substances. Compared to all of the drugs that owe their therapeutic actions to a drug–receptor complexation, the number of medications acting by non–receptor-mediated mechanisms is small.

Factors Modifying Drug Effects

In selecting the proper drug and dosage to use, it is important to understand that many factors can alter an individual's response to a drug. Several of these important factors follow.

Body Size and Weight

Drug dosages should be adjusted in proportion to body weight because the greater the body weight, the more the drug can become diluted in the body. In contrast, for patients with *lower* body weight, such as infants, small children, and elderly or debilitated people, drug doses—in general—should be *reduced*; if this is not done, a usual therapeutic dose can become a toxic one in such patients (see Chapters 8 and 9).

Age

In general, pediatric and geriatric patients are very sensitive to the effects of many drugs, principally because of reductions in biotransformation and elimination processes, and reduced body mass (see Chapters 8 and 9).

Sex

Female patients may be more susceptible to the actions of some drugs, exhibiting a more intense and/or a more prolonged effect. This may be due to their smaller body weight and greater proportion of body fat, which lead to the reduced biotransformation of drugs. Hormonal factors also may account for the decrease in drug metabolism. Clinical data indicate that women have a lower rate of biotransformation of alcohol than men (see Chapter 82).

Route and Time of Administration

Absorption is greatly affected by the route of administration (as discussed in Chapter 2) as well as the time of administration; for instance, absorption of most orally administered drugs is greater when the stomach is empty compared to when it is full (ie, after a meal).

Pathologic Conditions

Rates of drug absorption, biotransformation, and elimination can be markedly altered by changes in the normal physiologic state of the patient secondary to, for example, nutritional disorders, thyroid dysfunction (increased sensitivity toward epinephrine), cardiovascular, hepatic, or renal disease (delayed metabolism and clearance of drugs), and anxiety (decreased analgesic efficacy).

Pharmacogenetics

An unexpected abnormal response to a drug may occur because of a difference in a patient's genetic composition; this is termed a *pharmacogenetic* reaction. Genetically determined alterations in catabolic enzymes usually reduce the normal metabolism of drugs, and therefore increase the chance that the patient will experience adverse drug effects. As these genetic factors become known and categorized, drug therapy will be more appropriately individualized.

Allergic Reactions

Some patients exhibit allergic reactions to drugs. These reactions are not different from those seen in other types of allergies (eg, to a bee sting), and range from a minor skin rash to bronchoconstriction and anaphylactic shock. Because an allergic reaction to a drug *can be fatal*, a drug history is not complete unless patients have been asked if they have ever experienced such a reaction in the past. Patients who are allergic to a drug should *not* receive it again.

Psychological Factors

The attitude and expectations of a patient taking a drug can greatly influence its effectiveness. The most relevant example of this type of response is the placebo effect, in which a clinical effect is seen after an inactive substance (ie, one that has no pharmacologic effects) is given to a patient who believes that an active drug has been administered, and then reports "feeling better." Patients receiving placebos have even reported that they have experienced adverse reactions (eg, dizziness, nausea)! Reassuring and encouraging a patient in order to enhance the clinical effectiveness of a drug is a vital role of every health professional.

Repeated Dosage

Variations in the response to an individual drug over time may take several forms:

1. *Cumulative effect:* a progressively increasing response to repeated doses that occurs if the rate of drug administration exceeds the rate of elimination.
2. *Tolerance:* decreased response to a drug resulting from its repeated administration. Mechanisms by which tolerance occurs include an increase in biotransformation, and receptor adaptation. This latter process has been characterized as either "receptor downregulation" (reduction in number and/or affinity of receptors) or "receptor upregulation" (increase in number and/or affinity of receptors). It occurs with various types of agents including psychoactive (eg, benzodiazepines), cardiovascular (eg, propranolol) and abused (eg, cocaine) drugs. The *rapid* development of tolerance, such as exhibited during cocaine abuse, is known as *tachyphylaxis*.

3. *Resistance:* impaired response to a dose that normally is effective. It is a type of tolerance usually seen in connection with anti-infective drugs: The microorganism becomes resistant to the bactericidal effects of the antibiotic. The phenomenon of resistance is considered in greater detail in Chapter 58.

Combined Effects of Drugs

Effects of one drug may be modified in several ways by the presence of a second drug.

1. *Synergism:* an enhanced pharmacologic response resulting from the simultaneous use of two drugs.
   a. *Additive effect:* the total drug response *equals* the sum of the responses of all drugs that a patient is taking. In this instance, the drugs usually are of the same type and often have the same mechanism(s) of action (eg, narcotics).
   b. *Potentiation:* the total drug response is *greater* than the sum of the responses of all drugs being administered to a patient. It is usually seen when two drugs exert the same clinical effect by different mechanisms. For example, the combined antihypertensive effect of hydrochlorothiazide, a diuretic, and propranolol, a beta-blocker, is significantly greater than the sum of their individual antihypertensive actions.
2. *Antagonism:* a reduced or completely blocked effect of one drug that occurs after a second drug has been administered.
   a. *Competitive:* competition for the same receptor sites (eg, acetylcholine [agonist] and atropine [antagonist], or naloxone [antagonist] and morphine [agonist]).
   b. *Chemical:* inactivation of a drug by formation of a chemical complex (eg, chelating agents in metal poisoning, such as BAL used in the treatment of lead poisoning).
   c. *Physiologic:* use of two drugs having opposite biologic effects (eg, caffeine, a stimulant, to counteract the sedative effects of ethanol).

Mechanisms of Drug Action

Although the *clinical* effects of a drug can be described in terms of specific alterations in physiologic function, the underlying biochemical and biophysical mechanisms of many drug actions are not as well known. As discussed earlier, the interaction of a drug molecule with a receptor site is the initial event by which most drugs evoke their biologic responses. A drug–receptor interaction initiates a sequence of biochemical and/or physiologic events that produces the final therapeutic response to the drug. Several theories have been advanced to help explain how the combination of a drug molecule with a reactive site on a receptor can lead to a wide range of clinical effects.

Enzyme Inhibition

Many drugs have been shown to interfere with enzymes necessary for the normal functioning of tissues and organs. Because almost all biologic reactions are catalyzed by cellular enzymes, alteration of normal enzymatic activity can significantly accelerate or retard biologic functions.

Inhibition of tyrosine hydroxylase decarboxylase can decrease catecholamine synthesis, and drugs having these actions have been used as antihypertensive drugs. Cholinesterase inhibitors increase acetylcholine levels by slowing its enzymatic inactivation and are effective in treating glaucoma and myasthenia gravis.

Inhibitors of hepatic microsomal enzymes can increase the effects of those drugs whose activity usually is terminated—completely or in part—by these enzymes (eg, the effects of cimetidine on the actions of theophylline).

Enzyme Stimulation

Drugs that increase the action of adenylate cyclase, the enzyme that forms cyclic adenosine monophosphate, have a variety of actions in the body, including bronchodilation, lipolysis, and glycogenolysis. Certain drugs (eg, phenobarbital) can accelerate the activity of hepatic microsomal enzymes; this effect increases the biotransformation of other drugs and reduces their therapeutic activity (see Chapter 6).

Alterations in Membrane Permeability

Drugs can selectively increase (eg, benzodiazepines) *or* decrease (eg, local anesthetics) the permeability of cellular membranes to ions, or increase active transport processes (eg, insulin).

Interaction With Neurotransmitters

Most physiologic processes are regulated by the activity of neurotransmitters (eg, dopamine, epinephrine, acetylcholine). Drugs may modify the actions of neurotransmitters in several ways:

- Increase synthesis (eg, lecithin)
- Reduce synthesis (eg, metyrosine)
- Reduce presynaptic storage (eg, reserpine)
- Increase release (eg, amphetamine)
- Reduce release (eg, clonidine)
- Activate postsynaptic receptors (eg, pilocarpine)
- Block postsynaptic receptors (eg, atropine)
- Reduce reuptake at presynaptic membrane (eg, amitriptyline)
- Reduce enzymatic inactivation (eg, physostigmine)

Other mechanisms of drug action include—but are not limited to—chemical neutralization (eg, of gastric acid), detergent action (on bronchiolar mucus), adsorption (of toxins), and osmotic swelling (of muciloids to provide a laxative action). Specific details of the actions of these agents may be found in the respective chapters associated with the agents or agent groups.

Selected Bibliography

Bakris GL, Talbert R: Drug dosing in patients with renal insufficiency. Postgrad Med 94(8):153, 1993

Cheymol G: Clinical pharmacokinetics of drugs in obesity: An update. Clin Pharmacokinet 25(2):103, 1993

du Souich P, Verges J, Erill S: Plasma protein binding and pharmacological response. Clin Pharmacokinet 24(6):435, 1993
Edwards G, Weston AH: The pharmacology of ATP-sensitive potassium channels. Annu Rev Pharmacol Toxicol 33:597, 1993
Lee BL, Wong D, Benowitz NL, Sullam PM: Altered patterns of drug metabolism in patients with acquired immunodeficiency syndrome. Clin Pharmacol Ther 53:529, 1993
Mulder GJ: Glucuronidation and its role in regulation of biological activity of drugs. Annu Rev Pharmacol Toxicol 32:25, 1992
Scharf S, Christophidis N: Prescribing for the elderly: 1. Relevance of pharmacokinetics and pharmacodynamics. Med J Aust 158:395, 1993
Seeman P, Van Tol HHM: Dopamine receptor pharmacology. Curr Opin Neurol Neurosurg 6:602, 1993
Yost CS: G proteins: Basic characteristics and clinical potential for the practice of anesthesia. Anesth Analg 77:822, 1993
Zini R, Riant P, Barre J, Tillement J-P: Disease induced variations in plasma protein levels: Implications for drug dosage regimens (Part II). Clin Pharmacokinet 19(3)218, 1993

Nursing Bibliography

Payne R: Oral analgesics for cancer pain: Pharmacology, anatomy and physiology. American Journal of Hospice and Palliative Care 8(6): 19–26, 1991
Schwertz D: Basic principles of pharmacologic action. The Nursing Clinics of North America 26(2):273–290, 1991

5

Pharmacologic Basis of Adverse Drug Reactions

A primary goal of pharmaceutical research is to create a drug that will produce maximum therapeutic effects without causing any adverse reactions. Although many new medications are, in fact, less toxic than older ones, they still produce adverse drug reactions (ADRs).

Adverse reactions to drug therapy include any unwanted or potentially harmful effects resulting from drug administration. Not all ADRs are unexpected, however; some represent an extension of the pharmacologic actions of a drug. Other ADRs often can be predicted on the basis of the route of drug administration, presence of other drugs, and condition of the patient.

Minor ADRs are those classified as annoying; they are rarely serious. Examples are drowsiness, dry mouth, and nausea. In contrast, major ADRs are serious toxic effects that can be fatal. Examples include gastric ulceration, respiratory depression, hepatotoxicity, and blood dyscrasias. Changing the dose, dosage form, route of administration, and/or diet often can reduce or abolish minor ADRs. Major ADRs, however, are more difficult to control. Therefore, selection of a drug includes consideration of the types of ADRs that the drug can produce, and the frequency of their occurrence. That is, the possibility of serious toxicity resulting from drug usage usually is acceptable if the condition being treated is serious enough to warrant the risk. Conversely, drugs causing a high degree of adverse effects should not be used to treat trivial or psychosomatic illnesses. For example, chloramphenicol, a highly toxic antibacterial agent, is acceptable in the treatment of certain meningeal infections in which other agents were ineffective, but it should not be used to treat minor infections of the respiratory tract.

Classification of Adverse Drug Reactions

Classification of ADRs is difficult because a wide range of effects can occur. More than one category is needed to represent appropriately the many different types. The following classification will be used:

- I. Pharmacologic
  - A. Predictable
  - B. Drug Interactions
  - C. Drug Dependence
- II. Nonpharmacologic
  - A. Hypersensitivity
  - B. Pharmacogenetic
  - C. Photosensitivity
  - D. Carcinogenicity
  - E. Teratogenicity
- III. Disease Related

Pharmacologic Adverse Drug Reactions

Predictable

Overdosage with a therapeutic agent usually will elicit, among other effects, an excessive reaction to the *primary* effect of the drug. For example, antianxiety agents (eg, diazepam) often will produce drowsiness, possibly sufficient to cause the patient to fall asleep during the daytime. In this case, the adverse reaction often can be diminished or eliminated by reducing the dosage and/or the frequency of administration. Other common examples are hemorrhaging with anticoagulants, and excessive electrolyte depletion during diuretic therapy.

In many instances, adverse effects are related to one or more *secondary* actions produced by a drug. In some cases, secondary drug effects can be largely eliminated by adjusting the dosage carefully in each individual. Sometimes, however, secondary effects of a drug cannot be controlled by dosage reduction because minimal amounts already are being used. For example, even in small, therapeutic doses, anticholinergic agents used for relief of gastrointestinal (GI) spasm and hypermotility usually produce xerostomia (dry mouth), blurring of vision, and some degree of urinary retention and constipation. Another example of a drug-induced secondary reaction is constipation with narcotic analgesics.

Secondary adverse reactions may be quite serious, requiring careful patient monitoring and perhaps changes in the drug regimen. Potentially dangerous secondary effects of drugs include the following: thrombotic complications with oral contraceptives, arrhythmias with digitalis, and GI ulceration with aspirin and related drugs.

Many pharmacologic ADRs have been extensively documented. Thus, in assessing the suitability of a particular drug, its predictable toxicity should be weighed against its potential beneficial effects.

Drug Interactions

The presence of a second drug may greatly modify the actions of a concurrently administered drug. In many instances, drugs are used together to achieve a better clinical response than either drug could achieve alone. This is an example of a positive clinical interaction. On the other hand, indiscriminate multiple-drug therapy can be quite hazardous; the chance of untoward reactions increases dramatically as additional drugs are added to a therapeutic regimen. This problem becomes especially acute in the elderly or the seriously ill patient, for whom several different drugs may be administered concurrently. Adverse effects due to multiple-drug therapy can be manifested in several ways; this aspect of pharmacotherapy is examined further in Chapter 6.

Drug Dependence

Certain drugs are more likely to induce a state of psychological dependence ("addiction") and/or physical dependence. This serious issue is discussed more completely in Chapter 82.

Nonpharmacologic Adverse Drug Reactions

Another group of ADRs has no relationship to the pharmacologic actions of a drug. Rather, they are related to an abnormal sensitivity or reactivity to the drug on the patient's part. Principal hazards of the nonpharmacologic ADR are that it cannot be predicted from the profile of drug action, and it can occur abruptly, that is, without any warning signs or symptoms. Fortunately, these types of reactions develop in only a fraction of patients receiving the drug.

Hypersensitivity

Hypersensitivity or allergic reactions are perhaps the largest single group of untoward drug effects. Allergic reactions are not dose related and are largely independent of the pharmacologic properties of the drug molecule. These hypersensitivity reactions are associated with an altered reactivity or sensitization of the patient resulting from prior exposure to a drug that behaves like an allergen. The drug (or a metabolite) interacts with a tissue or plasma protein, activating the reticuloendothelial system, resulting in production of antibodies to the drug (or metabolite) molecule. A subsequent exposure to the same drug (or in some cases a similar one) elicits an antigen–antibody reaction that produces the symptoms of the allergic response (eg, itching, edema, congestion, wheezing).

Allergic drug reactions may be classified as either immediate (eg, anaphylaxis, urticaria) or delayed (eg, serum sickness).

Immediate

An immediate allergic drug reaction develops within minutes of drug exposure. The drug–antibody reaction probably releases several vasoactive substances, such as histamine and bradykinin, from their tissue stores. These substances can react with the smooth muscle of many body tissues (blood vessels, bronchioles, GI tract) to produce characteristic signs of the allergic reaction such as bronchoconstriction or vasodilation. The symptoms may be very mild (rash, itching, urticaria) or serious enough (respiratory distress, circulatory collapse) to require immediate attention and swift medical treatment to prevent death. In general, the severity of the reaction is independent of the drug itself, but probably depends to a large extent on a patient's sensitivity. It has been documented that even very small doses of common drugs such as aspirin and penicillin can produce violent hypersensitivity reactions in susceptible patients. The grave concern about these kinds of reactions is that often they are totally unpredictable, and quick recognition and proper treatment are essential to minimize serious consequences such as respiratory distress, hypotension, and cardiovascular collapse.

Delayed

A delayed allergic drug reaction develops slowly after drug challenge. The clinical picture of delayed hypersensitivity often includes a diffuse rash, fever, and swelling and stiffness of the joints. This syndrome is frequently referred to as *serum sickness*. This name derives from the fact that the allergic response results from damage produced by *circulating* immune complexes that may lodge in small vessels and cause the characteristic symptoms. Sometimes the liver, kidneys, and bone marrow may become damaged, although the factors that determine specific organ involvement are largely unknown.

Pharmacogenetics

Pharmacogenetics is a specialized field of study that deals with altered drug responses that are under hereditary control; great strides have been made in determining some of the genetic differences that predispose certain people to toxic drug effects. Many of these types of reactions alter the rate at which drugs are biotransformed, such as prolonged depression of respiration after administration of succinylcholine (skeletal muscle relaxant). Other types include the development of hemolytic anemia (toxic reaction linked to a genetic alteration of the enzyme glucose-6-phosphate dehydrogenase in red blood cells) after exposure to certain drugs (eg, primaquine).

Carcinogenicity

Some drugs can induce malignant changes in cells. Although the mechanisms are not clearly understood, there is some limited information as to which patients are more likely to develop cancer from certain drugs (eg, postmenopausal women appear to have an increased risk of endometrial cancer if they receive estrogen therapy for more than 1 year). There also is concern with regard to development of future malignancies in the treatment of pediatric leukemias and lymphomas with antineoplastics, which by their nature are potentially carcinogenic.

Teratogenicity

Alcohol and various drugs are known to produce anatomic, biochemical, and/or functional defects in the developing fetus, especially when they are consumed by the mother during her first trimester. The United States Food and Drug Administration (FDA) has established five categories indicating the potential of a drug for causing fetal damage (see Chapter 1). Drugs (both over-the-counter and prescription) should *not* be taken during pregnancy unless a physician has been consulted. There also is evidence that teratogenic effects may be produced by the *father's* use—or use in the recent past—of substances (eg, marijuana) that can damage sperm; this is a developing area of toxicologic study.

Photosensitivity

A unique type of dermatologic hypersensitivity reaction after use of many drugs is observed on exposure to sunlight and is termed *photosensitization*. Two principal types of reactions can occur in people whose skin has been sensitized by either topical or internal use of photosensitizing drugs. A *photoallergic* reaction presents as a papular eruption on sun-exposed areas, similar to that resulting from contact dermatitis. It is probably caused by the photosensitizing drug forming an antigen by absorption of sunlight, and subsequent combination with a skin protein. The resultant antibody formation sensitizes the patient to further synthesis of antigen by continued sun exposure.

A *phototoxic* reaction, on the other hand, is characterized by a severe sunburn; as such, it is not always viewed as a hypersensitivity reaction. Nevertheless, it is probably caused by a photosensitizing chemical that absorbs ultraviolet radiation energy to such an extent that it becomes toxic to epidermal cells.

A wide variety of clinically useful drugs can produce photosensitization. This fact is noted under the "Significant Adverse Reactions" heading for each of the offending drugs.

Disease-Related Adverse Effects

The pathophysiologic state of a patient is a major determinant of the potential for a drug to cause adverse effects. Underlying disease states, often unrecognized, can greatly increase the possibility of drug toxicity. The more common abnormalities are discussed briefly in the following.

Hepatic Disease

Because the liver plays a major role in the inactivation of many drugs, an impairment of hepatic function may increase blood levels of a drug. If normal dosing schedules are followed, accumulation of drug in the body can occur, resulting in symptoms of drug overdosage. Because of the large reserve capacity of the liver, however, hepatic activity will remain close to normal except in the most severe forms of hepatic disease.

Renal Disease

The presence of kidney disease can cause many ADRs to be produced by those drugs that are eliminated largely through the renal system. In the presence of renal disease, doses of potentially toxic drugs excreted by the kidney (eg, aminoglycoside antibiotics) must be reduced to avoid accumulation and subsequent toxicity. In progressive renal failure, there may be a decrease in plasma proteins (eg, albumin); this will increase the free (unbound) levels of many drugs, resulting in potentiation of their pharmacologic effects, possibly to the point of toxicity.

Emotional Disorders

Mentally unstable people should be monitored carefully during their drug therapy. Too often, emotionally disturbed patients do not comply with proper dosing instructions; this may then lead to overdosage of their prescribed drugs (eg, sedative/hypnotics) or use of other drugs that were not prescribed for them. A major problem exists with misuse of, or overmedication with, antipsychotic drugs. Because many patients taking these drugs are emotionally unstable to some extent, they represent an extremely high-risk group for potential adverse reactions.

Other Disease States

Many other existing diseases can increase the likelihood for a particular drug to elicit an ADR. Use of nonselective beta-adrenergic blockers (eg, nadolol, propranolol) in patients with asthma may worsen the already impaired ventilatory flow. Beta-adrenergic blockers, as well as the calcium channel blocker verapamil, also should not be given to patients with advanced heart block, because these drugs can reduce myocardial contractility and further slow atrioventricular conduction. Aspirin and other anti-inflammatory drugs are more likely to cause GI bleeding in a person with an active or recent gastric ulcer. Careful assessment of a patient's overall health status is important in ensuring the safest and most effective use of a drug.

Nursing Management

Pretherapy Assessment

Carefully assess the seriousness of the condition being treated before using any medications. The potential benefit should outweigh the apparent risk, and less toxic agents should be tried first, if at all possible.

Obtain a careful drug history, including any previous drug allergies, from each patient before administering any prescribed medication. This measure reduces the possibility of hypersensitivity reactions.

Nursing Interventions

Medication Administration

Recognize that any drug can be potentially toxic, and administer all drugs with respect for their adverse effects as well as their beneficial effects.

Plan to administer drugs to maximize their intended effects and to minimize their untoward reactions. For example, give diuretics in the morning to reduce the need to void at night, and give antihistamines at night to avoid daytime drowsiness.

Surveillance During Therapy

Always monitor the dose being given to ensure that it is within acceptable limits for the condition and patient being treated.

Adverse Drug Reactions—A Glossary

Alopecia: loss of hair, sometimes accompanied by extreme drying of the scalp. Alopecia is a side effect of many antineoplastic agents as well as anticoagulants, mephenytoin, methimazole, and others.

Anaphylactic reaction: a severe systemic allergic reaction that develops suddenly, progresses rapidly, and is frequently fatal if not treated. Symptoms range from itching, hives, nasal congestion, abdominal cramping, and diarrhea to dyspnea, hypotension, fainting, choking sensation, cardiovascular collapse, and possibly death. An anaphylactic reaction theoretically can occur with any drug, but it is most commonly observed with drugs that are frequently associated with drug allergies, such as penicillins, sulfonamides, and salicylates.

Blood dyscrasias: abnormal conditions of the formed elements or other clotting constituents of the blood. Several types commonly are observed:

Agranulocytosis: an acute febrile disease characterized by an absence of granulocytes and often a corresponding reduction in monocytes and lymphocytes. Clinical symptoms include chills, fever, and extreme weakness. Because of the lack of white blood cells, the body's defense mechanism is impaired, and severe infection can result. It is potentially fatal. Early warning signs are mucous membrane ulceration, sore throat, skin rash, and fever. Recovery normally occurs within 1 to 2 weeks after drug is withdrawn. Any existing infection should be vigorously treated. Agranulocytosis is the most common drug-induced blood dyscrasia.

Anemia: a reduction in the number of red blood cells, hemoglobin concentration, and volume of packed red cells. The result is a sharp curtailment in the oxygen-carrying capacity of the blood.

Aplastic: results from drug-induced damage to the bone marrow and is marked by a deficiency of red cells, hemoglobin, and granular cells, and a predominance of lymphocytes. Clinical signs include fatigue, tachycardia, bleeding, fever, and increased susceptibility to infection. Aplastic anemia is often fatal owing to hemorrhage and overwhelming infection.

Hemolytic: characterized by a short life span of the red cell. Circulating erythrocytes are destroyed owing to increased hemolytic activity induced by certain drugs or poisons. Especially common in people with a glucose-6-phosphate dehydrogenase deficiency. Withdrawal of offending agent usually corrects the condition.

Thrombocytopenia: a lowered blood platelet count, resulting from either platelet destruction or depression of the platelet-forming mechanism in the bone marrow. Onset may be sudden, and symptoms include purpura (petechiae; epistaxis; oral, vaginal, or GI bleeding) and easy bruising. The platelet count returns to normal within a few weeks after cessation of drug therapy, but the count may again rise briefly immediately after withdrawal of the drug. Most severe complications can result from excessive cerebral hemorrhage.

Erythema multiforme: an acute inflammatory skin disease characterized by lesions consisting of concentric circles of erythema, usually appearing on the neck, face, and legs. Occasionally blisters are observed. Often accompanied by fever, malaise, arthralgia, and gastric distress. The most severe variant, *Stevens-Johnson syndrome*, is characterized by high fever, headache, and inflammatory lesions of the mouth, eyes, and genitalia. Often the bronchial and visceral mucosa are involved. Death can occur because of renal impairment.

Exfoliative dermatitis: erythema and scaling of the skin over large parts of the body. Symptoms include itching, weakness, malaise, fever, and weight loss. Exfoliation may include loss of hair and nails as well as skin, and mucosal sloughing can occur. The reaction is generally unpredictable in its duration and recurrence. Relapses are frequent, and secondary infections can be serious. Exfoliative dermatitis may occur secondary to preexisting dermatoses or to contact dermatitis resulting from an underlying carcinoma, or can be caused by drug usage.

Hepatotoxicity: liver damage resulting from either infection or drug hypersensitivity. The most frequently observed drug-induced manifestation is *jaundice*, characterized by hyperbilirubinemia and deposition of bile pigments in the mucous membranes and skin; these pigments impart the typical yellow appearance. At least three main types of jaundice are recognized:

Cholestatic: due to interference with the normal secretion of bile by an obstruction of the biliary passages. It may result from gallstones, tumors, or drug-induced inflammation of the bile channels.

Hepatocellular: due to impairment of the function of liver cells. It is also termed *necrotic jaundice*, and closely resembles severe viral hepatitis.

Hemolytic: due to a drug hypersensitivity or a direct toxic effect of the drug on erythrocytes, possibly interference with normal glucose metabolism in the red cells. In addition, a hepatitis-like reaction may be elicited by several kinds of drugs, resulting from either a hypersensitivity to the drug or a direct toxic effect of the drug on liver cells.

Lupus erythematosus (LE): an autoimmune inflammatory disorder that can occur in two forms, one affecting only the skin (discoid LE) and the other, more serious, affecting multiple body organs (systemic LE). The etiology of the naturally occurring disease is unknown, but both forms occur predominantly in young women. Several drugs, for example hydralazine and procainamide, can also cause a lupus-like reaction. Among the many symptoms are diffuse rash; fever; malaise; alopecia; joint symptoms including stiffness, swelling, and synovitis; conjunctivitis; photophobia; pneumonitis; pleurisy; myocarditis; arrhythmias; lymphadenopathy; splenomegaly; and hemolytic anemia. Renal and neurologic features are absent in drug-induced lupus but are seen in the spontaneously occurring form of the disease. Clinical features generally revert slowly toward normal when the offending drug is withdrawn, but altered laboratory values (eg, elevated antinuclear antibody titer, leukopenia, thrombocytopenia) indicative of the disease may persist for many months.

Nephrotoxicity: damage to the functional units of the kidney, such as the glomerular filtration apparatus, blood vessels, or renal tubular cells, or a dysfunction of the components (eg, enzymes, transport carriers) involved in the tubular secretory and reabsorptive processes.

Neurotoxicity: damage to different nervous system structures, manifested as a wide range of central and peripheral disturbances. Some of the more important neurotoxic effects of drugs are the following:

Myasthenia-like reaction: extreme muscle weakness due to an impairment in the transmission of impulses at the neuromuscular junction.

Extrapyramidal reactions: disturbances of the extrapyramidal motor-regulating system in the central nervous system, resulting in abnormal motor function. Common manifestations include immobility (akinesia); fixed positioning of the limbs (rigidity); sudde lent movements of the arms and head (dyst restlessness (akathisia); and rhythmic, clon activity (tremor). Extrapyramidal reactions quently associated with use of antipsych

Ototoxicity: progressive hearing loss and by damage to the eighth cranial nerve panied by vertigo and nystagmus if t branch of the nerve is affected. It i aminoglycoside antibiotics and ce

Ocular toxicity: disturbances in the functioning of the eye. The most common manifestation is blurred vision, which can occur after use of many drugs, especially those with an anticholinergic action. Other drug-induced ocular disorders include myopia, scotomata, amblyopia, optic neuritis, corneal deposits, pigmentary retinopathy, and cataracts.

Photosensitivity: an altered responsiveness to light, usually eczematous in nature. Common manifestations are itching, scaling, urticaria, and in severe cases, multiform lesions.

Purpura: localized hemorrhaging, occurring in the skin, mucous membranes, or serous membranes. The lesions may be petechiae (small blood spots) or ecchymoses (larger areas of bleeding). Purpura is commonly seen in patients with thrombocytopenia caused by increased platelet destruction.

Selected Bibliography

Ganzini L, Millar SB, Walsh JR: Drug-induced mania in the elderly. Drugs & Aging 3(5):428, 1993

Hollinger MA: Drug-induced lung toxicity. J Am Coll Toxicol 12(1):31, 1993

Kessler DA: Introducing MEDWatch: A new approach to reporting medication and device adverse effects and product problems. JAMA 269(21):2765, 1993

Kulig K: Initial management of ingestions of toxic sustances. N Engl J Med 326(25):1677, 1992

Lennard MS: Genetically determined adverse drug reactions involving metabolism. Drug Saf 9(1):60, 1993

Liebelt EL, Shannon MW: Small doses, big problems: A selected review of highly toxic common medications. Pediatr Emerg Care 9(5):292, 1993

Montella KR, Powrie R: Critical illness in pregnancy: 4. Pharmacological considerations. Emerg Med 26(1):99, 1994

Reider MJ: Immunopharmacology and adverse drug reactions. J Clin Pharmacol 33:316, 1993

Sue Y-J, Shannon M: Pharmacokinetics of drugs in overdose. Clin Pharmacokinet 23(2):93, 1992

Nursing Bibliography

Cooke D: The use of CNS manifestation in the early detection of digitalis toxicity. Heart Lung 22(6):548–553, 1993

Cooke D: Shielding your patient from digitalis toxicity. Nursing '92 23(11):49–50, 1992

Haybach P: Tuning into ototoxicity. Nursing '93 23(6):34–41, 1993

Kessler D: Using Medwatch: A better way to report adverse events. Nursing '93 23(11):49–50, 1993

Murphy T: Digoxin toxicity: Ventricular dysrythmias to watch for. American Journal of Nursing 93(12):37–41, 1993

6 Drug Interactions

A *drug interaction* refers to an event in which the usual therapeutic effect of a drug is modified by other factors, such as diet, environment, or additional drugs. When two drugs are administered simultaneously—or within a short time of each other—an interaction can occur that may either increase or decrease the intended effect of one or both drugs. The result may be either a harmful or a beneficial action on the patient. Knowing the causes of drug interactions, and having the ability to predict their occurrence, can greatly minimize the toxicity resulting from simultaneous drug usage. The means by which the presence of a second drug can enhance or reduce the effects of an initial drug were briefly reviewed in Chapter 4 under "Combined Effects of Drugs."

The clinical significance of adverse drug interactions is too often minimized. For example, when a patient on multiple-drug therapy has an unusual reaction, it can be difficult to determine whether this effect is caused by some change in the patient's physiology, by the disease being treated, or by the addition of another drug that is now interacting with other drugs in the regimen. A significant drug interaction could be missed if the unusual reaction is viewed *only* as a deterioration in the patient's status or the appearance of a new disease. In fact, it is known that drug interactions have not been recognized immediately, especially when the reaction is mild. Nurses, when making a careful assessment of *any* change in a patient's condition, must have sufficient knowledge of pharmacology to recognize the possibility of a developing drug interaction problem.

The practice of multiple-drug therapy is becoming increasingly prevalent in geriatric patients, many of whom often have more than one chronic disease requiring drug treatment. As the number of drugs used simultaneously increases, the chance for drug interactions to occur also increases. Thus, the benefit-to-risk ratio is very important to assess when making decisions about the number—and types—of drugs to be used in the management of chronic diseases. For example, although occasional episodes of dizziness or tachycardia may be acceptable consequences of drug combinations used to control severe hypertension, the increased risk of hemorrhage produced by the use of aspirin for a headache in patients already on coumarin anticoagulant therapy is unacceptable.

Because drug interactions occur more often than they should, many can be eliminated, or at least minimized, by recognizing probable causative factors and then by *taking appropriate preventive action*. Some of the more common causes of drug interactions are:

1. *Insufficient knowledge:* Safe and effective combination drug therapy requires adequate understanding of the mechanisms of action and potential complications of each drug administered.
2. *Physiologic state of the patient:* A patient's age, sex, weight, and genetic abnormalities can greatly influence the frequency of drug interactions.
3. *Presence of disease states:* The likelihood of a drug interaction is higher in those patients whose pathologic condition (such as liver, kidney, or cardiovascular disease) may reduce the elimination of one or more drugs used to treat them.
4. *Dosage form of the drug:* Incompatibility of different dosage forms or improper pharmaceutical preparation of a drug may cause drug interactions on either a physical or a chemical level. Generally, the major concern in this regard is one of bioavailability—that is, what fraction of the dose will be available to the systemic circulation after absorption. Drugs that are rated as "generically equivalent" must have *no* significant differences in the rate and amount of drug absorbed. Unfortunately, this is not always the case, and when absorption is less than required, the desired therapeutic effect also will be reduced. Another example is when a patient is taking a sustained-release product and a second drug added to therapy increases gastrointestinal (GI) motility and shortens intestinal transit time; thus, the sustained-release dosage form is eliminated more quickly and may not release an adequate amount of drug into the blood.
5. *Dietary factors:* Aspects of a patient's diet can interact with certain drugs. In cases in which such interactions are documented, it is important that the patient be advised to avoid the offending dietary agents. For example, licorice produces hypokalemia, calcium (eg, in dairy products) can retard tetracycline absorption, and tyramine (eg, in cheeses) increases blood pressure in patients taking monoamine oxidase (MAO) inhibitors.
6. *Behavioral patterns of the patient:* The fairly common practice of seeing more than one physician concurrently can increase the risk of a drug interaction if each physician is not fully aware of all the drugs being taken by the patient. Self-medication is likewise responsible for a large number of drug interactions that could easily be avoided with proper counseling.
7. *Environmental factors:* Often overlooked as a contributory factor in drug interactions is the possibility of exposure to pollutants (industrial, agricultural) and other types of chemical agents that are pharmacologically active. Although little information exists about interactions with these substances, even small amounts of insecticides, fungicides, or industrial wastes can markedly alter the effects of certain therapeutic agents. For example, chlorinated insecticides may stimulate drug metabolism by liver enzymes, whereas pesticides containing cholinesterase inhibitors can cause respiratory distress, muscle weakness, and convulsions.

Drug Interactions—Classification and Mechanisms

An understanding of the basic mechanisms by which drug reactions develop will enable the health professional to *prevent* many interactions from occurring and, at minimum, to recognize a developing interaction before it becomes a serious problem. Some drug interactions are desirable, and therefore often purposely caused; most, however, are unwanted and are harmful to the patient.

Drug interactions occurring in the body can be categorized into several classes, depending on the mechanisms responsible for the interaction. The following classification is intended to serve only as an overview of this complex field; for information pertaining to a specific drug, review the relevant chapter in this text or consult the *latest edition* of the *Physicians' Desk Reference*.

- I. Physicochemical
  - A. Physical
  - B. Chemical
- II. Pharmacodynamic
  - A. Similar Pharmacologic Effects
  - B. Opposite Pharmacologic Effects
  - C. Competitive Receptor Antagonism
  - D. Blockade of Neuronal Uptake
  - E. Altered Receptor Sensitivity
- III. Pharmacokinetic
  - A. Absorption
    1. Gastric pH
    2. Intestinal Motility and Function
    3. Chemical Binding
    4. Sequestration
    5. Intestinal Flora
    6. Active Transport
    7. Other Factors
  - B. Distribution
    1. Plasma Protein Binding
    2. Blood Flow
  - C. Biotransformation
    1. Enzyme Inhibition
    2. Enzyme Induction
    3. Residual Enzyme Effects
  - D. Elimination
    1. Urinary pH
    2. Tubular Transport
    3. Fluid and Electrolyte Balance
- IV. Immunologic
- V. Chemotherapeutic

Physicochemical

The term *incompatibility* is often used to designate a physical or chemical interaction that occurs in a mixture of drugs *before* they are administered.

Physical

Drugs are physically incompatible if the physical state of either drug is altered when they are mixed. For example, amphotericin will precipitate if mixed with normal saline instead of 5% dextrose. Likewise, the anticoagulant effect of heparin, a negatively charged acid, is antagonized by protamine, a positively charged base.

Chemical

When drugs being mixed together interact to form chemically altered products, they are chemically incompatible. For example, chemical incompatibilities in solution exist between methicillin + kanamycin, aminophylline + chlorpromazine, and dopamine + sodium bicarbonate.

In most cases, physical and chemical incompatibilities are manifested by a visible change such as formation of a precipitate or change in color. Occasionally, however, these interactions may occur without any observable signs, possibly resulting in undetected loss of potency. Thus, the compatibility of two drugs always should be ascertained by reference to an appropriate source *before mixing* to ensure that the clinical efficacy of each will not be diminished. An intravenous compatibility chart is provided in the Appendix.

Pharmacodynamic

Several types of interactions result from alterations in the normal pharmacologic effects of one drug due to the presence of a second drug with similar or different pharmacologic effects.

Similar Pharmacologic Effects

Each of two drugs possessing similar pharmacologic actions will usually enhance the pharmacologic and toxicologic effects of the other. This synergistic interaction can result in either an additive effect or potentiation (see Chapter 4). For example, alcohol and barbiturates are central nervous system depressants having an additive effect when used in combination. Anticholinergics and tricyclic antidepressants, which also have significant anticholinergic action, can result in increased side effects such as dry mouth, blurred vision, and urinary retention if used concurrently.

Opposite Pharmacologic Effects

Simultaneous administration of two drugs with opposing actions usually reduces or abolishes the pharmacologic effects of each. This type of interaction generally is easy to predict when the mechanism of action of each drug is known. An example is the use of amphetamine, which raises blood pressure, by a patient who is taking antihypertensive drugs.

Competitive Receptor Antagonism

This form of drug interaction is similar to that occurring when drugs with opposing pharmacologic actions are administered. The effects of one drug can be cancelled by the concomitant use of a second drug that blocks the access of the first drug to its receptor site of action. Again, this kind of interaction usually can be avoided by an awareness of the mechanisms of action of the two agents. For example, anticholinergic drugs should not be used in patients with glaucoma because they would block the receptor actions of the cholinergic drugs (such as pilocarpine) used to treat this eye disorder. Propranolol, a beta-adrenergic blocking drug, would interfere with the bronchodilatory action of isoproterenol in the treatment of chronic obstructive pulmonary disease.

Blockade of Neuronal Uptake

Drugs interfering with the uptake of other medications by nerve endings can cause significant interactions that usually decrease the effects of one or both drugs. For example, tricyclic antidepressants inhibit the uptake of guanethidine by nerve endings; therefore, they decrease the antihypertensive effect of guanethidine, which must be taken up by the nerve endings to produce its intended effect.

Altered Receptor Sensitivity

The sensitivity of a receptor for a particular drug action can be modified by the presence of a second drug. For example, thyroxine may increase the sensitivity of receptors to the anticoagulant effect of the coumarins, so that a dosage adjustment is needed. Another example is the prolonged use of antipsychotic drugs, which can lead to hypersensitivity of central dopamine receptors. This supersensitivity to dopamine is thought to be responsible for the appearance of a series of chronic orofacial involuntary movements (known as tardive dyskinesias) that occur with chronic administration of antipsychotic drugs. As a general rule, receptor sensitivity decreases with prolonged stimulation and increases with chronic blockade. This phenomenon explains the action of many drugs that alter receptor sensitivity, and the terms *downregulation* and *upregulation* can be applied to drug-induced decreases or increases, respectively, in receptor sensitivity. This concept is explained more fully in relation to those drugs acting in this manner under the heading "Mechanism of Action" throughout this book.

Pharmacokinetic

Many interactions are the result of drug-induced alterations in the absorption, distribution, biotransformation, and/or elimination of other drugs.

Absorption

Any substance that alters the normal physiologic processes of the GI tract can markedly change drug absorption.

Gastric pH. Drugs that elevate the pH of gastric fluid (eg, antacids) can *decrease* the absorption of weakly acidic drugs and *increase* the absorption of weakly basic drugs. This is because ionized drug molecules are largely water soluble and will not readily cross biologic membranes. Acidic drugs, such as aspirin, barbiturates, and oral anticoagulants, are largely ionized at high pH and therefore are less efficiently absorbed. Conversely, basic drugs, such as narcotics, exist largely in the nonionized (lipid-soluble) state at a high pH, and thus are better absorbed in this case.

Intestinal Motility and Function. The faster a drug passes through the stomach and intestines, the less it is absorbed. Therefore, drugs that increase GI motility such as laxatives, cholinergic drugs, and metoclopramide, can reduce absorption of orally administered drugs—that is, these drugs will be in contact with the absorbing membrane for a shorter time. In contrast, drugs that decrease GI motility (eg, narcotics, anticholinergics) will increase the absorption and, consequently, the blood level, of some drugs; the result could be an increase in toxicity.

Chemical Binding. Several substances can form complexes with many orally administered drugs, thereby impairing their GI absorption. The absorption of tetracyclines is inhibited by the presence of drugs (eg, antacids) containing calcium, magnesium, or aluminum, or by foods (eg, milk, cheese) that contain calcium; unabsorbable complexes are formed. Cholestyramine (an ionic-exchange resin) can interfere with the absorption of drugs such as warfarin, digitoxin, and phenylbutazone, also by forming an unabsorbable chemical complex.

Sequestration. Fat-soluble drugs, including vitamins A, D, and K, will be taken up into fatty substances such as mineral oil, reducing their absorption.

Intestinal Flora. Alterations in the microbial population of the GI tract can occur with many antibiotics that kill organisms that synthesize vitamin K; this effect can increase the therapeutic effect of oral anticoagulants and therefore increase the chance of hemorrhage. Drug-induced diarrhea, also occurring in response to changes in intestinal flora, can reduce drug absorption (owing to an increase in speed through the GI tract).

Active Transport. Active transport mechanisms involved in the absorption of many drugs can be inhibited by pharmacologic agents that compete for these processes. Phenytoin, for example, impedes absorption of folic acid, leading to megaloblastic anemia in many instances. Certain amino acids compete for the same transport mechanisms involved in the absorption of levodopa.

Other Factors. Additional factors associated with altered absorption of one drug in the presence of a second drug include decreased mucosal blood flow, altered volume and content of GI secretions, and direct damage to the mucosal surface.

Distribution

The distribution of drugs within the body can be significantly altered by the presence of other drugs.

Plasma Protein Binding. Drugs bound to proteins in plasma are inactive. When released from these proteins, the free drug can produce its pharmacologic effect. Many drugs are extensively bound to plasma proteins; when two such drugs are administered simultaneously, a drug interaction is likely to occur. This interaction results from the fact that one protein-bound drug displaces the other (the drug with strongest affinity for the binding sites will displace the weaker one). This can increase the pharmacologic effects of the displaced drug, its elimination, or both (displaced drug now subject to increased biotransformation and excretion). This type of drug interaction becomes very significant with highly protein-bound drugs (>80%), because a minimal decrease in the bound fraction of such a drug can produce a substantial increase in pharmacologic effect. Examples of highly protein-bound drugs that are likely to interact are barbiturates, oral anticoagulants, oral hypoglycemics, sulfonamides, hydantoins, nonsteroidal anti-inflammatory drugs, calcium channel blockers, cyclophosphamide, clofibrate, diazoxide, chloral hydrate, and methotrexate.

Blood Flow. Pharmacologic agents capable of modifying blood flow to different body organs can greatly influence the distribution and handling of other drugs. For example, epinephrine is often combined with local anesthetics to restrict the spread of the anesthetic—and therefore increase its duration of action—by reducing local blood flow. Some cardiovascular drugs can alter blood volume and blood pressure by producing vasoconstriction, thereby restricting the access of other drugs to certain body organs. Reduction in hepatic blood flow by vasoconstrictors likewise can significantly reduce the rate and extent of drug metabolism.

Biotransformation

Biotransformation, the process of converting drugs to their respective metabolites, usually occurs in the liver. These reactions generally are mediated by enzymes; consequently, any drug capable of altering the enzymatic processes involved in the metabolism of other drugs can produce a drug interaction.

Enzyme Inhibition. There are many examples of compounds that interfere with the activity of inactivating enzymes, thereby potentiating other drugs. Monoamine oxidase (MAO) inhibitors, compounds that inhibit the normal functioning of the endogenous enzyme MAO, elevate levels of biogenic amines and may produce severe hypertensive reactions in the presence of pressor amines. Xanthine oxidase inhibitors such as allopurinol raise plasma levels of mercaptopurine by blocking its breakdown. Cholinesterase inhibitors such as physostigmine and neostigmine block degradation of choline esters and can enhance the effects of acetylcholine, succinylcholine, and other cholinergic drugs.

Enzyme Induction. Certain pharmacologic agents, including barbiturates, hydantoins, griseofulvin, and chlorinated hydrocarbon insecticides, can increase the levels of hepatic microsomal enzymes involved in the metabolic breakdown of many classes of drugs. This process, known as *enzyme induction*, decreases the therapeutic response to drugs that are metabolized by these enzymes because the drugs are now metabolized more rapidly. Many different drugs and chemicals can stimulate hepatic enzymes, and the number of potential drug interactions is large. For example, coumarin anticoagulants are metabolized at a much faster rate in the presence of a barbiturate; this interaction usually requires a dosage adjustment. Enzyme induction is responsible for development of tolerance to certain drugs because some drugs may stimulate their own liver metabolism; examples are barbiturates and glutethimide.

Residual Enzyme Effects. A potential source of drug interaction is the prolonged period of alteration of enzyme activity that can occur for days or weeks after the discontinuance of a drug. For example, antidepressants that are MAO inhibitors reduce the activity of MAO enzymes for as long as *2 weeks* after these drugs have been removed from a patient's therapy; if other types of antidepressants are given during this 14-day period, a severe hypertensive episode can occur. Enzyme induction will continue to exist for as long as 1 week after the withdrawal of barbiturate therapy.

Elimination

Drug interactions occurring with the excretion of drugs may involve any of the renal excretory processes (glomerular filtration, tubular reabsorption, active tubular secretion). Many clinically important drug interactions are caused by changes in urinary pH, tubular secretion, or fluid and electrolyte balance.

Urinary pH. Acidification of the urine (ie, to lower urinary pH) by use of ascorbic acid and ammonium chloride can reduce the effects of basic drugs (eg, narcotics, quinidine), which become largely ionized at the acidic pH; this change increases both water solubility and consequently urinary excretion. Conversely, renal elimination of acidic drugs, such as aspirin, barbiturates, and anticoagulants, will be increased by alkalinization of urine with sodium bicarbonate. Alteration of urinary pH is often an effective technique in treating drug overdosage.

Tubular Transport. Many drugs are actively secreted from the renal capillary network into the tubules of the kidney, where they are subsequently eliminated in the urine. When any two actively secreted drugs are used together, a drug interaction can occur because of competition for the active secretory mechanisms. Drugs that interact by this mechanism, leading to prolongation of therapeutic effects, include aspirin, sulfonamides, penicillins, thiazide diuretics, indomethacin, probenecid, oral hypoglycemics, acetazolamide, diazoxide, and methotrexate. Small doses of aspirin may impair the uricosuric effect (promotion of uric acid excretion) of probenecid by interfering with the active secretion of uric acid into the renal tubules. Aspirin also may inhibit the excretion of methotrexate. This type of drug interaction is used clinically for the specific enhancement of the pharmacologic therapeutic effects of some medications. For example, probenecid is employed to delay the rapid excretion of penicillin, thereby significantly prolonging the effective duration and therapeutic activity of this antibiotic.

Fluid and Electrolyte Balance. Changes in fluid and electrolyte levels induced by certain drugs can markedly affect the therapeutic effectiveness and toxicity of other drugs, particularly those that act on the heart, kidney, and/or skeletal muscles. Hypokalemia (low serum potassium levels), produced by many diuretic agents and corticosteroids, *increases* the likelihood of digitalis toxicity; potassium loss also may cause prolonged paralysis after use of antidepolarizing skeletal muscle relaxants. In contrast, hypokalemia can antagonize the antiarrhythmic effects of quinidine, lidocaine, procainamide, and phenytoin. Another interaction of clinical significance is the combined use of drugs that cause sodium and water retention (eg, corticosteroids) with antihypertensive or diuretic drugs; drugs that cause fluid retention can decrease the therapeutic effects of drugs in treatment of hypertension.

Immunologic

Certain drugs may alter antibody production. Vaccines and toxoids stimulate antibody production, whereas glucocorticoids such as hydrocortisone can markedly inhibit the immune response and should not be used with vaccines.

Chemotherapeutic

Although antibiotics are frequently given in combination, drug interactions can occur if bacteriostatic and bactericidal drugs are given together. For example, penicillins are bactericidal because they interfere with cell-wall synthesis in dividing bacteria. They are less effective, however, when used with tetracyclines—drugs that prevent cell division and bacterial growth. This mutual antagonism can cause serious complications when combination therapy is used to treat severe infections.

In conclusion, many drug interactions are not serious or life threatening, but ignoring them, either through lack of knowledge or because of inadequate observation, can produce harm to—and result in the death of—the patient.

Selected Bibliography

Ananth J, Johnson K: Psychotropic and medical drug interactions. Psychother Psychosom 58(3):178, 1992

Fassoulaki A, Farinotti R, Servin F, Desmonts JM : Chronic alcoholism increases the induction dose of propofol in humans. Anesth Analg 77:553, 1993

Gugler R, Allgayer H: Effects of antacids on the clinical pharmacokinetics of drugs. Clin Pharmacokinet 18(3):210, 1990

Hussar DA: Drug interactions. In Gennaro AT (ed): Remington's Pharmaceutical Sciences, 19th ed. Mack Publishing Easton, PA, 1995

Jankel CA, Fitterman LK: Epidemiology of drug–drug interactions as a cause of hospital admissions. Drug Saf 9(1):51, 1993

Schneider JK, Mion LC, Frengley JD: Adverse drug reactions in an elderly outpatient population. Am J Hosp Pharm 49:90, 1992

Tollefson GD: Adverse drug reactions/interactions in maintenance therapy. J Clin Psychiatry 54(8, suppl):48, 1993

Wix AR, Doering PL, Hatton RC: Drug–food interaction counseling programs in teaching hospitals. Am J Hosp Pharm 49:855, 1992

Nursing Bibliography

Hussar D: Reviewing drug interactions. Nursing '93 23(9):50–57, 1993

Kuhn M: Drug interactions and their nursing implications. Journal of the New York State Nurses' Association 24(2):10–16, 1993

7

Therapeutic Drug Monitoring

The process by which individualization of drug therapy is accomplished is termed *therapeutic drug monitoring*. Clinical research establishes the blood level range (target concentration) that a drug should achieve to provide a good therapeutic response with minimum toxicity. These target concentrations become goals to guide dosage adjustments in each patient, especially for drugs with a narrow margin of safety (small difference between the therapeutic dose and the toxic dose). The actual daily dose may be a less useful guide because the same dose of a drug may produce different blood levels in different patients. For example, a dose may be subtherapeutic (plasma concentrations too low) for one patient, but the exact same dose may result in toxicity (plasma concentrations too high) in another patient. One reason for this is that patients differ in their ability to biotransform (metabolize) drugs.

Within the therapeutic range, there usually is sufficient opportunity for "fine tuning" of drug dosage. For example, the patient requiring higher doses of a therapeutic agent because of a more severe form of a disease may be more effectively treated. Therefore, the rational use of serum or plasma drug concentrations can result in optimal dosage adjustments; this will provide greater efficacy and, consequently, better patient compliance with the drug regimen.

In addition to establishing the correct dose of a pharmacologic agent, periodic evaluations of plasma drug concentrations enable members of the healthcare team (physicians, nurses, and pharmacists) to identify those factors that can alter the plasma level of a drug (eg, changes in the absorption, distribution, biotransformation, and/or elimination of the drug).

The fields of analytical chemistry, drug metabolism, genetics, and computer technology provide part of the foundation for applications of therapeutic drug monitoring. Developments in laboratory instrumentation have resulted in a greatly simplified approach to the analysis of serum, plasma, and other types of biologic fluids for drugs; such assays are now in the reach of every clinical laboratory. Older methodologies requiring tedious isolation procedures for drug chemicals have given way to newer, "on-the-spot" techniques using immunologic assay methods, many of which possibly (in the future, probably) can be performed at the bedside. Such developments allow a rapid correlation between a patient's response to a drug and the drug's plasma concentration, thus providing better management of drug therapy.

Controlled clinical studies have generated reference therapeutic ranges for many drugs; many of these ranges are provided in Table 7-1.

Basic Pharmacokinetic Principles

Use of the therapeutic monitoring process requires an understanding of basic principles of pharmacokinetics. It is the adjustment in amount or frequency of dosage, based on pharmacokinetic concepts, that alters drug levels in the blood and allows individualization of therapy.

Bioavailability

Bioavailability is commonly defined as the *fraction* of an administered dose of a drug that reaches the systemic circulation; the *rate* at which a drug is absorbed also is a component of bioavailability. The intravenous route of administration affords 100% bioavailability for all agents and provides a basis for comparison to other routes of administration. All other routes of administration provide less than 100% bioavailability. For many drugs, the bioavailability after oral administration is reduced by the first-pass effect (in gastrointestinal [GI] tract or liver). Further, the bioavailability of a drug administered by mouth may vary greatly among patients; in some, reduced bioavailability may signify impairment of absorptive processes.

Pharmaceutical factors (eg, rate of disintegration of a tablet in the stomach and intestines) usually are not causes of variability in bioavailability because such are factors are under regulatory control of the Food and Drug Administration (FDA). The FDA, however, has recalled various products when it was discovered that they delivered amounts of drug to the blood that were *below* or—in some cases—*above* the desired therapeutic range.

Volume of Distribution

The extent of distribution of a drug in the body relative to its concentration in the blood or plasma is the *volume of distribution*; this is an artificial value. The *apparent* volume of distribution, V_d, is the relationship that exists at the same time between the amount of drug in the body (residual dose) and its plasma concentration:

$$V_d = \frac{\text{dose (mg/kg)}}{\text{plasma concentration (mg/L)}}$$

The units of a typical V_d are in liters/kilogram or simply liters. The volume of distribution of a drug is typically considered to be a fixed property of the drug but, in fact, is influenced by disease states, lean-to-fat tissue ratio, gender, age, and other patient characteristics.

Clearance

"Clearance" is the term used to describe the volume of blood (or plasma) that is completely cleared of the drug by metabolism and/or renal excretion per unit time (units = volume [mL]/time [min]). For some drugs, clearance is predominantly a function of the adequacy of hepatic function, whereas for others clearance is determined by renal processes. For many drugs, clearance rates are influenced by both processes. Clearance is an important consideration in the therapeutic drug monitoring

Table 7-1. **Therapeutic Monitoring Parameters for Selected Drugs**

Agent	*Pharmacologic Use*	*Therapeutic Range*	V_d *(L/kg)*	$T_{1/2}$ *(hr)*	*Comments*
Amikacin	Anti-infective	5–10 μg/mL (T) 20–30 (P)	0.25	2–3	V_d reduced in obesity; Cl inc in burned patients
Amiodarone	Antiarrhythmic	1–2.5 μg/mL	18–148	2.5–10 days	Long duration of clearance
Amitriptyline	Antidepressant	0.05–0.20 μg/mL	15.5	9–25	V_d and $T_{1/2}$ inc with age >65 y
Acetylsalicyclic acid	Anti-inflammatory	1–2 mg/dL (A) 15–25 mg/dL	0.14–0.18	0.2–0.3	Protein binding dec in uremia
Buspirone	Anxiolytic	0.09–0.15 μg/mL	5.3	2–4	Food dec first-pass effect $T_{1/2}$ inc with hepatic dysfunction
Carbamazepine	Anticonvulsant	4–12 μg/mL	1.2	12–17	Enhances own metabolism
Desipramine	Antidepressant	0.075–0.15 μg/mL	15–37	14–25	Cl dec with age >65 y
Digoxin	Inotropic	0.5–2.0 ng/mL	5.7–7.3	34–44	V_d dec in uremia; V_d and Cl inc in hyperthyroidism
Disopyramide	Antiarrhythmic	2–4 μg/mL	0.6–1.4	4–10	V_d dec in uremia
Doxepin	Antidepressant	0.03–0.17 μg/mL	2.0	6–8	Active metabolites
Encainide	Antiarrhythmic	0.1–0.3 μg/mL	3.6–4	 0.03–5.6 8–13	Two classes of metabolizers: extensive (90%) poor (10%)
Ethosuximide	Anticonvulsant	40–100 μg/mL	0.7	60	Principally pediatric use
Flecainide	Antiarrhythmic	0.2–1.0 μg/mL	5.5–10	11–16	Cl inc in acidic urine; active metabolites
Fluphenazine	Antipsychotic	0.9–17 ng/mL	20	14–20	
Flurazepam	Hypnotic	0.9–28 ng/mL	3.4	2.3	Active metabolites
Gentamicin	Anti-infective	0.5–2.0 μg/mL (T) 4–8 μg/mL (P)	0.22–0.3	1.5–4	V_d dec in obesity; Cl dec in renal dysfunction
Haloperidol	Antipsychotic	6–10 ng/mL	20	10–20	
Imipramine	Antidepressant	0.01–0.13 μg/mL	21	8–16	Cl dec with age >65 y; active metabolites
Lidocaine	Antiarrhythmic	1–5 μg/mL	3	1.5–2.0	V_d dec in CHF; inc in cirrhosis; Cl dec in CHF, shock
Lithium	Antimanic	0.4–1.3 mEq/L[a] 1.0–1.4 mEq/L[b]	0.7–1.0	20–27	a—in affective disorders b—mania
Maprotiline	Antidepressant	0.05–0.35 μg/mL	22–52	27–58	Active metabolites
Mexiletine	Antiarrhythmic	0.7–2.0 μg/mL	5.4	8–10	Cl dec with uremia; Cl inc with acidic urine
Nortriptyline	Antidepressant	0.05–0.15 μg/mL	21–27	18–35	Cl dec with age >65 y
Phenobarbital	Anticonvulsant	15–40 μg/mL	0.6–0.7	2–6 days	Hepatic enzyme inducer
Phenytoin	Anticonvulsant	10–20 μg/mL	0.4–0.8	7–26	V_d inc with uremia; Cl dose dependent
Primidone	Anticonvulsant	5–12 μg/mL	0.6	10–12	Cl dec with uremia; 15–25% metabolized to phenobarbital
Procainamide	Antiarrhythmic	4–8 μg/mL	2–3	2.5–4.7	Slow/fast acetylator dependent; V_d inc in CHF, obesity; Cl dec in MI, CHF
Propranolol	Beta blocker	0.01–0.34 μg/mL	2–8	3.4–6	V_d inc in hepatitis, hyperthyroidism; Cl inc in hyperthyroidism, smoking
Quinidine	Antiarrhythmic	0.3–0.6 μg/mL	2	6–8	V_d dec in CHF, inc in cirrhosis; Cl dec in CHF
Theophylline	Bronchodilator	10–20 μg/mL	0.465	3–9	Cl inc in smokers
Valproic acid	Anticonvulsant	50–100 μg/mL	0.13	10–16	Disrupts protein binding of other drugs

V_d, volume of distribution; $T_{1/2}$, half-life; T, trough concentration; P, peak concentration; Cl, clearance; A, Analgesic concentration; R, anti-inflammatory concentration; inc, increased; dec, decreased; CHF, congestive heart failure; MI, myocardial infarction.

process when hepatic and/or renal dysfunction are present secondary to disease.

Elimination Half-Life

The elimination half-life ($T_{1/2\beta}$) is the time required for the blood (plasma; serum) drug concentration to be reduced by 50%. Processes involved in this parameter are biotransformation and excretion. In healthy patients, this half-life is considered an unchangeable (fixed) characteristic of a drug; it is used to determine the appropriate *frequency* of administration of a drug. During repeat doses (eg, daily dosing of lithium in treating manic-depressive disorder), the elimination half-life is used as a measure of the time required for the drug level in the blood to reach the steady state.

Alterations in clearance due to disease or other factors can affect the elimination half-life of a drug. For example, a reduction in kidney function can reduce the excretion of a drug; this will increase both the half-life and duration of action of the drug. Further, under such conditions, drug accumulation will occur, leading to possible drug toxicity. Therefore, the elimination half-life is an important factor to consider in therapeutic drug monitoring.

Steady-State Concentration

The steady-state plasma drug concentration is reached when the amount of drug (dose) given by repetitive administration eventually equals the amount of drug lost from the body (due to biotransformation and/or elimination) during that time. A steady-state condition begins to develop when the drug is administered at an interval of time *equal* to its half-life; after approximately five half-lives, the steady-state condition usually will have been achieved. For example, assume that a drug has a half-life of 4 hours; when the drug is given once every 4 hours, the steady state will be reached at approximately 20 hours (4-hour half-life × 5).

Just because the steady state has been achieved does *not* automatically mean that the blood level is in the therapeutic range; the steady state may occur in the *subtherapeutic* or the *toxic* range.

In the process of therapeutic drug monitoring, the determination of whether a patient's blood level of a drug is in the therapeutically effective range must wait until the steady-state condition is achieved. This is necessary to ensure that equilibrium between drug availability and drug elimination has, in fact, occurred. Changes in the amount and/or frequency of drug dosage—designed to bring the patient's blood drug level into the therapeutic range—will initially disrupt the steady-state phase; achievement of the new steady-state level will require an additional three to five dose intervals. During this entire process, therapeutic monitoring can be used to avoid either underdosing or overdosing.

Loading Doses

A loading dose of a drug is the amount of the drug that must be administered to bring the drug level in the blood into the therapeutically effective range rapidly; this process is used when pharmacotherapy is initiated. Loading doses are typically administered parenterally for drugs that have a significant first-pass effect or produce significant GI side effects when large doses are given orally. Characteristically, loading doses are administered by intravenous infusion to achieve steady-state concentrations in a more rapid manner than that achievable by oral administration.

Maintenance Dosing

A maintenance dose of a drug is the amount of the drug (dose) that must be continually administered to maintain the steady-state condition (ie, to keep the blood level of drug fairly constant). Therefore, the goal is to establish the maintenance dose as approximately equal to the amount of drug lost from the body by clearance processes. Thus, in addition to evaluating a patient's clinical response to a drug, therapeutic monitoring is very useful in the process of adjusting maintenance doses of a drug to the individual needs and characteristics of a patient.

Dosing Interval

The dosing interval is defined as the amount of time that elapses between consecutive doses of a regularly administered drug. This is typically a number that easily divides into 24 hours (eg, a drug to be taken six times a day obviously translates into taking the drug once every 4 hours).

During the dosing interval, the concentration of a drug in the blood is expected to have a peak (maximum) and a trough (minimum); the trough level should occur in the time period just before the next dose is administered. Blood samples for the therapeutic monitoring process typically are obtained as "trough specimens." Peak concentrations of a drug usually are reached within 2 hours of oral administration; this depends, however, on many factors, including GI motility, the presence or absence of food in the GI tract, and—if the drug is given in tablet form—how fast the product goes into solution (dissolves) in the GI tract. In contrast, peak levels are achieved within a shorter time after subcutaneous or intramuscular injection. The exact time at which the peak concentration occurs is highly variable, even in the same patient.

Need for Therapeutic Drug Monitoring

During the past 30 years, clinical investigations have clearly demonstrated that there are large differences among patients in the clearance of drugs. Studies on identical (as compared to fraternal) twins have shown that differences in drug clearance are most often inherited (ie, are due to genetic factors). These differences are most likely related to drug metabolism (biotransformation), and less significant with regard to renal excretion *except* in cases in which renal excretion is the primary clearance process. In this latter case, individual differences in renal excretion rates become very important.

Drugs that are appropriate for the therapeutic monitoring process include those that:

- Have a relatively narrow margin of safety, that is, a small therapeutic index (eg, digoxin)
- Potentially can impair their own clearance process (eg, aminoglycosides)
- Exhibit wide variabilities among patients with regard to absorption, biotransformation, and/or excretion (eg, phenytoin)
- Are used to treat diseases on a protective (prophylactic) basis (eg, anticonvulsants)

Influence of Drug Absorption

For many medications administered orally, significant differences exist among patients in the speed and/or amount of drug absorption. Some patients cannot absorb drugs efficiently because of GI disorders, the presence of substances in the diet that interfere with the absorptive process, or simultaneous use of other medications that compete for absorptive sites. In some cases, coingested substances can absorb drug molecules and prevent their passage across the epithelium of the GI tract. Examples of this type of interference include the binding of digoxin to cholestyramine and the attachment of tetracyclines to calcium ions (from certain dairy products).

An important parameter that characterizes absorption is bioavailability. As discussed earlier in this chapter, the degree of bioavailability indicates the amount of drug that reaches the systemic circulation and thus becomes available for action at the desired target tissue. This parameter usually is calculated from measurements over time of the amount of drug in the blood. Different batches (lots) of a drug or different brands of a drug (eg, generic drugs) may vary in bioavailability to such a degree that the intended effect is not achieved (bioavailability too low) or unexpected toxicity occurs (bioavailability too high). The therapeutic drug monitoring process obviously is useful in such cases.

Patient compliance is another aspect of drug therapy related to drug absorption. Many drugs produce adverse reactions (ie, disagreeable side effects) that reduce patient motivation to follow correctly the therapeutic plan developed by the doctor; the patient may completely stop taking the drug. The therapeutic monitoring process can identify noncompliance and help to reinforce the need for adhering to the therapeutic regimen.

Drug Distribution

Differences among patients in the distribution of drugs throughout the body are known to exist. Such differences in distribution (or *volume of distribution*) are often the result of changes in the protein binding of drugs; they are reflected in the ratio between the protein-bound fraction and the non–protein-bound—or "free drug"—fraction. The degree of protein binding may be changed by many factors, including age, menstrual status, disease state (especially liver disease), nutritional status, and the simultaneous use of other drugs that compete for protein-binding sites. Variations in the volume of distribution also occur because of differences in the amount of adipose tissue compared to the amount of lean body tissue.

The therapeutic monitoring process can help to identify these problems through measurement of "free drug" fractions, which will detect *abnormally* low (the more likely event) or high degrees of protein binding of a drug.

Drug Metabolism (Biotransformation)

Differences in drug metabolism among patients have been demonstrated for a wide variety of drugs. In fact, metabolic variability is to be expected for all drugs that have systemic availability. That a genetic component (hereditary factor) underlies individual variability is documented by studies in which rates of drug metabolism were compared between fraternal and identical twins; fraternal twins showed more difference in biotransformation of drugs than identical twins. These variations in metabolic rate as observed in the general population are principally due to increased or decreased activities of enzymes involved in drug metabolism. Such differences become significant when they affect the half-life of a drug. The impact on drug half-life may become clinically apparent through the therapeutic drug monitoring process.

Criteria for Therapeutic Drug Monitoring

Concentration of drug in the serum and at the receptor site must be in equilibrium.

Because a blood specimen represents a measurement at a point in time, a necessary requirement for therapeutic monitoring of a drug is that its plasma concentration must be in dynamic equilibrium with all other compartments in the body. This occurs at the steady-state condition.

Drugs that act irreversibly or are stored for prolonged periods in peripheral compartments of the body become less acceptable candidates for therapeutic monitoring.

Intensity and duration of pharmacologic effects (therapeutic action and toxicity) must show a correlation with blood levels.

Drugs that show delayed effects are not good candidates in cases in which plasma drug concentrations are used for therapeutic monitoring. For example, antidepressants that are inhibitors of monoamine oxidase (MAO) disappear from the blood and concentrate in tissues containing this catabolic enzyme. Therefore, MAO inhibitors are poor candidates because the intensity and duration of the pharmacologic effect (reversal of clinical depression) do not correlate with plasma levels.

Methods for assay of the drug should have been validated for clinical use and should be available to the clinic.

For an agent to be monitored in the clinical setting, readily available assay methods (ie, optimally located on-site) should ensure rapid availability of plasma drug concentration results, before unwarranted toxic or adverse reactions occur.

Benefits of Therapeutic Drug Monitoring

At initiation of drug therapy, when rapid and effective treatment is needed, drug monitoring helps to determine the proper dose and dosing rate quickly.

During maintenance therapy in stable, chronically ill patients, drug monitoring can help determine the best possible regimen (ie, provides optimum therapeutic outcomes with minimum [or no] toxicity).

Drug monitoring can be used to evaluate any change in blood levels of one drug when other drugs are added to or removed from a therapeutic regimen (ie, monitor effects of drug interactions).

In patients with altered physiologic and/or pharmacokinetic parameters, therapeutic doses can be properly modified.

Sampling of Biologic Specimens

To gain information about the drug concentration in the body, various specimens can be obtained. *Invasive* methods include the sampling of blood or spinal fluid, tissue biopsy, or assessment of any biologic material that requires parenteral or surgical intervention in the patient. *Noninvasive* approaches to biologic sampling include the sampling of urine, saliva, feces, expired air, sweat, or any other biologic material that can be obtained without parenteral or surgical intervention. The measurement of drug concentrations in each of these biologic materials yields different information.

Drug concentration measurements in blood, serum, or plasma provide the most direct approach for assessing the pharmacokinetic and pharmacodynamic profile of a specific patient. Whole blood contains red blood cells, white blood cells, and platelets, which are the cellular elements, and proteins, which participate in the drug distribution process (primarily albumin for weak acids and alpha-1-acid glycoprotein for weak bases). To obtain serum, the collected blood is allowed to clot. The serum fraction is obtained as the supernatant fluid after centrifugation of the clotted blood specimen. Plasma is obtained in a similar manner, except the blood is collected in the presence of an anticoagulant such as heparin (also ethylenediaminetetraacetic acid [EDTA], oxalate, or other calcium binders). Serum differs from plasma in both the nature of its protein content (proteins that participate in the clotting process are not present in serum, but are present in plasma) and electrolyte content. From a practical point of view, assays for drug content yield similar results when plasma and serum samples are used. The important assumption in therapeutic drug monitoring is that plasma (and the in vitro correlate, serum) perfuses all the tissues of the body, including the cellular components in the blood. If it is assumed that the plasma is in dynamic equilibrium with the tissues, then changes in tissue drug concentrations will be immediately reflected in changes in the plasma or serum drug concentration.

Tissue biopsy specimens are obtained occasionally for the purpose of determining an accurate pathologic diagnosis, as in the case of neoplasia. With current laboratory methods, the small amount of tissue obtained by biopsy is sufficient to develop important target tissue pharmacodynamic and pharmacokinetic information. Drug concentrations in a tissue biopsy specimen may not reflect drug concentrations in any other tissue, but may be used to ascertain if the drug reached the tissues in a concentration sufficient to produce the desired effects. This information is therapeutically important, for example, in the treatment of solid tissue tumors with antineoplastic agents. An alternative approach to measuring tissue concentrations that is being evaluated is the use of microdialysis probes, which can be used to follow tissue drug concentrations over the dosing interval.

Measurement of a drug in urine also can have therapeutic monitoring relevance. Typically, urine drug concentrations constitute an indirect means of ascertaining bioavailability. The rate and extent of drug excretion in urine reflects the rate and extent of systemic availability of the drug. In addition, urine drug detection may play a role in enhancing therapeutic regimen compliance (as in substance abuse treatment program monitoring or in methadone maintenance programs). Urine drug detection approaches also have been used to detect noncompliance and drug substitution problems in the psychiatric setting. A newer approach to substance detection that is gaining popularity is the use of the sweat collection patch, which is worn over a 2-week period. Laboratory analysis of the sweat collection patch reflects drug use compliance and noncompliance over the surveillance period.

Measurement of drug in feces may reflect drug that has not been absorbed after an oral dose. In addition, however, fecal drug content also may reflect biliary secretion after systemic absorption. Fecal drug excretion is typically measured in mass balance studies in which efforts are taken to account for the entire dose administered to a patient. In such a study, both urine and feces are collected, and their drug content measured. In the case where the solid oral dosage form does not go through a disintegration–dissolution phase but simply leaches out the active ingredient, fecal collection may be performed in the interest of obtaining the dosage form itself. Subsequent assay of the dosage form will yield the amount of residual drug left and imply the actual dosage amount available systemically to the patient.

Saliva drug concentrations also have been studied for several drugs that are suitable for therapeutic drug monitoring. If the drug concentration in the saliva is considered to be in equilibrium with the plasma concentration, then the salivary concentration could be used to monitor the patient's drug therapy. In addition, an important feature associated with salivary monitoring is the observation that salivary drug concentrations reflect free drug (non–protein-bound fraction) content in the plasma, which should correlate better with both efficacy and toxicity. Two difficulties diminish the potential of this noninvasive approach:

The pH differential between saliva and plasma reduces the spectrum of agents assessable by this technique because of the problem of ion trapping.

Scientific data suggest that each patient may have a slightly different saliva:plasma concentration ratio (this would affect the interpretation of salivary drug concentrations).

Significance of Measuring Plasma Drug Concentrations

The intensity of a pharmacologic or toxicologic effect of a drug often is related to the concentration of the drug at the receptor sites, usually located in the tissue cells. Because most tissues are richly perfused with tissue fluids and plasma, measuring the plasma concentration of a drug is of significant value in evaluating the therapeutic response.

Clinically, variations among patients with regard to the pharmacokinetics of a drug are common. Monitoring and evaluating the plasma concentration of a drug provide assurance that the calculated dose actually provided a plasma concentration needed to produce a therapeutic response. With some agents, the variation in receptor sensitivity is so wide that plasma monitoring is necessary to differentiate the patient who needs a very low dose from the patient who requires a very large dose. In addition, the patient's physiologic function may be altered by disease, nutritional and environmental factors, concurrent drug therapy, and other factors.

In the absence of supporting information, the value of plasma drug concentration information is limited with respect to dosage adjustments. For example, assume that a single plasma sample obtained at some time during administration of a drug revealed a drug concentration of 10 μg/mL. Clinical data indicate that the upper limit of the therapeutic range for this drug is 15 μg/mL. To determine the significance of this, the following information is needed:

- Time at which the blood sample was obtained *in relation* to when the last dose drug was administered (the optimum time to take a blood sample is immediately before a dose; at this point the blood level will be at its lowest [trough level] between doses)
- Dose of the drug currently being administered
- Length of time the patient has been taking this particular dose (necessary to determine if the steady-state condition has been achieved)
- Route of administration
- Patient's response to the drug (whether the therapy appears ineffective [subtherapeutic], effective, or toxic)

In summary, monitoring drug plasma concentrations allows for adjustment of doses such that pharmacotherapy can be more effectively individualized and optimized. When physiologic function is altered because of disease and/or the presence of other drugs, therapeutic monitoring becomes even more valuable. Those health professionals (ie, physicians, nurses, pharmacists) involved in managing the patient can use it to modify drug dosage accordingly. Any therapeutic decision, however, never should be made on the basis of plasma drug concentrations alone; the primary diagnostic process is still the *direct* clinical examination and evaluation of the patient. For instance, electrocardiographic (ECG) data on digoxin-induced changes in electrophysiologic activity of the heart are complementary to the plasma digoxin concentration data in determining the therapeutic effectiveness of digoxin in congestive heart failure. As additional assays are developed, plasma drug monitoring will become a more routine process in the pharmacotherapeutic management of patients.

Selected Bibliography

Brown GR, Miyata M, McCormack JP: Drug concentration monitoring: An approach to rational use. Clin Pharmacokinet 24(3):187, 1993

Desoky EE, Klotz U: Value, limitations and clinical impact of therapeutic drug monitoring in adults. Drug Invest 6(3):127, 1993

Drobitch RK, Svensson, CK: Therapeutic drug monitoring in saliva. Clin Pharmacokinet 23(5):365, 1992

Greenblatt DJ: Basic pharmacokinetic principles and their application to psychotropic drugs. J Clin Psychiatry 54(9; Suppl):8, 1993

Janicak PG: The relevance of clinical pharmacokinetics and therapeutic drug monitoring: Anticonvulsant mood stabilizers and antipsychotics. J Clin Psychiatry 54(9; Suppl):35, 1993

Pacifici GM, Viani A: Methods of determining plasma and tissue binding of drugs: Pharmacokinetic consequences. Clin Pharmacokinet 23(6):449, 1992

Preskorn SH, Burke MJ, Fast GA: Therapeutic drug monitoring: Principles and practice. Psychiatr Clin North Am 16(3):611, 1993

Talbert RL: Drug dosing in renal insufficiency. J Clin Pharmacol 34:99, 1994

Nursing Bibliography

McPherson M: Home anticoagulation monitoring. Journal of Home Health Care Practice 4(1):63–77, 1991

Wild L: What is the role of the critical care nurse in using a peripheral nerve stimulator to determine the level of paralysis in a patient receiving neuromuscular blocking agents? Critical Care Nurse 13(2):70, 1993

Wilkes G: Polypharmacy: Dangers of multiple drug therapy in patients with human immunodeficiency virus infector. Home Health Nurse 10(5):30–46, 1992

8 Pediatric Pharmacology

The age span from infancy to adolescence and puberty represents a continuum of major anatomic, physiologic, and psychological changes that have a significant impact on pharmacotherapeutics. Even with adjustments in drug dosing based on weight (milligram per kilogram basis [mg/kg]), the pediatric patient cannot be considered as just a "little adult." Unique and potentially serious problems can occur during drug therapy if careful attention is not given. The selection of both dose and route of administration is crucial to the safe and appropriate use of therapeutic agents in this population. Unfortunately, specific guidelines for the safe and efficacious use of pharmaceuticals in pediatric patients are not always available; thus, the practitioner provides drug therapy to the child by reducing the recommended adult dose based on body weight or surface area. Compared to adults, however, children also have reduced absorption, biotransformation, and elimination mechanisms. There are many examples of cases in which an infant's impaired ability to biotransform and eliminate drugs has resulted in unexpected and sometimes fatal toxicity (for example, the *gray baby syndrome* observed with the use of the antibiotic, chlormphenicol).

Although it is difficult to classify the pediatric population arbitrarily according to age or developmental characteristics, certain stages in a child's growth appear to represent hallmark periods in drug handling. These may be described as:

1. *Neonatal period (0–1 month):* marked physiologic immaturity with rapid changes in physiologic function; generally considered a critical period in terms of drug administration.
2. *Infancy (1–12 months):* improvement in capacity to biotransform and eliminate drugs.
3. *Toddler period (1–3 years):* fairly well developed biotransformation elimination processes; child resists many medications when presented; use of rituals and routines facilitate medication compliance at this age.
4. *Preschool and adolescence (3 years and older):* few anatomic concerns but occasional behavioral problems associated with drug administration may occur; for safe drug therapy, dosage adjustment based on body weight is an important consideration; dosage requirements for many drugs may change with the onset of puberty.

Factors That Affect Therapeutic Response

Many factors are involved in selecting a correct dose and evaluating the subsequent therapeutic response in any patient (see Chapter 3); these factors are of even greater significance in children.

Absorption

In general, the absorption of orally administered drugs in infants younger than 6 to 9 months of age is slower than in adults. Young children exhibit reduced gastric motility, prolonged gastric emptying time, a lower gastric pH, decreased absorptive capacity, and differences in the composition of intestinal flora; all can affect the rate of drug absorption. In small infants, the processes responsible for transporting drugs across intestinal membranes may be underdeveloped; this leads to reduced absorption of certain nutrients and vitamins. The gastrointestinal tract of the infant is also more sensitive to chemical influences, leading to a greater incidence of nausea, vomiting, and diarrhea that can significantly alter the amount of drug absorbed from the intestinal tract.

Conversely, owing to a reduced keratin layer and thinner epithelium in the small child, the absorption of *topically* applied drugs is greatly enhanced compared to adults. This can be particularly significant with topically applied corticosteroids for conditions such as diaper rash and eczema; significant absorption can produce many undesired systemic reactions.

Absorption of drugs from intramuscular (IM) injection sites (eg, vastus lateralis muscles) may be more erratic in infants than in older children because of smaller muscle mass and the associated reduced intramuscular circulation. Drugs used to treat serious illness in hospitalized children often are given by the intravenous (IV) route (frontal or superficial scalp vein in very young infants).

Distribution

Factors that affect drug distribution among various pediatric age groups include differences in circulatory dynamics, amount of body water, binding of drugs to plasma proteins, membrane permeability, and specificity of drugs for tissue receptor sites.

Circulatory Dynamics

In general, drugs penetrate tissues according to the extent of blood flow to the tissues; highly perfused tissues (liver, kidney, brain) achieve higher concentrations of drugs than poorly perfused tissues (bone, muscle). The growth and development of these organs proceed at different rates in the developing child; therefore, the degree of drug distribution changes as the child matures. It is important to recognize that young infants may have poor peripheral circulation; this results in a reduced absorption rate of drugs given by IM or subcutaneous (SC) injection.

Body Water

The newborn has a higher percentage of both total body water and extracellular fluid volume (80%–85%) compared to the older child; conversely, fat content in the neonate is lower.

Therefore, water-soluble drugs diffuse to a greater extent in the very young, often resulting in reduced plasma concentrations compared to those observed in older children. Lipid-soluble drugs may be stored to a lesser degree as a result of the lower amount of adipose tissue.

An important consideration in the neonate is the occurrence of dehydration; in this condition, normal doses of a drug can result in very high plasma concentrations because of the reduction in overall extracellular fluid volume.

Binding

In the newborn, the binding of most drugs to plasma proteins such as albumin and the globulins is significantly less than that observed for adults. Factors causing this include:

- Lower levels of plasma proteins in the neonate (reduced hepatic synthesis)
- Altered binding characteristics of neonatal plasma proteins
- Presence of high concentrations of endogenous substances (eg, bilirubin, steroids, hormones, fatty acids) that compete for plasma protein-binding sites during the postpartum period.

Because a reduction in protein binding results in an increased amount of pharmacologically active (free; unbound) drug in plasma, toxic reactions are more likely to occur. There is an even greater chance of adverse reactions when multiple-drug therapy is undertaken. Among the more important drugs that may exhibit reduced plasma protein binding in the newborn are salicylates, barbiturates, penicillins, and phenytoin.

Membrane Permeability

Delayed maturation of the blood–brain barrier and other biologic membranes leads to increased distribution of drugs into certain areas of the body. Lipid-soluble drugs (eg, anesthetics, sedatives, analgesics, antibiotics) readily penetrate the central nervous system of the neonate, producing high concentrations that may cause serious harm (respiratory depression, brain damage). Other factors in the neonate that play a role in the penetration of drugs into the brain include changes in blood chemistry (acidosis, hypoxia, hyperglycemia), fluctuations in body temperature (hyperpyrexia), and abnormalities in development of the blood–brain barrier (incomplete myelination).

Drug Receptor Specificity

Observed differences in the responsiveness of infants and adults to certain drugs suggest that the sensitivity of some receptor sites is not equal. For example, therapeutic doses of atropine and epinephrine are proportionately greater on a mg/kg basis in the infant than in the adult, suggesting that the receptor responsiveness is lower in the infant.

Biotransformation

In the early neonatal period, hepatic drug metabolism is low because of the immaturity of the liver, as well as its focus on metabolism of endogenous substances such as fetal hemoglobin and estrogen. Drug-metabolizing enzymes in the liver mature at different rates. The functional capacity of the liver, therefore, changes very rapidly after birth; any major problems associated with reduced hepatic function usually occur in the first weeks after delivery. The major impact of this reduced hepatic biotransformational capacity occurs with drugs that exhibit significant first-pass metabolism. If the dose of such drugs is not appropriately reduced, serious toxic reactions may occur because of drug accumulation.

Enzyme induction can be produced in the neonate by drugs such as phenobarbital, a known inducer of hepatic cytochrome P450 enzymes. This effect becomes evident when multiple-drug therapy is undertaken; the addition of a second drug that causes enzyme induction can markedly reduce the duration of action—and consequently the efficacy—of the first (initial) drug. Exposure in utero to enzyme inducers during therapy for the mother (eg, phenobarbital for treatment of epilepsy) causes enzyme induction in the fetus. At birth, infants born to such women are capable of metabolizing many drugs at an accelerated rate.

The low hepatic function in the neonate results in a lower synthesis of plasma proteins, allowing larger quantities of a drug to circulate unbound (free) in the blood. As liver function matures and plasma protein levels increase (normalization of plasma protein concentrations), dramatic increases occur in the percentage binding of drugs, which can lead to a decrease in drug efficacy because of decreased concentrations of free drug.

Excretion

As with liver metabolic function, renal excretory capacity is immature at birth but gradually matures with advancing age. For example, a full-term newborn has approximately 33% of the glomerular filtration rate and renal tubular excretion capacity of an adult (in the premature neonate, this capacity is reduced even further). During the first month of life, the capacity to excrete solute load increases to about 50% of adult levels. This change is exemplified in changes in the half-life of drugs whose action is terminated primarily by the kidney. For drugs that depend on renal excretion for termination of their therapeutic activity (eg, penicillins, aminoglycosides, salicylates, acetaminophen, aminophylline, digoxin, thiazide diuretics), initial reductions in dose must be made for the neonate, with careful monitoring during prolonged therapy. For example, gentamicin is administered every 12 hours in the week-old neonate, but can be increased to every 8 hours at 2 to 4 weeks of age. Because of the newborn's rapidly changing characteristics, therapeutic drug monitoring should be used for aminoglycosides and, whenever possible, other drugs; therapeutic monitoring will minimize possible adverse effects. By 9 months of age, renal function is approximately proportional to that of the young adult; therefore, in the healthy child no adjustment for age is necessary as long as renal function is normal.

Drug Dosage and Administration

The pediatric population poses unique problems with regard to drug dosage and administration. Because many factors other than age and size can alter drug response in these patients, no single rule can be used to guide clinical decisions about dosage and route. In spite of this uncertainty, most pharmacotherapy is undertaken on the basis of proportionality of weight (dosage corrected by assessment of mg/kg of body weight). In most cases, this is probably the most appropriate method for determining pediatric dosage. For drugs that are very toxic (eg, cancer chemotherapeutic agents), however, dosage determined on the basis of surface area is more accurate and safer.

Dosage

Many rules for dosing in children are based on calculating the pediatric dose as a fraction of the adult dose using a measurable parameter such as weight or surface area. The four commonly cited pediatric dosage rules are given below; the first three are largely of theoretical interest:

1. *Young's rule* (2 years and older):

$$\frac{\text{Age (yr)}}{\text{Age (yr)} + 12} \times \text{ADULT dose}$$

2. *Clark's rule* (infants and young children)

$$\frac{\text{Weight (lb)}}{\text{150 lb}} \times \text{ADULT dose}$$

(150 lbs = weight of "average" adult)

3. *Fried's rule* (infants younger than 1 year)

$$\frac{\text{Age (months)}}{150} \times \text{ADULT dose}$$

4. *Surface area rule* (all children except for newborns)

$$\frac{\text{Surface area of child (m}^2\text{)}}{1.7} \times \text{ADULT dose}$$

The surface area is determined from the child's height and weight using standard nomograms found in many pharmacology and pediatric texts. It is the most accurate method of determining the correct pediatric dosage because surface area reflects the growth of body systems that influence metabolism and excretion.

There are essentially no clinical data, however, comparing the therapeutic response of drugs dosed in pediatric patients by surface area to the response in a patient dosed by body weight.

Dosage must be individualized for the patient, the drug, and the disease, whether the patient is a child or an adult. The difficulty with pediatric dosing is that when rules are based on age, variations in body weight among children are not used in the calculation. Similarly, rules based on body surface area do not take into account differences in percentage of body water. Rules based on weight *assume* an average adult weight of 150 lbs; for many drugs, infants would receive an *underdosage* if given mg/kg doses calculated by this method.

Although pediatric dosage rules can provide guidelines for the use of many drugs in children, no guarantee of safety or adequacy of dosage can be provided, especially in the newborn. Indeed, no rule can anticipate all the variables encountered in pediatric therapy, especially those attributable to individual differences in drug response. Thus, the determination of appropriate drug dosage in children must be critically evaluated and adjusted for each patient, and the pediatric patient carefully monitored during therapy to maximize drug efficacy and minimize toxicity.

Administration

The preferred method of drug administration in young children is the oral route in the form of a liquid preparation. This may not be the best method in certain conditions (eg, renal impairment and rapid or severe dehydration). A brief consideration of several routes of administration used in children is presented in the following.

Oral

This is *generally* the preferred route.

Liquid medications, especially if flavored, may facilitate administration, but also should be kept out of the child's reach to prevent self-administration and potential overdosage.

In small infants, medication may be placed along the side of the tongue by dropper or syringe to avoid its being pushed out by tongue movement.

Most tablets and capsules can be crushed and mixed with honey, syrup, jam, or fruit if the child is unable or unwilling to swallow them whole; because some tablets and capsules cannot be broken (eg, sustained-action formulations), parents should consult a pharmacist before using this procedure.

Rectal

Can be used when oral route is contraindicated or difficult (eg, cleft palate, nausea, or vomiting).

Many drugs are erratically absorbed rectally.

Diarrhea often makes rectal administration impractical.

Intramuscular

Often used for single-dose administration (eg, vaccines, antibiotics).

Buttocks and the deltoid muscle should *not* be used in infants and small children (younger than 2 years of age) because of danger of sciatic nerve damage and lack of sufficient muscle mass; vastus lateralis is the preferred site.

With repeated injections, sites should be rotated.

Absorption is generally good and fairly rapid.

Always use bony prominences to identify injection site.

Intravenous

Should be used in young children only when other routes have failed or are inappropriate.

Infants and small children should be restrained so needle is not dislodged once inserted.

Because of reduced peripheral circulation in the very young, veins in the extremities are difficult to locate; the superficial scalp or frontal veins are used.

Drug must be properly diluted and drug given at a slow rate (eg, 0.5–2 mL/min) because overdosage is most dangerous with IV administration, and adverse reactions can develop quickly.

Circulatory overload can occur more rapidly in children than in adults. As a general rule, never give more than 250 mL fluid to a child younger than 2 years, or 500 mL to an older child, unless special conditions warrant (eg, rapid or severe dehydration).

Topical and Local (Eye, Ear, Nose)

Possibility of significant percutaneous absorption into the systemic circulation (especially with repeated application of lipid-soluble agents).

Eye and ear drops may be warmed before instillation; solutions at room temperature are less irritating.

Oil-based preparations should *not* be used in the nose, because aspiration can lead to lipid pneumonia.

When nose drops are used in infants, instillation should be followed after a brief period with aspiration with a bulb syringe.

Regardless of the method of drug administration used, the most important single factor for successful pediatric pharmacotherapy is the relationship between the child and the practitioner. Successful, uncomplicated drug administration depends to a great extent on the cooperation between the child and the person administering the drug. Establishment of a secure, positive relationship between the drug-giver and the drug-receiver is, therefore, very important. Each child has an individual personality that must be used to maximum advantage in administering medications. Honest explanations are essential, and medications should never be portrayed as candy, rewards, or anything less serious than they really are. If the child is old enough, explanations relating to why the medications are being used and the importance of a proper dosage schedule (in a manner appropriate to the child's age and level of understanding) lead to a higher degree of cooperation on the part of the child. A child's fears should be understood and allayed if possible. Drug administration in the pediatric setting can be exceedingly difficult, and requires not only skill but patience, understanding, and recognition of the child's concerns and feelings.

Nursing Management

Pretherapy Assessment

Assess and record important baseline data (age and developmentally specific information) necessary for:
- a. detection of adverse effects of prescribed drug.
- b. selection of appropriate route of administration.
- c. selection of appropriate drug administration method.

Review past medical history and documents for evidence of existing or previous medical history related to conditions that:
- a. require cautious administration of a prescribed drug: age/physiologic development; medical history,
- b. contraindicate use of a drug: allergy to prescribed drug or drug family; patient age/physiologic development; patient medical history.

Nursing Interventions

Medication Administration

Plan the most convenient and individualized drug regimen (route of administration, dosage form, dosing schedule) that takes into account the child's age, developmental level, diagnosis, and expected outcomes of therapy.

Plan and implement individualized nursing interventions that:
- a. inform the patient/parents about the expected actions and adverse effects of a prescribed drug.
- b. identify the early onset of expected adverse effects and intervene appropriately.
- c. minimize the symptoms produced by the expected adverse effects of the prescribed drug.
- d. identify the safety needs of the patient and intervene appropriately to minimize environmental hazards and risk of injury.

Recognize the child's fears.

Answer questions honestly, providing information that is clear, accurate, developmentally appropriate, and specific to the question asked.

Ask parents and significant others to assist in medication administration regime if they are a positive influence and choose to be present.

Use caution in offering rewards (candy, toys) in conjunction with drug administration procedures. Instead, use strategies that make the experience as positive (pleasurable) as possible such as:
- a. Incorporate play techniques (appropriate to age and developmental level) to explain procedures, encourage cooperation and compliance, and evaluate response.
- b. Allow child choices (injection site, drink flavors) as appropriate.
- c. Use distraction (conversation, imagery, music, VCR tapes, hand-held games).
- d. Realize that topical (cream) anesthetics are available for application to site before injection (IM, SC) or IV insertion.

Do not force any drug orally. Rationale: risk of pulmonary aspiration.

Do not disguise disagreeable-tasting drugs by mixing with foods in child's normal diet. Rationale: child may associate the food with the drug and an eating problem may develop.

Consult pharmacy or practitioner–prescriber before crushing tablets or emptying capsules and mixing with juice, formula, milk, or food. Rationale: bioavailability may be altered.

Administer ear drops to children 3 years of age and younger by pulling the pinna of the ear *down and back* to straighten the external auditory canal.

Administer ear drops to children 3 years of age and older by pulling the pinna of the ear *up and out* to straighten the external auditory canal.

Administer nose drops 30 minutes before feeding children who nurse or use bottle. Rationale: facilitates suckling.

Administer IM injections into the vastus lateralis or rectus femoris muscle (avoid gluteal and deltoid muscles) in children younger than 18 to 24 months of age.

Use physical restraint judiciously.

Surveillance During Therapy

Use age and developmentally specific assessment techniques to monitor drug therapy. Rationale: children vary in their ability to communicate response to drug therapy (expected effects, adverse effects).

Always monitor the drug dose being administered. Rationale: to ensure that it is within acceptable limits for the diagnosis and patient being treated.

Compare current status with previous status to detect improvements, deterioration in the patient's condition.

Monitor patient for therapeutic drug effect.

Monitor for adverse effects, toxicity, and interactions.

Monitor for signs of hypersensitivity that may require discontinuation of drug.

Facilitate acquisition of diagnostic tests ordered for ongoing assessment of drug response.

Monitor diagnostic test results obtained over the course of therapy.

Interpret results of diagnostic tests and contact practitioner–prescriber as appropriate.
Monitor for possible drug–laboratory test interactions.
Monitor for possible drug–drug and drug–nutrient interactions.

Patient Teaching

Instruct patient/parents about medication administration (dose, dose frequency, administration equipment and technique) to ensure safety.
Instruct patient/parents about expected actions and possible adverse effects of prescribed drug.
Instruct patient/parents about appropriate action to take if adverse effects occur:

a. how to manage symptoms related to expected adverse effects of prescribed drug.
b. when to notify practitioner–prescriber.
c. under which conditions to discontinue administration of prescribed drug before notification of practitioner–prescriber.
d. under which conditions to seek immediate medical attention if adverse side effects develop.

Instruct patient/parents about the importance of completing the full course of therapy as prescribed; that is, not to discontinue the drug once signs and symptoms have subsided.
Inform patient/parents of the consequences of not taking or abruptly discontinuing a prescribed drug.
Instruct patient/parents that a prescribed drug is to be taken only in the manner and for the condition for which it is prescribed.
Instruct patient/parents to keep all medications out of the reach of children.

Selected Bibliography

Cloyd JC, Fischer JH, Kriel RL, Kraus DM: Valproic acid pharmacokinetics in children: IV. Effects of age and antiepileptic drugs on protein binding and intrinsic clearance. Clin Pharmacol Ther 53:22, 1993
Fawzi WW, Chalmers TC, Herrera MG, Mosteller F: Vitamin A supplementation and child mortality. JAMA 269(7):898, 1993
Greenberger PA, Odeh YK, Frederiksen MC, Atkinson AJ: Pharmacokinetics of prednisone transfer to breast milk. Clin Pharmacol Ther 53:324, 1993
Knight M: Adverse drug reactions in neonates. J Clin Pharmacol 34: 128, 1994
Walson PD, Getschman S, Koren G: Principles of drug prescribing in infants and children: A practical guide. Drugs 46(2):281, 1993
Ward RM: Drug therapy of the fetus. J Clin Pharmacol 33:780, 1993
Zenk KE: Challenges in providing pharmaceutical care to pediatric patients. Am J Hosp Pharm 51: 688, 1994

Nursing Bibliography

Dionne R, McManus C: Pediatric critical care pharmacodynamics. Critical Care Nursing Clinics of North America 5(2):367–376, 1993
Keegan-Wells D, Stewart J: The use of venous access devices in pediatric oncology nursing practice. Journal of Pediatric Oncology Nursing 9(4):159–169, 1992
Klein E: Premedicating children for painful invasive procedures. Journal of Pediatric Oncology Nursing 9(4): 170–179, 1992
Patterson K: Pain in the pediatric oncology patient. Journal of Pediatric Oncology Nursing 9(3):119–130, 1992
Walsh B: Meeting the challenge of infection. A case study. Journal of Pediatric Oncology Nursing 9(4):146–158, 1992

9
Geriatric Pharmacology

With advancing age, the number of cells in most body tissues diminishes and changes occur in metabolism, permeability, and respiration. Connective tissue and fat proliferate, and adaptation to stress becomes impaired. Muscle strength, oxygen use, and sensory perception decline. These changes in organ and tissue function (Table 9-1) may alter responsiveness to drugs, which can result in the development of unpredictable effects of pharmacotherapy in elderly patients; adverse reactions occur more frequently—and tend to be more serious—than in younger adults.

A progressive increase in life span has resulted in a greater proportion of the population reaching advanced age; distinctions are now being made between the "young-old" (age 65–75 years) and "old-old" (age 75 years and older). Each group has unique qualities and needs (physiologic and psychosocial) that should be addressed independently, especially with regard to pharmacotherapy.

Accompanying this increase in life span is a corresponding increase in chronic illness such as cardiovascular disease (hypertension, coronary artery disease, congestive heart failure, peripheral vascular disease), pulmonary disease, diabetes melitus, cerebrovascular disease, cancer, and arthritic conditions. Taken individually, the pharmacologic management of each of these conditions often is accomplished with the use of more than one drug. Because it is common for elderly patients to be diagnosed with more than one chronic illness, the potential for development of adverse effects and drug–drug interactions increases with multidrug therapy (polypharmacy). In many cases, geriatric patients are taking more than one drug; sometimes the number of medications is greater than six! This significantly increases the chance that an adverse reaction, possibly due to a drug–drug interaction, will occur. Over-the-counter (OTC) products (eg, aspirin) and "socially acceptable" drugs (eg, nicotine, caffeine, and alcohol) are used by this population and also may have an impact on therapeutic outcomes.

It has been estimated that in the United States, the elderly account for almost one third of all drugs used (almost 30% of all prescription drugs and 40% of all OTC preparations). Nearly 90% of geriatric patients experience one or more episodes of adverse reactions to these drugs. The goal of pharmacotherapy in the elderly is to achieve maximum benefit with minimal adverse effects. To achieve this, an individualized approach to assessment, planning, and intervention must be taken, given the uniqueness of each person in terms of physical and psychosocial issues.

Variables That Affect Drug Responses in Geriatric Patients

The presence of numerous pathophysiologic conditions in the elderly can make selection of the proper drug and/or dose difficult. Safe and effective use of drugs in geriatric patients depends on individually planned therapy and requires constant reevaluation. A number of variables influence the response to drugs in the geriatric population. Generally, they tend to be absorbed, distributed, biotransformed, and eliminated much less efficiently than in younger adults, and this increases the potential for the development of adverse effects and drug interactions (drug–drug, drug–nutrient). The following is a brief discussion of how age-related changes can alter the response to a drug.

Absorption

Many changes can occur in the gastrointestinal (GI) tract that can impair the capacity to absorb food as well as drugs; such changes include a loss of absorbing cells, decreased GI motility, impaired gastric secretory cell function, reduced intestinal blood flow, and elevated gastric pH. Such alterations can retard active and passive absorption of drugs. In the elderly, drugs generally are absorbed less consistently and at a slower rate; however, the *extent* to which drugs are absorbed is probably not significantly different from that in younger adults.

Distribution

Drug distribution in the elderly may be severely curtailed in response to age-related decreases in cardiac output and perfusion of body organs. Other factors such as compromised peripheral blood flow due to atherosclerosis, increased body fat, decreased total body water, and decreased plasma proteins (albumin) also serve to reduce the systemic distribution of drugs in this population.

Biotransformation

Significant changes in liver function generally do not occur until rather late in life (after age 70 years) because of the large reserve capacity of this organ. Some reduction in hepatic function, however, may develop at an earlier age secondary to the presence of chronic liver disease (eg, hepatitis, cirrhosis) or diminished hepatic blood flow (reduction of up to 50% can occur because of arteriosclerosis, congestive heart failure, or pulmonary hypertension). A decrease in the ability to metabolize drugs is often the result of the age-related progressive loss of liver cells and microsomal enzyme function, as well as decreased liver perfusion and the presence of chronic disease states. Collectively, these alterations increase the elimination half-life ($T_{1/2\beta}$) for most drugs, which prolongs the duration of action and increases the chance of drug accumulation. It is therefore necessary to evaluate these patients closely and continuously so that the dose can be altered in sufficient time to avoid an adverse reaction.

Table 9-1. **Potential Changes in Organ Function With Age**

Heart	***Lungs***
Size ↑	Loss of elasticity
Heart rate ↓	
Cardiac output ↓	***Kidneys***
Impaired adaptation to stress	Renal blood flow ↓
	Glomerular filtration rate ↓
Cardiovascular System	Loss of functioning nephrons
Peripheral blood flow ↓	
Systemic resistance ↑	***Liver***
Loss of vessel elasticity	Enzymatic activity ↓
	Impaired hepatic perfusion
Nervous System	
Loss of neuronal function	***Hormonal***
Brain weight ↓	Loss of gonadal steroidal function
Impaired neuronal conduction	Anabolic activity ↓
Sensory perception (vision, hearing) ↓	
	Gastrointestinal
Musculoskeletal System	Digestive secretions ↓
Osteoporosis	Motility and peristalsis ↓
Loss of muscle mass	Gastric acidity ↓

↓, decreased; ↑, increased

Elimination

The amount of drug that can be removed from the blood by the kidney depends primarily on the volume of blood presented to the glomeruli; this is a function of renal blood flow. It is estimated that blood flow to the kidney is reduced by approximately 50% in a person who reaches the age of 70 years. Consequently, glomerular filtration also will decrease. This impaired renal perfusion greatly limits the amount of drug that can be filtered and excreted; the $T_{1/2B}$ may be prolonged. Tubular reabsorption and active tubular secretion also are diminished to some degree. Dose adjustments may become necessary in the presence of altered creatinine clearance (24-hour urinary excretion) to prevent drug accumulation and subsequent toxicity.

Other Factors

Additional factors that contribute to altered drug responsiveness in the elderly population include the following.

Altered Tissue Sensitivity

Certain drugs such as benzodiazepines can produce effects that are more powerful than expected in geriatric patients. Although diminished drug metabolism may partially account for this effect, age-related alterations in receptor sensitivity to certain pharmacologic agents may be involved. Conversely, certain drugs (eg, beta-blockers) are less powerful in some elderly patients; this may reflect an age-related reduction in the number and/or sensitivity of receptor sites.

Presence of Chronic Disease States

As discussed earlier, many elderly patients are diagnosed with one or more chronic pathologic conditions such as cardiovascular disease (hypertension, coronary artery disease, congestive heart failure, peripheral vascular disease), liver disease, pulmonary disease, kidney disease, and diabetes mellitus. These often can markedly alter responsiveness to a particular drug. Changes in drug response may result from pharmacokinetic alterations (absorption, distribution, metabolism, and elimination) or from reduced compensatory reactions secondary to impaired homeostatic mechanisms. For example, hypotension is common in the elderly, resulting from blunted cardiovascular reflex responses normally responsible for maintaining blood pressure. Hypotension produced as a side effect of drugs (eg, certain antipsychotics) may therefore be more severe than in younger patients.

Hormonal Changes

Many drugs acting through hormonal mechanisms may produce unexpected responses because of age-related reductions in endocrine function (eg, changes in secretion of insulin, and thyroid and sex hormones). When hormonal replacement therapy is indicated in the geriatric patient, it must be initiated with caution because the response may be greatly enhanced owing to receptor site hypersensitivity. Age-related atrophic changes in certain structures (bone, genital organs) resulting from diminished endogenous hormones may greatly modify drug activity to the point of toxicity. For example, administration of corticosteroids in the elderly can produce marked glucose intolerance, increased susceptibility to infection, and osteoporosis.

Behavioral Changes

Often overlooked, but critically important as a major determinant of drug response in elderly patients, is the patient's mental condition (cognitive function). Acute mental confusion can be produced by many conditions, including the following: infections; cardiovascular, respiratory, and central nervous system (CNS) disorders; metabolic, nutritional, and fluid and electrolyte imbalances; physical trauma; surgery and general anesthesia; environmental changes; and clinical depression. In addition, pharmacotherapy, especially polypharmacy, is also a major cause of acute mental confusion in the aged. Drug categories that commonly produce this response include cardiovascular agents (cardiac glycosides, antihypertensives, diuretics), CNS agents (sedative–hypnotics, anxiolytics, narcotic and nonnarcotic analgesics, antihistamines, antiparkinson agents, antidepressants, anxiolytics, antipsychotics), glucocorticoids, and anticholinergic drugs. Cognitive changes produced by these drugs can markedly affect the life of a patient by reducing the ability to participate in activities of daily living, impairing interpersonal relationships, and causing poor compliance with the therapeutic drug regimen, which can lead to reduced effectiveness or accidental overdose.

Drug Therapy in the Elderly

Drug therapy in the elderly population often is difficult to manage and always potentially hazardous. An understanding of the normal process of aging, alterations in physiology and functional capacity, and age-related changes in pharmacodynamics and pharmacokinetics (absorption, distribution, metabolism, elimination) is essential to provide safe and effective pharmacologic management for this population.

It is extremely important to conduct an ongoing, detailed assessment of the drug regimen for every geriatric patient. The following aspects of patient care should therefore be considered:

Is the drug therapy necessary? It is not necessary to administer drugs to treat every health problem of an elderly person. The benefit-to-risk ratio assumes critical importance in planning and managing drug therapy in geriatric patients because this population is highly prone to development of adverse drug reactions.

Is the duration of therapy appropriate? Many diseases in the elderly require prolonged drug therapy, often with multiple drugs. It is important that the drug regimen be periodically reviewed for appropriateness and to identify actual and potential problems. In some cases, doses of drugs can be changed or drugs can discontinued (eliminated from the protocol) before harmful effects occur.

Is the drug therapy adequate? Approximately 80% of all elderly patients have more than one chronic illness. Therefore, drug therapy is complicated, but the overprescribing of medications can be as harmful as *inadequate* therapy. The large number of different drugs used in therapy and the resulting complex dosing schedules greatly increase the probability for development of drug–drug interactions and toxicity. Polypharmacy should be avoided whenever possible.

Is the patient compliant with prescribed drug therapy? The capacity of a geriatric patient to comply with the dosing schedule of prescribed drugs must be assessed. Factors such as chronic disease, chronic therapy, multiple drugs and doses, difficult-to-use dosage forms, physical disability (eg, reductions in vision, strength, and motor coordination), health beliefs, knowledge deficit (disease process, treatment plan, drugs), diminished cognitive function, and drug costs are factors that promote noncompliance with prescribed drug therapy. Ongoing assessment and follow-up, coupled with mutual goal setting and patient–family teaching, are interventions that help to increase compliance.

Nursing Management

Pretherapy Assessment

Assess and record important baseline data necessary for detection of adverse effects (perform a detailed, individualized nursing assessment).

Review past medical history and documents for evidence of existing or previous medical history related to conditions that:

a. require cautious administration of a prescribed drug: medical history.
b. contraindicate use of a drug, eg, allergy to prescribed drug or drug family; medical history.

Nursing Interventions

Medication Administration

Administer drugs to maximize their intended effects and minimize their adverse effects. For example, administer diuretics in the morning to reduce the need void at night.

Plan and implement individualized nursing interventions that:

a. inform the patient about the expected actions and adverse effects of a prescribed drug.
b. identify the early onset of expected and undesirable adverse effects and intervene appropriately.
c. minimize the symptoms produced by the expected adverse effects of the prescribed drug.
d. identify the safety needs of the patient and intervene appropriately to minimize environmental hazards and risk of injury.

Recognize factors (through detailed, individualized, ongoing nursing assessment) that promote noncompliance with drug therapy.

CAUTION

Factors that promote noncompliance in the elderly were presented in the previous section.

Plan and implement individualized, mutually derived nursing interventions directed at fostering compliance with drug therapy.

Surveillance During Therapy

Always monitor the drug dose being administered. Rationale: to ensure that it is within acceptable limits for the diagnosis and patient being treated.

Compare current status with previous status to detect improvements, deterioration in the patient's condition.

Monitor patient for therapeutic drug effect.

Monitor for adverse effects, toxicity, and interactions.

Monitor for signs of hypersensitivity that may require discontinuation of drug.

Facilitate acquisition of diagnostic tests ordered for ongoing assessment of drug response.

Monitor diagnostic test results obtained over the course of therapy.

Interpret results of diagnostic tests and contact practitioner–prescriber as appropriate.

Monitor for possible drug–laboratory test interactions.

Monitor for possible drug–drug and drug–nutrient interactions.

Monitor for compliance with drug therapy.

Patient Teaching

Instruct patient about expected actions and possible adverse effects of prescribed drug.

Teach patient/family drug administration techniques and safety measures to ensure that correct drug is taken in the correct dose, at the correct time.

Instruct patient about appropriate action to take if adverse effects occur:

a. How to manage symptoms related to expected adverse effects of prescribed drug.
b. When to notify practitioner–prescriber.
c. Conditions for discontinuing administration of prescribed drug before notification of practitioner–prescriber.
d. Under which conditions to seek immediate medical attention if adverse side effects develop.

Instruct patient regarding the importance of completing

the full course of therapy *as prescribed*; that is, *not* to discontinue the drug as soon as signs and symptoms have subsided.

Inform patient of the consequences of not taking or abruptly discontinuing a prescribed drug.

Instruct patient that a prescribed drug is to be taken only in the manner and for the condition for which it is prescribed.

Instruct patient to keep all medications out of the reach of children, especially those that have been dispensed without child-protective caps as per patient request.

Selected Bibliography

Beard K: Adverse reactions as a cause of hospital admission in the aged. Drugs and Aging 2(4):356, 1992

Creasey HM, Broe GA: Prescribing for the elderly: Parkinson's disease. Med J Aust 159:249, 1993

Cumming RG, Klineberg RJ: Psychotropics, thiazide diuretics and hip fractures in the elderly. Med J Aust 158:414, 1993

Ganzini L, Millar SB, Walsh JR: Drug-induced mania in the elderly. Drugs and Aging 3(5):428, 1993

Jones D: Characteristics of elderly people taking psychotropic medication. Drugs and Aging 2(5):389, 1992

Kolbeinsson H, Jonsson A: Delirium and dementia in acute medical admissions of elderly patients in Iceland. Acta Psychiatr Scand 87:123, 1993

Leslie C, Scott PJW, Caird FI: Principal alterations to drug kinetics and dynamics in the elderly. Med Lab Sci 49:319, 1992

Ritschel WA: Drug disposition in the elderly: Gerontokinetics. Methods Find Exp Clin Pharmacol 14(7):555, 1992

Shorr RI, Robin DW: Rational use of benzodiazepines in the elderly. Drugs and Aging 4(1):9, 1994

Thapa PB, Meador KG, Gideon P, Fought RL, Ray WA: Effects of antipsychotic withdrawal in elderly nursing home residents. J Am Geriatr Soc 42:280, 1994

Nursing Bibliography

Ali N: Promoting safe use of multiple meds by elderly persons. Geriatric Nursing 13(3):134–138, 1992

Brockopp D, Warden S, Colclough G, Brockopp G: Nursing knowledge: Acute postop pain management. Journal of Gerontologic Nursing 19(11):31–37, 1993

Hahn K, Weitor G: Helpful tools for medication screening. Geriatric Nursing 13(3):160–166, 1992

LeSage J: Polypharmacy in geriatric patients. The Nursing Clinics of North America 26(2):290, 1991

Linderborn K: Independently living seniors and vitamin therapy: What nurses should know. Journal Gerontological Nursing 19(8):10–20, 1993

Miller C: CHF—old and new drugs. Geriatric Nursing 14(4):190–199, 1993

Moore J, Johnson J: OTC drug use by rural elderly. Geriatric Nursing 14(4):190–199, 1993

Ryan P, Vortherms R, Ward S: Cancer pain: Knowledge attitudes of pharmacologic management. Journal Gerontological Nursing 20(1): 7–16, 1994

Shaefer M, Williams L: Poly pharmacy in geri patients. Nursing Clinics of North America 28(4):273–290, 1993

Wolfe S, Schirm V: Medication counseling for the elderly—effects on knowledge and compliance after hospital D/C. Geriatric Nursing 13(3):134–138, 1992

10
Legal Aspects of Drug Therapy

Various federal laws enacted during the 20th century were designed to protect the public from false claims of therapeutic benefit and to minimize the occurrence of toxic reactions—that is, to ensure both the *efficacy* and *safety* of available drug products. The first part of this chapter presents the most important federal drug laws, including narcotic drug regulations, followed by an examination of Canadian drug regulations. The remainder of the chapter examines the nurse's role and responsibility in the handling and administration of controlled substances.

United States Drug Legislation

The Pure Food and Drug Act

The first important federal law concerning drugs was the Wiley-Heyburn Act, more commonly known as the Pure Food and Drug Act, which took effect in 1907. It was an attempt to prohibit adulteration and misbranding of food and drugs distributed by interstate commerce. Sale of preparations containing any of the listed narcotic or habit-forming drugs without a proper label showing both the name and amount of the drug was prohibited. Under this law, however, accurate labeling was all that the federal government could require. Further provisions were the designation of the *United States Pharmacopeia* (USP) and the *National Formulary* (NF) as the official standards for establishing the strength, quality, and purity of all medications sold in interstate commerce; in addition, the U.S. Food and Drug Administration (FDA) was established as the regulatory agency to enforce this law.

Drugs listed in the USP or NF are designated as *official drugs* and conform to standards that include drug strength, purity, packaging safety, and labeling as established by these compendia. Drugs meeting these standards can be identified by the letters USP or NF after their name. In the past, the USP and NF were separate entities; however, because of their similarity in style and content, they are now combined into a single publication (USP-NF). Because this publication is revised only every 5 years, many new drugs do not appear in the USP-NF until several years after they have become available. Thus, it is important to understand that although a new drug may not be classified as *official* (because it may not currently appear in the official compendium), it should not be regarded as being ineffective or unsafe; the term *official* means *only* that a drug has been included in the USP-NF. The Sherley Amendment to the Pure Food and Drug Act, passed in 1912, prohibited use of false advertising claims. For over 30 years, these two laws comprised the only governmental regulation over the sale of drugs.

The Federal Food, Drug and Cosmetic Act

Increased concern about the safety of drug products eventually led to the passage of the Federal Food, Drug and Cosmetic Act of 1938. It was quite comprehensive in nature, and contained a number of provisions intended to ensure both the safety and the efficacy of drug products. Among the important requirements of this act were 1) new drugs had to be shown to be safe *before* being marketed, 2) *all* drugs (prescription and nonprescription [over-the-counter; OTC]) had to be properly labeled, 3) certain drugs that were known to be "habit forming" must be so labeled, and 4) "good manufacturing procedures" had to be followed in the processing of drugs according to FDA standards.

Durham-Humphrey Amendment

Although comprehensive, the 1938 Act had several deficiencies, and a number of amendments were added in later years. The first amendment, enacted in 1952, was the Durham-Humphrey Amendment. It designated certain drugs as being available by prescription only. These drugs, termed *legend* drugs, must have the following statement on their containers: "Caution: Federal law prohibits dispensing without prescription." This amendment also prohibited refilling of such drugs without authorization, and presented guidelines about oral and telephone orders for prescription drugs and refills. In addition, the Durham-Humphrey Amendment recognized another class of drugs, namely those that were safe for use without medical prescription (ie, OTC drugs). Proper labeling procedures for OTC drugs also were provided in this amendment.

Kefauver-Harris Amendment

Despite the existing drug laws, federal control over drug advertising and marketing practices was still inadequate according to many observers. In 1958, U.S. Senator Estes Kefauver launched a controversial Senate investigation of the drug industry that ultimately led to the passage in 1962 of the Kefauver-Harris Amendment to the Federal Food, Drug and Cosmetic Act. Among the important provisions of this amendment was the requirement that drugs be proved *effective* as well as safe before entering the market. The FDA was given authority to oversee and regulate the procedures by which new drugs were tested for safety and efficacy. Guidelines for advertising of prescription drugs were tightened considerably, as were guidelines for testing drugs on humans. Quality-control laws for drug manufacturing were upgraded, and the role of the FDA in registering, monitoring, and inspecting drug manufacturers was greatly increased.

Another provision of the 1962 amendment granted the FDA the authority to regulate the efficacy, as well as the safety, of all drugs marketed since 1938, not just those available from 1962. Thus, drug products marketed between 1938 and 1962 had to be reevaluated to determine their efficacy.

The Drug Efficacy Study Implementation

To facilitate this task, the FDA contracted with the National Academy of Sciences and its research division, the National Research Council, to evaluate efficacy data and therapeutic claims of drug products. This study was called the Drug Efficacy Study Implementation (DESI). Based on the results of the evaluation, every drug was classified into one of six categories as follows:

1. *Effective*: Considerable evidence of effectiveness for the designated indications
2. *Probably effective*: More evidence is necessary to conclusively demonstrate effectiveness
3. *Possibly effective*: Little evidence to suggest effectiveness for the recommended indications
4. *Ineffective*: No significant evidence of effectiveness
5. *Ineffective as a fixed combination*: No evidence to suggest all components of the combination are necessary for the claimed effect, although one or more components may be effective if given alone
6. *Effective but*: A restriction or qualification must be added to the labeling

Drugs rated as ineffective were withdrawn from the market. Those rated either **probably effective** or **possibly effective** had to carry their rating on the label, and their manufacturers were given additional time by the FDA either to substantiate their claims or to withdraw the drugs from the market.

Federal Narcotic Drug Laws

It was not until 1914 that the first federal law aimed at controlling traffic in so-called illicit drugs was enacted.

Harrison Narcotic Act

The Harrison Narcotic Act of 1914 established and legally defined the word *narcotic* and established regulations governing the importation, manufacture, sale, and use of opium, cocaine, and their derivatives. Subsequent revisions of the Harrison Narcotic Act added marijuana and many newer synthetic opiate drugs. This law, with minor periodic revisions, stood for over 50 years; unfortunately, it gradually became obsolete, and proved ineffective in controlling the expanding national drug abuse problem.

Controlled Substances Act

To tighten federal control of abused drugs, Congress passed the Comprehensive Drug Abuse Prevention and Control Act of 1970; it superseded all previous federal drug laws regulating narcotics and other dangerous drugs. This legislation, commonly referred to as the Controlled Substances Act, was designed to control the manufacturing, distribution, administration, and disposition of narcotics, depressants, stimulants, and other drugs having abuse potential as designated by the Drug Enforcement Administration (DEA), a government agency responsible for enforcing the provisions of the Controlled Substances Act.

Among its many provisions, the Controlled Substances Act classified the various drugs of abuse into five *schedules* according to their medical usefulness and potential for abuse. The drugs comprising the various schedules are given in Table 10-1. Regulations governing each group of drugs are as follows:

Schedule I: High abuse potential and no *accepted* medical use in the United States. Schedule I drugs are not available for routine prescription use, but may be obtained for investigational studies by proper application to the DEA.

Schedule II: Valid medical indications but have a high abuse potential. Misuse of these substances can lead to strong psychological and physical dependence.

Schedule III: Drugs in Schedule III have a moderate potential for abuse, less than that in Schedules I or II. Misuse, however, still can lead to some physical dependence and strong psychological dependence.

Schedule IV: Low abuse potential; less than that of Schedule III drugs. Misuse most often results in varying degrees of psychological dependence, with occasional reports of physical dependence.

Schedule V: Abuse potential less than in Schedule IV. Drugs in Schedule V consist mainly of preparations containing moderate amounts of opioid drugs, generally for antitussive or antidiarrheal use.

Each commercial container of a controlled substance bears on its label a symbol designating the schedule to which it belongs. Symbols are a large red C, either enclosing or followed by roman numeral I, II, III, IV, or V, referring to the schedule to which the drug belongs.

The following discussion pertains to the requirements for ordering and dispensing controlled substances. The pharmacology of these substances, together with a review of procedures for recognizing and treating drug abuse, is found in Chapter 82.

Prescribing and Dispensing Controlled Drugs

The requirements for dispensing a controlled drug outlined here are the currently mandated federal regulations. In many instances, however, individual *state* laws are more stringent than the *federal* law, and must be observed by all practitioners within a particular state. Health professionals handling controlled substances must therefore know the specific regulations of the state(s) in which they are employed, and which ones, if any, supersede the federal law.

All prescription orders for Schedule II drugs must be either typewritten or written in ink (or indelible pencil) and signed by the physician. Prescriptions for Schedule II drugs *cannot* be refilled; all records and inventory information must be maintained separately from other pharmacy records. A triplicate order form is necessary for ordering Schedule II drugs. Under certain emergency situations (outlined later), a Schedule II drug may be dispensed on oral authorization.

Orders for Schedule III and IV drugs and those Schedule V drugs requiring a prescription (see discussion later) can be issued either orally or in writing. They are valid for *only 6 months* after the date of the prescription; they can be refilled up to five times within this 6-month interval, if so authorized by the physician. Oral prescription orders must be immediately committed to writing. Prescriptions for drugs in Schedules III, IV, or V must be readily retrievable from the files; if they are filed with the

Table 10-1. **Schedules of Controlled Drugs**

Schedule I
benzylmorphine
cannabinols (eg, hashish, marijuana, tetrahydrocannabinol)
dihydromorphine
hallucinogens (eg, bufotenin, DET, DMT, DOB, DOM, ibogaine, LSD, MDA, mescaline, peyote, PMA, psilocybin, psilocyn)
ketobemidone
levomoramide
nicocodine
nicomorphine
racemoramide

Schedule II

Depressants
amobarbital
methaqualone
pentobarbital
phencyclidine
secobarbital

Narcotics
alfentanil
codeine
etorphine
fentanyl
hydromorphone
levomethadyl
levorphanol
meperidine
methadone
opium and opium alkaloids (eg, morphine, codeine)
oxycodone
oxymorphone
phenazocine
sufentanil

Stimulants
amphetamine
coca leaves
cocaine
dextroamphetamine
methamphetamine
methylphenidate
phenmetrazine

Cannabinoids
dronabinol
nabilone

Schedule III

Depressants
aprobarbital
butabarbital
glutethimide
hexobarbital
methyprylon
thiamylal
thiopental

Narcotics
opiates in combination with other nonnarcotic drugs (eg, Empirin with codeine, Tylenol with codeine, Hycodan)
paregoric

Stimulants
benzphetamine
chlorphentermine
phendimetrazine

Androgens/Anabolic Steroids
fluoxymesterone
methyltestosterone
nandrolone
oxandrolone
oxymetholone
stanozolol
testosterone

Schedule IV

Depressants
barbital
benzodiazepines (alprazolam, chlordiazepoxide, clonazepam, estazolam, clorazepate, diazepam, flurazepam, halazepam, lorazepam, midazolam, oxazepam, prazepam, quazepam, temazepam, triazolam)
chloral hydrate
ethchlorvynol
mephobarbital
meprobamate
methohexital
paraldehyde
phenobarbital
zolpidem

Narcotics
difenoxin and atropine (eg, Motofen)
pentazocine
propoxyphene

Stimulants
diethylpropion
fenfluramine
mazindol
pemoline
phentermine

Schedule V
buprenorphine
diphenoxylate and atropine (eg, Lomotil)
loperamide
narcotic drugs in combination with other nonnarcotic agents, generally used as antitussives, where the amount of narcotic (eg, codeine, dihydrocodeine) is limited

regular prescription orders (except Schedule II drugs), each must be marked with the letter "C" in red ink to facilitate retrieval. Records must be maintained for at least 2 years.

Each time a prescription for a Schedule III, IV, or V drug is refilled, the date and amount of drug dispensed must be noted on the back of the order blank, and initialed by the dispenser. The label of any controlled drug in Schedules II, III, or IV must contain the following statement "Caution: Federal law prohibits the transfer of this drug to any person other than the patient for whom it was prescribed."

Partial Distribution of Controlled Substances

If the full quantity of a Schedule II drug cannot be supplied with the original prescription order, the remaining portion may be dispensed within 72 hours provided the quantity dispensed with the initial order is noted on the face of the written prescription. Additional partial quantities can not be supplied after the 72-hour time limit; a new prescription order is required.

Partial dispensing of Schedule III and IV drugs is allowed provided the quantity dispensed is noted on the back of the prescription order. The balance of the partial quantities dispensed may not exceed the total amount authorized (that is, original quantity plus allowable refills), nor extend past the 6-month time limit.

Emergency Dispensation of Schedule II Drugs

In the event of an emergency situation, a Schedule II drug can be dispensed on oral authorization from the doctor provided that certain conditions are satisfied. An "emergency situation" is defined as:

Immediate administration of the drug is necessary for proper treatment.
No appropriate alternative treatment is available.
A written prescription cannot reasonably be provided by the prescribing physician before the drug is required.

The rules for dispensing a Schedule II drug in an emergency situation are as follows:

Quantity dispensed must be limited to the amount necessary to treat the patient during the emergency period.
Prescription order must be immediately put in writing.
All efforts to verify the identity of the prescriber should be made, in the event that he or she is not known to the dispenser.
A written prescription with the notation "Authorization for Emergency Dispensing" must be delivered to the dispenser within 72 hours of the oral authorization, or, if mailed, postmarked within 72 hours.

Nonprescription Dispensation of Schedule V Drugs

Certain Schedule V medications can be dispensed without a prescription providing the following conditions are satisfied:

The dispensing is done only by a pharmacist or pharmacist-intern.
The purchaser is at least 18 years of age (proof of age is necessary if the purchaser is unknown to the dispenser).

Not more than 240 mL or not more than 48 solid dosage units of any substance containing opium, nor more than 120 mL or not more than 24 solid dosage units of any other controlled substance may be distributed to the same purchaser within 48 hours.

The name and address of the purchaser, kind and quantity of substance purchased, date of sale, and pharmacist's initials must be recorded for each sale in a Schedule V record book, and records maintained for 2 years.

State and local laws, which often are more stringent with respect to retail distribution of Schedule V substances, must be observed instead of the federal law.

A practitioner (physician, dentist, veterinarian) must apply for permission to dispense controlled drugs by registering with the DEA and, on approval, receives a seven-digit registration number (DEA number) that must appear on *every* order for controlled substances. The DEA registration must be renewed annually. Likewise, every pharmacy that dispenses controlled drugs must register annually with the DEA, and its DEA number must be available for inspection at the location of business.

Canadian Drug Regulations

In Canada, two pieces of legislation, the Food and Drug Act and the Narcotic Control Act, form the basis of the drug laws. The laws are administered and overseen by the Health Protection Branch of the Department of National Health and Welfare.

The Food and Drug Act, which controls the manufacture, distribution, and sale of all drugs except narcotics, became law in 1953. The Narcotic Control Act, which performs a similar function with regard to narcotic drugs, was passed in 1961.

Nonprescription Drugs

In Canada, there are three groups of drugs that may be obtained without a prescription. *Proprietary medicines*, such as mild pain relievers, cough drops, and some topical preparations may be purchased at any retail outlet. Use of these medications does not require the counseling of a health professional. *Over-the-counter medications* are sold principally in pharmacies, and are intended for treating minor, self-limiting illnesses; however, professional advice is recommended before using these products. Examples are laxatives, cold and cough medications, and dietary supplements. *Medications available only in the pharmacy* is a self-explanatory term, referring to medications used on the recommendation of a physician or a pharmacist after consultation with the patient. Drugs such as insulin and nitroglycerin, as well as some codeine-containing analgesic or cough combinations, fall into this category.

Prescription Drugs

Drugs available by prescription fall into one of the following categories:

Schedule F: the largest group of prescription drugs; must be identified by the symbol *Pr* on the label.

Schedule G (Controlled Drugs): drugs having mood-altering effects that are likely to become habit forming; includes amphetamines, barbiturates, and some narcotics (eg, butorphanol, nalbuphine), but *not* most anxiolytics (eg, benzodiazepines); the symbol ◇C must appear on labels and all advertisements.

Narcotic Drugs: drugs classified legally as having potent addictive properties; includes most opiates as well as cannabis and phencyclidine; the letter *N* must appear on all labels and advertisements and these drugs are subject to stringent restrictions; only exception is codeine, when combined with at least two other drugs in amounts not in excess of 8 mg/tablet or 20 mg/ounce—these codeine-containing products are classified as *narcotic preparations* and may be purchased without a prescription.

Schedule H (Restricted Drugs): similar to Schedule I drugs in the United States; substances having no recognized medicinal properties but a high abuse potential and grave health risk; includes approximately 25 chemicals (eg, LSD, psilocybin, and mescaline).

Dispensation of Prescription Drugs

Schedule F drugs may be obtained by either oral or written prescription and refilled as often as indicated by the physician. Schedule G drugs also may be obtained by written or verbal order, but refilled only if indicated on a *written* prescription. Narcotic drugs may be dispensed only on a written prescription and cannot be refilled. As in the United States, provincial (or state) laws may supersede federal laws in Canada with regard to the restrictions placed on the classification and distribution of drugs. Provincial laws, however, may *not* remove a drug from the prescription-only list once it has been placed there by federal regulations.

Nurse's Role in Administration of Controlled Drugs

The nurse is guided in the administration of controlled substances by agency policies, which reflect state and federal regulations.

Administration Within Healthcare Institutions

In any institution, whether acute or extended care, controlled drugs must be kept in a locked cabinet with access to these medications limited to certain personnel. Agency policy states the frequency of counting the stock (usually every shift), who may give the drugs, how the drugs are to be obtained from the central pharmacy, and who has ultimate responsibility for loss of any of these drugs. Because state regulatory agencies generally investigate all losses of controlled substances, such incidents must be accurately reported.

Institutional policies also reflect the frequency with which controlled drugs are to be reordered. The nurse must comply with these policies and ensure that such drugs are reordered promptly. In acute care settings, it may be necessary to reorder some Schedule II drugs every 24 to 48 hours, whereas other drug orders may be valid for 7 days. In extended care facilities, orders may be written and renewed once every 30 days. Regardless of the time limitation, the nurse is responsible for monitoring the response to the drugs administered, and for reporting to the physician evidence of change in pain control, development of tolerance, addiction behaviors, or toxic reactions. Changes may occur rapidly, so the nurse should document the patient's response to the drug each time it is administered.

Administration in Home Care Settings

In the home care setting, patients and their families are responsible for obtaining the controlled medication through a local pharmacy. The nurse, however, must monitor the patient's response to the drug and report any changes to the doctor. If the patient or a family member is suspected of abusing the drug, the nurse should share this concern with both the physician and the dispensing pharmacist. The frequency of refill requests can then be monitored. Hospice nurses report that this problem occurs occasionally and is best dealt with by professionals—the physician, pharmacist, nurse, and regulatory agencies—rather than by a single person making an accusation.

Medication Orders

Proper ordering of medications is essential for safe and effective drug therapy. Transmission of the physician's wishes regarding drug treatment of the patient usually is accomplished by a written order kept in either a drug file or a patient chart (hospitalized patients), or in the form of a prescription (outpatient). Medication orders may be given by telephone, but it is important that such orders be put in writing as soon as possible to minimize chance of error.

Generally, people empowered by state law to write prescriptions include physicians, dentists, and veterinarians. In some states, however, the law has been modified to permit nurse practitioners and physicians' assistants to write prescription orders for certain types of drugs.

The Nurse's Role in Carrying Out Medication Orders

The nurse has several legal responsibilities in carrying out medication orders written in the hospital. Nurses must accurately transcribe orders to the medication record sheet, which provides a quick reference to all the medications a patient is receiving. This transcription should be clearly written so that all staff personnel will be able to read the order.

Clarifying and Evaluating Written Orders

If the order has not been clearly written, the nurse should seek clarification from the doctor. Legally, the standard against which nurses are judged is that they will give the *right* medication in the *right* dose, by the *right* route, at the *right* time, to the *right* patient. That standard makes the nurse liable for giving a wrong medication to a patient even if the physician who ordered it committed the error. Therefore, *when in doubt, question the order.*

There are two steps in the process of assessing the physician's order for a medication: first, an initial reading for clarity, and second, a reading for the appropriateness of the order. What has been written must be understandable and free of confusion. Any abbreviations, if used, must be correctly interpreted, and the order must contain all parts and information described above. Second, before dispensing the medication, the nurse must evaluate the order for appropriateness, determining, for example, whether the dosage form can be conveniently taken by the patient, whether the patient has any underlying condition (eg, liver or kidney disease) that may alter the effect of the drug, whether the patient is taking other drugs that may interact with the newly prescribed drug, and whether the patient has demonstrated previous allergies to the medication.

Telephone Orders

Occasionally, the nurse will be asked to take a telephone order. Institutional policies will identify the context in which this act is permitted. Many institutions require that two nurses listen to telephone orders as they are given to ensure accuracy and appropriateness, and to protect the nurse. Telephone orders are most appropriate in emergency situations when the physician cannot be present. The accuracy of a telephone order depends on communication between sender and receiver. To ensure that the order is clear, it is always a good idea to write it down and repeat it to the physician before hanging up the telephone. The physician must cosign the order within 24 hours of giving it. Telephone orders can involve risk if the physician later denies having given the order, or if the nurse misinterprets the order. Most institutions discourage the use of telephone orders for these reasons, and nurses should be cautious about accepting them.

Responsibility for Errors in Administration

A nurse who administers a drug has a legal responsibility to perform properly. If an error in medicating a patient occurs, the nurse can become the target of a malpractice suit. Therefore, in addition to providing a patient with maximum therapeutic benefits and minimum toxicity, the nurse also will reduce malpractice liability by being knowledgeable about the medications given, careful in administration, and alert to potential problems that may result in errors.

Many medication errors made by nurses involve failure to follow institutional policies. It is extremely important to know what such policies are because they are designed to protect both the health professional *and* the patient. The safe administration of a drug depends on coordinated, responsible action by a team of colleagues, all of whom are legally accountable. The interaction of all health professionals will increase the safety of patient care. Nurses should take an active role in ensuring patient safety by using caution in giving drugs and by participating in discussions of committees that formulate guidelines for patient care.

Selected Bibliography

Brushwood DB: Government liable for failure to monitor a patient's serum gentamicin concentration in an Army hospital. Am J Hosp Pharm 49:1748, 1992

Brushwood DB: Hospital's obligation to monitor medical services. Am J Hosp Pharm 50:1437, 1993

Calfee BE: Steering clear of trouble: Litigation lessons. Nursing '94 24(1):46, 1994

Falk KH (ed): *Legal Medicine: Legal Dynamics of Medical Encounters*, 2nd ed. St Louis, Mosby Year Book, 1991

Kessler DA: Introducing MEDWatch: A new approach to reporting medication and device adverse effects and product problems. JAMA 269(21):2765, 1993

Oddens BJ, Algra A, van Gijn J: Informing patients about clinical trials. Clin Invest 71:572, 1993

Parmley WW: Disciplinary actions: How often and why? J Am Coll Cardiol 23(1):278, 1994

Rhodes AM: Law versus ethics. Amer J Maternal/Child Nursing 18:311, 1993

Torres A: The use of Food and Drug Administration–approved medication for unlabeled (off-label) uses. Arch Dermatol 130:32, 1994

Nursing Bibliography

Cohen M, Senders J, Davis N: twelve ways to prevent medication errors. Nursing '94 24(2):34–42, 1994

Davis N: Confusion over illegible orders. American Journal of Nursing 1(1): 1994

Fennell K: Prescriptive authority for nurse–midwives: A historical review. Nursing Clinics of North America 26(2):511, 1991

Kilroy R, Iafrate R: Provision of pharmaceutical care in the intensive care unit. Critical Nursing Clinics of North America 5(2):221–226, 1993

Rafferty K, Henry J: Ethical considerations in drug administration for critically ill patients. Critical Care Nursing Clinics of North America 5(2):377–382, 1993

II

Drugs Acting on the Nervous System

11

The Nervous System: A Review

The human nervous system is an immensely complex functional unit, composed of nearly one trillion nerve cells or neurons, as well as trillions of supporting glial cells. In concert with the endocrine system, the nervous system regulates and coordinates the functioning of the organ systems of the body. Whereas the endocrine system provides a more slowly developing but long-lasting control, the nervous system evokes rapid responses of the body to changes in the internal and external environments, thereby providing moment-to-moment control.

The nervous system can be categorized in the following manner:

- I. **Anatomic divisions**
  - A. Central nervous system (CNS)
    - 1. Brain
    - 2. Spinal cord
  - B. Peripheral nervous system
    - 1. Cranial nerves (12 pairs)
    - 2. Spinal nerves (31 pairs)
- II. **Functional divisions**
  - A. Somatic nervous system
  - B. Autonomic nervous system
    - 1. Sympathetic division
    - 2. Parasympathetic division

The following brief review of important concepts related to the functioning of the nervous system is presented to provide background sufficient to promote understanding of the subsequent chapters dealing with those classes of drugs affecting neuronal functioning.

Peripheral Nervous System

Functionally, the peripheral nervous system is often subdivided into the somatic nervous system and the autonomic nervous system. Several important differences exist between these two systems, as outlined in Table 11-1.

Somatic Nervous System

The somatic nervous system conveys sensory information from cutaneous receptors, proprioceptors, and specialized sensory receptors to the CNS and mediates appropriate responses by the skeletal muscles. The somatic nervous system is generally viewed as a *voluntary* system, because the sensations usually are consciously perceived and movements may be consciously controlled.

Autonomic Nervous System

In contrast, the autonomic nervous system includes those sensory and motor nerves that primarily innervate internal organs (smooth muscle, heart, glands) that usually function independently of the individual's will. This system is therefore classified as an *involuntary* system. Although responses of the somatic system, such as contraction of skeletal muscle, are almost always excitatory, those of the autonomic system may be either excitatory (eg, vasoconstriction) or inhibitory (eg, bradycardia, bronchodilation), depending on the organ and neurotransmitter involved.

The autonomic system is further subclassified into *sympathetic* and *parasympathetic* divisions. The characteristics of each division are listed in Table 11-2.

The parasympathetic division is often referred to as a *cholinergic* system because the neurotransmitter at its postganglionic nerve endings is acetylcholine, whereas the sympathetic division may be termed an *adrenergic* system because its postganglionic neurotransmitter *in most cases* is norepinephrine. Activation of the sympathetic division of the autonomic nervous system allows a person to cope effectively with stressful "emergency" situations (Cannon's famous "flight or fight" response). In contrast, the parasympathetic division promotes the normal day-to-day activities of life. "Sympathetic" and "parasympathetic," however, are anatomic terms, and do not necessarily reflect the neurotransmitters released from nerve endings in every instance. This point is further discussed later.

Many effector structures are innervated by *both* divisions of the autonomic system, and in dually innervated structures the effects of the two divisions are usually opposed—that is, if sympathetic activation causes excitation, parasympathetic activation causes inhibition. The two divisions, however, do not always exert equal control over all dually innervated structures. For example, the sympathetic division influences blood vessel tone, and hence blood pressure, to a much greater degree than the parasympathetic system, whereas the reverse is true in the functioning of the gastrointestinal tract.

A few structures, however, are singly innervated, including the adrenal medulla, sweat glands, certain blood vessels, intrinsic eye muscles (eg, iris) and pilomotor muscles of the skin. The response of these structures is usually *excitatory*, regardless of their innervation. These differences are illustrated in Table 11-3, which outlines the effects of sympathetic versus parasympathetic stimulation on different structures of the body, clearly indicating the opposing nature of most responses as well as the excitatory nature of singly innervated structures. It should be noted that although the sweat glands and some skeletal muscle blood vessels are innervated by sympathetic fibers, the neurotransmitter released at the nerve ending is acetylcholine, not norepinephrine. Given these exceptions, peripheral nerves are probably best classified chemically—that is, on the basis of the principal neurotransmitter released from their nerve endings. Nerves releasing acetylcholine are thus termed *cholinergic*, and those releasing norepinephrine (or in some cases dopamine) are called *adrenergic* or *noradrenergic*. The mechanisms by which these neurotransmitters function at nerve endings are reviewed in the following sections.

Table 11-1. **Comparison of the Somatic and Autonomic Nervous Systems**

	Somatic	*Autonomic*
Nature of the Response	Voluntary	Involuntary
Centers of Neuronal Origin in the CNS	Cerebrum, cerebellum, midbrain, basal ganglia, spinal cord	Midbrain, hypothalamus, pons, medulla, spinal cord
Structures Innervated by Efferent Nerve Fibers	Skeletal muscles, sensory organs	Smooth muscle, cardiac muscle, exocrine and endocrine glands
Efferent Nerve Pathways	Single neuron with cell body in CNS and axon terminal at effector structure (eg, skeletal muscle fiber)	Two-neuron chain, with cell body of *pre*ganglionic neuron in CNS and axon terminal in a peripheral ganglia. *Post*ganglionic neuron has cell body in ganglia (synapses with *pre*ganglionic nerve ending) and axon terminal at effector structure (eg, heart, GI tract, bronchioles, glands)
Effect of Nerve Impulse on Innervated Structures	Excitation (eg, skeletal muscle contraction)	Excitation (eg, vasoconstriction, salivation) or inhibition (eg, bradycardia, bronchodilation)

Neurotransmitter Function

The functional cell of the nervous system is the *neuron*, a highly specialized, excitable cell capable of generating and propagating electrical impulses (action potentials). The passage of an impulse *along* a neuron, termed *conduction*, is an electrical process involving changes in the potential difference across the neuronal membrane caused by alterations in the flow of ions through the membrane. Drugs such as local anesthetics are capable of interrupting conduction of nerve impulses along a neuron by interfering with ionic flow across the membrane.

Communication *between* neurons occurs at specialized sites termed *synapses*. Although *electrical synapses* (or gap junctions) that allow direct transfer of ions do exist, most synapses are *chemical*, requiring the action of a chemical mediator, or *neurotransmitter*, such as acetylcholine or norepinephrine. Neurotransmitters diffuse across the synaptic cleft, bind to postsynaptic membrane receptors, and in so doing, open ion channels that eventually lead to changes in the potential of the postsynaptic membrane. Neurotransmitter-mediated communication also occurs at junctions between effector structures such as muscle fibers and glands.

The complex, multistep process of chemical neurotransmission can be readily affected by many different classes of drugs. To understand better how drugs can affect nerve impulse transmission, it is helpful to review the sequence of events that occur during chemical transmission.

Sequence of Neurotransmission

Biosynthesis of Neurotransmitter

Chemical substances that mediate transmission are formed from precursor substances within the neuron. Acetylcholine is synthesized from choline and acetyl coenzyme A by the action of the enzyme choline acetyltransferase. Norepinephrine is formed from the amino acid tyrosine through a series of enzymatic conversions. In the adrenal medulla, as well as in certain brain areas, norepinephrine is further converted to epinephrine.

Storage of Neurotransmitter

On formation, the neurotransmitter is taken up into specialized sites (vesicles) within the nerve ending by way of a carrier-mediated process and stored. This allows the neuron to build up

Table 11-2. **Comparison of the Parasympathetic and Sympathetic Divisions of the Autonomic Nervous System**

	Parasympathetic Division	*Sympathetic Division*
Outflow From CNS	Craniosacral	Thoracolumbar
	Cranial nerves (3, 7, 9, 10; ie, oculomotor, facial, glossopharyngeal, and vagus) and sacral (S2 to S4) segments of the spinal cord	Thoracic (T1 to T12) and lumbar (L1 to L3) segments of the spinal cord
Ganglia	Near or within structure innervated	Close to spinal cord
Preganglionic Fiber	Long and myelinated	Short and myelinated
Postganglionic Fiber	Short and nonmyelinated	Long and nonmyelinated
Response to Stimulation	Localized to a restricted area	Generalized and widespread
Neurotransmitter at all Ganglia	Acetylcholine	Acetylcholine
Neurotransmitter at Postganglionic Nerve Ending	Acetylcholine	Norepinephrine

Table 11-3. **Responses of Effector Structures to Autonomic Nervous System Activation**

Effector	Parasympathetic Activation: Action	Parasympathetic Activation: Receptor	Sympathetic Activation: Action	Sympathetic Activation: Receptor
Heart				
Rate	↓	M	↑	$beta_1$
Contractility	↓ (atria)	M	↑	$beta_1$
AV conduction	↓	M	↑	$beta_1$
Blood Vessels				
Coronary			Dilated	$beta_2$
Skeletal muscle*			Dilated	M, $beta_2$
Skin and mucosa			Constricted	$alpha_1$
Cerebral, pulmonary, abdominal viscera	Dilated		Constricted	$alpha_1$
Stomach and Intestine				
Motility and tone	↑	M	↓	$beta_2$, $alpha_2$ (?)
Sphincters	Relaxed	M	Contracted	$alpha_1$
Glandular secretion	↑	M		
Urinary Bladder				
Detrusor muscle	Contracted	M	Relaxed	$beta_2$
Trigone and sphincter	Relaxed	M	Contracted	$alpha_1$
Other Smooth Muscle				
Bronchial muscle, ureters, gallbladder, and ducts	Contracted	M	Relaxed	$beta_2$
Salivary Glands	Stimulated (profuse, watery secretion)	M	Stimulated (sparse, thick, mucinous secretion)	$alpha_1$
Eye				
Radial muscle of iris			Contracted (mydriasis)	$alpha_1$
Sphincter muscle of iris	Contracted (miosis)	M		
Ciliary muscle	Contracted (accommodated for near vision)	M	Relaxed (for far vision)	$beta_2$
Spleen Capsule			Contracted	$alpha_1$
Liver			Glycogenolysis; gluco-neogenesis	$alpha_1$, $beta_2$
Uterus (Pregnant)	Contracted	M	Relaxed	$beta_2$
Kidney			Renin secretion	$beta_1$
Skin				
Sweat glands†			Stimulated	M, alpha
Pilomotor muscles			Contracted	alpha
Pancreas				
Islet cells			Insulin secretion ↓	$alpha_2$
Acinar cells	Enzyme secretion ↑	M		
Adrenal Medulla	Secretion of epinephrine and norepinephrine	N		
Fat Cells			Lipolysis	$beta_{1,3}$

AV, atrioventricular; M, muscarinic; N, nicotinic; ↓, decreased; ↑, increased.
* Skeletal muscle blood vessels have sympathetic *cholinergic* dilator fibers as well as adrenergic fibers ($beta_2$).
† Sweat glands are stimulated by both cholinergic and adrenergic fibers of the sympathetic nervous system.

a surplus of the transmitter in anticipation of need. Acetylcholine is stored in the vesicle in conjunction with adenosine triphosphate (ATP) and possibly other peptides. Some norepinephrine also is stored in vesicles, bound to ATP as well, and this is referred to as the "reserve pool." Additional norepinephrine exists in a "protected" form in the cytoplasm of the nerve ending, but is *not* released by a nerve action potential (see next section); however, it can be expelled by a number of drugs.

Release of Neurotransmitter

With the arrival of a nerve action potential at the nerve ending, depolarization of the *presynaptic* membrane occurs, resulting in release of the neurotransmitter from its storage site into the synaptic junction. Release of the neurotransmitter is thought to occur in response to influx of calcium ions into the nerve ending, resulting in destabilization of the storage vesicles and their subsequent fusion with the terminal plasma membrane, followed by the extrusion of the neurotransmitter into the synaptic cleft.

The release of presynaptic stores of norepinephrine can be regulated by a feedback mechanism that is mediated by $alpha_2$- as well as beta-adrenergic receptor sites (Table 11-4) on the presynaptic nerve ending (see discussion under "Receptor Concept," later). As the level of norepinephrine released from the nerve ending rises, increased activation of presynaptic $alpha_2$ receptor sites on the terminal nerve ending occurs, slowing further release of norepinephrine. Conversely, activation of presynaptic beta receptors can increase neurotransmitter release. In this way, the neurotransmitter can regulate its own rate of release. A number of other clinically useful drugs also influence the release of norepinephrine by either activating or blocking presynaptic $alpha_2$ or beta receptor sites.

Prejunctional regulation of neurotransmitter release is probably not limited to norepinephrine. Evidence suggests that most substances that function as neurotransmitters, including acetylcholine, serotonin, histamine, and polypeptides, can regulate their own release through a feedback mechanism.

Interaction With Postsynaptic Membrane

The released neurotransmitter diffuses across the synaptic junction and interacts (complexes) with specific reactive areas (receptor sites) on the postsynaptic membrane. This interaction initiates a chain of biochemical events that results in a change in the function of the effector structure.

Inactivation of Neurotransmitter

Neurotransmitter action can be terminated in several ways:

1. *Diffusion of the released neurotransmitter away from the synaptic area* is probably important in removing excess or overflow, but is usually of little consequence for terminating the effects of physiologic quantities.
2. *Enzymatic breakdown of neurotransmitter* plays a relatively greater role for acetylcholine than for norepinephrine. Acetylcholinesterase cleaves acetylcholine into choline and acetate, thus terminating its action. Two enzymes, monoamine oxidase (MAO), which is found predominately in prejunctional nerve endings, and catechol-*O*-methyl transferase (COMT), which is located postjunctionally, inactivate norepinephrine, but are probably of little significance in *initially* terminating the action of the endogenously released hormone.
3. *Uptake of released neurotransmitter*, either into the presynaptic nerve terminal from which it was released (uptake I) or into surrounding nonneural glial or smooth muscle cells (uptake II), effectively terminates the activity of released neurotransmitter. Uptake I represents the principal means by which norepinephrine is inactivated after being extruded from the prejunctional nerve ending.

Repolarization of Postsynaptic Membrane

When neurotransmitter action ceases, the postsynaptic receptor area membrane is repolarized—that is, returned to its original ionic polarity and responsiveness.

Table 11-4. **Basic Characteristics of Autonomic Receptor Sites**

Type	*Locations*	*Activators*	*Blockers*
Cholinergic***			
Muscarinic (M)	Sites innervated by postganglionic parasympathetic fibers (heart, smooth muscle cells, exocrine glands); brain; autonomic ganglia (?)	Acetylcholine; pilocarpine	Atropine; bethanechol
Nicotinic (N)	Autonomic ganglia (NI); neuromuscular endplate of skeletal muscle (NII)	Acetylcholine; nicotine	Trimethaphan (ganglia); *d*-tubocurare (neuromuscular junction)
Adrenergic†			
$Alpha_1$	Most blood vessels, gastrointestinal tract, pancreas, eye, skin	Norepinephrine; epinephrine; phenylephrine	Phentolamine; prazosin
$Alpha_2$	Presynaptic terminal ending of adrenergic nerve fibers; platelets; fat cells; vascular smooth muscle	Norepinephrine; epinephrine; clonidine	Imipramine
$Beta_1$	Heart; gastrointestinal tract; urinary bladder; eye; adipose tissue; presynaptic sympathetic nerve endings	Epinephrine; isoproterenol	Propranolol; metoprolol
$Beta_2$	Bronchioles, uterus, skeletal muscle, blood vessels, liver	Epinephrine; isoproterenol; albuterol	Propranolol
Dopamine	Renal, visceral and coronary blood vessels; brain; presynaptic nerve terminals	Dopamine	Haloperidol

* There are at least three and possibly as many as five subtypes of muscarinic receptors, and two subtypes of nicotinic receptors.

† There are at least three subtypes each of alpha, beta, and dopaminergic receptors; only the best characterized of each type are listed here.

Mechanism of Drug Action on the Peripheral Nervous System

Drugs acting on the nervous system may affect the transmission of impulses at one or more of the preceding steps.

Types of Drug Action

Types of drug action at each step are listed below, along with examples of drugs described in the text that have the particular type of action specified.

- Inhibition of biosynthesis (eg, carbidopa, metyrosine)
- Interference with intraneuronal binding or storage (eg, reserpine)
- Interference with transmitter release (eg, guanethidine, clonidine)
- Enhancement of transmitter release (eg, amphetamine, amantadine, guanidine)
- Activation of postsynaptic receptor sites (eg, pilocarpine, isoproterenol, bromocriptine)
- Blockade of postsynaptic receptor sites (eg, atropine, propranolol, tubocurarine)
- Interference with neurotransmitter inactivation (eg, physostigmine, imipramine, tranylcypromine)
- Prevention of postsynaptic membrane repolarization (eg, succinylcholine)

Receptor Concept

A receptor site may be viewed as a chemically reactive area on the surface of a cell membrane or located intracellularly that is capable of complexing with specific chemical substances (eg, drugs, endogenous neurohormones). This interaction initiates a sequence of biochemical changes in the postsynaptic structure that either stimulates or inhibits the functional activity of the effector structure, such as a muscle fiber, gland, or neuron. A more extensive discussion of drug–receptor interactions can be found in Chapter 4.

Receptors may be classified on the basis of their location, their selective responsiveness to different ligands (ie, activators or blockers), and their differences in effector structure responses. Table 11-4 lists several criteria for categorizing the different kinds of cholinergic and adrenergic receptor sites found in the nervous system.

Cholinergic Receptors: M and N

Cholinergic receptors are differentiated primarily on the basis of their anatomic location and the relative selectivity of cholinergic antagonists. The cholinergic receptor subtypes are named after the alkaloids that were originally used in their identification, and are referred to as muscarinic (M) sites, which respond to the alkaloid muscarine, and nicotinic (N) sites, which are activated by nicotine. *M sites* are located on effector structures innervated by postganglionic parasympathetic and a few sympathetic fibers. They may be found typically in the heart, smooth muscle cells, some glands, and skeletal muscle blood vessels. In addition, M receptors also have been identified in the brain and in autonomic ganglia (see discussion later). *N sites* are situated on postjunctional membranes of all autonomic ganglia (these receptors also may be termed N-I sites) and in the neuromuscular end-plate of skeletal muscle (these receptors are also named N-II sites). The nicotinic receptors in autonomic ganglia are not identical to those in skeletal muscle, inasmuch as they respond differently to certain agonists and antagonists. Further complicating the picture is the existence of multiple subtypes of muscarinic receptors; there are at least three and possibly as many as five.

Adrenergic Receptors: Alpha, Beta, and Dopamine

Adrenergic receptors have traditionally been classified as *alpha* and *beta* receptor sites according to their location, their differential activation or blockade by various drugs, and the types of responses they mediate. Each receptor type is then further subdivided to reflect differences in location and function. $Alpha_1$ receptors are found postsynaptically in vascular smooth muscle; gastrointestinal and urinary sphincter muscles; and in the eye, skin, pancreas, and salivary glands. $Alpha_2$ receptors occur on presynaptic noradrenergic nerve endings (where they control the release of norepinephrine) as well as in platelets, fat cells, and possibly also in vascular smooth muscle. $Beta_1$ receptors occur primarily in the heart and adipose tissue, as well as on presynaptic noradrenergic nerve endings and in the brain; $beta_2$ sites are present in the bronchioles, uterus, skeletal muscle vasculature, liver, kidney, and urinary bladder.

A fifth type of adrenergic receptor responds selectively to the neurotransmitter dopamine and is located on visceral and renal blood vessels, in a number of brain areas, and probably also on presynaptic sympathetic nerve terminals. Dopamine receptors are further subclassified into at least four subtypes (D_1–D_4).

A review of the responses elicited by activation of the different adrenergic receptors is presented in Table 14-1.

Other Receptor Sites

In addition to the receptor sites for the cholinergic and adrenergic neurohormones outlined above, other specialized types of receptors exist in peripheral and central structures. For example, at least two types of histamine receptors (H_1 and H_2 sites) are present in various body tissues, and these receptors selectively mediate the diverse actions of endogenous histamine on different body organs. A further discussion of histamine receptor sites is found in Chapter 16, which deals with antihistamine drugs. Serotonin, another endogenous neurohormone, interacts with at least five kinds of specific reactive sites, which explains its diverse pharmacologic effects. Antiserotonin drugs also are discussed in Chapter 16. Many other putative neurotransmitters, including aspartic acid, glycine, glutamic acid, gamma-aminobutyric acid, bradykinin, endogenous opioids, eicosanoids, and several peptides also are believed to exert their effects by chemically combining with corresponding receptor sites.

Receptor Desensitization and Downregulation

Receptor sensitivity can be significantly altered depending on the degree of activity at a particular receptor site. Persistent activation of a receptor leads to a gradual loss of sensitivity over seconds or minutes, blunting the response. This desensitization usually is readily reversible, and shortly after removal of the initial agonist, a second exposure to the agonist results in the return of the original response. Other terms, such as "refractoriness" or "tolerance" have been used to describe the effects of receptor desensitization.

Prolonged receptor activation by an agonist also can result in an actual decrease in the *number* of available receptors sites. When this occurs at a rate faster than the rate at which new receptors can be synthesized, the total number of available receptors sites is reduced, as is the response to the agonist. This phenomenon, termed "downregulation" of receptors, is not as readily reversible as is receptor desensitization, and thus the effect of the agonist is decreased for some time. Conversely, persistent receptor *antagonism* can increase the number of receptors ("upregulation") at a particular site; when the antagonist level decreases, an exaggerated response to the presence of endogenous agonists can occur, frequently resulting in the appearance of adverse effects. For example, prolonged dopamine blockade by antipsychotic drugs results in upregulation of central dopamine receptors. This dopamine supersensitivity is believed to be responsible for the appearance of several involuntary movements with long-term antipsychotic drug usage, because endogenous dopamine is able to act on hypersensitive receptor sites to elicit altered muscle activity.

Central Nervous System

The CNS is composed of the brain and the spinal cord; together they serve to regulate a tremendous range of sensory, motor, and integrative activities. Consequently, drugs that affect central neuronal function have the potential to alter a person's behavior significantly. The mechanisms of action of centrally acting drugs are similar to those of peripherally acting drugs, and in fact many drugs exert simultaneous effects on both the central and peripheral nervous systems (eg, sedation, hypotension). Moreover, because of the complex neuronal interconnections among CNS areas, drugs acting at a specific central locus may exert widespread pharmacologic effects throughout the body and simultaneously alter the functioning of several physiologic systems.

The diversity of functions regulated by the CNS can be illustrated best by outlining the major subdivisions of the brain and the principal physiologic functions controlled by each area. Many of these bodily functions are considered in more detail in chapters of this book that deal with drugs capable of influencing one or more of the CNS areas that control the given functions.

I. **Prosencephalon (forebrain)**
  A. Telencephalon
    1. Cerebral cortex
      a. Conscious perception and interpretation of all sensory input
      b. Control of voluntary movements
      c. Language centers
      d. Complex integrative functions (eg, conscious thought elaboration, memory retrieval, personality, creativity)
    2. Basal nuclei (basal ganglia)—caudate, putamen, globus pallidus
      a. Planning, programming, and modulation of patterns of movement
      b. Regulation of muscle tone
    3. Corpus callosum
      a. Major commissural tract connecting the two cerebral hemispheres, permitting functional integration of information
  B. Diencephalon
    1. Thalamus
      a. Major relay center for sensory input to the cerebral cortex
      b. Crude awareness (and affect?) of sensations
      c. Modulation of motor activity
      d. Integration of emotional behavior
    2. Hypothalamus
      a. Integration of autonomic nervous system activity
      b. Regulation of body water via thirst and control of renal excretion of water
      c. Regulation of body temperature
      d. Regulation of food intake
      e. Neuroendocrine activity: production of neurohypophyseal hormones (oxytocin, vasopressin); control of adenohypophyseal activity
      f. Control of biologic rhythms and involvement in sleep—wakefulness mechanisms

II. **Mesencephalon (midbrain)**
  A. Corpora quadrigemina (superior and inferior colliculi)
    1. Integration centers for visual and auditory reflexes
  B. Cerebral peduncles
    1. Major connection between higher and lower brain centers; involved in conveying motor as well as sensory information
  C. Substantia nigra
    1. Control of subconscious motor functions
  D. Red nucleus
    1. Control of motor activities

III. **Rhombencephalon (hindbrain)**
  A. Metencephalon
    1. Cerebellum
      a. Planning and coordination of skilled voluntary motor activities
      b. Control and maintenance of equilibrium and posture
      c. Adjustment of muscle tone
    2. Pons
      a. Major link between medulla and higher brain centers for sensory and motor functions
      b. Regulation of respiration (pneumotaxic and apneustic centers)
  B. Myelencephalon
    1. Medulla oblongata
      a. Control of vital respiratory and cardiovascular functions
      b. Regulation of nonvital reflexes (eg, swallowing, vomiting, sneezing, coughing, and hiccuping)
      c. Maintenance of equilibrium (vestibular nuclei)
      d. Maintenance of alertness and control of sleep (reticular nuclei)

In addition, several groups of CNS structures function as integrated systems to control certain aspects of behavior and motor activity.

Reticular Activating System

The reticular activating system (RAS) is a complex, polysynaptic system principally concerned with such functions as alertness, arousal, and consciousness. Anatomically, the RAS includes the brain stem reticular formation (RF), a diffuse network of neurons and nuclei scattered throughout the medulla, pons, and midbrain, and extending into the thalamus. Impulses reaching the thalamus are then relayed to the neocortex and the limbic system. The RF receives ample afferent input from general sensory ascending tracts, as well as from special sensory systems (eg, auditory and visual), by way of collateral fibers. Several RF nuclei are involved in the regulation of muscle tone and postural reflexes, thereby functioning as part of the extrapyramidal motor system.

The RAS can be markedly impaired by many classes of drugs, including barbiturates, anesthetics, and antipsychotics, resulting in varying degrees of CNS depression that in some instances leads to unconsciousness.

Limbic System

Emotional behavior related to survival is integrated by several brain areas collectively termed the "limbic system." Anatomically, the limbic system is composed of several forebrain structures (limbic cortex, hippocampus, anterior thalamus, amygdala, septal nuclei, and parts of the hypothalamus) interconnected by complex circuits (eg, fornix, stria terminalis, and medial forebrain bundle).

The limbic system regulates biologic rhythms, sexual activity, feeding, and such emotional responses as fear, rage, and pleasure. Limbic stimulation often elicits autonomic responses, such as changes in blood pressure, respiration, or endocrine function. Limbic structures (notably the limbic cortex and hippocampus) also are essential for motivation, learning, and memory. Drugs such as antipsychotics, antidepressants, and lithium that are used in the treatment of emotional disorders exert at least a part of their action on the structures of the limbic system.

Basal Ganglia

The basal ganglia (basal nuclei) are composed of three paired masses of gray matter in the cerebrum—the caudate nucleus, putamen, and globus pallidus, as well as functionally related structures, including the subthalamic nuclei, the substantia nigra, and the red nucleus. Using numerous feedback loops, as well as extensive links with the cerebral cortex, thalamus, and brain stem, the basal ganglia collectively plan and program patterns of movement, regulate muscle tone, and influence locomotor activity and postural reflexes. Lesions in the basal ganglia (or associated tracts) result in marked disturbances of motor functions, which may be excitatory or inhibitory in nature. Disorders of the basal ganglia include Parkinson's disease, chorea, athetosis, and hemiballismus.

12
Cholinergic Drugs

Direct Acting (Stimulation of Cholinergic Receptors)

Synthetic

Acetylcholine
Carbachol
Bethanechol

Natural

Pilocarpine
Nicotine

Indirect Acting (Inhibition of Cholinesterase)

Reversible

Physostigmine
Demecarium
Ambenonium
Edrophonium
Neostigmine
Pyridostigmine

Irreversible

Echothiophate
Isoflurophate

Miscellaneous

Enhanced Release of Ach

Guanidine

Antidote

Pralidoxime

Alzheimer's Treatment

Lecithin
Tacrine

Cholinergic drugs are those that produce the same physiologic effects as the neurotransmitter acetylcholine (ACh) does when released after stimulation of cholinergic nerves; thus these drugs are termed *cholinomimetic agents*.

On the basis of their principal mechanisms of action, cholinergic drugs can be divided into two major groups, "direct acting" and "indirect acting."

I. *Direct acting*

These drugs produce their cholinomimetic effects by directly activating cholinergic receptor sites on postsynaptic membranes, and can be further categorized as:

A. *Synthetic*: esters of choline (eg, bethanechol)

B. *Natural*: cholinomimetic alkaloids (eg, pilocarpine)

II. *Indirect acting*

These compounds exert their effects by elevating the endogenous levels of ACh in the region of the cholinergic receptors. This is accomplished by reducing the activity of the cholinesterase enzymes that metabolize ACh or by enhancing the release of ACh from nerve cells. Cholinesterase inhibitors can be further subdivided based on the type of binding: *reversible inhibition*, which is transient (hours) or *irreversible inhibition*, which is prolonged (weeks).

A. *Reversible cholinesterase inhibitors* (eg, physostigmine): Competitive, short-lived inhibition of cholinesterase; enzymatic function is quickly restored when the drug is discontinued.

B. *Irreversible cholinesterase inhibitors* (eg, echothiophate): Extremely stable complexation with enzyme; restoration of enzymatic function requires synthesis of new enzyme, which takes several weeks.

III. *Antidote* (eg, pralidoxime)

Disrupts bond between phosphorus group of enzyme inhibitor and esteratic site of cholinesterase enzyme; displaces cholinesterase inhibitor from enzymatic binding sites and reactivates enzyme.

IV. *Enhanced release of acetylcholine* (eg, guanidine)

Increases the release of ACh from nerve cells that have been stimulated.

Acetylcholine given as a drug has little clinical usefulness because it is rapidly hydrolyzed by esterase enzymes and therefore has a very short duration of action. Moreover, it is nonspecific, exerting an action at all cholinergic receptor sites in the body, which produces a very wide range of pharmacologic effects (Table 12-1). The synthetic cholinergic agents are much more resistant to enzymatic hydrolysis, possess a much longer duration of action, and therefore are more therapeutically useful. In addition, they have a greater degree of selectivity with regard to the effects produced (Table 12-2).

Direct-Acting Cholinomimetic Drugs

Synthetic (Choline Esters)

The choline esters directly stimulate cholinergic receptors. They are primarily used for their local effects in the eye, although bethanechol can be administered systemically and has selective effects on the gastrointestinal (GI) and urinary tract.

Topical Administration

- **Acetylcholine, Intraocular**

Miochol

Mechanism

Contracts smooth muscle of iris sphincter so that pupil constricts and ciliary muscle contracts, accommodating the eye for near vision.

Uses

During ocular surgery (eg, cataracts, iridectomy, penetrating keratoplasty) for production of rapid, complete miosis.

Dosage

0.5 to 2 mL of 1% solution administered by instillation into the anterior chamber of the eye, before or after securing one or more sutures.

Table 12-1. **Pharmacologic Effects of Acetylcholine and Clinical Consequences**

Effect	***Clinical Consequence***
Gastrointestinal Tract	
Peristalsis ↑	Diarrhea
Relaxation of sphincter muscles	
Glandular secretions ↑	
Cardiovascular System	
Heart rate ↓	Hypotension
Vasodilation	
Urinary Tract	
Contraction of detrusor muscle	Urination
Relaxation of trigone and sphincter	
Other Smooth Muscle	
Contraction of bronchiolar smooth muscle	Bronchoconstriction
Contraction of gallbladder and ducts	
Contraction of ureter	
Contraction of sphincter muscle of iris	Miosis
Contraction of ciliary muscle	Accommodation for near vision
Glands	
Stimulation of exocrine gland secretion (lacrimal, sweat, salivary, bronchial)	Sweating Salivation

↓, decreased; ↑, increased.

Fate

Rapidly hydrolyzed (duration of action is 10–20 minutes), so that solution need not be removed from the eye by flushing with saline.

Common Side Effects

Burning, itching, headache.

- ***Carbachol, Intraocular***

Miostat

- ***Carbachol, Topical***

Isopto Carbachol

Mechanism

Constricts the pupil and contracts the ciliary muscle of the eye; in glaucoma, facilitates outflow of aqueous humor.

Uses

Pupillary miosis during surgery (Miostat)
Long-term treatment of open-angle glaucoma, especially in cases resistant to pilocarpine (Isopto Carbachol)

Dosage

Miostat: 0.5 mL into anterior chamber of the eye before securing sutures
Isopto Carbachol: 1 to 2 drops up to 3 times/day into lower conjunctival sac

Fate

Most potent of the direct-acting cholinergic drugs. Onset of miosis is 2 to 5 minutes. Effects persist for up to 8 hours; very slowly hydrolyzed.

Common Side Effects

Headache, hyperemia of conjunctival vessels, ciliary spasm with temporarily decreased vision.

Significant Adverse Reactions

Systemic absorption may cause flushing, sweating, cramping, urinary urgency, and severe headache; usually not present after ophthalmic use in small doses.

Contraindications

Corneal abrasions, acute iritis. *Cautious use* in the presence of asthma, peptic ulcer, GI or urinary distress, hyperthyroidism, cardiac failure, and parkinsonism.

Interactions

Miotic effects may be reversed by atropine or other anticholinergics.

Systemic Application

- ***Bethanechol***

Duvoid, Myotonachol, Urecholine

(CAN) PMS-Bethanechol, Urocarb

Mechanism

Activates muscarinic receptors, thereby increasing peristalsis and stimulating urination and defecation; increases tone of the detrusor muscle; little effect on heart rate, blood pressure, or peripheral circulation.

Uses

Treatment of acute, nonobstructive urinary retention and neurogenic atony of the urinary bladder
Relief of postoperative abdominal distention

Dosage

Should be individualized depending on type and severity of condition:

Table 12-2. **Pharmacologic Properties of Choline Esters**

	Muscarinic Receptor Activation			***Nicotinic Receptor Activation***	***Inactivation by Cholinesterase***
	GI/Urinary	*Cardiovascular*	*Ocular*		
Acetylcholine	Moderate	Moderate	Weak	Moderate	Yes
Bethanechol	Strong	Weak	Moderate	None	No
Carbamylcholine	Strong	Weak	Moderate	Strong	No

Adults: Oral (PO), 10 to 50 mg 2 to 4 times/day; subcutaneous (SC), 2.5 to 5 mg 3 or 4 times/day
Children: 0.6 mg/kg/day in divided doses

Fate

Effects appear within 30 to 90 minutes after oral dose and persist for up to 6 hours; SC administration is effective within 15 minutes.

Common Side Effects

Sweating, flushing, salivation, abdominal discomfort, nausea (usually due to excessive dosage).

Significant Adverse Reactions

Diarrhea, GI pain and cramping, headache, urinary urgency, hypotension, and asthma-like attacks.

Contraindications

Hyperthyroidism, hypertension, hypotension, peptic ulcer, bronchial asthma, coronary artery disease, atrioventricular (AV) conduction defects, pronounced bradycardia, urinary obstruction, GI anastomosis, epilepsy, parkinsonism, pregnancy. *Cautious use* after urinary bladder surgery, GI resection, and in the presence of spastic GI disturbances, acute inflammatory lesions of the GI tract, marked vagotonia, and peritonitis.

Interactions

Significant drop in blood pressure can occur if used with ganglionic blocking agents.
Quinidine and procainamide may antagonize the action of bethanechol.

Nursing Management

Pretherapy Assessment

Assess and record baseline data necessary for detection of adverse effects of choline esters: General: vital signs (VS), body weight, skin color and temperature; Central nervous system (CNS): reflexes, ophthalmologic examination; GI: salivation, bowel sounds; Genitourinary (GU): frequency, voiding pattern; Laboratory: urine glucose.

Review medical history and documents for existing or previous conditions that:

a. require cautious use of choline esters:
Systemic: after urinary bladder surgery; GI resection; spastic GI disturbances; acute inflammatory lesions of the GI tract; marked vagotonia; peritonitis.

b. contraindicate use of choline esters:
Systemic: allergy to echothiophate; hyperthyroidism; hypertension; hypotension; peptic ulcer; asthma; coronary artery disease; bradycardia; AV conduction defects; urinary obstruction; GI anastomosis; epilepsy; parkinsonism; inflammation of the iris or ciliary body; narrow-angle glaucoma; **pregnancy (Category C)**; lactation (safety not established, avoid use in nursing mothers).

Nursing Interventions

Medication Administration

Do not administer drug to a patient with a condition that contraindicates its use.

Administer oral forms of drugs 1 hour before or 2 hours after meals, with a full glass of water to minimize GI upset.

Have atropine sulfate available as an antidote–antagonist in event of cholinergic crisis or hypersensitivity reaction.

Arrange for decreased dosage of drug if excessive sweating or nausea occurs.

Surveillance During Therapy

Monitor for urination in a patient receiving bethanechol for acute urinary retention; urination should occur within 1 hour.

Monitor for symptoms of systemic absorption of ophthalmic preparation that require discontinuation of the drug: extreme salivation, vomiting, urination, or defecation.

Monitor for signs of bronchial constriction or spasm and pulmonary edema, such as wheezing, crackles, jugular vein distention, and shortness of breath.

Monitor hydration if patient experiences diarrhea.

Monitor for signs of hypersensitivity that may require discontinuation of drug (in the dark-skinned patient, depigmentation of eyelid skin).

Interpret results of diagnostic tests and contact practitioner as appropriate.

Monitor for possible drug–drug and drug–nutrient interactions: systemic effects of neuromuscular blocking agents and other choline esters potentiated by choline esters.

Provide for patient safety needs and initiate interventions to minimize environmental hazards and risk of injury if CNS side effects develop.

Patient Teaching

Instruct patient about the importance of completing the full course of therapy as prescribed.

Instruct patient about possible adverse side effects of choline esters: difficulty with adaptation to changes in light intensity; eye, brow, or eyelid pain.

Inform patient that vision may be impaired temporarily or localized twitching of the eyelid may occur after the instillation of the ophthalmic dosage form.

Instruct patient on appropriate action to take if side effects occur:

a. Notify practitioner if excessive salivation, nausea, excessive sweating, frequent urination, or diarrhea occurs.

b. Notify practitioner of conjunctival irritation or allergic dermatitis symptoms.

Natural (Cholinomimetic Alkaloids)

A cholinomimetic alkaloid is a natural product that produces effects similar to those of cholinergic nerve stimulation. The drugs of clinical importance in this group are pilocarpine, which is used almost exclusively in the eye, and nicotine, which is used as an aid in programs designed to help smokers terminate cigarette use.

• Pilocarpine

Isopto Carpine, Pilocar, Salagen, and various other preparations

(CAN) Minims, Miocarpine

Mechanism

Direct cholinergic receptor activation results in contraction of the ciliary muscle and ciliary body; miosis occurs and the outflow of aqueous humor from the anterior chamber is facilitated. Systemic effects include stimulation of sweat, lacrimal, and nasopharyngeal secretion, decreased heart rate, vasodilation, bronchoconstriction, and increased GI motility.

Uses

Open-angle glaucoma
Narrow-angle glaucoma before surgery (with other cholinergics or carbonic anhydrase inhibitors)
To reverse effects of cycloplegics and mydriatics after surgery or eye examinations
Treatment of xerostomia (Salagen, *orally*)

Dosage

1 or 2 drops of 1% to 2% solution up to 6 times/day; concentrations greater than 4% are rarely used, although solutions up to 10% are available
Patients with dark-pigmented eyes may require higher concentrations because pilocarpine is absorbed by melanin pigment
To reverse mydriatic–cycloplegic effects of other drugs: 1 drop of a 1% to 2% solution
1 tablet (5 mg) 3 times/day (Salagen)

Fate

Onset of miosis is within 10 to 20 minutes. Duration of miotic effect is 4 to 8 hours, although residual effects can last for 24 hours; excreted in urine as conjugates.

Common Side Effects

Ciliary spasm, headache, difficulty in focusing, local irritation. Sweating with oral use.

Significant Adverse Reactions

Allergic sensitivity, provocation of acute asthmatic attacks. Nausea, chills, flushing, urinary frequency with oral use.

Contraindications

Acute iritis and inflammatory conditions of the anterior chamber. *Cautious use* in the presence of asthma.

Interactions

Effects may be reduced by anticholinergics, adrenergics, corticosteroids, and phenothiazines.

Nursing Interventions

Patient Teaching

Instruct patient to avoid touching eyelid with dropper tip because contamination can occur.
Advise patient to protect solutions from light because they are unstable.
Instruct patient to report symptoms of sweating, salivation, cramping, and nausea immediately because they may signify onset of systemic toxicity.

• Pilocarpine Ocular Therapeutic System

Ocusert Pilo

This continuous-release form of pilocarpine (20 or 40 μg/h) is placed into the lower conjunctival cul-de-sac. It is used primarily for continuous therapy of open-angle glaucoma. A unit is inserted into the conjunctival sac once a week. Release rate of pilocarpine is not affected by presence of other locally acting drugs (eg, epinephrine, carbonic anhydrase inhibitors). Myopia can occur for several hours after insertion of the system, but usually is mild. Unit can be moved to upper conjunctival sac before sleep to aid in retention during the night.

The preparation should be used cautiously in the presence of infectious conjunctivitis or keratitis. Safety for use in presence of retinal detachments has not been established. Signs of conjunctival irritation, erythema, and increased secretions may occur when first used but tend to lessen after the first week or two. The system is poorly tolerated, however, by many patients, and its usefulness is somewhat limited.

• Nicotine *(Pregnancy Category D)*

Habitrol, Nicoderm, Nicorette, Nicotrol, ProStep

Nicotine is the principal alkaloid found in tobacco leaves. It is used as replacement therapy to reduce withdrawal signs and symptoms while a person is attempting to stop smoking cigarettes. The drug is available as a resin complex in the form of a chewing gum (Nicorette) and as a transdermal patch (Habitrol, Nicoderm, Nicotrol, ProStep). The patches, which provide a steady release of nicotine over a 24-hour period, are applied once per day to a skin site that is clean, dry, and free of hair; recommended areas are the trunk or upper, outer arm. They must be applied to the skin right after removal from package because the nicotine content will be reduced by evaporation.

Nicotine content varies among the available products. Each system, however, has the highest amount of nicotine in the patches that are applied during the first stage (range of 4–12 weeks). There is less nicotine in patches used during the second phase (approximately 2 weeks); the lowest content is in the patches applied in the third (and last) stage (approximately 2 weeks). ProStep has only two stages.

Mechanism

Activates cholinergic receptors in autonomic ganglia, the neuromuscular junction, adrenal medulla, and brain. Nicotine stimulates the cerebral cortex, probably via the locus ceruleus; this action increases alertness and cognitive performance. Also, the limbic system presumably is activated, which promotes feelings of increased pleasure (also known as the "reward" effect).

Uses

Aid in smoking cessation to relieve nicotine withdrawal symptoms.

Dosage

Depends on product used. Three-stage patches release 15 or 21 mg/day in the first, 10 or 14 mg/day in the second, and 5 or 7 mg/day in the third stage. The two-stage product releases 22 mg/day in the first, and 11 mg/day in the last stage.

Fate

The elimination half-life of nicotine is approximately 1 to 2 hours.
Peak levels of nicotine from the transdermal system vary (eg, between 6–12 hours for Habitrol and between 2–4 hours for Nicoderm). Steady-state conditions are achieved within approximately 2 days.

Common Side Effects

Chewing gum: mouth or throat soreness, hiccups, nausea
Transdermal patch: erythema, burning and itching at application site; headache

Significant Adverse Reactions

CV: peripheral vasoconstriction, tachycardia, increased BP
GI: diarrhea, constipation, belching, nausea and vomiting
CNS: headache, insomnia, dizziness, nervousness, paresthesia, confusion
GU: dysmenorrhea
Respiratory: cough, hoarseness, difficulty breathing, pharyngitis

Contraindications

Immediate period after myocardial infarction; life-threatening arrhythmias; pregnancy (gum, Category X; transdermal, Category D). *Cautious use* in patients with CV disease (eg, angina pectoris, arrhythmias, hypertension, Buerger's disease), hyperthyroidism, diabetes, severe hepatic or renal impairment, and in nursing mothers.

Interactions

Drinks (eg, cola, coffee) and foods that reduce salivary pH will decrease absorption of nicotine from the gum dosage form.
Increased levels of catecholamines from nicotine may require elevation of dose of beta-blockers.
Smoking cessation resulting from nicotine use can alter the handling of a wide range of drugs in the body, possibly requiring dosage adjustments during chronic drug therapy.

CAUTIONS

Because smokers are known to exhibit enzyme induction, metabolism will return to normal as the level of nicotine drops and finally reaches zero; the biotransformation of drugs also will decline. If a patient is currently taking drugs that are biotransformed (eg, imipramine, propranolol, theophylline), the doses may have to be *lowered*. Also, when nicotine is eliminated, patients with insulin-dependent diabetes may experience an *increase* in absorption of insulin from subcutaneous tissue sites of injection (absence of nicotine-induced vasoconstriction).

Indirect-Acting Cholinomimetic Drugs

Inhibition of Cholinesterase

Reversible Inhibitors

Drugs in this group generally are short-acting cholinergic drugs used both topically and systemically. They are capable of increasing the amounts of functional ACh at the postsynaptic receptor site and are indicated primarily for their local effects in the eye and for the diagnosis and treatment of myasthenia gravis. These drugs may be used as antidotes to curariform and atropine-like drugs, to relieve postoperative urinary bladder atony, and to suppress paroxysmal atrial tachycardia.

Topical and Systemic Use

- ***Physostigmine, Ophthalmic***

Eserine, Isopto-Eserine

- ***Physostigmine, Systemic***

Antilirium

Mechanism

Competes with ACh for active sites on cholinesterase enzyme, slowing the inactivation of ACh and prolonging its action at cholinergic receptors; highly lipid soluble and readily enters the CNS

Uses

Topical (eye)
Treatment of open-angle glaucoma (alternative to pilocarpine)
Reverses cycloplegia and mydriasis caused by anticholinergic drugs
Systemic (Antilirium only)
Antidote to toxic neurologic effects caused by drugs (eg, scopolamine, tricyclic antidepressants) having central anticholinergic activity

Dosage

Eserine: 2 drops (0.25%–0.5% solution) 3 or 4 times/day (ophthalmic ointment also available)
Antilirium: Adults, 0.5 to 2 mg intramuscularly (IM) or slowly intravenously (IV); repeat as necessary if life-threatening signs occur. Children, 0.5 mg over 1 minute by slow IV injection; repeat in 5 to 10 minutes if needed

Fate

After topical application, peak miotic effect occurs in 1 to 2 hours, lasting 12 to 24 hours. Systemic doses rapidly metabolized by cholinesterases. Intravenous effects seen in 5 minutes; duration of 1 to 4 hours. Drug readily enters the CNS. Hydrolyzed and inactivated by cholinesterase enzyme.

Common Side Effects

Ophthalmic: decreased visual acuity, eyelid twitching, increased tearing, mild headache
Systemic: sweating, nausea, urinary urgency, cramping, salivation

Significant Adverse Reactions

Ophthalmic: altered pigmentation of the iris, conjunctival irritation, allergic dermatitis
Systemic: vomiting, diarrhea, muscle weakness, hypotension, bradycardia, bronchospasm, convulsions; respiratory paralysis

Contraindications

Ophthalmic: inflammation of the iris or ciliary body, narrow-angle glaucoma
Systemic: asthma, gangrene, cardiovascular disease, diabetes, obstruction of intestine or bladder. *Cautious use* in patients with epilepsy, parkinsonism, or bradycardia

Interactions

Systemic effects may be potentiated by depolarizing neuromuscular blocking agents (eg, succinylcholine) and choline esters.

Nursing Management

Pretherapy Assessment

Assess and record baseline data necessary for detection of adverse effects of physostigmine: General: VS, body weight, skin color and temperature; CNS: reflexes, ophthalmologic examination; GI: salivation, bowel sounds; GU: frequency, voiding pattern; Laboratory: urine glucose.
Review medical history and documents for existing or previous conditions that:
a. require cautious use of physostigmine: epilepsy; parkinsonism; bradycardia.
b. contraindicate use of physostigmine:
Ophthalmic: inflammation of the iris or ciliary body; narrow angle glaucoma.
Systemic: allergy to physostigmine; asthma; gangrene; cardiovascular disease; diabetes; obstruction of intestine or bladder; peptic ulcer; vagotonic states; **pregnancy (Category C)**; lactation (safety not established, avoid use in nursing mothers).

Nursing Interventions

Medication Administration

Administer IV slowly; rapid administration can lead to bradycardia, hypersalivation, respiratory distress, and convulsions.
Have atropine sulfate available as an antidote–antagonist in event of cholinergic crisis or hypersensitivity reaction.
Arrange for decreased dosage of drug if excessive sweating or nausea occurs.

Surveillance During Therapy

Monitor for symptoms of systemic absorption of ophthalmic preparation that require discontinuation of the drug: extreme salivation, vomiting, urination, or defecation.
Monitor for presence of bradycardia, difficulty breathing, urinary incontinence, or seizures with systemic administration.
Monitor for signs of hypersensitivity that may require discontinuation of drug.
Interpret results of diagnostic tests and contact practitioner as appropriate.
Monitor for possible drug–drug and drug–nutrient interactions: systemic effects of neuromuscular blocking agents and other choline esters potentiated by physostigmine.
Provide for patient safety needs and initiate interventions to minimize environmental hazards and risk of injury if CNS side effects develop.

Patient Teaching

Instruct patient about the importance of completing the full course of therapy as prescribed.
Instruct patient about possible adverse side effects of physostigmine: difficulty with adaptation to changes in light intensity (ophthalmic preparation).
Inform patient that vision may be impaired temporarily or localized twitching of the eyelid may occur after the instillation of the ophthalmic dosage form.
Instruct patient on appropriate action to take if side effects occur:
a. Notify practitioner if excessive salivation, nausea, excessive sweating, frequent urination, or diarrhea occurs.
b. Notify practitioner of conjunctival irritation or allergic dermatitis symptoms.

Topical Use Only

- ***Demecarium Bromide*** *(Pregnancy Category X)*

Humorsol

Demecarium is an anticholinesterase agent with a duration of action significantly longer than that of other reversible inhibitors. It is a powerful miotic that is used occasionally for treatment of glaucoma and convergent strabismus (accommodative esotropia). Recommended dosage is 1 or 2 drops in conjunctival sac once or twice a day. Miosis develops within 30 minutes and is maximal within 2 or 3 hours. Effects are prolonged (up to 1 week after single administration). Common side effects are blurred vision, twitching of the eyelids, brow pain, and lacrimation. Other adverse effects include photophobia, elevated intraocular pressure, cysts on iris, conjunctival thickening, and lens opacities. Systemic absorption may produce symptoms of cholinergic overdose. Demecarium is contraindicated in narrow-angle glaucoma and inflammatory conditions of the eye. Refer to the "Nursing Management" section for physostigmine (earlier) for information pertaining to the ophthalmic use of cholinergic drugs.

Systemic Use Only

- ***Ambenonium***
- ***Edrophonium***
- ***Neostigmine***
- ***Pyridostigmine***

These reversible cholinesterase inhibitors are used primarily for the diagnosis and treatment of myasthenia gravis. They all function in a similar manner: By increasing cholinergic neurotransmission at the neuromuscular junction, they alleviate the muscle weakness characteristic of myasthenia. Significant differences exist among the four drugs, however, with regard to onset and duration of action and incidence and severity of side effects. Table 12-3 lists the onset and duration of each of these

Table 12-3. **Comparison of Onset and Duration of Action Among Antimyasthenic Cholinesterase Inhibitors**

Drug	*Route*	*Onset*	*Duration*
Ambenonium	PO	30 min	4–8 h
Edrophonium	IM	2–10 min	10–40 min
	IV	<1 min	5–20 min
Neostigmine	PO	30–60 min	2–4 h
	IM	15–30 min	2–4 h
	IV	5–10 min	2–4 h
Pyridostigmine	PO	20–40 min	3–6 h
	IM	10–15 min	2–4 h
	IV	2–5 min	2–4 h

drugs when administered by different routes. Because many similarities also exist among these four drugs, they are discussed here as a group. Individual characteristics and dosage ranges are presented in Table 12-4.

Mechanism

Inhibit cholinesterase enzymes, causing an intensification and prolongation of the actions of ACh at cholinergic receptors throughout the body, including the neuromuscular junction. Neostigmine also exhibits a direct ACh-like stimulating effect at cholinergic receptors on skeletal muscle and may increase the release of presynaptic stores of ACh. These drugs improve muscle strength and delay fatigue; generalized cholinergic responses frequently are noted at the outset of therapy and may require use of a muscarinic antagonist (see Chapter 13) to minimize disturbing side effects. Tolerance to the muscarinic effects frequently develops.

Uses

Diagnosis of myasthenia gravis (edrophonium)
Treatment of myasthenia gravis (ambenonium, neostigmine, pyridostigmine)
Symptomatic management of the symptoms of poisoning with nondepolarizing skeletal muscle relaxants (IV pyridostigmine, neostigmine, or edrophonium)
Relief of postoperative abdominal distention and urinary retention (neostigmine; infrequent use)

Dosage

See Table 12-4.

Fate

Oral absorption generally is poor and erratic. Edrophonium is given by injection only and has a rapid onset and short duration of action. Ambenonium exhibits the longest duration of action with oral administration (see Table 12-3), followed by pyridostigmine and neostigmine; entrance of all drugs into the CNS is minimal. Biotransformation occurs by way of hepatic enzymes; metabolites are eliminated by the kidneys.

Common Side Effects

Nausea, diarrhea, abdominal discomfort, salivation, sweating, urinary urgency, muscle twitching.

Significant Adverse Reactions

CNS: dysphonia, irritability, restlessness, convulsions
Respiratory: increased bronchial secretions, laryngospasm, bronchoconstriction, respiratory paralysis
Ocular: miosis, cycloplegia, diplopia, lacrimation
CV: bradycardia, arrhythmias, hypotension
GI: increased salivary, gastric, and intestinal secretions; dysphagia, cramping
Other: muscle weakness, urinary frequency or incontinence, skin rash (neostigmine, pyridostigmine), thrombophlebitis with IV use

Overdosage may lead to a cholinergic crisis characterized by nausea, diarrhea, sweating, increased bronchial and salivary secretions, bradycardia, and increasing muscle weakness. Death can occur due to bronchial airway obstruction and respiratory paralysis.

Contraindications

Intestinal or urinary obstruction, megacolon, peritonitis. In addition, neostigmine and pyridostigmine are bromide salts and are contraindicated in patients with bromide hypersensitivity. *Cautious use* in patients with bradycardia or bronchial asthma.

Interactions

The actions of these cholinesterase inhibitors can be antagonized by drugs with neuromuscular blocking effects, such as aminoglycoside antibiotics, general and local anesthetics, and certain antiarrhythmic agents (quinidine, procainamide).
Neostigmine may prolong the action of depolarizing muscle relaxants such as succinylcholine (see Chapter 17).
Neostigmine can antagonize the effects of nondepolarizing neuromuscular blocking agents, such as gallamine, pancuronium, and metocurine.
Magnesium can antagonize the effects of anticholinesterase drugs on skeletal muscle because it exerts a direct muscle-relaxing effect.

Nursing Management

Pretherapy Assessment

Assess and record baseline data necessary for detection of adverse effects of reversible cholinesterase inhibitors: General: VS, body weight, skin color and temperature; CNS: reflexes, bilateral grip strength; GI: salivation, bowel sounds, normal output; GU: frequency, voiding pattern, normal output; Laboratory: EEG, thyroid function.
Review medical history and documents for existing or previous conditions that:
a. require cautious use of reversible cholinesterase inhibitors: bradycardia, asthma, epilepsy, peptic ulcer, cardiac arrhythmias, vagotonia.
b. contraindicate use of reversible cholinesterase inhibitors:
Systemic: allergy to anticholinesterases, bromides; intestinal or urinary obstruction; megacolon; peritonitis; **pregnancy (Category C)**; lactation (safety not established, avoid use in nursing mothers).

Table 12-4. **Antimyasthenic Cholinesterase Inhibitors**

Drug	*Usual Dosage Range*	*Nursing Considerations*
Ambenonium Chloride *Mytelase*	Adults: 5–25 mg 3 or 4 times/day (up to 75 mg/dose has been used in certain instances but is highly dangerous) Children: 0.5–1.5 mg/kg day in 3 or 4 divided doses	Longest acting of the orally effective antimyasthenic drugs; lower incidence of GI, respiratory, and CV side effects than neostigmine; cumulative effects have occurred owing to prolonged action; thus, be alert for early signs of overdosage (eg, salivation, difficulty in chewing or swallowing, muscle weakness); warning of overdosage may be minimal; teach patient and family to contact physician at first sign of side effects; to maximize advantage of drug's prolonged duration of action, instruct patients to take last dose of drug at bedtime so they can sleep through the night without recurrence of symptoms.
Edrophonium Chloride *Enlon, Reversol, Tensilon*	*Diagnosis:* Adults: 2 mg IV over 15–30 sec. If no reaction in 45 sec, inject additional 8 mg; alternately, give 10 mg IM if veins are inaccessible. Children: IV—1 mg if weight is less than 75 lb; 2 mg if more than 75 lb; administer within 45 sec, titrate up to 5 mg in small children and up to 10 mg in larger children. IM—2 mg if weight is less than 75 lb; 5 mg if more than 75 lb *Curariform Antagonists* 10 mg IV over 30–45 sec; repeat as necessary to a maximum of 40 mg.	Short-acting drug primarily used for differential diagnosis of myasthenia and for reversing neuromuscular block produced by curariform drugs (eg, tubocurarine, gallamine); not indicated for *chronic* therapy of myasthenia; positive response to diagnostic test is a brief improvement in muscle strength without muscle fasciculations or autonomic side effects; nonmyasthenic patients may evidence transient fasciculations and temporary muscle weakness; patients in cholinergic crisis show further muscle weakness and marked increase in oropharyngeal secretions and abdominal cramping; atropine sulfate and facilities for respiratory assistance should be immediately available; transient bradycardia can occur, and cardiac arrest has been reported; check pulse frequently during therapy.
Neostigmine Bromide *Prostigmin* ***Neostigmine Methylsulfate*** *Prostigmin* *(CAN) PMS-Neostigmine*	*Oral:* Adults: 15–30 mg 3 or 4 times/day. Increase gradually until maximum benefit, up to 375 mg/day. Dosage interval must be individualized. Children: 2 mg/kg/day every 3–4 h *Treatment of Myasthenia SC, IM* Adults: 0.5 mg; repeat as necessary based on response. Children: 10–40 µg/kg every 2–3 h *Diagnosis of Myasthenia:* Adults: 0.022 mg/kg IM Children: 0.04 mg/kg IM *Curariform antidote:* Adults: 0.5–2 mg by slow IV injection. Repeat to a total dose of 5 mg. Children: 0.07–0.08 mg/kg/dose	Reversible cholinesterase inhibitor that also has a direct agonistic action on cholinergic receptor sites; parenteral form can be used to diagnose myasthenia, but edrophonium is preferred because of more rapid onset and shorter duration; also indicated for symptomatic treatment of curariform drug overdosage; poorly absorbed orally; higher incidence of muscarinic side effects than other orally effective antimyasthenics; monitor changes in muscle strength and side effects in relation to each dose and document accordingly; keep atropine on hand at all times and be prepared to support respiration; available in combination with atropine sulfate as Neostigmine Methylsulfate Min-I-Mix for IV injection as an antidote to curariform drugs.
Pyridostigmine Bromide *Mestinon, Regonol*	*Oral:* Adults: 60–120 mg every 3–4 h initially. Maintenance dose can range from 60 mg–1.5 g/day. Average is 600 mg daily. Children: 7 mg/kg/day in 5 or 6 divided doses *IM, IV:* *Curare antidote:* 10–20 mg *Myasthenia:* 2 mg every 2–3 h	Most commonly used antimyasthenic drug; shorter acting than ambenonium and has slower onset but longer duration of action than neostigmine; lower incidence of GI side effects, salivation, and bradycardia than neostigmine and ambenonium; long-acting tablets are used every 6 h for maintenance therapy but increase the risk of cholinergic crisis; when using sustained-release tablets, instruct patient to take drug at least every 6 h, at same time every day; first signs of overdose may be twitching of muscles around the eyes, mouth, or upper arms; these symptoms should be reported as soon as they occur.

Nursing Interventions

Medication Administration

Administer IV slowly; rapid administration can lead to bradycardia, hypersalivation, respiratory distress, and convulsions.
Administer oral form with meals, with a full glass of water.
Provide small, frequent meals in event of GI distress or dysphasia.
Have atropine sulfate available as an antidote–antagonist in event of cholinergic crisis or hypersensitivity reaction.
Be aware that overdosage with anticholinesterase agents can cause muscle weakness (cholinergic crisis), difficult to distinguish from myasthenic weakness.
Ensure ready access to bathroom facilities in event of GI, GU effects.
Arrange for decreased dosage of drug if excessive sweating or nausea occurs.

Surveillance During Therapy

Monitor for symptoms of systemic absorption that require discontinuation of the drug: extreme salivation, vomiting, urination, or defecation.
Monitor for signs of CNS toxicity (jitteriness, confusion, dizziness).
Monitor for presence of bradycardia, difficulty breathing, urinary incontinence, or seizures with systemic administration.
Monitor for signs of hypersensitivity that may require discontinuation of drug.
Interpret results of diagnostic tests and contact practitioner as appropriate.
Monitor for possible drug–drug and drug–nutrient interactions: systemic effects of neuromuscular blocking agents and other choline esters potentiated by neostigmine; antagonism of effect of nondepolarizing neuromuscular blocking agents; antagonism of anticholinesterase effects on skeletal muscle by magnesium; decreased effects and possible muscular depression when used with corticosteroids.
Provide for patient safety needs and initiate interventions to minimize environmental hazards and risk of injury if CNS or visual side effects develop.

Patient Teaching

Instruct patient regarding the importance of completing the full course of therapy as prescribed.
Instruct patient to take drug before meals if dysphagia occurs.
Assist patient to plan a dosing schedule that corresponds with normal periods of stress and fatigue.
Teach patient how to record daily condition carefully, noting changes in muscle strength, respiration, and blood pressure, to assist in developing an optimal therapeutic regimen.
Instruct patient about possible adverse side effects of reversible cholinesterase inhibitors: difficulty with adaptation to changes in light intensity; blurred vision; increased urinary frequency; abdominal cramps; sweating.
Instruct patient on appropriate action to take if side effects occur:
a. Notify practitioner if excessive salivation, nausea, excessive sweating, frequent urination, diarrhea, muscle weakness, severe abdominal pain, irregular heartbeat, or difficulty breathing occurs.

Irreversible Inhibitors

The irreversible cholinesterase inhibitors are organophosphate compounds that cause phosphorylation of the enzyme cholinesterase, permanently inactivating it. Enzymatic activity remains impaired until new supplies of enzyme can be synthesized, often requiring weeks or even months for full restoration. These compounds were originally developed as chemical warfare agents and are now extensively used as pesticides and insecticides. The major clinical application of the irreversible cholinesterase inhibitors is in the eye, for the production of prolonged miosis and treatment of glaucoma.

• Echothiophate

Phospholine Iodide

Uses

Treatment of glaucoma (chronic open-angle *and* angle-closure after iridectomy)
Diagnosis and treatment of accommodative convergent strabismus (often with epinephrine or carbonic anhydrase inhibitors)

Dosage

Glaucoma: 1 drop (0.03%–0.125%) 1 or 2 times/day, individualized to condition
Strabismus: 1 drop 0.06%/day or 0.125% every other day (maximum 0.125%/day)

Fate

Fairly rapid onset of miosis (10 minutes); effects may persist for several weeks. Intraocular pressure is lowered within 6 hours.

Common Side Effects

Stinging and burning in the eye, temporary blurred vision, eyelid twitching, hyperemia, browache.

Significant Adverse Reactions

Iris cysts, conjunctival thickening, lens opacities, iritis, retinal detachment (rare); systemic absorption may produce symptoms of cholinergic crisis.

Contraindications

Narrow-angle glaucoma before surgery, inflammatory conditions of the eye. *Cautious use* in patients with asthma, ulcers, hypotension, epilepsy, parkinsonism, cardiovascular disease, and vagotonia.

Interactions

May enhance systemic effects of succinylcholine and other cholinesterase inhibitors.
Effects in eye are readily reversed by atropine.

Nursing Management

Pretherapy Assessment

Assess and record baseline data necessary for detection of adverse effects of echothiophate: General: VS, body weight, skin color and temperature; CNS: reflexes, ophthalmologic examination; GI: salivation, bowel sounds; GU: frequency, voiding pattern; Laboratory: urine glucose.

Review medical history and documents for existing or previous conditions that:

a. require cautious use of echothiophate: after urinary bladder surgery; GI resection; spastic GI disturbances; acute inflammatory lesions of the GI tract; marked vagotonia; peritonitis.

b. contraindicate use of echothiophate: allergy to echothiophate; hyperthyroidism; hypertension; hypotension; peptic ulcer; asthma; coronary artery disease; bradycardia; AV conduction defects; urinary obstruction; GI anastomosis; epilepsy; parkinsonism; inflammation of the iris or ciliary body; narrow-angle glaucoma; **pregnancy (Category C)**; lactation (safety not established, avoid use in nursing mothers).

Nursing Interventions

Medication Administration

Do not administer drug to a patient with a condition that contraindicates its use.

Have atropine sulfate available as an antidote–antagonist in event of cholinergic crisis or hypersensitivity reaction.

Arrange for decreased dosage of drug if excessive sweating or nausea occurs.

Surveillance During Therapy

Monitor for toxicity.

Monitor for symptoms of systemic absorption of ophthalmic preparation that require discontinuation of the drug: extreme salivation, vomiting, urination, or defecation.

Monitor for signs of bronchial constriction or spasm and pulmonary edema, such as wheezing, crackles, jugular vein distention, and shortness of breath.

Monitor hydration if patient experiences diarrhea.

Monitor for signs of hypersensitivity that may require discontinuation of drug (in the dark-skinned patient, depigmentation of eyelid skin).

Interpret results of diagnostic tests and contact practitioner as appropriate.

Monitor for possible drug–drug and drug–nutrient interactions: systemic effects of neuromuscular blocking agents and other choline esters potentiated by echothiophate.

Provide for patient safety needs and initiate interventions to minimize environmental hazards and risk of injury if CNS side effects develop.

Patient Teaching

Instruct patient regarding the importance of completing the full course of therapy as prescribed.

Instruct patient about possible adverse side effects of echothiophate: difficulty with adaptation to changes in light intensity; eye, brow, or eyelid pain.

Inform patient that vision may be impaired temporarily or localized twitching of the eyelid may occur after the instillation of the ophthalmic dosage form.

Instruct patient on appropriate action to take if side effects occur:

a. Notify practitioner if excessive salivation, nausea, excessive sweating, frequent urination, or diarrhea occurs.

b. Notify practitioner of conjunctival irritation or allergic dermatitis symptoms.

• Isoflurophate *(Pregnancy Category X)*

Floropryl

Isoflurophate is similar to echothiophate in actions, indications, and toxicity. Because it is insoluble in water, however, it is available only as an ophthalmic ointment (0.25%) that many patients find inconvenient to use. After application to the lower conjunctival sac, miosis occurs within 15 to 30 minutes and becomes maximal within 4 hours. Effects may persist for several weeks because of the permanent inactivation of existing cholinesterase. Isoflurophate is unstable in water. Potency is lost if the ointment comes into contact with moisture; thus, the tip of the tube should not be allowed to come into contact with any moist surface. The drug is readily absorbed from the skin, and systemic effects have occurred after topical contact. Refer to the foregoing discussion of echothiophate for applicable adverse effects, cautions, and drug interactions.

Dosage

Glaucoma: 0.25-inch strip of 0.025% ointment every 8 to 12 hours. Frequency of application is then adjusted on the basis of tonometric readings of intraocular pressure. For maintenance therapy, the drug may be applied once every 8 to 72 hours.

Accommodative esotropia: not more than a 0.25-inch strip of ointment every night for 2 weeks. Dosage is then reduced gradually to once-a-week application as the patient's condition warrants. Therapy may need to be continued indefinitely.

Nursing Management

See "Nursing Management" section for echothiophate.

Enhanced Release of Acetylcholine

• Guanidine

Guanidine

Guanidine is a unique cholinergic agent that can alleviate the muscle weakness that occurs in myasthenia gravis. Because of its relatively high toxicity, however, its use generally is restricted to the myasthenic syndrome of Eaton-Lambert (carcinomatous myopathy), in which muscle weakness accompanies a malignant disease, particularly bronchogenic carcinoma.

Mechanism

Increases the release of acetylcholine after nerve cells have been stimulated.

Uses

Alleviation of the symptoms (muscle weakness, fatigability) of the myasthenic syndrome of Eaton-Lambert
Treatment of severe myasthenia gravis (investigational use only)

Dosage

Initially, 10 to 15 mg/kg/day in 3 or 4 divided doses. Increase dosage gradually up to a maximum of 35 mg/kg/day.

Common Side Effects

Gastric irritation, nausea, anorexia, flushing, sweating.

Significant Adverse Reactions

GI: diarrhea, abdominal cramping, vomiting
Neurologic: paresthesias, lightheadedness, irritability, nervousness, trembling, ataxia, tremor, confusion, mood changes, hallucinations
Dermatologic: rash, petechiae, purpura, ecchymoses, skin eruptions, scaling of skin
Hematologic: bone marrow depression, anemia, leukopenia, thrombocytopenia
Renal: elevation of creatinine, renal tubular necrosis, interstitial nephritis
CV: palpitations, tachycardia, hypotension, atrial fibrillation
Other: sore throat, fever

Nursing Management

Pretherapy Assessment

Obtain baseline complete blood cell count and differential counts, and perform routine follow-up counts. At first indication of bone marrow suppression, withhold drug and notify prescriber, because drug should be discontinued.

Nursing Interventions

Medication Administration

Be prepared for frequent dosage changes because dose must be carefully titrated in each patient to allow for the possibility of extreme variation in individual tolerance.
Ensure that IV atropine (for GI symptoms) and IV calcium gluconate (for neuromuscular and convulsive symptoms) are available to treat cases of overdosage.

Surveillance During Therapy

Monitor renal status, because abnormalities have occurred. Discuss changes with prescriber if indications of malfunction appear.
Check results of serum creatinine tests, which should be repeated periodically; drug-induced elevations have been noted. Discuss changes with prescriber.

Patient Teaching

Instruct patient to notify drug prescriber immediately if sore throat, skin rash, fever, or mucosal ulceration occurs (possible early signs of a developing blood dyscrasia).
Instruct patient to report appearance of GI disorders (eg, anorexia, diarrhea) to drug prescriber, because these often indicate that the dosage is too high and might need to be reduced.
Inform patient that the paresthesias that may occur shortly after a dose of guanidine do not indicate that the dosage is excessive.

Reversal of Cholinesterase Inhibition

A specific antidote, pralidoxime chloride (PAM), is available primarily for treating overdosage with organophosphate cholinesterase inhibitors, which usually occurs as a result of insecticide poisoning. PAM also can reverse the effects of the reversible cholinesterase inhibitors (eg, neostigmine) used in treatment of myasthenia gravis, although it is less effective. Therapy with PAM should be initiated promptly after poisoning because within hours, the enzyme–inhibitor complex becomes extremely stable and largely resistant to the antidotal action of the reactivator PAM.

• Pralidoxime Chloride

Protopam, PAM

Mechanism

Disrupts bond between the phosphorus group of the enzyme inhibitor and the esteratic site of the cholinesterase enzyme, thus separating the cholinesterase inhibitor from the enzyme. This action reactivates the enzyme and reduces respiratory paralysis due to organophosphate intoxication.

Uses

Antidote to poisoning with pesticides and insecticides of the organophosphate class (eg, diazinon, malathion)
Antidote to overdosage by anticholinesterase drugs used in treatment of myasthenia gravis

Dosage

Insecticide poisoning:
Adults: 1 to 2 g as IV infusion in 100 mL saline over 15 to 30 minutes, often with atropine (2 mg–4 mg IV); PO, 1 to 3 g every 5 hours
Children: 20 to 40 mg/kg IV infusion with 0.5 to 1 mg atropine (most effective if given within a few hours after exposure to poison; usually ineffective if 48 hours have elapsed)
Anticholinesterase overdosage: Initially, 1 to 2 g IV injection; increments of 250 mg every 5 minutes until symptoms subside

Fate

Slowly and erratically absorbed orally; peak plasma levels occur at 5 to 10 minutes IV and 10 to 20 minutes IM; not bound to plasma protein; relatively short acting (plasma half-life is 2 hours); metabolized in the liver and readily excreted in urine, partly as unchanged drug.

Common Side Effects

Dizziness, blurred vision, headache, drowsiness, nausea.

Significant Adverse Reactions

Tachycardia, hyperventilation, laryngospasm, muscle weakness. Excitement and hypomania may occur after recovery of consciousness.

Contraindications

Cautious use in patients with myasthenia gravis.

Interactions

Certain drugs should not be used concurrently with PAM in organophosphate poisoning (morphine, theophylline, succinylcholine, reserpine, and phenothiazines) because enzyme reactivator exerts a depolarizing effect at the neuromuscular junction.

Barbiturates may be potentiated by cholinesterase inhibitors.

Nursing Management

Pretherapy Assessment

Assess and record baseline data necessary for detection of adverse effects of pralidoxime: General: VS, body weight, skin color and temperature; CNS: reflexes, ophthalmologic examination, muscle strength; GI: liver function; CV: electrocardiogram; GU: frequency, voiding pattern; Laboratory: renal and liver function tests; nature of insecticide involved in poisoning (pralidoxime is ineffective in cases of carbamate [Sevin] poisoning and should not be used in poisonings that do not involve anticholinesterase substances).

Review medical history and documents for existing or previous conditions that:

a. require cautious use of pralidoxime: use in myasthenic disease.
b. contraindicate use of pralidoxime: allergy to any component of the drug; impaired renal function; **pregnancy (Category C)**; lactation (safety not established, avoid use in nursing mothers).

Nursing Interventions

Medication Administration

Administer IV slowly or use infusion control device; rapid administration can lead to tachycardia, larnygospasm, muscular rigidity.

Have IV sodium thiopental or diazepam available if convulsions interfere with respiration after organophosphate poisoning.

Monitor patient for indications of atropine toxicity (xerostomia, blurred vision, flushing, excitement) when used with atropine; these require termination of atropine treatment.

Surveillance During Therapy

Monitor patient for 72 hours after poisoning; monitor results of red blood cell and plasma cholinesterase determinations to determine patients progress.

Monitor for signs of hypersensitivity that may require discontinuation of drug.

Interpret results of diagnostic tests and contact practitioner as appropriate.

Monitor for possible drug–drug and drug–nutrient interactions: systemic effects of neuromuscular blocking agents and other choline esters potentiated by physostigmine.

Provide for patient safety needs and initiate interventions to minimize environmental hazards and risk of injury if CNS side effects develop.

Patient Teaching

Instruct patient/significant others about the importance of completing the full course of therapy as prescribed.

Cholinergic Drugs Used in Alzheimer's Disease

As humans approach the end of their life span, a decline in brain function occurs. In part, this change may be linked to lowered activity of CNS cholinergic neurons: reductions in choline acetyl transferase, synthesis of ACh, and responsiveness of postsynaptic cholinergic receptors in the frontal cortex and hippocampus. In addition, there are indications that an actual *loss* of cortical neurons occurs (>50% in some brain areas by 85 years of age).

In elderly patients presenting with Alzheimer's disease, *additional* neuronal changes have been noted: increased deposition of beta-amyloid protein (whether this is a cause or an effect of the disease has not been established), reduced number of synapses (there is, however, an increase in synaptic size, which may be compensatory), and reduced acetylcholinesterase activity (possible compensation for reduced ACh synthesis). Although the hereditary nature of Alzheimer's disease has been established, other factors can produce this condition in younger people (eg, head trauma as occurring in professional boxers). Also, there evidence that excessive exposure to aluminum may contribute to the development of the disease, possibly as a cofactor.

Neural transplants, successful to a limited degree in reducing the severity of Parkinson's disease, have not been adequately studied in Alzheimer's disease. There are, however, various pharmacologic approaches to its treatment, most of which are still in the investigational stage.

Enhancement of Central Cholinergic Activity

There is a probable limit to this method because deficits may be due to an actual loss of cholinergic neurons, not just to some decline in function.

Increase Synthesis of Acetylcholine

- **Lecithin (Phosphatidylcholine)**

This agent is a precursor of ACh; its administration increases ACh levels in central synapses, an effect supported by the fact that lecithin reduces tardive dyskinesias.

A dose of 26 g daily, PO, has been shown to increase plasma choline levels significantly. There was no demonstrable improvement in memory or cognition when it was used alone, however, possibly because the presynaptic uptake of choline may be impaired. Therapeutic effects of lecithin in Alzheimer's disease were observed only when it was combined with physostigmine or tacrine.

Increase Release of Acetylcholine

• 4-Aminopyridine

4-Aminopyridine, a K^+ channel blocker, is an investigational agent that has been used in clinical trials for treatment for Alzheimer's disease. K^+ channel blockers reduce K^+ efflux, increase Ca^{2+} influx, and increase the release of ACh.

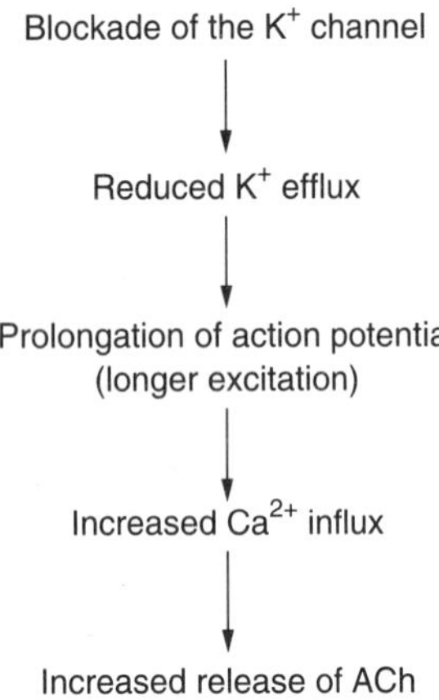

One study showed improvement in memory; another investigation reported no increase in cognition. Adverse reactions included xerostomia, disorientation, and confusion.

Reduce Catabolism of Acetylcholine

This method may be limited because of evidence of reduced levels of cholinesterase in Alzheimer's disease, possibly due to downregulation of cholinesterase as compensation for reduced levels of ACh.

• Physostigmine

Physostigmine is a centrally acting reversible anticholinesterase agent that was discussed earlier in this chapter. Physostigmine has a short $T_{1/2}$ (approximately 20 to 30 minutes) and requires administration throughout the day.

At a dose range of 2 to 16 mg daily, physostigmine produced only a slight increase in memory performance in a 6-week clinical trial. In this study, adverse reactions included bradycardia, diarrhea, nausea, vomiting, diaphoresis, dizziness, and headache.

• Tacrine

Cognex

Tacrine is a centrally acting, reversible cholinesterase inhibitor that is used in treating mild to moderate dementia due to Alzheimer's disease. Its effectiveness appears to be greatest in the early stages of therapy, and its effects lessen as the disease process advances. There is no conclusive evidence that tacrine alters the ultimate course of the underlying dementia.

Mechanism

Elevates endogenous ACh levels in the cerebral cortex by slowing the enzymatic breakdown of ACh released from functional cholinergic nerve endings.

Uses

Treatment of dementia of Alzheimer's disease.

Fate

Rapidly absorbed orally; maximal plasma levels occur in 1 to 2 hours; drug is approximately 50% protein bound; extensively metabolized in the liver; elimination half-life is 2 to 4 hours; average plasma concentrations are 50% higher in women than in men; smoking significantly reduces plasma concentrations.

Common Side Effects

Elevated serum transaminases (ALT), GI distress, anorexia, myalgia, ataxia.

Significant Adverse Reactions

GI: abdominal pain, diarrhea, hepatotoxicity (25% of patients exhibit significant [three times normal] elevations in ALT, which are reversible if discontinued promptly)
CNS: headache, dizziness, confusion, insomnia, tremor, agitation, depression
Respiratory: rhinitis, dyspnea, upper respiratory infection
Other: rash, urinary frequency, arthralgia, sweating, conjunctivitis

Note: A large number of other adverse reactions have been reported in patients receiving tacrine, but they are infrequent; a direct cause-and-effect relationship remains to be established.

Contraindications

Jaundice with elevated bilirubin above 3 mg/dL. *Cautious use* in patients with liver disease, ulcers, urinary hesitancy, seizure disorders, asthma.

Interactions

Tacrine can interfere with the action of anticholinergic drugs and enhance the activity of cholinomimetic agents.
Tacrine can increase theophylline plasma levels.
Cimetidine can increase the effects of tacrine, presumably by slowing its elimination.

Nursing Management

Pretherapy Assessment

Assess and record important baseline data necessary for detection of adverse effects of tacrine: vital signs (T, P, R, BP); CNS (orientation, reflexes); GI (output, liver function); laboratory (liver function tests, CBC).
Review past medical history and documents for evidence of existing or previous medical history related to conditions that:
a. require caution with tacrine: impaired renal or he-

patic function; ulcerative disease; seizure disorders; asthma.

b. contraindicate use with tacrine: allergy to tacrine; jaundice with bilirubin greater than 3 mg/dL; **pregnancy (Category C)**.

Nursing Interventions

Medication Administration

Administer oral form of drug **on an empty stomach (1 hour before or 2 hours after meals, with a full glass of water)**.
Initiate a meal schedule that provides small, frequent meals if GI upset occurs.
Provide ready access to bathrooms and interventions directed at symptom relief if diarrhea occurs.
Identify the safety needs of the patient and initiate interventions to minimize environmental hazards and risk of injury if CNS side effects develop.

Surveillance During Therapy

Monitor patient for therapeutic effects of tacrine therapy.
Compare current status with previous status to detect improvements or deterioration in the patient's condition.
Monitor for adverse effects, toxicity, and interactions.
Monitor for signs of hypersensitivity (including *photosensitivity*) that may require discontinuation of drug.
Facilitate acquisition of diagnostic tests ordered for ongoing assessment of drug response.
Monitor CBC, urinalysis, and liver and kidney function test results obtained over the course of therapy.
Interpret results of diagnostic tests and contact practitioner/prescriber as appropriate.
Monitor for possible drug–laboratory test interactions.

Patient Teaching

Instruct patient that the prescribed drug is to be taken for the condition for which it is prescribed.
Instruct patient to keep these drugs and all medications out of the reach of children.

Other Drugs Used in Alzheimer's Disease

Other, noncholinergic-related treatments have been used experimentally in patients with Alzheimer's disease. They include the following.

Reduction of Systemic Aluminum

Aluminum levels found in central neurons of patients with Alzheimer's disease can be five to nine times higher than in healthy, age-matched subjects. Some geographic areas with high aluminum concentrations in water have a higher-than-expected frequency of residents with cognitive impairment.

Deferoxamine (Desferal)

Approved uses of this parenteral iron chelator are for treatment of acute iron intoxication and chronic iron overload (see Chapter 81). Unlabeled (unapproved) uses of deferoxamine are as a chelator to reduce aluminum levels in bones of patients with renal failure and in patients presenting with dialysis-induced encephalopathy. In a long-term clinical trial, deferoxamine, given by IM injection 5 days per week for 2 years, slowed the rate of cognitive deterioration by 50%. Adverse reactions include hearing loss, impaired vision, diarrhea, leg cramps, and tachycardia; they generally are reversible on termination of therapy.

L-Deprenyl (Selegiline)

Alzheimer's disease, like Parkinson's disease, may be caused by increased production of oxygen free radicals, which promote the degeneration of neurons. L-Deprenyl, an irreversible inhibitor of the enzyme monoamine oxidase B, has been shown to delay for approximately 1 year the initiation of L-dopa therapy. This indicates the strong possibility that L-deprenyl has slowed the central neuronal degeneration in patients with Parkinson's disease (see Chapter 28 for additional details).

At a dose of 10 mg PO, daily, L-deprenyl was given in combination with tacrine or physostigmine in a 4-week clinical trial in patients with Alzheimer's disease; there was a noted improvement in cognition, but it was additive only with the cholinesterase inhibitors.

Selected Bibliography

D'Mello GD: Behavioural toxicity of anticholinesterases in humans and animals: A review. Human Exper Toxico 12:3, 1993
Johnson JT, Ferretti GA, Nethery WJ, et al: Oral pilocarpine for post-irradiation xerostomia in patients with head and neck cancer. N Engl J Med 329:390, 1993
Levy A, et al.: Transdermal physostigmine in the treatment of Alzheimer's disease. Alzheimer Dis Assoc Disord 8:15, 1994
Naguib M: Dose–response relationships for edrophonium and neostigmine antagonism of pipercuronium-induced neuromuscular block. Anesth Analg 78:306, 1994
Okayama M, Shen T, Midorikawa J, et al: Effect of pilocarpine on propranolol-induced bronchostriction in asthma. Am J Respir Crit Care Med 149:76, 1994
Pierce JR: Stroke following application of a nicotine patch. Ann Pharmacother 28:402, 1994
Rosen J, Pollock BG, Altieri LP, Jonas EA: Treatment of nortriptyline's side effects in elderly patients: A double-blind study of bethanechol. Am J Psychiatry 150:1249, 1993
Sano M, Bell K, Marder K, et al: Safety and efficacy of oral physostigmine in the treatment of Alzheimer disease. Clin Neuropharmacol 16:61, 1993
Smith EW, Smith KA, Maibach HI, et al: The local side effects of transdermally absorbed nicotine. Skin Pharmacol 5:69, 1992
Traub M, Freedman SB: The implication of current therapeutic approaches for the cholinergic hypothesis of dementia. Dementia 3:189, 1992
Van Wyk M, Sommers DK, Moncrieff J, Becker PJ: The influence of neostigmine and metoclopramide or their combination on gastric emptying. Curr Ther Res 54(3):300, 1993
Willems JL, De Bisschop HC, Verstraete AG, et al: Cholinesterase reactivation in organophosphorus poisoned patients depends on the plasma concentrations of the oxime pralidoxime methylsulphate and of the organophosphate. Arch Toxicol 67:79, 1993

Nursing Bibliography

Kopecky J: Ophthalmic drugs and anesthesia interactions. Current Reviews for Nurse Anesthetists 3(1):16–21, 1992

Oral physostigmine in Alzheimer's disease. Nurse's Drug Alert 15(12): 92, 1991

Ramsey F: Reversal of neuromuscular blockade. Current Reviews for Nurse Anesthetists 514(7):50–56, 1991

Reading P, St. John R: Aerosolized therapy for ventilator assisted patients. Critical Care Nursing Clinics of North America 5(2):271–280, 1993

13
Anticholinergic Drugs

Antimuscarinics

Atropine
L-Hyoscyamine
Scopolamine
Dicyclomine
Oxybutynin
Oxyphencyclimine
Cyclopentolate
Tropicamide
Benztropine
Biperiden
Diphenhydramine
Ethopropazine
Procyclidine
Trihexyphenidyl
Anisotropine
Clidinium
Glycopyrrolate
Homatropine
Ipratropium
Isopropamide
Mepenzolate
Methantheline
Methscopolamine
Propantheline
Tridihexethyl

Ganglionic Blocking Agents

Mecamylamine
Trimethaphan

Anticholinergic drugs block the action of acetylcholine (ACh) at cholinergic receptors throughout the body. This diverse group of drugs can divided into three subgroups based on their *relative* specificity for the different types of cholinergic receptor sites (see Chapter 11) as follows:

I. *Muscarinic blockers* (eg, atropine, propantheline). These comprise the "classic" group of anticholinergic agents that inhibit cholinergic transmission at postganglionic parasympathetic M (muscarinic) receptor sites (eg, on smooth muscle, cardiac muscle, and exocrine glands).
II. *Ganglionic blockers* (eg, mecamylamine, trimethaphan). These drugs block cholinergic transmission at N (nicotinic) I sites at autonomic ganglia in both parasympathetic and sympathetic nerve fibers.
III. *Neuromuscular blockers* (eg, pancuronium). This type inhibits the action of ACh at synapses between nerves and skeletal muscles (neuromuscular junction) or N II receptor sites (see Chapter 17).

The term *anticholinergic* is associated primarily with the muscarinic blockers because most of the commonly used anticholinergic drugs have a relatively selective blocking action at M sites in normal doses. Considerable overlap in receptor-blocking effects is observed, however, when large doses of any one of the three types of cholinergic blockers are administered. This extension of cholinergic blockade to all cholinergic receptors frequently is responsible for a disturbing range of side effects when any cholinergic blocking agent is used in large amounts.

Because parasympathetic cholinergic nerves are distributed throughout the body, anticholinergic drugs exert a wide range of pharmacologic effects. Major organs affected by these drugs include the eye, respiratory tract, heart, gastrointestinal (GI) tract, urinary bladder, most nonvascular smooth muscle, exocrine glands, and, to varying degrees, the central nervous system (CNS). The principal pharmacologic actions of the anticholinergic group of drugs are listed in Table 13-1.

Atropine and scopolamine represent the principal naturally occurring anticholinergic drugs; along with hyoscyamine, they are known as the *belladonna alkaloids* (Table 13-2). They are rapidly absorbed after oral administration, have a relatively selective blocking action at M receptor sites, and readily enter the CNS. The belladonna alkaloids, however, produce a wide range of undesirable peripheral and central effects that occur when the drugs are used therapeutically (ie, given in doses used to reduce GI motility and secretions). For this reason, several *tertiary* and *quaternary* ammonium compounds have been synthesized in an attempt to reduce the incidence of side effects while providing a degree of cholinergic receptor site specificity. These goals, however, have been only partially realized.

The synthetic *tertiary amines* may be further subdivided into antispasmodics, mydriatics, and antiparkinsonian drugs (see Table 13-2). The antispasmodics possess little cholinergic blocking action; rather, their effects appear to be related to a direct relaxant effect on GI smooth muscle. Thus, gastric acid secretion is relatively unimpaired, and these drugs are more properly termed *smooth muscle relaxants* rather than anticholinergics. In contrast, the antiparkinsonian tertiary amines are anticholinergic; this action occurs primarily in the CNS.

The *quaternary amine* anticholinergics (see Table 13-2), unlike the belladonna alkaloids and tertiary amines, are poorly and erratically absorbed after oral administration (they have a low lipid–water partition coefficient, ie, are less lipid soluble). Therefore, they do not readily cross lipid membranes and their distribution to the GI mucosa, eye, and CNS is limited. They are of little value in the eye as mydriatics, and their central effects are minimal. Compared to the tertiary compounds, the quaternary amines have greater blocking effects at peripheral ganglia and neuromuscular junctions.

Because many antimuscarinic drugs are similar with regard to therapeutic uses and side effects, their pharmacology will be discussed as a group. Dosage forms, indications, and specific characteristics for each drug are listed in Table 13-3. The two anticholinergic drugs that are primarily ganglionic blocking agents are reviewed separately at the end of this chapter. Finally, those anticholinergic drugs acting at N receptors on skeletal muscle (ie, at the neuromuscular junction) are discussed with other skeletal muscle relaxants in Chapter 17.

Antimuscarinics

Mechanism

Blockade (via competitive antagonism) of ACh (or direct-acting cholinergic drugs) at postsynaptic muscarinic receptor sites. Large doses may block cholinergic transmission at autonomic ganglia and the neuromuscular junction. Certain drugs (eg, antiparkinsonian agents) also may decrease uptake of dopamine into presynaptic nerve endings (see Chapter 28).

Table 13-1. **Pharmacologic Actions of Anticholinergics**

Effects	*Clinical Consequences*
Cardiovascular	
Heart rate ↓ initially in small doses (central vagal stimulation	
Heart rate ↑ in normal doses (peripheral vagal blockade)	Prevention of reflex bradycardia
Gastrointestinal Tract	
Mobility ↓ Smooth muscle tone ↓ Secretions ↓	Delayed gastric emptying, constipation
Urinary Tract	
Relaxation of detrusor muscle Contraction of sphincter muscle	Urinary retention
Eye	
Mydriasis (sphincter muscle response ↓) Cycloplegia (ciliary muscle response ↓)	Blurred vision
Smooth Muscle	
Slight relaxation of nonvascular smooth muscle (eg, biliary, bronchiolar, intestinal, uterine)	Relief of biliary or intestinal colic
Exocrine Glands	
Sweat gland secretion ↓ Salivation ↓ Mucous gland secretion ↓ (nasopharynx and bronchioles)	Anhidrosis, xerostomia, hyperthermia
Central Nervous System	
Drowsiness, disorientation, hallucinations (large doses)	
Tremor and rigidity of parkinsonism ↓	Treatment of Parkinson's disease
Vestibular activation ↓	Prevention of motion sickness

↓, decreased; ↑, increased.

Table 13-2. **Classification of Antimuscarinic Drugs**

Belladona Alkaloids
Atropine
L-Hyoscyamine
Scopolamine

Tertiary Amine Antispasmodics
Dicyclomine
Oxybutynin
Oxyphencyclimine

Tertiary Amine Mydriatics
Cyclopentolate
Tropicamide

Tertiary Amine Antiparkinsonian Agents
Benztropine
Biperiden
Diphenhydramine
Ethopropazine
Procyclidine
Trihexyphenidyl

Quaternary Amine Anticholinergics
Anisotropine
Clidinium
Glycopyrrolate
Homatropine
Ipratropium
Isopropamide
Mepenzolate
Methantheline
Methscopolamine
Propantheline
Tridihexethyl

Uses

Refer to Table 13-3 for specific uses of each agent.

Production of mydriasis and cycloplegia to facilitate eye examinations
Preoperative medication to reduce excess salivation and prevent bradycardia
Reduction of GI motility and secretions in cases of peptic ulcer, GI spasms, irritable bowel syndrome, or other GI disorders
Reduce muscarinic side effects associated with cholinesterase inhibitor treatment of myasthenia
Relief of nasopharyngeal and bronchial secretions accompanying upper respiratory and allergic disorders
Relief of bronchoconstriction due to excessive parasympathetic nerve activity in bronchial asthma, and other chronic obstructive pulmonary diseases
Prevention and relief of motion sickness
Treatment of enuresis in children and relief of urinary urgency or frequency
Treatment of sinus bradycardia and conduction block due to excessive vagal tone
Production of sedation and amnesia ("twilight sleep") in obstetrics (infrequent use)
Antidote to overdosage with cholinergic agents (anticholinesterases, organophosphate insecticides and pesticides)
Relief of symptoms of parkinsonism (especially tremor and rigidity), and control of extrapyramidal disorders resulting from antipsychotic drugs (see Chapter 28)

Dosage

See Table 13-3 for specific doses. The *general* dose response is:

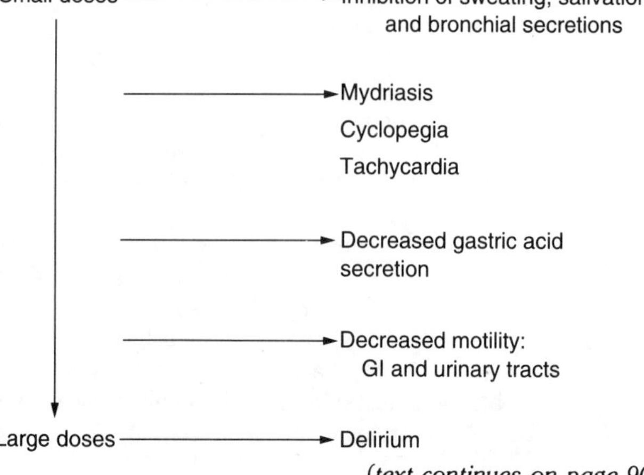

(*text continues on page 90*)

Table 13-3. **Antimuscarinics**

Drug	*Usual Dosage Range*	*Major Uses*	*Nursing Considerations*
BELLADONNA ALKALOIDS			
Atropine *Several manufacturers*	*Systemic* Adult: 0.4–0.6 mg every 4–6 h Children: 0.1–0.6 mg depending in weight *Ophthalmic* Adults: 1–2 drops 4 times/day Children: 1 drop 0.5%–1% 1–3 times/day *Refraction* 1–2 drops 1 h before examination *Inhalation (oral)* Adults: 0.025 mg/kg diluted with 3–5 mL saline by nebulizer 3–4 times/day Children: 0.05 mg/mL diluted in saline by nebulizer 3–4 times/day	See general discussion of anticholinergics in text.	Atropine flush due to peripheral vasodilation is a normal effect of the drug; when used in the eye, prevent systemic absorption by compressing lacrimal sac after installation; do not use in children under 6 yr of age; reduce systemic dose in elderly patients to minimize danger of tachycardia and elevated intraocular pressure; orally inhaled atropine produces a bronchodilatory effect with minimal tachycardia and drying of secretions; ophthalmic drops are available with prednisolone (Mydrapred); IV doses of more than 2 mg may initially cause bradycardia, which wil subside within minutes; give oral doses no less than 30 min before mealtimes for best response and give the nigthtime dose at least 2 h after the last meal.
Belladonna Alkaloids, Levorotatory *Bellafoline*	*Adults* Tablets: 0.25–0.5 mg 3 times/day *Children* Tablets: 0.125–0.25 mg 3 times/day	Preoperative medication, GI hypermotility, dysmenorrhea, respiratory hypersecretion and bronchial asthma, motion sickness, enuresis, nocturia	Infrequently used preparation; belladonna tincture is also available for GI disturbances (spasms, hypermotility); 0.6–1.0 mL 3–4 times/day; caution—tincture contains 65%–70% alcohol.
Hyoscyamine Sulfate *Anaspaz, Cystospaz, Cystospaz-M, Levsin, Levsinex, Neoquess (CAN) Bellaspaz*	Oral/Sublingual Adults: 0.125–0.25 mg 3–4 times/day Children 2–10 yr; 1/2 adult dose *Parenteral* SC, IM, or IV: 0.25–0.5 3–4 times/day	GI spasm and hypersecretion, cholinergic poisoning, dysmenorrhea, urinary spasm, acute rhinitis	Well absorbed orally; may be useful in controlling diarrhea; tablets, elixir, and drops are also available with phenobarbital (Levsin PB).
Scopolamine Hydrobromide *Isopto Hysocine, and several manufacturers*	*Systemic* Adults: (SC, IM) 0.3–0.6 mg Children: (SC, IM) 0.1–0.3 mg *Ophthalmic* 1–2 drops; adjust dosage to requirements	Preanesthetic medication, spastic states, obstetric analgesic (with narcotics), ophthalmic mydriatic and cycloplegic, hyperrhidrosis, excess salivation and secretion	CNS depression can occur with systemic use; overdosage results in excitement, confusion, and delerium; produces amnesia when given with narcotics; may produce delerium if used alone in severe pain; effects generally persist 4–6 h; neostigmine and physostigmine are effective antidotes; initial response to the drug may be a paradoxical excitation that will subside as the patient becomes more sedated; do not be misled by such activity; guard the patient's safety by using side rails and other protective measures as needed.
Scopolamine Transdermal Therapeutic System *Transderm-Scop*	Apply 1 system to the postauricular skin once every 3 days, several hours before exposure	Prevention of motion sickness	Circular adhesive patch that delivers steady-state blood levels of scopolamine over 3 days; most frequent side effects are dry mouth, blurred vision, and drowsiness; use with caution in the presence of glaucoma, urinary or GI obstruction, impaired liver or kidney function, and in the elderly; safe use in children has not been established; response to this drug will vary from person to person; best results are obtained when the disk is applied the night before motion is experienced; use a new site for a second application.

(*continued*)

Table 13-3. **Antimuscarinics (Continued)**

Drug	Usual Dosage Range	Major Uses	Nursing Considerations
TERTIARY AMINE ANTISPASMODICS			
Dicyclomine Hydrochloride *Bentyl, and several other manufacturers (CAN) Bentylol, Formulex, Lomine*	*Adults* Oral: 80–160 mg daily in 4 divided doses IM: 20 mg every 4–6 h *Children:* 5–10 mg 3–4 times/day	GI spasm and hyperirritability, ulcerative colitis, infant colic	Usually adminsistered with antacids in GI disorders, because it does not reduce gastric secretions; common side effects are dizziness, abdominal fullness, and slight euphoria; has fewer side effects than atropine but is still contraindicated for any patient with the potential for an adverse response to anticholinergics.
Oxybutynin Chloride *Ditropan*	Adults: 5 mg 2–4 times/day Children: 5 mg 2–3 times/day	Urinary incontinence (reflex neurogenic bladder)	Exhibits both a direct smooth muscle relaxing action and a weak antimuscarinic action on smooth muscle; has only one-fifth the anticholinergic activity of atropine but is 5–10 times as potent as an antispasmodic; delays desire to void; do not use in children under 5 y or in patients with paralytic ileus, intestinal atony, megacolon, myasthenia, or obstructive uropathy.
Oxyphencyclimine Hydrochloride *Daricon*	5–10 mg 2–3 times/day	Adjunctive treatment of peptic ulcer	May induce CNS stimulation; do not use in children under 12 y.
TERTIARY AMINE MYDRIATRICS			
Cyclopentolate Hydrochloride *Cyclogyl, AK-Pentolate*	*Refraction* Adults: 1 drop 1%–2% solution, followed by a second drop in 5 min Children: 1 drop 0.5%–1% solution, followed by a second drop in 5 min	Ophthalmic refraction for diagnostic purposes	Effects can persist for up to 24 h; pilocarpine (1–2 drops 1%–2% solution) reduces recovery time to 3–6 h; can produce behavioral disturbances in children (ataxia, disorientation, restlessness, incoherent speech) if absorbed systemically; ophthalmic drops available with phenylephrine (Cyclomydril) for increased mydriatic effect.
Tropicamide *Mydriacyl, Opticyl, Tropicacyl*	*Refraction* 1–2 drops of 1%; repeat in 5 min and every 20–30 min as needed to maintain mydriasis *Examination of Fundus* 1–2 drops 0.5% 20–30 min before examination	Ophthalmic refraction for diagnostic purposes	Effects occur in 20–30 min; recovery takes 4–6 h; larger doses may be necessary if iris is heavily pigmented; available in combination with hydroxyamphetamine as Paremyd.
TERTIARY AMINE ANTIPARKINSONIAN DRUGS			
Benzotropine Mesylate *Cogentin (CAN) Apo Benztropine Bensylate, PMS Benzotropine*	*Parkinsonism* 1–2 mg daily to a maximum of 6 mg *Extrapyramidal Reactions* 1–4 mg 1–2 times/day *Acute Dystonic Reactions* 1–2 mg IM or IV followed by 1–2 mg PO twice/day	Parkinsonism, extrapyramidal reactions	If used with L-dopa, adjust dose of each medication accordingly; start with low dose and gradually increase; no significant difference in onset of action IM or IV; sedative effect can occur; withdraw gradually (see Chapter 28).
Biperiden *Akineton*	*Parkinsonism* 2 mg 3–4 times/day with meals *Extrapyramidal Reactions* 2 mg 1–3 times/day PO or 2 mg IM or IV, repeated every half hour to a maximum of 4 doses	Parkinsonism, extrapyramidal reactions	Most effective on akinesia and rigidity. May elevate mood. Can produce incoordination after IV or IM use (see Chapter 28).

(*continued*)

Table 13-3. **Antimuscarinics (Continued)**

Drug	Usual Dosage Range	Major Uses	Nursing Considerations
Diphenhydramine *Benadryl and other manufacturers*	*Oral* Adults: 25–50 mg 3–4 times/day Children: 5 mg/kg/day in divided doses	Parkinsonism, extrapyramidal reactions	Occasionally used in milder forms of Parkinson's disease; widely used in dystonias; urinary retention is common, see also Chapter 16.
Ethopropazine Hydrochloride *Parsidol* *(CAN) Parsitan*	Initially 50 mg 1–2 times/day to a maximum of 600 mg/day in severe cases	Parkinsonism, extrapyramidal reactions	Does not potentiate CNS depressants; drug causes high incidence of dose related side effects, including drowsiness, hypotension, confusion, and GI distress (see Chapter 28).
Procyclidine *Kemadrin* *(CAN) PMS Procyclidine, Procyclid*	*Parkinsonism* 2.5–5 mg 3 times/day *Extrapyramidal Reactions* 2.5–5 mg 3–4 times/day	Parkinsonism, extrapyramidal reactions	Most effective against rigidity; may temporarily worsen tremor. In elderly, may induce confusion and psychotic reactions; note decreased urinary output and reduce dose if necessary (see Chapter 28).
Trihexyphenidyl Hydrochloride *Artane, Trihexy* *(CAN) Apo-Trihex, Novohexidyl, PMS-Trihexyphenidyl*	*Parkinsonism* 1 mg initially, increased by 2-mg increments every 3–5 days to a total dose of 6–10 mg/day; usual maintenace dosage is 6–12 mg daily in divided doses *Extrapyramidal Reactions* 5–15 mg in divided doses	Parkinsonism, extrapyramidal reactions	When used with L-dopa, reduce dose of each drug proportionately; major effect is on rigidity, with minimal effects on tremor; sustained-release capsules are *not* intended for initial therapy but may be used once patient is stabilized; may produce CNS stimulation and excessive drying of the mouth; often given before meals (see Chapter 28).
QUATERNARY AMINE ANTIMUSCARINICS			
Anisotropine Methyl Bromide	Adults: 50 mg 3 times/day	GI spasms, adjunctive therapy in peptic ulcer	Oral absorption is erratic; infrequently used.
Clidinium Bromide *Quarzan*	2.5–5 mg 3–4 times/day	GI hypermotility and hypersecretion	Erratically absorbed orally; reduce dosage in geriatric or debilitated patients; also available in combination with chlordiazepoxide as Librax.
Glycopyrrolate *Robinul, Robinul Forte*	*Oral* 1–2 mg 2–3 times/day *Parenteral* IM, IV: 0.1–0.2 mg 3–4 times/day *Reversal of Neuromuscular Blockade* 0.2 mg IV for every 1 mg neostigmine or equivalent received *Preanesthetic Medication* 0.004 mg/kg IM 30–60 min before anesthesia (children under 12 y of age—0.004–0.008 mg/kg)	GI disorders, preoperative medication	Not indicated in children under 12 y for GI disorders; used preoperatively to reduce salivary, bronchial, pharyngeal, and gastric secretions and to block vagal inhibition of cardiac reflexes during anesthesia; may cause burning at site of injection; do not mix with solutions of sodium chloride or bicarbonate; oral absorption is irregular.
Homatropine Hydrobromide *Homatrine, Isopto Homatropine* *(CAN) Ak-Homatropine*	*Refraction* 1–2 drops 2% every 10–15 min if necessary *Iritis* 1–2 drops 2%–5% every 3–4 h	Refraction, iritis, relief of ciliary spasm, preoperative, cycloplegic, and mydriatic	Cycloplegia may be prolonged and caution in driving is recommended.

(continued)

Table 13-3. **Antimuscarinics (Continued)**

Drug	*Usual Dosage Range*	*Major Uses*	*Nursing Considerations*
Ipratropium *Atrovent*	2 inhalations 4 times/day (maximum 12 inhalations/ 24 h)	Bronchospasm associated with chronic obstructive pulmonary disease	Orally inhaled anticholinergic that relaxes bronchiolar smooth muscle by inhibiting action of parasympathetic nervous system; does not affect volume or viscosity of respiratory secretions; systemic absorption is minimal; *not* indicated for *initial* treatment of *acute* episodes of bronchospasm; most frequent side effects are cough, dryness of oropharynx, and nervousness (see Chapter 57).
Isopropamide Iodide *Darbid*	5–10 mg twice a day (every 12 h)	GI spasm and hypersecretion, diarrhea	Not for use in children under 12 y; erratically absorbed orally; iodine skin rash may occur; may alter protein-bound iodine and ^{131}I tests, because drug is an iodide salt.
Mepenzolate *Cantil*	25–50 mg 4 times/day	GI hypermotility, diarrhea, ulcerative colitis	Urinary hesitancy and constipation can occur, especially at larger doses; erratically absorbed orally.
Mathantheline Bromide *Banthine*	Adults: 50–100 mg 4 times/ day Children (less than 1 y): 12–25 mg 4 times/day over 1 y: 25–50 mg 4 times/ day	Adjunctive therapy in peptic ulcer	Less effective than many other similar agents; tablets are very bitter; poorly absorbed orally.
Methscopolamine Bromide *Pamine*	2.5 mg 3 times/day and 2.5–5 mg at bedtime	GI hypermotility, adjunctive therapy in peptic ulcer	Take drug 30 min before meals; may exert curare-like relaxant effect on smooth muscle
Propantheline Bromide *Pro-Banthine* *(CAN) Banlin, Novopropanthil, Propanthel*	*Oral* 7.5–15 mg 3 times/day and 30 mg at bedtime Children: 1.5–3 mg/kg/day in 3–4 divided doses	GI spasm and hypersecretion, adjunctive therapy in peptic ulcer	Increased fluid intake may minimize fecal impaction and urinary hesitancy; blurring of vision and dizziness can occur.
Tridihexethyl Chloride *Pathilon*	Adults: 25–50 mg 3–4 times/ day	Adjunctive therapy in peptic ulcer	Infrequently used.

Fate

Belladonna alkaloids and most tertiary amines are well absorbed in the eye and GI tract. Scopolamine is also absorbed significantly through the skin behind the ear (postauricular) when applied as a transdermal patch (see Table 13-3). Quaternary amines are poorly and erratically absorbed orally. The extent of distribution largely depends on lipid solubility; the more lipid-soluble alkaloids and tertiary amines are widely distributed peripherally and centrally, whereas quaternary amines have a more limited peripheral distribution. The duration of action of quaternary amines is somewhat longer than that of tertiary amines.

Common Side Effects

Dry mouth, blurred vision, urinary hesitancy, constipation, palpitations, flushing.

Significant Adverse Reactions

GI: vomiting, dysphagia, bloating, paralytic ileus, and possibly gastroesophageal reflux
CV: tachycardia, hypertension
CNS: headache, nervousness, drowsiness, confusion, restlessness, insomnia, delirium, hallucinations, elevated body temperature
Ocular: photophobia, cycloplegia, increased intraocular tension
Dermatologic: rash, urticaria, systemic allergic reactions
Other: urinary retention, dysuria, impotence, suppression of lactation, respiratory difficulties, muscular incoordination

Contraindications

Narrow-angle glaucoma, severe coronary artery disease, urinary or GI obstruction, intestinal atony, paralytic ileus, myasthenia gravis, ulcerative colitis, hiatal hernia, serious hepatic or renal disease. *Cautious use* in patients with glaucoma, asthma, duodenal ulcer, coronary artery disease, arrhythmias, hyperthyroidism, chronic lung disease, and prostatic hypertrophy.

Interactions

The following drugs may increase the side effects of antimuscarinics: antihistamines, tricyclic antidepressants, antipsychotics, antianxiety drugs, meperidine, nitrites and nitrates, methylphenidate, quinidine, procainamide, disopyramide, primidone, monoamine oxidase (MAO) inhibitors, and amantadine.

Guanethidine, histamine, and reserpine can antagonize the inhibitory effects of antimuscarinics on gastric acid secretion.

Antimuscarinics may enhance the actions of bronchodilators (eg, adrenergics, theophylline), isoniazid, and methotrimeprazine.

Antacids may impair the GI absorption of antimuscarinics.

Antimuscarinics may decrease the effects of cholinergics (eg, pilocarpine or physostigmine) used locally in the eye. Antimuscarinics, when used with haloperidol or corticosteroids, may elevate intraocular pressure.

The effect of levodopa may be decreased by antimuscarinics owing to accelerated gastric breakdown.

The effect of metoclopramide on GI motility is antagonized by antimuscarinics.

Nursing Management

Pretherapy Assessment

Assess and record baseline data necessary for detection of adverse effects of antimuscarinics: General: vital signs (VS), body weight, skin color and temperature; CNS: reflexes, bilateral grip strength, ophthalmologic examination; GI: bowel sounds, normal output; Genitourinary (GU): prostate palpation, normal output; Laboratory: electrocardiogram (ECG), renal and liver function.

Review medical history and documents for existing or previous conditions that:

a. require cautious use of antimuscarinics: glaucoma; asthma; duodenal ulcer; coronary artery disease; arrhythmias; hyperthyroidism; Down's syndrome; brain damage; spasticity; chronic lung disease; prostatic hypertrophy.
b. contraindicate use of antimuscarinics: allergy to antimuscarinics; narrow-angle glaucoma; urinary or GI obstruction; megacolon; intestinal atony; paralytic ileus; myasthenia gravis; ulcerative colitis; hiatal hernia; serious hepatic or renal disease; **pregnancy (Category C)**; lactation (secreted in breast milk, may reduce milk production, safety not established, avoid use in nursing mothers).

Nursing Interventions

Medication Administration

Administer oral medication 30 minutes before meals to reduce GI distress.

Administer intravenously (IV) slowly; rapid administration can lead to tachycardia, hypertension, respiratory distress, and convulsions.

Provide small, frequent meals in event of GI distress or dysphasia.

Provide measures to prevent constipation, such as increased intake of fluid and dietary fiber.

Have antidotal measures (cholinesterase inhibitors, barbiturates, levarterenol, respiratory aids, oxygen) available in case of overdosage or hypersensitivity reaction, especially with parenteral use.

Expect to prepare unusual doses; many are small (eg, atropine 0.4–0.6 mg), and it is easy to administer an overdose.

Ensure ready access to bathroom facilities in event of GI, GU effects.

Surveillance During Therapy

Monitor urinary output and bowel regularity.

Monitor pulse and respiration; report changes immediately.

Monitor for symptoms of systemic absorption of ophthalmic dosages forms: dry mouth, urinary retention, constipation.

Monitor for signs of CNS toxicity (blurred vision, mydriasis, mental confusion or excitement), especially in the elderly, that indicate the need for dosage reduction or consideration of an alternative medication.

Monitor for signs of hypersensitivity that may require discontinuation of drug.

Interpret results of diagnostic tests and contact practitioner as appropriate.

Monitor for possible drug–drug and drug–nutrient interactions: increased anticholinergic effects when given with other drugs having anticholinergic activity: certain antihistamines, certain antiparkinsonian agents, meperidine, tricyclic antidepressants (TCAs), MAO inhibitors; decreased antipsychotic effectiveness of haloperidol and phenothiazine derivatives; guanethidine, histamine, and reserpine can antagonize the inhibitory effects on gastric acid secretion; can enhance the actions of bronchodilators, isoniazid, and methotrimeprazine; when used with haloperidol or corticosteroids can increase intraocular pressure; effects of levodopa decreased as a result of accelerated gastric breakdown; effect of metoclopramide on GI motility antagonized; induction of ventricular arrhythmias in patients receiving cyclopropane.

Provide for patient safety needs and initiate interventions to minimize environmental hazards and risk of injury if CNS, visual, or hyperpyrexic side effects develop.

Patient Teaching

Instruct patient about the importance of completing the full course of therapy as prescribed.

Instruct patient to take drug before meals if dysphagia occurs.

Instruct patient to avoid use of over-the-counter (OTC) preparations when using antimuscarinics, because serious reactions may result.

Instruct patient, especially the elderly, to take special care during physical activity because antimuscarinic agents may impair coordination.

Instruct patient about possible adverse side effects of antimuscarinic agents: dizziness, confusion, constipation, dry mouth, blurred vision, sensitivity to light, impotence, difficulty in urination.

Instruct patient on appropriate action to take if side effects occur:

a. Notify practitioner if skin rash, flushing, eye pain, difficulty breathing, tremors, loss of conditioning, irregular heartbeat, palpitations, headache, abdominal distention, hallucinations, severe or persistent dry mouth, difficulty swallowing, difficulty in urination, constipation, or sensitivity to light, occurs.

Ganglionic Blocking Agents

Synaptic transmission in ganglia of the autonomic nervous system is mediated by ACh and thus can be reduced by drugs that block ACh at postganglionic cholinergic receptor sites. Specific anticholinergic drugs that act primarily at autonomic ganglia are termed *ganglionic blocking agents*. Only two such drugs are available for therapeutic use: mecamylamine and trimethaphan. Their clinical applicability is restricted to producing hypotension for specialized circumstances. Because these agents are nonselective in their blocking action, they reduce neurotransmission in both sympathetic and parasympathetic ganglia. Thus, in addition to interfering with sympathetic impulses that constrict vascular smooth muscle, they block nerve signals to many other body organs; the result is a wide range of side effects. Typical effects caused by parasympathetic blockade include decreased GI motility and secretions, dry mouth, urinary retention, constipation, paralysis of ocular accommodation, mydriasis, and impotence. These adverse reactions limit the clinical use of these drugs.

Ganglionic blocking agents can be categorized by their mechanism of action as either *depolarizing* or *antidepolarizing* blocking agents. *Depolarizing* blockers, of which the alkaloid nicotine is an example, initially stimulate the postganglionic receptors, then block further receptor activation by persistently occupying the site and preventing repolarization of the postsynaptic membrane. Although of no therapeutic value, nicotine is of considerable toxicologic importance because it is systemically absorbed from tobacco smoke and may be accidentally inhaled from nicotine-containing insecticides. The pharmacologic effects of nicotine are quite variable and depend largely on the amount absorbed, the extent and level of exposure, and the physiologic state of the individual—that is, the presence of underlying pathologic conditions such as peripheral vascular disorders, hypertension, coronary artery disease, or congestive heart failure. Nicotine is used as a smoking deterrent in the form of chewing gum or a transdermal patch, and is reviewed in Chapter 12.

The clinically useful ganglionic blocking agents are *antidepolarizing*, that is, they block (competitive antagonism) ACh at postganglionic receptor sites. Their predominant effect is to reduce sympathetic vascular tone, producing marked vasodilation and hypotension (primarily orthostatic), and decreasing venous return to the heart and consequently cardiac output. They are *powerful* blood pressure-lowering agents but are infrequently used because of their extensive side effects.

• Mecamylamine

Inversine

Mechanism

Competitive antagonism of ACh at cholinergic receptors in autonomic ganglia, producing prolonged (6–12 hours) lowering of blood pressure predominantly of the postural type, in both normotensive and hypertensive subjects.

Uses

Management of moderately severe to severe essential hypertension and uncomplicated malignant hypertension when other antihypertensive drugs have failed.

Dosage

Initially 2.5 mg twice a day orally, increased by 2.5-mg increments every 2 days until optimal effect is obtained (average dosage 25 mg/day in 2 to 4 divided doses).

Fate

Completely absorbed orally; onset in 30 to 90 minutes; duration 6 to 12 hours; widely distributed; enters CNS; excreted slowly through kidneys, largely in unchanged form; excretion is enhanced in an acidic urine.

Common Side Effects

Dryness of the mouth, constipation, anorexia, weakness, fatigue, mydriasis, and blurred vision.

Significant Adverse Reactions

Abdominal distention, ileus, orthostatic hypotension, dizziness, syncope, urinary retention, and impotence; tremor, confusion, convulsions, and mental confusion are rare occurrences.

Contraindications

Coronary or renal insufficiency, recent myocardial infarction, uremia, chronic pyelonephritis, pyloric stenosis, and glaucoma. *Cautious use* in patients with cerebral insufficiency; bladder neck or urethral obstruction; prostatic hypertrophy; elevated blood urea nitrogen (BUN) levels.

Interactions

Hypotensive effect of mecamylamine can be enhanced by alcohol, other antihypertensive agents, diuretics, anesthetics, MAO inhibitors, and bethanechol.

Mecamylamine may potentiate sympathomimetic drugs.

Effects of mecamylamine can be prolonged by urinary alkalinizers (eg, sodium bicarbonate).

Nursing Management

Pretherapy Assessment

Assess and record baseline data necessary for detection of adverse effects of mecamylamine: General: VS, body weight, skin color and temperature; CNS: reflexes, bilateral grip strength, ophthalmologic examination including tonometry; CVS: orthostatic blood pressure (BP), supine BP, edema; GI: bowel sounds, normal output; GU: prostate palpation, normal output; Laboratory: ECG, renal and liver function.

Review medical history and documents for evidence of existing or previous conditions that:

a. require cautious use of mecamylamine: cerebral insufficiency; bladder neck or urethral obstruction; prostatic hypertrophy; renal insufficiency; fever; infection; hemorrhage; surgery; vigorous exercise; salt depletion.

b. contraindicate use of mecamylamine: allergy to mecamylamine; coronary or renal insufficiency; recent myocardial infarction; chronic pyelonephritis; pyloric stenosis; glaucoma; **pregnancy (Category C)**; lactation (secreted in breast milk, safety not established, discontinuing nursing if drug is required).

Nursing Interventions

Medication Administration

Administer oral medication after meals to permit smoother control. Smaller doses are prescribed in the mornings, whereas larger doses are used in the afternoon. Rationale: response to drug is greater in the morning.

Provide small, frequent meals in event of GI distress or dysphasia.

Determine initial and maintenance dosage by BP readings in the erect position at the time of maximal drug effect, as well as by signs and symptoms of orthostatic hypotension.

Discontinue the drug gradually, substituting another antihypertensive as mecamylamine dose is decreased. Rationale: abrupt discontinuation may result in the return of severe hypertension, the occurrence of a fatal cerebrovascular event, or the precipitation of congestive heart failure.

Provide measures to prevent constipation, such as increased intake of fluid and dietary fiber.

Arrange to decrease dosage in the presence of fever, infection, or salt depletion.

Ensure ready access to bathroom facilities in event of GI, GU effects.

Surveillance During Therapy

Monitor urinary output and bowel regularity: paralytic ileus has occurred; constipation may be prevented when used with neostigmine, treated with milk of magnesia.

Monitor pulse and respiration; report changes immediately.

Monitor patient for orthostatic hypotension, most marked in the morning and accentuated by hot weather, alcohol, exercise.

Monitor salt intake.

Monitor for signs of CNS toxicity (blurred vision, mydriasis, mental confusion or excitement, weakness, fatigue, or sedation), especially in the elderly, that indicate the need for dosage reduction or consideration of an alternative medication.

Monitor for signs of hypersensitivity that may require discontinuation of drug.

Interpret results of diagnostic tests and contact practitioner as appropriate.

Monitor for possible drug–drug and drug–nutrient interactions: enhanced hypotensive effect induced by alcohol, other antihypertensives, diuretics, anesthetics, MAO inhibitors, and bethanechol; potentiation of sympathomimetic drug effects; prolongation of effects with urinary alkalinizers.

Provide for patient safety needs and initiate interventions to minimize environmental hazards and risk of injury if CNS, visual, or hyperpyrexic side effects develop.

Patient Teaching

Patient teaching and patient cooperation are crucial to the safe and effective use of mecamylamine:

Instruct patient about the importance of completing the full course of therapy as prescribed.

Instruct patient as to the dose; take this drug exactly as prescribed.

Inform the patient that monitoring of BP is necessary for the safe, efficacious therapy with this agent.

Instruct patient to take drug before meals if dysphagia occurs.

Instruct the patient about the importance of not discontinuing this drug without the approval of the practitioner.

Instruct patient to avoid substances that increase urinary pH (eg, sodium bicarbonate). Rationale: increased urinary pH retards mecamylamine excretion, increasing the risk for a toxic effect.

Instruct patient that bulk laxatives are ineffective in the treatment of drug-induced constipation.

Instruct patient to avoid use of alcohol or OTC preparations when using mecamylamine, because serious reactions may result.

Instruct patients, especially the elderly, to take special care during physical activity because mecamylamine agents may impair coordination.

Instruct patient to maintain an adequate salt intake, especially in hot weather, with exercising, or excessive sweating.

Instruct patient about possible adverse side effects of mecamylamine: dizziness, weakness; blurred vision, dilated pupils, sensitivity to bright light; constipation; dry mouth; GI upset; impotence, decreased libido.

Instruct patient on appropriate action to take if side effects occur:

a. Notify practitioner if tremor, seizure, frequent dizziness or fainting; or severe or persistent constipation, frequent loose stools with abdominal distention, occurs.

• Trimethaphan

Arfonad

Mechanism

Short-lived blockade (competitive antagonism) of ACh at ganglionic receptor sites; also may exert direct relaxant effect on vascular smooth muscle; causes pooling of blood in peripheral and splanchnic vessels; also may release histamine; blood pressure is markedly reduced and peripheral blood flow is improved.

Uses

Production of controlled hypotension during surgery
Acute control of blood pressure in hypertensive emergencies
Emergency treatment of pulmonary edema resulting from pulmonary hypertension

Dosage

Only by IV infusion: 500 mg (10 mL) diluted to 500 mL in 5% dextrose; begin IV drip at 3 mL/min to 4 mL/min and adjust to individual needs; may range from 0.3 to 6 mL/min.

Fate

Onset of action is immediate; duration approximately 10 to 30 minutes; excreted by the kidneys largely as intact drug.

Significant Adverse Reactions

Primarily due to overdose: excessive hypotension, rapid pulse, cyanosis, angina-like pain, and vascular collapse.

Contraindications

Conditions in which hypotension may subject the patient to undue risks such as hypovolemia, shock, asphyxia, anemia, respiratory insufficiency, impaired renal function, severe arteriosclerosis, or severe cardiac disease. *Cautious use* in patients with arteriosclerosis; cardiac, hepatic, or renal disease; Addison's disease; degenerative CNS disease; diabetes; allergies; and in the elderly, debilitated, or the very young.

Interactions

Hypotensive effects can be potentiated by antihypertensive agents, anesthetics, vasodilators, and diuretics.

Nursing Management

Pretherapy Assessment

Assess and record baseline data necessary for detection of adverse effects of trimethaphan: General: VS, body weight, skin color and temperature; CNS: reflexes, pupil size; CVS: orthostatic BP, supine BP, edema; GI: bowel sounds, normal output; GU: prostate palpation, normal output; Laboratory: renal and liver function, blood and urine glucose.
Review medical history and documents for existing or previous conditions that:
a. require cautious use of trimethaphan: arteriosclerosis; cardiac, hepatic, or renal disease; Addison's disease; degenerative CNS disease; diabetes; allergies; use in the elderly, the debilitated, or the very young.
b. contraindicate use of trimethaphan: allergy to trimethaphan; conditions in which hypotension may subject the patient to undue risks: hypovolemia, shock, asphyxia, anemia, respiratory insufficiency, severe cardiac disease; **pregnancy (Category C)**; lactation (secreted in breast milk, safety not established, discontinuing nursing if drug is required).

Nursing Interventions

Medication Administration

Do not use infusion fluid for administration of any other drugs.
Always dilute drug immediately before use; discard unused portion.
Ensure adequate oxygenation during treatment (maintenance of cerebral and coronary tissue oxygenation).

Surveillance During Therapy

Monitor pulse and respiration; report changes immediately.
Monitor patient for orthostatic hypotension.
Monitor salt intake.
Monitor for signs of CNS toxicity (blurred vision, mental confusion or excitement, weakness, fatigue, or sedation), especially in the elderly, that indicate the need for dosage reduction.
Monitor for signs of hypersensitivity that may require discontinuation of drug.
Interpret results of diagnostic tests and contact practitioner as appropriate.
Monitor for possible drug–drug and drug–nutrient interactions: enhanced hypotensive effect induced by alcohol, other antihypertensives, diuretics, and anesthetics.

Patient Teaching

In most situations, the patient will be completely unaware that the drug is being used; however, if the patient is awake or is in the company of significant others:

Instruct patient about the importance of completing the full course of therapy as prescribed.
Instruct patient about possible adverse side effects of trimethaphan: dry mouth; blurred vision.
Instruct patient on appropriate action to take if side effects occur:
a. Notify practitioner if pain at the injection site, difficulty breathing, or skin rash or itching occur.

Selected Bibliography

Amitai Y, Almog S, Singer R, Hammer R, Bentur Y, Danon YL: Atropine poisoning in children during the Persian Gulf crisis. JAMA 268:630, 1992
Flicker C, Ferris SH, Serby M: Hypersensitivity to scopolamine in the elderly. Psychopharmacology 107:437, 1992
Hoffstein V, Zamel N, McClean P, Chapman KR: Changes in pulmonary function and cross-sectional area of trachea and bronchi in asthmatics following inhalation of procaterol hydrochloride and ipratropium bromide. J Respir Crit Care Med 149:81, 1994
Levin SL: Salivatory responses to classical and nontraditional parasympatholytic agents in human subjects: Critical comments. J Clin Pharmacol 32:1013, 1992
Monane M, Avorn J, Beers MH, Everitt DE: Anticholinergic drug use and bowel function in nursing home patients. Arch Intern Med 153:633, 1993
Peters NL: Snipping the thread of life: Antimuscarinic side effects of medications in the elderly. Arch Intern Med 149:2414, 1989
Takakura K, Harada J, Mizogami M, Goto Y: Prophylactic effects of pirenzepine (M_1-blocker) on intraoperative stress ulcer: Comparison with an H_2-blocker. Anesth Analg 78:84, 1994
Tune L, Carr S, Hoag E, Cooper T: Anticholinergic effects of drugs commonly prescribed for the elderly: Potential means for assessing risk of delirium. Am J Psychiatry 149(10):1393, 1992
Walkup J: Increased anticholinergic levels, memory and judgment. Hum Psychopharmacology 6:189, 1991

Wood CD, Stewart JJ, Wood MJ, Mims M: Effectiveness and duration of intramuscular antimotion sickness medications. J Clin Pharmacol 32:1008, 1992

Nursing Bibliography

Countering IV erythromycin's ill effect. Emergency Medicine 24(9):49, 52, 1992

Johanson G: Use of anticholinergics in palliative care. American Journal of Hospice and Palliative Care 9(1):1, 1992

McCormick K, et al.: Urinary incontinence in adults. American Journal of Nursing 92(10):75, 1992

Nicto J, et al.: Transdermal scopolamine as treatment of bradyarrhythmias. Chest 101(6):1588–1590, 1992

Transdermal scopolamine to control drooling. Chest 16(1):3, 1992

14 Adrenergic Drugs

Endogenous Catecholamines
- Epinephrine
- Norepinephrine
- Dopamine

Synthetic Catecholamines
- Isoproterenol
- Dobutamine

Vasopressor Amines
- Mephentermine
- Metaraminol
- Methoxamine
- Phenylephrine

Nasal Decongestants

Ophthalmic Decongestants

Sympathomimetic Bronchodilators
- Ephedrine
- Ethylnorepinephrine
- Selective $beta_2$ agonists

Smooth Muscle Relaxants
- Isoxsuprine
- Ritodrine

CNS Stimulants and Anorexiants

Adrenergic drugs—either naturally occurring or synthetic—produce physiologic responses similar to those caused by stimulation of the adrenal medulla or of sympathetic nervous system. For this reason, they are also called *sympathomimetic drugs*, that is, drugs that mimic stimulation of sympathetic neurons.

The principal adrenergic compounds naturally occurring in the body are the endogenous catecholamines epinephrine, norepinephrine, and dopamine. *Epinephrine*, the major secretory product of the adrenal medulla, is released during periods of physical or emotional stress and plays an important role in the body's adaptation to stress. It also is found in other organs of the body, where its role is less clear. *Norepinephrine*, the principal mediator of transmission at adrenergic neuroeffector junctions, is found in adrenergic nerve endings. In addition, norepinephrine is found in certain brain regions and in peripheral sympathetic ganglia, where it probably serves a modulatory function. *Dopamine* is a neurotransmitter involved in central regulation of both motor function and pituitary hormone secretion. It also acts peripherally in certain vascular beds to cause dilation of mesenteric and renal blood vessels.

The adrenergic agents in clinical use comprise a large and diverse group of drugs with a wide spectrum of pharmacologic actions. Based on their major mechanism of action, adrenergic drugs can be divided into three groups:

I. *Direct acting*: bind to and activate postsynaptic adrenergic receptor sites (eg, dopamine, norepinephrine).
II. *Indirect acting*: promote release of stored adrenergic neurotransmitters from presynaptic adrenergic nerve terminals (eg, tyramine).
III. *Dual acting*: agents having both direct and indirect actions (eg, amphetamine, ephedrine).

There are different kinds of adrenergic receptor sites (see Chapter 11 for more complete discussion). Most adrenergic receptor sites are of two basic types, alpha and beta, which can be further subdivided based on their location (Table 14-1). Of clinical importance are two types of alpha receptors—$alpha_1$ and $alpha_2$—and two types of beta receptors—$beta_1$ and $beta_2$. (These names sometimes are written with the Greek letters for which they are named: α_1, β_1, and so on.) In addition, there are receptors specific to dopamine; these dopaminergic (DA) sites, found in the brain and on certain blood vessels, are further subdivided into DA_1, DA_2, DA_3 and DA_4 sites. Dopamine also can interact with certain alpha and beta receptor sites. The major *peripheral* pharmacologic effects elicited by activation of the various adrenergic and dopaminergic receptor sites are listed in Table 14-2.

In addition to their peripheral actions, many adrenergic compounds exert profound effects on the central nervous system (CNS). Alterations in catecholamine activity in many brain structures are responsible for many affective (eg, psychosis) and motor (eg, Parkinson's disease) disorders. Drugs useful in treating these conditions function largely by modifying the availability or action of endogenous adrenergic amines. Many noncatecholamine adrenergic drugs (eg, amphetamine, ephedrine) can easily penetrate the CNS and elicit marked stimulatory effects; these agents, often abused and potentially dangerous, are considered in Chapter 29 with other CNS stimulants.

The following classification is used to discuss adrenergic drugs in this chapter (remember that many adrenergic agents fall into more than one of these categories):

I. Endogenous catecholamines (eg, dopamine, epinephrine, norepinephrine)
II. Synthetic catecholamines (eg, dobutamine, isoproterenol)
III. Vasopressor amines (eg, metaraminol)
IV. Nasal decongestants (eg, phenylephrine)
V. Ophthalmic decongestants (eg, naphazoline)
VI. Bronchodilators (eg, ephedrine, metaproterenol)
VII. Smooth muscle relaxants (eg, isoxsuprine, ritodrine)
VIII. CNS stimulants and anorexiants (eg, amphetamine)

Endogenous Catecholamines

The three major endogenous catecholamines, epinephrine, norepinephrine, and dopamine, serve as neurotransmitters and modulators of the sympathetic nervous system; they are found widely distributed throughout the body. Moreover, many categories of drugs (eg, antihypertensives, vasopressors) produce their pharmacologic effects by blocking or simulating the action of these catecholamines. Thus, catecholamines participate in the action of a wide range of drugs. Because catecholamines also can be prepared synthetically, they are widely used in

Table 14-1. **Adrenergic Receptor Sites**

Alpha$_1$	*Alpha$_2$*	*Beta$_1$*	*Beta$_2$*	*Dopaminergic*
Principal Agonists				
Epinephrine Norepinephrine	Epinephrine Norepinephrine	Epinephrine Isoproterenol	Epinephrine Isoproterenol	Dopamine*
Major Peripheral Locations				
Vascular smooth muscle GI and urinary sphincters Eye (radial muscles) Spleen Salivary glands Skin (sweat glands, pilomotor muscles)	Presynaptic adrenergic and cholinergic nerve terminals Platelets Fat cells Pancreas Vascular smooth muscle GI tract (?)	Heart Intestinal smooth muscle Adipose tissue Kidney	Smooth muscle (bronchiolar, GI, uterine, urinary) Skeletal muscle blood vessels Liver	Renal, coronary, and visceral blood vessels
Responses				
Vasoconstriction (rapid onset—short lived) Contraction of GI and urinary sphincters Mydriasis (contraction of radial muscle) Salivary and sweat gland secretion	Platelet aggregation Vasoconstriction (slow onset—long lived)	Cardiac stimulation Lipolysis Increased renin secretion	Glycogenolysis, gluconeogenesis	
Pancreatic secretions ↓	Neurotransmitter release ↓ Inhibition of lipolysis GI motility ↓	GI motility ↓	Bronchodilation Uterine relaxation GI motility ↓ Relaxation of urinary bladder Dilation of skeletal muscle blood vessels	Dilation of renal, coronary, and visceral blood vessels

* Dopamine also can activate cardiac beta$_1$ receptors and vascular alpha$_1$ receptors in higher doses.

treating many clinical disorders. The therapeutic indications of the catecholamines are based primarily on their cardiac stimulatory, vasoconstrictive, and bronchodilating actions.

Epinephrine

Parenteral: Adrenalin, Sus-Phrine
Inhalation: Asthmahaler, Asthmanefrin, Bronitin Mist, Bronkaid Mist, Medihaler-Epi, Micronefrin, Primatene, Vaponefrin, ***(CAN)*** Dysne-Inhal, Epipen
Nasal: Adrenalin
Ophthalmic: Adrenalin, Epifrin, Epinal, Eppy/N, Glaucon

Mechanism

Direct nonspecific activation of alpha- and beta-adrenergic receptor sites; alpha activation elicits vasoconstriction in many vascular beds; beta$_1$ activation increases heart rate and the force of myocardial contraction. Beta$_2$ activation evokes bronchodilation and dilation of vessels in skeletal muscles through formation of cyclic adenosine monophosphate (AMP); uterine smooth muscle usually is contracted except in the latter stages of pregnancy, when myometrial tone is decreased (beta$_2$ activation); blood glucose is elevated because of glycogenolysis and gluconeogenesis. In the eye, epinephrine induces mydriasis but lowers intraocular pressure by inhibiting formation and stimulating outflow of aqueous humor; effects on the CNS are minimal at normal doses because epinephrine does not significantly penetrate the blood–brain barrier.

Uses

Symptomatic relief of anaphylactic, allergic, and other hypersensitivity reactions
Pressor agent for acute hypotensive states
Nasal decongestion
Bronchodilation and pulmonary decongestion (relaxes bronchial smooth muscle and constricts mucosal blood vessels)
Restoration of normal cardiac rhythm in cases of cardiac arrest
Management of simple, open-angle glaucoma (decreases production and increases outflow of aqueous humor)
Ocular decongestion (vasoconstriction) and production of mydriasis
Topical hemostasis (controls superficial bleeding)
Potentiation and prolongation of the action of local anesthetics

Dosage

I. *Parenteral*
  A. Cardiac arrest: 5 to 10 mL 1:10,000 IV, repeated at 5-minute intervals as required
  B. Intracardiac: 3 to 5 mL 1:10,000

Table 14-2. Adrenergic Drug Effects

Structure	Response	Receptor Type
Cardiovascular System		
Heart	Rate ↑	$Beta_1$
	Force ↑	$Beta_1$
	AV conduction velocity ↑	$Beta_1$
Blood Vessels		
Skeletal	Vasoconstriction	$Alpha_1$, $alpha_2$
	Vasodilation	$Beta_2$
Mucosal	Vasoconstriction	$Alpha_1$
Mesenteric	Vasoconstriction	$Alpha_1$
	Vasodilation	Dopaminergic
Coronary and renal	Vasodilation	Dopaminergic
Bronchioles	Smooth muscle relaxation	$Beta_2$
GI Tract		
Smooth muscle	Relaxation	$Beta_2$
Sphincter	Contraction	$Alpha_1$
Uterus		
Smooth muscle	Relaxation	$Beta_2$
Eye		
Radial muscle	Contraction	$Alpha_1$
Ciliary muscle	Relaxation (weak)	$Beta_1$
Skin		
Pilomotor muscles	Contraction	$Alpha_1$
Sweat glands	Secretion (weak)	$Alpha_1$
Liver	Glycogenolysis	$Beta_2$
	Gluconeogenesis	$Beta_2$
Adipose Tissue	Lipolysis	$Beta_1$
	Inhibition of lipolysis	$Alpha_2$
Pancreas	Insulin secretion ↓	$Alpha_2$
Kidney	Secretion of renin	$Beta_1$
Platelets	Aggregation	$Alpha_2$

C. Intraspinal: 0.2 to 0.4 mL 1:1000 added to anesthetic solution

D. Bronchospasm:

Adults: 0.3 to 0.5 mL 1:1000 subcutaneous (SC) or intramuscular (IM); repeat every 20 minutes up to 4 hours, *or* 0.1 to 0.3 mL of a 1:200 suspension SC

Children: 0.01 mg/kg 1:1000 SC; repeat every 20 minutes up to 4 hours

E. With local anesthetic: 1:20,000 to 1:100,000

II. *Inhalation*

A. Aerosol: 8 to 15 drops 1% to 2% solution from metered aerosol or nebulizer. Allow 1 to 5 minutes between inhalations, and use least number of inhalations that are effective

III. *Topical*

A. Nasal: 1 to 2 drops 0.1% solution every 4 to 6 hours

B. Hemostatic: 1:1000 to 1:10,000 applied locally

IV. *Ophthalmic*

A. Glaucoma: 1 to 2 drops 0.25% to 2% solution (individualized to patient needs)

B. Ocular mydriasis and hemostasis: 1 to 2 drops 0.1% solution

Fate

Ineffective orally because it is rapidly destroyed by digestive enzymes.

Readily absorbed by mucous membranes. Aqueous solutions are very unstable, oxidize readily (amber or yellow color in solution), and should be used immediately. Effects occur quickly when given by inhalation or via SC, IM, or intraocular administration. Suspension forms provide more prolonged actions (6–12 hours). Drug usually is rapidly inactivated by uptake into adrenergic nerve endings or through enzymatic (monoamine oxidase [MAO], catecholoxymethyltransferase [COMT]) hydrolysis. Circulating drug is hydrolyzed in the liver, and metabolites (chiefly vanillylmandelic acid [VMA]) are excreted in the urine.

Common Side Effects

Systemic: nervousness, anxiety, nausea, sweating, pallor, palpitations, headache, insomnia

Ophthalmic: headache, stinging, lacrimation, rebound hyperemia

Nasal: burning, mucosal dryness, sneezing, rebound congestion

Significant Adverse Reactions

Systemic: weakness, dizziness, hypertension, anginal pain (especially in patients with coronary insufficiency), tachycardia and arrhythmias, pulmonary edema, dyspnea, urinary retention, cerebral or subarachnoid hemorrhage, delusions, tremor, psychoses, lactic acidosis

Ophthalmic: conjunctival irritation; pigmentation of eyelids, cornea, or conjunctiva; iritis; shedding of eyelashes; scotomas

Contraindications

Severe hypertension, arrhythmias, coronary artery disease, shock, porphyria, narrow-angle glaucoma, organic brain damage, during labor (delays second stage), and in combination with general anesthetics, especially halogenated hydrocarbons (increased risk of arrhythmias). *Cautious use* in patients with hypertension, hyperthyroidism, diabetes, parkinsonism, cardiovascular disease, emphysema, psychoneuroses, prostatic hypertrophy, or tuberculosis, and in infants and elderly patients.

Interactions

Epinephrine may be potentiated by other sympathomimetic agents (eg, phenylephrine, mephentermine), tricyclic antidepressants, MAO inhibitors, antihistamines, thyroxine, guanethidine.

Epinephrine may produce toxic effects when used in combination with digitalis (arrhythmias), general anesthetics (arrhythmias), isoproterenol (arrhythmias), or propranolol (bradycardia).

Epinephrine may induce hyperglycemia, altering the requirements for insulin or oral hypoglycemic agents.

Cardiac and bronchodilatory effects of epinephrine are antagonized by propranolol. Pressor effects are blocked by vasodilators such as nitrites or alpha-adrenergic blockers (eg, phentolamine) but may be intensified by beta-blockers (eg, propranolol).

Diuretics may increase the vascular pressor response to epinephrine.

Nursing Management

Pretherapy Assessment

Assess and record baseline data necessary for detection of adverse effects of epinephrine: General: VS, body weight, skin color and temperature; CNS: orientation, reflexes, ophthalmologic examination; intraocular pressure (glaucoma); cardiovascular system (CVS): pulse, blood pressure (BP); gastrointestinal (GI): bowel sounds, normal output; genitourinary (GU): prostate palpation, normal output; Laboratory: electrocardiogram (ECG), renal and liver function, blood and urine glucose, serum electrolytes, thyroid function.

Review medical history and documents for existing or previous conditions that:

a. require cautious use of epinephrine: hypertension; hyperthyroidism; diabetes; parkinsonism; cardiovascular disease; emphysema; psychoneuroses; prostatic hypertrophy; tuberculosis; use in the elderly and in infants.

b. contraindicate use of epinephrine: allergy to epinephrine, components of drug preparation (inhalant or ophthalmic mixtures containing sulfites); narrow-angle glaucoma; severe hypertension; arrhythmias; coronary artery disease; shock (other than anaphylactic); porphyria; organic brain damage; general anesthetics; **pregnancy (Category C)**; labor and delivery (may delay the second stage of labor, accelerate fetal heart rate, cause fetal and maternal hypoglycemia, *do not use* if maternal BP > 130/80); lactation (secreted in breast milk, may reduce milk production, safety not established, avoid use in nursing mothers).

With ophthalmics: do not use while wearing soft contact lens; in aphakic patients, maculopathy with decreased visual acuity may occur; promptly discontinue use.

Nursing Interventions

Medication Administration

When drug is given intravenously (IV), check BP and pulse frequently (use cardiac monitor if possible) while a small amount is slowly injected. Injections are repeated only as needed to obtain desired effect. Check BP every 3 to 5 minutes until patient is fully stabilized. Observe for signs of shock (eg, cyanosis, pallor), and ensure that all emergency equipment and drugs are readily available.

Check solution *strength* and required dosage carefully before administration. A tuberculin syringe may help ensure dosage accuracy.

Massage SC or IM injection site to hasten absorption, and rotate injection sites to prevent tissue necrosis related to localized vasoconstriction.

Use topical nasal solutions for acute states only (not longer than 3–5 days).

Avoid simultaneous administration with isoproterenol; serious cardiac arrhythmias can result.

Avoid exposing solution to heat, light, or air because deterioration rapidly ensues.

Discard solution if it is yellow or amber or contains a precipitate. Drug is readily destroyed by numerous chemical agents.

Use minimal doses for minimal periods of time. Rationale: "epinephrine-fastness" (drug tolerance) can occur with prolonged use.

Have available:

a. a rapid-acting alpha-adrenergic blocker or a vasodilator in case of excessive hypertensive reaction.

b. facilities for intermittent positive pressure breathing (IPPB) in case pulmonary edema occurs.

c. a beta-blocker in case cardiac arrhythmias occur.

Surveillance During Therapy

Monitor for adverse effects.

Monitor for signs of CNS toxicity (anxiety, restlessness, dizziness, psychologic disturbances, convulsions, blurred vision, symptoms of paranoid schizophrenia).

Interpret results of diagnostic tests and contact practitioner as appropriate.

Monitor for possible drug–drug and drug–nutrient interactions: increased sympathomimetic effects when given with tricyclic antidepressants, *Rauwolfia* alkaloids; may produce toxic effects when given with digitalis, general anesthetics, isoproterenol, or propranolol; may induce hyperglycemia, increasing the requirements for hypoglycemic agents; cardiac and bronchodilatory effects diminished by propranolol; pressor effects blocked by nitrites or alpha-adrenergic blockers, but may be enhanced by beta-blockers; vascular pressor response may be increased by diuretics.

Provide for patient safety needs and initiate interventions to minimize environmental hazards and risk of injury if CNS, visual, or hyperpyrexic side effects develop.

Patient Teaching

General

Instruct patient regarding the importance of completing the full course of therapy as prescribed.

Instruct patient to avoid use of over-the-counter (OTC) preparations when using epinephrine because serious reactions may result.

Instruct patient about possible adverse side effects of epinephrine: dizziness, drowsiness, fatigue, anxiety, emotional changes, nausea, vomiting, change in taste, fast heart rate.

Instruct patient on appropriate action to take if side effects occur:

a. notify practitioner if chest pain, dizziness, insomnia, weakness, tremor, irregular heartbeat, difficulty breathing, or decrease in visual acuity occurs.

Systemic

Teach patient with a history of acute bronchial asthmatic attacks how to administer epinephrine SC.

Inhalation

Instruct patient to use the least number of inhalations needed to relieve symptoms, and allow 1 or 2 min-

utes between them. Excessive use can produce severe adverse systemic effects.
Urge patient to consult practitioner immediately if symptoms are not relieved within 15 to 30 minutes.
Instruct patient to reduce dosage if bronchial irritation, nervousness, or insomnia is noted.
Instruct patient to rinse mouth with water after inhalation to avoid swallowing residual drug and to prevent excessive mouth-drying effects.

Ophthalmic

Suggest taking drug at bedtime, if possible, to minimize photophobia (sensitivity to light) and blurred vision related to mydriasis. Visual perception may be impaired, especially at night.
Instruct patient to inform drug prescriber if localized symptoms (stinging, burning, headache, tearing) persist with continued drug use.
Instruct patient to stop using drug and consult practitioner if allergic reaction develops (eg, itching, edema, watery discharge).
Instruct patient to inform the practitioner in charge of drug use if general surgery is planned. With certain anesthetics (eg, halothane, other halogenated hydrocarbons), epinephrine should be discontinued before surgery to prevent arrhythmias associated with systemic absorption.

Nasal

Instruct patient to avoid excessive use because rebound congestion and hyperemia frequently occur.
Advise cautious use with elderly person or infant because systemic absorption can produce untoward reactions (eg, tachycardia, hypertension, anxiety).
Inform patient that instillation will sting but discomfort will be temporary.

• **Norepinephrine** *(Pregnancy Category D)*

Levarterenol, Levophed

Mechanism

Direct activation of alpha-adrenergic receptor sites on blood vessels, producing powerful vasoconstriction; also possesses slight inotropic action on cardiac beta receptors (increased force of contraction). Increases BP and coronary artery blood flow, but also increases workload of the heart; in normal doses, little effect on the CNS or on metabolic activity.

Uses

Restoration of BP in acute hypotensive states
Adjunctive treatment of cardiac arrest and extreme hypotension

Dosage

Used by IV infusion—initially, 8 to 12 μg/min (2–3 mL/min) of a 4-μg/mL dilution (4 mg norepinephrine/1000 mL 5% dextrose); maintenance dose—2 to 4 μg/min (0.5–1 mL/min)

Fate

Rapid acting; effects disappear within 2 minutes after termination of IV infusion; rapidly inactivated by uptake into sympathetic nerve endings and also by enzymatic hydrolysis; excreted in the urine largely as metabolites.

Common Side Effects

Bradycardia (reflex), headache, palpitation, nervousness.

Significant Adverse Reactions

Hypertension, respiratory distress, tremors, arrhythmias in the presence of certain anesthetics, tissue necrosis after extravasation; large doses may cause chest pain, photophobia, hyperglycemia, vomiting, severe hypertension, cerebral hemorrhage, and convulsions.

Contraindications

Hypovolemic shock, vascular thrombosis; extreme hypoxia or hypercapnia; pregnancy; during general anesthesia when halogenated hydrocarbons (eg, halothane) are used. *Cautious use* in patients with hypertension, heart disease, hyperthyroidism, peripheral vascular disorders, and in the elderly.

Interactions

The pressor effects of norepinephrine may be potentiated in the presence of tricyclic antidepressants, MAO inhibitors, other sympathomimetic drugs, beta-blockers, antihistamines, guanethidine, and methyldopa.
Norepinephrine, together with oxytocic drugs, can cause severe hypertension.
Norepinephrine may precipitate cardiac arrhythmias in the presence of halogenated hydrocarbon general anesthetics.
Thiazide and high-ceiling (eg, bumetanide, furosemide) diuretics may reduce arterial responsiveness to norepinephrine.

Nursing Management

Pretherapy Assessment

Assess and record baseline data necessary for detection of adverse effects of norepinephrine: General: VS, body weight, skin color and temperature; CVS: pulse, BP; GI: bowel sounds, normal output; GU: normal output; Laboratory: ECG, serum electrolytes.
Review medical history and documents for existing or previous conditions that:
a. require cautious use of norepinephrine: hypertension; hyperthyroidism; cardiovascular disease; use in the elderly.
b. contraindicate use of norepinephrine: allergy to norepinephrine; hypovolemic shock; vascular thrombosis; extreme hypoxia or hypercaphia; during general anesthesia with halogenated hydrocarbons; **pregnancy (Category D)**; lactation (secreted in breast milk, avoid use in nursing mothers).

Nursing Interventions

Medication Administration

Administer IV infusions into a large vein, preferably of the antecubital fossa, to prevent extravasation.
Do not infuse into femoral vein in the elderly or those with occlusive vascular disease.
Check BP every 2 to 5 minutes during and after infusion. Attend patient constantly and carefully monitor skin color and temperature.
Use microdrip IV administration set and an infusion control device to ensure accuracy. Monitor flow rate continuously.

Monitor cardiac rate and rhythm. Atropine should be available to treat bradycardia; propranolol to treat other arrhythmias.
Administer whole blood or plasma separately. Both are incompatible with norepinephrine.
Discard solutions that are colored or contain precipitate.
Seek clarification before adding to saline *alone* because oxidation and loss of potency can occur rapidly. A 5% dextrose vehicle should be used.

Surveillance During Therapy

Monitor for signs of CNS toxicity (headache, secondary to overdosage and extreme hypertension).
Monitor patient for other early signs of overdosage (vomiting, blurred vision, anginal symptoms) so that dosage can be adjusted appropriately.
Monitor intake and output. Urinary output should be determined frequently to assess renal perfusion.
Report indications of blood volume depletion. Adequate blood volume must be maintained to prevent tissue ischemia resulting from vasoconstrictive effect of the drug.
If extravasation occurs (blanching of skin, swelling, hardness), stop infusion. The area should be infiltrated with 10 to 15 mL saline containing 5 to 10 mg phentolamine as soon as possible. Once BP and tissue perfusion can be self-maintained, continue monitoring vital signs to ensure circulatory adequacy while therapy is discontinued by *gradual* reduction of infusion rate.
Interpret results of diagnostic tests and contact practitioner as appropriate.
Monitor for possible drug–drug and drug–nutrient interactions: pressor effects may be potentiated in presence of tricyclic antidepressants, MAO inhibitors, other sympathomimetics, beta-blockers, antihistamines, guanethidine, and methyldopa; use with oxytocic drugs can cause severe hypertension; use in presence of cyclopropane and halogenated hydrocarbon general anesthetics may precipitate cardiac arrhythmias; arterial responsiveness may be reduced by thiazide and loop diuretics; decreased vasopressor effects may be seen when used with phenothiazine derivatives.
Provide for patient safety needs and initiate interventions to minimize environmental hazards and risk of injury if CNS, visual, or hyperpyrexic side effects develop.

Patient Teaching

Because norepinephrine is used only in acute emergency situations, patient teaching depends on patient awareness and focuses on issues of patient status rather than aspects of pharmacotherapy.

• Dopamine

Dopastat, Intropin

(CAN) Revimine

Mechanism

Direct activation of specific dopaminergic receptors in mesenteric and renal vasculature, resulting in vasodilation and increased renal blood flow; also stimulates myocardial beta receptors, enhancing force of contraction and increasing cardiac output with minimal cardioaccelerator action. In high doses, activates alpha receptors in other vascular beds, causing constriction. Produces less oxygen demand on the myocardium and has a lower incidence of arrhythmias than other catecholamines.

Uses

Correction of the hemodynamic imbalances associated with different forms of shock (eg, trauma, heart surgery, myocardial infarction, renal failure, septicemia).

Dosage

Initially—2 to 5 μg/kg/min of diluted solution by IV infusion. May increase by increments of 5 to 10 μg/kg/min up to 20 to 50 μg/kg/min in severely ill patients.

Fate

Rapid onset (5 min) and short duration of action (5–10 min); largely inactivated by liver and plasma enzymes and excreted chiefly in the urine as metabolites. A portion is converted to norepinephrine in adrenergic nerve endings; does not cross the blood–brain barrier.

Common Side Effects

Nausea, vomiting, palpitations, tachycardia, slight hypotension, mild respiratory difficulty, and headache.

Significant Adverse Reactions

Usually occur with high doses: hypertension, conduction irregularities, azotemia, decreased urinary outflow. Necrosis and tissue sloughing may occur after extravasation.

Contraindications

Ventricular arrhythmias, pheochromocytoma. *Cautious use* in patients with occlusive vascular disease.

Interactions

Pressor effects of dopamine may be potentiated by MAO inhibitors, tricyclic antidepressants, other sympathomimetics, oxytocics, ergot alkaloids, and furazolidone.
Actions of dopamine and diuretics may be mutually additive.
Dopamine may produce arrhythmias in the presence of halogenated hydrocarbon anesthetics.
Use of phenytoin with dopamine may lead to hypotension, bradycardia, and seizures.

Nursing Management

Pretherapy Assessment

Assess and record important baseline data necessary for detection of adverse effects of dopamine: General: VS, body weight, skin color and temperature; CVS: pulse, BP, pulse pressure; GU: normal output; Laboratory: ECG, serum electrolytes, hematocrit.
Review medical history and documents for existing or previous conditions that:

a. require cautious use of dopamine: use in people with occlusive vascular disease.
b. contraindicate use of dopamine: hypovolemic shock; pheochromocytoma; tachyarrhythmias; general anesthesia with cyclopropane or halogenated

hydrocarbon anesthetics; ventricular fibrillation; **pregnancy (Category C)**; labor, delivery; lactation (safety not established).

Nursing Interventions

Medication Administration

Administer IV infusions into a large vein, preferably of the antecubital fossa, to prevent extravasation.

Do not infuse into femoral vein in the elderly or those with occlusive vascular disease.

Check BP every 2 to 5 minutes during and after infusion. Attend patient constantly and carefully monitor skin color and temperature.

Dilute the solution in the dopamine ampule before using. Add it to a sterile diluent solution (250 or 500 mL of sodium chloride, sodium lactate, dextrose 5%, lactated Ringer's), according to package instructions.

Protect dopamine solutions from light and discard if discolored.

Administer whole blood or plasma separately. Both are incompatible with norepinephrine.

Discard solutions that are colored or contain precipitated matter.

Seek clarification before adding to alkaline IV solutions because inactivation and loss of potency can occur rapidly.

Use microdrip IV administration set and an infusion control device to ensure accuracy. Monitor flow rate continuously.

Surveillance During Therapy

Carefully monitor BP, heart rate and rhythm, and urine flow during infusion. Rate of flow must be adjusted to maintain desired hemodynamic and renal responses.

Monitor cardiac rate and rhythm. Atropine should be available to treat bradycardia; propranolol to treat other arrhythmias.

Monitor for signs of CNS toxicity (headache, secondary to overdosage and extreme hypertension).

Monitor patient for other early signs of overdosage (headache, vomiting, blurred vision, anginal symptoms) so that dosage can be adjusted appropriately.

Monitor for changes in color, temperature, and texture of skin at injection site, indications of possible extravasation. If extravasation occurs, infiltration with 10 to 15 mL saline containing 5 to 10 mg phentolamine helps prevent necrosis.

Check continually for reduced urine output and monitor for other symptoms of overdosage (hypertension, arrhythmias, change in color of extremities) if high dosages are used. The dosage must be reduced if such symptoms are noted.

Monitor intake and output. Urinary output should be determined frequently to assess renal perfusion.

Report indications of blood volume depletion. Adequate blood volume must be maintained to prevent tissue ischemia resulting from vasoconstrictive effect of the drug.

If extravasation occurs (blanching of skin, swelling, hardness), stop infusion. The area should be infiltrated with 10 to 15 mL saline containing 5 to 10 mg phentolamine as soon as possible to help prevent necrosis. Once BP and tissue perfusion can be self-maintained, continue monitoring vital signs to ensure circulatory adequacy while therapy is discontinued by *gradual* reduction of infusion rate.

Interpret results of diagnostic tests and contact practitioner as appropriate.

Monitor for possible drug–drug and drug–nutrient interactions: pressor effects may be potentiated in presence of tricyclic antidepressants, MAO inhibitors, other sympathomimetics, beta-blockers, antihistamines, guanethidine, and methyldopa; use together with oxytocic drugs can cause severe hypertension; use in presence of cyclopropane and halogenated hydrocarbon general anesthetics may precipitate cardiac arrhythmias; arterial responsiveness may be reduced by thiazide and loop diuretics; decreased vasopressor effects may be seen when used with phenothiazine derivatives.

Provide for patient safety needs and initiate interventions to minimize environmental hazards and risk of injury if CNS, visual, or hyperpyrexic side effects develop.

Patient Teaching

Because dopamine is used only in acute emergency situations, patient teaching depends on patient awareness and focuses on issues of patient status rather than aspects of pharmacotherapy.

Synthetic Catecholamines

Two synthetic catecholamines, isoproterenol and dobutamine, are available for clinical use; their only significant pharmacologic action is stimulation of beta-adrenergic receptor sites. Isoproterenol is nonselective (activates all beta receptors) and dobutamine is relatively specific (activation of cardiac $beta_1$ receptors).

• Isoproterenol

Sublingual or parenteral: Isuprel
Inhalation: Medihaler-Iso

Mechanism

Direct beta-adrenergic receptor activation, resulting in cardiac stimulation, vasodilation, and bronchodilation; also relaxes smooth muscle of the GI tract and uterus, releases free fatty acids, stimulates insulin secretion, and increases glycogenolysis

Uses

Relief of bronchospasm associated with respiratory disorders and general anesthesia

Adjunct in management of shock, cardiac arrest, Adams-Stokes syndrome, atrioventricular (AV) block, and carotid sinus hypersensitivity

Dosage

I. *Parenteral*
   A. Bronchospasm (during anesthesia): 0.01 to 0.02 mg IV of a 1:50,000 solution in saline or dextrose 5%

B. Shock: 0.25 to 2.5 mL/min of 1:500,000 dilution in dextrose 5% by IV infusion (0.5–5 μg/min)
C. Cardiac arrest: IV (injection)—1 to 3 mL of a 1:50,000 dilution (0.02–0.06 mg); IV (infusion)—1.25 mL of 1:250,000 dilution per minute (5 μg/min); IM, SC—1 mL of 1:5000 solution undiluted (0.2 mg); Intracardiac—0.1 mL of 1:5000 solution (0.02 mg)

II. *Sublingual*
A. Bronchospasm: 10 to 20 mg 3 or 4 times/day (children—5 to 10 mg 3 or 4 times/day)
B. Heart block: 10 mg initially (range 5–50 mg); maintenance therapy *only*

III. *Inhalation*
A. Solution: 3 to 7 inhalations of 1:100 solution or 5 to 15 inhalations of 1:200 solution in a hand-held nebulizer; repeat in 5 to 10 min, if needed; may be given up to 5 times/day.
B. Aerosol: 1 to 2 inhalations of metered dose aerosol 4 to 6 times/day.

Fate

Readily absorbed when given parenterally or as aerosol; sublingual absorption is unreliable; duration after most forms of administration is 2 to 4 hours (1–2 h with inhalation); metabolites are excreted largely in the urine, within 24 hours after biotransformation in the GI tract, liver, lungs, and other tissues.

Common Side Effects

Nervousness, headache, palpitations, flushing, nausea, dizziness, mild tremors, and dryness of the oropharynx.

Significant Adverse Reactions

Buccal ulcerations (sublingual), bronchial irritation and edema, cardiac distress (tachycardia, dysrhythmias, anginal pain), parotid gland enlargement (rare); overdosage may result in severe bronchoconstriction, cardiac excitability, and possibly cardiac arrest.

Contraindications

Arrhythmias associated with tachycardia, concurrent administration of epinephrine. *Cautious use* in patients with coronary artery disease, hypertension, hyperthyroidism, diabetes.

Interactions

Combined use with epinephrine may lead to serious arrhythmias.
Arrhythmias may develop if used with halogenated hydrocarbon anesthetics.
Effects are specifically antagonized by propranolol and other beta-adrenergic blockers.

Nursing Management

Pretherapy Assessment

Assess and record baseline data necessary for detection of adverse effects of isoproterenol: General: VS, body weight, skin color and temperature; CVS: pulse, BP, pulse pressure; CNS: orientation, reflexes; Laboratory: ECG, serum electrolytes, blood and urine glucose, thyroid function tests.

Review medical history and documents for existing or previous conditions that:
a. require cautious use of isoproterenol: hypertension; cardiac disease; hyperthyroidism; diabetes; history of seizure disorder.
b. contraindicate use of isoproterenol: hypersensitivity to isoproterenol; tachyarrhythmias; pheochromocytoma; general anesthesia with cyclopropane or halogenated hydrocarbon anesthetics; ventricular fibrillation; **pregnancy (Category C)**; labor, delivery; lactation (safety not established).

Nursing Interventions

Medication Administration

Check type of solution carefully while preparing drug. Those intended for oral inhalation cannot be injected.
Discard discolored or cloudy solutions.
If drug is to be given rectally, use *sublingual tablets* only.
Carefully check dosage and method of inhalation prescribed (eg, nebulizer, aerosol, powder).
Have a beta-blocker available in case cardiac arrhythmias occur.
Do not exceed recommended dosage of inhalation products; if a second inhalation is needed, administer at peak effect of previous dose (3–5 min later).
Ensure that oxygen and other respiratory aids are available.
Use microdrip IV administration set and an infusion control device to ensure accuracy. Monitor flow rate continuously.

Surveillance During Therapy

Monitor BP, heart rate and rhythm, and urine flow during infusion and note blood pH and P_{CO_2} results. Rate of flow must be adjusted to maintain stability of these parameters.
Closely assess patient in shock during infusion. If heart rate exceeds 110 beats/min, infusion should be reduced or terminated because of the danger of arrhythmias.
Monitor cardiac rate and rhythm. Atropine should be available to treat bradycardia; propranolol to treat other arrhythmias.
Monitor for signs of CNS toxicity (headache, secondary to overdosage and extreme hypertension).
Interpret results of diagnostic tests and contact practitioner as appropriate.
Monitor for possible drug–drug and drug–nutrient interactions: combined use with epinephrine may lead to serious arrhythmias; use with cyclopropane or halogenated hydrocarbon anesthetics may lead to arrhythmias; effects antagonized by propranolol or other beta-adrenergic blockers.
Provide for patient safety needs and initiate interventions to minimize environmental hazards and risk of injury if CNS, visual, or hyperpyrexic side effects develop.

Patient Teaching

Sublingual
Instruct patient to allow sublingual tablet to dissolve under tongue without sucking tablet or swallowing saliva until drug has been absorbed.

Inform patient that mild systemic effects (eg, flushing, palpitations) may be experienced with sublingual use.
Advise patient that prolonged use of sublingual tablets can damage teeth. Suggest rinsing mouth thoroughly after each administration.
Inhalation
Teach patient how to use the form of inhalation prescribed.
Instruct patient to breathe with normal force and depth, *not* deeply, when using powdered inhalant.
Suggest that patient rinse mouth after inhalation to minimize dryness.
Inform patient that saliva may appear pink or red after inhalation.
Warn patient to avoid excessive use (3–5 treatments within 6–12 h) of inhalation products because tolerance can develop and sudden deaths have been reported.
Instruct patient to place no more than a 1-day supply of drug in nebulizer and to rinse mouthpiece thoroughly every day.
Instruct patient to notify practitioner immediately if usual doses do not produce desired relief.

• Dobutamine

Dobutrex

Mechanism

Direct activation of $beta_1$-adrenergic receptors on the myocardium, with minimal action at alpha or $beta_2$ sites; increases contractile force but induces less increase in heart rate and less decrease in peripheral vascular resistance than comparably effective doses of isoproterenol.

Uses

Short-term treatment of acute heart failure related to depressed contractility.

Dosage

2.5 to 10 μg/kg/min IV infusion of a 250-, 500-, or 1000-μg/mL solution in sterile water or 5% dextrose. Occasionally, infusion rates up to 40 μg/kg/min are required.

Fate

Onset of action within 1 to 2 minutes; short duration of action; plasma half-life of 2 minutes; metabolized in the liver and excreted in urine as conjugates.

Common Side Effects

Tachycardia (5–15 beats/min increase), palpitations, mild hypertension (10–20 mm Hg increase in systolic pressure).

Significant Adverse Reactions

Premature ventricular beats, anginal pain, headache, dyspnea, nausea, pronounced tachycardia, marked hypertension.

Contraindications

Idiopathic hypertrophic subaortic stenosis. *Cautious use* in persons with arrhythmias, hypertension, or after a recent myocardial infarction.

Interactions

Halogenated hydrocarbons may increase the incidence of arrhythmias with dobutamine.
Pressor effects of dobutamine can be enhanced by MAO inhibitors, tricyclic antidepressants, other sympathomimetic amines, and oxytocic drugs.
In patients with diabetes, insulin requirements may be increased by dobutamine.

Nursing Management

Pretherapy Assessment

Assess and record baseline data necessary for detection of adverse effects of dobutamine: General: VS, body weight, skin color and temperature; CVS: pulse, BP, pulse pressure; GU: urine output; Laboratory: ECG, serum electrolytes, hematocrit.
Review medical history and documents for existing or previous conditions that:
a. require cautious use of dobutamine: arrhythmias; hypertension; recent myocardial infarction; diabetes.
b. contraindicate use of dobutamine: hypersensitivity to dobutamine; tachyarrhythmias; cyclopropane or halogenated hydrocarbon anesthetics; idiopathic hypertrophic subaortic stenosis; **pregnancy (Category C)**; labor, delivery; lactation (safety not established).

Nursing Interventions

Medication Administration

Be prepared to administer volume expanders (eg, Dextran) to the hypovolemic patient before dobutamine is started because hypovolemia should be corrected before initiating dobutamine therapy.
Be prepared to administer digoxin before dobutamine in the patient with existing atrial fibrillation and rapid ventricular response.
Expect drug effects to terminate shortly after discontinuation of therapy. The drug's duration of action is very brief.
Use dilutions for IV use within 24 hours. A color change in the solution during this period indicates slight oxidation, but there is no significant loss of potency during the first 24 hours.
Seek clarification before diluting in an alkaline solution (eg, sodium bicarbonate injection) because of potential incompatibility.
Do not mix with hydrocortisone, sodium succinate, cefazolin, cefamandole, neutral cephalothin, penicillin, sodium ethacrynate, sodium heparin.
May be administered through common IV tubing with dopamine, lidocaine, tobramycin, nitroprusside, KCl, or protamine sulfate.
Use microdrip IV administration set and an infusion

control device to ensure accuracy. Monitor flow rate continuously.

Surveillance During Therapy

Continually monitor BP, heart rate and rhythm, and, where possible, cardiac output and pulmonary capillary wedge pressure during infusion. Volume of infusion should be adjusted by coordinating concentration of the solution with patient's fluid requirements.

Monitor for adverse effects and toxicity.

Interpret results of diagnostic tests and contact practitioner as appropriate.

Monitor for possible drug–drug and drug–nutrient interactions: use with cyclopropane or halogenated hydrocarbon anesthetics may lead to arrhythmias; enhanced pressor effects with MAO inhibitors, tricyclic antidepressants, other sympathomimetics, and oxytocic drugs; risk of severe hypertension when used with *Rauwolfia* alkaloids, beta-blockers; decreases effectiveness of guanethidine.

Provide for patient safety needs and initiate interventions to minimize environmental hazards and risk of injury if CNS, visual, or hyperpyrexic side effects develop.

Patient Teaching

Because this drug is used only in acute emergency situations, teaching depends on patient's awareness and focuses on the patient's clinical condition rather than the drug itself.

Vasopressor Amines

Sympathomimetic vasopressor amines are drugs that have both direct and indirect adrenergic activity. Their predominant pharmacologic effect is production of systemic vasoconstriction, and they are indicated primarily for management of acute hypotensive situations (eg, cardiac arrest, circulatory shock, and those associated with drug reactions and complications of general anesthesia). Vasopressor amines are powerful drugs and must be used with extreme care.

• **Mephentermine** *(Pregnancy Category D)*

Wyamine

Mechanism

Produces both direct adrenergic receptor activation (primarily alpha$_1$) and an indirect action (release of norepinephrine). Pressor effect involves both increased cardiac output (beta activation of the heart) and peripheral vasoconstriction (alpha activation of blood vessels).

Uses

Hypotension secondary to ganglionic blockade or spinal anesthesia

Maintenance of BP in shock after hemorrhage while fluid replacement is accomplished

Dosage

IM, IV: 30 to 45 mg in a single injection (30-mg supplements as needed to maintain BP)

IV infusion: 0.1% (1.0 mg/mL) in 5% dextrose by continuous infusion at a rate of 1.0 mg/min; two 10-mL vials (30 mg/mL) added to 500 mL of 5% dextrose in water

Fate

Rapid onset after IM or IV administration; duration of pressor effect is 2 to 3 hours IM and 30 to 60 minutes IV; readily excreted as metabolites in the urine; minimal effects on the CNS.

Common Side Effects

Occasional anxiety.

Significant Adverse Reactions

Occasionally with large doses: tremor, arrhythmias, drowsiness, hypertension, incoherence, and convulsions.

Contraindications

Patients receiving MAO inhibitors, halothane or related anesthetics, or chlorpromazine. *Cautious use* in the presence of hypertension, cardiovascular disease, hyperthyroidism, or occlusive vascular disease, and in severe illness or debilitated state.

Interactions

Pressor effects may be potentiated by MAO inhibitors, tricyclic antidepressants, sympathomimetic amines, and oxytocic drugs.

May cause arrhythmias if used in combination with cyclopropane, halothane, or digitalis.

Pressor effects can be antagonized by guanethidine and reserpine

Hypotensive effects of chlorpromazine may be potentiated by mephentermine

Nursing Management

Pretherapy Assessment

Assess and record baseline data necessary for detection of adverse effects of mephentermine: General: VS, body weight, skin color and temperature; CVS: pulse, BP, pulse pressure; GU: urine output; Laboratory: ECG, serum electrolytes, hematocrit, blood and urine glucose, thyroid function tests.

Review medical history and documents for existing or previous conditions that:

a. require cautious use of mephentermine: hypertension; cardiovascular disease; hyperthyroidism; occlusive vascular disease; severe illness or debilitated state.
b. contraindicate use of mephentermine: hypersensitivity to mephentermine; cyclopropane or halogenated hydrocarbon anesthetics; MAO inhibitors; chlorpromazine; hypovolemia; **pregnancy (Category D)**; labor, delivery; lactation (safety not established).

Nursing Interventions

Medication Administration

Be prepared to administer volume expanders (eg, Dextran) to the hypovolemic patient before mephenter-

mine is started, because hypovolemia should be corrected before initiating mephentermine therapy.
Evaluate patient response with repeated injections to detect development of tolerance. Dosage should *not* be increased to compensate.
Give prescribed IM injection 10 to 20 minutes before spinal anesthesia to prevent hypotension.
Administer IV infusions into a large vein, preferably of the antecubital fossa, to prevent extravasation.
Have phentolamine available in case extravasation occurs.
Do not infuse into veins of the ankle or dorsum of the hand in patients with peripheral vascular disease, diabetes mellitus, or hypercoagulability states.
Use microdrip IV administration set and an infusion control device to ensure accuracy. Monitor flow rate continuously.

Surveillance During Therapy

Monitor BP, pulse, and ECG constantly during IV administration (every 2 min until stabilized, then every 5–15 min for duration of drug action). Rate of infusion and duration of therapy are regulated according to patient response. Used to treat hemorrhagic shock only until blood volume is replaced.
Monitor for adverse effects and toxicity.
Interpret results of diagnostic tests and contact practitioner as appropriate.
Monitor for possible drug–drug and drug–nutrient interactions: use with cyclopropane or halogenated hydrocarbon anesthetics may lead to arrhythmias; enhanced pressor effects with MAO inhibitors, tricyclic antidepressants, other sympathomimetics, and oxytocic drugs; risk of severe hypertension when used with *Rauwolfia* alkaloids, beta-blockers; decreases effectiveness of guanethidine.
Provide for patient safety needs and initiate interventions to minimize environmental hazards and risk of injury if CNS, visual, or hyperpyrexic side effects develop.

Patient Teaching

Because this drug is used only in acute emergency situations, teaching depends on patient's awareness and focuses on the patient's clinical condition rather than the drug itself.

• *Metaraminol* (Pregnancy Category D)

Aramine

Mechanism

Pressor effect is largely caused by peripheral vasoconstriction resulting from a direct alpha-adrenergic receptor agonistic action; cardiac beta stimulation probably plays only a minor role in pressor response; reflex bradycardia is common. Drug also can deplete norepinephrine stores in adrenergic nerve endings. Systolic and diastolic BP rises, but perfusion of vital organs may decrease.

Uses

Acute hypotensive states associated with spinal anesthesia
Adjunctive management of hypotension caused by brain damage, hemorrhage, surgery, drug reactions, septicemia, or cardiogenic shock

Dosage

IM, SC: 2 to 10 mg (prevention of hypotension)
IV injection: 0.5 to 5 mg followed by infusion of 15 to 100 mg in 500 mL 5% dextrose
IV infusion (preferred in shock): 15 mg/500 mL to 100 mg/500 mL 5% dextrose; rate adjusted to maintain desired BP (pediatric: 0.01 mg/kg IV; as a single dose)

Fate

Onset 1 to 2 minutes with IV infusion, 10 minutes with IM, and 10 to 20 minutes with SC; effects persist 15 to 60 minutes; partly excreted in the urine and partly taken up by adrenergic nerve endings; weak CNS stimulatory effect.

Common Side Effects

Restlessness, headache, flushing, sweating, palpitations.

Significant Adverse Reactions

Usually with large doses: tachycardia, anginal pain, arrhythmias, severe hypertension, convulsions, cardiac arrest, and cerebral hemorrhage. Prolonged use may perpetuate the shock state by preventing volume expansion; hypotension may occur after termination of the drug.

Contraindications

Combined use with halothane or related halogenated hydrocarbon anesthetics or MAO inhibitors (increased risk of arrhythmias), pulmonary edema, metabolic acidosis, use as the sole treatment in cases of hypovolemic shock. *Cautious use* in patients with hypertension, hyperthyroidism, diabetes, cirrhosis, and in patients taking digitalis drugs.

Interactions

Pressor effects may be enhanced by sympathomimetics, MAO inhibitors, tricyclic antidepressants, guanethidine, reserpine, oxytocics, and ergot alkaloids.
Arrhythmias may develop in combination with halogenated hydrocarbon anesthetics or digitalis.

Nursing Management

Pretherapy Assessment

Assess and record baseline data necessary for detection of adverse effects of metaraminol: General: VS, body weight, skin color and temperature; CVS: pulse, BP, pulse pressure; GU: urine output; Laboratory: ECG, serum electrolytes, hematocrit, blood and urine glucose, thyroid function tests.
Review medical history and documents for existing or previous conditions that:

a. require cautious use of metaraminol: hypertension; cardiovascular disease; hyperthyroidism; occlusive vascular disease; severe illness of debilitated state; cirrhosis; digitalis glycosides.
b. contraindicate use of metaraminol: hypersensitivity to metaraminol; cyclopropane or halogenated hydrocarbon anesthetics; MAO inhibitors; metabolic acidosis; hypovolemia; **pregnancy (Category D)**; labor, delivery; lactation (safety not established).

Nursing Interventions

Medication Administration

Be prepared to administer volume expanders (eg, Dextran) to the hypovolemic patient before mephentermine is started, because hypovolemia should be corrected before initiating metaraminol therapy.
Administer IV infusions into a large vein, preferably of the antecubital fossa, to prevent extravasation.
Have phentolamine available in case extravasation occurs.
Ensure that atropine is readily available to treat reflex bradycardia.
Seek clarification if prescribed for SC administration because necrosis is likely to occur if given SC.
Do not infuse into veins of the ankle or dorsum of the hand in patients with peripheral vascular disease, diabetes mellitus, or hypercoagulability states.
Use microdrip IV administration set and an infusion control device to ensure accuracy. Monitor flow rate continuously.

Surveillance During Therapy

Withdraw drug gradually because severe hypotension often occurs after abrupt termination.
Monitor BP, pulse, and ECG constantly during IV administration (every 2 min until stabilized, then every 5–15 min for duration of drug action). Rate of infusion and duration of therapy are regulated according to patient response. Used to treat hemorrhagic shock only until blood volume is replaced.
Monitor intake and output because renal response may fluctuate. Monitor patient with cirrhosis for excessive water, sodium, and potassium loss because drug may cause diuresis.
Monitor for adverse effects and interactions.
Ascertain whether blood volume is to be corrected before initiating administration because response may be erratic when shock and acidosis coexist.
Interpret results of diagnostic tests and contact practitioner as appropriate.
Monitor for possible drug–drug and drug–nutrient interactions: use with cyclopropane or halogenated hydrocarbon anesthetics or digitalis may lead to arrhythmias; enhanced pressor effects with MAO inhibitors, tricyclic antidepressants, other sympathomimetics, and oxytocic drugs; risk of severe hypertension when used with *Rauwolfia* alkaloids, beta-blockers; decreases effectiveness of guanethidine.
Provide for patient safety needs and initiate interventions to minimize environmental hazards and risk of injury if CNS, visual, or hyperpyrexic side effects develop.

Patient Teaching

Because this drug is used only in acute emergency situations, teaching depends on patient's awareness and focuses on the patient's clinical condition rather than the drug itself.

• **Methoxamine** *(Pregnancy Category D)*

Vasoxyl

Mechanism

Direct alpha-adrenergic receptor stimulant, producing extensive vasoconstriction with little or no effects on the heart or the CNS; may induce reflex bradycardia, which is abolished by atropine; reduces renal blood flow.

Uses

Restoration or maintenance of BP during anesthesia
Termination of paroxysmal supraventricular tachycardia

Dosage

I. *Hypotension*
   A. IV: 3 to 5 mg by slow injection
   B. IM (usual route): 10 to 15 mg just before anesthesia; repeat if necessary in 15 minutes
II. *Paroxysmal supraventricular tachycardia*
   A. IV: 10 mg by slow injection

Fate

Onset is 10 to 15 minutes after IM injection; immediately with IV use; duration 1 to 2 hours; not distributed to CNS; excretion is by way of the kidneys.

Common Side Effects

Paresthesias, pilomotor stimulation, bradycardia, coldness in the extremities.

Significant Adverse Reactions

Sustained hypertension, urinary urgency, severe headache, and vomiting.

Contraindications

With local anesthetics to prolong their action; advanced cardiovascular disease. *Cautious use* in patients with hypertension, hyperthyroidism, or myocardial damage, and after parenteral injection of the ergot alkaloids.

Interactions

See metaraminol.

Nursing Management

See metaraminol.

• **Phenylephrine** *(Pregnancy Category D)*

Neo-Synephrine

Mechanism

Direct, powerful activation of alpha-adrenergic receptors, resulting in marked vasoconstriction and reflex bradycardia; little direct effect on the heart or the CNS; most vascular beds are constricted.

Uses

Maintenance of BP during spinal and inhalation anesthesia
Treatment of shock- or drug-induced hypotension
Treatment of paroxysmal supraventricular tachycardia

Production of vasoconstriction for regional analgesia (added to local anesthetic solution)

Dosage

I. *Hypotension*
   A. SC, IM: 2 to 5 mg of a 1% solution
   B. IV: 0.1 to 0.5 mg of a 0.1% solution (may repeat in 15 min)
   C. IV infusion: 100 to 200 drops/min of a 1:50,000 solution until pressure is stabilized, then 40 to 60 drops/min for maintenance
   D. Pediatric: 0.1 mg/kg SC or IM

II. *To prolong spinal anesthesia*: 2 to 5 mg added to anesthetic solution

III. *Tachycardia*: 0.5-mg IV injection over 20 to 30 seconds; may increase by 0.1-mg increments as needed

Fate

Rapid acting after injection; duration of effects is 20 to 30 minutes with IV and 45 to 90 minutes with SC and IM.

Common Side Effects

Palpitations, tingling in extremities, reflex bradycardia, and lightheadedness.

Significant Adverse Reactions

Tachycardia, arrhythmias, tremor, dizziness, hypertension, and weakness.

Contraindications

Severe hypertension, ventricular arrhythmias. *Cautious use* in patients with hyperthyroidism, myocardial damage, partial heart block, bradycardia, severe arteriosclerosis, and in elderly patients.

Interactions

See metaraminol.

Nursing Management

See metaraminol.

Nasal Decongestants

Certain adrenergic drugs are given via the oral or intranasal route to relieve nasal congestion. They provide a prompt decongestant effect—especially when applied topically to the nasal mucosa—by a direct vasoconstrictive action on mucosal arterioles; this action reduces local blood flow, fluid exudation, and mucosal edema. Tolerance to the decongestant effect develops rapidly, particularly with use of nasal sprays. Prolonged use often leads to "rebound congestion," a condition characterized by hyperemia and edema of the mucosal membrane that can result in a continual "runny nose." Rebound congestion can occur in as short a period as 1 week. Most of the clinically important nasal decongestants have a reasonably long duration of action and usually are used only twice a day. A general discussion of adrenergic nasal decongestants is accompanied by more specific prescribing information for each drug in Table 14-3.

Mechanism

Direct activation of alpha-adrenergic receptor sites on smooth muscle of the nasal mucosal blood vessels; vasoconstriction reduces engorgement of mucosa and fluid exudation, thereby relieving congestion; mucus secretion also may be reduced; orally effective nasal decongestants exert a more generalized vasoconstrictive action and a less intense nasal mucosal decongestant action.

Uses

Relief of nasal congestion associated with allergic reactions, colds, acute and chronic inflammatory states, and hay fever

Adjunctive therapy in middle ear infections (reduces congestion around eustachian tubes)

Relief of pressure and pain due to ear block during air travel

Dosage

See Table 14-3.

Fate

Topically applied drugs exert a rapid effect that persists for several hours, up to 12 hours; readily absorbed through mucous membranes; large doses may exert systemic effects.

Common Side Effects

Stinging and burning of the nasal mucosa, sneezing, dryness of mucosa, and headache; prolonged use results in rebound congestion.

Significant Adverse Reactions

Usually observed after systemic absorption of topically applied drugs or with oral use: palpitations, tachycardia, hypertension, arrhythmias, nervousness, insomnia, dizziness, blurred vision. Severe overdosage and significant absorption may cause marked somnolence, sedation, hypotension, bradycardia, and coma.

Contraindications

Narrow-angle glaucoma, use with MAO inhibitors or tricyclic antidepressants. *Cautious use* in the presence of hypertension, angina, hyperthyroidism, diabetes, and arteriosclerosis.

Interactions

Systemic effects may be potentiated by other sympathomimetics, MAO inhibitors, tricyclic antidepressants, antihistamines, and thyroxine.

Nursing Management

Pretherapy Assessment

Assess and record baseline data necessary for detection of adverse effects of nasal decongestants: General: VS, body weight, skin color and temperature; CVS: pulse, BP; GU: urine output; Laboratory: ECG.

Review medical history and documents for existing or previous conditions that:

a. require cautious use of nasal decongestants: hypertension (be aware that nasal decongestants can diminish effectiveness of antihypertensive therapy); angina; hyperthyroidism; diabetes; arteriosclerosis;

Table 14-3. **Nasal Decongestants**

Drug	*Usual Dosage Range*	*Nursing Considerations*
Desoxyephedrine *Vicks inhaler*	1 to 2 inhalations as needed	Avoid excessive use; headache may occur
Ephedrine *Kondon's Nasal, Pretz-D, Vicks Vatronol*	*Topical:* 2 to 3 drops of 0.5% or small amount of jelly every 3 to 4 h *Oral:* 25 to 50 mg every 3 to 4 h	Avoid swallowing nose drops because systemic effects may occur; do not use drops or jelly longer than 4 days; other uses are discussed under Bronchodilators, Table 14-5
Epinephrine *Adrenalin*	1 to 2 drops of 0.1% every 4 to 6 h	Do not use in children younger than 6 y; avoid prolonged or excessive use; *see also* epinephrine under Endogenous Catecholamines
Naphazoline *Privine*	2 drops or sprays of 0.05% each nostril every 3 to 6 h	Insomnia is not a problem, so drug may be given at bedtime; naphazoline is incompatible with aluminum; may produce CNS depression; ophthalmic drops also available; *see* Table 14-4
Oxymetazoline *Afrin, Dristan Long Lasting, Neosynephrine 12 Hour, Sinex Long Acting, and other manufacturers* *(CAN) Nafrine*	*Adults:* 2 to 3 drops or sprays of 0.05% twice a day *Children <6 y:* 2 to 3 drops of 0.025% twice a day	Long-acting preparation; do not exceed twice-a-day dosage; do not use in children younger than 2 y; limit usage to 14 days maximum
Phenylephrine *Several manufacturers*	*Adults:* 0.25% to 1.0% solution or spray every 3 to 4 h *Children (6–12 y):* 0.25% solution every 3 to 4 h *Infants:* 0.125% to 0.2% solution every 2 to 4 h	Available in five different strengths; do not use for prolonged periods, especially in children; avoid swallowing solution because systemic effects can occur
Phenylpropanolamine *Propagest*	*Adults:* 25 mg orally every 4 h *or* 50 mg every 8 h *or* 75 mg every 12 h *Children (6–12 y):* 12.5 mg every 8 h, (2–6 yr) 6.25 mg every 8 h	Do not exceed recommended dosage, especially in children, because side effects are likely to occur; reserpine can antagonize effects of phenylpropanolamine; also available over the counter as an anorexiant of questionable efficacy, either alone or in combination with caffeine
Propylhexedrine *Benzedrex Inhaler*	1 to 2 inhalations as needed	Do not overuse because CNS stimulation can occur; may induce headache and temporary elevation of blood pressure
Pseudoephedrine *Novafed, Sudafed, and several other manufacturers* *(CAN) Eltor-120, Maxenal, Robidrine*	*Adults:* 60 mg orally every 4 to 6 h *or* 120 mg every 12 h *Children:* 15 to 30 mg every 4 to 6 h	Fewer side effects, less pressor action, and longer duration than ephedrine; rebound congestion is minimal; avoid taking drug near bedtime because stimulation can occur; do not use if restlessness, dizziness, tremors, or other signs of CNS excitation are present
Tetrahydrozoline *Tyzine*	*Adults:* 2 to 4 drops 0.1% every 3 to 4 h *Children (2–6 y):* 2 to 3 drops 0.5% every 3 to 4 h	Large doses may induce CNS depression; not recommended in children younger than 2 y; ophthalmic drops also available; *see* Table 14-4
Xylometazoline *Otrivin* *(CAN) Sinutab Sinus Spray*	*Adults:* 2 to 3 drops or sprays every 8 to 10 h *Children:* 2 to 3 drops 0.05% every 8 to 10 h	Effects persist 4 to 8 h; do not use in aluminum containers; do not exceed recommended dosage because systemic effects are likely

prostatic hypertrophy; unstable vasomotor syndrome.

b. contraindicate use of nasal decongestants: hypersensitivity; MAO inhibitors; tricyclic antidepressants; narrow-angle glaucoma; severe hypertension; ventricular tachycardia; **pregnancy (Category C)**; labor, delivery; lactation (safety not established).

Nursing Interventions

Medication Administration

Instill drops with patient in lateral, head-low position to minimize possibility of swallowing solution and consequent systemic absorption.

Surveillance During Therapy

Monitor for adverse effects and toxicity.
Interpret results of diagnostic tests and contact practitioner as appropriate.
Monitor for possible drug–drug and drug–nutrient interactions: systemic effects potentiated by other sympathomimetics, MAO inhibitors, tricyclic antidepressants, antihistamines, and thyroxine; impairment of hypotensive effects of antihypertensives.
Provide for patient safety needs and initiate interventions to minimize environmental hazards and risk of injury if CNS, visual, or hyperpyrexic side effects develop.

Patient Teaching

Explain the importance of adhering to recommended dosage and avoiding prolonged treatment with topical nasal decongestants because rebound congestion is likely to occur. Suggest patient consult healthcare provider if relief is not obtained within 5 days.
Instruct patient to stop using drug and notify healthcare provider promptly if anxiety, irregular or very fast heartbeat, change in BP, or difficulty in breathing occurs (signs of developing systemic toxicity).
Teach patient to keep spray bottle upright to ensure that a fine mist is expelled rather than a liquid stream that can cause overdosage.
Instruct patient to blow nose before nasal instillation to clear nasal passages.
Instruct patient using an inhaler to close one nostril while inhaling through open nostril.
Instruct patient to rinse spray or dropper tip in hot water after nasal instillation to prevent contamination from nasal secretions. The same container should never be used for more than one person.

Ophthalmic Decongestants

Sympathomimetics are used in ophthalmology primarily to produce arteriolar vasoconstriction and pupillary dilation; these pharmacologic effects occur by means of their powerful activation of alpha$_1$-adrenergic receptors. The specific clinical use depends on the strength of the different preparations. The strongest solutions of phenylephrine (2.5% and 10%) and hydroxyamphetamine (1%) are used mainly in diagnostic eye examinations, during ocular surgery, and to prevent synechiae formation in uveitis. Medium-strength solutions of epinephrine (0.5%, 1%, and 2%) are indicated in open-angle glaucoma. Weaker solutions of epinephrine (0.1%), naphazoline (0.012% and 0.02%), phenylephrine (0.08%, 0.12%, and 0.15%), and tetrahydrazoline (0.05%) are principally used for symptomatic relief of minor eye irritations caused by, for example, allergies, colds, wind, and pollen. The weaker solutions are available as over-the-counter (OTC) preparations, whereas the stronger solutions require a prescription.

Unlike anticholinergic agents, sympathomimetic ophthalmic decongestants cause neither cycloplegia (ie, paralysis of accommodation) nor an increase in intraocular pressure (IOP). Because of their mydriatic effect, however, they—like anticholinergics—are contraindicated in *narrow-angle* glaucoma; dilation of the pupil would occlude the drainage channels and further reduce the exit of aqueous humor. A general review of this class of drugs is accompanied by a listing of individual drugs in Table 14-4.

Mechanism

Direct activation of alpha-adrenergic receptor sites leading to constriction of small blood vessels and contraction of the radial muscle, producing pupillary dilation (mydriasis); epinephrine also possesses a beta-adrenergic action, which decreases formation of aqueous humor.

Uses

Not all drugs used for each indication; see Table 14-4.

Facilitate examination of the fundus of the eye
Reduce the incidence of synechiae formation in uveitis
Treatment of open-angle glaucoma (increases outflow and decreases production of aqueous humor)
Symptomatic relief of minor eye irritations due to colds, hay fever, dust, wind, and so forth
Dilation of the pupil before intraocular surgery

Dosage

See Table 14-4.

Fate

Onset of mydriatic effect is rapid and persists for several hours.

Common Side Effects

Stinging and burning in the eyes, headache, and blurred vision.

Significant Adverse Reactions

Conjunctival irritation; pigmentation of the eyelids, cornea or conjunctiva; maculopathy with a central scotoma; systemic absorption of significant amounts may lead to palpitations, tachycardia, hypertension, anxiety, sweating, insomnia, dizziness, and pallor.

Contraindications

Narrow-angle glaucoma. *Cautious use* in patients with hypertension, heart disease, diabetes, or cerebral arteriosclerosis.

Interactions

Effects may be potentiated by MAO inhibitors, tricyclic antidepressants, or other sympathomimetic drugs.
Mydriatic effects can be reduced by levodopa.
Arrhythmias with digitalis drugs and halogenated hydrocarbon anesthetics (eg, cyclopropane, halothane) can occur in the presence of sympathomimetics, although the incidence with ophthalmic application is rare.

• Dipivefrin

Propine

Dipivefrin is a lipid-soluble *pro-drug* of epinephrine, that is, it is *converted* to epinephrine by enzymatic hydrolysis after being instilled into the eye. Because of its highly lipophilic nature, dipivefrin penetration into the cornea is much greater than that of epinephrine; onset of activity occurs within 30 minutes. Dipivefrin is indicated for the control of intraocular pressure in chronic open-angle glaucoma; its use is associated with fewer side effects than direct epinephrine therapy because less drug is

Table 14-4. **Ophthalmic Decongestants**

Drug	Usual Dosage Range	Nursing Considerations
Dipivefrin *Propine (An epinephrine prodrug)*	1 drop every 12 h	May produce burning and stinging on application
Epinephrine *Several manufacturers*	1 to 2 drops 0.1% to 0.25% individualized to condition	*See* general discussion of epinephrine
Hydroxyamphetamine *Paredrine*	1 to 2 drops of 1% as needed	Pupillary dilation persists for several hours; used for eye exams, ocular surgery, and uveitis
Naphazoline *Ak-Con, Albalon, Allerest, Clear-Eyes Comfort, Degest-2, Muro's Opcon, Nafazair, Naphcon, VasoClear, Vasocon*	1 to 2 drops every 3 to 4 h	Mainly used as an ocular decongestant; 0.012% to 0.05% solutions available over the counter, 0.1% by prescription only; available in combination with pheniramine (Naphcon-A) and antazoline (Vasocon-A)
Oxymetazoline *OcuClear Visine L.R.*	1 to 2 drops of 0.025% 2 to 4 times/day (at least 6 h apart)	Long-acting preparation; for pediatric use, child must be 7 y of age or older
Phenylephrine *Ak-Dilate, Ak-Nefrin, Isopto Frin, Mydfrin, Neo-Synephrine*	10%: uveitis, open-angle glaucoma, before intraocular surgery 2.5%: refraction, ophthalmic exams 0.02% to 0.15%: ocular decongestion, relief of minor eye irritations	Do not use 10% solution in children; prior instillation of a local anesthetic in the eye may alleviate much of the stinging and burning caused by phenylephrine; the 2.5% solution may be used as a diagnostic test for narrow-angle glaucoma; also available over the counter combined with zinc sulfate (eg, Zincfrin), or by prescription only combined with pyrilamine (Prefrin-A); drug has a narrow safety margin; may cause rebound miosis in the elderly; readministration may be less effective
Tetrahydrozoline *Collyrium Fresh Eye Drops, Eyesine, Murine Plus, Optigene 3, Soothe, Visine*	1 to 2 drops of 0.05% up to 4 times/day	Mainly used to relieve minor symptoms of eye irritation; available without prescription

required (because of better absorption). The therapeutic response to twice-daily administration of dipivefrin approximately equals that of 2% pilocarpine given four times a day and, unlike with pilocarpine, miosis and cycloplegia (characteristic of cholinergic drugs) do not occur. The response is somewhat less than that produced by 2% epinephrine. Because of its mydriatic action, dipivefrin, like epinephrine, is contraindicated in narrow-angle glaucoma.

Adverse reactions associated with dipivefrin therapy are similar to those noted for ophthalmic epinephrine administration, but occur less often. Burning and stinging after instillation are the most common side effects. In addition, the systemic effects (tachycardia, increased BP, arrhythmias) that can develop after ocular administration of epinephrine also can develop with dipivefrin (see Table 14-4 for dosage).

Nursing Management

Pretherapy Assessment

Assess and record baseline data necessary for detection of adverse effects of ophthalmic decongestants: General: VS, body weight, skin color and temperature; CVS: pulse, BP; GU: urine output; Laboratory: ECG.

Review medical history and documents for existing or previous conditions that:

a. require cautious use of ophthalmic decongestants: hypertension (be aware that ophthalmic decongestants can diminish effectiveness of antihypertensive therapy); angina; hyperthyroidism; arteriosclerosis; prostatic hypertrophy; unstable vasomotor syndrome.
b. contraindicate use of ophthalmic decongestants: hypersensitivity; MAO inhibitors; tricyclic antidepressants; narrow-angle glaucoma; severe hypertension; ventricular tachycardia; **pregnancy (Category C)**; labor, delivery; lactation (safety not established).

Nursing Interventions

Medication Administration

Check concentration of drops carefully before administration. Stronger concentrations (2.5%–10%) are used for diagnostic eye examinations and during ocular surgery; intermediate strengths (0.5%–2%) are used to treat glaucoma; and weaker concentrations (0.05%–0.1%) are used to treat minor eye irritations.

Surveillance During Therapy

Monitor for adverse effects and toxicity.

Interpret results of diagnostic tests and contact practitioner as appropriate.

Monitor for possible drug–drug and drug–nutrient interactions: systemic effects potentiated by other sympathomimetics, MAO inhibitors, tricyclic antidepressants, antihistamines, and thyroxine; impairment of hypotensive effects of antihypertensives; mydriatic effects reduced by levodopa.

Provide for patient safety needs and initiate interventions to minimize environmental hazards and risk of injury if CNS, visual, or hyperpyrexic side effects develop.

Patient Teaching

Instruct patient to adhere to recommended dosage because systemic absorption can occur.

Inform older patient that blurred vision (ie, rebound miosis) can occur within 1 day after termination of drug use. If the drug is used again, it may be less effective in eliciting mydriasis.

Advise patient that some preparations may stain contact lenses.

Instruct patient to discard cloudy or discolored solution.

Bronchodilators

Sympathomimetic bronchodilators are used in the treatment of bronchial asthma and other chronic obstructive pulmonary diseases (COPDs). Parenteral (ie, SC, IM) injections of epinephrine usually are effective in relieving respiratory distress (dyspnea, wheezing, chest tightness) during an acute asthmatic attack. Some patients, however, respond poorly to epinephrine during an acute attack; such patients often are successfully treated by IV infusion of aminophylline, a xanthine bronchodilator discussed in Chapter 57. Continual symptomatic management of chronic asthma may be accomplished with oral or inhaled use of one of the adrenergic bronchodilators, although several other types of drugs (eg, theophylline, corticosteroids, ipratropium, cromolyn) may be used as well. These other drugs also are considered in Chapter 57.

Sympathomimetic agents used as bronchodilators possess prominent beta-adrenergic activity that elicits relaxation of the smooth muscle of the bronchioles. This action is primarily caused by an elevation in the levels of cyclic AMP resulting from activation of the enzyme adenylyl cyclase, which catalyzes formation of cyclic AMP from adenosine triphosphate (ATP).

Some drugs in this category (epinephrine, isoproterenol) activate all beta-adrenergic receptor sites, and their use often is associated with a disturbing range of side effects, particularly involving cardiac stimulation. Other adrenergic bronchodilators (eg, albuterol, metaproterenol) exhibit a greater degree of selectivity with regard to the $beta_2$ receptors located on bronchiolar smooth muscle, and thus elicit a lower incidence of cardiac side effects, although *complete* separation of $beta_1$ and $beta_2$ activity still has not been realized, especially at elevated doses. The relative popularity of the adrenergic bronchodilators is determined by many factors, including the type and severity of the condition being treated, practitioner preference, patient acceptance, and cost. Epinephrine and isoproterenol are potent bronchodilators whose use is somewhat restricted by their tendency to cause a considerable amount of cardiac excitation in many patients. They have been discussed previously in this chapter. Ephedrine is a less potent bronchodilator that exhibits more pronounced central excitatory effects than other adrenergic drugs. It is discussed in the following section, as is ethylnorepinephrine, another nonselective beta agonist. Finally, the selective $beta_2$ agonists are considered as a group and listed in Table 14-5. Other types of drugs used as bronchodilators (eg, theophylline) are discussed in Chapter 57.

There is mounting evidence that the *chronic* administration of inhaled adrenergic bronchodilators is unsafe. Increased morbidity and mortality have been reported in some studies after repeated, frequent use of these products. Their use should be closely monitored, and patients requiring frequent dosing of these products should be reevaluated and appropriate changes made in their therapeutic regimen if necessary.

• Ephedrine

Mechanism

Direct activation of both alpha- and beta-adrenergic receptor sites; indirect action through release of norepinephrine from presynaptic nerve terminals; effects include tachycardia, increased BP and cardiac output, mydriasis, and relaxation of bronchiolar and GI smooth muscle; bronchodilation is less intense than that produced by epinephrine but is more prolonged; central stimulatory effects are more pronounced than with epinephrine. Contracts urinary sphincter; may potentiate cholinergic neurotransmission at the neuromuscular junction.

Uses

Bronchodilation in milder forms of chronic pulmonary diseases (eg, bronchial asthma, bronchitis)

Relief of nasal mucosal congestion (see Table 14-3).

Maintenance of BP during spinal anesthesia, and control of postural hypotension (injection only)

Treatment of enuresis (with atropine)

Treatment of narcolepsy

Support of ventricular rate in Adams-Stokes syndrome

Adjunctive treatment of myasthenia gravis (with cholinesterase inhibitor)

Dosage

Adults: 25 to 50 mg PO, SC, IM, or slow IV injection every 3 to 4 hours as necessary (not to exceed 150 mg/24 h).

Children: 2 to 3 mg/kg/day in 4 to 6 divided doses PO, SC, or IV.

Fate

Readily absorbed orally or parenterally; onset of bronchodilation is 30 minutes orally and 10 minutes IM or SC; effects persist 3 to 5 hours orally and 1 to 2 hours IM or SC; crosses blood-brain barrier and exerts a central stimulating effect; excreted largely unchanged in the urine.

Common Side Effects

Similar to epinephrine; in addition, nervousness, anxiety, and insomnia due to central stimulatory properties are common.

Significant Adverse Reactions

Tachycardia, confusion, delirium, tremors (usually observed with large doses); vertigo, sweating, palpitations, urinary retention, arrhythmias; CNS and respiratory depression can occur with overdosage.

Contraindications

Narrow-angle glaucoma, patients receiving MAO inhibitors, severe hypertension, or severe coronary artery disease. *Cautious*

Table 14-5. **Selective $Beta_2$-Adrenergic Bronchodilators**

Drug	Usual Dosage Range	Nursing Considerations
Albuterol *Proventil, Ventolin* *(CAN) Novo-Salmol, Ventodisk, Volmax*	*Inhalation:* 1 to 2 inhalations every 4 to 6 h *Prevention of exercise-induced bronchospasm:* 2 inhalations 15 min before exercise *Oral:* 2 mg to 4 mg 3 to 4 times/day (maximum 32 mg/day) Children (2–6 y): 0.1 mg/kg 3 times/day Children (6–14 y): 2 mg 3 or 4 times/day	Gradually absorbed from the bronchioles; onset occurs within 15 min after inhalation and persists for 3 to 4 h; with oral use, onset is 30 min and effects persist for 4 to 6 h; most common side effects are nervousness and tremor (20%), headache (7%), and tachycardia (5%); may delay preterm labor; drug has displayed a tumorogenic potential in animals at high doses; do not use with other sympathomimetic drugs (danger of increased CV side effects)
Bitolterol *Tornalate*	2 inhalations at an interval of 1 to 3 min; a third inhalation may be given if necessary Prevention of bronchospasm: 2 inhalations every 8 h	Used for prophylaxis or treatment of bronchospasm; effects occur within 5 min and persist up to 8 h; may be used with theophylline or corticosteroids
Isoetharine *Arm-a-Med Isoetharine, Beta-2, Bronkometer, Bronkosol*	*Solution:* 3 to 7 inhalations of undiluted solution by a hand nebulizer *or* 0.25 to 0.5 mL of a 0.5% or 1% solution diluted 1:3 with saline or other diluent (lower-strength solutions are given undiluted) by oxygen aerosolization or IPPB apparatus *Aerosol nebulizer:* 1 to 2 inhalations as needed	Relaxes bronchial smooth muscle by an action on $beta_2$ receptors; also may inhibit histamine release; can be administered by IPPB apparatus—see package instructions; do not use if solution is brown or contains a precipitate; avoid contact with the eyes; oxygen flow rate is adjusted to 4 to 6 L/min over 15 to 20 min for oxygen aerosolization; pediatric dosage has not been established
Metaproterenol *Alupent, Metaprel*	*Oral:* Adults: 20 mg 3 or 4 times/day Children (6–9 y): 10 mg 3 or 4 times/day Children (<6 y): 1.3 to 2.6 mg/kg/day *Inhalation:* 10 inhalations of 5% solution by hand nebulizer or 2 or 3 inhalations of metered-dose aerosol inhaler every 3 to 4 h to a maximum of 12 inhalations/day	Effects appear almost immediately with inhalation and within 15 to 30 min orally. Duration is 2 to 4 h with inhaler and 4 to 5 h orally; nervousness, tremor, and weakness are common with oral administration of 20 mg; bad taste can occur with oral inhalation but will gradually disappear with repeated use; overdose can lead to cardiac arrest; encourage adherence to prescribed dose
Pirbuterol *Maxair*	2 inhalations every 4 to 6 h (maximum 12 inhalations/day)	Rapid-acting bronchodilator; effects occur within 5 min; duration of action is 5 to 6 h
Salmeterol *Serevent*	2 inhalations twice daily, 12 h apart	Longest acting sympathomimetic bronchodilator; onset of action is 20–30 min; effects persist for up to 12 h; may be used together with corticosteroids; effective in controlling nocturnal asthmatic attacks.
Terbutaline *Brethaire, Brethine, Bricanyl*	*Oral:* Adults: 2.5 to 5 mg 3 times/day (maximum 15 mg/day) Children >12 y: 2.5 mg 3 times/day *SC:* 0.25 mg; repeat in 15 to 30 min if needed; if no response after 2 doses, seek alternate measures *Aerosol:* 2 inhalations, 1 min apart, every 4 to 6 h	Slowly absorbed orally and parenterally. Effects appear within 15 to 30 min and persist 2 to 4 h with SC injection, up to 6 h with inhalation, and 4 to 8 h with oral administration; muscle tremor common with 5-mg oral dose; cardiovascular side effects more common with SC injection

IPPB, intermittent positive pressure breathing.

use in people with chronic heart disease, diabetes, hypertension, and hyperthyroidism.

Interactions

Pressor effects may be increased by ergot alkaloids, MAO inhibitors, furazolidone, and oxytocics.
Ephedrine may reduce the action of guanethidine.
Ephedrine may be less effective in the presence of methyldopa or reserpine.
Arrhythmias can occur if used in combination with halothane and related anesthetics or digitalis drugs.

Nursing Management

Pretherapy Assessment

Assess and record baseline data necessary for detection of adverse effects of ephedrine: General: VS, body weight, skin color and temperature; CNS: orientation, reflexes, peripheral sensation, vision; CVS: pulse, BP, peripheral perfusion; GU: urine output, bladder percussion, prostate palpation.
Review medical history and documents for existing or previous conditions that:
a. require cautious use of ephedrine: hypertension; hyperthyroidism; arteriosclerosis; prostatic hypertrophy; unstable vasomotor syndrome.
b. contraindicate use of ephedrine: hypersensitivity; narrow-angle glaucoma; MAO inhibitors; tricyclic antidepressants; thyrotoxicosis; severe hypertension; ventricular tachycardia; diabetes; **pregnancy (Category C)**; labor and delivery (may accelerate fetal heart rate, avoid use in women whose BP exceeds 130/80); lactation (safety not established).

Nursing Interventions

Medication Administration

Monitor BP frequently until patient is stabilized when drug is given IV.
Clarify prescription of prolonged-acting forms of high dosages for the elderly because they are more prone to develop hallucinations, convulsions, and CNS depression.

Surveillance During Therapy

Monitor for adverse effects and toxicity.
Interpret results of diagnostic tests and contact practitioner as appropriate.
Monitor for possible drug–drug and drug–nutrient interactions: systemic effects potentiated by other sympathomimetics, MAO inhibitors, tricyclic antidepressants, furazolidone, and oxytocics; impairment of hypotensive effects of antihypertensives.
Provide for patient safety needs and initiate interventions to minimize environmental hazards and risk of injury if CNS, visual, or hyperpyrexic side effects develop.

Patient Teaching

Explain the importance of adhering carefully to recommended dosage because central stimulatory effects can lead to abuse.
Inform patient that drug effects may diminish with prolonged use. A drug-free interval of several days may be needed to restore effectiveness.
Suggest that patient discuss insomnia with drug prescriber if it becomes a problem. Nighttime doses and long-acting preparations should be avoided if possible.
Instruct patient to avoid OTC preparations while taking this drug, because serious hypertensive interaction can occur.
Instruct the patient as to the types of side effects expected: dizziness, weakness, restlessness, lightheadedness, tremor, urinary retention.
Instruct patient regarding side effects, which if experienced should be reported to the practitioner: nervousness; palpitations; sleeplessness; sweating.
Urge older patient to notify drug prescriber immediately if difficulty in urinating occurs.

• Ethylnorepinephrine

Bronkephrine

Ethylnorepinephrine is an adrenergic bronchodilator similar in most respects to isoproterenol. It primarily activates beta-adrenergic receptor sites; its alpha effect is considerably less than that of epinephrine, hence the effect on BP is less marked.

The principal application of ethylnorepinephrine is relief of bronchospasm; however, it usually is reserved for acute attacks, inasmuch as it must be administered IM or SC. Onset of action is 5 to 10 minutes, and effects last 1 to 2 hours. The adult dose is 1 to 2 mg (0.5–1.0 mL), whereas children receive 0.1 to 0.5 mL according to weight. Refer to the discussion of isoproterenol earlier in this chapter for additional information.

• Selective Beta$_2$ Agonists

The selective beta$_2$ bronchodilators preferentially activate beta$_2$ receptor sites on bronchiolar and other smooth muscle at normal dosage levels, leading to relaxation. The absence of significant beta$_1$ receptor activity at recommended dosage reduces the degree of cardiac excitability frequently observed with nonselective beta agonists such as isoproterenol or epinephrine. When beta agonists are administered by inhalation, bronchodilation is comparable to that seen with isoproterenol. Certain beta$_2$ agonists are also available for oral or parenteral use for either acute (SC) or long-term (oral) symptomatic management of bronchial asthma. The beta$_2$ agonists are reviewed as a group, then detailed individually in Table 14-5.

Mechanism

In recommended doses, preferentially activate beta$_2$-adrenergic receptors, thereby relaxing bronchiolar, vascular, and uterine smooth muscle to varying degrees; action at cardiac beta$_1$ receptors is generally minimal, thus tachycardia and increased cardiac output rarely are significant.

Uses

Relief of reversible bronchospasm associated with asthma and other bronchospastic disorders
Delay premature labor

Dosage

See Table 14-5.

Fate

Inhaled drugs have a rapid onset of action, generally within 5 minutes; after oral or SC administration, effects are noted within 15 to 30 minutes; duration of action ranges from 2 to 4 hours with inhalation (up to 8 hours with bitolterol); effects persist 4 to 8 hours after oral administration; excretion is largely by the kidney, both as unchanged drug and metabolites.

Common Side Effects

Usually with oral dosage: nervousness, mild tremor, flushing, sweating, irritability, insomnia, headache, weakness.

Significant Adverse Reactions

Palpitations, tachycardia, arrhythmias, increased BP, dysuria, nausea, muscle cramping, coughing, chest discomfort, pulmonary edema and death (in women receiving ritodrine for management or preterm labor).

Contraindications

Tachyarrhythmias, severe coronary artery disease; use in combination with halogenated hydrocarbon general anesthetics. *Cautious use* in patients with mild to moderate coronary artery disease, hypertension, hyperthyroidism, diabetes; also in elderly or debilitated patients.

Interactions

Effects of selective $beta_2$ agonists may be potentiated by other sympathomimetics, MAO inhibitors, and tricyclic antidepressants, and inhibited by nonselective beta-adrenergic blocking agents (see Chapter 15).

Nursing Management

Pretherapy Assessment

Assess and record baseline data necessary for detection of adverse effects of selective $beta_2$ agonists: General: VS, body weight, skin color and temperature; CNS: orientation, reflexes; CVS: pulse, BP; Laboratory: blood and urine glucose, serum electrolytes, thyroid function tests, ECG.

Review medical history and documents for existing or previous conditions that:

a. require cautious use of selective $beta_2$ agonists: hypertension; hyperthyroidism; arteriosclerosis; prostatic hypertrophy; unstable vasomotor syndrome.

b. contraindicate use of selective $beta_2$ agonists: hypersensitivity; tachyarrhythmias; severe coronary artery disease; diabetes; **pregnancy (Category C)**; labor, delivery (oral use has delayed second stage of labor, parenteral use can accelerate fetal heart rate, cause hypoglycemia, hypokalemia, pulmonary edema in the mother, hypoglycemia in the neonate); lactation (safety not established, tumorigenicity in animals, nursing mothers should avoid these drugs).

Nursing Interventions

Medication Administration

Assess cardiovascular status periodically because toxicity can occur when drug is used parenterally. Specificity for $beta_2$ sites is observed principally after oral administration.

Ensure that administration times are alternated if more than one sympathomimetic agent is prescribed. Excessive tachycardia can occur if more than one drug is administered at the same time.

Seek clarification before administering more than two SC injections 15 to 30 minutes apart. Other measures should be used if patient does not respond to second injection.

Use minimal doses for minimal periods of time because drug tolerance can occur.

Provide small, frequent meals if GI upset occurs.

Surveillance During Therapy

Monitor for adverse effects.

Interpret results of diagnostic tests and contact practitioner as appropriate.

Monitor for possible drug–drug and drug–nutrient interactions: systemic effects potentiated by other sympathomimetics, MAO inhibitors, tricyclic antidepressants, and inhibited by nonselective beta-adrenergic blocking agents; increased risk of toxicity, especially cardiac when used in combination with theophylline derivatives; decreased effectiveness of insulin and oral hypoglycemics.

Patient Teaching

Explain the importance of adhering carefully to recommended dosage because central stimulatory effects can lead to abuse.

Inform patient that drug effects may diminish with prolonged use. A drug-free interval of several days may be needed to restore effectiveness.

Suggest that patient discuss insomnia with drug prescriber if it becomes a problem. Nighttime doses and long-acting preparations should be avoided if possible.

Instruct patient to avoid OTC preparations while taking this drug, because serious hypertensive interaction can occur.

Instruct the patient as to the types side effects expected: dizziness, weakness, restlessness, lightheadedness, tremor, urinary retention.

Teach patient how to administer an aerosol dose.

Stress the importance of adhering to recommended dosage and frequency of use because excess use can result in drug toxicity with serious complications such as acute asthmatic crisis or cardiac arrest.

Instruct patient to use only one inhaled medication at a time unless others are specifically prescribed.

Instruct patient to notify drug prescriber and stop using drug immediately if breathing difficulty increases with drug use, because severe side effects can develop. Increased airway resistance (paradoxical bronchospasm) sometimes develops after repeated use.

Advise patient to notify prescriber if usual dose does not provide relief for a sufficient period. Prolonged use may lead to shorter duration of action (tolerance).

Inform patient that a bad taste can occur with oral inhalation, but this will gradually disappear with repeated use.

Instruct patient regarding side effects, which if experienced should be reported to the practitioner: nervousness; palpitations; sleeplessness; sweating.

Urge older patient to notify drug prescriber immediately if difficulty in urinating occurs.

Smooth Muscle Relaxants

The ability of several adrenergic drugs to relax smooth muscle has led to their use in treating peripheral vascular insufficiency and premature labor.

Isoxsuprine is an orally effective sympathomimetic that exhibits a beta-adrenergic receptor agonistic action. Activation of $beta_2$ receptor sites in skeletal muscle vasculature can lead to vasodilation of normal vessels; however, the vasodilator effects of isoxsuprine on muscle blood flow are *not* prevented by beta-blockers. Thus, it probably also exerts a direct relaxant effect on vascular smooth muscle in addition to its beta-agonistic action. Although blood flow in normal resting skeletal muscle can be increased by isoxsuprine, there is no conclusive evidence that it has a beneficial effect in chronic occlusive vascular conditions such as arteriosclerosis or thromboangiitis obliterans. Skeletal muscle and cerebral vascular beds probably are dilated by reflexes stimulated by ischemia resulting from a vascular occlusion. This means that peripheral vasodilator drugs primarily increase blood supply to *nondilated, nonischemic* areas that are not in critical need of improved perfusion. Further compromising the efficacy of peripheral vasodilators is the fall in BP that frequently accompanies their administration. Thus, their hypotensive effect actually may *reduce* cerebral blood flow and perfusion of vital organs. Therefore, use of isoxsuprine for treating peripheral and cerebral vascular insufficiency should be discouraged.

Isoxsuprine also has been used to delay premature labor, because it exerts a relaxant effect on uterine smooth muscle. Its effects are nonselective, however, and side effects secondary to beta receptor activation elsewhere in the body are frequent. Use of isoxsuprine as a uterine relaxant has been largely supplanted by ritodrine, another beta agonist that exerts a somewhat more selective effect on $beta_2$ receptors in the uterus. These two sympathomimetic smooth muscle relaxants are discussed in the following section.

• Isoxsuprine

Vasodilan

Mechanism

Activation of beta-adrenergic receptor sites on vascular smooth muscle, diminishing vascular resistance, and increasing resting blood flow in skeletal muscles; also exerts a direct relaxant effect on vascular smooth muscle; exhibits some alpha-adrenergic blocking action, and high doses may inhibit platelet aggregation and lower blood viscosity; increases heart rate and contractile force and relaxes uterine smooth muscle.

Uses

Clinical effectiveness has not been demonstrated conclusively.

Symptomatic treatment of peripheral vascular insufficiency (eg, Raynaud's disease, thromboangiitis obliterans) or cerebrovascular insufficiency

Treatment of dysmenorrhea, premature labor, and threatened abortion (experimental uses only)

Dosage

Orally: 10 to 20 mg 3 or 4 times/day.

Fate

Peak effects occur in about 1 hour and persist 2 to 3 hours; largely excreted in the urine.

Common Side Effects

Lightheadedness, lethargy, and flushing.

Significant Adverse Reactions

Hypotension (primarily orthostatic), palpitations, tachycardia, dizziness, nausea, anxiety, abdominal distress, vomiting, and rash.

Contraindications

Arterial bleeding; immediate postpartum use. *Cautious use* in patients with coronary artery insufficiency, thyrotoxicosis, paroxysmal tachycardia, also after a myocardial infarction.

Interactions

Effects may be antagonized by other sympathomimetic drugs (particularly those possessing significant alpha activity).

Nursing Management

Pretherapy Assessment

Assess and record baseline data necessary for detection of adverse effects of isoxsuprine: General: VS, body weight, skin color and temperature; CNS: orientation, reflexes; CVS: pulse, BP, peripheral perfusion.

Review medical history and documents for existing or previous conditions that:

a. require cautious use of isoxsuprine: coronary artery insufficiency, thyrotoxicosis, paroxysmal tachycardia, recent myocardial infarction.
b. contraindicate use of isoxsuprine: allergy to isoxsuprine; hypotension; arterial bleeding; use in the immediate postpartum period; **pregnancy (Category C)**; lactation (safety not established, nursing mothers should avoid these drugs).

Nursing Interventions

Medication Administration

Assess peripheral vascular status periodically. People with extensive circulatory impairment may not respond to the drug. Inform practitioner if condition deteriorates (eg, numbness, coldness, paresthesias).

Carefully monitor pattern of contractions when drug is used for relief of premature labor (experimental use only). Dosage and rate of administration are adjusted accordingly.

Monitor BP and pulse in standing and lying positions frequently during treatment, especially with IM use.

Provide small, frequent meals if GI upset occurs.

Surveillance During Therapy

Monitor for adverse effects and toxicity.

Monitor pulse, BP, orthostatic BP with long-term use.
Interpret results of diagnostic tests and contact practitioner as appropriate.
Monitor for possible drug–drug and drug–nutrient interactions: effects may be antagonized by other sympathomimetic drugs (particularly those with strong alpha-adrenergic activity).
Provide for patient safety needs if CNS effects or hypotension occur.

Patient Teaching

Teach measures to help control postural hypotension if it occurs.
Instruct patient to notify drug prescriber promptly at first sign of a skin rash or fainting, chest pain, shortness of breath.
Teach patient about the types of side effects expected with therapy: flushing, palpitations, dizziness, weakness, dizziness on changing positions.
Inform patient that beneficial effects may not appear for several weeks. They usually are indicated by cessation of numbness, coldness, or tingling in the extremities.
Teach patient how to care for feet and legs (hygiene, measures to minimize trauma).
Teach adjunctive measures that may help alleviate condition (eg, exercise, cessation of smoking, proper footwear).

• Ritodrine

Yutopar

Ritodrine is a fairly selective $beta_2$-adrenergic receptor agonist that can inhibit uterine contractions. It is used in the management of premature labor. It is administered initially by IV infusion to arrest contractions, then orally for as long as necessary to prolong pregnancy to the desired extent. Its overall toxicity is somewhat lower than that of other agents used in premature labor (alcohol, magnesium sulfate, isoxsuprine).

Mechanism

Activates $beta_2$ receptor sites on uterine smooth muscle, thus reducing the contractile response; also affects $beta_1$ receptors when given in larger doses, resulting in tachycardia and BP changes.

Uses

Management of preterm labor in suitable patients, if the gestation is longer than 20 weeks.

Dosage

Initially, 0.1 mg/min by IV infusion. May be increased by 50 mg/min every 10 minutes to a maximum of 350 mg/min. Continue infusion for 12 hours after labor has ceased. Administer an oral dose of 10 mg 30 minutes before terminating infusion, then 10 mg every 2 hours for 24 hours, then 10 to 20 mg every 4 to 6 hours for as long as necessary. Maximum oral dose is 120 mg/day.

Fate

Oral bioavailability is approximately 30% of IV dose. Maximum serum levels after oral ingestion occur in 30 to 60 minutes; effective half-life is 1.5 to 2 hours; metabolized in the liver and excreted primarily in the urine, 90% within 24 hours; crosses placental barrier.

Common Side Effects

Especially with IV infusion: alterations in maternal and fetal heart rates and BP, transient elevations in blood glucose and insulin levels, hypokalemia, palpitations, nausea, tremors, headache, and erythema.

Significant Adverse Reactions

Especially with IV infusion: vomiting, anxiety, nervousness, chest pain, arrhythmias, dyspnea, sweating, chills, weakness, diarrhea, bloating, rash, anaphylactic shock, lactic acidosis, glycosuria, possibly fatal pulmonary edema.

Contraindications

Before the 20th week of pregnancy, any condition of mother or fetus in which continuation of pregnancy is dangerous (eg, antepartum hemorrhage, fetal death, eclampsia, pulmonary hypertension), cardiac arrhythmias, severe bronchial asthma, and pheochromocytoma. *Cautious use* in people with hypertension, diabetes, or cardiac disease.

Interactions

Combined administration of ritodrine and corticosteroids may lead to potentially fatal pulmonary edema.
Effects of other adrenergic amines may be potentiated by ritodrine.
Nonselective beta-blockers reduce the effectiveness of ritodrine.
Ritodrine may increase the diuretic-induced hypokalemia

Nursing Management

Pretherapy Assessment

Assess and record baseline data necessary for detection of adverse effects of ritodrine: General: VS, body weight, skin color and temperature; CNS: orientation, reflexes; CVS: pulse, BP, peripheral perfusion; Laboratory: thyroid function tests.
Review medical history and documents for existing or previous conditions that:
a. require cautious use of ritodrine: hypertension; cardiac disease; diabetes.
b. contraindicate use of ritodrine: allergy to ritodrine, components of the ritodrine formulation (metabisulfite); **pregnancy (Category B)**; lactation (safety not established, nursing mothers should avoid this drug).

Nursing Interventions

Medication Administration

Administer oral drug 1 hour before or 2 hours after meals; food may interfere with absorption.
Be prepared to initiate IV infusion if labor recurs during oral drug therapy.
Seek clarification if prescribed earlier than the 20th week of gestation because many fetuses are abnormal when labor begins before this time.
Discard solution if it is discolored, cloudy, or contains a precipitate.

Provide small, frequent meals if GI upset occurs.

Surveillance During Therapy

Closely monitor maternal pulse rate and BP as well as fetal heart rate, and observe for indications of maternal pulmonary edema (chest pain, dyspnea, sweating).
Carefully monitor infusion rate to avoid circulatory overload. Use an infusion control device if available.
Monitor for toxicity.
Interpret results of diagnostic tests and contact practitioner as appropriate.
Monitor for possible drug–drug and drug–nutrient interactions: combined use with corticosteroids may lead to pulmonary edema; potentiates effects of other adrenergic amines; effectiveness reduced by nonselective beta-blockers; may increase diuretic induced hypokalemia.
Provide for patient safety needs if CNS effects or hypotension occur.

Patient Teaching

Teach measures to help control postural hypotension if it occurs.
Instruct the patient to avoid OTC preparations.
Instruct patient to notify practitioner promptly at first sign of a skin rash; severe weakness; trembling; irregular heartbeat; shortness of breath; chest pain.
Instruct patient to report the development of palpitations. If they do not subside during therapy, dosage should be reduced.
Teach patient about the types of side effects expected with therapy: dizziness, weakness, trembling, nervousness.
Instruct patient to keep these drugs and all medications out of the reach of children.

Central Nervous System Stimulants and Anorexiants

The principal adrenergic drugs used for their central stimulatory effects are the amphetamine derivatives and ephedrine. The major indications for these compounds are control of obesity (reduction of appetite; anorexiant), relief of depression, and treatment of the attention deficit disorder syndrome in children. Because of their strong central excitatory action, they are a widely abused class of drugs. These agents are discussed in Chapter 29, and aspects of their abuse potential are reviewed in Chapter 82.

A number of products containing phenylpropanolamine, a sympathomimetic decongestant, in amounts ranging from 25 to 75 mg, are promoted as OTC nonprescription diet aids (eg, Acutrim, Control, Dexatrim, Prolamine). Many of these preparations contain other substances as well, such as vitamins, minerals, and grapefruit extract. Phenylpropanolamine is claimed to produce its anorexiant effect by a central action at the level of the appetite control center in the hypothalamus. Many health professionals doubt its efficacy as an appetite suppressant, however, and use of the drug, especially at high dosages, should be strictly controlled. Because of its cardiac-stimulating and BP-elevating effects, phenylpropanolamine should not be used by patients with cardiovascular disease, hypertension, diabetes, hyperthyroidism, glaucoma, or renal impairment. Combined use with other sympathomimetics, MAO inhibitors, and tricyclic antidepressants also should be avoided. In addition, because of its central stimulatory effect, coupled with the fact that it is readily available OTC, it often is abused. Phenylpropanolamine administration must be discontinued at once should palpitations, dizziness, or rapid pulse occur. Recommended doses are 25 mg phenylpropanolamine three times a day or 50 to 75 mg of the long-acting preparations once daily. Continuous use for longer than 3 months is not recommended. The drug must be used in conjunction with a restricted caloric intake.

Selected Bibliography

Cheung D, Timmers MC, Zwinderman AH, Bel EH, Dijkman JH, Sterk PJ: Long-term effects of a long-acting beta$_2$-adrenoceptor agonist, salmetrol, on airway hyperresponsiveness in patients with mild asthma. N Engl J Med 327:1198, 1992
Fukuda T, Dohi S, Naito H: Comparisons of tetracaine spinal anesthesia with clonidine or phenylephrine in normotensive and hypertensive humans. Anesth Analg 78:106, 1994
Kozlik-Feldmann R, Kramer H-H, Wicht H, Feldmann R, Netz H, Reinhardt D: Distribution of myocardial beta-adrenoceptor subtypes and coupling to the adenylate cyclase in children with congenital heart disease and implications for treatment. J Clin Pharmacol 33:588, 1993
Montastruc JL, Rascol O, Senard JM: Current status of dopamine agonists in Parkinson's disease management. Drugs 46(3):384, 1993
Moutquin J-M: Treatment of preterm labor with the beta-adrenergic agonist ritodrine: The Canadian Preterm Labor Investigators Group. N Engl J Med 327:308, 1992
Schteingart DE: Effectiveness of phenylpropanolamine in the management of moderate obesity. Int J Obes 16:487, 1992
Stein M, Deegan R, Wood AJJ: Long-term exposure to beta$_2$-receptor agonist specifically desensitizes beta-receptor-mediated venodilation. Clin Pharmacol Ther 54:187, 1993

Nursing Bibliography

Levin R: Advances in pediatric drug therapy of asthma. Nursing Clinics of North America 26(2):263–272, 1991

15 Adrenergic Blocking Agents

Alpha-Adrenergic Blocking Agents

Nonselective

- Phenoxybenzamine
- Phentolamine
- Tolazoline

Selective

Alpha$_1$

- Doxazosin
- Prazosin
- Terazosin

Alpha$_2$

- Yohimbine

Beta-Adrenergic Blocking Agents

Nonselective

- Carteolol
- Levobunolol
- Metipranolol
- Nadolol
- Penbutolol
- Pindolol
- Propranolol
- Sotalol
- Timolol

Selective (Beta$_1$)

- Acebutolol
- Atenolol
- Betaxolol
- Bisoprolol
- Esmolol
- Metoprolol

Alpha and Beta-Blocking Agent

- Labetalol

Drugs that antagonize the actions of neurotransmitters released from sympathetic nerve endings (eg, norepinephrine, epinephrine) at adrenergic receptor sites in body tissues are termed *adrenergic blocking agents*; they also are effective antagonists of exogenously administered adrenergic drugs.

Reflecting the accepted classification of adrenergic receptor sites into alpha and beta types, adrenergic receptor blockers also are divided into alpha-adrenergic and beta-adrenergic blocking agents. Adrenergic blocking drugs, however, have been developed with greater selectivity, that is, ability to block alpha and beta receptor *subtypes*. Thus, whereas some alpha blockers (eg, phentolamine, tolazoline) are *nonselective* (block both alpha$_1$ and alpha$_2$ receptors), others (eg, doxazosin, prazosin and terazosin) are *selective* (ie, block alpha$_1$ sites). Similarly, beta-adrenergic blocking agents can be grouped into nonselective antagonists (block beta$_1$ *and* beta$_2$ sites) such as nadolol, propranolol, pindolol, and timolol, and selective antagonists (ie, block only beta$_1$ sites) such as atenolol and metoprolol. This greater selectivity reduces some adverse reactions associated with nonselective adrenergic blockade.

Alpha-Adrenergic Blocking Agents

Drugs that block alpha-adrenergic receptor sites are termed *alpha blockers*. Nonselective alpha blockers act primarily on those alpha$_1$ sites located postsynaptically on vascular smooth muscle to antagonize the vasopressor (vasoconstrictive) effects of epinephrine and norepinephrine. They also block alpha$_2$ sites on the presynaptic membrane of sympathetic nerve endings, an action that can result in an increased release of neurotransmitters. In addition, some nonselective alpha blockers exert a direct relaxant effect on vascular smooth muscle that contributes to the peripheral vasodilation seen with these drugs. They also exert a cardiac stimulant action that may cause tachycardia. Conversely, some newer agents selectively block either alpha$_1$ or alpha$_2$ receptors.

Nonselective Alpha Blockers

• Phenoxybenzamine

Dibenzyline

Mechanism

Long-acting, essentially noncompetitive irreversible alpha-adrenergic blockade exerted at both presynaptic alpha$_2$ and postsynaptic alpha$_1$ sites; forms stable covalent bond with receptor site, possibly inducing structural alterations; increases blood flow to skin, mucosa, and viscera; induces orthostatic hypotension; may exhibit antihistaminic and antiserotonin activity at high dosages.

Uses

Control hypertension and sweating associated with pheochromocytoma

Investigational uses include symptomatic treatment of neurogenic bladder and prostatic obstruction

Dosage

Individually titrated to obtain symptomatic relief with minimal side effects. Initially: 10 mg orally twice daily. Increase by 10 mg every 4 days. Usual range 20 to 40 mg 2 to 3 times a day (may require several weeks to obtain optimal effect).

Fate

Oral absorption is erratic (20%–30% absorbed in active form); peak effects occur in 4 to 6 hours; may accumulate in adipose tissue at high dosages; excreted largely through the kidney and bile, mostly within 24 hours.

Common Side Effects

Lightheadedness, nasal congestion, dryness of the mouth, flushing, tachycardia, miosis, and gastrointestinal (GI) irritation if given on empty stomach.

Significant Adverse Reactions

Dizziness, orthostatic hypotension, weakness, failure of ejaculation; overdosage can cause vomiting, central nervous system (CNS) stimulation, and shock.

Contraindications

Congestive heart failure or other conditions when a drop in blood pressure might be dangerous. *Cautious use* in the presence of cerebral, coronary, or renal insufficiency.

Interactions

May increase blood pressure–lowering effects of antihypertensive agents.

May enhance the hypotensive and cardiac stimulant effects of epinephrine.

Nursing Management

Pretherapy Assessment

Assess and record baseline data necessary for detection of adverse effects of phenoxybenzamine: General: VS, body weight, skin color and temperature; CNS: orientation, reflexes, ophthalmic examination; Cardiovascular system (CVS): orthostatic BP, supine BP, peripheral perfusion, edema; GI: bowel sounds, normal output.

Review medical history and documents for existing or previous conditions that:

a. require cautious use of phenoxybenzamine: presence of cerebral, coronary, or renal insufficiency.

b. contraindicate use of phenoxybenzamine: allergy to phenoxybenzamine; conditions where a drop in BP is dangerous (congestive heart failure, myocardial infarction, angina); **pregnancy (Category C)**; lactation (safety not established, nursing mothers should avoid this drug).

Nursing Interventions

Medication Administration

Oral drug may be administered with or without food.

Provide ready access to bathroom facilities if GI effects occur.

Provide small, frequent meals if GI upset occurs.

Surveillance During Therapy

Monitor BP and heart rate and rhythm in both erect and recumbent positions during periods of dosage adjustment and for at least 4 days thereafter. Dosage should not be increased sooner than 4 days after previous increase.

Keep patient flat for 24 hours if severe hypotension occurs and norepinephrine infusion is used; apply abdominal binder and support hose or bandages to legs as necessary. Epinephrine should *not* be used because a further drop in blood pressure can occur owing to unmasking of the beta effect.

Use precautions for postural hypotension.

Monitor patient for signs of clinical improvement (eg, increased skin color and temperature, less sensitivity to cold). In patients with pheochromocytoma, reductions in BP and pulse are indications of effectiveness.

Monitor for toxicity.

Interpret results of diagnostic tests and contact practitioner as appropriate.

Monitor for possible drug–drug and drug–nutrient interactions: may increase BP-lowering effects of antihypertensive agents; may enhance the hypotensive, cardiac-stimulant effects of epinephrine.

Provide for patient safety needs if CNS effects or hypotension occur.

Patient Teaching

Teach measures to help control postural hypotension if it occurs.

Instruct the patient to avoid over-the-counter (OTC) preparations.

Inform patient that palpitations, rapid heart rate, and postural hypotension will disappear with continued therapy.

Inform patient that beneficial effects may not appear for several weeks.

Suggest taking drug with meals to minimize GI irritation.

Warn patient that symptoms of respiratory infection may be aggravated by the drug and must be treated with appropriate therapy. The healthcare provider should be contacted for treatment.

Instruct patient to notify practitioner promptly at first sign of a skin rash; increased heart rate; rapid weight gain; unusual swelling of the extremities; difficulty in breathing, especially when lying down; new or aggravated symptoms of angina (chest, arm, or shoulder pain); severe indigestion; dizziness, lightheadedness, or fainting.

Teach patient about the types of side effects expected with therapy: dizziness when changing position; drowsiness, fatigue; GI upset; nasal stuffiness; constricted pupils and difficulty with far vision; inhibition of ejaculation.

• Phentolamine

Regitine

(CAN) Rogitine

Mechanism

Reversible, competitive antagonism at presynaptic and postsynaptic alpha receptor sites and direct relaxant action on vascular smooth muscle; decreases peripheral vascular resistance and pulmonary pressure; slightly increases heart rate and cardiac output; GI motility may be stimulated (parasympathomimetic action), and secretion of pepsin and hydrochloric acid (histamine-like action) can be increased.

Uses

Control of hypertension in patients with pheochromocytoma during stress periods and before or during surgical excision of tumor

Prevention of tissue necrosis and sloughing associated with extravasation of norepinephrine or other vasopressors

Investigational uses include treatment of hypertensive crises due to monoamine oxidase (MAO) inhibitor interactions or rebound hypertension after withdrawal of antihypertensive drugs

Dosage

Hypertension: intravenous (IV), intramuscular (IM)—5 mg (adults), 1 mg (children)

Prevent necrosis: 10 mg added to each liter IV infusion *or* 5 to 10 mg in 10 mL saline infiltrated into area within 12 hours

Fate

Onset is rapid after IV or IM use; effects persist for 15 minutes with IV use and several hours after IM injection; excreted largely as metabolites in the urine.

Common Side Effects

Flushing, nasal congestion, and GI distress.

Significant Adverse Reactions

Usually after parenteral use: tachycardia, hypotension, arrhythmias, anginal pain, myocardial infarction, shock, and cerebrovascular occlusion.

Contraindications

Recent myocardial infarction, coronary insufficiency, and angina. *Cautious use* in patients with peptic ulcer, gastritis, coronary artery disease, or congestive heart failure.

Interactions

See phenoxybenzamine.

Nursing Management

Pretherapy Assessment

Assess and record baseline data necessary for detection of adverse effects of phentolamine: General: VS, body weight, skin color and temperature; CNS: orientation, reflexes, ophthalmic examination; CVS: orthostatic BP, supine BP, peripheral perfusion, edema; GI: bowel sounds, normal output.

Review medical history and documents for existing or previous conditions that:

a. require cautious use of phentolamine: presence of cerebral, coronary, or renal insufficiency; peptic ulcer; gastritis.

b. contraindicate use of phentolamine: allergy to phentolamine, conditions in which a drop in BP is dangerous (congestive heart failure, myocardial infarction, angina); **pregnancy (Category C)**; lactation (safety not established, nursing mothers should avoid this drug).

Nursing Interventions

Medication Administration

Oral drug may be administered with or without food.

Provide ready access to bathroom facilities if GI effects occur.

Provide small, frequent meals if GI upset occurs.

Surveillance During Therapy

Keep patient supine while drug is given IV. Monitor BP and pulse frequently until stabilized. Overdosage should be treated vigorously and promptly.

Monitor BP and heart rate and rhythm in both erect and recumbent positions during periods of dosage adjustment and for at least 4 days thereafter. Dosage should not be increased sooner than 4 days after previous increase.

Keep patient flat for 24 hours if severe hypotension occurs and norepinephrine infusion is used; apply abdominal binder and support hose or bandages to legs as necessary. Epinephrine should *not* be used because a further drop in BP can occur owing to unmasking of the beta effect.

Use precautions for postural hypotension.

Monitor patient for signs of clinical improvement (eg, increased skin color and temperature, less sensitivity to cold). In patients with pheochromocytoma, reductions in BP and pulse are indications of effectiveness.

Monitor for toxicity.

Interpret results of diagnostic tests and contact practitioner as appropriate.

Monitor for possible drug–drug and drug–nutrient interactions: may increase BP-lowering effects of antihypertensive agents; may enhance the hypotensive, cardiac-stimulant effects of epinephrine.

Provide for patient safety needs if CNS effects or hypotension occur.

Patient Teaching

Teach measures to help control postural hypotension if it occurs.

Instruct the patient to avoid OTC preparations.

Inform patient that palpitations, rapid heart rate, and postural hypotension will disappear with continued therapy.

Inform patient that beneficial effects may not appear for several weeks.

Suggest taking drug with meals to minimize GI irritation.

Warn patient that symptoms of respiratory infection may be aggravated by the drug and must be treated with appropriate therapy. The healthcare provider should be contacted for treatment.

Instruct patient to notify practitioner promptly at the first sign of a skin rash; increased heart rate; rapid weight gain; unusual swelling of the extremities; difficulty in breathing, especially when lying down; new or aggravated symptoms of angina (chest, arm, or shoulder pain); severe indigestion; dizziness, lightheadedness, or fainting.

Teach patient about the types of side effects expected with therapy: dizziness when changing position; drowsiness, fatigue; GI upset; nasal stuffiness; constricted pupils and difficulty with far vision; inhibition of ejaculation.

• Tolazoline

Priscoline

Mechanism

Reversible, nonselective blockade of alpha-adrenergic receptor sites and direct relaxant effect on vascular smooth muscle; also exhibits significant beta-adrenergic activity (increased cardiac rate, force, and output), cholinergic activity (increased GI motility), and histaminergic activity (increased gastric secretions).

Uses

Adjunctive management of persistent pulmonary hypertension in the newborn when sufficient oxygenation cannot be maintained by usual supportive care.

Dosage

Pulmonary hypertension: 1 to 2 mg/kg through scalp vein; follow with infusion of 1 to 2 mg/kg/h until arterial oxygen has risen sufficiently; the response, if it occurs, is evident within 30 minutes after the first dose; little experience with infusions lasting more than 36 to 48 hours.

Fate

Excreted largely unchanged by the kidney.

Common Side Effects

Flushing, tingling or loss of sensation in extremities, nausea, and reflex tachycardia.

Significant Adverse Reactions

Arrhythmias, anginal pain, orthostatic hypotension, ulcer-like pain, vomiting, epigastric distress, duodenal perforation, apprehension, rash, edema, oliguria, hematuria, pulmonary hemorrhage.

Contraindications

Patients hypersensitive to tolazoline.

Interactions

See phenoxybenzamine.

Nursing Management

See phentolamine. In addition:

Assess status of patient's skin periodically: Flushing in extremities, increased temperature, and piloerection indicate optimal dosage.

Place patient flat if hypotension occurs because of overdosage. The best treatment consists of IV fluids and infusion of ephedrine, not epinephrine or norepinephrine

Selective Alpha$_1$ Blockers

Certain newer alpha antagonists (doxazosin, prazosin, and terazosin) selectively block postsynaptic alpha$_1$ receptor sites on blood vessels; this action causes dilation of both arterioles and veins. Blood pressure is reduced even when the patient is supine. A significant hypotensive effect can occur during the initial doses; this phenomenon is termed the "first-dose" effect. These drugs are indicated for treatment of hypertension, either alone or combined with other antihypertensive drugs. Further information about these drugs is found in Chapter 33.

Selective Alpha$_2$ Blockers

• Yohimbine

Aphrodyne, Yocon, Yohimex

Yohimbine is the only available drug that selectively blocks presynaptic alpha$_2$ sites, receptors that reduce the release of catecholamines—especially norepinephrine. Thus, blockade of alpha$_2$ receptors promotes an *increased* release of catecholamines, primarily norepinephrine at peripheral sites. The mechanism of action of yohimbine is complex because the drug also appears to increase peripheral cholinergic activity; in addition, yohimbine has central stimulatory activity that can produce excitation, elevated BP and heart rate, irritability, and tremor. Other side effects include decreased urination, dizziness, and skin flushing.

Conclusive clinical data are lacking, but yohimbine has been used for treatment of orthostatic hypotension and impotence (especially when this sexual dysfunction may be caused by vascular problems, such as observed in patients with diabetes). The dose is 1 tablet (5.4 mg) 3 times a day. Yohimbine should not be used in patients with renal dysfunction or a history of GI ulcers, or in geriatric or psychiatric patients. It also is not recommended for use in children or pregnant women. Concurrent administration with other mood-altering drugs (eg, antidepressants, antipsychotics) may increase the incidence of adverse CNS effects.

Beta-Adrenergic Blocking Agents

Drugs that produce a reversible, competitive blocking action at beta-adrenergic receptor sites can antagonize the effects of catecholamines released from both adrenergic nerve endings and the adrenal medulla. Beta-blocking agents effectively reduce the myocardial stimulant, vasodilator, bronchodilator, and metabolic (glycogenolytic, lipolytic) actions of the catecholamines.

Beta-blockers may be classified as nonselective or selective. *Nonselective* beta antagonists (eg, carteolol, levobunolol, nadolol, pindolol, propranolol, sotalol, timolol) block both beta$_1$ and beta$_2$ receptor sites; *selective* beta-blockers (eg, acebutolol, betaxolol, esmolol, metoprolol) *predominantly* block beta$_1$ receptors. The selectivity of certain drugs for cardiac beta$_1$ sites is both relative and dose dependent; that is, in high concentrations, their beta-blocking action may extend to beta$_2$ receptors such as those in the bronchioles.

All available beta receptor blockers are effective competitive antagonists at beta receptors, but differences exist in the properties of the individual drugs. A brief comparison of some of the pharmacologic and pharmacokinetic properties of the beta-blockers is presented in Table 15-1. Labetalol, a combined beta and alpha blocker, is included in the table but is considered in greater detail in Chapter 33, because it is used exclusively as an antihypertensive agent. Esmolol, a rapid-acting beta-blocker used to control excessive heart rate, also is discussed along with the other beta-blockers.

Additional details relating to their therapeutic uses (eg, antianginal, antihypertensive, antiarrhythmic) can be found in the relevant chapters. A listing of approved and investigational uses of beta-blockers is presented in Table 15-2. Although the beta-blockers are discussed as a group, characteristics of individual drugs are noted where differences are important. Beta-blockers are individually listed in Table 15-3 with their respective dose ranges and other pertinent information.

Mechanism

Reversible competitive blocking action at beta-adrenergic receptor sites (see Table 15-1 for site specificity), resulting in decreased heart rate and force of contraction, slowed atrioventricular conduction, decreased plasma renin, and lowered BP; a quinidine-like membrane-stabilizing action is exhibited by propranolol and to a lesser extent by metoprolol and pindolol. Pindolol and carteolol also possess intrinsic sympathomimetic

Table 15-1. **Pharmacologic and Pharmacokinetic Properties of Beta-Blockers**

Drug	*Receptor Activity*	*Oral Absorption*	*Protein Binding*	*Elimination Half-Life*	*Membrane-Stabilizing Activity**	*Intrinsic Sympathomimetic Activity**
Acebutolol	$Beta_1$	90%	25%	3–4 h	0	+
Atenolol	$Beta_1$	50%	5%–15%	6–9 h	0	0
Betaxolol	$Beta_1$	99%	50%	14–22 h	0	+
Bisoprolol	$Beta_1$	90%	30%	9–12 h	0	0
Carteolol	$Beta_1$, $beta_2$	80%	20%–30%	6 h	0	+ +
Esmolol	$Beta_1$		50%–60%	10–20 min	0	0
Labetalol†	$Beta_1$, $beta_2$	100%	50%	6–8 h	+	0
Levobunolol	$Beta_1$, $beta_2$	(ophthalmic use only)				
Metipranolol	$Beta_1$, $beta_2$	(ophthalmic use only)				
Metoprolol	$Beta_1$	95%–100%	10%–15%	3–6 h	+	0
Nadolol	$Beta_1$, $beta_2$	30%	30%	20–24 h	0	0
Penbutolol	$Beta_1$, $beta_2$	95%–100%	80%–100%	4–6 h	0	+
Pindolol	$Beta_1$, $beta_2$	95%–100%	40%–50%	3–4 h	+	+ + +
Propranolol	$Beta_1$ $beta_2$	90%–100%	90%–95%	3–6 h	+ +	0
Sotalol	$Beta_1$, $beta_2$		0	12 h	0	0
Timolol	$Beta_1$, $beta_2$	100%	50%	6–8 h	0	0

* Refer to the discussion of mechanism of beta-blockers in the text for an explanation of these characteristics.
† Also possesses $alpha_1$ blocking activity and $beta_2$ agonistic activity.

activity and consequently reduce the heart rate less than other beta-blockers. Central effects of beta-blockers are exerted at the level of the vasomotor center in the brain stem to retard the outflow of tonic sympathetic nerve impulses. In the eye, beta-blockers reduce formation of aqueous humor without inducing miosis or hyperemia. Platelet aggregation may be impaired, possibly through inhibition of thromboxane A_2 synthesis.

Dosage

See Table 15-3.

Fate

Oral absorption usually is good for most beta-blockers. First-pass hepatic metabolism is significant for acebutolol, metoprolol, propranolol, and timolol; thus, interpatient plasma levels vary widely for these agents. Food enhances the bioavailability of propranolol and metoprolol. Protein binding is minimal with the exception of penbutolol and propranolol. Acebutolol, atenolol, carteolol, and nadolol do not readily pass the blood–brain barrier because their lipid solubility is low. Carteolol and nadolol are excreted largely unchanged by the kidney. The remaining beta-blockers are metabolized in the liver and are excreted as metabolites and unchanged drug by the kidney. Elimination half-lives range between 3 to 9 hours; longer-acting agents include betaxolol (14–22 hours), nadolol (20–24 hours), and sotalol (12 hours).

Common Side Effects

Not all effects seen with all drugs: drowsiness, lightheadedness, lethargy, nausea, paresthesias, cramping, and bradycardia.

Significant Adverse Reactions

Not all reactions seen with all drugs:

CV: tachyarrhythmias, chest pain, atrioventricular (AV) block, sinoatrial block, peripheral arterial insufficiency, pulmonary edema, syncope, cerebrovascular accident, cardiac failure
CNS: (decreased incidence with acebutolol, atenolol, carteolol, and nadolol) dizziness, vertigo, depression, weakness, behavioral disturbances, agitation, disorientation, memory loss, emotional instability, sleep disturbances, bizarre dreams, hallucinations, catatonia
GI: diarrhea, vomiting, gastric pain, anorexia, bloating, dry mouth, ischemic colitis, hepatomegaly
Respiratory: bronchospasm, dyspnea, cough, rales, nasal congestion
Musculoskeletal: joint pain, muscle cramping

Table 15-2. **Approved and Investigational Uses for Beta-Blockers**

Indication	Drugs
Approved Uses	
Angina	Atenolol, metoprolol, nadolol, propranolol
Arrhythmias	Acebutolol, esmolol, propranolol, sotalol
Glaucoma	Carteolol, betaxolol, levobunolol, metipranolol, timolol
Hypertension	*All except* esmolol, levobunolol, metipranolol, sotalol
Hypertrophic subaortic stenosis	Propranolol
Migraine prophylaxis	Propranolol, timolol
Myocardial infarction	Betaxolol, metoprolol, propranolol, timolol
Pheochromocytoma	Propranolol
Tremor, essential	Propranolol

Investigational Uses

One or more of the beta-blockers has been reported to be of benefit in the following conditions:

Aggressive behavior	Anxiety (eg, "stage fright")	Schizophrenia/acute panic episodes
Akathisia (induced by antipsychotics)	Gastric bleeding in portal hypertension	Thyrotoxicosis
Alcohol withdrawal	Rebleeding from esophageal varices in patients with cirrhosis	
Angina pectoris		

Dermatologic: rash, pruritus, skin irritation, sweating, dry skin, increased pigmentation

Other: hypoglycemia, alopecia, acute pancreatitis, agranulocytosis, thrombocytopenia, eosinophilia, urinary difficulty, fever, sore throat, psoriasis-like rash, blurred vision; elevated blood urea nitrogen, serum transaminase, alkaline phosphatase, and lactic dehydrogenase

Contraindications

Sinus bradycardia, greater than first-degree heart block, right ventricular failure, severe congestive heart failure, cardiogenic shock, in combination with drugs potentiating adrenergic amines (such as MAO inhibitors or tricyclic antidepressants); in addition, nonselective beta-blockers are contraindicated in bronchial asthma. *Cautious use* in patients with nonallergic bronchospasm (eg, chronic bronchitis, emphysema), peripheral vascular insufficiency, history of allergies, allergic rhinitis (especially during the pollen season), impaired renal or hepatic function, diabetes, or myasthenia gravis.

Interactions

Beta-blockers can have additive cardiac-depressant effects with digitalis, phenytoin, verapamil, and quinidine.

The effects of beta-blockers can be reversed by norepinephrine, isoproterenol, dopamine, dobutamine, and other sympathomimetic drugs.

Plasma levels of propranolol and possibly other beta-blockers can be elevated by chlorpromazine, cimetidine, furosemide, and hydralazine.

Beta-blockers can antagonize the bronchodilating action of theophylline and may reduce its clearance.

The hypotensive action of beta-blockers can be increased by diuretics and other antihypertensives, and reduced by indomethacin or salicylates.

Phenobarbital and phenytoin can reduce plasma levels of beta-blockers metabolized in the liver by accelerating their hepatic metabolism.

Beta-blockers may prolong insulin-induced hypoglycemia and mask the symptoms of lowered blood glucose.

Beta-adrenergic blockade may increase the incidence of the first-dose orthostatic hypotensive response to prazosin (see Chapter 31).

Propranolol or metoprolol may decrease the clearance of lidocaine.

Beta-blockers may enhance the muscle-relaxing actions of neuromuscular blocking agents.

Nursing Management

Pretherapy Assessment

Assess and record baseline data necessary for detection of adverse effects of beta-adrenergic blockers: General: VS, body weight, edema, skin color, and temperature; CNS: orientation, reflexes, vision, hearing; CVS: peripheral perfusion; GI: bowel sounds, normal output; Genitourinary: bladder palpation; Laboratory: liver and thyroid function tests, blood and urine glucose.

Review medical history and documents for existing or previous conditions that:

a. require cautious use of beta-adrenergic blockers: nonallergic bronchospasm (chronic bronchitis, emphysema); peripheral vascular insufficiency; history of allergies; allergic rhinitis; impaired renal or hepatic function; diabetes; myasthenia gravis.

b. contraindicate use of beta-adrenergic blockers: allergy to beta-adrenergic blockers, sinus bradycardia; second- or third-degree heart block; cardiogenic shock; congestive heart failure; MAO inhibitors; tricyclic antidepressants; bronchial asthma (nonselective agents); thyrotoxicosis; **pregnancy (Category**

Table 15-3. **Beta-Adrenergic Blocking Agents**

Drug	*Usual Dosage Range*	*Nursing Considerations*
Acebutolol *Sectral* *(CAN) Monitan, Rhotral*	*Hypertension:* Initially 400 mg daily in 1 single or 2 divided doses; usual maintenance dose range is 400–800 mg daily *Ventricular arrhythmias:* 200 mg twice a day initially; increase gradually until optimal response; usual dosage range is 600–1200 mg daily	Selective $beta_1$ blocker used for hypertension and controlling ventricular premature beats; may be taken without regard to meals; reduce dosage in elderly people because plasma levels are higher; use cautiously in impaired renal or hepatic function; low lipid solubility; does not significantly pass blood–brain barrier
Atenolol *Tenormin* *(CAN) Apo-Atenol, Novo-Atenol, Nu-Atenol*	*Hypertension:* Initially, 50 mg once a day; increase to 100 mg once a day if necessary after 1–2 wk *Angina:* 50 mg once a day; may increase to 100 mg once a day if necessary	Long-acting, selective $beta_1$ antagonist; minimal protein binding; dosage may have to be reduced in patients with significant renal failure because drug is excreted unchanged in the urine; does not pass blood–brain barrier; long half-life allows once-daily dosing—drug should be taken same time every day; available with chlorthalidone as Tenoretic
Betaxolol *Betoptic, Kerlone*	*Hypertension:* 10 mg once a day *Glaucoma:* 1 drop of 0.5% twice a day	Used for treating ocular hypertension and chronic open-angle glaucoma; may be given alone or in combination with other antiglaucoma drugs; onset of action is 30 min and effects persist up to 12 h; little effect on pupil size or accommodation; discomfort and tearing may occur on instillation; virtually devoid of systemic side effects
Bisoprolol *Zebeta*	*Hypertension:* 5 mg once a day; may be increased to a maximum of 20 mg daily	Long-acting, selective $beta_1$ blocker; use with caution in patients with hepatic or renal dysfunction; available with hydrochlorothiazide (6.25 mg) as Ziac
Carteolol Oral: *Cartrol* Ophthalmic: *Ocupress*	*Hypertension:* 2.5–5 mg once daily *Glaucoma:* 1 drop twice a day	Nonselective beta-blocker used for treatment of mild to moderate hypertension and chronic open-angle glaucoma; possesses intrinsic sympathomimetic activty, thus heart rate and cardiac output are reduced to a smaller extent than with most other beta-blockers; excreted largely unchanged in the urine—caution in people with kidney impairment
Esmolol *Brevibloc*	*Supraventricular tachycardia:* 50–200 μg/kg/min after a loading dose infusion of 500 μg/kg/min for 1 min	Short-acting cardioselective beta blocker indicated for rapid control of ventricular rate in patients with atrial fibrillation or flutter where short-term control of ventricular rate is desirable; usually administered for 24–48 h; venous irritation is associated with infusion concentrations greater than 10 mg/mL; rapidly metabolized by enzymes in red blood cells; plasma half-life is 10–15 min
Labetalol *Normodyne, Trandate*	*Hypertension:* *Oral:* Initially, 100 mg twice a day; increase in 100-mg twice-daily increments until desired response; usual maintenance dose is 200–400 mg, twice daily *IV:* 20 mg by slow IV injection initially; repeat at 10-min intervals with 40 or 80 mg to a maximum of 300 mg; *or* 2 mg/min of a 1-mg/mL dilution by IV infusion to a maximum of 300 mg (usual dosage range is 50–200 mg)	Combined nonselective beta blocker and $alpha_1$ blocker; may also exhibit $beta_2$ agonistic activity; used as an antihypertensive in both acute (IV) and chronic situations; does not elicit marked changes in heart rate, renal function, or cardiac output; postural hypotension can occur; complete discussion of the drug is found in Chapter 33
Levobunolol *Betagan Liquifilm*	*Glaucoma:* 1 drop of 0.25% or 0.50% in affected eye(s) 1 or 2 times/day	Long-acting, nonselective beta blocker; frequently causes stinging and burning on instillation
Metipranolol *OptiPranolol*	1 drop of 0.30% in affected eye(s) twice a day	Causes discomfort on instillation; also may induce local allergic reactions and headache; larger doses do *not* appear to provide increased effect
Metoprolol *Lopressor, Toprol XL* *(CAN) Apo-Metoprolol, Betaloc, Novo-Metoprol, Nu-Metop*	*Hypertension:* Initially, 50 mg orally, twice a day; increase at weekly intervals until optimum effect is attained; usual maintenance dose is 100 mg twice a day (range 100–450 mg/day)	Selective $beta_1$ blocker; well absorbed orally but undergoes significant first-pass hepatic metabolism; weakly protein bound; readily enters the CNS; if twice-daily administration does not provide sufficient blood pressure control owing to short half-life of drug, give 3 times/day in divided doses; ingestion of food enhances oral absorption; during early phase of myocardial

(continued)

Table 15-3. **Beta-Adrenergic Blocking Agents (Continued)**

Drug	Usual Dosage Range	Nursing Considerations
	Myocardial infarction: Three IV bolus injections of 5 mg each at 2-min intervals; then 50 mg orally every 6 h thereafter for 48 h, then 100 mg twice a day *Angina:* 100 mg/day in 2 divided doses; may increase to 400 mg/day	infarction, treatment should be initiated as soon as possible; if immediate IV administration is not possible or not tolerated, begin oral therapy (100 mg twice/day) as soon as clinical condition allows; treatment may be continued for months if deemed beneficial; prevention of reinfarction is most dramatic in patients suffering first infarction and presenting with left ventricular failure, cardiomegaly, or atrial fibrillation
Nadolol *Corgard* *(CAN) Apo-Nadol, Syn-Nadolol*	*Hypertension:* Initially, 40 mg once daily; increase gradually in 40–80 mg increments; usual dosage range 40–80 mg once daily; maximum dose is 320 mg/day *Angina:* Initially, 40 mg once daily; increase at 3–7 day intervals until desired effect; usual dosage range is 40–80 mg once daily; maximum dose is 240 mg/day	Long-acting, nonselective beta blocker; does not enter CNS; excreted essentially unchanged by kidney, therefore dosage may need to be reduced in renal failure; presence of food does not affect rate or extent (approximately 30%) of absorption; if drug is to be discontinued, taper dosage gradually over 1–2 wk; do not administer more often than once a day
Penbutolol *Levatol*	*Hypertension:* 20 mg once daily	Nonselective beta agonist used for treating mild to moderate hypertension; effects occur within 2–4 wk; larger doses do not seem to provide greater antihypertensive effect
Pindolol *Visken* *(CAN) Apo-Pindol, Novo-Pindol, Nu-Pindol, Syn-Pindolol*	*Hypertension:* Initially 5 mg 2 or 3 times/day; adjust dosage at 2–3-week intervals in increments of 10 mg to obtain desired reduction in pressure; maximum dose is 60 mg/day	Nonselective beta antagonist with intrinsic sympathomimetic activity, thus exhibits slightly less slowing of heart rate than other beta blockers; rapidly absorbed orally; peak plasma levels in 1 h; short acting; excreted both as unchanged drug and metabolites; no significant first-pass hepatic metabolism; use is frequently associated with slight weight gain
Propranolol *Inderal* *(CAN) Apo-Propranolol, Novo-Pranol, PMS Propranolol*	*Hypertension:* Initially, 40 mg twice a day *or* 80 mg sustained-release (SR) once daily; increase gradually until desired response; usual dosage range is 120–240 mg/day in 2 or 3 divided doses *or* 120–160 mg SR once daily *Angina:* Initially, 10–20 mg 3 or 4 times/day *or* 80 mg SR once daily; increase at 3–7-day intervals; usual dose is 160 mg/day in single or divided doses *Arrhythmias:* 10–30 mg 3 or 4 times/day *Hypertrophic subaortic stenosis:* 20–40 mg 3 or 4 times day *or* 80–160 mg once daily *Migraine:* Initially, 80 mg once daily or in divided doses; usual dosage range is 160–240 mg/day	Widely used, nonselective beta blocker; well absorbed orally (food enhances absorption), but undergoes extensive first-pass hepatic metabolism, and variations in plasma levels among patients are wide; highly protein bound; excreted largely as metabolites in urine; if treatment of angina is to be discontinued, reduce dose gradually because severe angina or myocardial infarction can be precipitated by abrupt termination; if a satisfactory response in treatment of migraine is not achieved within 4–6 wk after reaching the maximum dose (ie, 240 mg/day), drug should be discontinued; IV injection should be undertaken with extreme caution, and central venous pressure and ECG closely monitored; transfer to oral therapy as soon as possible
Sotalol *Betapace*	*Initial:* Orally, 160 mg/day in 2 divided doses; may increase to 320 mg/day	Nonselective beta-blocker used for treatment of documented *life-threatening* ventricular arrhythmias; *not* recommended for asymptomatic ventricular arrhythmias; 2–3 days should elapse between dose increments; arrhythmias may occur initially and with *each* dose increase (see also Chapter 32)
Timolol Oral: *Blocadren* Ophthalmic: *Timoptic* *(CAN) Apo-Timol (oral), Apo-Timop (ophthalmic)*	*Oral:* *Hypertension:* Initially, 10 mg twice a day; usual maintenance range is 20–40 mg/day in 2 divided doses *Myocardial infarction:* 10 mg twice a day for long-term prophylaxis after acute phase *Ophthalmic:* *Glaucoma:* 1 drop of 0.25%–0.5% solution twice a day	Nonselective beta antagonist used orally for hypertension, as prophylaxis after an acute myocardial infarction, and as eye drops for the management of chronic open-angle glaucoma; oral absorption is good and protein binding is minimal; oral drug is short acting and may have to be given 3 times/day if response is inadequate; effects in eye begin in 30 min, peak in 1–2 h, and persist up to 24 h; do not give more than 1 drop 0.5% twice a day; add other antiglaucoma drugs if necessary (see Chapter 12); when used intraocularly, systemic effects can occur frequently, especially with prolonged use; systemic absorption can be minimized by instructing patients to press gently on the lacrimal duct after drug administraton; ocular use is contraindicated in patients with bradycardia, second- or third-degree heart block, congestive heart failure, pulmonary edema, or bronchial asthma

C); lactation (secreted in breast milk, safety not established, nursing mothers should avoid this drug).

Nursing Interventions

Medication Administration

Before initiating administration, determine whether patient has any condition (eg, asthma, allergies, congestive heart failure) that might be aggravated by beta-blockers.
Use infusion control device and carefully monitor electrocardiogram and BP when drugs are administered IV. Have on hand atropine (for bradycardia), vasopressors (for hypotension), and bronchodilators for emergency use. Patient should be transferred to oral therapy as soon as possible.
Oral drug may be administered with food to facilitate absorption.
Withhold drug and seek clarification if prescribed for patient who received an MAO inhibitor drug within past 2 weeks.
Seek clarification if prescription exceeds recommended doses of bisoprolol, carteolol, nadolol, and atenolol because accumulation can occur. These drugs have long half-lives that permit once-daily dosing.
Do not discontinue these drugs abruptly after chronic therapy; taper drug gradually over 2 weeks with monitoring.
Provide small, frequent meals if GI upset occurs.
Ensure that alpha-adrenergic blocker has been given before beta-adrenergic blocker when treating patients with pheochromocytoma.

Surveillance During Therapy

Provide continual cardiac and BP monitoring when IV beta-adrenergic blockers are used.
Monitor for adverse effects and toxicity.
Interpret results of diagnostic tests and contact practitioner as appropriate.
Monitor for possible drug–drug and drug–nutrient interactions: additive cardiac-depressant effects with digitalis, phenytoin, verapamil, and quinidine; effects reversed with norepinephrine, isoproterenol, dopamine, dobutamine, and other sympathomimetic drugs; plasma levels may be elevated by chlorpromazine, cimetidine, furosemide, and hydralazine; can antagonize the bronchodilating effect of theophylline; enhancement of hypotensive action by diuretics and other antihypertensives; decreased effects with indomethacin, ibuprofen, piroxicam, sulindac, barbiturates; prolongation of hypoglycemic effects of insulin; peripheral ischemia possible with ergot alkaloids; increased first dose response with prazosin; increased serum levels and effects when used with lidocaine.
Monitor for possible drug–laboratory test interactions: interference with glucose or insulin tolerance tests, glaucoma screening tests.
Provide for patient safety needs if CNS effects or hypotension occur.

Patient Teaching

Instruct the patient to avoid OTC preparations.
Suggest taking drug with meals to minimize GI irritation.
Advise patient that if drugs are used for prolonged periods, tests may be performed periodically to assess blood, kidney, and liver function.
Explain that heart rate and rhythm and exercise capacity may be routinely monitored if angina is present. Beta-blockers should not be continued in patients with angina unless they reduce pain and increase work capacity.
Inform the patient with diabetes that the normal signs of hypoglycemia (tachycardia, sweating) may be blocked by these drugs.
Instruct patient to take propranolol and metoprolol during meals; other beta-blockers should be taken before meals.
Instruct patient to notify practitioner promptly at first sign of a skin rash; difficulty breathing, night cough; swelling of extremities; slow pulse; confusion, depression; fever, sore throat.
Teach patient about the types of side effects expected with therapy: dizziness, drowsiness, lightheadedness, blurred vision; nausea, loss of appetite; nightmares, depression; sexual impotence.

Selected Bibliography

Carruthers SG: The place of alpha blockers in the antihypertensive armamentarium. J Clin Pharmacol 33:260, 1993
Kaila T, Iisalo E: Selectivity of acebutolol, atenolol and metoprolol in healthy volunteers estimated by the extent the drugs occupy $beta_2$-receptors in the circulating plasma. J Clin Pharmacol 33:959, 1993
Penner SB, Stanko CK, Smyth DD: Selective $alpha_1$-adrenoceptor blockade and renal sodium handling in humans. J Clin Pharmacol 33: 1110, 1993
Rabkin SW: Mechanisms of action of adrenergic receptor blockers on lipids during antihypertensive drug treatment. J Clin Pharmacol 33:286, 1993
Saotome T, Minoura S, Terashi K, Sato T, Echizen H, Ishizaki T: Labetalol in hypertension during the third trimester of pregnancy: Its antihypertensive effect and pharmacokinetic analysis. J Clin Pharmacol 33:979, 1993
Schiffrin EL, Deng LY, Larochelle P: Effects of a beta-blocker or a converting enzyme inhibitor on resistance arteries in essential hypertension. Hypertension 23:83, 1994

Nursing Bibliography

Darnoff R, Frishman W, Lederman R, Stewart W: Beta-blockers: Beyond cardiology. Patient Care: 47–70, 1993

16

Antihistamine and Antiserotonin Agents

Antihistamine Agents

H_1 Receptor Antagonists

Astemizole
Azatadine*
Brompheniramine
Buclizine
Chlorpheniramine
Clemastine
Cyclizine
Cyproheptadine*
Dexchlorpheniramine
Dimenhydrinate
Diphenhydramine
Doxylamine
Loratadine
Meclizine
Methdilazine
Phenindamine
Promethazine
Pyrilamine
Terfenadine
Trimeprazine*
Tripelennamine
Triprolidine

H_2 Receptor Antagonists

Cimetidine
Famotidine
Nizatidine
Ranitidine

Antiserotonin Agents

Dihydroergotamine
Ergotamine
Methysergide
Ondansetron

** Also has antiserotonin activity.*

Antihistamines

Drugs that competitively block the effects of histamine at various receptor sites in the body are termed "antihistamines." They do *not* interfere with the *release* of histamine, production of antibodies, or interactions between antigens and antibodies.

Histamine is present in virtually all mammalian tissues, arising from the decarboxylation of the amino acid histidine. Sites of highest histamine concentration in the body include:

Mast cells and basophils, the fixed-tissue and circulating histaminocytes, respectively, where histamine is thought to be bound in an inactive complex with heparin and an acidic protein.

Gastric mucosal cells, where histamine is not extensively bound.

Certain central nervous system (CNS) cells, located primarily in the hypothalamus.

The major actions of histamine are centered on the cardiovascular system (CVS), nonvascular smooth muscle, exocrine glands, and the adrenal medulla; they include the following:

- Arteriolar and venular dilation
- Increased capillary permeability
- Increased heart rate
- Contraction of nonvascular smooth muscle (eg, bronchoconstriction, gastrointestinal [GI] hypermotility)
- Stimulation of gastric hydrochloric acid secretion
- Release of catecholamines from the adrenal medulla

These effects of histamine are mediated by an action on two distinct receptors, termed H_1 and H_2 receptor sites. H_1 receptors are those associated with the smooth muscle of the blood vessels, bronchioles, and GI tract; thus, contraction of nonvascular smooth muscle is an H_1 receptor effect. H_2 receptors are found on gastric parietal cells, the myocardium, and certain blood vessels; activation of H_2 receptors promotes secretion of gastric acid and tachycardia. Vascular dilation and increased permeability result from a combined action of histamine on both H_1 and H_2 sites.

The role of histamine in allergic (acute and chronic) and hypersensitivity reactions also is established. Because histamine release from cells can be triggered by chemical agents, a variety of drugs and toxins, and antigen–antibody reactions, it plays a critical role in the symptomatology of many allergic, anaphylactic, and hypersensitivity reactions. On release from binding sites or tissue stores, histamine can elicit a wide range of unwanted effects, from mild itching to circulatory shock.

The clinical use of histamine largely has been superseded by other drugs. Histamine and its structural analogue betazole were once commonly used in testing for functional achlorhydria (lack of gastric hydrochloric acid); they have now been replaced by a more effective and less toxic diagnostic agent, pentagastrin (Peptavlon), which is discussed in Chapter 80. Histamine phosphate (by injection) is occasionally used for diagnosis of pheochromocytoma (see Chapter 80); this is a dangerous procedure and should be used only by people trained in its technique.

Although antihistamines are classified as either H_1 or H_2 receptor antagonists, H_1 blockers comprise most of this class of drugs; therefore, the term *antihistamine* has come to be used synonymously with H_1 antagonists. In contrast, H_2 blockers exert a specific blocking effect on histamine receptor sites of gastric parietal cells, markedly reducing the output of hydrochloric acid. The clinically available H_2 antagonists are reviewed separately (after discussion of H_1 blockers).

H_1 Receptor Antagonists

H_1 receptor blockers can be categorized into one of several groups on the basis of their chemical composition (Table 16-1). Certain differences exist among the various groups of H_1 antagonists with regard to the incidence and type of side effects they elicit; these differences also are illustrated in Table 16-1. Clinical efficacy differs significantly from group to group, and certain patients may respond much better to one group of H_1 antagonists than to others.

Although H_1 antagonists can block cell responses to both exogenous and endogenous histamine, they are significantly more effective against the former. *Endogenous* histamine, however, is the main cause of most allergic reactions. Moreover, antihistamines are much more useful when given before a histamine challenge rather than after an allergic attack has begun. Finally, antihistamines are effective only to the extent that histamine is the primary causative factor in the allergic response. Therefore, H_1 antagonists are most effective in prevention of seasonal pollinosis and urticaria; somewhat less effective in

Table 16-1. **Classification of Antihistamines**

Chemical Category	Drugs	Characteristics
Alkylamines	Brompheniramine Chlorpheniramine Dexchlorpheniramine Triprolidine	Low incidence of drowsiness and moderate GI upset; widely used antihistamine group
Ethanolamines	Clemastine Dimenhydrinate Diphenhydramine Doxylamine	Moderate to high incidence of drowsiness; minimal GI upset; dimenhydrinate is used for prophylaxis of motion sickness; diphenhydramine and doxylamine used in OTC sleep aids
Ethylenediamines	Pyrilamine Tripelennamine	Moderately sedating; high incidence of GI upset; pyrilamine used in some OTC sleep aids
Phenothiazines	Methdilazine Promethazine Trimeprazine	High degree of drowsiness; trimeprazine also blocks serotonin; many side effects and contraindications; can be used for motion sickness
Piperazines	Cyclizine Meclizine	Used principally for prophylaxis of motion sickness
Piperidines	Azatadine Cyproheptadine Phenindamine	Sedation is moderate with cyproheptadine and azatadine which also block serotonin
Miscellaneous	Astemizole Loratidine Terfenadine	Nonsedating at recommended dosage; long-acting; weak anticholinergic action

allergic dermatoses, contact dermatitis, vasomotor rhinitis, serum sickness, and allergic transfusion reactions; and seldom useful alone in bronchial asthma, GI allergies, and systemic anaphylactic reactions.

H_1 receptor antagonists are remarkably similar in most of their actions; therefore, their pharmacology is discussed collectively. A listing of individual drugs is given in Table 16-2.

Mechanism

Competitive blockade of the actions of histamine at H_1 receptor sites on effector structures (eg, vascular and nonvascular smooth muscle, salivary and respiratory mucosal glands); also exert anticholinergic (eg, dry mouth), antiserotonergic, local anesthetic, and CNS depressant (eg, sedative) actions. Astemizole, loratadine, and terfenadine bind more selectively to peripheral H_1 receptors than to central H_1 sites; these antihistamines have minimal or no anticholinergic and sedative actions.

Uses

Not all H_1 blockers have *all* of the following indications; refer to Table 16-2 for uses of individual drugs.

- Relief of symptoms of certain allergic disorders (eg, allergic rhinitis, vasomotor rhinitis, uncomplicated urticaria and angioedema, allergic reactions to blood or plasma)
- Adjunctive treatment in anaphylactic reactions (with epinephrine and other measures)
- Prevention and treatment of motion sickness
- Temporary relief of insomnia
- Adjunctive therapy for parkinsonism and extrapyramidal reactions due to antipsychotic drug therapy
- Relief of coughs caused by colds, allergies, or minor throat irritations
- Prevention and control of nausea and vomiting associated with anesthesia or surgery
- Adjunct to analgesics for obstetrics and postoperative pain, and for preoperative sedation and relief of apprehension

Dosage

See Table 16-2.

Fate

Most drugs are used orally and are well absorbed; onset is normally within 10 to 30 minutes; duration is 3 to 4 hours (sustained-action forms, 8 to 12 hours); metabolized by liver and kidney and excreted largely in the urine, usually as metabolites; readily enter CNS and produce depression; effectiveness not significantly enhanced by parenteral administration; topical forms involve risk of sensitization.

Adverse Reactions

Frequency and severity vary among different preparations.

CV: hypotension, palpitations, tachycardia, arrhythmias: astemizole and terfenadine may produce prolongation of the QT interval leading to possible ventricular arrhythmias and death

GI: epigastric distress, dryness of mouth, thickened bronchial secretions, anorexia, nausea, vomiting, diarrhea or constipation

CNS: sedation (less with astemizole, loratadine, and terfenadine), confusion, dizziness, restlessness, impaired coordination, blurred vision, vertigo, tinnitus, heaviness and weakness of the hands, nervousness, tremors, paresthesias, irritability, excitation, insomnia, hysteria

Hematologic: hemolytic anemia, thrombocytopenia, leukopenia, pancytopenia, agranulocytosis

(*text continues on page 132*)

Table 16-2. **Antihistamines**

Drug	*Usual Dosage Range*	*Major Uses*	*Nursing Considerations*
Astemizole *Hismanal*	Adults and children >12 y: 10 mg once a day	Allergic disorders	Long-acting, largely nonsedating drug; minimal anticholinergic activity; taken on an empty stomach; not recommended in children younger than 12 y; can cause headache
Azatadine *Optimine*	1–2 mg twice a day	Allergic disorders	Do not use in children younger than age 12 y; has antiserotonin effects as well
Brompheniramine *Bromphen, Dimetane, and several other manufacturers*	*Oral:* Adults: 4–8 mg 3–4 times/day or 8–12 mg timed-release twice a day Children >6 y: 2–4 mg 3–4 times/day Children <6 y: 0.5 mg/kg daily in divided doses *Parenteral:* Adults: 5–20 mg IV, IM, or SC twice a day (maximum 40 mg/day) Children: 0.5 mg/kg/day	Allergic disorders; cough	Keep patient lying down during IV administration; sweating, hypotension, and faintness may occur with IV use; do not use solutions with preservatives IV; may induce agranulocytosis; perform blood counts during prolonged therapy
Buclizine *Bucladin-S*	*Nausea:* 50–150 mg/day *Motion sickness:* 50 mg 30 min before travel, and 50 mg every 4–6 h as needed	Nausea, vomiting, and vertigo; prevention of motion sickness	Tablets may be chewed or swallowed whole—also can be dissolved under tongue; do not use during pregnancy or in small children; may induce headache, nervousness, drowsiness, and dryness of mouth
Chlorpheniramine *Chlor-Trimeton, Teldrin, and other manufacturers* *(CAN) Chlorphen, Chlor-Tripolon, Novopheniram*	*Oral:* Adults: 4 mg 3–6 times day or 8–12 mg twice a day (timed-release) Children 6–12 y: 2 mg 3–6 times/day Children 2–6 y: 1 mg 3 or 4 times/day *Parenteral* Allergy: 5–20 mg IM, SC (maximum 40 mg/day) Anaphylaxis: 10–20 mg IV	Allergic disorders; transfusion and drug reactions; anaphylactic reactions	May be used prophylactically for blood transfusion; only injection solution used IV is 10 mg/mL; when given IV or added directly to stored blood, do not use solution with preservatives; low incidence of drowsiness and other side effects; has antiemetic, antitussive, and some local anesthetic action; timed-release preparations not recommended in children younger than age 12 y; may produce increased sedation in elderly people
Clemastine *Tavist*	Adults: 1.34–2.68 mg 2 or 3 times/day (maximum 3 tablets daily)	Allergic disorders	Not recommended in children younger than age 12 y; monitor blood levels; can produce hemolytic anemia; use cautiously in the elderly; available OTC
Cyclizine *Marezine* *(CAN) Marzine*	*Oral:* 50 mg 30 min before travel; repeat every 4–6 h to a maximum of 300 mg/day (children 6–10 y—1/2 adult dose) *IM:* 50 mg every 4–6 h	Prevention and treatment of motion sickness and postoperative nausea and vomiting	Do not use in pregnancy or in children younger than age 6 y; produces frequent drowsiness; for postoperative nausea and vomiting give 20–30 min before end of surgery; overdosage may produce hyperexcitability and convulsions; claimed to reduce the sensitivity of the labyrinthine apparatus to motion; store in a cool place; injection may discolor to light yellow—does not affect potency
Cyproheptadine *Periactin*	*Adults:* 4 mg 3 or 4 times/day (usual range 12–16 mg/day; maximum 32 mg/day) *Children (2–6 y):* 2 mg 2 or 3 times/day; maximum 12 mg/day; (7–14 y): 4 mg 2 or 3 times/day; maximum 16 mg/day	Allergic rhinitis; vasomotor rhinitis	Has atropine-like action; use with caution in patients with bronchial asthma, glaucoma, and cardiovascular disease

(*continued*)

Table 16-2. **Antihistamines (Continued)**

Drug	*Usual Dosage Range*	*Major Uses*	*Nursing Considerations*
Dexchlorphenira-mine *Dexchlor, Poladex, T.D. Polaramine, Polargen*	*Adults:* 2 mg 3–4 times a day or 4–6 mg repeat-action tablets twice a day *Child:* 1/2 adult dose *Infant:* 1/4 adult dose	Allergic disorders	Low incidence of many common side effects; do not use repeat-action tablets in children; available as an expectorant with pseudoephedrine and guaifenesin
Dimenhydrinate *Dramamine, and several other manufacturers* *(CAN) Gravol, Nauseatol, Travamine*	*Oral* Adults: 50–100 mg every 4 h Children (6–12 y): 25–50 mg 3 times/day Children (2–6 y): up to 25 mg every 6–8 h *IM:* Adults: 50 mg as needed Children: 1.25 mg/kg 4 times/day up to 300 mg/day *IV* (adults only): 50 mg in 10 mL sodium chloride given over 2 min	Prevention and treatment of nausea, vomiting and vertigo of motion sickness, radiation sickness, or anesthesia	Drowsiness is common, especially at higher dosages; caution when used in combination with aminoglycoside antibiotics, because it may mask signs of ototoxicity, leading to permanent damage; tolerance develops with continued use; do not mix parenteral solutions with other drugs because many are incompatible; dilute IV solutions with maximum allowable fluid—drug is irritating to veins.
Diphenhydramine *Benadryl, and other manufacturers* *(CAN) Allerdryl, PMS-Diphenhydramine, Insomnal*	*Oral* Adults: 25–50 mg 3–4 times/day Children (over 20 lb): 5 mg/kg/day in divided doses *Parenteral—IV or deep IM* Adults: 10–50 mg as needed (maximum 400 mg/day) Children: 5 mg/kg/day in 4 divided doses	Allergic disorders, motion sickness, adjunctive therapy in anaphylactic reactions, prevention of reactions to blood or plasma, sedative in pediatric patients, cough due to colds or allergies, treatment of insomnia, oral anesthesia in dental practice, parkinsonism, acute dystonias	Topical preparations may cause hypersensitivity reactions; high incidence of drowsiness initially, which decreases with use; monitor blood pressure carefully with parenteral use; very low incidence of GI disturbances; found in several OTC sleep aids (Sleep-EZE, Sominex 2, Twilite); solution is irritating to tissue—give deep IM and rotate injection sites with every dose.
Doxylamine *Unisom*	*Adults:* 25 mg 20–30 min before bedtime	Insomnia	Drowsiness is common; indicated as a non-prescription sleep aid
Loratadine *Claritin*	*Adults and children (12 y or older):* 10 mg once a day	Nasal and nonnasal symptoms of seasonal allergic rhinitis	In patient with hepatic dysfunction use 10 mg every *other* day; lower degree of sedation compared to most other antihistamines
Meclizine *Antivert, Antrizine, Bonine, Dizmiss, Ru-Vert M, Vergon* *(CAN) Bonamine*	*Motion sickness:* 25–50 mg 1 h before travel; repeat every 24 h *Vertigo:* 25–100 mg daily in divided doses as needed	Motion sickness, vertigo due to disease of the vestibular system	Do not use in pregnancy or young children; commonly causes dry mouth and drowsiness; weak anticholinergic action; tablets are oral or chewable; this drug has a slower onset and longer duration than many others; watch for delayed development of side effects
Methdilazine *Tacaryl* *(CAN) Dilosyn*	*Adults:* 8 mg 2–4 times/day *Children:* 4 mg 2–4 times/day	Pruritus, urticaria	Tablets may be chewed (4 mg) or swallowed whole (8 mg); structurally a phenothiazine (see Chapter 24 for possible adverse reactions); strong anticholinergic and antiemetic; do not use in children younger than age 3 y
Phenidamine *Nolahist*	*Adults:* 25 mg every 4–6 h; maximum of 150 mg every 24 h *Children (6 to 11 y old):* 12.5 mg every 4–6 h; maximum of 75 mg every 24 h	Symptomatic relief of hay fever, other respiratory allergies, or allergic rhinitis	CNS stimulation may occur

(continued)

Table 16-2. Antihistamines (Continued)

Drug	Usual Dosage Range	Major Uses	Nursing Considerations
Promethazine *Phenergan and other manufacturers* *(CAN) Histantil, PMS Promethazine*	*Oral:* Adults: 12.5–50 mg every 4–6 h as necessary Children: 6.25–12.5 mg 3 times/day as needed *Rectal:* 12.5–25 mg every 4–6 h as necessary *Parenteral (usually IM):* 12.5–25 mg individualized to condition Children: 0.6–1.2 mg/kg When used IV, maximum concentration is 25 mg/mL/min	Allergic disorders and reactions to blood plasma; motion sickness; nausea and vomiting due to anesthesia, drugs, or surgery; preoperative and obstetrical sedation; adjunct to analgesics in postoperative or chronic pain; sedation and light sleep; cough	Phenothiazine derivative (see Chapter 24); potent antihistamine and sedative with prolonged effects; may cause false-positive result on urine pregnancy tests (immunologic type); avoid intra-arterial injection because severe arteriospasm can result; irritating to tissue if given SC; give deep IM and rotate sites with every dose; photosensitivity is a problem; caution patient to use dark glasses and avoid bright light; reduce dose of analgesics and other sedative-hypnotics if used in combination with promethazine; injection is incompatible with alkaline drugs; should be diluted with saline before injection; flush heparin lock with saline before and after injecting drug because it is incompatible with heparin; avoid contact with skin or eyes; good antiemetic but may mask vomiting caused by other drugs; protect injectible form from light and do not use if cloudy or darkened; available with expectorant, either plain or with codeine or decongestants
Pyrilamine *Dormarex*	*Adults:* 25–50 mg 3 times/day *Insomnia:* 50 mg at bedtime	Allergic disorders, insomnia	Not recommended in children younger than age 6 y; found in several OTC cough formulations; drug is only mildly sedating and weakly anticholinergic
Terfenadine *Seldane*	*Adults and children >12 y:* 60 mg twice a day	Allergic disorders (especially rhinitis)	Long-acting oral antihistamine used for control of chronic allergic disorders; very minimally sedating; available in combination with pseudoephedrine as Seldane-D
Trimeprazine *Temaril* *(CAN) Panectyl*	*Adults:* 2.5 mg 4 times/day or 5 mg every 12 h *Children:* (>3 y) 2.5 mg 3 times/day; (6 mo to 3 y) 1.25 mg 3 times/day	Relief of itching in many allergic and nonallergic conditions including poison ivy and drug rash	A phenothiazine derivative; geriatric patients are more likely to develop hypotension, syncope, confusional states, parkinsonian reactions, and significant sedation
Tripelennamine *Pyribenzamine, Pelamine, PBZ*	*Adults:* 25–50 mg every 4–6 h (maximum 600 mg/day or 100 mg 2–3 times/day) *Children:* 5 mg/kg/day in 4–6 doses (maximum 300 mg/day)	Allergic disorders and reactions to blood or plasma; pruritis and other topical skin disorders; mucous membrane analgesia and anesthesia in the mouth; cough	Do not use 100-mg sustained-acting form in children; used as mouthwash for herpetic gingivostomatitis in children; caution in elderly because dizziness, sedation, and hypotension are more likely to occur; possesses some antitussive and local anesthetic activity
Triprolidine *Actidil, Myidil*	*Adults:* 2.5 mg 3–4 times/day *Children (6–12 y):* 1.25 mg 3–4 times/day *Children (2–6 y):* 0.6 mg 3–4 times/day *Children (<2 y):* 0.3 mg 3–4 times/day	Allergic disorders	Low degree of drowsiness and most other side effects; rapid onset of action; may cause paradoxical excitation and irritability; combined with pseudoephedrine as Actifed—this combination also is available with codeine and guaifenensin as Actifed-C; children younger than age 6 y should be given syrup only

Urinary: urinary frequency or retention, dysuria
Respiratory: wheezing, chest tightness, nasal congestion
Hypersensitivity: urticaria, drug rash, photosensitivity, anaphylactic shock
Other: headache, diplopia, sweating, pallor, stinging, or burning at site of injection
With overdosage: fever, ataxia, hallucinations, convulsions, coma, cardiovascular and respiratory collapse (children are especially susceptible)

Contraindications

Narrow-angle glaucoma, peptic ulcer, prostatic hypertrophy, GI or bladder obstruction; in premature or nursing infants, elderly or debilitated patients, pregnant or nursing women, patients on monoamine oxidase (MAO) inhibitor therapy.

Phenothiazine antihistamines (methdilazine, promethazine, trimeprazine) are contraindicated in comatose patients, states of CNS depression due to drug overdosage, jaundice, bone marrow depression, and in acutely ill or dehydrated children.

Astemizole and terfenadine are contraindicated in patients presenting with significant hepatic dysfunction *and* in patients taking erythromycin or the antifungal agents itraconazole and ketoconazole (see section on Interactions for a discussion of the mechanism of this interaction).

Cautious use in patients with cardiovascular disease, convulsive disorders, renal or hepatic impairment, hypertension, urinary retention, glaucoma, diabetes, asthma, or other chronic lower respiratory disease, and hyperthyroidism, and in young children, elderly, or debilitated patients, and pregnant women.

Interactions

Astemizole and terfenadine (and possibly loratadine) may result in serious cardiovascular reactions, including ventricular arrhythmias and cardiac arrest if given together with macrolide antibiotics (eg, azithromycin, clarithromycin, erythromycin, and troleandomycin) or oral antifungal agents (eg, fluconazole, ketoconazole, itraconazole, or miconazole). This interaction apparently is caused by inhibition of astemizole and terfenadine biotransformation by these antibiotics and antifungal agents, leading to higher blood levels that subsequently cause QT prolongation and ventricular arrhythmias.

Sedative effects may be enhanced when used with other CNS depressants (eg, alcohol, barbiturates, narcotics, antianxiety drugs).

Atropine-like side effects (eg, dryness of mouth, blurred vision, urinary retention, constipation) are potentiated by other anticholinergics, tricyclic antidepressants, and MAO inhibitors.

Effects of epinephrine can be increased by several antihistamines (eg, diphenhydramine, chlorpheniramine, tripelennamine).

Nursing Management

Pretherapy Assessment

Assess and record baseline data necessary for detection of adverse effects of antihistamines (H_1): General: vital signs (VS) body weight, skin color and temperature; CNS: orientation, reflexes, vision; GI: bowel sounds, normal output; Genitourinary (GU): prostate palpation; Laboratory: complete blood count (CBC) with differential.

Review medical history and documents for existing or previous conditions that:

a. require cautious use of antihistamines (H_1): cardiovascular disease; convulsive disorders; renal or hepatic impairment; hypertension; urinary retention; glaucoma; diabetes; asthma or other chronic lower respiratory disease; hyperthyroidism; and in young children, and elderly or debilitated patients.

b. contraindicate use of antihistamines (H_1): allergy to antihistamines; narrow-angle glaucoma; peptic ulcer; prostatic hypertrophy; GI or bladder obstruction; patients on MAO inhibitor therapy.

Phenothiazine antihistamines (methdilazine, promethazine, trimeprazine) are contraindicated in comatose patients; states of CNS depression due to drug overdosage; jaundice; bone marrow depression; and in acutely ill or dehydrated children.

Astemizole and terfenadine are contraindicated in patients presenting with significant hepatic dysfunction *and* in patients taking macrolide antibiotics (eg, erythromycin) or oral antifungal agents such as itraconazole and ketoconazole (see Interactions for a discussion of the mechanism); **pregnancy (Category B or C)**; lactation (secreted in breast milk, contraindicated in nursing mothers because of possible adverse effects to the neonate; may inhibit lactation; nursing mothers should avoid this drug).

Nursing Interventions

Medication Administration

Determine whether patient has any contraindicated condition before initiating administration.

Oral drug may be administered with food to facilitate absorption.

Administer syrup form if patient is unable to take tablets.

Give intramuscular (IM) antihistamine deep into large muscle mass to reduce tissue irritation. Subcutaneous injection should not be used.

Apply topical preparation only to intact skin. Avoid broken, exposed, or weeping areas.

Withhold drug and seek clarification if prescribed for patient who received an MAO inhibitor drug within past 2 weeks.

Provide small, frequent meals if GI upset occurs.

Surveillance During Therapy

Monitor for toxicity.

Withhold topical application of antihistamine-containing preparation at earliest sign of dermatologic toxicity. Serious hypersensitivity reactions can occur.

Observe patient closely during parenteral use. Hypersensitivity reactions are more likely to occur with parenteral rather than with oral administration. Inform patient that brief stinging sensation may occur.

Interpret results of diagnostic tests and contact practitioner as appropriate.

Monitor for possible drug–drug and drug–nutrient interactions: sedative effects enhanced when used with other CNS depressants; atropinic side effects enhanced by other anticholinergics, tricyclic antidepressants; effects of epinephrine increased by several antihistamines (diphenhydramine, chlorpheniramine, tripelenamine).

Provide for patient safety needs if CNS effects or hypotension occur.

Patient Teaching

Instruct the patient to avoid over-the-counter (OTC) preparations.

Suggest taking drug with meals to minimize GI irritation.

Instruct patient with severe allergy to carry identification stating type of allergy, medication being used, and name of practitioner.

Advise patient that if drugs are used for prolonged periods, tests may be performed periodically to assess blood, kidney, and liver function.

Instruct patient to notify practitioner promptly at first sign of a skin rash; difficulty breathing; night cough; hallucinations, tremors, loss of coordination; unusual bleeding or bruising; visual disturbances; irregular heartbeat.

Teach patient about the types of side effects expected with therapy: dizziness; drowsiness; epigastric distress, diarrhea, or constipation; dry mouth; thickening of bronchial secretions; dryness of nasal mucosa.

• Cyproheptadine

Periactin

Mechanism

Competitive antagonism of serotonin (5-hydroxytryptamine [5-HT]), histamine, and possibly acetylcholine at postsynaptic receptor sites; structural analogue of the phenothiazines; exhibits mild CNS depressant activity; may impair platelet aggregation; may stimulate the appetite, possibly by acting on the hypothalamus.

Uses

Relief of several allergic disorders, especially rhinitis, allergic conjunctivitis, and allergic skin manifestations (eg, cold urticaria, pruritus, angioedema)

Prevention or reduction of allergic reactions to blood and plasma

Adjunctive therapy for anaphylactic reactions

Relief of pruritus resulting from drug or serum reactions, physical allergies, or insect bites

Treatment of carcinoid syndrome

Unlabeled uses include appetite stimulation in underweight or anorectic patients, treatment of vascular cluster headaches, and prophylaxis of migraine

Dosage

See Table 16-2.

Fate

Absorption is adequate; onset of action is within 60 minutes; duration 4 to 6 hours.

Common Side Effects

Sedation; dryness of mouth, nose, and throat; dizziness; gastric distress; thickening of bronchial secretions.

Significant Adverse Reactions

Urinary difficulty, skin rash, excitation, impaired coordination, tremor, irritability, confusion, ataxia (CNS effects occur especially in children), hypotension, and tachycardia.

Contraindications

Urinary retention, bladder obstruction, lower respiratory disease, narrow-angle glaucoma, peptic ulcer, prostatic hypertrophy, elderly or debilitated patients, newborn or premature infants, nursing mothers, and combination with MAO inhibitors. *Cautious use* in bronchial asthma, glaucoma, hypertension, hyperthyroidism, cardiovascular disease, and in young children, pregnant or nursing women.

Interactions

MAO inhibitors or anticholinergics may intensify many of the side effects of cyproheptadine.

Cyproheptadine has additive CNS depressant effects with other depressants (eg, alcohols, narcotics, barbiturates).

Nursing Management

Pretherapy Assessment

Assess and record baseline data necessary for detection of adverse effects of cyproheptadine: General: VS, body weight, skin color and temperature; CNS: orientation, reflexes, vision; GI: bowel sounds, normal output; GU: prostate palpation; Laboratory: CBC with differential.

Review medical history and documents for existing or previous conditions that:

a. require cautious use of cyproheptadine: bronchial asthma; glaucoma; hypertension; hyperthyroidism; cardiovascular disease; and in young children.
b. contraindicate use of cyproheptadine: allergy to antihistamines; urinary retention; bladder obstruction; lower respiratory disease; narrow-angle glaucoma; peptic ulcer; prostatic hypertrophy; elderly or debilitated patients; newborn or premature infants; MAO inhibitors; **pregnancy (Category B)**; lactation (secreted in breast milk, contraindicated in nursing mothers because of possible adverse effects to the neonate; may inhibit lactation; nursing mothers should avoid this drug).

Nursing Interventions

Medication Administration

Determine whether patient has any contraindicated condition before initiating administration.

Oral drug may be administered with food to facilitate absorption.

Administer syrup form if patient is unable to take tablets.

Withhold drug and seek clarification if prescribed for patient who received an MAO inhibitor drug within past 2 weeks.

Provide small, frequent meals if GI upset occurs.

Surveillance During Therapy

Monitor for adverse effects and toxicity.

Interpret results of diagnostic tests and contact practitioner as appropriate.

Monitor for possible drug–drug and drug–nutrient interactions: MAO inhibitors or anticholinergics may intensify many of the side effects of cyproheptadine; cyproheptadine has additive CNS depressant effects with other depressants (eg, alcohol, narcotics, barbiturates).

Provide for patient safety needs if CNS effects or hypotension occur.

Patient Teaching

Instruct the patient to avoid OTC preparations.

Suggest taking drug with meals to minimize GI irritation.

Instruct patient with severe allergy to carry identification stating type of allergy, medication being used, and name of practitioner.

Warn patient to avoid activities requiring alertness and coordination in early stages of therapy because drowsiness is common, although it usually disappears in several days.
Caution patient to guard against injury resulting from dizziness and hypotension, which also may occur, particularly in the elderly.
Warn patient to avoid using other substances that add to CNS depressant effects (eg, alcohol, narcotics, barbiturates).
Advise parents to observe children for early signs of stimulation. They may experience an excitatory state (eg, agitation, confusion, possibly hallucinations).
Advise patient that if drugs are used for prolonged periods, tests may be performed periodically to assess blood, kidney, and liver function.
Instruct patient to notify practitioner promptly at first sign of a skin rash; difficulty breathing; night cough; hallucinations; tremors; loss of coordination; unusual bleeding or bruising; visual disturbances; irregular heartbeat.
Teach patient about the types of side effects expected with therapy: dizziness; drowsiness; epigastric distress, diarrhea, or constipation; dry mouth; thickening of bronchial secretions; dryness of nasal mucosa.

• Trimeprazine

Temaril

(CAN) Panectyl

Mechanism

Antagonism of the receptor actions of histamine and serotonin; structurally related to the phenothiazines (see Chapter 24); exerts some anticholinergic activity.

Uses

Relief of pruritus in urticaria and other dermatologic disorders
Preoperative sedation in children (investigational)

Dosage

See Table 16-2.

Fate

Onset of action in 30 to 60 minutes; duration is 3 to 6 hours; sustained-release forms persist for 8 to 12 hours; excreted in the urine as metabolites and intact drug.

Common Side Effects

Drowsiness, lightheadedness, dryness of the mouth, blurred vision, GI distress, and weakness.

Significant Adverse Reactions

Allergic skin reactions, extrapyramidal reactions, orthostatic hypotension, tachycardia, urinary difficulty, blurred vision, dryness of bronchial and other secretions, respiratory difficulties; see also phenothiazines (see Chapter 24).

Contraindications

Excess CNS depression, bone marrow depression, newborn or premature infants, pregnancy, acutely ill or dehydrated children (danger of adverse effects [eg, dystonias] is increased). *Cautious use* in patients with renal or hepatic disease, asthma, CNS disorders, hypertension, prostatic hypertrophy, history of convulsive disorders, narrow-angle glaucoma.

Interactions

Anticholinergic effects are intensified by MAO inhibitors, tricyclic antidepressants, thiazide diuretics.
Phenothiazine-related adverse effects may be intensified by reserpine, oral contraceptives, progesterone.
Drug may potentiate depressant and analgesic effects of narcotics, barbiturates, alcohol, and similarly acting drugs.

Nursing Management

Pretherapy Assessment

Assess and record baseline data necessary for detection of adverse effects of trimeprazine: General: VS, body weight, skin color and temperature; CNS: orientation, reflexes, vision, intraocular pressure; CVS: orthostatic blood pressure; GI: liver evaluation, bowel sounds, normal output; GU: urinary output, prostate palpation; Laboratory: CBC with differential, urinalysis, thyroid, liver and kidney function tests.
Review medical history and documents for existing or previous conditions that:

a. require cautious use of trimeprazine: renal or hepatic disease; asthma; CNS disorders; hypertension; prostatic hypertrophy; history of convulsive disorders; narrow-angle glaucoma.
b. contraindicate use of trimeprazine: allergy to antihistamines, phenothiazines; excess CNS depression; bone marrow depression; newborn or premature infants; acutely ill or dehydrated children (danger of adverse effects [eg, dystonias] is increased); **pregnancy (Category C)**; lactation (secreted in breast milk, contraindicated in nursing mothers because of possible adverse effects to the neonate; may inhibit lactation; nursing mothers should avoid this drug).

Nursing Interventions

Medication Administration

Determine whether patient has any contraindicated condition before initiating administration.
Oral drug may be administered with food to facilitate absorption.
Provide small, frequent meals if GI upset occurs.

Surveillance During Therapy

Monitor for possible phenothiazine-related toxic effects (see Chapter 24) because drug is a structural analogue of the phenothiazines.
Monitor for adverse effects.
Interpret results of diagnostic tests and contact practitioner as appropriate.
Monitor for possible drug–drug and drug–nutrient interactions: anticholinergic effects are intensified by MAO inhibitors, tricyclic antidepressants, thiazide diuretics; phenothiazine-related adverse effects may be inten-

sified by reserpine, oral contraceptives, progesterone; may potentiate depressant and analgesic effects of narcotics, barbiturates, alcohol, and similarly acting drugs.
Provide for patient safety needs if CNS effects or hypotension occur.

Patient Teaching

Instruct the patient to avoid OTC preparations.
Suggest taking drug with meals to minimize GI irritation.
Instruct patient with severe allergy to carry identification stating type of allergy, medication being used, and name of practitioner.
Warn patient to avoid activities requiring alertness and coordination in early stages of therapy because drowsiness is common, although it usually disappears in several days.
Warn patient to avoid hazardous activities because drug induces marked drowsiness, especially during first few days. Advise particular caution for elderly patient because hypertension, syncope, confusion, and excessive sedation may occur.
Explain that depressive effects of other drugs can be potentiated by trimeprazine.
Caution patient to guard against injury resulting from dizziness and hypotension, which may occur particularly in the elderly.
Warn patient to avoid using other substances that add to CNS depressant effects (eg, alcohol, narcotics, barbiturates).
Advise parents to observe children for early signs of stimulation. They may experience an excitatory state (eg, agitation, confusion, possibly hallucinations).
Advise patient that if drugs are used for prolonged periods, tests may be performed periodically to assess blood, kidney, and liver function.
Instruct patient to notify practitioner promptly at first sign of a skin rash; sore throat; fever; unusual bleeding or bruising; weakness; tremors; impaired vision; dark-colored urine; pale-colored stools; yellowing of the eyes or skin.
Teach patient about the types of side effects expected with therapy: drowsiness, lightheadedness, dryness of the mouth, blurred vision, GI distress, and weakness.

H_2 Receptor Antagonists

These drugs are competitive antagonists of histamine at H_2 receptors, sites that mediate gastric acid secretion and cardiac stimulation. Because H_2 antagonists can effectively (ie, almost completely) block the secretion of gastric hydrochloric acid in response to most stimuli, it appears that histamine plays a major role in acid secretion from gastric mucosal parietal cells. Clinical studies show substantial reductions in gastric secretory volume, total acidity, and pepsin activity after administration of an H_2 blocker. Therefore, these drugs have an important role in the therapeutic management of peptic ulcers and certain other gastric hypersecretory states.

The clinically available H_2 receptor antagonists are similar in many aspects and are discussed as a group. Certain important differences among the drugs exist, however, particularly with regard to their potential for causing some serious side effects and for interacting with other drugs. These differences are highlighted during the general discussion of the drugs. The individual drugs are listed in Table 16-3, with specific information about their dosages.

Mechanism

Selective antagonism of the actions of histamine at H_2 receptor sites, especially those in the gastric mucosa; reduce daytime and nocturnal basal gastric acid secretion by 90% to 100%, as well as acid secretion stimulated by food, caffeine, pentagastrin, and insulin; increase gastric pH to 5 or greater for 3 to 4 hours and decrease total pepsin output.

Uses

Short-term treatment of gastric and duodenal ulcers (up to 8 weeks)
Maintenance therapy for duodenal ulcer at reduced dosage after healing of an active ulcer
Treatment of gastroesophageal reflux disease and erosive esophagitis
Treatment of pathologic hypersecretory conditions (eg, Zollinger-Ellison syndrome, systemic mastocytosis, multiple endocrine adenomas)
Unlabeled uses include prevention of stress-induced ulcers (eg, in hospitalized patients), upper GI bleeding, and aspiration pneumonitis during general anesthesia; in addition, cimetidine has been used to treat hirsutism in women because of its antiandrogenic action (see Significant Adverse Reactions)

Dosage

See Table 16-3.

Fate

Oral absorption is generally good, although bioavailability can vary among the different drugs. Peak serum levels usually occur within 1 to 2 hours. Duration of action ranges from 4 to 5 hours with cimetidine and up to 12 hours with nizatidine and ranitidine. Plasma protein binding for all drugs is minimal (15%–35%); elimination half-life is short (2 to 3 hours), and the major route of excretion is in the urine as both unchanged drug and metabolites; the half-life may be significantly prolonged in patients with renal impairment.

Adverse Reactions

Not all reactions have been noted with each drug:

CNS: headache (especially with famotidine), dizziness, insomnia, malaise, ataxia; in addition, confusion, agitation, disorientation, hallucinations, and delirium, especially with cimetidine
GI: diarrhea, nausea, constipation, abdominal pain, increased serum transaminases
CV: altered heartbeat
Musculoskeletal: muscle pain, arthralgia

In addition, *cimetidine* has been associated with skin rash, blood dyscrasias (rarely), alopecia, gynecomastia, galactorrhea, impotence, and decreased sperm count because of its antiandrogenic activity.

Contraindications

No absolute contraindications. *Cautious use* in the presence of impaired renal or hepatic function, in very ill or debilitated

Table 16-3. **H_2 Receptor Antagonists**

Drug	Usual Dosage Range	Nursing Considerations
Cimetidine *Tagamet* *(CAN) Apo-Cimetidine, Novo-Cimetidine, Nu-Cimet, Peptol*	*Oral* *Duodenal ulcer:* Initially, 300 mg 4 times/day *or* 400 mg twice a day *or* 800 mg at bedtime for 4–6 wk; reduce to 400 mg at bedtime for maintenance therapy as necessary to prevent recurrence *Hypersecretory conditions:* 300 mg 4–6 times/day to a maximum of 2400 mg/day *Reflux disease:* 400 mg 4 times/day for 12 wk *Parenteral* IM injection: 300 mg every 6 h IV injection: 300 mg diluted to 20 mL in saline and injected over 1–2 min every 6 h IV infusion: 300 mg in 50 mL 5% dextrose, infused over 15–20 min every 6 h (maximum 2400 mg/day)	Used in treating both acute and chronic gastric and duodenal ulcers; drug has been administered up to 5 y in some patients; not recommended in children younger than 16 y; possesses antiandrogenic action that may cause some side effects over time (eg, gynecomastia, impotence); reduces hepatic metabolism of many drugs (*see* Interactions) by impairing cytochrome P-450 pathway in the liver; antacids should *not* be taken concurrently; injectable solutions stable up to 48 h at room temperature; reduce dosage in patients with severely impaired renal function
Famotidine *Pepcid*	*Oral* Duodenal ulcer: 40 mg once a day for 6–8 wk; maintenance therapy: 20 mg once a day Hypersecretory conditions: 20 mg every 6 h *Reflux disease:* 20–40 mg twice a day for 6–12 wk *IV:* 20 mg every 12 h *IM:* 40 mg before anesthesia	Long-acting H_2 receptor antagonist used for short–long-term treatment of duodenal ulcer; antacids may be given concomitantly if needed; does not affect hepatic metabolism of other drugs (as seen with cimetidine); no antiandrogenic activity has been reported; IV solutions stable for 48 h at room temperature
Nizatidine *Axid*	*Active duodenal ulcer or reflux disease:* 300 mg once daily at bedtime *or* 150 mg twice daily *Maintenance therapy:* 150 mg once daily at bedtime	Long-acting competitive H_2 receptor antagonist; dosage must be reduced in patients with renal insufficiency; does *not* inhibit hepatic enzymes nor possess antiandrogenic activity; most common side effects are drowsiness and sweating
Ranitidine *Zantac* *(CAN) Apo-Ranitidine, Novo-Ranidine, Nu-Ranit, Zantac-C*	*Oral* Initially: 150 mg twice a day *or* 300 mg once daily at bedtime Maintenance therapy: 150 mg at bedtime *IM:* 50 mg undiluted every 6 h *IV injection:* 50 mg every 6–8 h diluted to a volume of 20 mL and given over 5 min *IV infusion:* 50 mg in 100 mL given over 15–20 min every 6–8 h	Used to treat gastric and duodenal ulcers and other hypersecretory conditions; may be given without regard to meals and with antacids; does not generally reduce hepatic metabolism of other drugs; may slow clearance of warfarin or procainamide; no reported antiandrogenic activity; reduce dosage in persons with severely impaired renal function; transient pain can occur at injection sites; solutions stable for 48 h

patients, and in pregnant or nursing women. In addition, cimetidine must be used cautiously in patients with altered endocrine function.

Interactions

Numerous interactions have been reported with use of H_2 receptor antagonists; the following list presents some of the more commonly reported; however, it is *not* a complete listing.

Antacids and metoclopramide may impair oral absorption of H_2 blockers if administered simultaneously.

By reducing hepatic biotransformation, cimetidine may lengthen the half-life of many drugs, such as certain benzodiazepines, beta-blockers, caffeine, calcium channel blockers, carbamazepine, lidocaine, metronidazole, pentoxifylline, phenytoin, quinidine, sulfonylurea antidiabetics, theophylline, tricyclic antidepressants, and warfarin.

Cimetidine or ranitidine may increase the pharmacologic effects of procainamide by reducing its renal clearance.

Concurrent use of cimetidine and morphine may lead to increased respiratory depression.

The effectiveness of sucralfate may be reduced by H_2 blockers because sucralfate requires an acid medium to be most effective.

Decreased oral absorption of fluconazole and ketoconazole may occur in the presence of H_2 blockers because of increased gastric pH.

Concurrent administration of cimetidine and digoxin has reduced serum levels of digoxin.

Nursing Management

Pretherapy Assessment

Assess and record baseline data necessary for detection of adverse effects of H_2 receptor blockers: General: VS, body weight, skin color and temperature; CNS: orientation; CVS: baseline electrocardiogram (continuous with IV use); GI: liver evaluation, bowel sounds, normal output; Laboratory: CBC with differential, urinalysis, thyroid, liver and kidney function tests.

Review medical history and documents for existing or previous conditions that:

a. require cautious use of H_2 receptor blockers: presence of impaired renal or hepatic function; in severe illness of debilitated state; altered endocrine function

b. contraindicate use of H_2 receptor blockers: allergy to cimetidine and derivatives; **pregnancy (Category B)**; lactation (secreted and concentrated in breast milk, contraindicated in nursing mothers because of possible adverse effects to the neonate; nursing mothers should avoid this drug).

Nursing Interventions

Medication Administration

Determine whether patient has any contraindicated condition before initiating administration.

Oral drug may be administered with food and at bedtime.

Provide ready access to bathroom facilities.

Screen patient's medication record for potential drug interactions before administering cimetidine because it increases the half-life of many drugs.

Monitor patient receiving cimetidine and interacting drugs for possible overdosage. Dosage of potentiated drugs may need to be reduced.

Observe patient with renal impairment for signs of overdosage. Dosage should be reduced in patient with renal failure.

Discard injectable form added to commonly used IV solutions after it has been at normal room temperature for 48 hours, the length of time it remains stable.

Provide small, frequent meals if GI upset occurs.

Surveillance During Therapy

Monitor for adverse effects and toxicity.

Interpret results of diagnostic tests and contact practitioner as appropriate.

Monitor for possible drug–drug and drug–nutrient interactions: antacids and metoclopramide may impair oral absorption of H_2 blockers if administered simultaneously; by reducing hepatic biotransformation, cimetidine may lengthen the half-life of certain benzodiazepine drugs (alprazolam, chlordiazepoxide, diazepam, flurazepam, triazolam), beta-blockers, caffeine, theophylline, lidocaine, salicylates, phenytoin, quinidine, and other drugs metabolized in the liver; cimetidine or ranitidine may increase the pharmacologic effects of procainamide by reducing its renal clearance; cimetidine when used with morphine may lead to increased respiratory depression; the effectiveness of sucralfate may be reduced by H_2 blockers because sucralfate requires an acid medium to be most effective; decreased oral absorption of fluconazole and ketoconazole may occur in the presence of H_2 blockers because of increased gastric pH; increased effects of carbamazepine have been reported when given in conjunction with cimetidine; cimetidine when used with digoxin has reduced serum levels of digoxin.

Provide for patient safety needs if CNS effects or hypotension occur.

Patient Teaching

Instruct the patient to avoid OTC preparations.

Suggest taking drug with meals to minimize GI irritation.

Warn patient to avoid activities requiring alertness and coordination in early stages of therapy because drowsiness is common, although it usually disappears in several days.

Warn patient to avoid hazardous activities because drug induces marked drowsiness, especially during first few days. Advise particular caution for elderly patient because hypertension, syncope, confusion, and excessive sedation may occur.

Caution patient to guard against injury resulting from dizziness and hypotension, which may occur particularly in the elderly.

Warn patient to avoid using other substances that add to CNS depressant effects (eg, alcohol, narcotics, barbiturates).

Advise patient that if drugs are used for prolonged periods, tests may be performed periodically to assess blood, kidney, and liver function.

Instruct patient to notify practitioner promptly at first sign of a skin rash; sore throat; fever; unusual bleeding or bruising; tarry stools; confusion; hallucinations; muscle or joint pain.

Teach patient about the types of side effects expected with therapy: drowsiness, lightheadedness, GI distress, and weakness.

Antiserotonin Agents

Many antihistamine drugs exert varying degrees of serotonin-blocking activity, although, in most cases, this activity is too weak to be clinically significant. A few agents, however, exert considerable serotonin antagonism, and they are used in several disease states in which overactivity of serotonin may be the primary etiologic factor. Because drugs classified as antiserotonin agents possess many other pharmacologic actions (eg, antihistaminic, anticholinergic, local anesthetic, oxytocic, vasoconstrictor), their clinical effects are not always related just to their serotonin-blocking action. Antiserotonin drugs are used mainly for symptomatic management of allergic conditions, especially to relieve itching, for prophylaxis of migraine and other vascular headaches, to reduce diarrhea and abdominal cramping in the treatment of the carcinoid syndrome, and to decrease nausea and vomiting caused by certain antineoplastic agents.

• **Ergotamine** *(Pregnancy Category X)*

Ergostat (Sublingual)

(CAN) Gynergen

Ergotamine is an ergot alkaloid used principally for relief of pain associated with vascular headaches. It is reviewed in the following, together with its structural analogue dihydroergotamine and another ergot alkaloid, methysergide. Additional ergot alkaloids discussed elsewhere in this text are ergonovine (Chapter 41), bromocriptine (Chapter 28), and LSD (Chapter 82).

Because prolonged use of ergotamine is not recommended, and migraine is usually a chronically recurring condition, it is important to identify the underlying psychological and physical factors that contribute to the etiology of a migraine attack. Owing to a wide range of adverse reactions, drug therapy alone often is dangerous and rarely curative. Alternative measures such as relaxation therapies, stress-reduction techniques, and changes in diet should be explored.

Mechanism

Direct spasmogenic effect on smooth muscle of peripheral and cerebral arteries; constricts the vessels and thereby reduces the pressure exerted on sensory nerve endings by the strong pulsations of the dilated arteries; also exhibits an alpha-adrenergic blocking and a serotonin-blocking action; *not* a true analgesic and specific only for the pain of vascular headaches; large doses have an oxytocic effect on the myometrium.

Uses

Prevention or reduction in frequency of vascular headaches, such as migraine and cluster headache (histamine cephalgia)

Relief of pain associated with migraine and cluster headaches (most effective if given early in an attack)

Dosage

Sublingual: 1 tablet (2 mg) at onset of attack; repeat at 30-minute intervals to a maximum of 3 tablets/24 h or 10 tablets/wk

Ergotamine also is available with caffeine as oral tablets and suppositories (eg, Cafergot, Wigraine). These products do *not* provide as rapid relief as sublingual administration.

Fate

Incompletely and erratically absorbed from GI tract; sublingual absorption is more predictable; prolonged duration of action, up to 24 hours; metabolized in the liver and excreted in the bile.

Common Side Effects

Numbness or tingling in extremities, muscle weakness, cold hands or feet, GI discomfort, diarrhea.

Significant Adverse Reactions

Hypertension, bradycardia, angina-like pain, intermittent claudication, depression. Prolonged use of high doses can lead to ergotism, with vomiting, convulsions, weak pulse, confusion, cold and cyanotic skin, or gangrene due to severe peripheral vasoconstriction. Severe vasoconstriction can be overcome by a vasodilator such as nitroprusside (Nipride; see Chapter 33).

Contraindications

Pregnancy (Category X), occlusive or vasospastic coronary or peripheral vascular disease, hepatic or renal disease, hypertension, severe pruritus, sepsis, infectious states and malnutrition, and young children. *Cautious use* in elderly patients and in nursing mothers (nausea and vomiting can develop in infants breastfeeding from a woman taking ergotamine).

Interactions

Vasoconstrictor action of ergotamine may be enhanced by beta-blockers, vasopressor amines, alpha$_1$-adrenergic agonists, and other peripheral vasoconstrictors, possibly resulting in peripheral ischemia.

Effects of ergotamine may be potentiated by nitroglycerin (increased bioavailability) and macrolide antibiotics (eg, erythromycin, azithromycin).

Nursing Management

Pretherapy Assessment

Assess and record baseline data necessary for detection of adverse effects of ergot alkaloids: General: VS, body weight, skin color and temperature; CNS: peripheral sensation; CVS: peripheral pulses, peripheral perfusion; GI: liver evaluation, bowel sounds, normal output; Laboratory: CBC with differential, liver and kidney function tests.

Review medical history and documents for existing or previous conditions that:

a. require cautious use of ergot alkaloids: use in elderly people.
b. contraindicate use of ergot alkaloids: allergy to ergot and derivatives; occlusive or vasospastic coronary or peripheral vascular disease; hepatic or renal disease; hypertension; severe pruritus; sepsis; infectious states and malnutrition; and young children; **pregnancy (Category X)**; lactation (secreted in breast milk, can cause neonatal ergotism [vomiting, diarrhea, seizures]; contraindicated in nursing mothers because of possible adverse effects to the neonate; nursing mothers should avoid this drug).

Nursing Interventions

Medication Administration

Determine whether patient has any contraindicated condition before initiating administration.

Drug should be administered as soon as possible after first symptoms of a migraine attack.

Provide ready access to bathroom facilities.

Provide small, frequent meals if GI upset occurs.

Surveillance During Therapy

Monitor for adverse effects and toxicity.

Interpret results of diagnostic tests and contact practitioner as appropriate.

Monitor for possible drug–drug and drug–nutrient interactions: vasoconstrictor action of ergotamine may be enhanced by beta-blockers, vasopressor amines, alpha$_1$-adrenergic agonists, and other peripheral vasoconstrictors; effects of ergotamine may be potentiated by nitroglycerin (increased bioavailability) and troleandomycin (decreased metabolism).

Provide for patient safety needs if CNS effects or hypotension occur.

Patient Teaching

Inform the female patient that this drug cannot be used during pregnancy.

Explain that the drug is more effective if taken early in an attack. If visual impairment, paresthesias, nausea, or other early symptoms ("aura") of vascular headache occur, the initial dose should be taken right away.

Suggest using sublingual tablets, if possible, early in an attack to provide rapid relief of headache pain.

Instruct patient to watch for onset of early signs of drug induced vascular insufficiency, such as numbness, coldness, and weakness in extremities, or a tingling sensation. Stopping the drug for 2 or 3 days usually overcomes circulatory problems.

Urge patient to adhere to recommended dosage because adverse reactions are much more common at high dosage levels.

Suggest that, when feasible, patient lie down in a dark, quiet room after taking drug to expedite pain relief.

Discuss relaxation and coping techniques, avoidance of stress, importance of diet, and adequate rest to deter onset of headaches.

Instruct patient to notify practitioner promptly at first sign of irregular heartbeat; pain or weakness of extremities; severe nausea or vomiting; numbness or tingling of fingers or toes.

Teach patient about the types of side effects expected with therapy: nausea, vomiting, numbness, tingling, loss of sensation in the extremities.

• **Dihydroergotamine** *(Pregnancy Category X)*

D.H.E. 45

An ergot alkaloid possessing pharmacologic and toxicologic properties similar to those of ergotamine but having less vasoconstrictive, oxytocic, and emetic effects; given IM in a dose of 1 mg (1 mL), repeated at 1-hour intervals to a total dose of 3 mg, or IV for a more rapid onset in a dose of 1 mg, to be repeated once. Effects occur within 15 to 30 minutes after IM injection and persist for up to 4 hours.

Nursing Management

See **ergotamine**.

• **Methysergide** *(Pregnancy Category X)*

Sansert

(CAN) Deseril

Mechanism

Primarily acts as a serotonin receptor antagonist; also possesses moderate agonistic action at serotonin receptors and may exert direct smooth muscle stimulation as well; has little direct vasoconstrictive action itself but appears to interact with serotonin in such a way as to facilitate its vasoconstrictive activity on cranial arteries, thus reducing excessive pulsations; strictly a prophylactic drug; does not abort an acute attack of migraine.

Uses

Prevention or reduction in frequency of vascular (migraine-type) headaches, especially if frequency exceeds once a week or if severity is intense.

Dosage

Not for use in children.

Adults: 4 to 8 mg daily in divided doses (if no response in 3 weeks, effects are unlikely to develop)

Discontinue drug in 3- to 4-week intervals every 6 months in patients on long-term therapy to minimize danger of fibrotic complications (see Significant Adverse Reactions)

Fate

Well absorbed orally; onset of optimal effect is 1 to 2 days; metabolic fate not clearly established.

Common Side Effects

Gastrointestinal distress, abdominal pain, drowsiness, lightheadedness, flushing, muscle and joint pains.

Significant Adverse Reactions

CAUTION

Fibrotic complications may occur with prolonged use of methysergide; these include retroperitoneal fibrosis (associated with fatigue, weight loss, fever, backache, urinary obstruction, lower limb vascular insufficiency), pleural fibrosis (dyspnea, chest tightness, pleural effusion), and cardiac fibrosis (thickening of aortic root, aortic and mitral valves). Therapy must be suspended for a 3- to 4-week interval every 6 months to minimize the danger of fibrotic complications.

CV: chest or abdominal pain, numbness in extremities, paresthesias, peripheral edema, postural hypotension, tachycardia, thrombophlebitis, claudication

GI: nausea, vomiting, constipation, increased gastric acid

CNS: insomnia, euphoria, feelings of dissociation, hallucinations, nightmares (may be related to vascular headache and not the drug)

Dermatologic and hematologic: nonspecific rash, telangiectasia, alopecia, neutropenia, eosinophilia

Other: weight gain, weakness, scotomas

Contraindications

Peripheral vascular disease, phlebitis, arteriosclerosis, hypertension, coronary artery disease, pulmonary disease, impaired liver or renal function, collagen diseases, valvular heart disorders, pregnancy, debilitated states, and serious infections. *Cautious use* in patients with cardiac or renal disease and in nursing mothers.

Interactions

Concurrent use of methysergide and beta-blockers may result in peripheral ischemia.

Nursing Management

Pretherapy Assessment

Assess and record baseline data necessary for detection of adverse effects of methysergide: General: VS, body weight, skin color and temperature; CNS: orientation, gait, peripheral sensation; CVS: peripheral pulses, peripheral perfusion; GI: liver evaluation, bowel sounds, normal output; Laboratory: CBC with differential, liver and kidney function tests.

Review medical history and documents for existing or previous conditions that:

a. require cautious use of methysergide: cardiac or renal disease
b. contraindicate use of methysergide: allergy to methysergide, tartrazine, aspirin; peripheral vascular disease; phlebitis; arteriosclerosis; hypertension; coronary artery disease; pulmonary disease; impaired liver or renal function; collagen diseases; valvular heart disorders; pregnancy; debilitated states; and serious infections; **pregnancy (Category X)**; lactation (secreted in breast milk, can cause neonatal ergotism [vomiting, diarrhea, seizures]; contraindicated in nursing mothers because of possible adverse effects to the neonate; nursing mothers should avoid this drug).

Nursing Interventions

Medication Administration

Determine whether patient has any contraindicated condition before initiating administration.

Administer with food to prevent GI upset.

Do not administer continuously for longer than 6 months; provide a 3- to 4-week drug-free interval after each 6-month course.

Carefully evaluate patient's understanding of instructions. This is a very dangerous drug. Fibrotic complications (formation of scar tissue) can occur in any patient on long-term therapy.

Provide ready access to bathroom facilities.

Provide small, frequent meals if GI upset occurs.

Surveillance During Therapy

Monitor for adverse effects and toxicity.

Interpret results of diagnostic tests and contact practitioner as appropriate.

Monitor for possible drug–drug and drug–nutrient interactions: antimigraine effects may be antagonized by cerebral vasodilators (eg, isoxsuprine, papaverine).

Provide for patient safety needs if CNS effects or hypotension occur.

Patient Teaching

Suggest taking drug with meals to minimize GI distress.

Stress the urgency of reporting any sign of coldness or numbness in extremities; leg cramps; edema; girdle, flank, or chest pain; dysuria; or other early signs of developing toxicity.

Teach patient how to check for edema, and instruct to maintain low salt intake and adjust caloric intake if edema or weight gain is noted.

Advise patient that cardiac status, kidney function, blood status, and pulmonary function are carefully monitored during therapy because adverse effects usually are reversible if drug is discontinued early enough.

Teach measures to control orthostatic hypotension.

Inform patient that abrupt discontinuation of drug may cause headache rebound. The drug should be withdrawn *gradually* over a period of 2 to 3 weeks.

Discuss the importance of adjunctive measures (eg, relaxation, proper exercise, avoidance of stressful situations) in dealing with migraine-type headaches.

Inform the female patient that this drug cannot be used during pregnancy.

Instruct patient to watch for onset of early signs of drug-induced vascular insufficiency, such as numbness, coldness, and weakness in extremities, or a tingling sensation. Stopping the drug for 2 or 3 days usually overcomes circulatory problems.

Urge patient to adhere to recommended dosage because adverse reactions are much more common at high dosage levels.

Suggest that, when feasible, patient lie down in a dark, quiet room after taking drug to expedite pain relief.

Discuss relaxation and coping techniques, avoidance of stress, importance of diet, and adequate rest to deter onset of headaches.

Instruct patient to notify practitioner promptly at first sign of cold, numb, painful extremities; leg cramps when walking; girdle, flank or chest pain; painful urination; shortness of breath.

Teach patient about the types of side effects expected with therapy: nausea, vomiting, numbness, tingling, loss of sensation in the extremities.

• Ondansetron

Zofran

Ondansetron, a selective serotonin antagonist, is used for the prevention and reduction of nausea and vomiting that often occur during therapy with certain cancer chemotherapeutic agents.

Mechanism

Blocks $5HT_3$ subtype of serotonin receptor, both peripherally on vagal nerve terminals and centrally in the chemoreceptor trigger zone in the medulla, thus decreasing the effects of serotonin released by cytotoxic cancer chemotherapeutic drugs.

Uses

Prevention of nausea and vomiting due to emetogenic cancer chemotherapy, especially with drugs such as cisplatin, carmustine, dacarbazine, dactinomycin, mechlorethamine, and streptozocin

Prevention of postoperative nausea and vomiting

Dosage

Prevention of nausea and vomiting due to cancer chemotherapy; give 30 minutes *before* start of chemotherapy, diluted in 50 mL of 5% dextrose or 0.9% NaCl as follows:

IV: Adults and children 4 to 18 years old—three doses of 0.15 mg/kg *each* or a single dose of 32 mg.

Oral:

Adults and children 12 years and older—8 mg three times a day; begin 30 minutes before start of chemotherapy, with subsequent doses at 4 and 8 hours after first dose. Continue dosing 3 times a day for 1 to 2 days after chemotherapy.

Children 4 to 12 years old—4 mg three times a day, administered as outlined above.

Fate

Oral absorption is good; drug undergoes limited first-pass metabolism but extensive systemic biotransformation—only approximately 5% of a dose is eliminated unchanged in urine; half-life is 3.5 hours in younger patients, but up to 5.5 hours in older patients; plasma protein binding is approximately 75%; oral absorption significantly increased (17%) by food but does not appear to be a clinically significant interaction; metabolized by cytochrome P-450 enzymes; inducers or inhibitors may affect biotransformation.

Common Side Effects

Diarrhea, headache, fever, dizziness, drowsiness, musculoskeletal pain.

Significant Adverse Reactions

CV: hypotension, chest pain
GI: xerostomia, abdominal pain, constipation
GU: dysuria, urinary retention
CNS: fatigue, weakness, anxiety, agitation, extrapyramidal reaction
Dermatologic: pruritus, paresthesia

Contraindications

No absolute contraindications. *Cautious use* in pregnant or nursing women and in young children.

Nursing Management

Pretherapy Assessment

Assess and record important baseline data necessary for detection of adverse effects of ondansetron: General: VS (T, P, R, BP), skin integrity; CNS: orientation, reflexes; CVS: peripheral perfusion; GI: liver function, output; GU: renal function; Laboratory: renal function tests, CBC.

Review past medical history and documents for evidence of existing or previous medical history related to conditions that:

a. require caution with ondansetron: pregnancy, breast feeding.
b. contraindicate use of ondansetron: allergy to ondansetron; **pregnancy (Category B)**.

Nursing Interventions

Medication Administration

Administer **intravenously through a freely running infusion set; initial recommended dose is 32 mg infused 30 minutes prior to the start of emetogenic chemotherapy**.

Ondansetron should be mixed with 5% dextrose injection or 0.9% sodium chloride injection; it should not be mixed with alkaline solutions as precipitation may occur.

Oral dosage form should be administered 30 minutes prior to the start of emetogenic chemotherapy, with subsequent doses 4 and 8 hours after the first dose.

Surveillance During Therapy

Monitor patient for therapeutic effect of ondansetron therapy.

Compare current status with previous status to detect improvements or deterioration in the patient's condition.

Monitor for adverse effects, toxicity, and interactions.

Monitor for signs of hypersensitivity that may require discontinuation of drug.

Patient Teaching

Patients should be informed of the actions of this drug as it pertains to the possible antiemetogenic activity.

Selected Bibliography

Berthold CW, Dionne RA: Clinical evaluation of H_1-receptor and H_2-receptor antagonists for acute postoperative pain. J Clin Pharmacol 33:944, 1993

Cubeddu LX, Hoffmann IS: Participation of serotonin on early and delayed emesis induced by initial and subsequent cycles of cisplatinum-based chemotherapy: Effects of antiemetics. J Clin Pharmacol 33:691, 1993

Dauncey H, Chesher GB, Palmer RH: Cimetidine and ranitidine: Lack of effect on the pharmacokinetics of an acute ethanol dose. J Clin Gastroenterol 17(3):189, 1993

Gladziwa U, Klotz U: Pharmacokinetics and pharmacodynamics of H_2-receptor antagonists in patients with renal insufficiency. Clin Pharmacokinet 24(4):319, 1993

Koppa SD: H_2 antagonists and alcohol. Drug Ther 23(12):52, 1993

Monroe EW: Nonsedating H_1 antihistamines in chronic urticaria. Ann Allergy 71:585, 1993

Sanders LD, Whitehead C, Gildersleve CD, Rosen M, Robinson JO: Interaction of H_2-receptor antagonists and benzodiazepine sedation. Anaesthesia 48:286, 1993

Simons FER: H_1-receptor antagonists: Does a dose–response relationship exist? Ann Allergy 71:592, 1993

Susi D, Neri M, Ballone E, Mezzetti A, Cuccurullo F: Five year maintenance treatment with ranitidine: Effects on the natural history of duodenal ulcer disease. Am J Gastroenterol 89(1):26, 1994

Nursing Bibliography

Nursing guide to OTC allergy products. Nursing '93 23(9):67–72, 1993

Weiss J: Assessment and management of clients with headaches. The Nurse Practitioner 18(4):44, 1993

17

Skeletal Muscle Relaxants

Peripherally Acting Skeletal Muscle Relaxants

Antidepolarizing

Atracurium
Doxacurium
Gallamine
Metocurine
Mivacurium
Pancuronium
Pipecuronium
Tubocurarine
Vecuronium

Depolarizing

Succinylcholine

Direct-Acting Skeletal Muscle Relaxant

Dantrolene

Centrally Acting Skeletal Muscle Relaxants

Baclofen
Carisoprodol
Chlorphenesin
Chlorzoxazone
Cyclobenzaprine
Diazepam
Metaxalone
Methocarbamol
Orphenadrine

Skeletal muscle activity can be reduced by a diverse group of pharmacologic agents. Those agents classified as *peripherally acting* interfere with transmission of cholinergic impulses at the neuromuscular junction or act directly to inhibit the contractile mechanism of the skeletal musculature. They cause *paralysis* of skeletal muscles and are used primarily as adjuncts to general anesthetics; they also are used in minor surgical procedures and shock therapy. The other type, classified as *centrally acting*, reduces signal transmission within spinal cord motor reflex pathways. Drugs in this group produce varying degrees of skeletal muscle *relaxation*; they are used to reduce the muscle spasms and hyperreflexia associated with inflammatory conditions or anxiety, stress, and neurologic disorders.

According to their site of action, skeletal muscle relaxants may be classified in the following manner:

- I. Peripherally acting muscle relaxants
  - A. Neuromuscular blocking agents
    - 1. Antidepolarizing blockers (eg, pancuronium, tubocurarine)
    - 2. Depolarizing blockers (eg, succinylcholine)
  - B. Direct-acting myotropic agent (eg, dantrolene)
- II. Centrally acting muscle relaxants (eg, carisoprodol, methocarbamol)
  - A. Treatment of spasms (eg, carisoprodol)
  - B. Treatment of spasticity (eg, baclofen)
  - C. Treatment of spasms and spasticity (eg, diazepam)

Peripherally Acting Muscle Relaxants

Neuromuscular Blocking Agents

Neuromuscular blocking agents are anticholinergic agents; however, their effects at the neuromuscular junction occur only at therapeutic dosages. At higher amounts, their blockade extends to other cholinergic receptors—the autonomic ganglia and postganglionic parasympathetic sites. This extension of cholinergic blockade causes adverse reactions such as tachycardia and hypotension. Neuromuscular blockers do release histamine from intracellular stores; the increased levels of circulating histamine can produce increased salivary and mucosal secretions, bronchospasm, hypotension, and other unwanted effects. Because these drugs do *not* effectively penetrate the blood–brain barrier at therapeutic concentrations, their central nervous system (CNS) effects are minimal.

Two mechanisms are involved in the inhibition of transmission at the neuromuscular junction; both involve postsynaptic receptor sites. One group, typified by d-tubocurarine, is *antidepolarizing*, that is, they compete with acetylcholine (ACh) for the receptor site and prevent depolarization of the postsynaptic membrane. The second group of drugs, exemplified by succinylcholine, are *depolarizing* agents; they produce an initial activation (depolarization) of the receptor, followed by a persistent occupation that markedly delays repolarization and prevents further receptor stimulation.

Skeletal muscles are not equally susceptible to the paralytic effects of neuromuscular blocking agents:

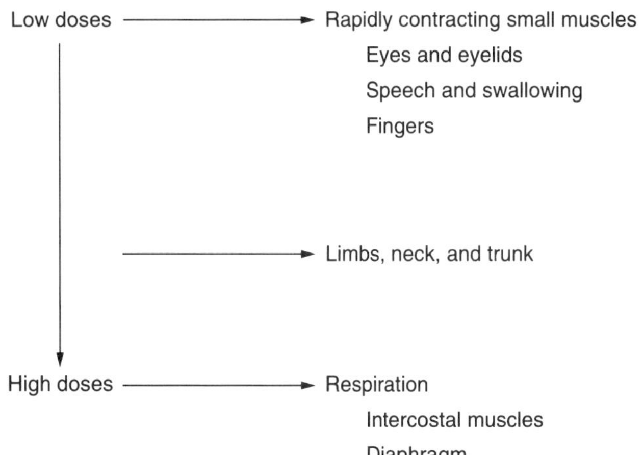

Recovery occurs in reverse order.

Because differences in sensitivity among these muscles are very slight, the margin between the effective dose and the toxic dose of neuromuscular blocking drugs is quite small; a slight overdose can cause severe hypotension and respiratory depression. Overdosage with neuromuscular blocking agents is therefore treated with vasopressors (eg, levarterenol) and artificial respiration with oxygen. Cholinesterase inhibitors (eg, edrophonium) may be used in cases of poisoning with *anti*depolarizing blockers to overcome the competitive blockade; they are *contraindicated* in treating overdosage caused by depolarizing blockers because they would further stimulate cholinergic receptors and intensify the muscle paralysis.

Nondepolarizing Blockers

This group also is referred to as the antidepolarizing, stabilizing, or curariform drugs. The latter designation derives from the fact that the first antidepolarizing muscle relaxant was the alkaloid *d*-tubocurarine, the active chemical found in a group of South American arrow poisons collectively called *curare*. Several synthetic and semisynthetic products have been developed, all of which possess, like *d*-tubocurarine, a quaternary nitrogen similar to that in the molecular structure of ACh.

Because the nondepolarizing blockers share a common mechanism of action and many of the same uses, these are listed below, followed by a section on Nursing Management common to all nondepolarizing blockers. The pharmacology of the individual drugs is then discussed.

Common Mechanism

These quaternary nitrogen drugs function as reversible competitive antagonists of ACh at postsynaptic receptors of the neuromuscular junction (nicotinic II sites). Because ACh cannot enter the receptor, depolarization does not occur. Thus, skeletal muscles can not contract, and a temporary state of muscle paralysis is produced. There is no initial contraction—that is, a flaccid paralysis develops.

Common Uses

Provide skeletal muscle relaxation:

- during surgery performed under general anesthesia
- to facilitate intubation
- to improve respiration in patients on mechanical ventilation
- to reduce injury in shock therapy

Common Interactions

Additive muscle relaxant effects can occur with concurrent use of certain antibiotics (eg, aminogylcosides, lincosamides, polymixins), inhalation general anesthetics (enflurane > isoflurane > halothane), ketamine, local anesthetics, lithium and quinidine.

The pharmacologic effects of nondepolarizing blockers can be decreased by cholinergic drugs, corticosteroids, ranitidine and theophylline.

Common Treatment of Overdosage

Depending on the status of the patient, treated by:

- artificial respiration with oxygen
- vasopressors (eg, levarterenol)
- cholinesterase inhibitors (eg, edrophonium) for poisoning with nondepolarizing blockers (tubocurarine, gallamine, metocurine, pancuronium) to overcome the competitive blockade

CAUTION

Cholinesterase inhibitors are *contraindicated* for overdosage with depolarizing blockers (eg, succinylcholine): They stimulate cholinergic receptors further and can intensify the muscle paralysis.

General Nursing Management: Nondepolarizing Blockers

Pretherapy Assessment

Assess and record baseline data necessary for detection of adverse effects of nondepolarizing blockers: General: vital signs (VS), body weight, skin color and temperature; CNS: reflexes, bilateral grip strength; Gastrointestinal (GI): bowel sounds, liver palpation; Laboratory: renal and liver function tests, serum electrolytes, urinalysis, hemoglobin, complete blood count (CBC).

Review medical history and documents for existing or previous conditions that:

a. require cautious use of nondepolarizing blockers: reduced pulmonary, renal, cardiovascular, endocrine or hepatic function; hypotension; thyroid disorders; history of allergies; debilitated or dehydrated patients.
b. contraindicate use of nondepolarizing blockers: allergy to any of these drugs; myasthenia gravis; patients in whom histamine release is a hazard; electrolyte imbalance; acidosis; **pregnancy (Category C)**; lactation (safety not established, avoid use in nursing mothers).

Nursing Interventions

Medication Administration

Agents should be administered by trained personnel (anesthesiologist/nurse anesthetist).

Administer by slow intravenous (IV) or intramuscular (IM) injection.

Verify results of renal function tests and serum electrolyte studies before administering. Drug effects may be increased in the presence of hypokalemia, hypermagnesemia, or decreased renal clearance.

Do not mix with alkaline barbiturate solutions; may form precipitates.

Have neostigmine or edrophonium available to overcome excessive or prolonged neuromuscular blockade.

Have a peripheral nerve stimulator available to assess degree of neuromuscular block, if appropriate.

Have atropine or glycopyrrolate available to deal with parasympathomimetic effects of cholinesterase inhibitors.

Provide fluids and vasopressors to deal with hypotension.

Surveillance During Therapy

Monitor vital signs continuously until recovery from drug effect is complete. Use precautions for possible residual muscle weakness caused by the accumulation of drug in some patients.

Monitor for toxicity.

Monitor for signs of pain or distress that the patient may not be able to communicate.

Reassure the conscious patient that personnel are aware of the patient's helplessness.

Change patient's position frequently to prevent venous stasis, decubitus ulcer formation.

Monitor for signs of hypersensitivity, which may require discontinuation of drug.

Interpret results of diagnostic tests and contact practitioner as appropriate.
Monitor for possible drug–drug and drug–nutrient interactions: a nondepolarizing blocker when used with diazepam may increase the possibility of malignant hyperthermia; muscle-relaxing effect can be enhanced by volatile anesthetics, aminoglycosides, polymyxins, lithium, magnesium salts, quinidine, and procainamide; may be antagonized by cholinergic drugs, cholinesterase inhibitors, and potassium.

Patient Teaching

Only patients who are conscious (such as those suffering from tetanus and needing ventilatory assistance) while receiving these drugs will need teaching about the drug.
Carefully explain to patient all procedures; remember that the patient cannot ask questions or express fears or concerns.

• Atracurium

Tracrium

Uses

Relaxation of skeletal muscles during surgery, as an adjunct to general anesthesia
Facilitation of endotracheal intubation or mechanical ventilation

Dosage

Initially, 0.4 to 0.5 mg/kg as an IV bolus injection; maintenance doses during prolonged surgical procedures are 0.08 to 0.2 mg/kg given every 15 to 45 minutes; alternatively, maintenance during prolonged procedures may be accomplished by IV infusion at a rate of 5 to 10 μg/kg/min. If atracurium is administered under isoflurane or enflurane anesthesia, the dosage should be reduced by one third.

Fate

Maximum neuromuscular blockade occurs within 2 to 5 minutes of IV injection; recovery begins within 20 to 30 minutes and is nearly complete within 1 hour after injection. Time of onset is shorter and duration of effect is longer as dosage increases; repeated doses have no cumulative effect on the duration of neuromuscular blockade if recommended dosage intervals are followed; rapidly inactivated in the plasma, with an elimination half-life of about 20 minutes; half-life is *not* altered by impaired renal function.

Common Side Effects

Especially at high doses: flushing, mild hypotension.

Significant Adverse Reactions

Mostly caused by histamine release at high doses: erythema, itching, urticaria, wheezing, hypotension, tachycardia; rarely, apnea and cyanosis.

Contraindications

No absolute contraindications. *Cautious use* in patients with myasthenia gravis, electrolyte disturbances, asthma, cardiovascular disease, or systemic allergies, and in pregnant or nursing women.

Interactions

The muscle-relaxing action of atracurium can be *enhanced* by halothane, enflurane, isoflurane, aminoglycosides, polymyxins, lithium, magnesium salts, quinidine, and procainamide.
The muscle-relaxing effects of atracurium may be *antagonized* by cholinergic drugs, cholinesterase inhibitors, and potassium.
Concurrent administration of succinylcholine with atracurium may accelerate the onset and increase the depth of neuromuscular blockade.

Nursing Management

See General Nursing Management.

• Doxacurium

Numorax

Uses

Facilitate endotracheal intubation and mechanical ventilation
Reduce intensity of skeletal muscle contractions during chemoshock and electroshock therapy

Dosage

Administered only by IV route. When used with narcotics and thiopental, 0.05 mg/kg; maintenance doses range from 0.005 to 0.01 mg/kg.

Fate

The half-life is approximately 100 minutes, depending on dose and status of patient (eg, $T_{1/2}$ is twice as long in patients who have received a kidney transplant).

Significant Adverse Reactions

Little or no release of histamine. Hypotension, flushing, tachycardia, bronchospasm, wheezing, urticaria, diplopia.

Contraindications

See gallamine.

Interactions

See gallamine.

Nursing Management

See General Nursing Management.

• Gallamine

Flaxedil

Uses

Produce skeletal muscle relaxation as an adjunct to general anesthesia
Facilitate management of patients undergoing mechanical ventilation
Reduce intensity of muscle contractions during electroshock or chemoshock therapy

Dosage

1 mg/kg by slow IV injection to a maximum of 100 mg; may be reinjected after 30 to 40 minutes at a dose of 0.5 to 1 mg/kg, depending on patient status.

Fate

Onset of action is immediate; maximal effect in 2 to 3 minutes; duration is 20 to 30 minutes; drug may accumulate in the body with repeated injections; excreted largely unchanged in urine.

Common Side Effects

Tachycardia, dizziness.

Significant Adverse Reactions

Usually an extension of its pharmacologic action: profound muscle weakness, respiratory depression, apnea, and hypersensitivity reactions.

Contraindications

Myasthenia gravis, shock, impaired renal function, severe cardiac disease or hypertension, hyperthyroidism, sensitivity to iodides (drug is the triethiodide salt), infants weighing less than 11 pounds (5 kg). *Cautious use* in the presence of impaired pulmonary function, collagen diseases, angina, or history of allergies, and in elderly, debilitated, or dehydrated patients.

Interactions

Muscle-relaxant effects may be potentiated by inhalation anesthetics, aminoglycoside antibiotics, amphotericin, clindamycin, lincomycin, lithium, potassium-depleting diuretics, antiarrhythmics (quinidine, procainamide, propranolol), phenothiazines, diazepam, calcium and magnesium salts, and trimethaphan.
Effects may be antagonized by cholinergic drugs, anticholinesterases, and potassium.
Tachycardia may be enhanced by anticholinergic agents (eg, atropine, phenothiazines, antihistamines, tricyclic antidepressants).

Nursing Management

See General Nursing Management.

• Metocurine

Metubine

Approximately two to three times more potent than *d*-tubocurarine; releases histamine on IV injection less frequently than *d*-tubocurarine, and produces minimal ganglionic blockade.

Uses

Adjunct to general anesthesia to induce adequate skeletal muscle relaxation
Assist patients undergoing mechanical respiration
Reduce intensity of muscle contractions during chemoshock and electroshock therapy

Dosage

Anesthesia adjunct: size of initial dose depends on general anesthetic used; usual range 0.2 to 0.4 mg/kg by IV injection over 30 to 60 seconds; repeat at 0.5 to 1 mg every 60 minutes as needed
Electroshock–chemoshock: 2 to 3 mg IV, injected slowly

Fate

Onset within 3 minutes; duration of effect 30 to 90 minutes (average 60 minutes); half-life is 3 to 4 hours; excreted rapidly by the kidney, approximately 50% unchanged.

Common Side Effects

Dizziness.

Significant Adverse Reactions

Bronchospasm, hypotension, profound muscle weakness, respiratory depression, apnea, circulatory depression, hypersensitivity reactions, and increased secretions.

Contraindications

Patients in whom histamine release poses a definite hazard (eg, asthmatic patients, those with allergies), myasthenia gravis, and sensitivity to iodides. *Cautious use* in patients with impaired pulmonary, cardiovascular, renal, endocrine, or hepatic function, hypotension, thyroid or collagen disorders, or history of allergies, and in elderly or debilitated patients and pregnant or nursing women.

Interactions

See gallamine. In addition, precipitate may form whenever drug is combined with thiopental or methohexital because drug is unstable in alkaline solutions.

Nursing Management

See General Nursing Management.

• Mivacurium

Mivacron

Uses

Skeletal muscle relaxation during general anesthesia or mechanical ventilation
Facilitation of tracheal intubation

Dosage

0.15 mg/kg over 5 to 15 seconds for intubation; maintenance dose of 0.10 mg/kg every 15 minutes.

Fate

Onset of activity in approximately 2 minutes; single dose has duration of action of about 7 minutes.

Common Side Effects

Flushing, mild hypotension.

Significant Adverse Reactions

Possible release of histamine; amount released increases with dose and speed of injection. See gallamine.

Contraindications

Use of multidose vials in people allergic to benzyl alcohol. *Cautious use* in patients with renal or hepatic impairment; in addition, skeletal muscle blockade may be significantly increased in patients with reduced plasma cholinesterase (eg, patients with malignant tumors, infections, severe burns, anemia, peptic ulcer, hypothyroidism).

Interactions

See gallamine.

Nursing Management

See General Nursing Management.

• Pancuronium

Pavulon

Approximately five times as potent as *d*-tubocurarine; little ganglionic blockade or histamine release; high doses produce tachycardia and mild hypertension, probably through a vagal blocking action.

Uses

Adjunct to anesthesia during surgery
Assist patients receiving mechanical ventilation

Dosage

Initially 0.04 to 0.1 mg/kg IV; increments of 0.01 mg/kg given as needed; children's dose same as adults, except for neonates, who should receive a test dose of 0.02 mg/kg to measure sensitivity.

Fate

Onset about 1 minute; maximal effects in 5 minutes, persisting approximately 60 minutes; excreted largely unchanged by the kidneys.

Common Side Effects

Tachycardia, muscle weakness, salivation.

Significant Adverse Reactions

Profound muscle weakness, apnea, acne-like skin rash, hypertension.

Contraindications

Myasthenia gravis, bromide hypersensitivity, severe coronary artery disease, and other conditions in which tachycardia is undesirable. *Cautious use* in patients with impaired pulmonary, renal, or cardiovascular function or electrolyte imbalances, in debilitated or dehydrated patients, and in children.

Interactions

See gallamine. In addition, use with cardiac glycosides may result in additive cardiotoxic effects.

Nursing Management

See General Nursing Management.

• Pipecuronium

Arduan

Uses

Relax skeletal muscles for endotracheal intubation and during general surgery; recommended for procedures lasting for 90 or more minutes.

Dosage

Endotracheal intubation: 70 to 85 μg/kg
Maintenance dose: 10 to 15 μg/kg produces skeletal muscle relaxation for approximately 50 minutes

Fate

Drug is eliminated primarily by the kidneys; in healthy patients, half-life is 1.7 hours; in patients who have received a kidney transplant, half-life is 4.0 hours.

Significant Adverse Reactions

Little or no release of histamine.

CV: hypotension, bradycardia, myocardial ischemia, hypertension, cerebrovascular accident (CVA), thrombosis
CNS: hypesthesia, depression
Genitourinary: anuria
Metabolic: hypoglycemia, hyperkalemia
Respiratory: dyspnea, respiratory depression

Interactions

See gallamine.

Nursing Management

See General Nursing Management.

• Tubocurarine

Tubocurarine

(CAN) Tubarine

In addition to its neuromuscular blocking action, tubocurarine possesses ganglionic blocking and histamine-releasing effects, which can lead to hypotension and bronchospasm.

Uses

Adjunct to general anesthesia to provide adequate muscle relaxation
Reduction in intensity of muscle contractions during shock therapy
Facilitation of mechanical ventilation
Diagnosis of myasthenia gravis (when results of other tests are inconclusive)

Dosage

Anesthesia adjunct: 40 to 60 units (6–9 mg) IV at time of incision; supplements of 20 to 30 units (3–4.5 mg) as needed
Shock therapy: 0.5 units/lb (1.1 units/kg) of body weight by slow IV injection before induction of shock
Diagnosis of myasthenia: 6.7% to 20% of average adult electroshock dose IV

Fate

Immediate onset of action; duration of paralysis 30 to 90 minutes; has a cumulative effect in the body; half-life is 1 to 3 hours; moderately (40%) bound to plasma proteins; irregular and unpredictable absorption when given IM; excreted largely through the kidney, approximately half in unchanged form.

Common Side Effects

Dizziness, muscle weakness, sensation of warmth.

Significant Adverse Reactions

Bronchospasm, hypotension, profound muscle weakness, respiratory and circulatory depression, increased bronchial and salivary secretions, hypersensitivity reactions, and malignant hyperthermia.

Contraindications

Myasthenia gravis, patients in whom release of histamine is a hazard, hyperthermia, and electrolyte imbalance or acidosis. *Cautious use* in the presence of reduced pulmonary, renal, cardiovascular, endocrine, or hepatic function; hypotension; thyroid disorders; or history of allergies, and in debilitated or dehydrated patients.

Interactions

See gallamine. In addition, concurrent use of tubocurarine and diazepam may increase the risk for malignant hyperthermia

Nursing Management

See General Nursing Management.

• Vecuronium

Norcuron

Onset of action is faster and duration of paralysis is longer with increasing doses; hemodynamic function is largely unchanged at recommended dosage.

Uses

Adjunct to general anesthesia to provide skeletal muscle relaxation during surgery or mechanical intubation.

Dosage

Initial adult dosage: 0.08 to 0.1 mg/kg given as an IV bolus; during prolonged procedures, additional doses of 0.01 to 0.015 mg/kg may be given at 15- to 25-minute intervals as necessary
Children older than 10 years: same as adult dosage
Children younger than 10 years: may require a slightly higher initial dosage and more frequent supplementation
Not recommended for neonates

Fate

Maximal neuromuscular blockade occurs within 3 to 5 minutes; recovery is nearly complete within 45 to 60 minutes; repeated doses have little cumulative effect; drug is approximately 75% protein bound; elimination half-life is 60 to 75 minutes, and vecuronium is eliminated in both urine and bile.

Significant Adverse Reactions

Excessive muscle weakness, respiratory insufficiency, apnea.

Contraindications

No absolute contraindications. *Cautious use* in patients with myasthenia gravis or other neuromuscular disorders, hepatic disease (prolongs recovery time), electrolyte imbalances, obesity (may impair normal ventilation), cardiovascular disease, edema, and in elderly patients and pregnant or nursing women.

Interactions

See gallamine.

Nursing Management

See General Nursing Management.

Depolarizing Blockers

The action of the depolarizing neuromuscular blocking agents is biphasic: an initial depolarization of the muscle end-plate, inducing an immediate but short-lived activation (depolarization) of the muscle fibers followed by a persistent occupation of the receptor site, which prevents repolarization and essentially desensitizes the receptor site to ACh. This "second-phase" block persists for 10 to 30 minutes, depending on the drug and dose used. During this time, the muscle remains paralyzed to motor nerve stimulation. The major difference between these drugs and the antidepolarizing blockers discussed previously is that, owing to the initial depolarization phase, transient muscle contractions (fasciculations) occur immediately after administration of the depolarizing drug. Contractions are followed rapidly by a flaccid paralysis similar to that observed with the antidepolarizing agents. There also is some evidence that the neuromuscular blockade after administration of a depolarizing drug may persist beyond the actual presence of the drug at the receptor; this suggests the possibility of desensitization of the receptor caused by conformational changes of the reactive area.

• Succinylcholine

Anectine, Quelicin, Sucostrin

Mechanism

Depolarizing neuromuscular blockade leading to initial muscle contraction (fasciculations), followed quickly by flaccid paralysis; rapidly hydrolyzed by plasma cholinesterases; slightly increases intraocular pressure; may produce altered heart rhythm and slightly elevated blood pressure.

Uses

Skeletal muscle relaxation as an adjunct to general anesthesia
Reduction of the intensity of muscle contractions during shock therapy
Facilitation of intubation procedures
Assistance with mechanical respiration

Dosage

Adults: 0.3 to 1.1 mg/kg IV given over 10 to 30 seconds, which produces muscle paralysis lasting approximately 5 to 10 minutes; prolonged muscle relaxation is achieved by subsequent IV injections of 0.04 to 0.07 mg/kg at appropriate intervals
Children: 1 to 2 mg/kg by IV injection *or* 2.5 to 4 mg/kg IM; IM injections should be given deep into the deltoid muscle

Fate

Onset after IV use within 1 minute; maximum effects last 2 to 4 minutes and disappear within 8 to 10 minutes; quickly hydrolyzed by plasma cholinesterases; onset with IM injection 2 to 3 minutes; duration 10 to 20 minutes; excreted through kidneys, both as metabolites and small amounts of unchanged drug.

Common Side Effects

Muscle twitching, bradycardia (especially in children).

Significant Adverse Reactions

Prolonged muscle weakness, muscle pain, tachycardia, hypertension, arrhythmias, respiratory depression, apnea, excessive salivation, increased intraocular pressure, hyperkalemia, rash, myoglobinemia, decreased GI motility, anaphylactoid reactions, and cardiac arrest; abrupt onset of malignant hyperthermia, a hypermetabolic disease of skeletal muscle, can occur with succinylcholine; early signs include muscle rigidity, tachycardia, rising body temperature, and metabolic acidosis.

Contraindications

History of malignant hyperthermia, severe respiratory depression, acute narrow-angle glaucoma, penetrating eye injury, and genetically determined deficiency of plasma pseudocholinesterase. *Cautious use* in patients with renal, cardiovascular, hepatic, pulmonary, or metabolic disorders; severe burns, electrolyte imbalance, glaucoma, spinal cord injury, degenerative neuromuscular diseases, fractures, respiratory depression, or in patients with low levels of plasma pseudocholinesterase (eg, dehydrated or anemic patients; patients exposed to neurotoxic insecticides; patients with liver disease, cancer, collagen disorders, or myxedema; and patients receiving certain other drugs (see Interactions).

Interactions

Neuromuscular blocking action of succinylcholine may be enhanced by aminoglycosides, beta-blockers, chloroquine, furosemide, lidocaine, lithium, isoflurane, magnesium salts, oxytocin, phenothiazines, polymyxin antibiotics, procainamide, quinidine, and trimethaphan.

Effects of succinylcholine may be prolonged and intensified by drugs that interfere with the action of plasma pseudocholinesterase enzyme (eg, cholinesterase inhibitors, cyclophosphamide, thiotepa, monoamine oxidase [MAO] inhibitors, procaine, antimalarial drugs, oral contraceptives, pancuronium, and chlorpromazine).

Diazepam may reduce duration of neuromuscular blockade elicited by succinylcholine.

Succinylcholine may cause arrhythmias in the patient receiving digitalis or quinidine by causing a sudden release of potassium from muscle cells.

Concurrent administration of an antidepolarizing muscle relaxant may reduce the effectiveness of succinylcholine.

Nursing Management

Pretherapy Assessment

Assess and record baseline data necessary for detection of adverse effects of succinylcholine: General: VS, body weight, skin color and temperature; CNS: reflexes, bilateral grip strength; GI: bowel sounds, liver palpation; Laboratory: renal and liver function tests, serum electrolytes, urinalysis, hemoglobin, CBC.

Review medical history and documents for existing or previous conditions that:

a. require cautious use of succinylcholine: reduced pulmonary, renal, cardiovascular, endocrine or hepatic function; severe burns; electrolyte imbalance; glaucoma; spinal cord injury; degenerative neuromuscular disorders; fractures; respiratory depression; patients with a low plasma pseudocholinesterase level.
b. contraindicate use of succinylcholine: allergy to succinylcholine; severe respiratory depression; acute narrow-angle glaucoma; penetrating eye injury; genetically determined deficiency of plasma pseudocholinesterase; **pregnancy (Category C)**; lactation (safety not established, avoid use in nursing mothers).

Nursing Interventions

Medication Administration

Agent should be administered by trained personnel (anesthesiologist/nurse anesthetist).

Administer a test dose to patients with a low plasma pseudocholinesterase level.

Use only freshly prepared solutions.

Administer a small dose of tubocurarine before succinylcholine injection to reduce the severity of muscle fasciculations.

Administer by slow IV or IM injection.

Verify results of renal function tests and serum electrolyte studies before administering. Drug effects may be increased in the presence of dehydration, hypothermia, hypokalemia, hypermagnesemia, or decreased renal clearance.

Do not mix with alkaline barbiturate solutions.

Have a peripheral nerve stimulator available to assess degree of neuromuscular block, if appropriate.

Administer only after unconsciousness has been attained with anesthesia to avoid patient distress.

Provide fluids and vasopressors to deal with hypotension.

Surveillance During Therapy

Monitor vital signs continuously until recovery from drug effect is complete. Use precautions for possible residual muscle weakness caused by the accumulation of drug or metabolite in some patients.

Monitor for toxicity.

Monitor for signs of pain or distress that the patient may not be able to communicate.

Reassure the conscious patient that personnel are aware of the patient's helplessness.

Change patient's position frequently to prevent venous stasis, decubitus ulcer formation.

Monitor for signs of tachyphylaxis (loss of drug response) with repeated use.

Monitor for signs of hypersensitivity, which may require discontinuation of drug.

Interpret results of diagnostic tests and contact practitioner as appropriate.

Monitor for possible drug–drug and drug–nutrient interactions: actions may be enhanced by aminoglycosides, beta-blockers, chloroquine, furosemide, lidocaine, lithium, volatile anesthetics, oxytocin, magnesium salts, phenothiazines, polymyxins, procainamide, quinidine, and trimethaphan; effects prolonged by agents that impair the action of plasma pseudocholinesterase (cholinesterase inhibitors, cyclophosphamide, MAO inhibitors, procaine, antimalarials, oral contraceptives, pancuronium, and chlorpromazine); diazepam may reduce depolarizing neuromuscular blockade; succinylcholine may cause arrhythmias in patients receiving digitalis or quinidine.

Patient Teaching

Only patients who are conscious (such as those suffering from tetanus and needing ventilatory assistance) while receiving these drugs will need teaching about the drug. Carefully explain to patient all procedures; remember that the patient cannot ask questions or express fears or concerns.

Direct-Acting Skeletal Muscle Relaxant

A different type of peripherally acting skeletal muscle relaxant is typified by the drug dantrolene; unlike the classic neuromuscular blocking agents, dantrolene does not interfere with transmission of impulses between somatic motor nerves and skeletal muscle. Its action appears to occur through a direct effect on the skeletal muscle fibers that interferes with their contractile mechanisms. Specifically, the drug retards the release of a contraction-activating substance, probably calcium, from its binding sites in the sarcoplasmic reticulum. Dantrolene is available in oral form for treatment of muscle spasticity resulting from chronic neurologic disorders such as cerebral palsy, multiple sclerosis, or stroke, and as an IV injection for the emergency management of malignant hyperthermia such as that resulting from general anesthesia.

The principal danger with dantrolene therapy is hepatotoxicity, especially with high doses (ie, above 400 mg/day) or long-term treatment. The risk of hepatic injury appears to be greater in women, in patients older than 35 years of age, and in patients taking additional medications.

• Dantrolene

Dantrium

Mechanism

Direct relaxation of skeletal muscle fibers through interference with the release of calcium ions from the sarcoplasmic reticulum; impairs catabolism within muscle cells by blocking increases in myoplasmic calcium and therefore prevents abnormal rise in body temperature; may possess some CNS action as well, resulting in drowsiness, dizziness, and weakness

Uses

Relief of muscle spasticity associated with chronic neurologic disorders—cerebral palsy, stroke, spinal cord injury, or multiple sclerosis (most effective where spasticity is painful and limits muscle performance)

Emergency treatment of malignant hyperthermia (IV injection)

Preoperative prophylaxis of malignant hyperthermia in high-risk patients (orally)

Dosage

Muscle spasticity

Adults: initially 25 mg orally once daily; increase gradually in 25-mg increments to a maximum of 100 mg 2 to 4 times/day; maintain each dose for 4 to 7 days before increasing

Children: initially 0.5 mg/kg orally twice a day; increase by 0.5-mg/kg increments to a maximum of 3 mg/kg 2 to 4 times/day

Malignant hyperthermia (adults and children)

Treatment: initially 1 mg/kg IV; if abnormalities persist or reappear, repeat up to a cumulative dose of 10 mg/kg; usual required dose is 2 to 5 mg/kg

Prophylaxis: 4 to 8 mg/kg/day orally in 3 or 4 divided doses for 1 to 2 days before surgery (last dose given 3–4 hours before start of surgery)

Fate

Oral absorption is slow and incomplete but consistent; significantly bound to plasma proteins; optimal effects with oral use may take several days to become manifest; half-life is 8 to 9 hours with oral administration and 5 hours after IV injection; metabolized primarily in the liver, and both metabolites and unaltered drug are excreted in the urine.

Common Side Effects

Oral use only: drowsiness, dizziness, weakness, malaise, fatigue, diarrhea.

Significant Adverse Reactions

Oral use only:

GI: constipation, bleeding, cramping, anorexia, difficulty in swallowing, gastric irritation, severe diarrhea

CNS: headache, lightheadedness, insomnia, visual and speech disturbances, taste alterations, seizures, depression, confusion, nervousness

CV: tachycardia, phlebitis, erratic blood pressure

Urinary: urinary frequency, crystalluria, incontinence, nocturia, urinary retention, impotence

Dermatologic: abnormal hair growth, rash, pruritus, urticaria, eczema-like reaction, photosensitization

Other: hepatitis, backache, myalgia, lacrimation, chills, fever, respiratory distress

Contraindications

Hepatic disease, conditions in which spasticity is necessary to sustain upright position or balance. *Cautious use* in presence of impaired pulmonary function, cardiac impairment caused by myocardial disease, a history of hepatic dysfunction, in pregnant or lactating women, children younger than 5 years of age, and in patients older than 35 years of age at high risk for development of hepatotoxicity.

Interactions

Estrogens may increase the danger of hepatotoxicity.

CNS depression may be potentiated by other tranquilizing agents.

Warfarin and clofibrate reduce the protein binding of dantrolene and may potentiate its effects.

Nursing Management

Pretherapy Assessment

Assess and record baseline data necessary for detection of adverse effects of dantrolene: General: VS, body weight, skin color and temperature; CNS: reflexes, bilateral grip strength; GI: bowel sounds, normal output; GU: prostate palpation, normal output, voiding pattern; Laboratory: renal and liver function tests, total bilirubin, urinalysis, hemoglobin, CBC.

Review medical history and documents for existing or previous conditions that:

a. require cautious use of dantrolene: impaired pulmonary function; cardiac impairment secondary to myocardial disease; history of hepatic dysfunction; children younger than 5 years of age.
b. contraindicate use of dantrolene: allergy to dantrolene; acute hepatic disease (hepatitis, cirrhosis); conditions in which spasticity is necessary to sustain upright position or balance; **pregnancy (Category C)**; lactation (safety not established, avoid use in nursing mothers).

Nursing Interventions

Medication Administration

Ensure ready access to bathroom facilities if GI effects occur.

Arrange to discontinue drug if diarrhea is severe; it may be possible to readminister at a lower dose level.

Monitor IV injection sites and ensure that extravasation does not occur; drug is very alkaline and irritating to tissues.

Provide small, frequent meals and frequent mouth care if GI upset occurs.

Provide control over lighting if vision effects occur.

Surveillance During Therapy

Monitor for signs of developing hepatotoxicity (elevations in alanine aminotransferase, aspartate aminotransferase, alkaline phosphatase, total bilirubin).

Monitor for signs of renewed spasticity if drug is withdrawn for 2 to 4 days to confirm subtle improvement.

Monitor for signs of hypersensitivity, which may require discontinuation of drug.

Interpret results of diagnostic tests and contact practitioner as appropriate.

Monitor for possible drug–drug and drug–nutrient interactions: estrogens may increase danger of hepatotoxicity; CNS depression potentiated by other tranquilizing agents; protein binding reduced by oral anticoagulants.

Patient Teaching

Inform patient that beneficial effects may be delayed 1 to 2 weeks and that side effects will lessen with time.

Inform the patient of typical side effects related to dantrolene therapy: drowsiness; dizziness; blurred vision; nausea; difficulty urinating, increased urinary frequency, urinary incontinence; headache; malaise; photosensitivity.

Teach the patient that the following signs and symptoms should be reported to the practitioner if they occur: skin rash, itching; bloody or black tarry stools, pale stools, severe diarrhea; yellowing of the skin or eyes.

Centrally Acting Muscle Relaxants

The purpose of the centrally acting muscle relaxants is to decrease skeletal muscle tone and involuntary movement without loss of voluntary motor function or consciousness. Most CNS depressants (eg, barbiturates) produce muscle relaxation but are of little use clinically because they also cause marked sedation and other undesirable effects. Attempts to develop centrally acting muscle relaxants that produce no sedation have not been very successful; most central muscle relaxants evoke a degree of sedation that makes long-term use undesirable.

Treatment of Spasms

Based on their mechanism of action, these agents have been termed *interneuronal* or *polysynaptic* blocking drugs. They act at different levels within the CNS (ie, brain stem or spinal cord interneurons) to depress synaptic transmission in motor reflex pathways. They appear to exert a weak synaptic blocking action between neurons of these motor circuits, the degree of impairment being proportional to the number of synapses involved in the pathway. In addition to their neuronal blocking action, most of these drugs also directly depress higher centers (eg, basal ganglia) that regulate motor activity. This CNS-depressant action probably contributes significantly to the muscle-relaxant effects of most of the centrally acting drugs. With the exception of baclofen and diazepam (see Chapter 25), the drugs comprising the centrally acting muscle relaxants are remarkably similar in their pharmacologic and toxicologic effects. No single agent possesses a significant therapeutic advantage over any other agent, and for the most part, choice of a drug is a personal preference. Because they share many common properties, they are discussed as a group; individual drugs are described in Table 17-1.

Mechanism

Interfere with transmission of impulses in polysynaptic motor reflex pathways at the level of the spinal cord, brain stem, and probably basal ganglia; prolong synaptic recovery time and decrease repetitive spinal interneuronal discharges; no effect on contractile mechanism of muscle fibers or on the motor endplate of skeletal muscles; CNS-depressant action probably contributes to the muscle-relaxant effect.

Uses

Relief of pain and discomfort of muscle spasms associated with acute musculoskeletal disorders (eg, inflammatory states, peripheral injury [sprains, strains], connective tissue disorders).

Dosage

See Table 17-1.

Fate

Well absorbed orally; maximum effects usually occur in 1 to 4 hours and persist for several hours; most of these drugs are metabolized by the liver and are excreted in the urine.

Table 17-1. **Centrally Acting Skeletal Muscle Relaxants**

Drug	Usual Dosage Range	Nursing Considerations
Baclofen *Lioresal*	5 mg 3 times/day; increase by 5 mg every 3 days to optimal effect (maximum 80 mg/day)	Primarily used orally for relief of spasticity due to multiple sclerosis or spinal cord diseases; sedation is common but is usually transient; absorption is variable and reduced at higher doses; give with food to decrease GI distress; may increase urinary frequency; do not use in patients with stroke or rheumatic disorders, in children younger than 12 y, pregnant women, nursing mothers; cautious use in epileptics and in presence of renal impairment; reduce dose slowly to avoid possibility of hallucinations on abrupt withdrawal; may alter laboratory tests for AST, alkaline phosphatase, and blood glucose; also used by intrathecal pump for *severe* spasticity of spinal cord origin and possibly for reducing spasticity in cerebral palsy
Carisoprodol *Soma*	350 mg 3 or 4 times/day	Also available in combination with aspirin as Soma Compound; and with aspirin and codeine as Soma Compound w/Codeine (C-III); contraindicated in acute intermittent porphyria, children younger than 12 y, and meprobamate sensitivity; allergic reactions may develop early in regimen (rash, erythema, pruritus, eosinophilia)—stop drug and treat symptomatically; carefully monitor urine output and avoid overhydration; use cautiously in addiction-prone people; withdrawal symptoms can occur after prolonged use
Chlorphenesin *Maolate* *(CAN) Mycil*	Initially 800 mg 3 times/day; may reduce to 400 mg 3 or 4 times/day if effective	Do not use in pregnancy, children, liver disease, or for periods exceeding 8 wk; discontinue at first sign of allergic reaction; paradoxical excitation may occur but usually is controlled by dosage reduction; blood dyscrasias may occur—instruct patient to have routine blood counts
Chlorzoxazone *Paraflex, Parafon Forte DSC, Remular-S*	Adults: 250–500 mg 3 or 4 times/day; reduce gradually as improvement is noted; maximum dose is 750 mg 3 or 4 times/day	Use cautiously in pregnancy, history of drug allergy, hepatic dysfunction; may discolor urine but is *not* nephrotoxic; give with meals to minimize GI irritation; may cause drowsiness or lightheadedness
Cyclobenzaprine *Flexeril*	10 mg 3 times/day to a maximum of 60 mg/day (not in children younger than 15 y)	Do not use for longer than 2 to 3 wk; *not* effective in spasticity due to cerebral or spinal cord disease or cerebral palsy; contraindicated in hyperthyroidism, arrhythmias, congestive heart failure, acute recovery phase of myocardial infarction, or with MAO inhibitors; similar to tricyclic antidepressants in action (see Chapter 26), and may have similar central effects; high incidence of drowsiness, dry mouth, and dizziness; possesses anticholinergic activity, responsible for atropine-like side effects and interactions (see Chapter 13); caution in glaucoma and urinary retention; reduce dose slowly—withdrawal symptoms can occur
Diazepam *Valium, Zetran*	Adults: 2–10 mg 3 to 4 times/day Geriatric patients: 2–2.5 mg 1 to 2 times/day Children: 1–2.5 mg 3 to 4 times/day	Adjunct for relief of skeletal muscle spasm resulting from inflammation, trauma, or upper motor neuron disorders; may impair psychomotor skills and cause drowsiness; psychological and physical dependence have occurred; see also Chapter 25
Metaxalone *Skelaxin*	800 mg 3 or 4 times/day (not in children younger than 12 y)	Contraindicated in anemia, renal or hepatic impairment, nursing mothers; liver function studies should be done regularly; cautious use in epilepsy, pregnancy, allergic states; GI upset is common as are headache, nervousness, and irritability; may interfere with Benedict's and cephalin flocculation tests
Methocarbamol *Robaxin*	*Oral* Adults: 1.5 g 4 times/day initially; reduce to 750–1000 mg 4 times/day Children: 60–75 mg/kg/day *IM:* 0.5–1 g every 8 h *IV:* 300 mg/min to a total daily dose of 1–3 g for maximum 3 days *IV infusion:* 1 g (10 mL) diluted to 250 mL saline or 5% dextrose given by IV drip *Tetanus:* 1–3 g directly into IV tubing every 6 h (children 15 mg/kg every 6 h)	IV use may control neuromuscular manifestations of tetanus; substitute oral administration as soon as possible; avoid extravasation because irritation and thrombophlebitis can result; do *not* give SC; contraindicated in renal dysfunction (vehicle may cause acidosis and urea retention), children younger than 12 y, epilepsy (especially IV); keep patient recumbent during and at least 15 min after IV use to minimize orthostatic hypotension and other side effects; may interfere with laboratory tests for 5-HIAA and VMA; too-rapid IV injection may cause CNS side effects (eg, dizziness, vertigo, syncope, headache, blurred vision) as well as bradycardia, hypotension, flushing, and anaphylactic reaction; cautious use in myasthenia gravis; check IV infusion for proper flow to minimize danger of thrombophlebitis and sloughing; may darken urine; also available with aspirin as Robaxisal

(*continued*)

Table 17-1. **Centrally Acting Skeletal Muscle Relaxants (Continued)**

Drug	Usual Dosage Range	Nursing Considerations
Orphenadrine citrate *Banflex, Flexon, Flexoject, Myolin, Norflex*	*Oral:* 100 mg twice a day *IV, IM:* 60 mg every 12 h (give IV over 5 min with patient supine)	Available with aspirin and caffeine as Norgesic; strong anticholinergic with high incidence of atropine-like side effets (see Chapter 13); contraindicated in glaucoma, myasthenia gravis, duodenal obstruction, ulcers, prostatic hypertrophy, bladder obstruction, pregnancy, children; periodic monitoring of blood, renal, and liver function recommended with prolonged use; caution in urinary retention, tachycardia, coronary insufficiency, arrhythmias; narrow safety margin—monitor for signs of toxicity (eg, flushing, fever, blurred vision, dry mouth)

AST, Asparate aminotransferase; MAO, monoamine oxidase; 5-HIAA, hydroxyindole acetic acid; VMA, vanillylmandelic acid.

Common Side Effects

Drowsiness, fatigue, dizziness, lightheadedness, dry mouth, and GI upset; in addition, other anticholinergic side effects (eg, blurred vision, urinary hesitancy) are common with cyclobenzaprine and orphenadrine.

Significant Adverse Reactions

Not all effects noted with all drugs:

GI: anorexia, nausea, diarrhea, hiccups, bleeding, abdominal pain
CNS: ataxia, headache, blurred vision, insomnia, confusion, irritability, paresthesias
CV: tachycardia, hypotension, flushing, thrombophlebitis, chest pain, palpitations, syncope
Urinary: urinary retention, dysuria, enuresis
Hematologic: petechiae, leukopenia, pancytopenia, thrombocytopenia, agranulocytosis, hemolytic anemia
Hypersensitivity: rash, erythema, pruritus, fever, asthma-like reaction, dermatoses, angioedema, anaphylactic reactions
Hepatic: abnormal liver function tests, jaundice
Respiratory: nasal congestion, dyspnea
Other: dysarthria, dyspepsia, tremors, euphoria, metallic taste, pain or sloughing at site of injection, increased intraocular tension, conjunctivitis, tinnitus, slurred speech

Contraindications

See Table 17-1. *Cautious use* in patients with impaired renal or hepatic function or respiratory depression, in patients who must drive or operate machinery, in patients taking other CNS depressants, in young children, in elderly or debilitated patients, and in pregnant or lactating women; in addition, orphenadrine and cyclobenzaprine should be used cautiously in the presence of glaucoma, urinary retention, arrhythmias, and tachycardia, because they possess significant anticholinergic activity.

Interactions

CNS-depressive effects of centrally acting muscle relaxants and other CNS depressants (eg, alcohol, barbiturates, narcotics, antianxiety agents) are additive.

MAO inhibitors may increase the toxicity of cyclobenzaprine.

Atropine-like side effects may be intensified by use of anticholinergic drugs with cyclobenzaprine and orphenadrine.

Cyclobenzaprine may interfere with the antihypertensive action of guanethidine and similarly acting compounds.

Nursing Management

Pretherapy Assessment

Assess and record baseline data necessary for detection of adverse effects of central muscle relaxants: General: VS, body weight, skin color and temperature; CNS: reflexes, ophthalmic examination; GI: bowel sounds, normal output; GU: prostate palpation, normal output, voiding pattern; Laboratory: renal and liver function tests, thyroid function tests, blood and urine glucose.

Review medical history and documents for existing or previous conditions that:

a. require cautious use of central muscle relaxants: renal or hepatic dysfunction; respiratory depression; other CNS depressants; use in young children or the elderly.
b. contraindicate use of central muscle relaxants: allergy to the muscle relaxant prescribed; hyperthyroidism; arrhythmias; **pregnancy (Category C)**, lactation (safety not established, avoid use in nursing mothers).

Nursing Interventions

Medication Administration

Ensure ready access to bathroom facilities if GI effects occur.

Arrange to discontinue drug if diarrhea is severe; it may be possible to readminister at a lower dose level.

Provide small, frequent meals and frequent mouth care if GI upset occurs.

Provide analgesics if headache occurs.

Surveillance During Therapy

Monitor for toxicity.

Monitor for signs of hypersensitivity, which may require discontinuation of drug.

Interpret results of diagnostic tests and contact practitioner as appropriate.

Monitor for possible drug–drug and drug–nutrient interactions: additive CNS effects with other CNS depressants; MAO inhibitors increase the toxicity of cyclobenzaprine; cyclobenzaprine may interfere with antihypertensive actions of guanethidine.

Patient Teaching

Teach the patient to avoid the use of alcohol and sleep-inducing or over-the-counter compounds.

Caution patient to avoid engaging in hazardous activities because drug-induced drowsiness is common.

Inform the patient of typical side effects related to central muscle-relaxant therapy: drowsiness, dizziness, blurred vision, dyspepsia, dry mouth.

Teach the patient that the following signs and symptoms should be reported to the practitioner if they occur: skin rash, itching, pale stools, yellowing of the skin or eyes, urinary retention, fever, sore throat, easy bruising.

Treatment of Spasticity

Pharmacologic management of spasticity in patients presenting with multiple sclerosis, spinal cord injury, or other types of spinal cord disorders can be accomplished with the drug baclofen. It may be given orally or intrathecally to provide a degree of muscle relaxation in some of these cases.

• Baclofen

Lioresal

Mechanism

Has a molecular structure similar to that of gamma-aminobutyric acid (GABA), an inhibitory neurotransmitter of the CNS; produces hyperpolarization of afferent nerve terminals; inhibits both monosynaptic and polysynaptic spinal reflexes; may have some supraspinal actions that may contribute to its therapeutic effect as well as its adverse reactions.

Uses

Alleviation of spasticity resulting from multiple sclerosis; best response occurs in patients with multiple sclerosis with *reversible* spasticity

Treatment of spinal cord injuries and other spinal cord diseases

Investigational oral uses include treatment of tardive dyskinesias and trigeminal neuralgia; intrathecally, has been used to reduce spasticity of cerebral palsy in children

Dosage

Oral: Initiate therapy with approximately 15 mg daily for 3 days; increase dosage slowly (eg, every 3 days) up to a maximum of 80 mg/day

Intrathecal: for patients who do not respond to oral therapy; test doses of 50 to 100 μg are used; patients not responding to 100 μg should not receive any further treatment; in patients in whom a therapeutic effect did occur, the average maintenance doses ranged from 300 to 800 μg per day

Fate

Rapidly and extensively absorbed orally; half-life is 3 to 4 hours; eliminated primarily by the kidney in unchanged form; onset of action after intrathecal administration is 0.5 to 1 hour; effects may last 4 to 8 hours.

Common Side Effects

Oral and intrathecal: drowsiness, muscle weakness, dizziness.

Significant Adverse Reactions

CV: hypotension, chest pain

CNS: dizziness, headaches, insomnia, paresthesia, tremor, euphoria, depression; hallucinations and seizures have occurred on abrupt withdrawal

GI: dry mouth, constipation, diarrhea

GU: urinary retention, enuresis, reduced ability to ejaculate; may cause ovarian cysts

Contraindications

Treatment of skeletal muscle spasm resulting from stroke, rheumatic disorders or Parkinson's disease; injection should not be given IV, IM, SC, or epidurally; oral use is not recommended in children. *Cautious use* in patients with impaired renal function, infections, epilepsy, psychotic disorders, and in pregnant or nursing mothers.

Interactions

Additive depressant effects on brain function can occur in combination with other CNS depressants.

Nursing Management

See Nursing Management for Central Muscle Relaxants.

Selected Bibliography

Albright AL, Cervi A, Singletary J: Intrathecal baclofen for spasticity in cerebral palsy. JAMA 265:1418, 1991

Ding Y, Fredman B, White PF: Use of mivacurium during laparoscopic surgery: Effect of reversal drugs on postoperative recovery. Anesth Analg 78:450, 1994

Feldman S, Fauvel N: Potentiation and antagonism of vecuronium by decamethonium. Anesth Analg 76:631, 1993

Fiacchino F, Gemma M, Bricchi M, Giombini S, Regi B: Sensitivity to curare in patients with upper and lower motor neurone dysfunction. Anaesthesia 46:980, 1991

Gariepy LP, Varin F, Donati F, Salib Y, Bevan DR: Influence of aging on the pharmacokinetics and pharmacodynamics of doxacurium. Clin Pharmacol Ther 53:340, 1993

Jensen FS, Viby-Mogensen J: Reaction to succinylcholine in two patients segregating for the plasma cholinesterase allele E^k. Acta Anaesthesiol Scand 36:753, 1992

Meyer KC, Prielipp RC, Grossman JE, Coursin DB: Prolonged weakness after infusion on atracurium in two intensive care unit patients. Anesth Analg 78:772, 1994

Prielipp RC, Jackson MJ, Coursin DB: Comparison of the neuromuscular recovery after paralysis with atracurium versus vecuronium in ICU patient with renal insufficiency. Anesth Analg 78:775, 1994

Rhee KJ, O'Malley RJ: Neuromuscular blockade-assisted oral intubation versus nasotracheal intubation in the prehospital care of inured patients. Ann Emerg Med 23:37, 1994

Nursing Bibliography

Davidson J, Dattolo J, Goskowicz R, et al.: Neuromuscular blockade: Nursing interventions and case studies from infancy to adulthood. Critical Care Nursing Quarterly 15(4):53–67, 1993

Semorin-Holleran R: The use of neuromuscular blocking agents in critical care nursing practice. Critical Care Nursing Clinics of North America 16(1):37–44, 1993

Van Sickel A, Spadaccia K: Muscle relaxants and reversal agents. Critical Care Nursing Clinics of North America 3(1):151–158, 1991

18

Local Anesthetics

Antidepolarizing

Esters of Benzoic or Aminobenzoic Acid

- Benoxinate
- Benzocaine
- Butamben
- Chloroprocaine
- Cocaine
- Cyclomethycaine
- Dyclonine
- Procaine
- Proparacaine
- Propoxycaine
- Tetracaine

Amides

- Bupivacaine
- Dibucaine
- Etidocaine
- Lidocaine
- Mepivacaine
- Prilocaine

Ether

- Pramoxine

Coolants

- Chloroethane
- Dichlorodifluoromethane
- Dichlorotetrafluoroethane
- Ethyl chloride
- Trichloromonofluoromethane

Antidepolarizing Agents

These local anesthetic agents induce a reversible blockade of impulse conduction along all sensory, motor, and autonomic nerve fibers. Loss of sensation may be accompanied by other physiologic changes as well, such as muscle relaxation (motor nerve paralysis) and hypotension (sympathetic nerve blockade). When these agents are administered in the region of mixed nerve fibers, differences in onset and recovery occur, depending on the size and state of myelination of the nerve fibers. In general, small, nonmyelinated C fibers (eg, dorsal root and sympathetic postganglionic) mediating pain and vasoconstrictor impulses are affected first by local anesthetics, followed by the small, myelinated A-delta fibers mediating pain and temperature. Larger fibers carrying sensory impulses (eg, A-alpha, A-beta) are blocked next, and finally motor nerves (eg, A-gamma) are anesthetized, resulting in decreased skeletal muscle tone. Recovery proceeds in the opposite direction: motor function is restored before sensory function.

Although the primary effects of antidepolarizing local anesthetics develop in the area of topical application or at the injection site, *systemic* absorption does occur to varying degrees, and may produce adverse reactions. Large doses—or inadvertent injection into a blood vessel—of local anesthetics may lead to cardiovascular effects such as hypotension or cardiac depression, or to central nervous system (CNS) effects such as excitation and convulsions followed by depression. Systemic absorption of local anesthetics can be minimized by adding a local vasoconstrictor (eg, 1:200,000 epinephrine) to the drug solution to constrict the vessels in the immediate area of the injection; this will prevent spread of the administered anesthetic. Vasoconstrictors also prolong the duration of local anesthesia and reduce the amount of drug needed. If surgery is performed, they may reduce local hemorrhaging.

Antidepolarizing local anesthetics must be able to *penetrate* the nerve membrane before they can exert any pharmacologic action; they have to be in the nonionized state to do this. Because local anesthetics are weak bases, they are produced in the form of water-soluble cationic salts. At the site of application or injection, they are converted to the free base (nonionic, lipid-soluble form) by the local biologic fluids. In this form, they diffuse across the nerve membrane and reach their sites of action. This uncharged, nonionic form is then converted back to the cationic form and produces local anesthesia—it is the cationic (ionized) form of the drug that *acts* within the nerve fiber.

The cationic form of these local anesthetics stabilizes the nerve membrane by decreasing its permeability to sodium; this action increases the threshold for excitation. It does so by competing with calcium ions bound to phospholipids for a site in the nerve membrane that controls the passage of sodium across the membrane and into the cell. Thus, the initial event in the generation of a nerve action potential (ie, depolarization) is blocked.

Classifications of antidepolarizing local anesthetics are based on chemical structure or clinical use. Structurally, most belong to one of three categories:

I. Esters of benzoic or aminobenzoic acid (eg, procaine)
II. Amides (eg, lidocaine)
III. Ethers (eg, pramoxine)

The ester types usually are short acting because they are rapidly hydrolyzed by plasma cholinesterases. Amide drugs, primarily inactivated in the liver, are much longer acting; thus, procaine provides local anesthesia for approximately 30 minutes, whereas bupivacaine has a significantly longer duration, from 2 to 4 hours. Because amide local anesthetics depend on the liver for metabolism, impairment of hepatic function can greatly prolong their half-lives, and can result in a higher incidence of adverse effects if they enter the systemic circulation.

Although some local anesthetics are used only by a single route of administration, several are given by more than one route; examples of this clinically applicable classification are as follows:

I. *Surface anesthetics*: skin, mucous membranes (eg, throat, rectal), eye, ear (eg, benzocaine, cocaine, dibucaine)
II. *Infiltration anesthetics*: local intradermal or subcutaneous injection (eg, procaine, lidocaine)
III. *Spinal anesthetics*: subarachnoid injection (eg, bupivacaine, procaine, tetracaine)
IV. *Epidural anesthetics*: injection into area surrounding the dura mater of spinal cord (eg, bupivacaine, lidocaine, mepivacaine)

Because the general pharmacologic actions and clinical implications of antidepolarizing local anesthetics are similar, they are discussed as a group. Specific characteristics of individual agents are detailed in Table 18-1, along with prescribing information (including the recommended routes of administration).

Table 18-1. **Local Anesthetics**

Drug	Usual Dosage Range	Nursing Considerations
ANTIDEPOLARIZING AGENTS		
Benoxinate and Sodium Fluorescein *Fluress*	Tonometry and removal of sutures and foreign bodies: 1–2 drops before operation Ophthalmic anesthesia: 2 drops 90 sec apart for 3 instillations.	Short-acting anesthetic with possible bacteriostatic action; no effect on pupil size or accommodation; minimal stinging or burning; fluorescein sodium stains abraded or ulcerated areas, facilitating visualization of foreign bodies
Benzocaine *Several manufacturers*	Apply to area several times a day as required; *rectal ointment* given morning and night, and after each bowel movement *Gel:* used as a lubricant (eg, catheters, specula) *Liquid, gel, or aerosol* for oral mucous membrane anesthesia in dentistry or topical anesthesia *Candy/gum* as an aid in weight loss: 6–15 mg just before food consumption (maximum 45 mg/day)	Slowly absorbed from mucous membranes—exerts a fairly prolonged action; drug is a component of many combination products (eg, oral, anorectal, otic, topical); produces hypersensitivity reactions in some people; stop drug at first sign of allergic response; avoid contact with eyes; may be used for temporary relief of toothache and in dental procedures; not recommended for use in teething child; used to lubricate catheters, endoscopic tubes, sigmoidoscopes, proctoscopes, and vaginal specula; also used as gum or candy (Ayds, Slim-Mint) to decrease taste sensation as an adjunct in weight-reduction programs
Bupivacaine *Marcaine, Sensorcaine (CAN) Marcain*	Infiltration: 0.25% Epidural/caudal: 0.25%–0.5% Peripheral nerve block: 0.25%–0.5% Retrobulbar block: 0.75% Sympathetic block: 0.25% Dental block: 0.5%	Onset slower than lidocaine, but more prolonged duration; widely used for nerve block, epidural or caudal, for long surgical or obstetrical procedures, and relief of pain during labor (*caution:* 0.75% concentration should not be used for obstetric anesthesia; cardiac arrest and death have occurred); maximum dose 400 mg (with epinephrine) in 24 h; do not use for spinal block; not for use in children younger than 12 y
Butamben *Butesin*	Apply 2 or 3 times/day as needed	Used mainly for minor burns and skin irritations
Chloroprocaine *Nesacaine*	Infiltration/nerve block: 1%–2% Caudal/epidural: 2%–3%	Onset within 10 min; effects persist 30–90 min; available without preservatives for caudal or epidural block; more rapid acting and less toxic than procaine; intravenous use may cause thrombophlebitis; prior use of chloroprocaine may interfere with subsequent use of bupivacaine
Cocaine (C-II) *Several manufacturers*	Surface anesthesia: 1%–4%	Central stimulant that can lead to overwhelming psychological dependence when repeatedly inhaled, smoked, or ingested; causes vasoconstriction when applied to mucous membrane; not used by injection or in the eyes; onset of acton is rapid when applied locally, and duration is about 1–2 h; widely abused drug (see Chapter 82)
Dibucaine *Nupercainal*	Apply locally 2–3 times/day	Onset about 15 min and duration 3–4 h
Dyclonine *Dyclone*	Apply topically to skin or mucous membranes	Used before endoscopic procedures to block the gag reflex; also used to relieve pain of oral or anogenital lesions; onset is about 10 min, duration approximately 60 min; may be used in patients hypersensitive to other local anesthetics
Etidocaine *Duranest*	Infiltration: lumbar, central nerve block—1% Caudal: 1% Cesarean, intra-abdominal: 1%–1.5% Maxillary: 1.5%	Onset of action within 3–5 min; duration up to 8 h with epinephrine (caution in ambulatory patients); induces profound motor blockade when given peridurally; not for use in children younger than 14 y; use caution in elderly patients
Lidocaine *Xylocaine, and several other manufacturers (CAN) Xylocard*	Apply topically as needed; solution for pain and inflammation of mouth, throat, pharynx, and urethra, as needed Injection: Infiltration—0.5%–1% Nerve block: Dental—2%; intercostal—1%; brachial—1.5%; paracervical—1% Epidural: thoracic—1%; lumbar—1%–2% Caudal: obstetric—1%; surgical—1.5%; spinal—5% with glucose; saddle block—1.5% with dextrose	Slightly more potent than procaine; rapid onset of action (1–2 min) lasting up to 2 h; widely used as antiarrhythmic agent (see Chapter 32); do not use solution with epinephrine for arrhythmias or solutions with preservatives for spinal or epidural block; oral solutions can interfere with swallowing reflex; caution in pediatric and geriatric patients; can enhance muscle relaxing action of neuromuscular blocking agents; contraindicated in patients with blood dyscrasias

(continued)

Table 18-1. **Local Anesthetics (Continued)**

Drug	Usual Dosage Range	Nursing Considerations
Mepivacaine *Carbocaine, Isocaine, Polocaine*	Nerve block: 1%–2% Paracervical block: 1% Caudal/epidural: 1%–2% Infiltration: 1% Analgesia: 1%–2% Dental block—3% alone or 2% with levonordefrin	Twice as potent as procaine, with comparable onset but more prolonged duration of action; possesses some vasoconstrictive action, so usually does not require a vasoconstrictor; injection containing levonordefrin used in dental procedures *only;* not used topically; less drowsiness and depression than observed with lidocaine; use with caution in renal dysfunction and with elderly patients
Pramoxine *Phicon, Pramegel, Prax, ProctoFoam, Tronothane, Tronolane*	Apply topically or rectally 2 or 3 times/day as needed.	Not used by injection, or applied to the eye or nasal mucosa; component of many anorectal preparations (eg, ointments, foams, suppositories); used mainly to relieve pain and itching, especially of hemorrhoids, and to facilitate endotracheal, intragastric, and rectal intubation procedures
Prilocaine *Citanest*	Nerve block infiltration in dental procedures: 4%	Similar to lidocaine in its actions, but has a slower onset; may induce drowsiness and sleepiness; associated with some cases of methemoglobinemia; use is largely restricted to dental procedures
Procaine *Novocain*	Infiltration: 0.25%–0.5% Nerve block: 0.5%–2% Spinal block: 10%	Not used topically; rapidly eliminated, short-acting (30–60 min), little central stimulation; relatively nontoxic but fairly high incidence of allergic reactions; metabolic product may interfere with actions of sulfonamides, and other local anesthetics should be used in presence of sulfonamide antibiotics; amide of procaine is an effective antiarrhythmic agent (see Chapter 32)
Proparacaine *Aktaine, Alcaine, Ophthaine, Ophthetic*	Cataract surgery: 1 drop every 5–10 min Removal of sutures: 1–2 drops 2–3 min before surgery Foreign bodies: 1–2 drops before extraction Tonometry: 1–2 drops before measurement	Used in the eye exclusively; causes minimal irritation; may produce allergic contact dermatitis with drying and fissuring of fingertips; also available with 0.25% fluorescein for short corneal or conjunctival procedures
Propoxycaine *Ravocaine*	Nerve block or infiltration: 7.2 mg	Used in fixed combination with procaine for local anesthesia in dental procedures; preparations also contain norepinephrine or levonordefrin as local vasoconstrictors
Tetracaine *Pontocaine*	Apply locally (0.5%–2%) as needed for pain, burning, itching Cataract surgery: 1 drop (0.5%) every 5–10 min Suture removal: 1 or 2 drops (0.5%) 2–3 min before procedure Foreign bodies: 1–2 drops before operating Tonometry: 1–2 drops before measurement Ophthalmic inflammation: apply ointment 2–3 times/day Spinal anesthesia: 0.2%–1% Caudal anesthesia: 0.2%–0.3% with dextrose Nasal or pharyngeal anesthesia: 2% solution	More potent (8–10 times) and longer acting than procaine, but more toxic; onset of action relatively slow with duration 2–3 h; used in rather low concentrations for surface anesthesia of eye, nose, and throat, as well as spinal and caudal anesthesia; induces prolonged spinal anesthesia for operations requiring 2–3 h; doses exceeding 15 mg are rarely required; do not reuse leftover autoclaved ampules because crystals may form; product should be stored under refrigeration
TOPICAL COOLANTS		
Chloroethane *Ethyl Chloride*	Sports injuries: spray for only a few seconds until tissue begins to frost and turn white Preinjection anesthesia: spray for only 3–5 sec; do *not* frost skin	Topical coolant used to relieve pain associated with minor surgical procedures (eg, lancing, drainage), athletic injuries, injections, and myofascial pain; avoid inhalation because drug may produce coma or respiratory or cardiac arrest
Dichlorotetrafluoroethane + Ethyl Chloride *Fluoro-Ethyl*	Preinjection anesthesia: spray from about 4 inches above target skin area for 2–3 sec	See chloroethane
Dichlorodifluoromethane + trichloromonofluoromethane *Fluori-Methane*	Preinjection anesthesia: spray from 12 inches above target skin area for 3–5 sec	Do not inhale vapors; *do not frost* the target skin area; see chloroethane

Uses

See Table 18-1 for indications for individual drugs.

Relief of pain, soreness, irritation, and itching associated with skin and mucous membrane disorders (eg, minor burns, rashes, wounds, allergic conditions, fungus infections, skin ulcers, hemorrhoids, fissures)
Production of corneal and conjunctival anesthesia to facilitate ophthalmic procedures such as tonometry, gonioscopy, removal of foreign bodies, and minor ocular surgery
Production of infiltration, nerve block, spinal, epidural, or caudal anesthesia in surgery, obstetrics, or dental work
Management of cardiac arrhythmias (see Chapter 32)

Dosage

See Table 18-1.

Fate

See Table 18-1 for specific information.

Absorption depends largely on site of administration, dosage, degree of vasoconstriction, and blood flow to the area. Onset of action is usually rapid (5–10 minutes with most injections); duration is variable and may range from 1 hour (procaine) to 4 to 6 hours (bupivacaine, dibucaine, etidocaine). Some agents are rapidly hydrolyzed by plasma cholinesterases (eg, procaine) or liver enzymes (eg, lidocaine), whereas others are more resistant to inactivation. Excreted primarily in the urine mainly as metabolites, but some unchanged drug as well.

Common Side Effects

Topical: sensitization reactions, stinging or burning in the eyes
Injection: (rare at low doses) slight hypotension, anxiety

Significant Adverse Reactions

Varies among drugs; usually related to excessive dosage or sensitivity to a specific drug or group of drugs.

Topical: hyperallergenic corneal reaction, keratitis, corneal opacities, allergic contact dermatitis with fissuring of fingertips, urticaria, cutaneous lesions, edema, anaphylactic reactions, urethritis with swelling, irritation, sloughing, and necrosis
Injection: (mainly due to systemic absorption) CNS stimulation (dizziness, blurred vision, confusion, irritability, tinnitus, tremors, convulsions) followed by CNS depression (drowsiness, unconsciousness, respiratory arrest), difficulty in speaking, hearing, swallowing, or breathing, muscle twitching, hypotension, myocardial depression, bradycardia, cardiac arrest
Epidural or caudal injection: may provoke spinal block, urinary retention, incontinence, loss of sexual function, paresthesias, headache, or backache
Spinal anesthesia: may cause hypotension, severe headache or backache, respiratory depression, or nerve root damage

Contraindications

Spinal: inflammatory conditions of the spine, septicemia, meningitis, lumbar tuberculosis, metastatic lesions of the spine
Epidural: placenta previa, abruptio placentae
Other: prilocaine is contraindicated in methemoglobinemia; bupivacaine should not be used for obstetric paracervical block (also see Table 18-1)
Cautious use in patients with heart block, liver or kidney disease, hyperthyroidism shock, malignant hyperthermia, and inflammation at the intended site of injection; vasoconstrictor-containing preparations should be used cautiously in patients with hypertension or peripheral vascular disease; caution also is warranted when performing spinal anesthesia in patients with chronic backache, frequent headache, or a history of migraine or hypotension

Interactions

Certain anesthetic drugs (eg, lidocaine) may enhance muscle-relaxing effects of neuromuscular blocking agents.
Additive cardiac-depressant effects may occur when some local anesthetics and other cardiac-depressant drugs (eg, quinidine, propranolol, phenytoin) are given together.
Solutions of local anesthetics containing a vasoconstrictor such as epinephrine may produce blood pressure alterations in combination with monoamine oxidase (MAO) inhibitors, tricyclic antidepressants, phenothiazines, and pressor agents.
Vasoconstrictors in local anesthetic solutions may precipitate arrhythmias in combination with halothane and related general anesthetics.
Procaine, chloroprocaine, and tetracaine may retard action of sulfonamide antibiotics.
Injected local anesthetics may have additive effects with sedatives or other CNS depressants.
The metabolism of the ester-type local anesthetics may be slowed by cholinesterase inhibitors.

Nursing Management

Pretherapy Assessment

Assess and record baseline data necessary for detection of adverse effects of local anesthetics: General: vital signs (VS),body weight, skin color and temperature; CNS: reflexes, pupil size; Laboratory: electrocardiogram.
Review medical history and documents for existing or previous conditions that:
a. require cautious use of local anesthetics: reduced level of plasma esterases, heart block, liver or kidney disease, hyperthyroidism, shock, malignant hyperthermia, inflammation at the intended site of injection; vasoconstrictor-containing preparations should be used with caution in patients with hypertension.
b. contraindicate use of local anesthetics: allergy to the local anesthetic to be used, para-aminobenzoic

acid (PABA), or parabens; *spinal*: inflammatory conditions of the spine, septicemia, meningitis, lumbar tuberculosis, metastatic lesions of the spine; *epidural*: placenta previa; abruptio placentae; **pregnancy (Category C)**; labor and delivery (fetal bradycardia, neonatal depression or seizures observed); lactation (safety not established, avoid use in nursing mothers).

Nursing Interventions

Medication Administration

Administration generally performed by anesthesiologist/ nurse anesthetist.

Ensure that resuscitative equipment and antidotal medications are readily available.

Surveillance During Therapy

Monitor for toxicity.

Monitor for signs of hypersensitivity, which may require discontinuation of drug.

Interpret results of diagnostic tests and contact practitioner as appropriate.

Monitor for possible drug–drug and drug–nutrient interactions: enhancement of neuromuscular blockade; enhancement of cardiotoxic effects of cardiac depressants (quinidine, propranolol, phenytoin); local anesthetic solutions containing epinephrine may enhance blood pressure alterations in combination with MAO inhibitors, tricyclic antidepressants, phenothiazines, pressor agents; PABA-based anesthetics may impair the actions of sulfonamides; metabolism of ester-type anesthetics may be slowed by cholinesterase inhibitors.

Patient Teaching

Advise the patient to avoid prolonged use of any local anesthetic preparation.

Inform the patient of typical side effects related to local anesthetic therapy: sensitization reactions, slight hypotension, anxiety.

Teach the patient that the following signs and symptoms should be reported to the practitioner if they occur: hyperallergenic corneal reaction; allergic contact dermatitis; urethritis with swelling, sloughing, and necrosis.

Coolants

Several agents produce local anesthesia by rapid and deep cooling of the skin surface; they also are known as "vapocoolants." The skin temperature is reduced to approximately −20°C, a level at which sensory stimuli are not transmitted by peripheral nerve endings; the result is a localized analgesia. Vapocoolants are available in spray form; when applied properly, the anesthesia is brief (duration of about 1 minute) and reversible. Improper application can easily result in freezing of skin and underlying tissues, which can cause permanent damage.

Chlorofluoroalkanes

Fluori-Methane

This product is a combination of **di**chloro**di**fluoromethane (15%) plus **tri**chloro**mono**fluoromethane (85%). It is used to reduce pain induced by injections, for relief of muscle spasms, for management of myofascial pain ("spray-and-stretch" technique), and as an adjunct for the management of restricted motion. Fluori-Methane should not be used in patients with vascular impairment of the extremities. Inhalation of the vapors should be minimized, and contact with the eyes should be avoided. Formation of frost on exposed areas also should be avoided.

Ethyl Chloride

Ethyl Chloride (chloroethane) is a spray used to produce topical anesthesia to reduce pain of injections and for minor surgery (eg, incision and drainage of small abscesses, lancing of boils). It is also used to decrease initial trauma of sports injuries and as a counterirritant in the management of muscle spasms (eg, those associated with osteoarthritis, myofascial pain, and restricted motion). It is applied from approximately 12 inches above the area to be treated. When the target site is on or near the face, the patient's mouth, nose, and eyes must be covered. Systemic absorption can occur after *topical application*. Freezing of tissue can reduce resistance to local infection, slow the rate of healing, and alter pigmentation of skin; areas adjacent to the intended site of application can be protected by applying petrolatum. Thawing of frozen tissue often is painful. Chloroethane is potentially nephrotoxic and hepatotoxic, especially after prolonged exposure. Inhalation can produce narcosis, general anesthesia, coma, respiratory arrest, and cardiac arrest. The drug should not be used in patients with vascular impairment of the extremities.

Chlorofluoroalkane + Ethyl Chloride Combination: Fluoro-Ethyl

A product composed of **di**chloro**tetra**fluoroethane (75%) plus ethyl chloride (25%), Fluoro-Ethyl is used to reduce pain caused by injections, minor surgical procedures, bruises, contusions, minor sprains, and dermabrasion. Refer to the discussions of ethyl chloride and Fluori-Methane.

Selected Bibliography

Armel HE, Horowitz M: Alkalinization of local anesthesia with sodium bicarbonate: Preferred method of local anesthesia. Urology 43(1): 101, 1994

den Hartigh J, Hilders CGJM, Schoemaker RC, Hulshof JH, Cohen AF, Vermeij P: Tinnitus suppression by intravenous lidocaine in relation to its plasma concentration. Clin Pharmacol Ther 54:415, 1993

Edmonson EA, Simpson RK, Stubler DK, Beric A: Systemic lidocaine therapy for poststroke pain. J Southern Med Assoc 86(10):1093, 1993
Fukuda T, Dohi S, Naito H: Comparisons of tetracaine spinal anesthesia with clonidine or phenylephrine in normotensive and hypertensive humans. Anesth Analg 78:106, 1994
Joyce TH: Topical anesthesia and pain management before venipuncture. J Pediatr 122:S24, 1993
Palmer CM, Voulgaropoulos D: Management of the parturient with a history of local anesthetic allergy. Anesth Analg 77:625, 1993
Steward DJ: Eutectic mixture of local anesthetics (EMLA). J Pediatr 122:S21, 1993
Thomas AD, Caunt JA: Anaphylactoid reaction following local anesthesia for epidural block. Anaesthesia 48:50, 1993

Nursing Bibliography

Luberow T, Ivankovich A: Post op epidural analgesia. Critical Care Nursing Clinics of North America 3(1):25–34, 1991
Paice J, Magolan J: Intraspinal drug therapy. Critical Care Nursing Clinics of North America 26(2):477–498, 1991

19
General Anesthetics

Inhalation Anesthetics
- ***Gas***
  - Nitrous oxide
- ***Volatile Liquids***
  - Desflurane
  - Enflurane
  - Halothane
  - Isoflurane
  - Methoxyflurane

Intravenous Anesthetics
- ***Ultrashort-Acting Barbiturates***
  - Methohexital
  - Thiamylal
  - Thiopental
- ***Nonbarbiturates***
  - Etomidate
  - Propofol
- ***Dissociative Agent***
  - Ketamine
- ***Neuroleptanalgetic Agent***
  - Droperidol/fentanyl combination

General anesthetics are drugs that produce three major pharmacologic effects: analgesia, reduced muscle activity, and loss of consciousness. They have different advantages and disadvantages, as well as varying degrees of potency. Because no currently available agent is an "ideal" general anesthetic, several other drugs—or "adjuncts"—are often used in combination to provide smooth induction, a sufficient depth and duration of anesthesia, adequate muscle relaxation, and minimal toxicity.

Although several theories have been proposed, there is no single hypothesis that explains the **mechanism** of action of all general anesthetics. They do increase the threshold for cell stimulation and, therefore, reduce neuronal excitability; these alterations are reversible. Possible mechanisms of action include: 1) reduced entrance of Na^+ (which prevents depolarization), 2) reduced entrance of Ca^{2+} (which decreases release of excitatory neurotransmitters), and 3) increased entrance of Cl^- (which causes hyperpolarization) by enhancing activity of the gamma-aminobutyric acid $(GABA)_A$ receptor. This last mechanism is of current interest because the $GABA_A$ receptor complex appears to have multiple sites to which general anesthetics having **very different molecular structures** can bind.

An important **site** of action of general anesthetics is the reticular formation in the brain stem; this is the first area of the central nervous system (CNS) to be affected.

By reducing the number of impulses transmitted from this area of the brain stem to the cerebral cortex, these drugs progressively reduce sensory awareness; when a sufficient concentration of anesthetic is present, consciousness is lost. Cells of the dorsal horn of the spinal cord are also quite sensitive to general anesthetics, resulting in an interruption of incoming sensory (eg, pain) impulses.

As the degree of general anesthesia deepens, a series of physiologic changes ensue. These provide an indication of the depth of depression of the CNS. Traditionally, these changes have been categorized into four stages (I–IV), which were originally described for diethyl ether, a drug having a very slow onset of action and thus exhibiting a distinct separation between the succeeding stages. In anesthesiology of today, however, the distinctive signs of each stage of anesthesia are not observed because many currently used general anesthetics have a rapid onset of action, moving the patient very quickly through the early stages. In addition, mechanical respiratory assistance eliminates the variability in respiratory rate and depth seen with progressive deepening of anesthesia. Finally, certain characteristic signs of the different stages (eg, pupillary diameter, tear secretion, and muscle relaxation) can be influenced by the use of preanesthetic medications like anticholinergics and skeletal muscle relaxants.

The principal physiologic changes that occur as the patient passes through the stages of general anesthesia are presented in Table 19-1. Most surgery is performed at plane 2 or 3 of stage III, because muscle relaxation is usually optimal at this depth.

Safe, effective general anesthesia depends in part on proper preparation of the patient. In addition to the anesthetic drug itself, several other drugs ("adjuncts") are used routinely before, during, and after surgical procedures.

Preanesthetic Medication

The purposes of preanesthetic medication and examples of drugs used are as follows:

I. Relief of anxiety (benzodiazepines, eg, diazepam)
II. Sedation (benzodiazepines eg, midazolam)
III. Reduction in salivary and mucous secretions (anticholinergics)
IV. Inhibition of undesirable side effects (eg, bradycardia and muscle spasms) produced by general anesthetics (anticholinergics; peripherally acting skeletal muscle relaxants)

The use of narcotics for preoperative sedation and analgesia is subject to some controversy because they depress respiration and cough, prolong the anesthetic state, and induce postoperative nausea and vomiting. Administration of opioids before surgery, however, or "preemptive analgesia," has been shown to reduce both postoperative pain and the use of analgesics. This concept, although still being evaluated by anesthesiologists, anesthetists, and other health professionals involved in pain management, will probably be employed to a greater extent in the future.

Antibiotics (eg, cefazolin; metronidazole) are often administered before (and for a brief period after) certain types of surgery (eg, intra-abdominal, vaginal hysterectomy, cesarean section) associated with a higher than average likelihood of infection.

Table 19-1. **Stages and Characteristics of General Anesthesia**

Stage/ Plane	*Respiration*	*Cardiovascular*	*Muscle Tone*	*Reflexes*	*Other*
Stage I	Regular	Normal	Normal	Normal	Analgesia, euphoria, amnesia
Stage II	Rapid, irregular	Heart rate ↑ Blood pressure ↑	Tense Struggling	Swallowing Retching Gagging Vomiting	Mydriasis, roving eyeballs, loss of consciousness, diminished eyelid reflex
Stage III					
Plane 1	Regular	Heart rate and blood pressure normal	Smaller muscles relaxed	Lid and pharyngeal (gag) reflexes absent	Increased lacrimation, miosis, some eye movement, increased respiration and blood pressure with incision
Plane 2	Regular but shallow	Normal	Large muscles relaxed	Corneal and laryngeal reflexes absent	Eyes stilled, miosis, decreased lacrimation, no response to incision
Plane 3	Shallow and mainly abdominal	Blood pressure falls slightly; some tachycardia	Complete relaxation	Pupillary (light) and cough reflex disappear	Mydriasis, decreased lacrimation
Plane 4	Abdominal and very shallow	Hypotension and some tachycardia	Complete relaxation	No reflexes	Mydriasis; no lacrimation
Stage IV	Respiratory paralysis	Marked hypotension and failing circulation	Complete relaxation	No reflexes	Extreme mydriasis, medullary paralysis, and eventual death

Intraoperative Medication

Drugs are given **during** surgery based on the procedure (type and length) and status of the patient. Neuromuscular blocking agents (eg, succinylcholine) are commonly administered while the patient is still at a relatively light level of anesthesia. By producing skeletal muscle relaxation, neuromuscular blocking agents allow a lower dose of general anesthetic to be used, thus reducing the incidence of adverse reactions. Because all these agents have a relatively short duration of action, good control of skeletal muscle activity can be maintained by an experienced anesthesiologist or anesthetist. For a more complete description of the peripherally acting skeletal muscle relaxants, see Chapter 17.

Postoperative Medication

Principal indications for use of drugs postoperatively are:

I. Nausea and vomiting (antiemetics, eg, prochlorperazine)
II. Abdominal distention and urinary retention (cholinergic agents, eg, bethanechol)
III. Pain (analgesics)
IV. Constipation (laxatives and stool softeners, eg, docusate, bisacodyl)

In summary, careful use of preoperative, intraoperative, and postoperative anesthetic adjuncts can greatly facilitate induction and maintenance of—and recovery from—the anesthetic state.

Clinically useful general anesthetics may be classified in the following manner:

I. Inhalation anesthetics
  A. Gas (nitrous oxide)
  B. Volatile liquids (eg, halothane, isoflurane)
II. Intravenous anesthetics
  A. Ultrashort-acting barbiturates (eg, thiopental, methohexital)
  B. Nonbarbiturates (eg, etomidate, propfol)
  C. Dissociative agent (ketamine)
  D. Neuroleptanalgesia (droperidol/fentanyl combination)

Although the clinical pharmacology of each general anesthetic drug is reviewed briefly here, anyone who routinely handles these drugs should become thoroughly familiar with the advantages and disadvantages of each preparation and the procedures for its proper administration (ie, open-drop, semiclosed, or complete rebreathing methods) by consulting specific literature pertaining to each agent. The following discussions of the more widely used drugs should not be viewed as a complete description of the pharmacologic properties and clinical implications of the compounds.

Inhalation Anesthetics

Inhalation anesthetics include gases and volatile liquids. Both types enter the circulation rapidly on inhalation; they are quickly transported through the lungs to the bloodstream and then to the CNS. They are returned to the lungs and eliminated (exhaled). Most leave the body unchanged (ie, not significantly biotransformed). Halothane and methoxyflurane, however, are metabolized to a significant extent in the liver. A potential danger with most of the potent, lipid-soluble inhalational anesthetics is *malignant hyperthermia*, an acute condition characterized by a sudden, drastic elevation in body temperature that is often fatal unless treated immediately and vigorously. This condition is also associated with the use of many neuromuscular blocking agents, especially when given concurrently with inhalation anesthetics. When these drugs are used together, the patient must be carefully monitored. Treatment consists of injections of dantrolene (see Chapter 17) or a calcium channel blocker (see Chapter 34).

General Nursing Management for Inhalation Anesthetics

Pretherapy Assessment

Assess and record baseline data necessary for detection of adverse effects of inhalation general anesthetics: General: vital sounds (VS), body weight, skin color and temperature; CNS: orientation, affect; GI: bowel sounds, normal output; GU: normal output, voiding pattern; Laboratory: renal and liver function tests, urinalysis, Hgb, CBC.

Review medical history and documents for existing or previous conditions that:

a. require cautious use of inhalation anesthetic: impaired pulmonary function, cardiac impairment secondary to myocardial disease, history of hepatic dysfunction.
b. contraindicate use of inhalation anesthetic: allergy to the anesthetic, acute hepatic disease (hepatitis, cirrhosis), malignant hyperthermia, **pregnancy (Category C)**, lactation (safety not established, avoid use in nursing mothers).

Nursing Interventions

Medication Administration

Assure ready access to bathroom facilities if GI effects occur.

Have oxygen available for use with nitrous oxide.

Have anticholinergics available in event of bradycardia.

Review patients's medication history to identify drugs that may interact with the inhalation anesthetic, such as labetalol, alcohol, CNS depressants, xanthines, and neuromuscular blocking agents.

Surveillance During Therapy

Monitor for adverse effects, toxicity and interactions, such as exaggerated response, hypotension, prolonged respiratory depression, confusion, ataxia, or nausea and vomiting.

Interpret results of diagnostic tests and contact practitioner as appropriate.

Monitor patient for fluid intake and output.

Monitor patient for temperature changes.

Monitor for possible drug–drug and drug–nutrient interactions: increased potential for arrhythmias with halogenated volatile anesthetics; additive myocardial depression with beta blockers, quinidine, procainamide, disopyramide, digitalis, and verapamil; potentiation of effects of neuromuscular blocking drugs.

Patient Teaching

Inform the patient that dizziness, confusion, vivid dreams, and hallucinations can occur with nitrous oxide use.

Advise the patient not to eat for at least 8 hours before surgery to prevent aspiration of stomach contents during anesthesia.

Inform the patient of typical side effects related to inhalation anesthetic therapy: impaired psychomotor function, nausea, vomiting, shivering.

Gases

Nitrous oxide is one of the most widely used of all general anesthetics, most often as part of a total anesthetic regimen that also includes sedatives, other anesthetics, narcotics, barbiturates, and muscle relaxants; such a regimen is termed *balanced anesthesia*. This type of drug combination usually produces rapid induction with minimal adverse effects, and it allows a significant reduction in the amount of each drug required.

• Nitrous Oxide (N_2O)

Nitrous oxide, also known as "laughing gas," is a nonexplosive gas that displays a rapid onset of action and correspondingly short duration of action. It is a poor skeletal muscle relaxant and, because of its lack of potency, can induce only a very light plane of anesthesia. It cannot elicit sufficient depth of anesthesia to allow performance of most surgical procedures when used alone. Nitrous oxide is most often employed as a component of balanced anesthesia in conjunction with other, more potent inhalational anesthetics and preanesthetic medication

Uses

Induction of anesthesia

Maintenance (supplement) of general anesthesia

Production of analgesia for minor surgical or dental procedures (analgesia approximately equivalent to morphine)

Dosage

Always used in an oxygen mixture

Induction anesthesia: 70% to 80% N_2O for brief periods

Maintenance anesthesia: 50% to 70% N_2O to prolong anesthetic state

Analgesia: 20% to 30% N_2O

CAUTION

Hypoxia will occur if concentrations of N_2O greater than 80% are used for any length of time; at minimum, 20% oxygen must be given whenever N_2O is used.

Fate

Nitrous oxide has a rapid onset and short duration of action; it is excreted primarily by exhalation from the lungs.

Significant Adverse Reactions

CAUTION

Nitrous oxide is considerably more soluble in blood than is nitrogen; thus it will enter pockets of trapped gas, replacing nitrogen and expanding the volume of gas. This situation can occur in the bowel, lung, or middle ear, leading to possible damage to the organs as a consequence of rapid expansion. Likewise, a significant elevation in cerebrospinal fluid pressure has occurred with nitrous oxide after injection of air into the cerebral ventricles during a pneumoencephalogram.

Dizziness
Vivid dreaming, and possibly hallucinations
If a state of hypoxia persists for any length of time, cyanosis, convulsions, leukopenia, and bone marrow depression can occur
Very high concentrations of nitrous oxide may cause vomiting, myocardial and respiratory depression, and ultimately death
Chronic exposure, as occurs during the career of dental surgeons and their technicians, has produced leg weakness and ataxia, which is probably caused by peripheral neuropathy; impotence has also been reported.

Nursing Management

(See also General Nursing Management for Inhalation Anesthetics.)

Nursing Interventions

Medication Administration

Ensure that oxygen is available for use with N_2O. No more than a few undiluted (without oxygen) breaths should be administered. Hypoxia occurs if concentrations greater than 80% are employed for any length of time.
Expect supplemental drugs (muscle relaxants, barbiturates, other general anesthetics) to be administered when N_2O is employed in anesthesia because it is a rather weak anesthetic and muscle relaxant.

Patient Teaching

Warn patient that dizziness, confusion, vivid dreams, and hallucinations may occur with N_2O use but will disappear when the drug is stopped.
Caution patient receiving N_2O to use care in driving car or operating other machinery until effects of drug have completely disappeared.

Volatile Liquids

Volatile liquid anesthetics are administered by inhalation of the vapors given off by the liquid along with adequate amounts of oxygen. The depth of anesthesia can be fairly well controlled by varying the concentration, because these agents are generally short acting. Recovery begins as soon as the drug is removed because most drugs are excreted largely through the lungs. These agents must be used cautiously in patients with pulmonary diseases, because excretion may be impaired and accumulation toxicity can result.

• Desflurane

Suprane

A relatively new general anesthetic that provides skeletal muscle relaxant activity but often elicits respiratory irritation on administration.

Uses

Induction of anesthesia
Maintenance of general anesthesia for inpatients and outpatients

Not recommended for induction of pediatric patients.

Dosage

Induction: initial 3% to 11%
Maintenance: 2.5% to 8.5%

Fate

Induction of anesthesia occurs within 2 to 4 minutes; there is minimal biotransformation (<0.02%).

Significant Adverse Reactions

Hypotension, tachycardia, frequent irritation of respiratory tract causing coughing and holding of breath (which will delay induction), increased production of secretions and laryngospasm

Nursing Management

See General Nursing Management for Inhalational Anesthetics

• Enflurane

Ethrane

A potent, volatile liquid anesthetic widely used for many surgical procedures; induction and recovery are rapid, skeletal muscle relaxation is good (only minimal amounts of muscle relaxants are needed for more extensive surgery), and the drug is nonflammable; salivary and bronchial secretions are increased; myocardial contractility is somewhat depressed but heart rate is unchanged; blood pressure is usually reduced; high concentrations of enflurane have a CNS stimulant effect and can lead to increased muscle contractions and seizures; frequently given in combination with nitrous oxide, which allows use of a smaller amount of enflurane and hence less danger of CNS excitation; releases fluoride ion, and thus large amounts may damage kidneys.

Uses

Induction and maintenance of general anesthesia, usually in combination with minimal amounts of skeletal muscle relaxants
Provide analgesia for vaginal delivery or supplement other anesthetics for cesarean section (high levels may relax uterus)

Dosage

Induction: 2.0% to 4.5% for 7 to 10 minutes
Maintenance: 0.5% to 3.0%

Fate

Rapid onset of action and recovery; excreted largely (85%–90%) through the lungs, the remainder metabolized by the liver and excreted in the kidney.

Significant Adverse Reactions

Decreased myocardial contractility, hypotension, CNS stimulation with prolonged use, renal damage, malignant hyperthermia

Contraindications

There are no absolute contraindications. *Cautious use* is advised in patients with impaired kidney function, history of epilepsy or other convulsive states, cardiac disease, or arrhythmias.

Interactions

An increased potential for arrhythmias related to effects of catecholamines on the myocardium may occur in the presence of enflurane.
Additive myocardial depression can occur when enflurane is used in combination with beta-blockers, quinidine, procainamide, disopyramide, digitalis drugs, and verapamil.
Enflurane may potentiate the muscle-relaxing effects of antidepolarizing neuromuscular blockers.

Nursing Management

See General Nursing Management for Inhalational Anesthetics.

• Halothane

Fluothane

(CAN) Somnothane

A potent, nonflammable, pleasant-smelling volatile liquid anesthetic, halothane is one of the most widely used anesthetic drugs. It is nonirritating to the respiratory tract and does not increase salivary or bronchial secretions. Muscle relaxation is only fair with halothane, however, and a skeletal muscle relaxant is almost always used. Cardiac output, contractile force, and blood pressure all decrease after administration; in addition, the drug sensitizes the myocardium to the arrhythmogenic effects of catecholamines, and serious arrhythmias can result if a catecholamine (eg, epinephrine) is used in the presence of halothane. Respiratory depression is marked, and apnea, hypoxia, and acidosis may develop during deep anesthesia. Postanesthetic nausea and vomiting are rare. Halothane has been associated with liver dysfunction (hepatitis, jaundice), especially in persons with prior hepatic disease or previous exposure to halothane.

Uses

Induction and maintenance of general anesthesia

Dosage

(Usually with oxygen or oxygen–nitrous oxide mixture)

Induction: 1% to 4%
Maintenance: 0.5% to 1.5%

Fate

Quickly absorbed; largely excreted through the lungs, but up to 20% may be converted to metabolites and excreted in the urine

Significant Adverse Reactions

Arrhythmias (in presence of sympathomimetic agents), hypotension, rapid and shallow respiration, vomiting, hypoxia, respiratory difficulty, postoperative shivering, liver damage, increased intracranial pressure, malignant hyperthermia (rare)

Contraindications

Obstetrical anesthesia (drug is a potent uterine relaxant), severe hepatic or biliary disease. *Cautious use* is advised in persons with cardiac disease or preexisting liver damage, and during pregnancy.

Interactions

Halothane may potentiate the effects of antidepolarizing muscle relaxants (eg, curare, gallamine) and ganglionic blocking agents.
Arrhythmias may be produced by the combination of halothane and catecholamines

Nursing Management

See General Nursing Management for Inhalational Anesthetics

• Isoflurane

Forane

A volatile liquid anesthetic structurally similar to enflurane, isoflurane has a rapid onset and quick recovery. It does not sensitize the heart to catecholamines, and produces good muscle relaxation. CNS excitation is minimal, but respiratory depression may be significant, and blood pressure progressively decreases with depth of anesthesia.

Uses

Induction and maintenance of general anesthesia

Dosage

Induction: 1.5% to 3% for 5 to 10 minutes
Maintenance: 1.0% to 2.5% with nitrous oxide

Fate

Induction and recovery are rapid; less than 1% of the total dose absorbed systemically is metabolized; primarily excreted through the lungs

Significant Adverse Reactions

Respiratory depression, mild hypotension, tachycardia, malignant hyperthermia

Contraindications

No absolute contraindications. *Cautious use* in patients with respiratory disease or congestive heart failure

Interactions

The muscle relaxant effect of isoflurane can be increased by concomitant use of other skeletal muscle relaxants.

Increased respiratory depression can occur in combination with barbiturates, narcotics, and other respiratory depressants.

Nursing Management

See General Nursing Management for Inhalational Anesthetics

• Methoxyflurane

Penthrane

A very potent inhalation anesthetic, with slow onset and recovery, methoxyflurane produces fair muscle relaxation and significant analgesia at light levels of anesthesia. Incidence of arrhythmias is low, but profound circulatory depression can occur at higher concentrations. The drug is associated with liver and especially kidney damage caused by accumulation of free fluoride ion as a metabolic by-product of methoxyflurane. It is not widely used.

Uses

Maintenance of surgical anesthesia of less than 4-hour duration (usually with nitrous oxide and oxygen)

Production of analgesia in obstetrics and minor surgical procedures

Dosage

Analgesia: 0.3% to 0.8% (may be used with hand-held inhalers, eg, Analgizer, Cyprane)

Anesthesia

Induction: up to 2% for 2 to 5 minutes

Maintenance: 0.1% to 2.0% with at least 50% nitrous oxide

(Use lowest effective concentration at all times)

Fate

Slow onset often associated with excitement; high lipid solubility leads to prolonged emergence if not discontinued 30 to 40 minutes before end of surgery; up to 70% of the drug is metabolized in the liver; the remainder is excreted through lungs and kidneys

Significant Adverse Reactions

Mild hypotension, nausea, postanesthetic drowsiness, renal dysfunction, hepatic dysfunction (jaundice, necrosis), respiratory depression, prolonged postoperative sedation, delirium, malignant hyperthermia, cardiac arrest (rare)

Contraindications

Renal disease, vascular surgery near the renal vessels, patients receiving the drug within the previous month, cirrhosis, viral hepatitis, and patients showing jaundice or unexplained fever with other inhalation anesthetics. *Cautious use* in patients with liver disease, diabetes, for surgical procedure lasting more than 4 hours (increased likelihood of fluoride ion accumulation), and during pregnancy

Interactions

Use of methoxyflurane with certain nephrotoxic antibiotics (eg, vancomycin, aminoglycosides, amphotericin) may cause fatal renal toxicity

Muscle-relaxing action of antidepolarizing neuromuscular blocking agents may be augmented by methoxyflurane. Reduce dose of each accordingly

Nursing Management

See General Nursing Management for Inhalational Anesthetics

Intravenous Anesthetics

These agents are used mainly for induction of anesthesia but may also be employed as the sole anesthetic agent in short surgical procedures associated with minimal pain, and to supplement other anesthetic agents during longer procedures.

Ultrashort-Acting Barbiturates

The barbiturates employed in general anesthesia are those having an extremely rapid onset—and relatively short duration (15–30 min)—of action. They are rapidly taken up by the brain after IV injection; peak levels occur in the brain shortly (30–45 sec) after injection. Within 5 minutes after injection, the brain level of the barbiturate has declined to about 50% of the peak. At 30 minutes after injection, only approximately 10% remains in the brain because the drug has been redistributed to other fatty stores in the body.

The response of the CNS to these drugs is essentially the same as that after an inhalation anesthetic: in succeeding order, loss of consciousness, diminished reflexes, loss of motor tone, and ultimately failure of the vital medullary centers. Recovery occurs in the reverse sequence and is caused by redistribution because the rate of metabolism and elimination from the body is slow (approximately 10%–15% per hour).

The major advantages of intravenous barbiturates compared with many inhalation anesthetics are rapidity and smoothness of onset, absence of salivation, greater patient acceptance (no occlusive face mask), short duration (allowing better control), speedy recovery, nonflammability, lower degree of irritation, and little danger of arrhythmias.

Disadvantages include respiratory and circulatory depression (Large doses decrease cardiac output and blood pressure by means of direct myocardial depressant action.), poor analgesia, laryngospasm, bronchospasm, poor skeletal muscle relaxant activity, and if leakage occurs, possible tissue necrosis.

Prolonged or repeated administration may lead to cumulative toxicity (eg, overdose) because the drugs are removed slowly from the body.

Because there are many similarities among the three anesthetic barbiturates, they are discussed as a group. Dosages and specific information pertaining to each drug are given in Table 19-2.

- **Methohexital**
- **Thiamylal**
- **Thiopental**

Uses

Induction of anesthesia
Supplementation of other general anesthetics
Production of anesthesia for short surgical procedures with minimal painful stimuli
Induction of hypnosis
Control of convulsive states during and after general or local anesthesia or other causes (thiopental)

Dosage

See Table 19-2.

Fate

Induction is smooth and rapid; onset of anesthesia occurs within 30 to 60 seconds after intravenous injection; drugs quickly cross blood–brain barrier and then rapidly redistributed to other parts of the body (first to highly vascular organs and subsequently to fatty tissue, where they are stored); duration of anesthesia with methohexital is 5 to 8 minutes, compared with 15 to 30 minutes with thiamylal and thiopental; rectal absorption of thiopental is good, and onset occurs within 10 minutes; plasma half-life of the drugs ranges between 4 and 8 hours; repeated dosing or continuous infusion leads to accumulation of the drug in lipid storage sites, causing prolonged drowsiness and respiratory or circulatory depression.

Adverse Reactions

(Not all reactions occur with all drugs; most are noted with prolonged administration.)

CV: Myocardial and circulatory depression, hypotension, arrhythmias, thrombophlebitis, pain on injection, necrosis or sloughing of tissue on extravasation, arteriospasm on inadvertent intra-arterial injection
Respiratory: Laryngospasm, bronchospasm, respiratory depresion, apnea, dyspnea
CNS: Prolonged somnolence, headache, emergence delirium, anxiety
Other: Nausea, vomiting, allergic reactions (pruritus, urticaria, rhinitis), abdominal pain, salivation, shivering, muscle twitching

Contraindications

Latent or manifest porphyria, absence of suitable veins for intravenous administration; thiopental contraindicated in status

Table 19-2. **Intravenous Barbiturate Anesthetics**

Drug	*Usual Dosage Range*	*Nursing Considerations*
Methohexital *Brevital* *(CAN) Brietal*	*Induction:* 5 mL–12 mL of 1% solution by infusion at 1 mL/5 sec *Maintenance:* 2 mL–4 mL of 1% solution every 4–7 min	Shortest-acting IV barbiturate, poor muscle-relaxing ability; proper preanesthetic medication should be given; sterile water for injection is the preferred diluent; do *not* use dilutions that are not clear and colorless; dilutions in sterile water are stable at room temperature for 6 wk; do *not* mix with acid solutions or allow contact with silicone; incompatible with lactated Ringer's solution
Thiamylal *Surital*	*Induction:* 3 mL–6 mL of 2.5% solution at a rate of 1 mL/5 sec *Maintenance:* 2.5% solution by intermittent IV injection as needed *or* 0.3% solution by continuous drip	Similar to methohexital with a longer duration of action (10–30 min); do not mix with atropine, tubocurarine, or succinylcholine; do not reconstitute with Ringer's solution or solutions containing bacteriostatic agents or buffers; sterile water for injection is the preferred diluent for IV injection solutions; continuous-drip solutions are prepared with 5% dextrose or isotonic sodium chloride to avoid hypotonicity; use only clear solutions; stable at room temperature for 24 h and refrigerated for 6 days
Thiopental *Pentothal*	Anesthesia: *Induction:* 2 mL–3 mL of 2.5% solution IV at 20–40 sec intervals *Maintenance:* 1 mL–2 mL 2.5% solution as needed (IV drip—0.2%–0.4%) Convulsions: 3 mL–5 mL of 2.5% solution Psychiatry: 4 mL–5mL 2.5% solution (IV drip—0.2% at 50 mL/min) Preanesthetic sedation: 1 g/75 lb (30 mg/kg) rectally to a maximum of 1.5 g for children and 4 g for adults	Most widely used IV barbiturate anesthetic; rectal administration may cause irritation, diarrhea, cramping, and bleeding; do not give rectally in presence of inflammatory, ulcerative, or bleeding lesions of the lower bowel; do not use concentrations less than 2% in sterile water for injection for IV administration, because hemolysis can occur; use freshly prepared solutions; discard unused portions after 24 h; avoid mixing with other solutions having an acid pH (eg, tubocurarine or succinylcholine solutions)

asthmaticus. *Cautious use* in persons with severe cardiovascular disease, bronchial asthma, hypotension, shock, Addison's disease, hepatic or renal dysfunction, myxedema, increased blood urea, severe anemia, increased intracranial pressure, and myasthenia gravis

Interactions

CNS depressant effects may be additive to those of other depressants, including alcohol, sedatives, and narcotics.

Orthostatic hypotension may be elicited by combined use with bumetanide, furosemide, or ethacrynic acid.

Nursing Management for Injection Anesthetics

Pretherapy Assessment

Assess and record baseline data necessary for detection of adverse effects of injection anesthetics: General: vital signs, body weight, skin color, and temperature; CNS: orientation, affect; GI: bowel sounds, normal output; GU: normal output, voiding pattern; Lab: renal and liver function tests, urinalysis, hemoglobin, complete blood count.

Review medical history and documents for existing or previous conditions that:

a. require cautious use of injection anesthetic: cardiovascular disease, increased intracranial pressure, bronchial asthma, severe anemia, myasthenia gravis
b. contraindicate use of injection anesthetic: allergy to the anesthetic; acute hepatic disease (hepatitis, cirrhosis); latent or manifest prophyria; status asthmaticus; absence of suitable veins for intravenous administration; children younger than 2 years; monoamine oxidase inhibitors; **pregnancy (Category C)**, lactation (safety not established, avoid use in nursing mothers).

Nursing Interventions

Medication Administration

Keep resuscitative equipment and emergency drugs readily available.

Keep intravenous fluids and vasopressors available to treat hypotension.

Assure ready access to anticholinergics in event of bradycardia.

Review patients' medication history to identify drugs that may interact with the injection anesthetic, such as labetalol, alcohol, CNS depressants, xanthines, and neuromuscular blocking agents.

Surveillance During Therapy

Monitor injection sites for irritation, extravasation; solutions may be alkaline, irritating, and cause necrosis.

Monitor for adverse effects, toxicity, and interactions, such as exaggerated response, myoclonic movements (with etomidate), hypotension, prolonged respiratory depression, confusion, ataxia, or nausea and vomiting.

Interpret results of diagnostic tests and contact practitioner as appropriate.

Monitor patient for fluid intake and output.

Monitor patient for temperature changes.

Monitor for possible drug–drug and drug–nutrient interactions: CNS depressants may have additive CNS effects with intravenous barbiturates; severe hypertension and tachycardia (ketamine and thyroid drugs); orthostatic hypotension elicited by combined use of a loop diuretic and intravenous barbiturate.

Patient Teaching

Incorporate teaching about the injection anesthetic with other preoperative teaching.

Inform the patient about what to expect (rapid onset of sleep), what they will feel (with rectal or intravenous administration) and how they will feel when they wake up.

Stress the importance of notifying the practitioner of any unusual symptoms up to 24 hours after the injection anesthetic.

Inform the patient of typical side effects related to injection anesthetic therapy: impaired psychomotor function, nausea, vomiting, shivering.

Nonbarbiturates

• Etomidate

Amidate

Etomidate is a rapid-acting hypnotic but, like barbiturates, has no analgetic action. It is used principally for induction of general anesthesia. The drug has minimal effects on heart rate, cardiac output, or peripheral circulation, but produces frequent myoclonic muscle movements and transient venous pain on injection

Uses

Induction of general anesthesia

Supplemental anesthesia during short operative procedures

Prolonged sedation of critically ill patients (investigational use)

Dosage

Induction: 0.2 mg/kg to 0.6 mg/kg IV over 30 to 60 seconds

Maintenance: 0.1 mg/kg to 0.3 mg/kg as needed in combination with nitrous oxide and oxygen

Fate

Onset is usually within 1 minute, and effects persist for 3 to 5 minutes; rapidly metabolized in the liver and primarily excreted by the kidney; highly lipid soluble and widely distributed in the body

Common Side Effects

Transient venous pain, myoclonic skeletal muscle movements, tonic muscle activity, eye movements

Significant Adverse Reactions

Hypotension, tachycardia, arrhythmias, hyperventilation, transient apnea, laryngospasm, hiccups, postoperative nausea and vomiting

Contraindications

Children under 10 years of age. *Cautious use* in patients with respiratory disease or skeletal muscle hyperactivity states and pregnant or nursing women.

Interactions

An additive CNS depressant effect can occur in combination with narcotics, sedatives, and other depressants.

Nursing Management

See Nursing Management for Injection Anesthetics

• *Propofol*

Diprivan

This agent is a rapidly acting nonbarbiturate that is employed by intravenous injection for induction and maintenance of general anesthesia; it may possess a slight degree of analgetic action. Hypnosis occurs approximately 40 seconds—and induction of anesthesia within 1 to 3 minutes—after injection.

Uses

Continuous sedation in patients who are intubated or who are on mechanical ventilation in the intensive care unit (ICU)
Induction of general anesthesia
Maintenance of general anesthesia when used in "balanced anesthesia"

Dosage

Anesthesia:
Induction: adults (<55 years old), 2 to 2.5 mg/kg
Maintenance: 100 to 200 mcg/kg/min
Sedation:
Induction: adults (<55 years old), 100 to 150 mcg/kg/min
Maintenance: 25 to 75 mcg/kg/min

Patients awaken at plasma levels of approximately 0.5 μg/mL.

Fate

Widely distributed in tissues; high degree of biotransformation to inactive metabolites, primarily a glucuronide conjugate; recovery from sedation or anesthesia is rapid; patients are oriented and respond to verbal commands approximately 8 minutes after terminating the infusion; the elimination half-life ranges from 300 to 700 minutes; prolonged infusions may increase half-life to longer than 700 minutes.

Common Side Effects

Bradycardia, hypotension, burning or stinging at injection site

Significant Adverse Reactions

Dermatologic: rash, pruritis
CNS: clonic/myoclonic movement, seizures, rigidity, thrashing, confusion, delirium, hallucinations
CV: arrhythmias, hemorrhage
GI: hypersalivation, diarrhea
Respiratory: bronchospasm, cough, hyperventilation
GU: green urine, urinary retention

Contraindications

Whenever general anesthesia is contraindicated. *Cautious use* in patients with increased intracranial pressure or impaired cerebral circulation; not recommended for use during delivery, because neonatal depression may occur; fatalities have occurred when used to provide ICU sedation in pediatric patients presenting with infections of the respiratory tract. (Most deaths were correlated with doses above those used for adults.)

Interactions

Simultaneous use of other CNS depressants can increase the degree of depression induced by propofol.

Nursing Management

See Nursing Management for Injection Anesthetics

Dissociative Agent

• *Ketamine*

Ketalar

Ketamine is a rapid-acting drug that produces general anesthesia with good analgesia, normal or slightly increased skeletal muscle tone, normal pharyngeal-laryngeal reflexes, and variable effects on the cardiovascular and respiratory systems. This agent differs from other general anesthetics in that the patient is "dissociated" or "disconnected" from the immediate environment (eg, the room in which the patient is placed), exhibiting a trancelike state; the term used is "dissociative anesthesia." It occurs because ketamine appears to block association pathways of the brain before it reduces somesthetic sensory input. In addition, ketamine may inhibit the thalamo-neocortical system before it blocks the reticular activating system and the limbic system. Thus, the patient may not remember the experience.

Ketamine possesses a wide margin of safety and is compatible with commonly used general and local anesthetics. Emergence from ketamine anesthesia is prolonged (several hours), and in 10% to 15% of patients is marked by psychological manifestations ranging from pleasant (dreamlike states, vivid imagery) to quite disagreeable (nightmarelike effects, hallucinations). These may be accompanied by confusion, excitement, and irrational behavior. Emergence reactions can be reduced by co-administration of IV diazepam.

Uses

Diagnostic and short surgical procedures not requiring skeletal muscle relaxation (eg, treatment of burns)
Induction of anesthesia before administration of other general anesthetics
Supplementation of low-potency agents such as nitrous oxide

Dosage

Induction: 1 mg/kg to 4.5 mg/kg IV injection over 60 seconds, or 6.5 mg/kg to 13 mg/kg IM. Alternatively, 1 mg/kg to 2 mg/kg by slow IV injection (0.5 mg/kg/min) in combination with diazepam (2 mg–5 mg intravenously over 60 sec) in a separate syringe

Maintenance: increments of one-half to full induction doses repeated as needed, titrated to patient's needs

Fate

Onset of surgical anesthesia is 30 seconds with IV injection and 3 to 4 minutes for IM; duration lasts 5 to 10 minutes IV and 15 to 25 minutes IM. Recovery time is dose-dependent; metabolites are excreted primarily in the urine.

Common Side Effects

Increased blood pressure (usually elevated within a few minutes after injection but returns to normal within 15 minutes), tachycardia, respiratory stimulation.

Significant Adverse Reactions

Laryngospasm; increased muscle tone (may progress to tonic or clonic convulsions); pain at injection site, rash, diplopia, nystagmus; large doses may produce respiratory depression, hypotension, or arrhythmias; on recovery, CNS effects such as excitement, delirium, hallucinations, vivid dreams, nightmares, confusion, and irrational behavior may occur.

CAUTION

During recovery period, minimize verbal, visual, and tactile stimulation to reduce danger of irrational behavior and other disturbing psychological manifestations. A rapid-acting barbiturate may be given to control severe emergence reactions, which are less likely to occur in the very young (younger than 15 years of age), the elderly (older than 65 years), and when the drug is used IM rather than IV.

Contraindications

Individuals for whom an elevation in blood pressure may prove dangerous; drug should not be used without additional muscle relaxants in surgical or diagnostic procedures involving the pharynx, larynx, or bronchial tree. *Cautious use* in patients with hypertension, elevated cerebrospinal fluid pressure, in alcoholics, and in pregnant women.

Interactions

Barbiturates or narcotics may prolong ketamine recovery time

Severe hypertension and tachycardia can occur in the presence of thyroid drugs

Ketamine may increase the neuromuscular blocking effects of nondepolarizing muscle relaxants (eg, tubocurarine, atracurium, vecuronium)

Nursing Management

See Nursing Management for Injection Anesthetics

Neuroleptanalgetic Agent

• Droperidol/Fentanyl

Innovar

This agent is a combination of two drugs: a neuroleptic or major tranquilizer (droperidol) and a potent narcotic (fentanyl). The effect that is produced is termed *neuroleptanalgesia*, characterized by general quiescence, reduced motor activity, and profound analgesia; complete loss of consciousness usually does not occur. It can elicit mild to moderate hypotension and bradycardia, respiratory depression, and muscle rigidity. Anesthesia can be induced by co-administration of 65% nitrous oxide in oxygen.

Uses

Production of tranquilization and analgesia for diagnostic and minor surgical procedures

Pre-anesthetic tranquilization

Induction of anesthesia

Adjunct for the maintenance of general and regional anesthesia, with nitrous oxide and oxygen

Dosage

Each milliliter contains 50 μg fentanyl and 2.5 mg droperidol.

Premedication: 0.5 mL to 2.0 mL IM 45 to 60 minutes before surgery (Children, 0.25 mL/20 lb IM)

Induction: 1 mL/20 to 25 lb by slow IV injection (3–5 min), or 10 mL/250 mL 5% dextrose by IV drip (Children, 0.5 mL/20 lb IM; initial dose should be reduced in elderly, debilitated, or other poor-risk patients)

Diagnostic: 0.5 mL to 2.0 mL IM 45 to 60 minutes before procedure; increments of 0.5 mL to 1.0 mL IV may be used for prolonged procedures as needed. Dosage must be individually determined and then adjusted according to need. Vital signs must be monitored during administration

Fate

The drug combination exhibits a fairly slow onset and prolonged duration, although each component has different characteristics. Fentanyl possesses an onset of 5 to 10 minutes and a duration of 30 to 60 minutes. Droperidol has a slower onset (30 min) and prolonged action (up to 6 h)

Common Side Effects

Drowsiness, mild hypotension

Significant Adverse Reactions

Extrapyramidal symptoms, muscle rigidity, dizziness, laryngospasm, bronchospasm, respiratory depression, shivering, tachycardia, vomiting, delirium, hallucinations

Contraindications

Presence of monoamine oxidase (MAO) inhibitors, children younger than 2 years of age, and parkinsonism. *Cautious use* in persons with arrhythmias, chronic obstructive pulmonary disease, liver or kidney dysfunction, and in trauma patients (increased likelihood of muscle rigidity)

Interactions

CNS depressants (eg, barbiturates, narcotics, alcohol) may have additive CNS effects with Innovar

Nursing Management

See Nursing Management for Injection Anesthetics

Selected Bibliography

Carstoniu J et al: Nitrous oxide in early labor. Anesthesiology 80(1):30, 1994

Elliott RH, Strunin L: Hepatotoxicity of volatile anesthetics. Br J Anaesth 70:339, 1993

Frenkel C, Duch DS, Urban BW: Effects of IV anaesthetics on human brain sodium channels. Br J Anaesth 71:15, 1993

Miller RD (ed): Anesthesia. 3rd ed. New York, Churchill Livingstone, 1990

Moneret-Vautrin DA, Laxenaire MC: The risk of allergy related to general anesthesia. Clin Exp Allergy 23:629, 1993

Moerman N, Bonke B, Oosting J: Awareness and recall during general anesthesia. Anesthesiology 79:454, 1993

Ramsay DS, Brown AC, Woods SC: Acute tolerance to nitrous oxide in humans. Pain 51:367, 1992

Wessen A, Persson PM, Nilsson A, Hartvig P: Concentration-effect relationships of propofol after total intravenous anesthesia. Anesth Analg 77:1000, 1993

Yost CS: G proteins: Basic characteristics and clinical potential for the practice of anesthesia. Anesth Analg 77:822, 1993

Nursing Bibliography

Rivellini D: Local and regional anesthesia: Nursing implications. Nursing Clinics of North America 28(3):547–572, 1993

Strong N: Assessing the post anesthesia patient. Critical Care Nursing Clinics of North America 16(1):1–7, 1993

Tomasa G, Faut-Callahan M: The anesthetic management of the trauma patient. Critical Care Nursing Quarterly 15(4):47–52, 1993

Waugaman W, Foster S: New advances in anesthesia. Nursing Clinics of North America 26(2):451–476, 1991

20

Narcotic Analgesics (Agonists) and Antagonists

Narcotic Analgesics: Agonists

- ***Phenanthrenes***
  - *Naturally occurring opium alkloids*
    - Codeine
    - Morphine
  - *Semisynthetic derivatives of morphine*
    - Hydromorphone
    - Oxymorphone
  - *Semisynthetic derivatives of codeine*
    - Hydrocodone
    - Oxycodone
- ***Methadones***
  - Levomethadyl
  - Methadone
  - Propoxyphene
- ***Morphinan***
  - Levorphanol
- ***Phenylpiperidines***
  - Alfentanil
  - Fentanyl
  - Meperidine
  - Sufentanil

Narcotic Analgesics: Agonist–Antagonists

- ***Aminotetralin***
  - Dezocine
- ***Benzomorphan***
  - Pentazocine
- ***Morphinan***
  - Butorphanol
- ***Phenanthrenes***
  - Buprenorphine
  - Nalbuphine

Narcotic Antagonists

- Naloxone
- Naltrexone

Narcotic analgesics—or "opioids"—include both naturally occurring and synthetic drugs that interact with opioid receptors in the central nervous system (CNS) to relieve severe pain. Conversely, narcotic **antagonists** are drugs that occupy—but do not activate—these same receptors; they are used primarily to reverse the effects of overdoses of narcotics.

Narcotic Analgesics

Morphine and codeine are naturally occurring alkaloids obtained from the opium poppy. Morphine is the prototypical narcotic analgesic and is more potent than codeine. Other commonly used narcotics are either (a) **semisynthetic** derivatives (ie, chemical modifications of morphine or codeine) or (b) **synthetic** agents (ie, completely created in the chemical laboratory); many drugs in these two groups are more potent than morphine and some differ slightly in their respective pharmacologic actions.

Classification of Narcotic Analgesics

Drugs possessing an opioid activity may be classified as either **narcotic agonists** or **narcotic agonist–antagonists**. The agonists consist of narcotics that only activate opioid receptor sites (see discussion below). The agonist–antagonist compounds are more complex; they activate some opioid receptors *and* partially block other sites. Within each of these broad categories, subclassifications are based on the chemical structure of the individual drugs. Even within each subclass, representative drugs are characterized by different potencies and toxicities. For example, morphine and codeine belong to the same chemical grouping (ie, phenanthrenes), but morphine is more potent and toxic.

Pharmacologic Actions of Opioids

At therapeutic doses, narcotic analgesics produce many pharmacologic effects on different systems of the body; the more important actions are outlined in Table 20-1. Not all of these effects occur to the same degree (see Table 20-3), however; moreover, many actions are dose dependent and become more intense at high dosages.

Narcotics exert their effects by combining with opioid receptors in the CNS, each receptor mediating distinctive actions. Sites of high receptor concentration include the dorsal horn of the spinal cord and several subcortical brain areas, such as the periaqueductal gray matter, hypothalamus, thalamus, locus coeruleus, and raphe nuclei. The narcotics bind to these different receptors to varying degrees; the relative preference of an opiate for certain receptor types over others determines the overall pharmacologic profile of the drug (Table 20-2). Of great clinical importance is the finding that receptors responsible for many opioid side effects *differ* from those that mediate the analgesic actions of these drugs; thus it may be possible to separate undesirable from desired opiate effects. For example, most narcotic agonists have agonistic activity at *mu* (μ), *kappa* (κ), and possibly also *delta* (δ) receptors; The mixed agonist–antagonists, however, appear to bind preferentially to the *kappa* and possibly *sigma* (σ) receptors and may act as partial *antagonists* at the *mu* sites. This differential receptor action of the mixed agonist–antagonist narcotics may help explain their lower abuse potential, reduced euphoric effects, and greater sedative action compared with the narcotic agonists. In addition, antagonism of *mu* receptors by mixed agonist–antagonists can 1) partially reverse the effects of other narcotic agonists acting at these sites; and 2) induce withdrawal reactions when given to a patient who has been taking—for a prolonged time—a narcotic agonist.

Recent evidence has suggested the presence of subtypes of μ receptors; for example, respiratory depression and constipation are thought to be mediated by the μ_2 receptor, whereas supraspinal analgesia is believed to result from μ_1 receptor interaction. Morphine is capable of activating both μ_1 and μ_2 receptors. Conversely, some endogenous opiates (see below), such as enkephalins, activate only μ_1 sites and may not be associated with the degree of respiratory depression noted with morphine and its analogs.

Table 20-1. **Pharmacologic Effects of Analgesics**

CNS

Analgesia
Sedation
Euphoria
Emesis (*anti*emetic at very high doses)
Depressed cough reflex
Respiratory depression (depression of medullary respiratory center)

Cardiovascular

Orthostatic hypotension (depression of medullary vasomotor center; peripheral vascular dilation)

GI Tract

Peristalsis and stomach motility decreased
Delayed gastric emptying time
Constipation

Smooth Muscle

Increased tone of most nonvascular smooth muscle (eg, GI, urinary, biliary)

Urinary System

Urinary tract spasm
Contraction of urinary sphincter
Release of antidiuretic hormone
Decreased renal blood flow (?)

Eye

Miosis

Neuroendocrine

Release of prolactin and somatotropin
Decreased release of luteinizing hormone and thyrotropin

Table 20-2. **Opiate Receptors**

Receptor	Pharmacologic Effects
mu (μ)	Supraspinal analgesia (μ_1) Euphoria (μ_1) Respiratory depression (μ_2) Physical dependence (μ_2) Constipation (μ_2)
kappa (κ)	Spinal analgesia Sedation Miosis
delta (δ)	Spinal analgesia Affective behavior
sigma (σ)	Dysphoria Hallucinations Respiratory/vasomotor stimulation

Endogenous Opioids

Electrical stimulation of certain CNS areas evokes potent analgesia that can be attenuated by administration of narcotic antagonist drugs. This phenomenon suggests the presence of endogenous substances that interact with opiate receptors to produce effects similar to those of exogenously administered opiates.

The three distinct groups of endogenous opioidlike peptides that have been isolated are called *endorphins, enkephalins*, and *dynorphins*. Each group is derived from a distinct precursor polypeptide and exhibits a characteristic distribution pattern in the CNS.

Beta-endorphin is a 31-amino-acid peptide derived from a larger peptide that also produces adrenocorticotropic hormone (ACTH) and α-melanocyte–stimulating hormone. It occurs predominantly in the pituitary gland and may influence a variety of behavioral and physiologic responses to pain.

Enkephalins are pentapeptides; the two most extensively studied are methionine-enkephalin (met-enkephalin) and leucine-enkephalin (leu-enkephalin). The enkephalins are located in nerve endings throughout the CNS and are particularly abundant in the brainstem and the dorsal horn of the spinal cord, as well as in the basal ganglia and portions of the limbic system. Enkephalins are believed to reduce the transmission of pain signals by binding to opiate receptors in the spinal cord and decreasing the release of Substance P, a neurotransmitter at afferent nerve endings carrying pain impulses. Enkephalins may be released by a variety of stimuli, providing the body with a natural mechanism for pain control and other behavioral modifications.

Dynorphins are derived from still another precursor and are located in neurons throughout the brain. Their precise role in pain modulation or behavior remains to be established.

Endogenous opioid peptides display differing affinities for opioid receptor sites. For example, enkephalins appear to bind to both δ and μ_1 sites with approximately equal affinity. Beta-endorphin likewise binds predominantly to μ and δ sites, although it can interact with more specialized sites as well. Dynorphins appear to interact primarily at κ sites, although some may bind to μ and δ receptors as well. The clinical significance of this differential receptor interaction among the endogenous opiates remains to be established.

Endorphins and enkephalins are of little clinical value, however, because they are not absorbed orally and are rapidly degraded by metabolizing enzymes in the brain, blood, and other tissues. Several synthetic enkephalins are being tested for their analgesic activity.

Narcotic analgesics can modify the actual *sensation* of pain through their effect on pain pathways in the spinal cord and brain. They can also modify the *perception* of pain through their effect on higher cortical areas. Thus, the transmission of a painful stimulus from the site of origin to the sensory cortex is reduced, whereas the painful sensation is perceived as being less intense or bothersome. The resultant tranquility and release from tension often lead to a state of euphoria and an exaggerated sense of well-being; it is this euphoric state that causes drug addicts to develop a tendency to abuse narcotics. **In marked contrast**, legitimate patients who require narcotic drugs to relieve their severe pain (eg, cancer pain) do *NOT* become drug addicts! If the source of pain can be eliminated (eg, removal of a tumor by surgery), the normal patient can be withdrawn from the narcotic and will *NOT* want to continue taking it. It must be understood that the causes of drug addiction are psychological, social, and, possibly, genetic; the pharmacology of a drug is of minor influence in **creating** an addict (See Chapter 82 for a more complete discussion of this important issue in pain management).

The principal *acute* toxic effect of morphine and related narcotic agonists is respiratory depression, characterized by slow, shallow, irregular respiration and cyanosis. Other important adverse effects include hypotension, decreased urinary output, and hypothermia. Treatment includes mechanical ventilation and use of a narcotic antagonist. Conversely, use of narcotic agonist–antagonists may induce sedation at normal doses, and higher doses may elicit sweating, nausea, and dizziness. However, the extent of respiratory depression is less at elevated doses than with comparable doses of pure narcotic agonists.

Long-term use of narcotics leads to the development of tolerance and, eventually, physical dependence in both legitimate patients and addicts. In the drug abuser, useful diagnostic signs of dependence are miosis, constipation, superficial infections, itching, needle marks, scars, and abscesses. In both patients and drug addicts who are using narcotics for prolonged periods (weeks → months → years), abrupt and complete termination of narcotic therapy **or** administration of a narcotic antagonist induces a fairly predictable pattern of withdrawal reactions. Lacrimation, rhinorrhea, sweating, yawning, chills, and goose pimples usually occur within 8 to 16 hours after the last dose. Peak withdrawal effects are generally observed within 36 to 48 hours; they include abdominal cramping, muscle aching, nausea, vomiting, diarrhea, hyperthermia, and hyperventilation. Most symptoms subside within 3 to 5 days, but some may persist for much longer periods. The longer the interval that the narcotics are used, and the higher the daily doses, the more severe the withdrawal reactions will be. Further attention is directed to the problem of narcotic abuse in Chapter 82.

Most narcotic drugs are similar in the **type** of clinical actions and adverse effects that they produce; they differ primarily in potency and the **frequency** of causing toxicity. A comparison of the properties of the opiates is presented in Table 20-3. Specific information relating to preparations, dosage, and characteristics of individual drugs is given in Table 20-4.

Mechanism

Actions of narcotic drugs are complex and involve multiple sites and several mechanisms of action: elevation of the pain threshold, alteration in perception of pain, blunting of the anxiety or apprehension associated with the presence of pain, and induction of somnolence and clouding of mentation. Possible mechanisms include 1) direct activation of opiate receptor sites in the spinal cord, brain stem, and subcortical brain nuclei; 2) potentiation of the effects of endogenous opioids; and 3) activation of descending spinal cord pathways, which dampens incoming sensory pain impulses. By reducing the entrance of calcium

(continued)

Table 20-3. **Comparative Pharmacologic Properties of Opiates**

	*Equianalgesic Doses (mg)**		*Onset of Action (min)†*	*Duration of Action (h)†*	*Analgesic Efficacy*	*Addictive Liability*	*Antitussive Activity*	*Respiratory Depression*	*Sedation*	*Emesis*
	PO	*SC, IM*								
Agonists										
Morphine	60	10	10–20	4–6	High	High	Strong	Moderate	Moderate	Moderate
Alfentanil	—	—	2–4 (IV)	0.5–1	High	High	—	—	—	—
Codeine	200	120	15–30	3–5	Low	Medium	Strong	Weak	Weak	Weak
Fentanyl	—	0.1–0.2	5–15	1–2	High	High	—	Weak	—	—
Hydrocodone	30	—	—	4–8	Medium	Medium	Strong	Moderate	Weak	Weak
Hydromorphone	7	1–2	15–30	4–5	High	High	Strong	Moderate	Moderate	Weak
Levorphanol	4	2	15–30	4–6	High	High	Moderate	Moderate	Moderate	Weak
Meperidine	300–400	80–100	10–20	2–4	Medium	High	Weak	Moderate	Weak	—
Methadone	10–20	10	10–15	4–6	High	High	Moderate	Moderate	Moderate	Weak
Oxycodone	30	15	15–30	3–5	Medium	Medium–High	Strong	Moderate	Moderate	Moderate
Oxymorphone	6	1–1.5	5–10	3–5	High	High	Weak	Strong	—	Strong
Propoxyphene‡	—	—	15–30 (PO)	4–6	Low	Low	—	Weak	Weak	Weak
Sufentanil	—	—	2–4 (IV)	0.5–1	High	High	—	—	—	—
Agonist–Antagonists										
Buprenorphine		0.3	10–15	4–6	High	Low	—	Moderate	Moderate	Weak
Butorphanol		2–4	5–10	3–4	High	Low	—	Weak	Moderate	Weak
Dezocine		10	15–30	2–4	High	Low	—	Moderate	Moderate	Weak
Nalbuphine		10	10–15	3–6	High	Low	—	Moderate	Moderate	—
Pentazocine	150	30–60	15–30	3–4	Medium	Medium–Low	—	Moderate	Moderate	Weak

* All doses as stated are approximately equivalent to 10 mg morphine IM or SC; note that long-term administration of narcotics alters pharmacokinetics and reduces the oral:parenteral dose ratio; for example, with morphine the ratio is reduced from 6:1 to 3:1 during long-term use.
† Onset and duration of action based on IM or SC administration.
‡ Propoxyphene is a very weak analgesic that cannot be compared to other opiates in equianalgesic doses.

Table 20-4. Narcotic Analgesics

Drug	*Usual Dosage Range*	*Nursing Considerations*
NARCOTIC AGONISTS		
Phenanthrenes		
Codeine (C-II) *(CAN) Paveral*	*Analgesia* Adults: 15–60 mg 4 times/day orally; SC, IM, or IV Children: 0.5 mg/kg every 4–6 h orally, SC, or IM *Antitussive* Adults: 10–20 mg/4–6 h to a maximum of 120 mg/24 h Children: (6–12 y) 5–10 mg/4–6 h (maximum 60 mg/day); (2–6 y) 2.5–5 mg/4–6 h (maximum 30 mg/day)	Less potent and less abuse potential than morphine; widely used in cough medications; suppresses cough by direct depressant effect on medullary cough center; as an analgesic, most frequently used in combination with aspirin, acetaminophen, or other analgesics; high doses (eg, 60 mg) may cause restlessness and excitement; rapid onset of action after oral administration (10–15 min) and effects persist for up to 6 h; used in combination with centrally acting muscle relaxants for pain of muscle spasm and rigidity
Hydromorphone (C-II) *Dilaudid* *(CAN) PMS-Hydromorphone*	*SC, IM:* 2–4 mg/4–6 h (may also be given by slow IV injection) *Oral:* 2–4 mg/4–6 h *Rectal:* 1 suppository every 6 h–8 h	Very potent (8–10× morphine) analgesic, producing less sedation, vomiting, and nausea than morphine; elicits marked respiratory depression; therefore, use smallest dose possible; suppositories may give prolonged effect; high abuse potential and popular "street drug" because of extreme potency and lack of strong hypnotic effect; oral form useful in treating severe chronic pain but drug is relatively short-acting.
Morphine (C-II) *Astramorph PF, Duramorph, Infumorph, MS Contin, MSIR, OMS Concentrate, Oramorph SR, Roxanol, RMS* *(CAN) Epimorph, Morphitec, M.O.S., Statex*	*Oral:* 10–30 mg/4–6 h *or* 30–60 mg sustained release every 8–12 h *SC, IM:* (Adults) 5–20 mg/4 h (usual 10 mg); (Children) 0.1–0.2 mg/kg *IV:* 4–10 mg injected slowly *Rectal:* 10–20 mg/4 h *Epidural:* 5 mg in lumbar region once daily or 2–4 mg by continuous infusion over 24 h *Intrathecal:* 1/10 of epidural dose	Principal opium alkaloid, and standard with which other opiates are compared; most effective parenterally because oral availability may be somewhat limited; commonly produces drowsiness and relief from anxiety—large doses induce deep sleep and profound respiratory depression; oral form (especially sustained release tablets) is very effective in controlling chronic pain when given on a regular dosing schedule; oral solution may be combined with other medications (sedatives, alcohol, amphetamine, phenothiazines) as a "cocktail" for relief of severe pain—such mixtures have been termed Brompton's mixtures; however, use of a single opiate in sufficient dosage is as effective in controlling pain with fewer side effects
Opium (C-II) *Paregoric, Pantopon*	*Injection* IM, SC: 5–20 mg/4–5 h *Tincture* 0.6 mL (6 mg morphine) 4 times/day *Camphorated tincture:* Adults: 5–10 mL (2–4 mg morphine) 1–4 times/day Children: 0.25–0.5 mL/kg 1–4 times/day	Activity is primarily due to morphine content; has been largely replaced by morphine or other narcotics, except for paregoric, which is widely used orally for cramps and diarrhea and also topically for teething pain in infants; discontinue drug once diarrhea has been controlled to prevent excessive dosage; do *not* confuse paregoric (camphorated opium tincture containing 2 mg morphine/5 mL) with opium tincture itself (50 mg morphine/5 mL); absorption of drug from GI tract is improved if diluted in a little water (injection and tincture are schedule II; camphorated tincture is schedule III)
Oxycodone (C-II) *Roxicodone* *(CAN) Supeudol*	5 mg/6 h	Moderately potent, orally effective narcotic, commonly used in fixed combinations with aspirin (Percodan) or acetaminophen (Percocet, Tylox)
Oxymorphone (C-II) *Numorphan*	*SC, IM:* 1–1.5 mg/4–6 h *IV:* 0.5 mg as needed *Rectal:* 5 mg/4–6 h *Analgesic during labor:* 0.5–1 mg IM/4–6 h	Rapid-acting potent (5–10× morphine) analgesic; used for preoperative sedation, obstetrical analgesia, and relief of anxiety in patients with dyspnea due to pulmonary edema or left ventricular failure; high incidence of nausea, vomiting, and euphoria; little constipation or antitussive action; not recommended in children younger than 12 years
METHADONES		
Levomethadyl (C-II) *ORLAAM*	*Initial:* 20–40 mg orally every 48–72 h *Maintenance:* usually 60–90 mg orally 3 times/wk	Dosage must be individualized and *carefully* titrated; usual schedule is a dose given every Monday, Wednesday, and Friday

(*continued*)

Table 20-4. **Narcotic Analgesics** **(Continued)**

Drug	*Usual Dosage Range*	*Nursing Considerations*
Methadone (C-II) *Dolophine*	*Analgesia* IM, SC, orally: 2.5–10 mg/3–4 h (Children: 0.7 mg/kg/day) *Chronic pain regimen:* 5 mg every 12 h to 20 mg every 5 h; start with 5 mg every 5–6 h and titrate according to patient's needs *Narcotic detoxification* (highly individualized depending on severity of withdrawal symptoms): 15–20 mg orally (up to 40 mg) to suppress symptoms; treatment not to exceed 21 days, during which time the dosage is gradually reduced *Maintenance therapy:* 20–120 mg daily, individualized to control abstinence symptoms without inducing sedation or respiratory depression	May be used to relieve severe pain, usually orally or IM; SC administration may be painful; longer acting and less sedating than morphine, especially when given long-term; exerts a similar degree of respiratory depression and addiction liability as morphine; not recommended for obstetrics or as an analgesic in young children except in cancer-related pain, for which it is very effective; also used for detoxification and maintenance in approved programs for narcotic addiction; administered orally on a daily basis—abstinence syndrome is qualitatively similar to that of morphine, but onset is slower, course is more prolonged, and symptoms are less severe; with prolonged oral use, most side effects disappear, but constipation and sweating often persist; euphoria is much less prominent with methadone, and addict may eventually overcome compulsive need for the narcotic "high"; should be used in combination with psychiatric and social counseling (see Chap. 82)
Propoxyphene (C-IV) *Darvon, Darvon-N, Dolene* *(CAN) Novopropoxyn, 642 Tablets*	*Adults:* 65 mg–100 mg every 4 h *Note:* 65 mg of the HCl salt (Darvon) is equivalent to 100 mg of the napsylate salt (Darvon-N)	*Very weak* analgesic, structurally related to methadone; little antitussive activity; has many of the side effects of narcotics and is associated with habituation and physical dependence to approximately the same degree as codeine; restlessness, tremor, and mild euphoria commonly occur; usually administered in fixed combination with aspirin and caffeine (eg, Darvon Compound) or with acetaminophen (eg, Darvocet, E-Lor, Wygesic); will potentiate CNS depressant effects of alcohol and tranquilizers—such combinations are a major cause of drug-related fatalities; avoid prolonged or excessive dosage and concurrent use of tranquilizers or alcohol; maximum recommended doses are 390 mg/day of the HCl salt and 600 mg/day of the napsylate salt
MORPHINAN		
Levorphanol (C-II) *Levo-Dromoran*	2–3 mg orally or SC/4–6 h	Very potent analgesic (4–5× morphine); almost as effective orally as parenterally; used preoperatively to potentiate and prolong general anesthesia and to shorten recovery time; also is a useful supplement to nitrous oxide–oxygen anesthesia; low incidence of nausea, vomiting, and constipation but strong sedative and respiratory depressant; slow onset of peak effect (60–90 min) but prolonged duration (6–8 h); reduce dose in pediatric and geriatric population and in poor-risk patients; has a bitter taste; protect from light
PHENYLPIPERIDINES		
Alfentanil (C-II) *Alfenta*	*Analgesia adjunct* 8–50 μg/kg IV, followed by increments of 3–15 μg/kg as required (maximum 75 μg/kg) *Induction anesthetic* 130–245 μg/kg IV followed by 0.5–1.5 μg/kg/min IV infusion	Rapid-acting narcotic used IV as an analgesic adjunct during N_2O/O_2 barbiturate anesthesia; also used as a primary induction anesthetic in general surgery if intubation and mechanical ventilation are required; base dosage on *lean* body weight in obese individuals; reduce dosage in elderly or debilitated persons; not recommended in children younger than 12; vital signs must be closely monitored
Fentanyl (C-II) *Duragesic, Sublimaze*	*Preoperative* 0.05–0.1 mg IM *General anesthesia* Induction: 0.05–0.1 mg IV (repeat at 2–3 min intervals) Maintenance: 0.025–0.1 mg IV or IM as needed *Adjunct to general anesthesia* 0.002–0.05 mg/kg as needed *Postoperative* 0.05–0.1 mg IM/1–2 h for pain, tachypnea, and delirium Children (2–12 y): 0.02–0.03 mg/20–25 lb Transdermal system (Duragesic): Apply one patch every 72 h	Very potent (100× morphine) analgesic used for short durations (eg, preoperative, intraoperative, or postoperative to relieve pain and anxiety and as an anesthetic agent with oxygen in selected high-risk operations such as open-heart surgery, complicated neurologic procedures); rapid onset (10–15 min IM) and short duration (1–2 h); respiratory depression often outlasts analgesia; have antidotal measures (eg, oxygen, endotracheal tube, narcotic antagonist, muscle relaxant) on hand; rapid IV administration may cause muscle spasm or rigidity; also available as a transdermal patch in 4 strengths (25 μg/h, 50 μg/h, 75 μg/h, 100 μg/h) for management of *chronic pain* requiring opioids; transdermal dose is based on 24-hour oral or IM morphine-equivalent dose; available in combination with the neuroleptic droperidol as Innovar, which is used for analgesia and tranquilization (neuroleptanalgesia) for short surgical and diagnostic procedures (see Chap. 19); combination may cause restlessness, hallucinations, extrapyramidal symptoms, and postoperative drowsiness; vital signs should be monitored continually during use

(continued)

Table 20-4. **Narcotic Analgesics (Continued)**

Drug	Usual Dosage Range	Nursing Considerations
Meperidine (C-II) *Demerol*	*Analgesia* IM, SC, orally: 50–150 mg/3–4 h Children: 1–2 mg/kg IM, SC, or orally every 3–4 h *Preoperative medication* Adults: 50–100 mg IM or SC 30–90 min before anesthesia Children: 1–2 mg/kg IM or SC *Obstetrical analgesia* 50–100 mg IM or SC; repeat at 1–3 h intervals	Moderately potent analgesic (1/10 morphine) with weak antitussive activity; less spasmogenic and constipating than most other narcotics; more rapid onset and shorter duration of action (2–4 h) compared with morphine; significantly less effective orally than parenterally; frequent dizziness and occasional tremors, uncoordinated muscle movements, and other signs of CNS excitation can occur; attains high levels in breast milk; used for moderate pain, often associated with diagnostic procedures, minor surgical procedures, or obstetrics; also for preanesthetic medication and by slow IV infusion (1 mg/mL) for support of anesthesia; solutions of meperidine and barbiturates are incompatible; prolonged therapy may cause elevated normeperidine levels (detectable by plasma sample) which can lead to CNS symptoms ranging from shakiness to seizures
Sufentanil (C-II) *Sufenta*	*Adults* For general surgery in which intubation and mechanical ventilation are required: 1–2 μg/kg with N_2O/O_2; maintenance dose of 10 μg–25 μg as analgesia lightens For more complicated surgery: 2–8 μg/kg with N_2O/O_2; maintenance doses of 25–50 μg as needed For complete anesthesia: 8–30 μg/kg with 100% O_2 and a muscle relaxant; maintenance doses of 25–50 μg as anesthesia lightens *Children* (younger than 12 y) 10–25 μg/kg with 100% O_2 for general anesthesia in children undergoing cardiovascular surgery	Can induce and maintain anesthesia with 100% O_2 in patients undergoing major surgical procedures such as cardiovascular surgery or neurosurgery in the sitting position; also used as an analgesic adjunct at doses less than 8 μg/kg to maintain balanced general anesthesia; dosage should be based on lean body weight and reduced in the elderly or debilitated; doses above 8 μg/kg induce sleep; catecholamine release is suppressed at doses up to 25 μg/kg, and sympathetic responses are attenuated at doses between 25 μg/kg and 35 μg/kg; postoperative mechanical ventilation required because of extended respiratory depression
NARCOTIC AGONIST–ANTAGONISTS		
Aminotetralin		
Dezocine *Dalgan*	IM: 10 mg (range: 5–20 mg); can repeat every 3–6 h (maximum, 120 mg/day) IV: 5 mg (range: 2.5–10 mg)	SC injection is not recommended—produces irritation; overdose can produce respiratory depression; not a controlled drug
Benzomorphan		
Pentazocine (C-IV) *Talwin*	Oral: 50 mg/3–4 h (maximum dose—600 mg/day) IM, SC, IV: 30 mg every 3–4 h (maximum, 360 mg/day) Obstetrics: 30 mg IM *or* 20 mg IV/2–3 h	One-third as potent as morphine parenterally; possesses some narcotic antagonist activity as well, therefore, can antagonize effects of other opiates and may elicit withdrawal symptoms in patients who have been taking other narcotics regularly; onset is 15–30 min after IM, SC, or oral use and 2–3 min IV; duration from 2–3 h parenterally and up to 5 h with oral use; has sedative activity and may be used preoperatively in obstetrics as well as for moderate to severe pain; addiction liability about equal to codeine; tablets are marketed as Talwin-Nx and contain 0.5 mg naloxone, a potent narcotic antagonist; although inactive orally, naloxone has profound antagonistic actions against narcotics when injected, and its inclusion in the tablet is intended to curb a form of pentazocine abuse in which the tablets are dissolved and injected; can induce tachycardia, hypertension, confusion, hallucinations, bizarre thought processes, and other CNS effects in large doses; abrupt discontinuation of drug may lead to muscle cramping, chills, restlessness, anxiety, and other symptoms of narcotic withdrawal; do *not* mix with soluble barbiturates because a precipitate will form; rotate injection sites if used chronically to minimize sclerosis of skin and subcutaneous tissues; severe respiratory depression is treated with naloxone and other supportive measures
Morphinan		
Butorphanol *Stadol*	IM: 2 mg/3–4 h (maximum 4 mg/dose) IV: 1 mg/3–4 h Nasal Spray: 1 spray (1 mg) in one nostril or in both nostrils as necessary; repeat in 3–4 h as needed	Potent analgesic (4–7× morphine on a weight basis); respiratory depression with 2-mg dose is equivalent to that achieved with 10 mg morphine, but does not increase appreciably at 4 mg; nasal spray is used for management of pain including migraine; possesses weak narcotic antagonistic activity (considerably less than that of naloxone); use with

(*continued*)

Table 20-4. **Narcotic Analgesics** **(Continued)**

Drug	*Usual Dosage Range*	*Nursing Considerations*
		caution in patients dependent on narcotics because withdrawal symptoms can occur; most frequent side effect is sedation; peak analgesia occurs in 1 h with IM use (1–2 h with nasal spray) and persists for 3–4 h; not recommended in children younger than 18 y or in nursing mothers; use cautiously in the presence of liver or kidney disease, coronary artery insufficiency (increases cardiac workload) and respiratory impairment; not a controlled substance
PHENANTHRENES		
Buprenorphine *Buprenex*	*Adults and children older than 12 y:* 0.3–0.6 mg IM *or* slow IV every 6 h as needed	Semisynthetic derivative of thebaine that has a high affinity for mu receptors and dissociates from them slowly; exhibits a long duration of action (up to 6 h) and low degree of dependence; approximately 20–30 times more potent than morphine; possesses antagonist activity equal to that of naloxone; may reduce blood pressure and heart rate and produces respiratory depression equal to that of morphine at normal dosage ranges; sedation is very common; use cautiously in elderly or debilitated patients, or patients with impaired hepatic, renal, or pulmonary function; may precipitate withdrawal symptoms in narcotic-dependent patients
Nalbuphine *Nubain*	*SC, IM, IV:* 10 mg/70 kg individual; repeat every 3–6 h as necessary; maximum, 160 mg/day	Chemically related to oxycodone and naloxone, and possesses both agonistic activity at kappa and delta receptors and weak antagonistic activity at mu receptors; analgesia is approximately equivalent to morphine on a milligram basis, with somewhat lower abuse potential (less than that of codeine or propoxyphene); may precipitate withdrawal symptoms in patients on chronic narcotic therapy; use 1/4 normal dose initially in these patients; high incidence of sedation; does not increase systemic vascular resistance or cardiac workload like other narcotic agonist–antagonists; at usual adult dose, respiratory depression is equal to that seen with morphine—larger doses (ie, above 30 mg), however, do not appreciably increase respiratory depression, unlike morphine; duration of analgesia ranges from 3 to 6 h; do not use in pregnant women or in children younger than 18 y (Not a controlled drug)

into neuronal cells, narcotics decrease the release of Substance P found in primary sensory afferent nerve endings, especially in the spinal cord, Substance P appears to function as an excitatory neurotransmitter at nerve endings, transmitting pain signals to higher centers in the CNS. Narcotics also decrease sensitivity of the medullary respiratory center to carbon dioxide, resulting in dose-dependent respiratory depression. They also depress responsiveness of α-adrenergic receptors, leading to visceral pooling of blood and orthostatic hypotension. Other effects include reduction of gastrointestinal (GI) peristalsis by a direct relaxant effect on intestinal smooth muscle, increased tone of the urinary bladder sphincter, and stimulation of the chemoreceptor trigger zone in the brain stem, causing nausea and vomiting.

Uses

Relief of moderate to severe pain (eg, myocardial infarction, carcinomas, burns, fractures, postsurgical trauma)

As **pre**operative medication to provide a synergistic effect to that of the general anesthetics **and** to improve pain relief in the **post**operative period

Relief of persistent nonproductive cough (especially codeine and hydrocodone)

Relief of severe diarrhea

Immediate (short-term) relief of dyspnea associated with pulmonary edema or left ventricular failure by reduction of left ventricular workload

Improve respiration in patients on mechanical ventilators (decrease tendency of such patients to "fight" the assisted breathing)

Obstetric analgesia

Dosage

See Table 20-4.

Fate

Absorption from subcutaneous and intramuscular injection sites as well as GI mucosa is generally good. Some drugs (eg, morphine) undergo significant first-pass hepatic metabolism; their effective oral dose is considerably higher than the parenteral dose (see Table 20-3). Widely distributed in the body and localize in highest amounts in the liver, kidneys, lungs, and spleen. Brain concentrations are usually low as compared with other body organs; highly lipophilic drugs (eg, fentanyl) cross the blood–brain barrier more readily than do weakly lipophilic agents such as morphine. Analgesic effects are noted within 30 minutes after oral administration and 5 to 15 minutes after parenteral injection. Duration of analgesia differs among individuals with narcotic drugs (see Table 20-3). Drugs are mostly converted to polar metabolites, which are readily excreted by the kidneys. Small quantities of unchanged drug may also be eliminated in the urine and feces.

Common Side Effects

Dizziness, lightheadedness, sedation, nausea, sweating, flushing

Significant Adverse Reactions

CNS: euphoria or dysphoria, headache, agitation, tremor, disorientation, delirium, uncoordinated movements, and transient hallucinations

CV: bradycardia, palpitations, hypotension, syncope, and phlebitis (intravenous injection only)

GI: dry mouth, anorexia, constipation, vomiting, biliary tract spasm

Respiratory: respiratory depression (observed in fetus and newborn as well)

Genitourinary: urinary hesitancy or retention, dysuria, antidiuretic effect, loss of potency or libido

Hypersensitivity: urticaria, pruritus, sneezing, edema, hemorrhagic urticaria, wheal and flare at IV injection site

Other: pain at injection site, local tissue irritation, porphyria

Acute overdose: extreme miosis, hypothermia, oliguria, bradycardia, hypotension, deep sleep, marked respiratory depression, pulmonary edema, coma, cardiac arrest

Contraindications

Convulsive states, severe respiratory depression, increased intracranial pressure, acute asthma, undiagnosed acute abdominal conditions, severe ulcerative colitis, and hepatic cirrhosis. *Cautious use* in persons with adrenal insufficiency, hypothyroidism, cerebral arteriosclerosis, prostatic hypertrophy, acute alcoholism, impaired renal or hepatic function, supraventricular tachycardia, diabetic acidosis, severe obesity, and in elderly, debilitated, pregnant, or lactating patients

Interactions

Central nervous system depressant effects of narcotics may be potentiated or prolonged by concurrent use of other CNS depressants (eg, barbiturates, alcohol, anesthetics, phenothiazines, sedatives, tricyclic antidepressants).

Muscle relaxation and respiratory depression may be intensified by concurrent use of narcotics and neuromuscular blocking agents (eg, succinylcholine).

Symptoms of acute narcotic overdose, possibly causing death, may occur with use of *meperidine* within 14 days of a monoamine oxidase (MAO) inhibitor.

Withdrawal symptoms may occur in patients addicted to narcotics if the narcotic agonist–antagonists (see Table 20-3) are added, because they may antagonize the effects of the pure agonists.

Meperidine has anticholinergic effects that may be additive with those of other drugs (eg, atropinelike agents, tricyclic antidepressants, quinidine).

Phenytoin or rifampin may reduce blood concentrations of methadone to such an extent as to precipitate withdrawal symptoms.

Orthostatic hypotension may be intensified by concurrent use of narcotic analgesics and high-ceiling diuretics such as furosemide, bumetanide, and ethacrynic acid.

The analgesic efficacy of opiates may be enhanced by concurrent use of hydroxyzine and tricyclic antidepressants.

Nursing Management

Pretherapy Assessment

Assess and record baseline data necessary for detection of adverse effects of opiate narcotic analgesics: General: vital signs, body weight, skin color and temperature; CNS: orientation, affect, bilateral grip strength; cardiovascular (CVS): orthostatic blood pressure (BP); GI: bowel sounds, normal output; genitourinary (GU): normal output, voiding pattern; laboratory: renal, thyroid, and liver function tests, urinalysis, electrocardiogram (ECG), electroencephalogram (EEG).

Review medical history and documents for existing or previous conditions that:

a. require cautious use of opiate narcotic analgesics: adrenal insufficiency; hypothyroidism; cerebral arteriosclerosis; prostatic hypertrophy; acute alcoholism; impaired renal or hepatic function; supraventricular tachycardia; use in the elderly
b. contraindicate use of opiate narcotic analgesics: allergy to the narcotic analgesic; convulsive states; severe respiratory depression; increased intracranial pressure; acute asthma, chronic obstructive pulmonary disease (COPD), cor pulmonale, hypoxia, hypercapnia; undiagnosed acute abdominal conditions; severe ulcerative colitis; hepatic cirrhosis; **pregnancy (Category C)**, labor (administration of narcotics to the mother can cause respiratory depression in the neonate, may prolong labor), lactation (secreted in breast milk, wait 4 to 6 hours after administration to nurse baby)

Nursing Interventions

Medication Administration

Have resuscitative equipment and emergency drugs readily available.

Have intravenous fluids and vasopressors available to treat hypotension.

Collaborate with patient and health care team to plan dosing schedule that will optimally provide desired degree of pain relief. Usage at fixed intervals usually provides better control with smaller total dosage than administration only on request (PRN).

Administer *before* pain becomes intense to attain maximal analgesic effect.

Check rate and depth of respirations, pupil size, and degree of alertness before administration. If early signs of toxicity (respiratory rate below 12/min and shallow; miosis, deep sleep) are observed, withhold drug, advise practitioner, and be prepared to administer narcotic antagonist.

Give dilute solution by *slow* injection, when administering intravenous bolus, because severe toxic effects (eg, respiratory depression, hypotension, circulatory collapse, cardiac arrest) can occur quickly with rapid injection. A narcotic antagonist and measures for respiratory assistance should always be at hand.

Use microdrip intravenous administration set and an infusion control device to ensure accuracy. Monitor flow rate continuously.

Continually evaluate adequacy of drug regimen. Dosage and timing should be carefully titrated to correspond with response to drug and need for pain control.

Advocate dosage increases in appropriate situations. Repeated requests for more medication may signal development of tolerance, increased pain, or different pain, all of which may require additional drug.

Be prepared to assist with management of severe withdrawal symptoms when an antagonist is administered to a drug-dependent individual. Supportive measures (eg, oxygen, IV fluids, vasopressors) should be at hand, and the smallest possible dose of antagonist should be used.

Administer cautiously in obstetrics because drugs easily cross the placental barrier and can induce respiratory depression in the fetus and neonate.

Administer narcotics frequently during first 24 hours after major surgery to prevent pain from interfering with rest, increasing anxiety, and decreasing ability to engage in important activities (eg, turning, coughing, ambulating).

Protect patient from injury. Ambulation may induce dizziness and transient hypotension. Assist with ambulation; keep side rails up while patient is in bed.

If nausea and vomiting occur, assist patient to lie flat and still to avoid the exacerbation caused by motion and an upright position.

Learn regulations governing handling and dispensing of all classes of controlled substances (see Chapter 10). Keep proper records of all narcotic drugs used.

Surveillance During Therapy

Monitor for adverse effects, toxicity, and interactions, such as exaggerated response, hypotension, prolonged respiratory depression, confusion, ataxia, or nausea and vomiting.

Interpret results of diagnostic tests and contact practitioner as appropriate.

Assess pain experience (eg, patient's mood, affect, and functional ability, the process eliciting pain, characteristics of the pain) before administration. Appropriate use varies greatly in different circumstances (eg, acute, chronic, terminal illness).

Maintain balanced perspective toward drug dependence, which may occur with repeated administration of opiates. Excessive fear of dependence on the part of both patient and clinicians is often manifested by undermedication. Patients *rarely* abuse drugs as a result of hospital experiences, and dependence is irrelevant in terminal illness.

Maintain appropriate concern about toxicity. Tolerance develops to nearly all drug effects, including side effects (except constipation and miosis), although at different rates.

Monitor patient blood pressure; vasopressors should be at hand, and the smallest possible dose of antagonist should be used.

Closely observe patient dependent on opiates if a narcotic agonist–antagonist (eg, pentazocine) is administered because the drug's antagonist properties may precipitate withdrawal.

Assess need for analgesic in patient unable to speak or nonalert (especially postsurgically). Signs include elevated respiratory rate and pulse, grimacing, restlessness.

Assist postoperative patient receiving narcotic to cough, deep breathe, and change positions frequently to prevent atelectasis and other respiratory difficulties. Drugs depress cough and sigh reflexes.

Employ appropriate nursing interventions (eg, anxiety reduction, touch, positioning) for pain relief as adjuncts to medication.

Monitor intake and output, periodically remind or assist patient to void (eg, help male to stand), and notify practitioner if patient is unable to void: urinary retention can occur.

Use preventive measures for constipation (eg, ambulation, increased intake of fluid and dietary fiber), and monitor bowel regularity and bowel sounds because constipation and paralytic ileus can occur.

If flushing, sweating, itching, feelings of warmth, visual or auditory distortions, or dysphoria occur, reassure patient that they are not uncommon, they will disappear shortly, and they are not a cause for alarm. Keep patient quiet and reduce sensory stimulation as much as possible.

Discuss possible fear of dependence if patient is reluctant to take appropriate analgesic. Reassure as needed, explain risks and benefits of opiate use and pain reduction.

Monitor patient for fluid intake and output.

Monitor patient for temperature changes.

Monitor for possible drug–drug and drug–nutrient interactions: CNS depressant effects potentiated by other CNS depressants; muscle relaxant and respiratory depressant activities intensified by neuromuscular blockers; potentiation of toxicity with MAO inhibitors; reduction in blood concentrations by phenytoin or rifampin; analgesic efficacy enhanced by hydroxyzine, amphetamines, tricyclic antidepressants.

Patient Teaching

Inform the patient of typical side effects related to narcotic analgesic therapy: dizziness, sedation, drowsiness, impaired visual acuity.

Caution patient that mental or physical abilities may be impaired, making tasks involving use of machinery (eg, driving) hazardous.

Explain that other CNS depressants should not be used with narcotic drugs without professional consultation because of their additive effects.

Inform patient that orthostatic hypotension can occur. Advise gradual rising to sitting and standing positions to minimize dizziness.

Alert patient that the following adverse effects should be reported to their practitioner if they occur: severe nausea, vomiting, constipation, shortness of breath, difficulty breathing, skin rash.

Narcotic Agonists–Antagonists

The *narcotic agonist–antagonist* type of analgesic (see Tables 20-3 and 20-4) was designed to be less addictive than narcotic agonists, with a comparable degree of analgesia in most cases; these goals may have been accomplished to a certain degree, but cases of abuse of these drugs are known.

Mechanism

Most narcotic agonist–antagonists stimulate κ opioid receptors with antagonist effects at μ receptors. In contrast, buprenorphine, which has also been classified as a *"partial agonist,"* stimulates μ receptors but to a lesser degree than narcotic agonists and can also produce antagonist activity. In general, these agents elicit less respiratory depression than narcotic agonists (eg, morphine) in large doses.

Uses

Management of pain (eg, postoperative; obstetric analgesia)

Common Side Effects

Sedation, lightheadedness, GI upset

Significant Adverse Reactions

CV: hypotension, tachycardia, hypertension
GI: vomiting, dry mouth, constipation; diarrhea; anorexia
CNS: dizziness, headache, hallucinations (pentazocine)
Respiratory: respiratory depression
Dermatologic: irritaton at injection site, pruritus
GU: urinary retention, urinary frequency

Contraindications

No absolute contraindications. *Cautious use* in patients physically dependent on narcotic agonists (eg, morphine). Also, the cautions outlined for the narcotic agonists, above, should be heeded for the agonist–antagonists as well.

Interactions

Additive depressant effects can occur when given in the presence of other CNS depressants (eg, general anesthetics, barbiturates, benzodiazepines, alcohol)

Nursing Management

See Nursing Management for Narcotic Agonists, above

Narcotic Antagonists

Drugs capable of reversing the effects of the narcotic agonists are termed *narcotic antagonists*. Both drugs in this category, naloxone and naltrexone, are viewed as "pure" antagonists because they produce **no** agonist activity; this is different from mixed agonist–antagonist narcotics, which do possess agonistic activity.

Naloxone is a rapid-acting drug given parenterally to reverse (or prevent, in some cases) the effects of opioid drugs, especially in the event of overdosage. It reverses the respiratory-depressant, sedative, hypotensive, analgesic, and psychotomimetic effects of opiate drugs. In the absence of narcotics, naloxone exhibits essentially no pharmacologic activity. The drug is specific for treating overdoses of opioids and will **not** reverse respiratory depression induced by other types of CNS depressants (eg, barbiturates, anesthetics). Naloxone is relatively short-acting (ie, 15–30 min) and must be administered at frequent intervals if the patient is severely intoxicated.

Naltrexone is an orally administered narcotic antagonist that can attenuate or block the subjective effects of opioid drugs and reduce the physical dependence on these agents. It is used as an adjunct in maintaining an opioid-free state in detoxified former addicts.

• Naloxone

Narcan

Mechanism

Competitive antagonism of narcotic drugs at opiate receptor sites; displaces opiate drugs from receptor sites, thereby reversing respiratory depression, sedation, hypotension, and analgesia seen with opiates; can also reverse the dysphoric effects of agonist–antagonist narcotic drugs such as pentazocine; when administered in the **absence** of narcotics, produces no analgesia, respiratory depression, miosis, or other effects noted with narcotic drugs; no tolerance or dependence has been reported

Uses

Reversal of respiratory depression and other untoward effects induced by narcotic agonists and narcotic agonists–antagonists
Diagnosis of suspected narcotic overdosage
Investigational uses include reversal of alcoholic coma and improvement of circulation in refractory shock

Dosage

Narcotic overdosage (known or suspected)
Adults: 0.4 mg to 2.0 mg IV (preferred), IM, or SC; may be repeated IV at 2- to 3-minute intervals for 2 to 3 doses, then at 1- to 2-hour intervals as needed to a total of 10 mg
Children and neonates: 0.01 mg/kg IV, IM, or SC initially; may repeat with 0.1 mg/kg if needed
Postoperative narcotic depression: 0.1 mg to 0.2 mg IV at 2- to 3-minute intervals until desired degree of reversal is attained

Fate

Onset of action is 2 to 5 minutes; duration of action depends on dosage and route of administration, but effects generally last from 1 to 4 hours; metabolized in the liver and excreted as conjugated products in the urine; virtually inactive when given orally.

Significant Adverse Reactions

(Occur with excessive dose or too rapid reversal of narcotic depression)

Nausea, vomiting, hypertension, tachycardia, hyperventilation, tremors

Contraindications

Respiratory depression due to nonnarcotic drugs. *Cautious use* in the presence of cardiac instability, during pregnancy, and in known or suspected narcotic addicts

Nursing Management

Pretherapy Assessment

Assess and record baseline data necessary for detection of adverse effects of naloxone: General: vital signs, body weight, skin color and temperature, sweating; CNS: reflexes, pupil size; CVS: orthostatic BP; GI: bowel sounds, normal output; GU: normal output, voiding pattern.

Review medical history and documents for existing or previous conditions that:

a. require cautious use of naloxone: cardiac instability; use in known or suspected narcotic dependency.
b. contraindicate use of naloxone: allergy to the narcotic antagonists; respiratory depression due to nonnarcotic drugs; **pregnancy (Category B)**, lactation (safety not established).

Nursing Interventions

Medication Administration

Do not mix naloxone with preparations containing bisulfite, metabisulfite, high–molecular-weight anions, or alkaline pH solutions.

Be prepared to assist with management of severe withdrawal symptoms when an antagonist is administered to a drug-dependent individual. Supportive measures (eg, oxygen, intravenous fluids, vasopressors) should be at hand, and the smallest possible dose of antagonist should be used.

Ensure that additional supportive measures (eg, respiratory assistance, vasopressors) are available when drug is used.

Be prepared for administration of up to three doses. After three doses, lack of significant improvement suggests that depressant effects may be partly or wholly due to drugs other than narcotics (eg, barbiturates).

Administer diagnostic test for narcotic dependence only in presence of a practitioner, and inform patient of risks involved and possible untoward reactions.

Maintain open airway, provide artificial respiration, cardiac massage, vasopressors if needed to counteract acute narcotic overdosage.

Learn regulations governing handling and dispensing of all classes of controlled substances (see Chapter 8). Keep proper records of all narcotic drugs used.

Surveillance During Therapy

Monitor patient for signs of pain (eg, sweating, tachycardia, grimacing, vomiting). If these are noted, the antagonist should be stopped. Large doses may reverse the analgesic as well as the respiratory-depressant effect of narcotics. Dose should be titrated according to patient response.

Expect severity of withdrawal symptoms to vary with amount and type of opiate used. They are particularly severe with methadone. In contrast, they will not occur when a narcotic antagonist is administered to a meperidine abuser unless person is habituated to extremely large doses (1.6 g or more/day).

Monitor patient carefully after positive response. Naloxone has relatively short duration of action, and its effect may wear off before effects of the opiate have been sufficiently reversed.

Monitor for adverse effects, toxicity, and interactions, such as nausea, vomiting, hypertension, tachycardia, hyperventilation, and tremors.

Interpret results of diagnostic tests and contact practitioner as appropriate.

Provide comfort measures to help patient deal with withdrawal symptoms.

Patient Teaching

Inform the patient of typical side effects related to narcotic antagonist therapy: nausea, vomiting, sweating, tachycardia, tremulousness if patient is narcotic dependent; little or no side effects if patient is not dependent on narcotics.

Alert patient that the following adverse effects should be reported to their practitioner if they occur: sweating, feelings of tremulousness.

• Naltrexone

Trexan

Mechanism

Competitively blocks the effects of opiates at opioid receptor sites; attenuates the euphoria and other subjective effects of opiate drugs and assists in maintaining an opioid-free state; blockade can be surmounted by large doses of opiates; therefore drug is only used in conjunction with proper counseling and other supportive measures.

Uses

Adjunctive therapy, as an aid in the maintenance of an opioid-free state in detoxified former addicts

Dosage

Note: Naltrexone should not be administered until a person has remained opioid free for **at least 7 days** to prevent precipitation of withdrawal symptoms.

Initially, 25 mg orally; if no withdrawal signs are noted, an additional 25 mg is given; thereafter, 50 mg once daily. Alternatively, 100 mg every 2 days or 150 mg every 3 days if patient is stabilized.

A 50 mg dose will block—for 24 hours—the euphoric effects of a 25-mg IV dose of heroin.

Fate

After oral administration, peak blood levels occur within 1 hour. Naltrexone undergoes extensive first-pass hepatic metabolism, and some of the metabolites are active antagonists as well. Effects persist from 24 hours to 72 hours and are apparently independent of dosage. Naltrexone and its metabolites are excreted principally by the kidneys.

Significant Adverse Reactions

(Result from withdrawal from opiate effects)

Anxiety, nervousness, insomnia, abdominal pain and cramping, nausea, vomiting, joint and muscle pain, nasal congestion, liver damage, skin rash, anorexia, dizziness, chills, increased thirst

Contraindications

Persons receiving opioid drugs or in acute opioid withdrawal, acute hepatitis, or liver failure. *Cautious use* in persons with liver dysfunction and in pregnant women or nursing mothers.

Nursing Management

Pretherapy Assessment

Assess and record baseline data necessary for detection of adverse effects of naltrexone: General: vital signs, body weight, skin color and temperature, sweating; CNS: reflexes, pupil size; CVS: edema, baseline ECG; GI: bowel sounds, liver evaluation, normal output; GU: normal output, voiding pattern; Laboratory: urine screen for opioids, liver function tests

Review medical history and documents for existing or previous conditions that:

a. require cautious use of naltrexone: liver dysfunction.

b. contraindicate use of naltrexone: allergy to the narcotic antagonists; persons receiving opioid drugs; acute opioid withdrawal syndrome; acute hepatitis; **pregnancy (Category C)**, lactation (safety not established, use caution in nursing mothers)

Nursing Interventions

Medication Administration

Administer only after withdrawal program and 7- to 10-day opioid-free interval have been completed. Check urine opioid levels.

Do not administer until patient has passed a naloxone challenge.

Monitor environment to help patient deal with headache, fever, chills, CNS effects of the drug.

Provide ready access to bathroom facilities if diarrhea occurs.

Expect small initial amount to be used. If no withdrawal symptoms occur, remainder of dose is given. Maintenance doses may be administered every 1 to 3 days.

Be prepared to assist with management of severe withdrawal symptoms when an antagonist is administered to a drug-dependent individual. Supportive measures (eg, oxygen, intravenous fluids, vasopressors) should be at hand, and the smallest possible dose of antagonist should be used.

Learn regulations governing handling and dispensing of all classes of controlled substances (see Chapter 10). Keep proper records of all narcotic drugs used.

Surveillance During Therapy

Monitor patient for signs of pain (eg, sweating, tachycardia, grimacing, vomiting). If these are noted, the antagonist should be stopped. Large doses may reverse the analgesic as well as the respiratory-depressant effect of narcotics. Dose should be titrated according to patient response.

Monitor for adverse effects, toxicity, and interactions, such as nausea, vomiting, diarrhea; blurred vision; anxiety; decreased sexual function.

Interpret results of diagnostic tests and contact practitioner as appropriate.

Provide comfort measure to help patient deal with withdrawal symptoms.

Patient Teaching

Inform the patient of typical side effects related to narcotic antagonist therapy: nausea, vomiting, sweating, tachycardia, tremulousness if patient is narcotic dependent; little or no side effects if patient is not dependent on narcotics.

Notify practitioner if any of the following adverse effects occur: unusual bleeding or bruising; dark, tarry stools; yellowing of the eyes or skin; running nose; tearing; sweating; chills; joint or muscle pain.

Support and encourage patient's attempt to remain opiate-free. Effective therapy requires very high motivation because drug does not suppress urge to experience opiate-induced euphoria ("high").

Discuss danger of overdosing with an opiate. A dose large enough to produce a "high" by overcoming naltrexone action would be dangerous, possibly fatal.

Instruct patient to promptly report signs of liver damage (eg, jaundice, dark urine, itching) because drug is a direct hepatotoxin.

Instruct patient to inform practitioner of naltrexone use. If administration of an opioid is unavoidable, dosage will need to be high, and respiratory depression will be deeper and more prolonged than usual.

Instruct patient to wear identification tag indicating naltrexone use.

Selected Bibliography

Ashburn MA, Lipman AG: Management of pain in the cancer patient. Anesth Analg 76:402, 1993

Barsan WG et al: Safety assessment of high-dose narcotic analgesia for emergency department procedures. Ann Emerg Med 22(9):1444, 1993

Ferrell BR, McCaffery M, Rhiner M: Pain and addiction: an urgent need for change in nursing education. J Pain Symptom Manage 7(2):117, 1992

Homan RV: Transnasal butorphanol. Am Fam Physician 49(1):188, 1994

Howe CJ: A new standard of care for pediatric pain management. Amer J Maternal/Child Nurs 18(6):325, 1993

McNicol R: Postoperative analgesia in children using continuous s.c. morphine. Br J Anaesth 71:752, 1993

Pasternak GW: Pharmacological mechanisms of opioid analgesics. Clin Neuropharmacol 16(1):1, 1993

Richmond CE, Bromley LM, Woolf CJ: Preoperative morphine pre-empts postoperative pain. Lancet 342:73, 1993

Stein C: Peripheral mechanisms of opioid analgesia. Anesth Analg 76:182, 1993

Zimmermann DL, Stewart J: Postoperative pain management and acute pain service activity in Canada. Can J Anaesth 40(6):568, 1993

Nursing Bibliography

Donnelly A, Lamb R: Analgesic agents in critical care. Critical Care Nursing Clinics of North America 5(2):281, 1993

Fulton J, Johnson G: Using high dose morphine to relieve cancer pain. Nursing '93 23(2):34–39, 1993

Jurf J, Nirschl A: Acute post operative pain management: A comprehensive review and update. Critical Care Nursing Quarterly 16(1):8–25, 1993

Morgan A, Lindley C, Berry J: Assessment of pain and patterns of analgesic use in hospice patients. American Journal of Hospice and Palliative Care 11(1):13–25, 1994

Narcotics and implications for post anesthesia care unit. Nursing Clinics of North America 2(3): 1993

Portenoy R: Drug therapy for cancer pain. American Journal of Hospice and Palliative Care 9(6):22–31, 1992

Vissering T: Pharmacologic agents for pain management. Critical Care Nursing Clinics of North America 3(1):17–24, 1991

21

Nonnarcotic Analgesic and Anti-inflammatory Drugs

Salicylates

- Aspirin (acetylsalicylic acid)
- Choline salicylate
- Diflunisal
- Magnesium salicylate
- Methyl salicylate
- Salicylamide
- Salicylic acid
- Salsalate (salicylsalicylic acid)
- Sodium salicylate
- Sodium thiosalicylate

Para-aminophenol Derivative

- Acetaminophen

Pyrazolones

- Oxyphenbutazone
- Phenylbutazone

Nonsteroidal Anti-inflammatory Drugs (NSAIDs)

Acetic acids

- Diclofenac
- Etodolac
- Indomethacin
- Ketorolac
- Nabumetone
- Sulindac
- Tolmetin

Fenamates

- Meclofenamate
- Mefenamic acid

Oxicams

- Piroxicam

Proprionic Acids

- Fenoprofen
- Flurbiprofen
- Ibuprofen
- Ketoprofen
- Naproxen
- Oxaprozin
- Suprofen

Gold Compounds

- Auranofin
- Aurothioglucose
- Gold sodium thiomalate

Miscellaneous Anti-inflammatory Agent

- Penicillamine

Antigout Drugs

- Allopurinol
- Colchicine
- Probenecid
- Sulfinpyrazone

Nonnarcotic analgesics reduce inflammation (anti-inflammatory action) and are also called nonsteroidal anti-inflammatory drugs (NSAIDs). They also relieve pain but are not as powerful as narcotics (eg, morphine) and are less dangerous (eg, life-threatening respiratory depression does not occur except in an overdose). Nonnarcotic agents are used to relieve mild to moderate pain, reduce elevated body temperatures (antipyretic action) and reduce inflammation. Aspirin (acetylsalicylic acid; ASA) is effective in prevention of recurrent transient ischemic attacks (TIAs) and other thromboembolic conditions that can cause serious disorders, for example, myocardial infarction. In addition, certain members of this group (eg, salicyclic acid, methyl salicylate) are employed topically as keratolytics, counterirritants, and astringents.

Aspirin is the most widely used and least expensive of the nonnarcotic analgesics. Because it is so readily available (ie, does not require a prescription and can be purchased in supermarkets), aspirin does not receive the same respect given to other important therapeutic drugs. Other nonnarcotic analgesics (eg, acetaminophen) may offer some advantages over aspirin (eg, decreased gastrointestinal [GI] irritation, reduced effect on blood coagulation) and are frequently used in its place, especially in small children and in aspirin-sensitive patients.

Salicylates

Drugs in this category are derivatives of salicylic acid and possess analgesic, antipyretic, and anti-inflammatory actions. In addition, some of these drugs are capable of inhibiting platelet aggregation and, in large doses, can decrease prothrombin production and impair renal tubular reabsorption of uric acid.

Because most differences among the salicylates are largely quantitative, they are considered as a group. Characteristics of individual drugs are given in Table 21-1.

Mechanism

Analgesia: block prostaglandin synthesis by interfering with the activity of the enzyme cyclooxygenase (Fig. 21-1), thus reducing sensitivity of peripheral pain receptors to mechanical or chemical activation; may enhance reabsorption of fluid from swollen, inflamed tissues and possibly interfere with transmission of pain impulses at subcortical brain centers (eg, thalamus)

Antipyresis: reduce outflow of vasoconstrictor impulses from hypothalamus, thus promoting vasodilation, sweating, and heat loss; decrease production of prostaglandin E in response to endogenous pyrogens

Anti-inflammatory: reduce vascular leakage of fluids and neutrophils, secretory cells that release various substances (enzymes, reactive oxygen radicals) that provoke tissue injury; interfere with release of tissue-destructive lysosomal enzymes; inhibit synthesis of prostaglandins, endogenous substances thought to mediate the inflammatory reaction by causing tissue swelling and sensitization of peripheral pain receptors

Reduced platelet aggregation: block formation of platelet thromboxane A_2, a prostaglandin derivative that facilitates platelet aggregation and causes vasoconstriction. Platelet aggregation appears to be markedly inhibited by aspirin but not by other salicylates. This difference is due to the acetyl group in the aspirin molecule, which *irreversibly* inhibits platelet cyclooxygenase and thereby thromboxane synthesis; this effect persists for the life of the platelet. Low doses of aspirin are apparently more effective in reducing platelet aggregation than are higher doses. It is thought that this dosage-related difference in effectiveness is related to a greater inhibitory action on the formation of platelet thromboxane A_2 than on the formation of vessel-wall prostacyclin (a prostaglandin vasodilator and inhibitor

Table 21-1. **Salicylates**

Drug	*Usual Dosage Range*	*Nursing Considerations*
Aspirin *Several manufacturers*	*Adults:* Pain, fever: 325–650 mg every 4 h Inflammation: 3.6–5.4 g/day Transient ischemic attacks; 40–325 mg/day (highly variable–see text) Prevention of myocardial infarction: 40–325 mg 1–2 days *Children:* Pain, fever: 65 mg/kg/day in divided doses Inflammation: 90–130 mg/kg/day in divided doses at 4–6-h intervals	*See* general discussion of salicylates. In addtion: keep in a cool, dry place; do not use if vinegarlike odor is detectable because potency is likely to be reduced; use of suppositories may be best route if patient is vomiting, but absorption will be more variable; do not use controlled-release preparations for short-term analgesia or antipyresis, because the onset of action is slow.
Choline salicylate *Arthropan* *(CAN) Teejel*	890–1740 mg 4 times/day	Liquid preparation provides more rapid absorption and less gastric irritation than aspirin; useful in patients with difficulty in swallowing tablets or capsules, in patients who experience gastric distress with regular aspirin, and in patients who should avoid sodium-containing salicylates; taste may be objectionable—drug can be mixed with fruit juice or other vehicle if desired; do not give with antacids; available in combination with magnesium salicylate as Trilisate (tablets and liquid).
Diflunisal *Dolobid*	Pain: 500 mg–1 g initially, followed by 250–500 mg every 8–12 h Rheumatoid arthritis/osteoarthritis: 500 mg–1 g daily in 2 divided doses (maximum, 1,500 mg/day)	A salicylic acid derivative *not* metabolized to salicylic acid; used for mild to moderate pain and osteoarthritis; long-acting (used twice a day) analgesic comparable in potency to aspirin or acetaminophen at a dose of 500 mg and equivalent to acetaminophen plus codeine at a dose of 1 g; platelet-inhibitory effect is dose-related and usually transient and reversible; at 1 g/day, bleeding time is only slightly increased; anti-inflammatory efficacy is equal to 2–3 g/day of aspirin, with less GI distress in some patients; do *not* use in children younger than age 12; *use cautiously* in patients with impaired cardiac function or hypertension, because fluid retention can occur; do not administer or take aspirin, acetaminophen, or a nonsteroidal anti-inflammatory drug with diflunisal
Magnesium salicylate *Doan's Pills, Magan, Mobidin and other manufacturers*	650 mg 4 times/day *or* 1,090 mg 3 times/day; increase to 3.6–4.8 g/day in 3 or 4 divided doses as needed; up to 9.6 g/day has been used in rheumatic fever	*Not* recommended in children under age 12; a sodium-free salicylate having a somewhat lower incidence of GI upset than regular aspirin; use with caution in patients with impaired renal function; contraindicated in advanced renal insufficiency; also see choline salicylate (above)
Methyl salicylate *(oil of wintergreen)*	Applied topically as a counterirritant to relieve pain associated with muscular and rheumatic conditions	Significant absorption can occur through the skin and may produce untoward effects; toxic if orally ingested, especially by children; liquids containing more than 5% methylsalicylate must be in child-resistant containers; use cautiously on irritated skin
Salicylic Acid *Compound W, Freezone, Occlusal, and other manufacturers* *(CAN) Saligel, Sebcur, Soluver*	Applied to affected area, usually at night, and washed off in the morning; after remission, used occasionally to maintain clearing effect	Primarily used topically as a keratolytic agent for conditions such as psoriasis, keratosis, acne, fungal infections, or any other condition requiring removal of excessive dead skin; skin should be hydrated with wet packs or soaks at least 5 min before use; may cause irritation and burning of skin; systemic absorption can occur to a significant extent; also may be applied as an ether-alcohol or a colloidian solution (Freezone, Compound W, Occlusal, Off-Ezy, Wart-off) for removal of corns, warts, and calluses; *use cautiously* in children younger than 12; avoid contact with eyes or mucous membranes
Salsalate *Amigesic, Artha-G, Disalcid, Marthritic, Mono-Gesic, Salsitab, Salflex*	3 g/day in divided doses	Primarily used for relief of signs and symptoms of rheumatoid arthritis and other rheumatic conditions; minimal effect on platelet aggregation; after absorption, drug is hydrolyzed to two molecules of salicylic acid; drug is insoluble in gastric juice and not absorbed until it reaches small intestine; low incidence of GI upset; not for use in children younger than age 12; do *not* combine with other salicylates
Sodium salicylate	325–650 mg/4 h as needed	Less effective than an equal dose of aspirin; irritating to GI mucosa because free salicylic acid is liberated; use cautiously in renal dysfunction or in individuals on a low-sodium diet; infrequently used product
Sodium thiosalicylate *Rexolate, Tusal*	Analgesia: 50–100 mg IM daily or alternate days Rheumatic fever: 100–150 mg IM every 4–6 h for 3 days, then 100 mg twice/day Acute gout: 100 mg IM every 3–4 h for 2 days, then 100 mg/day	Readily absorbed after IM administration; infrequently used in inflammatory conditions and acute stages of rheumatic fever

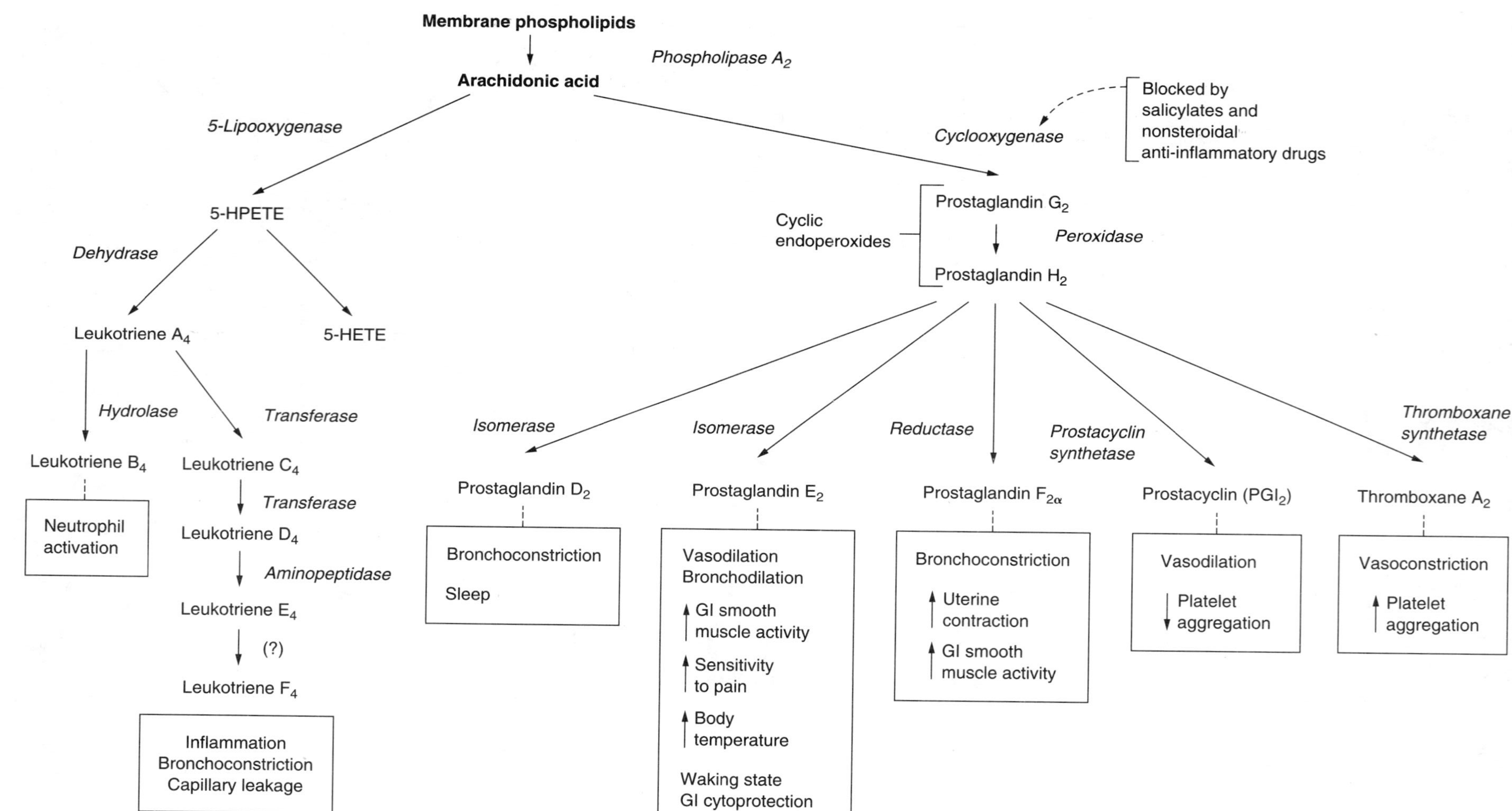

Figure 21-1 Synthesis of eicosanoids (prostaglandins, thromboxanes, leukotrienes) and their principal physiologic actions.

of platelet aggregation). Further, the *prolonged* effect of aspirin suggests that *daily* dosing may be too frequent. The *precise dose* of aspirin that is most effective in blocking platelet aggregation remains to be definitively established, but appears to be significantly lower than the analgesic or antipyretic dose. The effects on platelet aggregation suggest a potential clinical value for these compounds in protecting against certain thrombotic events thought to be associated with cerebrovascular and ischemic heart diseases

Other actions: decrease prothrombin formation (high doses only), decrease excretion of uric acid (small doses), increase excretion of uric acid (high doses), and decrease glucose tolerance

Uses

Relief of mild to moderate pain, especially that associated with inflammatory states (eg, myalgia, neuralgia, cephalalgia)

Reduction of elevated body temperature

Symptomatic treatment of certain inflammatory conditions (eg, rheumatoid and osteoarthritis, bursitis, rheumatic fever)

Prophylaxis of thromboembolic complications (eg, venous emboli, cerebral ischemia) associated with cardiovascular disorders and reduction in the risk of recurrent transient ischemic attacks (*no* benefit in treating completed strokes)

Prevention of acute myocardial infarction (investigational use for aspirin)

Dosage

See Table 21-1

Fate

Absorbed essentially intact from stomach and upper intestine; peak serum levels occur within 1 to 2 hours; rapidly hydrolyzed to salicylic acid (except diflunisal) and excreted either free or as conjugates in the urine; rate of excretion is inversely related to blood level, larger doses being eliminated more slowly than small doses; salicylic acid is highly (70%–90%) protein bound; alkalinization of the urine increases the rate of excretion of salicylates by favoring ionization in the renal tubules, which decreases reabsorption

Common Side Effects

Gastric distress, heartburn, occasional nausea

Significant Adverse Reactions

CAUTION

Use of salicylates, especially aspirin, in children with influenza or chickenpox has been associated with occasional development of Reye's syndrome, an acute, life-threatening condition marked by initial severe vomiting and lethargy and progressing to delirium, coma, and death. Mortality rate is 20% to 30%, and permanent brain damage frequently occurs in survivors. Although a *definite* causal relationship to salicylates has not been confirmed, aspirin and other salicylates should *NOT* be given to children with influenza or chickenpox.

The following reactions generally are dose related and are more common at high doses or with prolonged use.

Salicylism (a syndrome consisting of headache, nausea, tinnitus, dizziness, confusion, sweating, palpitations, hyperventilation, diarrhea, impaired hearing or vision)

Idiosyncratic hypersensitivity reactions (bronchoconstriction, urticaria, edema, asthma-like attacks, shock)

Renal or hepatic impairment

GI bleeding or ulceration

Anemia

Anorexia

Elevations in serum amylase, aspartate aminotransferase (AST) (serum glutamic-oxaloacetic transaminase; SGOT) and alanine aminotransferase (ALT) (serum glutamic-pyruvic transaminase; SGPT)

Severe intoxication may lead to central nervous system (CNS) stimulation (delirium, hallucinations), respiratory alkalosis followed by acidosis, acid–base disturbances, petechial hemorrhaging, hyperthermia, hypokalemia, oliguria, convulsions, respiratory failure, and coma.

Contraindications

History of severe GI disorders (ulcer, hemorrhage, gastritis), severe anemia, deficiency of vitamin K, and hemophilia. *Cautious use* in persons with gastric ulcers, anemia, impaired hepatic function, chronic renal insufficiency, asthma or nasal polyps, in persons taking anticoagulants, and in pregnant or nursing women

Interactions

Effects of aspirin may be enhanced or prolonged by drugs that acidify the urine (eg, ammonium chloride, ascorbic acid), and may be decreased by urinary alkalinizers (eg, absorbable antacids, sodium bicarbonate).

By competing for protein binding sites, the salicylate metabolite of aspirin may enhance the actions and toxicity of oral anticoagulants, heparin, naproxen, oral hypoglycemic drugs, phenytoin, thiopental, indomethacin, methotrexate, thyroid hormones, sulfonamide antibiotics, valproic acid, and penicillins.

Aspirin in small doses can inhibit the uricosuric effects of probenecid and sulfinpyrazone.

Aspirin may increase the risk of bleeding in persons taking anticoagulants and drugs that interfere with platelet aggregation.

Phenobarbital may decrease aspirin's efficacy by enzyme induction.

The antihypertensive action of beta-blockers may be blunted when used with salicylates, possibly because of prostaglandin inhibition.

The incidence of GI distress and bleeding may be increased by steroids, alcohol, indomethacin, pyrazolones, and other anti-inflammatory drugs.

Furosemide may decrease salicylate excretion so that toxicity occurs at lower doses.

Salicylates in high doses have a hypoglycemic action and may potentiate the effects of insulin and sulfonylurea hypoglycemics.

Antacids and activated charcoal reduce the oral absorption of aspirin.

Aspirin may lower the clinical effectiveness of NSAIDs.

Nursing Management

Pretherapy Assessment

Assess and record baseline data necessary for detection of adverse effects of salicylates: General: vital signs (VS), body weight, skin color and temperature; CNS: eighth cranial nerve function, orientation, reflexes; cardiovascular system (CVS): perfusion; GI: bowel sounds, liver evaluation; Lab: renal and liver function tests, urinalysis, complete blood count (CBC), clotting times, stool guaiac.

Review medical history and documents for existing or previous conditions that:

a. require cautious use of salicylate: gastric ulcer; anemia; impaired hepatic function; chronic renal insufficiency; asthma; nasal polyps; oral anticoagulants
b. contraindicate use of salicylate: allergy to salicylate, tartrazine; history of severe GI disorders (ulcer, hemorrhage, gastritis); severe anemia; vitamin K deficiency; hemophilia; chickenpox; influenza; **pregnancy (Category D)**, lactation (secreted in breast milk, risk of adverse effect on neonatal platelets, avoid use in nursing mothers).

Nursing Interventions

Medication Administration

Administer with food or after meals if GI upset occurs.

Administer with a full glass of water to reduce risk of tablet or capsule being trapped in the esophagus.

Do not use salicylate preparations that have a strong vinegar-like odor.

Be prepared for possible development of hypersensitivity reactions, especially in patient with asthma, polyps, or a history of allergic reactions. Have epinephrine, antihistamines, and other supportive measures (eg, oxygen, respiratory aids) at hand.

Be prepared to assist with treatment in cases of aspirin intoxication: prompt emesis or gastric lavage, administration of fluids and electrolytes, oxygen with artificial respiration, and dialysis in cases of *severe* intoxication.

Administer carefully and do not give for prolonged periods to children with fever and dehydration because they may be especially likely to develop toxic effects even with small doses.

Inform practitioner if patient is vomiting or otherwise incapable of taking drug orally. Suppositories may be used, but absorption is more variable than with oral route.

Surveillance During Therapy

Monitor for adverse effects and toxicity.

Interpret results of diagnostic tests and contact practitioner as appropriate.

Monitor for possible drug–drug and drug–nutrient interactions: effects may be enhanced or prolonged by drugs that acidify the urine (eg, ammonium chloride, ascorbic acid), and decreased by urinary alkalinizers (eg, absorbable antacids, sodium bicarbonate); may enhance the actions and toxicity of oral anticoagulants, heparin, naproxen, oral hypoglycemic drugs, phenytoin, thiopental, indomethacin, methotrexate, thyroid hormones, sulfonamide antibiotics, valproic acid, and penicillins; can inhibit the uricosuric effects of probenecid and sulfinpyrazone; may increase the risk of bleeding in persons taking anticoagulants and drugs that interfere with platelet aggregation; phenobarbital may decrease efficacy by enzyme induction; antihypertensive action of beta-blockers may be blunted when used with salicylates, possibly because of prostaglandin inhibition; incidence of GI distress and bleeding may be increased by steroids, alcohol, indomethacin, pyrazolones, and other anti-inflammatory drugs; furosemide may decrease excretion so that toxicity occurs at lower doses; have a hypoglycemic action and may potentiate the effects of insulin and sulfonylurea hypoglycemics; antacids and activated charcoal reduce the oral absorption; may lower the clinical effectiveness of NSAIDs

Patient Teaching

Instruct patient to be alert for early signs of overdose when high doses are used (eg, tinnitus, dizziness, impaired vision or hearing) and to report their occurrence to appropriate healthcare provider.

Instruct patient taking large doses of aspirin for its anti-inflammatory effects to maintain a constant dosage schedule to minimize fluctuations in plasma levels.

Caution individual with aspirin hypersensitivity to read labels of over-the-counter (OTC) medications (eg, cold preparations) carefully because many contain aspirin or other salicylates.

Inform patient on anticoagulant therapy to use aspirin cautiously. Teach patient to observe carefully for appearance of signs of increased anticoagulant effects (eg, mucous membrane bleeding, bruising, petechiae). If signs appear, practitioner should be notified because the anticoagulant dosage may need to be reduced.

Inform patient that continual self-medication with aspirin for fever or pain may obscure more serious underlying conditions. Advise against prolonged use unless directed by a healthcare professional.

Advise cardiac patient that, although effervescent preparations (eg, Alka Seltzer) may be more rapidly absorbed and less irritating to the GI tract, repeated use may be hazardous because of their high sodium content. They also may alkalinize the urine.

Inform patient who experiences GI upset with aspirin, even when taken with food or milk, that enteric-coated tablets are available (eg, Easprin, Ecotrin) that resist breakdown in the stomach and therefore may eliminate much gastric distress.

Explain that combinations of aspirin and other nonnarcotic analgesics (eg, acetaminophen, salicylamide) are probably no more effective than aspirin alone and may result in a higher incidence of adverse effects. Such combinations should be avoided.

Inform patient that commercially buffered aspirin is probably no less irritating to gastric mucosa than plain aspirin taken with food, milk, or a full glass of water.

Instruct patient to keep tablets in a cool, dry place. Exposure to moisture or excessive heat hastens hydrolysis and causes loss of potency. Tablets should not be used if a vinegar-like odor is detectable.

CAUTION

See *Caution* under **Significant Adverse Reactions.**

Para-aminophenol Derivative

• Acetaminophen

Tempra, Tylenol, and various other manufacturers

(CAN) Atasol, Neo-Dol, PMS Acetaminophen, Robigesic, Rounox

The only para-aminophenol derivative of interest in clinical medicine is acetaminophen, a widely used analgesic and antipyretic. Acetaminophen is commonly used as an aspirin substitute and has several advantages over aspirin:

- Lower incidence of GI upset and bleeding
- Lower incidence of hypersensitivity reactions
- No significant interaction with oral anticoagulants or uricosuric drugs
- Availability in a palatable liquid form for pediatric use

The principal disadvantage of acetaminophen relative to aspirin is that acetaminophen possesses no significant anti-inflammatory action, presumably because it has no inhibitory effect on prostaglandin synthesis in the periphery. In addition, excessive doses of acetaminophen can cause hepatotoxicity, and liver damage may occur with long-term use in alcoholics and patients with impaired hepatic function (see **Significant Adverse Reactions**).

Mechanism

The precise analgesic mechanism of action has not been completely established; elevates the pain threshold, possibly by blocking prostaglandin synthesis in the CNS; reduces elevated body temperature by an action on the hypothalamic heat-regulating center, leading to vasodilation and sweating, and also possibly by inhibiting the action of endogenous pyrogens; possesses no significant anti-inflammatory action, presumably because it has no inhibitory effect on *peripheral* prostaglandin synthesis; unlike aspirin, exhibits no uricosuric, platelet antiaggregatory, ulcerative, or prothrombin-inhibitory activity

Uses

Relief of mild to moderate pain, such as that of musculoskeletal origin, headache, toothache, teething, dysmenorrhea, "flu," tonsillectomy

Reduction of elevated temperatures associated with colds and other bacterial and viral infections

Dosage

Adults: 325 mg to 650 mg 3 to 4 times/day (maximum 4.0 g/day for short-term therapy)

Children:

Younger than 1 year: 40 to 80 mg 4 to 5 times/day
1 to 3 years: 120 to 160 mg 4 to 5 times/day
4 to 8 years: 240 to 320 mg 4 to 5 times/day
9 to 12 years: 400 to 480 mg 4 to 5 times/day

Fate

Well absorbed from the GI tract; onset 15 to 30 minutes; duration 3 to 5 hours; protein binding is variable but usually not clinically significant; metabolized in the liver, and 80% to 90% is excreted in the urine as conjugated metabolites; a minor intermediate metabolite is converted to a hepatotoxic substance but is normally rapidly detoxified by conjugation with glutathione by sulfhydryl groups and excreted as the conjugated product; large acute doses or chronic dosing with acetaminophen can deplete hepatic stores of glutathione, the substance that quickly detoxifies the potentially hepatotoxic intermediate; in these situations, hepatic necrosis can occur (see below)

Common Side Effects

None with occasional usage

Significant Adverse Reactions

(Usually with long-term use of high doses)

Urticaria, hypoglycemia, CNS stimulation, cyanosis, methemoglobinemia, hemolytic anemia, leukopenia, kidney damage, psychological changes

Acute poisoning is characterized by

Chills, diarrhea, emesis, fever, skin eruptions, palpitations, weakness, sweating, CNS stimulation (excitement, delirium, toxic psychosis) followed by CNS depression, vascular collapse, convulsions, and coma

Hepatotoxicity can occur with overdosage or long-term high dosage (5 to 8 g/day), especially in adults. Initial signs are nausea, vomiting, malaise, sweating, diarrhea, and abdominal pain.

The degree of liver damage after acute overdosage can be estimated by determining the serum half-life ($T_{1/2}$) or the plasma levels of acetaminophen. Hepatic damage is likely if the $T_{1/2}$ is greater than 4 hours *or* if plasma levels exceed 250 to 300 μg/mL 4 hours after ingestion or 50 μg/mL 12 hours after ingestion

Treatment of acute overdosage includes emesis, gastric lavage, and activated charcoal. Hepatic damage can be minimized or prevented by administration of acetylcysteine *within the first 10 to 12 hours* after ingestion of acetaminophen (see Chapter 56). A loading dose of 140 mg/kg is given initially, either intravenously or orally followed by 70 mg/kg orally every 4 hours for 17 doses

Contraindications

Glucose-6-phosphate dehydrogenase deficiency. *Cautious use* in patients with impaired liver or kidney function or for periods longer than 10 days

Interactions

The rate of absorption of acetaminophen may be slowed by anticholinergics, narcotics, activated charcoal, and antacids.

Oral contraceptives may increase the hepatic metabolism of acetaminophen.

Increased plasma levels of acetaminophen have resulted when used with diflunisal.

Chronic alcohol ingestion increases the likelihood of toxicity with large doses of acetaminophen.

Caffeine increases the analgesic effectiveness of acetaminophen

Nursing Management

Pretherapy Assessment

Assess and record baseline data necessary for detection of adverse effects of acetaminophen: General: VS, body weight, skin color and temperature; GI: liver evaluation; Lab: renal and liver function tests, CBC.
Review medical history and documents for existing or previous conditions that:

a. require cautious use of acetaminophen: impaired liver and renal function.
b. contraindicate use of acetaminophen: allergy to acetaminophen; glucose-6-phosphate dehydrogenase deficiency; **pregnancy (Category C)**, lactation (secreted in breast milk, no adverse effects reported).

Nursing Interventions

Medication Administration

Administer with food or after meals if GI upset occurs. Administer with a full glass of water to reduce risk of tablet or capsule being trapped in the esophagus.

Do not exceed recommended dosage.

Monitor acetaminophen serum concentrations beginning at 4 hours after ingestion if overdosage occurs (determine acetaminophen toxicity); *N*-acetylcysteine (antidote) should be available and used within the first 12 hours of ingestion if toxic serum levels are present or serum levels are not available.

Surveillance During Therapy

Monitor for toxicity.

Observe prolonged users of the drug for possible signs of methemoglobinemia (cyanosis, dyspnea, vertigo, weakness, angina-like pain), hemolytic anemia (pallor, palpitations), and kidney damage (albuminuria, hematuria).

Interpret results of diagnostic tests and contact practitioner.

Monitor for possible drug–drug and drug–nutrient interactions: increased toxicity if taken with chronic, excessive alcohol ingestion; increased hypothrombinemia with oral anticoagulants; increased risk of hepatotoxicity with barbiturates, carbamazepine, hydantoins, rifampin, or sulfinpyrazone.

Patient Teaching

Caution against indiscriminate, excessive, or prolonged use. Urge patient to keep drug away from children because many liquid preparations are pleasantly flavored and may be consumed in large amounts.

Explain that drug should be used cautiously in arthritis or rheumatic conditions because it lacks anti-inflammatory action. If pain persists for more than 10 days or if redness is present, a practitioner should be consulted because additional medication may be indicated.

Teach patient that at recommended doses there are few adverse effects.

Teach patient to notify practitioner if skin rash, unusual bleeding or bruising, yellowing of eyes or skin, or changes in voiding patterns occur.

Pyrazolones

- **Phenylbutazone**
- **Oxyphenbutazone**

The pyrazolones are currently represented by three drugs (phenylbutazone, oxyphenbutazone, and sulfinpyrazone) that have pharmacologic effects similar to those of the salicylates, but are more potent anti-inflammatory agents. Sulfinpyrazone, however, is a much more effective uricosuric drug than it is an anti-inflammatory agent and is employed in the maintenance therapy of gout. It is discussed later in this chapter.

Phenylbutazone and oxyphenbutazone are very effective anti-inflammatory agents, but they are highly toxic compounds and are infrequently used today. They are occasionally employed for *short-term* therapy of severe acute inflammatory conditions not alleviated by other less toxic agents such as the salicylates. Although they possess analgesic and antipyretic actions as well, the pyrazolones should never be used in place of aspirin or acetaminophen as general-purpose pain relievers or fever reducers.

Phenylbutazone and its metabolite oxyphenbutazone are quite similar in their actions and are reviewed together.

Mechanism

Not completely established; interfere with the synthesis of prostaglandins and mucopolysaccharides in cartilage; inhibit leukocyte migration and activity of lysosomal enzymes; exert a weak blocking effect on uric acid reabsorption by renal tubular cells; produce significant retention of sodium and water

Uses

Relief of acute symptoms of active rheumatoid arthritis, ankylosing spondylitis, osteoarthritis, psoriatic arthritis, and painful shoulder conditions (eg, peritendinitis, bursitis, capsulitis) *not responding to other anti-inflammatory drugs*

Symptomatic treatment of acute superficial thrombophlebitis

Short-term treatment of acute attacks of degenerative joint disease of the hips and knees

Treatment of acute gout (short-term use only; not for maintenance therapy)

Dosage

(For both drugs)

Arthritis, spondylitis, painful shoulder: initially, 300 to 600 mg in divided doses (maximum 600 mg/day); maintenance dose, 100 to 400 mg/day

Acute gout: 400 mg initially, then 100 mg every 4 hours for up to 4 days

Fate

Rapidly and completely absorbed from GI tract; onset of action in 30 minutes; highly bound (90%–98%) to plasma proteins with a $T_{1/2}$ of 75 to 85 hours; therefore, prolonged duration (3–5 days); slowly metabolized in the liver and excreted in the urine

Common Side Effects

Nausea, vomiting, gastric discomfort, skin rash, diarrhea, vertigo, insomnia, nervousness, blurred vision, water and electrolyte retention

Significant Adverse Reactions

CAUTION

Aplastic anemia and agranulocytosis can occur with use of these drugs, especially with prolonged administration or in elderly patients; regular hematologic examinations must be performed in all patients receiving the drugs for an interval longer than 1 week.

GI: ulceration of the esophagus, stomach, small intestine, and bowel; occult GI bleeding, gastritis, abdominal distention; hematemesis

Hematologic: blood dyscrasias, bone marrow depression

Allergic/dermatologic: (requires prompt withdrawal of drug) petechiae, toxic pruritus, erythema nodosum, erythema multiforme, exfoliative dermatitis, Stevens-Johnson syndrome (see Chapter 5), serum sickness, polyarteritis, urticaria, arthralgia, fever, anaphylactic shock

Renal/metabolic: proteinuria, hematuria, oliguria, anuria, glomerulonephritis, renal stones, tubular necrosis, ureteral obstruction, sodium and chloride retention, edema, metabolic acidosis, hyperglycemia, thyroid hyperplasia, toxic goiter

CV: hypertension, pericarditis, myocarditis with muscle necrosis, cardiac decompensation

Ocular/otic: diplopial optic neuritis, retinal hemorrhage, retinal detachment, hearing loss

CNS: (seen primarily with overdose): agitation, confusion, lethargy, depression, hallucinations, convulsions, psychosis, hyperventilation

Contraindications

GI inflammation; ulceration or persistent dyspepsia; blood dyscrasias; hypertension; thyroid disease; renal, hepatic, or cardiac dysfunction; temporal arteritis; polymyalgia rheumatica; patients receiving anticoagulants or potent chemotherapeutic agents; children younger than 14 years; senile patients. *Cautious use* in alcoholics (in presence of alcohol, increased GI adverse effects can occur, including in patients with chronic obstructive respiratory disease, visual disturbances, edema, unexplained bleeding, or glaucoma); during pregnancy or nursing; and in older persons

Interactions

Pyrazolones may potentiate the effects of other protein-bound drugs (oral anticoagulants, sulfonamides, phenytoin, oral hypoglycemics, and other anti-inflammatory drugs such as salicylates and indomethacin).

Pyrazolones may decrease the effects of digitoxin.

Effects of pyrazolones may be decreased by tricyclic antidepressants and by cholestyramine, which inhibits pyrazolone absorption.

The effects of insulin and oral hypoglycemics can be enhanced by pyrazolones

Enzyme inducers (eg, phenobarbital, phenytoin) may shorten the $T_{1/2}$ of the pyrazolones

Nursing Management

Pretherapy Assessment

Assess and record baseline data necessary for detection of adverse effects of pyrazolones: General: VS, body weight, skin color and temperature; CNS: reflexes, ophthalmic and audiometric evaluations, peripheral sensation; GI: liver evaluation, bowel sounds, mucous membranes; Lab: renal and liver function tests, CBC, clotting times, serum electrolytes.

Review medical history and documents for existing or previous conditions that:

a. require cautious use of pyrazolones: alcoholism; chronic obstructive pulmonary disease (COPD); edema; glaucoma; elderly; unexplained bleeding
b. contraindicate use of pyrazolones: allergy to pyrazolones, aspirin, or other NSAIDs; GI inflammation; GI ulceration; blood dyscrasias; hypertension; thyroid disease; renal, hepatic, or cardiac dysfunction; temporal arteritis; polymyalgia rheumatica; oral anticoagulant therapy; antineoplastics; **pregnancy (Category C)**, lactation (secreted in breast milk, potential risk to neonate, do not use in nursing mothers).

Nursing Interventions

Medication Administration

Ensure that a detailed history and complete physical and laboratory examinations have been performed before initiating administration. Laboratory examinations should be repeated at regular, frequent intervals during therapy.

Administer with food or with milk to avoid GI upset.

These drugs should not be used as *first choice* in inflammatory states; they are indicated only when other less toxic agents are ineffective or poorly tolerated, and they should be discontinued if any sigvificant change in white cell count occurs.

Arrange for reduced dosage as soon as therapeutic effect is achieved.

Surveillance During Therapy

Arrange for discontinuation of the drug if blood dyscrasia, signs of hepatic toxicity, or eye changes occur.

Carefully monitor laboratory studies and patient for indications of adverse reactions. Hematologic status should be monitored for several weeks after termination of therapy because the occurrence of blood dyscrasias remains a possibility for some time after discontinuation.

Interpret results of diagnostic tests and contact practitioner as appropriate.

Monitor for possible drug–drug and drug–nutrient interactions: potentiate the effects of other protein-bound acidic drugs (oral anticoagulants, sulfonamides, phenytoin, oral hypoglycemics, salicylate, indomethacin); decrease the effectiveness of digitoxin; effects decreased by tricyclic antidepressants; $T_{1/2}$ shortened by hepatic enzyme inducers (phenobarbital).

Provide for patient safety needs if CNS or other visual effects occur.

Patient Teaching

Stress importance of adhering to recommended dosage because incidence of adverse effects increases *sharply* at high dosage levels.

Suggest taking with meals or milk to minimize gastric irritation.

Instruct patient to restrict salt intake to avoid edema, especially if patient is hypertensive, because drugs induce sodium retention.

Urge patient to report appearance of early signs of possible blood dyscrasias (fever, sore throat, mouth ulceration), as well as epigastric pain, unusual bruising or bleeding, black or tarry stools, skin rash, blurred vision, pruritus, or significant edema or weight gain. If any of these appear, the drug should be discontinued immediately.

Advise patient that drug will probably be discontinued if no therapeutic effect is observed within 1 week. If improvement is noted, dosage should be reduced promptly to lowest effective level.

Explain the need to comply with frequent requests for blood tests. Hematologic status should be monitored frequently during prolonged therapy, especially in patients older than 40.

Teach patient to notify practitioner if the following occur: skin rash, itching; mouth sores; sore throat; fever; weight gain; swelling in ankles or fingers; unusual bleeding or bruising; yellowing of eyes or skin; changes in vision; black, tarry stools.

Nonsteroidal Anti-inflammatory Agents

Effective anti-inflammatory drugs that are less toxic than many of the older, established agents have long been sought. Several organic acids have demonstrated a somewhat *lower incidence* of side effects (eg, tinnitus, GI distress) than comparably effective doses of the salicylates or pyrazolones. These compounds have been termed the *nonsteroidal anti-inflammatory drugs* (NSAIDs). They are approximately equal to large doses of aspirin in relieving most types of inflammation; however, they have been reported to be *more* effective in certain inflammatory states such as psoriatic arthropathy or ankylosing spondylitis.

Like aspirin, NSAIDs also possess analgesic and antipyretic activity, but they should not be used for the relief of minor headache pain or reduction of elevated body temperature in place of more commonly prescribed drugs (aspirin, acetaminophen). However, with the exception of indomethacin and meclofenamate, they are often quite effective in relieving other types of mild to moderate pain such as dysmenorrhea, postextraction dental pain, postsurgical episiotomy, and soft-tissue athletic injuries.

Their action in inflammatory states is to reduce joint swelling, pain, and stiffness, and to improve the functional capacity of the joint; however, they do *not* alter the progressive course of the underlying pathologic condition. Many of these compounds are expensive, and it may be difficult to completely justify their use in treating inflammatory conditions in persons who can tolerate the large daily doses of salicylates needed to control inflammation and who are capable of complying with such a regimen. Rather, these compounds are logical alternatives to the salicylates in patients unable to take large doses of aspirin-like drugs on a continual basis. They should be used as aspirin substitutes instead of the more toxic pyrazolones and corticosteroids. The long duration of action of several of the NSAIDs permits once- or twice-daily dosing, facilitating patient compliance, another advantage over the multiple daily doses of aspirin.

These drugs (other than indomethacin, ketorolac, and meclofenamate) exhibit a somewhat lower incidence of the *milder* forms of GI distress than commonly occur with high-dose salicylate use. It must be noted, however, that most of the other untoward reactions and drug interactions associated with large doses of aspirin and related compounds are also evident to a similar degree with the NSAIDs. In addition, aspirin itself should not be given with these nonsteroidal drugs because it can reduce their levels in the blood and their activity. Likewise, combinations of the nonsteroidal drugs with low doses of corticosteroids are probably not significantly more effective than either drug alone, in most patients.

Ketorolac is an NSAID that, unlike others in this group, produces pain relief equal to morphine but without the severe respiratory depression and constipation; it can, however, cause severe gastric irritation, a toxic effect that limits the duration of its use (eg, maximum of 5 days postoperatively).

The NSAIDs are discussed as a group; individual drugs are listed in Table 21-2.

Mechanism

Inhibit prostaglandin synthetase and, like aspirin, block the synthesis of prostaglandins, thereby lowering sensitivity of peripheral pain receptors and reducing capillary leakage; also appear to decrease accumulation of neutrophils at inflammatory sites; reduce sensitivity of hypothalamic temperature-regulating center; decrease contractions of the myometrium by inhibiting prostaglandin activity in the uterus

Uses

Relief of symptoms of rheumatoid arthritis, osteoarthritis, ankylosing spondylitis, and psoriatic arthropathy (not recommended in class IV disease, in which patient is incapacitated, largely bedridden, and capable of little or no self-care)

Relief of mild to moderate pain associated with dysmenorrhea, dental extractions, episiotomy, and athletic injuries such as strains and sprains (*except* meclofenamate and indomethacin)

Treatment of acute gout and gouty arthritis (especially naproxen or indomethacin)

Treatment of juvenile rheumatoid arthritis (tolmetin and naproxen are the *only* agents approved.)

Dosage

See Table 21-2.

Table 21-2. **Nonsteroidal Anti-inflammatory Drugs**

Drug	*Usual Dosage Range*	*Nursing Considerations*
Diclofenac *Cataflam, Voltaren (CAN) Apo-Diclo, Novo-difenac, Nu-Diclo*	*Oral:* 100–200 mg/day in 3 or 4 divided doses *Ophthalmic* 1 drop 4 times/day	Chemically unique drug used orally for rheumatoid and osteoarthritis and ankylosing spondylitis; also used in the eye after cataract surgery to prevent inflammation; short plasma half-life, but drug persists for extended period in synovial fluid; may inhibit synthesis of leukotrienes as well as prostaglandins (see Fig. 21-1); incidence of side effects is similar to that of most other nonsteroidal drugs; may be useful in mild to moderate pain, acute painful shoulder and juvenile rheumatoid arthritis
Etodolac *Lodine*	Osteoarthritis: 800–1,200 mg/day in divided doses Mild–moderate pain: 200–400 mg/6–8 h	Duration of analgesia from 4 to 12 h; can be used for prolonged period in management of osteoarthritis
Fenoprofen *Nalfon*	Arthritis: 300–600 mg 4 times/day (maximum 3200 mg/day) Mild to moderate pain: 200 mg/4–6 h	Administer 30 min before or 2 h after meals unless GI distress occurs, then give with milk; perform periodic auditory function tests during chronic therapy; *not* recommended for children younger than 14; periodic liver function tests are advised, because drug can elevate serum transaminase, LDH, and alkaline phosphatase; drowsiness and headache are common; urinary toxicity is more common than with other similar drugs
Flurbiprofen *Ansaid, Ocufen (CAN) Apo-Flurbiprofen, Froben*	Rheumatoid and osteoarthritis: 200–300 mg/day in 2–4 divided doses Prevention of intraoperative miosis—1 drop every 3 min beginning 2 h before surgery	Used orally for treating arthritis and also as an eye drop for preventing miosis due to contraction of iris sphincter during surgery; may also be useful in mild to moderate pain and primary dysmenorrhea; low doses have been shown to retard bone loss in periodontal disease; side effects are similar to those observed with other nonsteroidal drugs
Ibuprofen *Advil, Motrin, Nuprin and several other manufacturers (CAN) Actiprofen, Apo-Ibuprofen, Amersol, Novoprofen*	Arthritis: 400–800 mg 3–4 times/day (maximum—3,200 mg/day) Mild–moderate pain: 400 mg/4–6 h Dysmenorrhea: 400 mg/4 h OTC for aches, pain, fever: 200 mg every 4–6 h to a maximum of 1,200 mg/day	Available OTC (200-mg tablets) and for prescription-only use (all other strengths); not to be used more than 10 days for pain or 3 days for fever; slightly more effective than aspirin as an anti-inflammatory drug and for relief of dysmenorrhea; minimal interaction with oral anticoagulants; if blurred or diminished vision occurs, discontinue drug; perform periodic ophthalmologic examination
Indomethacin *Indameth, Indochron-ER, Indocin (CAN) Apo-Indomethacin, Indocid, Novo-methacin, Nu-Indo*	Chronic inflammation: 25 mg 2–3 times/day to a maximum daily dose of 200 mg; 75 mg sustained-release capsules may be used once or twice daily Acute gout: 50 mg 3 times/day for 3–5 days Patent ductus arteriosus: 0.2 mg/kg initially IV, followed by 0.1–0.25 mg/kg for 2 succeeding doses at intervals 12–24 h	Potent anti-inflammatory agent used in moderate to severe rheumatoid and osteoarthritis and acute gouty arthritis; also for aiding closure of patent ductus arteriosus in premature infants; most frequent side effects are headache, stomach pain (always given with meals) nausea; discontinue drug if significant improvement has not occurred in 2–3 wk; give largest portion of dose at bedtime if morning stiffness or persistent night pain is encountered; drug is given IV *only* in infants for closure of ductus and only if, 48 h after birth, usual medical management is ineffective; IV administration may significantly reduce urinary output and can precipitate renal insufficiency
Ketoprofen *Orudis, Oruvail (CAN) Apo-Keto, Rhodis*	Arthritis: 75 mg 3 times/day or 50 mg 4 times/day (maximum, 300 mg/day); alternately 200 mg sustained-release tablet (Oruvail) once daily. Mild–moderate pain; dysmenorrhea: 50 mg 3–4 times/day	Principally indicated for rheumatoid arthritis and osteoarthritis; recurrent peptic ulcers have occurred during prolonged use; dyspepsia, GI distress, and headache are quite common; initial dose should be reduced 1/3 to 1/2 in elderly patients with impaired renal function; drug may be removed by dialysis in cases of poisoning with renal failure
Ketorolac *Toradol (oral) Acular (ophthalmic)*	*Oral:* Moderate–severe pain 10 mg/4–6 h for limited duration (maximum, 40 mg per/day) *IM:* Initially 30–60 mg; followed by 1/2 dose every 6 hours; maximum—150 mg/day (5 days maximum).	Used orally for short-term pain relief; high incidence of gastric irritation and headache; reduce dose in patients with decreased kidney function or persons older than age 65; ophthalmic drops used for relief of itching due to seasonal allergies

(*continued*)

Table 21-2. **Nonsteroidal Anti-inflammatory Drugs (Continued)**

Drug	*Usual Dosage Range*	*Nursing Considerations*
	Ophthalmic: 1 drop 4 times/day	
Meclofenamate *Meclomen*	Arthritis: 200–400 mg/day in 3–4 divided doses Mild–moderate pain: 50–100 mg every 4–6 h	*Not* recommended for children younger than 14; should *not* be used as initial therapy for rheumatoid arthritis or osteoarthritis because of high incidence of diarrhea (10%–30%), vomiting (10%–12%), and other GI disorders (10%); administer with meals, milk, or antacids; periodic hemoglobin/hematocrit determinations are recommended during extended therapy
Mefenamic acid *Ponstel* *(CAN) Ponstan*	Acute pain: Initially 500 mg; then 250 mg/6 h Dysmenorrhea: Initially 500 mg, then 250 mg every 6 h for 2–4 days	Short-acting drug used to relieve moderate pain of brief duration and to treat symptoms of primary dysmenorrhea; diarrhea occurs frequently and necessitates discontinuation of therapy; administer with food and do not exceed 1 wk of treatment; maximum duration for dysmenorrhea is 3–4 days; *do not* use in patients with a history of renal impairment or chronic inflammation or ulceration of the GI tract, discontinue drug if skin rash, petechiae, dark stools, or hematemesis is noted; *contraindicated* in children younger than 14
Nabumetone *Relafen*	1,500–2,000 mg/day	Prolonged half-life (23–30 h) allows once daily administration; may elicit *fewer* GI adverse affects than most other comparable drugs
Naproxen *Naprosyn* *(CAN) Apo-Naproxen, Naxen, Novonaprox, Nu-Naprox*	Arthritis: 250–500 mg twice a day (maximum—1000 mg/day) Mild–moderate pain: 550 mg (sodium salt) initially, then 275 mg every 6–8 h Acute gout: 750 mg followed by 250 mg every 8 h until attack has subsided Juvenile rheumatoid arthritis: 10 mg/kg/day in 2 divided doses	Prolonged half-life (13 h) in the body allows only twice-a-day administration, which may aid in patient compliance; sodium salt is more quickly absorbed, giving a faster onset of action; duration of action is equal to base, however; drug may have to be used for up to 1 month to obtain a significant clinical response; readily crosses placental barrier and is excreted in significant concentrations in breast milk: 200 mg tablet is available over-the-counter for temporary relief of head ache, muscle aches, menstrual cramping, and minor pain of arthritis
Naproxen sodium *Aleve, Anaprox* *(CAN) Apo-Napro-Na, Neo-Prox, Synflex*	*OTC* (Aleve): 200 mg every 8–12 h	
Oxaprozin *Daypro*	Arthritis: 1,200 mg once per day	Prolonged half-life (42–50 h) allows once daily administration
Piroxicam *Feldene* *(CAN) Apo-Piroxicam, Novapirocam, Nu-Pirox*	Initially, 20 mg once daily; maintenance dosage is 10–20 mg once daily	Long-acting drug used in rheumatoid and osteoarthritis; steady-state plasma levels are generally attained within 1–2 wk; antacids do not affect plasma levels, but aspirin can reduce blood levels of piroxicam to 80% of normal; GI side effects are experienced by 20% of patients; *not* recommended for use in children
Sulindac *Clinoril* *(CAN) Apo-Sulin, Novo-Sudac*	150–200 mg twice a day (maximum, 400 mg/day)	Long-acting drug used twice a day; useful in rheumatoid arthritis, osteoarthritis and gouty arthritis, spondylitis, and acute painful shoulder; may allow a gradual reduction in corticosteroid dosage if used concurrently; liver function test abnormalities can occur; *not* indicated for use in children; high incidence (10%) of GI pain and other GI symptoms; administer with food
Suprofen *Profenal*	2 drops into conjunctival sac 3 h, 2 h, and 1 h before surgery; may use 2 drops every 4 h day before surgery	Used for prevention of intraoperative miosis; do not use in presence of herpes simplex infection; local irritation, redness and photophobia can occur.
Tolmetin *Tolectin*	Adults: Initially, 400 mg 3 times/day (maximum—2,000 mg/day); maintenance doses are 600–1800 mg/day in 3–4 divided doses. Children (older than 2 yr): 20 mg/kg/day in 3–4 divided doses (maximum, 30 mg/kg/day)	May be used in juvenile rheumatoid arthritis in children older than 2; minimal interaction with oral anticoagulants; if GI intolerance occurs, give with food, milk, or antacids other than sodium bicarbonate; sodium and water retention can occur; *caution* in cardiac patients; headache is observed in 10% of patients

Fate

Rapidly and almost completely absorbed; food generally delays absorption but does not affect total amount absorbed. Peak serum levels are usually attained within 1 to 3 hours, except oxaprozin and piroxicam (3–5 hours). Half-lives differ greatly, with nabumetone, oxaprozin, and piroxicam having the longest (24–48 hours), and diclofenac, ibuprofen, and tolmetin possessing the shortest (1–2 hours). All drugs are highly bound to plasma proteins and are excreted largely as metabolites through the kidney. Some biliary excretion also occurs.

Common Side Effects

GI upset, dizziness, headache, tinnitus, constipation

Significant Adverse Reactions

(Incidence and severity differ among individual drugs; see Table 21-2)

GI: nausea, vomiting, cramping, diarrhea, bloating, epigastric pain, peptic ulceration, ulcerative stomatitis, bleeding, proctitis
Allergic: pruritus, skin rash, urticaria, erythema multiforme (rare), purpura (rare)
CNS: drowsiness, nervousness, insomnia, confusion, depression, tremor, muscle weakness
Eye/ear: blurred vision, diplopia, diminished hearing
CV: palpitation, tachycardia, edema, prolonged bleeding time, arrhythmias, chest pain
Hepatic: cholestatic hepatitis, jaundice
Renal: dysuria, proteinuria, cystitis, oliguria, fluid retention, glomerular and interstitial nephritis, renal papillary necrosis (*Note*: Indomethacin and fenoprofen appear to be the most nephrotoxic)

Contraindications

Aspirin sensitivity, active peptic ulcer; in addition, mefenamic acid is contraindicated in patients with ulceration or chronic inflammation of the GI tract and in those with significantly impaired renal function. *Cautious use* in the presence of epilepsy, parkinsonism, psychotic disturbances, GI pain or bleeding, coagulation defects, hypertension, infections, and in elderly or debilitated patients

Interactions

Effects of other protein-bound drugs (eg, hydantoins, sulfonamidms, oral hypoglycemics, oral anticoagulants, pyrazolones) may be increased by NSAIDs.
Gastrointestinal adverse reactions may be intensified when used with indomethacin, pyrazolones, salicylates, and corticosteroids.
Aspirin and other salicylates may reduce the blood level of nonsteroidal drugs.
Barbiturates may lower the effects of fenoprofen by promoting its metabolism by the liver.
Plasma levels of NSAIDs can be increased by probenecid.
Diuretics and antihypertensive drugs may be less effective because of the fluid retention associated with some NSAIDs

Nursing Management

Pretherapy Assessment

Assess and record baseline data necessary for detection of adverse effects of NSAIDs: General: VS, body weight, skin color, and temperature; CNS: reflexes, ophthalmic and audiometric evaluations, peripheral sensation; GI: liver evaluation, bowel sounds, mucous membranes; Lab: renal and liver function tests, CBC, clotting times, serum electrolytes, stool guaiac.
Review medical history and documents for existing or previous conditions that:
a. require cautious use of NSAIDs: epilepsy; parkinsonism; psychotic disturbances; GI pain or bleeding; coagulation defects; hypertension; infections; in the elderly.
b. contraindicate use of NSAIDs: allergy to pyrazolones, aspirin, or other NSAIDs; GI inflammation; GI ulceration; blood dyscrasias; hypertension; renal, hepatic, or cardiac dysfunction; **pregnancy (Category B or C)**, lactation (secreted in breast milk, potential risk to neonate; do not use in nursing mothers).

Nursing Interventions

Medication Administration

Administer with food or with milk to avoid GI upset.

Surveillance During Therapy

Arrange for discontinuation of the drug if signs of hepatic toxicity, renal impairment, or eye changes occur.
Monitor results of creatinine clearance tests, which should be performed often, if renal function is impaired. These drugs should be used very cautiously in patients with renal impairment.
Carefully monitor laboratory studies and patient for indications of adverse reactions.
Interpret results of diagnostic tests and contact practitioner as appropriate.
Monitor for possible drug–drug and drug–nutrient interactions: potentiate the effects of other protein-bound acidic drugs (oral anticoagulants, sulfonamides, phenytoin, oral hypoglycemics, salicylate, indomethacin); plasma levels increased by probenecid; blood levels reduced by salicylate; reduced effectiveness of antihypertensives and diuretics; $T_{1/2}$ shortened by hepatic enzyme inducers (phenobarbital).
Provide for patient safety needs if CNS, visual effects occur.

Patient Teaching

Suggest taking with meals or milk to minimize gastric irritation.
Instruct patient to restrict salt intake to avoid edema because drugs induce sodium retention, especially if patient is hypertensive.
Urge patient to report appearance of early signs of possible blood dyscrasias (fever, sore throat, mouth ulceration), as well as epigastric pain, unusual bruising or bleeding, black or tarry stools, skin rash, blurred vision, pruritus, or significant edema or weight gain. If

any of these appear, the drug should be discontinued immediately.

Teach patient to notify practitioner if skin rash, itching, mouth sores, sore throat, fever, weight gain, swelling in ankles or fingers, unusual bleeding or bruising, yellowing of eyes or skin, changes in vision, or black, tarry stools occur.

Gold Compounds

Injectable preparations containing approximately 50% elemental gold have been used for many years as part of the regimen for treating severe rheumatoid arthritis. Aurothioglucose and gold sodium thiomalate are two preparations used primarily in active arthritis that progresses despite adequate rest, physical therapy, and other drug treatment. In addition, auranofin is an orally effective compound containing 29% gold used for the management of active severe rheumatoid arthritis. These gold compounds can temporarily arrest the progression of bone destruction in involved joints, but there is no substantial evidence that they can repair damage caused by previously active disease. Gold compounds are potentially highly toxic, so persons receiving them must be carefully and continually observed for adverse reactions.

Injections are normally given at weekly or longer intervals for prolonged periods, occasionally with rest periods if remission has occurred. Because of the long course of therapy, the need for repeated injections, and the necessity for periodic laboratory tests to detect toxicity, patients often have difficulty complying with this form of therapy. The oral gold preparation appears to be nearly as effective as the injectable drugs, with the advantage of a lower incidence of adverse reactions and better patient compliance.

- ***Auranofin***

  Ridaura

- ***Aurothioglucose***

  Solganal

- ***Gold Sodium Thiomalate***

  Myochrysine

Mechanism

Largely speculative; in animals, gold reduces macrophage phagocytosis, increases collagen cross-linkages, inhibits lysosomal enzymes, decreases formation of glucosamine-6-phosphate in connective tissue, inactivates the first component of complement, prevents prostaglandin synthesis, interferes with binding of tryptophan to plasma proteins, and suppresses the anaphylactic release of histamine

Uses

Adjunctive treatment of active adult and juvenile rheumatoid arthritis not adequately controlled by other less toxic agents (greatest benefit in the early, active stages)

Investigational uses include treatment of pemphigus (with steroids) or psoriatic arthritis in persons for whom NSAIDs are ineffective.

Dosage

Aurothioglucose

Adults: Weekly IM injections; first week, 10 mg; second and third week, 25 mg; thereafter, 50 mg. If improvement is noted, continue with 50-mg injections at 2- to 4-week intervals as necessary. Cessation of treatment depends on individual response.

Children (6–12 years): One-fourth of adult dose; maximum, 25 mg/week to children younger than 12

Gold Sodium Thiomalate

Adults: weekly injections; first week, 10 mg; second week, 25 mg; third and subsequent weeks, 25 to 50 mg until major clinical improvement or toxicity occurs. Injections of 25 to 50 mg may be given every third or fourth week indefinitely if clinical improvement remains stable.

Children: 1 mg/kg, not to exceed 50 mg on a single injection; schedule is same as for adults.

Auranofin

6 mg a day orally, in a single or divided dosage; may increase to 3 mg 3 times/day after 6 months if response is inadequate

Fate

Injectable drugs show slow absorption from injection site; peak effects occur in 4 to 6 hours after IM administration and within 1 or 2 hours of oral ingestion; serum $T_{1/2}$s vary but increase up to several months with repeated injections; gold is well distributed throughout the body; arthritic joints appear to concentrate more gold than nonarthritic joints; injected gold is excreted mainly in the urine (70%), whereas gold administered orally is eliminated predominantly in the feces

Common Side Effects

(25%–50% incidence)

Erythema, dermatitis, pruritus, stomatitis, metallic taste, flushing, dizziness, sweating, proteinuria

In addition, diarrhea occurs in more than half of patients receiving oral gold.

Significant Adverse Reactions

Dermatologic: papular, vesicular, or exfoliative dermatitis; alopecia, chrysiasis

Mucous membrane: gingivitis, pharyngitis, gastritis, colitis, upper respiratory tract inflammation, vaginitis

Hematologic: blood dyscrasias (rare)

Renal: glomerulitis, hematuria, nephritis

Allergic: syncope, bradycardia, angioedema, difficulty in swallowing or breathing, anaphylactic shock

Other: GI distress (nausea, cramping, vomiting, colic), iritis, corneal ulcers (rare), hepatitis, acute yellow atrophy, peripheral neuritis, synovial destruction, electroencephalogram (EEG) abnormalities, pulmonary fibrosis

Laboratory signs of gold toxicity include leukopenia (less than 4,000 white blood cells [WBC]/mm^3), decrease in hemoglobin, proteinuria, platelet count less than 100,000/mm^3, and a granulocyte count less than 1,500/mm^3. Close monitoring of laboratory values is essential to ensure safe and effective therapy.

Contraindications

Uncontrolled diabetes, renal disease, hepatic dysfunction, severe hypertension, cardiac failure, systemic lupus, history of blood dyscrasias, eczema, colitis, severe illness of debilitated state, recent radiation therapy, elderly patients, and pregnancy. *Cautious use* in individuals with a history of allergies, compromised cerebral or coronary circulation, or moderate hypertension

Interactions

Incidence of blood dyscrasias or hematologic toxicity may be increased when used with pyrazolones, antimalarial drugs (eg, hydroxychloroquine), immunosuppressants (eg, azathioprine), or cytotoxic drugs.

Corticosteroids can reduce the effectiveness and increase the toxicity of gold salts.

Nursing Management

Pretherapy Assessment

Assess and record baseline data necessary for detection of adverse effects of gold salts: General: VS, body weight, skin color and temperature; GI: liver evaluation, bowel sounds, mucous membranes; Lab: renal and liver function tests, CBC, chest x-ray.

Review medical history and documents for existing or previous conditions that:

a. require cautious use of gold salts: history of allergies; compromised cerebral, coronary circulation; moderate hypertension

b. contraindicate use of gold salts: allergy to gold preparations; uncontrolled diabetes; renal disease; hepatic dysfunction; severe hypertension; cardiac failure; systemic lupus; history of blood dyscrasias; eczema; colitis; recent radiation therapy; **pregnancy (Category C)**, lactation (secreted in breast milk, toxic effects to neonate; do not use in nursing mothers).

Nursing Interventions

Medication Administration

Assess patient carefully before beginning therapy.

Do not administer to patients with history of idiosyncratic or severe reactions to gold therapy.

Have dimercaprol (BAL) available as a specific antidote to gold overdosage.

Shake vial well, and do not use if color is darker than pale yellow. Inject deep into gluteal muscle with patient lying down. Instruct patient to remain lying for 20 minutes after injection to eliminate possibility of dizziness.

Administer with food or with milk to avoid GI upset.

Assure ready access to bathroom facilities if diarrhea occurs; arrange for reduced dosage if diarrhea becomes severe.

Provide frequent mouth care for stomatitis.

Surveillance During Therapy

Arrange for discontinuation of the drug at first signs of toxicity.

Carefully monitor laboratory studies and patient for indications of adverse reactions.

Monitor results of laboratory studies. Differential, white blood cell, erythrocyte, and platelet counts; hemoglobin determination; and urinalysis should be performed before therapy is initiated and after every second injection. The drug should be discontinued if proteinuria, hematuria, markedly reduced hemoglobin, leukopenia, or platelet count below 100,000/mm^3 occurs.

Interpret results of diagnostic tests and contact practitioner as appropriate.

Monitor for possible drug–drug and drug–nutrient interactions: incidence of hematologic toxicity increased when used with pyrazolones, antimalarials, immunosuppressants, or cytotoxic drugs; effectiveness reduced and toxicity potential increased by corticosteroids.

Provide for patient safety needs and protect from exposure to sunlight to decrease risk of chrysiasis.

Patient Teaching

Carefully explain the need to be aware of early signs of developing toxicity (eg, mouth sores, pruritus, GI upset, dermatitis, rash, bleeding gums, petechiae, fever, chills, weakness, sore throat, dysphagia) and the need to immediately report any signs to drug prescriber.

Inform patient that periodic blood and urine tests will be required.

Inform patient that beneficial effects may take several months to become evident, but that their duration will be prolonged once they occur.

Discuss use of proper oral hygiene to reduce risk of stomatitis and other mouth disorders.

Suggest that patient avoid exposure to sunlight as much as possible during therapy because dermatologic toxicity may be increased.

Advise patient to continue to observe closely for possible adverse effects after therapy has been completed because toxic effects can occur for months afterwards.

Miscellaneous Anti-inflammatory Agent

• Penicillamine

Cuprimine, Depen

Penicillamine is a chelating agent that has been successfully used to remove excess copper in patients with Wilson's disease and to decrease cystine excretion in cystinuria. It is also approved for the treatment of severe forms of rheumatoid arthritis. Because of its potential to elicit *serious* adverse effects, however, its use should be restricted to those patients with progressive rheumatoid disease that is unresponsive to other less toxic anti-inflammatory agents.

Mechanism

Largely unknown; may inhibit lysosomal enzyme release in connective tissue; suppresses T cell activity in vitro, and lowers gamma M immunoglobulin (IgM) rheumatoid factor titer. Other actions ascribed to penicillamine are degradation of collagen, inhibition of lymphocyte transformation, and reduction of circulating immune complexes. Drug is also capable of combining with copper, thus removing excess amounts of the substance from patients with Wilson's disease. It reduces cystine excretion in cystinuria, probably by forming a substance more soluble and hence more readily excretable than cystine.

Uses

Treatment of severe, active rheumatoid arthritis resistant to other conventional forms of therapy such as rest, exercise, salicylates, NSAIDs, and corticosteroids (up to several months may be needed to obtain a suitable clinical response).
Promotion of copper excretion in patients with Wilson's disease (hepatolenticular degeneration)
Promotion of cystine excretion in patients with cystinuria
Investigational uses include treatment of primary biliary cirrhosis and scleroderma.

Dosage

Rheumatoid arthritis: initially, 125 to 250 mg/day for 4 weeks; increase at 4- to 12-week intervals by 125 to 250 mg/day depending on response and tolerance; maximum 1,000 to 1,500 mg/day for 3 to 4 months; if no response at this level, discontinue drug; usual maintenance range is 500 to 750 mg/day (dosage may be reduced *gradually* if patient has been in remission for at least 6 months)
Wilson's disease: Initially, 250 mg 4 times/day, increased to 500 mg 4 times/day as needed
Cystinuria: Adults: 250 to 500 mg 4 times/day; Children: 30 mg/kg/day

Fate

Well absorbed orally if given on an empty stomach; peak plasma level in 1 to 2 hours; serum $T_{1/2}$ is approximately 2 hours; excreted in the urine, almost completely within 24 hours

Common Side Effects

Loss of sense of taste, indigestion, epigastric pain, nausea, anorexia, rash, pruritus, proteinuria

Significant Adverse Reactions

GI: vomiting, diarrhea, oral ulceration, activation of peptic ulcer
Hematologic: leukopenia, thrombocytopenia, bone marrow depression, agranulocytosis, aplastic anemia
Allergic: arthralgia, lymphadenopathy, pemphigoid reaction, urticaria, exfoliative dermatitis, colitis, synovitis, thyroiditis
Renal/hepatic: hematuria, hepatic dysfunction, cholestatic jaundice, pancreatitis, glomerulonephritis (Goodpasture's syndrome)
CNS: tinnitus, optic neuritis
Other: thrombophlebitis, myasthenia-like reaction, hyperpyrexia, polymyositis, systemic lupus–like syndrome, mammary hyperplasia, epidermal necrolysis, alveolitis, obliterative bronchiolitis

Contraindications

Renal insufficiency; pregnancy; young children; history of penicillin sensitivity or blood dyscrasias; when used with other anti-inflammatory drugs (pyrazolones, gold compounds), antimalarials, or cytotoxic agents. *Cautious use* in persons with a history of allergies or respiratory disease.

Interactions

Penicillamine may potentiate the neurotoxicity of isoniazid.
Effects of penicillamine can be reduced by the presence of iron, antacids, or food, which can decrease absorption.
Risk of blood dyscrasias and renal toxicity may be increased by concomitant use of antimalarial drugs, antineoplastics, gold compounds, or pyrazolones.
Penicillamine can lower serum levels of digoxin

Nursing Management

Pretherapy Assessment

Assess and record baseline data necessary for detection of adverse effects of penicillamine: General: VS, body weight, skin color and temperature; CNS: reflexes, ophthalmic/audiometric examination, peripheral sensation; GI: liver evaluation, bowel sounds, mucous membranes; Lab: renal and liver function tests, CBC, clotting times, x-ray for renal stones.
Review medical history and documents for existing or previous conditions that:
a. require cautious use of penicillamine: history of allergies; respiratory disease
b. contraindicate use of penicillamine: allergy to penicillamine, penicillin; renal insufficiency; history of penicillamine-related aplastic anemia or agranulocytosis; when used with other anti-inflammatory drugs (pyrazolones, gold salts), antimalarials, or cytotoxic drugs; **pregnancy (Category C)**, lactation (secreted in breast milk, toxic effects to neonate; do not use in nursing mothers).

Nursing Interventions

Medication Administration

Assess patient carefully before beginning therapy.
Administer drug on an empty stomach; 1 hour before or 2 hours after meals and at least 1 hour from any other drug, food, or milk. Wilson's disease: administer drug 30 to 60 minutes before meals and at bedtime. Cystinuria: administer in 4 equal doses (bedtime dose most important); ensure that patient drinks 1 pint of fluid at bedtime and 1 pint of fluid during the night.
Provide frequent mouthcare as needed.
Arrange for nutritional consultation; hypogeusia may lead to anorexia or inappropriate eating habits.

Surveillance During Therapy

Discontinue the drug if fever occurs.
Carefully monitor laboratory studies and patient for indications of adverse reactions.
Monitor results of laboratory studies. Urinalyses, differential blood cell counts, hemoglobin determinations,

and direct platelet counts should be performed every 2 weeks for the first 6 months of therapy and monthly thereafter. If WBC counts are below 3,500 or platelet counts are below 100,000, therapy should be discontinued.

Monitor patient carefully for indications of proteinuria or hematuria, possible early signs of developing glomerulonephritis. Drug should be discontinued if proteinuria exceeds 2 g/24 hours, or if gross or persistent microscopic hematuria develops.

Interpret results of diagnostic tests and contact practitioner as appropriate.

Monitor for possible drug–drug and drug–nutrient interactions: may potentiate neurotoxicity of isoniazid; effectiveness reduced by presence of iron, antacids, or food; risk of blood dyscrasias and renal toxicity increased by antimalarials, gold salts, or pyrazolones; lowers serum digoxin concentrations.

Patient Teaching

Assist patient to plan dosing schedule so that drug is taken on an empty stomach, at least 1 hour apart from any other drug, food, antacid, or milk.

Instruct patient to promptly report early signs of possible developing blood dyscrasias (eg, fever, sore throat, chills, bruising, abnormal bleeding, malaise) to appropriate person. Blood studies should be performed immediately. Drug-induced fever is an indication for discontinuing the drug.

Instruct patient to be alert for appearance of allergic manifestations (eg, fever, arthralgia, lymphadenopathy, rash, intense pruritus) and to advise practitioner immediately. Reduction in dosage and use of antihistamines can usually eliminate early rash and pruritus.

Prepare patient for the possibility of increased skin friability, especially at pressure points (eg, elbows, knees, buttocks), because the drug increases soluble collagen. External bleeding or vesicles containing blood may appear, and skin wrinkling can occur. These effects are not progressive and do not require discontinuance of drug; they may disappear with dosage reduction.

Instruct patient to watch for signs of increasing muscle weakness because drug can cause a myasthenia-like syndrome. Symptoms will usually disappear after drug withdrawal.

Discuss use of proper oral hygiene to reduce risk of stomatitis and other mouth disorders.

Antigout Drugs

Gout is a metabolic disorder of purine metabolism characterized by an excess of uric acid in the blood (hyperuricemia) that results from either overproduction or a defect in elimination. When the solubility of uric acid salts is exceeded in body fluids, monosodium urate crystals begin to precipitate out of the blood and are deposited in joints, skin, kidney, and other tissues, resulting in the appearance of symptoms of acute gout pain, swelling, tenderness, and other signs of inflammation. The pharmacotherapy of gout, therefore, involves controlling the serum levels of uric acid to prevent attacks, and providing relief of the symptoms of an acute attack of gouty arthritis. Drugs used as antigout agents may be classified as one of the following:

- *Anti-inflammatory agents*: relieve the pain and inflammation associated with an acute attack of gout
- *Hypouricemic (uricosuric) agents*: reduce the blood levels of uric acid with prolonged administration

The drugs that may be used to relieve the symptoms of an acute attack are indomethacin, phenylbutazone, oxyphenbutazone, naproxen, sulindac, and colchicine. The first five were discussed previously in this chapter, because they are also used to control symptoms of rheumatoid arthritis and osteoarthritis. Colchicine is reviewed in detail in this section. Hypouricemic agents either interfere with the synthesis of uric acid (eg, allopurinol) or promote the urinary excretion of uric acid by blocking its renal tubular reabsorption (eg, probenecid, sulfinpyrazone). These drugs are also discussed in this section.

• Colchicine

An alkaloid capable of dramatically relieving pain and inflammation associated with acute attacks of gouty arthritis within 12 hours to 24 hours, colchicine is also useful but somewhat less effective in the treatment of chondrocalcinosis (pseudogout). It is nonanalgesic and nonuricosuric, and is specific for the symptoms of gout, being effective in up to 90% of patients if given at the first sign of an attack. Although once it was exclusively the drug of choice, colchicine has now been largely replaced by indomethacin, sulindac, or phenylbutazone because of its extremely high incidence of GI side effects.

Mechanism

Reduces leukocytic production of lactic acid, thereby decreasing acid deposition; impairs phagocytic breakdown of WBC membrane and release of tissue-damaging enzymes; also binds to microtubular cellular proteins, thereby arresting mitosis at metaphase and interfering with movement of mobile cells (eg, leukocytes)

Uses

Relief of pain and inflammation of acute gout and pseudogout

Limiting the destruction of joint cartilage and reducing the incidence of acute attacks (not an approved indication)

Other experimental uses include symptomatic treatment of leukemia, adenocarcinoma, sarcoid arthritis, mycosis fungoides, acute calcium-dependent tendinitis, and familial Mediterranean fever

Dosage

Oral: 1 to 1.2 mg initially, at earliest sign of acute attack, followed by 0.5 to 1.2 mg every 1 to 2 hours until pain is relieved or diarrhea occurs (4–8 mg total dose usually required for acute attack; prophylaxis, 0.5–0.6 mg orally 3 or 4 times/week; severe cases, 0.5–1.8 mg daily)

IV: 1 to 2 mg initially, followed by 0.5 mg every 6 hours (maximum, 4 mg/24 h)

Fate

Rapidly absorbed orally; relatively short-acting ($T_{1/2}$ 20 minutes); partially metabolized in the liver; both metabolites and unchanged drug are recycled into the GI tract through the bile and intestinal secretions; mainly eliminated in the feces, with 10% to 20% excreted in the urine; drug may persist for up to 9 days in leukocytes after single intravenous dose

Common Side Effects

Nausea, vomiting, abdominal pain, diarrhea

Significant Adverse Reactions

Usually observed at high doses or with hepatic dysfunction

Severe diarrhea, muscle weakness, dermatitis, hematuria, oliguria, generalized vascular damage, alopecia
Prolonged use may lead to:
Agranulocytosis, aplastic anemia, peripheral neuritis
Overdose may be characterized by:
Vomiting, diarrhea (profuse and bloody), burning in the throat, stomach, or skin, hematuria, shock caused by extensive vascular damage, marked muscle weakness, delirium, convulsions

Contraindications

Severe renal, GI, cardiac, or hepatic disease; intravenous use contraindicated with vascular damage. *Cautious use* in elderly or debilitated patients, especially those with renal, hepatic, GI, or heart disease

Interactions

Effects of colchicine are enhanced by alkalinizing agents (eg, sodium bicarbonate) and inhibited by acidifying agents (eg, ascorbic acid).
Colchicine may increase the response to CNS depressants and sympathomimetics.
Prolonged use of colchicine may reduce GI absorption of vitamin B_{12}.

Nursing Management

Pretherapy Assessment

Assess and record baseline data necessary for detection of adverse effects of colchicine: General: VS, body weight, skin color and temperature; CNS: reflexes; GI: liver evaluation, bowel sounds, normal output; GU: normal output; Lab: renal and liver function tests, CBC, urinalysis.
Review medical history and documents for existing or previous conditions that:
a. require cautious use of colchicine: use in the elderly, especially those with renal, hepatic, GI, or heart disease.
b. contraindicate use of colchicine: allergy to colchicine; blood dyscrasias, severe renal, cardiac, GI, or hepatic disease; **pregnancy (Category C), (parenteral: Category D)**, lactation (safety not established).

Nursing Interventions

Medication Administration

Use intravenous route only, not subcutaneous or intramuscular, if parenterally administered. Observe injection site for signs of localized irritation (pain, swelling, erythema) because thrombophlebitis may occur.
Arrange for opiate antidiarrheal medication if diarrhea is severe.
Adminstration should begin at first warning of an acute attack; delay can decrease the effectiveness of the drug.

Surveillance During Therapy

Inform practitioner if oral administration is associated with excessive GI toxicity. The intravenous route may be used, but overdose occurs more commonly with intravenous use, and extravasation can cause pain and necrosis of tissues.
Monitor intake and output, and force fluids to maintain urine output of at least 2 L/day to promote urate excretion and reduce danger of uric acid deposition in kidneys and ureters.
Advocate use of fixed combination (Col-Benemid, Proben-C), if appropriate, to increase likelihood of compliance when colchicine is used with probenecid to treat chronic gouty arthritis complicated by frequent, recurrent attacks.
Monitor for adverse effects.
Carefully monitor laboratory studies and patient for indications of adverse reactions.
Interpret results of diagnostic tests and contact practitioner as appropriate.
Monitor for possible drug–drug and drug–nutrient interactions: effects enhanced by alkalinizing agents and impaired by acidifying agents; increases responsiveness to CNS depressants and sympathomimetics; prolonged use may reduce GI absorption of vitamin B_{12}.

Patient Teaching

Instruct patient to take with meals or milk to reduce GI irritation.
Instruct patient to note and report early signs of toxicity (nausea, vomiting, diarrhea, abdominal discomfort, weakness). Drug should be discontinued until symptoms subside, then carefully resumed.
Instruct patient to note and report early signs of bone marrow depression. Drug should be discontinued if sore throat, bleeding gums, fever, or weakness occurs.
Instruct patient to immobilize affected joints and avoid applying heat or pressure to involved areas during an acute attack.
Instruct patient to inform practitioner of diagnosis of gout before any surgery. Before and after any surgical procedure (including dental), 0.5 to 0.6 mg should be administered 3 times a day for 3 days because surgery may precipitate an acute attack of gout.
Explain that colchicine may be needed in the *initial stages* of therapy with uricosuric agents because these drugs can mobilize large quantities of uric acid and thus can increase the incidence of acute attacks during the early phase of therapy.
Discuss adjunctive measures (eg, diet control, weight reduction, increased fluid intake, avoidance of alcoholic beverages in large amounts) that may help reduce the incidence and severity of attacks.

• Probenecid

Benemid, Probalan

(CAN) Benuryp

A uricosuric agent that enhances the excretion of uric acid through the kidneys, probenecid has no analgesic or anti-inflammatory action and thus is of no value in treating acute attacks. The drug also inhibits renal tubular *secretion* of penicillins and cephalosporins and is often used to increase the plasma level of penicillins by 2 to 4 times, thus enhancing their effects.

Mechanism

Inhibits the renal tubular reabsorption of urates, increasing excretion of uric acid and reducing plasma uric acid levels; decreased serum urate concentration retards further urate deposition and increases resorption of urate deposits in tissues; competitively inhibits tubular secretion (ie, plasma to renal tubule) of many weak organic acids, especially penicillins

Uses

Treatment of hyperuricemia associated with gout and gouty arthritis

Adjuvant to therapy with penicillins and cephalosporins to elevate and prolong plasma levels of antimicrobial

Dosage

Gout: 0.25 g twice a day for 1 week, then 0.5 g twice a day thereafter; may increase if necessary by 0.5 g/day every 4 weeks to a maximum of 2 g/day

Penicillin therapy:

Adult: 2 g daily in divided doses

Children: 40 mg/kg/day in divided doses; (in children weighing more than 50 kg, adult dosage may be given)

Gonorrhea: 1 g probenecid given together with 4.8 million units penicillin G or 3.5 g ampicillin

Fate

Completely absorbed orally; peak effects in 2 to 4 hours; $T_{1/2}$ is 8 to 10 hours; highly bound to plasma protein (85%–95%), metabolized in the liver; slowly excreted in urine primarily as metabolites and some unchanged drug; excretion increased by alkalinization of the urine

Common Side Effects

GI irritation, nausea, skin rash, headache, worsening of symptoms of acute gout for first few days

Significant Adverse Reactions

Abdominal discomfort, diarrhea, sore gums, urinary frequency, flushing, dizziness, hypersensitivity reactions (dermatitis, fever, pruritus, anaphylaxis), anemia, hepatic necrosis, nephrotic syndrome, and aplastic anemia are rare.

Contraindications

Patients younger than 2 years, blood dyscrasias, uric acid kidney stones, an acute gouty arthritis attack, severe renal impairment. *Cautious use* in persons with peptic ulcer, acute intermittent porphyria, and glucose-6-phosphatase deficiency

Interactions

Probenecid prolongs the action of penicillins and cephalosporins and may enhance the action of methotrexate, clofibrate, oral anticoagulants, oral hypoglycemics, naproxen, indomethacin, sulfinpyrazone, sulfonamides, and thiazide diuretics.

Salicylates can antagonize the uricosuric effect of probenecid, especially in small analgesic doses.

Xanthines (eg, caffeine, theophylline) and pyrazinamide may antagonize the uricosuric effect of probenecid.

Nursing Management

Pretherapy Assessment

Assess and record baseline data necessary for detection of adverse effects of probenecid: General: VS, body weight, skin color and temperature; CNS: reflexes, gait; GI: liver evaluation, bowel sounds, normal output, gums; GU: normal output; Lab: renal and liver function tests, CBC, urinalysis.

Review medical history and documents for existing or previous conditions that:

a. require cautious use of probenecid: peptic ulcer; acute intermittent porphyria; glucose-6-phosphate dehydrogenase deficiency; chronic renal insufficiency
b. contraindicate use of probenecid: allergy to probenecid; blood dyscrasias; uric acid kidney stones; acute gouty arthritis attack; age younger than 2 years; **pregnancy (Category C)**, lactation (safety not established)

Nursing Interventions

Medication Administratimn

Administer drug with meals or antacids if GI upset occurs.

Double-check any analgesics ordered for pain; salicylates must be avoided.

Provide frequent mouth care if sore gums develop.

Provide comfort measures if headache develops.

Surveillance During Therapy

Monitor intake and output, and force fluids to maintain urine output of at least 2 L/day to promote urate excretion and reduce danger of uric acid deposition in kidneys and ureters.

Monitor for toxicity.

Carefully monitor laboratory studies and patient for indications of adverse reactions.

Interpret results of diagnostic tests and contact practitioner as appropriate.

Monitor for possible drug–drug and drug–nutrient interactions: prolongs action of penicillins, cephalosporins; enhances actions of methotrexate, clofibrate, oral anticoagulants, oral hypoglycemics, naproxen, indomethacin, sulfinpyrazone, sulfonamides, and thiazides; uricosuric effect antagonized by salicylate, xanthines and pyrazinamide

Provide for patient safety needs if dizziness occurs.

Patient Teaching

Instruct patient to take drug with milk or meals to minimize GI upset.

Caution patient to follow prescribed dosage regimen carefully. Reduction in dosage level may lead to sharp elevation of serum uric acid levels and precipitation of acute attacks.

Inform patient that frequency of acute attacks may increase during first few months of therapy with probenecid. Prophylactic doses of colchicine or indomethacin may be indicated during initial stages of probenecid therapy (Colchicine and probenecid are available in combined form as Col-Benemid or Proben-C.).

Discuss the need to maintain a high fluid intake (2–3 L/day) and to alkalinize the urine to help retard formation of uric acid kidney stones. Sodium bicarbonate, potassium citrate, or other urinary alkalinizers may be prescribed.

Inform patient of the danger of taking aspirin or related drugs while on probenecid therapy: clinical effects of the uricosuric drug may be greatly reduced.

Instruct patient to notify practitioner if an acute attack occurs while taking the drug. The drug should not be discontinued, but colchicine or indomethacin may be added to the regimen. Therapy with probenecid should not, however, be initiated during an acute attack because symptoms may worsen.

Although there is no firm evidence that excessive dietary intake of purines is a primary cause of gout, suggest that patient restrict high-purine foods such as liver, meat extracts, peas, meat soups, broth, and alcohol during early stages of therapy, at least until uric acid levels have stabilized.

• Sulfinpyrazone

Anturane

A pyrazolone derivative with relatively weak anti-inflammatory action, indicated primarily for the maintenance therapy of hyperuricemia, this drug also inhibits platelet aggregation, and some studies suggest that it is effective in reducing the incidence of cardiac death in patients with recent myocardial infarction. This effect may be related to an inhibition of platelet synthesis of thromboxane A_2, protection of the vascular endothelium from injury, and diminished release of adenosine diphosphate (ADP) and possibly serotonin.

Mechanism

Inhibits the active renal tubular reabsorption of uric acid, thereby increasing its urinary excretion and reducing serum urate levels; decreases platelet aggregation, although the mechanism is not completely established (see above); very small doses may interfere with active tubular *secretion* of uric acid (transport from blood to renal tubule), thereby causing retention of serum urates

Uses

Maintenance therapy in hyperuricemia to reduce the incidence and severity of acute attacks of gouty arthritis

Prevention of cerebrovascular and ischemic heart disease and transient ischemic attacks, and reduction in fatalities after myocardial infarction (experimental use only)

Dosage

Initially: 200 to 400 mg daily in divided doses; increase gradually to an optimal dose (maximum, 800 mg/day); continue without interruption, even during an acute attack, which can be treated with colchicine, phenylbutazone, or indomethacin

To decrease platelet aggregation: a dosage of 200 mg 4 times/day is recommended

Fate

Well absorbed orally; onset in 30 to 60 minutes; duration, 4 to 6 hours, perhaps up to 10 hours; highly bound to plasma proteins (98%–99%); excreted primarily unchanged (90%) in the urine

Common Side Effects

Nausea, epigastric pain, burning, dyspepsia

Significant Adverse Reactions

Activation of peptic ulcer, dizziness, tinnitus, skin rash, fever, blood dyscrasias, jaundice, precipitation of acute gout (early stages of therapy), urolithiasis, renal colic

Contraindications

Active peptic ulcer or GI inflammation. *Cautious use* in impaired renal function, unexplained GI pain, pregnancy

Interactions

Sulfinpyrazone may potentiate the effects of anticoagulants, sulfonylurea hypoglycemic agents, sulfonamides, penicillins, insulin, allopurinol, indomethacin, and nitrofurantoin.

The uricosuric effects of sulfinpyrazone may be reduced by salicylates (low doses) and xanthines (eg, caffeine, theophylline).

Serum urate levels may be elevated by diuretics, alcohol, diazoxide, and mecamylamine, necessitating higher sulfinpyrazone dosage.

Incidence of blood dyscrasias may be increased with combined use of sulfinpyrazone and colchicine, other pyrazolones, or indomethacin.

Nursing Management

Pretherapy Assessment

Assess and record baseline data necessary for detection of adverse effects of sulfinpyrazone: General: VS, body weight, skin color and temperature; GI: liver evaluation, bowel sounds, normal output, gums; GU: normal output; Lab: renal and liver function tests, CBC, urinalysis.

Review medical history and documents for existing or previous conditions that:

a. require cautious use of sulfinpyrazone: renal and hepatic disease; blood dyscrasias
b. contraindicate use of sulfinpyrazone: allergy to sulfinpyrazone, phenylbutazone, or other pyrazoles; ac-

tive peptic ulcer or GI inflammation; **pregnancy (Category C)**, lactation (safety not established)

Nursing Interventions

Medication Administration

Administer drug with food or milk to reduce GI upset.
Force fluids: 2 to 3 L/d to decrease risk of renal stone development.
Check urine alkalinity; urates cystallize in acid urine; arrange for urinary alkalinizers.
Double-check any analgesics ordered for pain; salicylates should be avoided.

Surveillance During Therapy

Monitor intake and output, and force fluids to maintain urine output of at least 2 L/day to promote urate excretion and reduce danger of uric acid deposition in kidneys and ureters.
Monitor for toxicity.
Monitor results of prothrombin times carefully in patient taking sulfinpyrazone and an oral anticoagulant. Adjustment in dosage may be needed.
Carefully monitor laboratory studies and patient for indications of adverse reactions.
Interpret results of diagnostic tests and contact practitioner.
Monitor for possible drug–drug and drug–nutrient interactions: potentiates activity of oral anticoagulants, oral hypoglcemic agents, azathioprine, and 6-mercaptopurine; effects reduced by thiazide and loop diuretics, salicylate, probenecid, and xanthines; increased risk of blood dyscrasias with combined use with colchicine, other pyrazolones, or indomethacin
Provide for patient safety needs if CNS changes occur.

Patient Teaching

Instruct patient to take drug with food or milk to reduce GI irritation.
Inform patient that rigid adherence to dosage schedule is important because *minor* fluctuations in serum levels can lead to untoward reactions.
Discuss the need to maintain a fluid intake of at least 2,000 mL/day to reduce danger of urate deposition and to alkalinize the urine to increase uric acid solubility (Sodium bicarbonate, potassium citrate, or other urinary alkalinizers may be prescribed.).
Instruct patient to be alert for appearance of fever, sore throat, mucosal lesions, malaise, joint pains, sudden bleeding, or skin rash. Often early signs of blood dyscrasias, these are indications for discontinuing the drug.
Instruct patient not to alter sulfinpyrazone dosage schedule during an acute attack. Colchicine or other anti-inflammatory drugs should be *added* to the regimen.
Caution patient to avoid aspirin-containing medications because effects of sulfinpyrazone may be reduced.
Explain to patient on long-term therapy that blood counts and renal function tests should be performed periodically to avert blood dyscrasias and renal colic.

• Allopurinol

Zyloprim

(CAN) Apo-Allopurinol, Purinol

The drug of choice for controlling hyperuricemia resulting from *overproduction* of uric acid, allopurinol is especially effective in preventing development of uric acid stones. By reducing the serum urate level, reabsorption of deposits of urate crystals from tissues is enhanced. Use of allopurinol must be undertaken cautiously because the incidence of untoward reactions, some rather severe, is fairly high.

Mechanism

Competitively inhibits the action of xanthine oxidase, the enzyme responsible for converting the natural purine hypoxanthine to xanthine, and xanthine to uric acid; substantially reduces both serum and urinary levels of uric acid even in the presence of renal damage; has no analgesic, anti-inflammatory, or uricosuric activity

Uses

Treatment of gout, either primary or secondary to the hyperuricemia associated with blood dyscrasias and their treatment
Treatment of primary or secondary uric acid nephropathy
Treatment of recurrent uric acid stone formation
Prevention of urate deposition and uric acid nephropathy in patients receiving cancer chemotherapy (see Nursing Alerts) or radiation for leukemia and other malignancies

Note: Usually given with colchicine or a uricosuric drug at the outset of therapy to prevent acute attacks of gouty arthritis (see under Significant Adverse Reactions)

Dosage

Chronic gout/hyperuricemia: 200 to 600 mg/day in divided doses depending on severity of condition
Prevention of uric acid nephropathy during antineoplastic therapy: 600 to 800 mg/day for 2 to 3 days with high fluid intake; reduce slowly to minimum effective maintenance levels
Children (hyperuricemia secondary to malignancy only): 6 to 10 years of age, 300 mg/day; younger than 6 years, 150 mg/day

Fate

Fairly rapidly absorbed orally; peak plasma levels in 2 to 6 hours; short $T_{1/2}$ (2–3 hours) of the parent compound in plasma; widely distributed in body, except for the brain; largely converted to oxypurinol (also a xanthine oxidase inhibitor) that is slowly excreted in the urine ($T_{1/2}$ of 18–30 hours); small amounts excreted unchanged in urine (10%–30%) and feces (10%–20%)

Common Side Effects

Skin rash, pruritus

Significant Adverse Reactions

Acute attacks of gouty arthritis may occur early in the course of therapy with allopurinol because urate crystals are mobilized from tissues when plasma urate levels are reduced. Mobilization is followed by recrystallization in the plasma and precipitation in joints. Colchicine may be given during the initial period of allopurinol therapy to minimize these acute attacks.

Hypersensitivity reactions (fever, chills, malaise, nausea, muscle pain, eosinophilia, leukopenia, reversible acute interstitial nephritis)

Dermatologic: exfoliative, urticarial, or purpuric skin lesions; erythema multiforme; toxic epidermal necrolysis; alopecia; dermatitis

Hematologic: blood dyscrasias, bone marrow depression, vasculitis, necrotizing angiitis

GI: vomiting, diarrhea, abdominal pain

Other: peripheral neuritis, cataract formation, acute gouty attacks (early in therapy), hepatotoxicity, drowsiness, vertigo

Contraindications

Children other than those with hyperuricemia secondary to malignancy, and nursing mothers. *Cautious use* in patients with liver or kidney disease and during pregnancy

Interactions

Allopurinol may potentiate the action of oral anticoagulants, oral hypoglycemic agents, azathioprine, and 6-mercaptopurine. The drug is a *nonspecific* enzyme inhibitor and therefore can potentially alter the metabolism of a wide range of drugs dependent on hepatic metabolism for clearance.

The effects of allopurinol may be reduced by thiazide and loop diuretics, salicylates, sulfinpyrazone, probenecid, and xanthines.

Allopurinol may increase iron absorption and hepatic iron stores. Do not administer oral iron to patients taking allopurinol or use the two drugs together.

Increased incidence of skin rash may occur with combinations of ampicillin (and possibly other penicillins) and allopurinol.

Allopurinol may increase serum levels of theophylline.

Nursing Management

Pretherapy Assessment

Assess and record baseline data necessary for detection of adverse effects of allopurinol: General: VS, body weight, skin color and temperature; CNS: reflexes, orientation: GI: liver evaluation, bowel sounds, normal output, gums; GU: normal output; Lab: renal and liver function tests, CBC, urinalysis.

Review medical history and documents for existing or previous conditions that:

a. require cautious use of allopurinol: renal and hepatic disease; blood dyscrasias
b. contraindicate use of allopurinol: allergy to allopurinol; children other than those with hyperuricemia secondary to malignancy; **pregnancy (Category C)**, lactation (safety not established)

Nursing Interventions

Medication Administration

Administer drug after meals.

Force fluids: 2–3 L/day to decrease risk of renal stone development.

Check urine alkalinity; urates cystallize in acid urine; arrange for urinary alkalinizers.

Although allopurinol is employed during cancer chemotherapy to prevent hyperuricemia and uric acid nephropathy caused by certain antineoplastic agents, expect the dosage of purine analogs (eg, 6-mercaptopurine) to be reduced when it is used with them. Allopurinol retards inactivation of these particular antineoplastic drugs and thus increases their toxicity.

Surveillance During Therapy

Monitor intake and output, and force fluids to maintain urine output of at least 2 L/day to promote urate excretion and reduce danger of uric acid deposition in kidneys and ureters.

Monitor for toxicity.

Carefully monitor laboratory studies and patient for indications of adverse reactions.

Interpret results of diagnostic tests and contact practitioner as appropriate.

Monitor for possible drug–drug and drug–nutrient interactions: potentiates activity of oral anticoagulants, oral hypoglcemic agents, azathioprine, and 6-mercaptopurine; effects reduced by thiazide and loop diuretics, salicylate, probenecid, and xanthines; may increase iron absorption; may increase serum theophylline concentrations; may increase the incidence of rash with penicillins.

Provide for patient safety needs if CNS changes occur.

Patient Teaching

Instruct patient to *continually* observe for signs of skin rash, often an early sign of hypersensitivity. Rash may be followed by severe allergic or more serious dermatologic disorders (eg, exfoliative dermatitis, Stevens-Johnson syndrome, toxic epidermal necrolysis). Patient should discontinue drug and notify practitioner if rash develops.

Discuss the need to maintain a fluid intake of at least 2 L/day to reduce danger of urate deposition and to alkalinize the urine, thereby increasing uric acid solubility (Sodium bicarbonate, potassium citrate, or other urinary alkalinizers may be prescribed.).

Caution user against engaging in activities requiring alertness because drug may cause drowsiness and vertigo during early stages of therapy.

Inform patient that effects may take several weeks to develop. Caution against changing dosage levels unless instructed to do so.

Explain the need for blood counts and liver and kidney function tests, which should be performed before therapy is initiated and periodically during therapy, particularly if patient has preexisting liver disease.

Inform patient that the transfer will probably be gradual when allopurinol is substituted for a uricosuric agent.

Dosage of the uricosuric should be reduced slowly while the dose of allopurinol is simultaneously increased over several weeks.

Suggest that patient restrict high-purine foods (eg, kidney, liver, dried beans, meat extracts) and reduce weight as adjunctive measures to control hyperuricemia. Dietary intake of purines has *not*, however, been firmly linked to the causation of gout.

Selected Bibliography

Brien J: Ototoxicity associated with salicylates. Drug Safety 9(2):143, 1993

Gittelman DK: Chronic salicylate intoxication. J Southern Med Assoc 86(6):683, 1993

Joos S: The use of glucocorticoids and non-steroidal anti-inflammatory drugs for preventive postsurgical pain relief. Bailliere's Clin Anaesth 7(3):615, 1993

Kaplan BH, Nevitt MP, Pach JM, Herman DC: Aseptic meningitis and iridocyclitis related to ibuprofen. Am J Ophthamal 117(1):119, 1994

Kaufman DW et al: Nonsteroidal anti-inflammatory drug use in relation to major upper gastrointestinal bleeding. Clin Pharmacol Ther 53: 485, 1993

Lanza FL: Gastrointestinal toxicity of newer NSAIDs. Am J Gastroenterol 88(9):1318, 1993

Nuutinen LS, Laitinen JO, Salomaki TE: A risk-benefit appraisal of injectable NSAIDs in the management of postoperative pain. Drug Safety 9(5):380, 1993

Parker RK, Holtmann B, Smith I, White PF: Use of ketorolac after lower abdominal surgery. Anesthesiology 80:6, 1994

Taha AS et al: Duodenal histology, ulceration and Helicobacter pylori in the presence or absence of non-steroidal anti-inflammatory drugs. Gut 34:1162, 1993

Turner D, Berkel HJ: Nonsteroidal anti-inflammatory drugs for the prevention of colon cancer. Can Med Assoc J 149(5):595, 1993

Nursing Bibliography

McCaffery M, Beebe A: Do you know the value of a non-narcotic? Nursing '92, 22(10):48–49, 1992

Nursing guide to OTC analgesics. Nursing '93 23(3):66–75, 1993

22

Barbiturate Sedative-Hypnotics

Amobarbital
Aprobarbital
Butabarbital
Butalbital
Mephobarbital
Pentobarbital
Phenobarbital
Secobarbital

Barbiturates produce nonspecific depression of the central nervous system (CNS); the intensity of this action depends on the dose. The central effects associated with these drugs range—with increasing doses—from mild sedation to induction of sleep (hypnosis) to complete loss of consciousness (anesthesia). Although occasionally employed as sedative-hypnotics (small doses for daytime sedation and larger doses for induction of sleep), the primary uses of barbiturates today are as anticonvulsants (see Chapter 27) and general anesthetics (see Chapter 19).

The major pharmacologic action of barbiturates is a reduction in overall CNS alertness. They act at several levels of the CNS; with increasing dosage they can depress many centrally mediated functions, including motor activity and respiration. Barbiturates are effective anticonvulsants, and longer-acting derivatives such as phenobarbital are employed as specific antiepileptic agents. They are *not* effective analgesics in subanesthetic doses and generally do not produce significant hypnosis in patients with severe pain. Conversely, when combined with powerful analgesics, barbiturates enhance pain relief.

The most important adverse reactions occur with either acute overdose or chronic use of the drugs. *Acute overdose* of barbiturates is a medical emergency and is characterized by marked respiratory depression, reduced body temperature and blood pressure, and eventually coma. The principal dangers associated with *prolonged* use of the barbiturates are addiction and physical dependence. Withdrawal from barbiturates should be accomplished gradually because sudden termination can produce anxiety, tremors, delirium, and life-threatening convulsive seizures. Repeated use of barbiturates also decreases the time spent in REM (rapid eye movement) sleep, the phase associated with dreaming. Personality changes have been noted in persons deprived of REM sleep for long periods, and signs of irritability, confusion, aggressiveness, and decreased attention may be observed with prolonged use of barbiturates. Conversely, cessation of barbiturate use after prolonged periods can lead to "rebound REM," manifested by increased dreaming (often of a bizarre nature), nightmares, and hallucinations; this "rebound REM" is not restful and is a major reason why legitimate patients who are chronic users have difficulty in stopping the use of these drugs.

The clinically useful barbiturates have been categorized into one of four groups based on their duration of action. These groups are:

- Long-acting (10–12 hours): mephobarbital, phenobarbital
- Intermediate-acting: (6–8 hours): amobarbital, aprobarbital, butabarbital
- Short-acting (3–4 hours): pentobarbital, secobarbital
- Ultrashort-acting (10–30 minutes): methohexital, thiamylal, thiopental

Although this classification is convenient, remember that differences in duration of action among the first three categories depend on several factors other than the drug itself, such as dosage form, route of administration, presence of pathologic conditions (eg, liver or kidney dysfunction), and length of treatment.

The ultrashort-acting barbiturates are indicated principally as induction anesthetics and are discussed in Chapter 19. The remaining barbiturates are reviewed as a group, and specific information relating to each drug is given in Table 22-1.

Mechanism

Act at several sites in the CNS; interfere with the transmission of impulses at synapses in the reticular formation of the brain stem and thalamus, thereby decreasing overall impulse transmission to the cortex; may increase the threshold for electrical excitation of the motor cortex; appear to enhance gamma-aminobutyric acid (GABA)-induced depression of CNS neurons (barbiturates increase the **duration** of the opening of the $GABA_A$-activated Cl^- channel; more Cl^- flows inside the cell, causing hyperpolarization—and stabilization—of the cell membrane); in large doses, barbiturates can increase Cl^- influx irrespective of GABA action; they produce no analgesia alone and may intensify reaction to painful stimuli in small doses; reduce analgesic requirements by approximately 50% when combined with potent analgesics and administered together; have minimal effects on autonomic or cardiovascular system in normal therapeutic doses; depress the respiratory center in a dose-dependent fashion.

Uses

Short-term treatment of insomnia (tolerance develops within 2 weeks)
Control of acute convulsive states (IV, IM)
Treatment of various forms of epilepsy
Preoperative and postoperative sedation
Daytime sedation for the relief of anxiety, tension, and nervousness (obsolete use)
Induction anesthesia and brief, minor surgical procedures (ultrashort-acting drugs; see Chapter 19)
As aid in psychoanalysis (narcoanalysis and narcotherapy)
Management of catatonic and manic reactions (intravenous, intramuscular)

Dosage

See Table 22-1

Table 22-1. **Barbiturates**

Drug	Usual Dosage Range	Nursing Considerations
SHORT-ACTING		
Pentobarbital (C-II) *Nembutal* *(CAN) Carbrital, Nova-Rectal, Novopentobarb*	Oral Sedation: *Adults*—20 mg 3–4 times/day *Children*—2–6 mg/kg/day in divided doses Hypnosis: (*Adults*)—100 mg Rectal: *Adults:*—120–200 mg *Children*—30–120 mg based on age and weight IM *Adults*—150–200 mg *Children*— 25–80 mg IV *Adults*—100-mg initially; repeat at 50–100 mg increments to a maximum of 500 mg	Used for preoperative sedation, for minor diagnostic or surgical procedures, and for emergency control of convulsions; hypnotic effects show rapid tolerance; parenteral solution is highly alkaline; avoid extravasation because necrosis can occur; do *not* give more than 5 mL at one IM site; administer slowly IV, and wait at least 1 min before giving subsequent injections; potent respiratory depressant; can cause bronchospasm, hypotension, and apnea if injection is too rapid; IM injections should be made deep into large muscle mass (eg, gluteus); suppositories are Schedule III
Secobarbital (C-II) *Seconal* *(CAN) Novo-Secobarb*	Oral Preoperative: *Adults*—200 mg–300 mg 1–2 h before surgery *Children*—50–100 mg Hypnosis: *Adults*—100 mg Rectal *Adults*—120–200 mg *Children*—15–120 mg based on age and weight IM Hypnosis: *Adults*—100–200 mg *Children*—3–5 mg/kg IV Convulsions: 5.5 mg/kg at a rate of 50 mg/15 sec; repeat every 3–4 h as needed Anesthesia: 50 mg/15 sec slow IV injection until effect is attained (maximum, 250 mg)	Used for insomnia, to provide basal hypnosis for anesthesia, in the emergency control of convulsions, and for dental and minor surgical procedures; tolerance develops quickly (within 2 wk) to the hypnotic effect; aqueous solutions for injection must be freshly prepared with sterile water for injection; make sure drug dissolves completely, and use solution within 30 minutes because it is very unstable; injectable form is also available in a more stable aqueous-polyethylene glycol vehicle that should be refrigerated; use of this latter vehicle is contraindicated in patients with renal dysfunction or insufficiency because it is irritating to the kidneys; give *slowly* IV and monitor patient continually; also available in fixed combination with amobarbital as Tuinal (see below)
INTERMEDIATE-ACTING		
Amobarbital (C-II) *Amytal* *(CAN) Isobec, Novamobarb*	Oral Sedation: 30–50 mg 2–3 times/day Hypnosis: 100–200 mg Preoperative: 200 mg 1–2 h before surgery Labor: 200–400 mg initially; repeat at 1–3-h intervals to a maximum of 1 g IM and IV Individually titrated according to condition, age, weight; usual adult range is 65–500 mg by deep IM injection or slow IV injection	Used as sedative, hypnotic, preanesthetic medication, as anticonvulsant, and for the management of catatonic or manic reactions; prepare solutions with sterile water and use within 30 min after opening vial; do not use if solution is not clear; inject deeply IM or by slow IV (1 mL/min maximum IV rate) available in fixed combination with secobarbital as Tuinal (see below)
Aprobarbital (C-III) *Alurate*	Sedation: 40 mg 3 times/day Hypnosis: 40–160 mg depending on severity	Infrequently used for daytime sedation or relief of insomnia
Butabarbital (C-III) *Butalan, Buticaps, Butisol, Sarisol* *(CAN) Barbased, Day-Barb*	Sedation: *Adults:* 15–30 mg 3–4 times/day *Children:* 7.5–30 mg/day Hypnosis: *Adults:* 50–100 mg *Children:* based on age and weight	Used as mild sedative, for insomnia, and preoperatively; similar to phenobarbital in most respects
LONG-ACTING		
Mephobarbital (C-IV) *Mebaral*	Sedation: *Adults:* 32–100 mg 3–4 times/day *Children:* 16–32 mg 3–4 times/day Epilepsy: *Adults:* 400–600 mg/day *Children:* 16–64 mg 3–4 times/day depending on age	Used for daytime sedation in various anxiety states, and primarily as adjunctive treatment of grand mal and petit mal epilepsy (see Chapter 27); similar to phenobarbital in most respects but is very weak hypnotic and produces minimal drowsiness; dosage alterations should be made gradually in epileptic states to avoid precipitation of convulsions

(continued)

Table 22-1. **Barbiturates (Continued)**

Drug	Usual Dosage Range	Nursing Considerations
Phenobarbital (C-IV) *Several manufacturers* *(CAN) Ancalixir*	Oral Sedation: *Adults:* 16–32 mg 2–4 times/day *Children:* 1–3 mg/kg/day Hypnosis: *Adults:* 100–320 mg Epilepsy: *Adults:* 100–300 mg/day *Children:* 3–5 mg/kg/day IV Convulsions: *Adults:* 300 mg to 800 mg initially, then 120 mg to 240 mg every 20 min, as needed (maximum 2 g/24 h) *Children:* 20 mg/kg initially, then 6 mg/kg every 20 min as needed IM Preoperative and postoperative: *Adults:* 32–200 mg *Children:* 8 mg–100 mg	Widely used for sedation and in grand mal and focal seizures, either alone or combined with other antiepileptic drugs; used IV in acute convulsive states (see Chapter 27); solutions should be freshly prepared with sterile water for injection, and used within 30 min after preparation; do *not* use if solution is not clear after 5 min of mixing; some injectable forms contain alcohol and propylene glycol and are more stable than aqueous solutions; drug has a long half-life (2–5 days), and too-frequent dosing can cause accumulation toxicity
COMBINATION PRODUCT		
Amobarbital (+) Secobarbital (C-II) *Tuinal*	Hypnosis: 1 capsule at bedtime	Fixed combination of either 50 mg or 100 mg of *each* barbituate; widely abused drug

Fate

Variably absorbed from gastrointestinal (GI) tract and intramuscular injection sites; soluble sodium salts are absorbed more rapidly than free bases, especially on an empty stomach; widely distributed in the body and bound to plasma proteins to varying degrees; lipid solubility is a major determinant of distribution—highly lipid-soluble barbiturates (eg, pentobarbital) more readily penetrate body tissues, have a rapid onset and a short duration of action, whereas those with low lipid solubility (eg, phenobarbital) have a slow onset and long duration. However, highly lipid-soluble drugs are quickly redistributed from active CNS sites to fatty tissue stores from which the drug is then slowly released over many hours. Doses that are given too frequently can produce cumulation toxicity. Most drugs are extensively metabolized in the liver and excreted in the urine; aprobarbital and phenobarbital are excreted, in large part, unchanged.

Common Side Effects

Drowsiness, ataxia, hangover (especially with longer-acting derivatives)

Significant Adverse Reactions

Oral:

Skin rash, vertigo, lethargy, nausea, diarrhea, jaundice (rare), hypersensitivity reactions (fever, urticaria, hives, serum sickness), muscle and joint pain, paradoxical excitation occasionally seen, especially in children and older people

Chronic use causes tolerance and physical dependence

IV: see *Oral*; in addition,

Respiratory depression, coughing, hiccuping, laryngospasm, bronchospasm, hypotension, pain at injection site, thrombophlebitis, blood dyscrasias (rare)

Overdose:

Respiratory depression, hypothermia, depressed reflexes, anuria, rapid pulse, pulmonary edema, anoxia, cyanotic skin, stupor, coma

Contraindications

Latent or manifest porphyria, marked liver impairment, severe respiratory disease or obstruction, uncontrolled pain, impaired renal function, and early pregnancy. *Cautious use* in pediatric, elderly, debilitated, or nursing patients or in the presence of fever; hyperthyroidism; diabetes; hepatic, renal, or cardiac impairment; as well as in severe anemia and alcoholism.

Interactions

Potentiate CNS depression—including respiratory—produced by other sedative-hypnotics, alcohol, narcotics, phenothiazine and other antipsychotic drugs, antihistamines, general anesthetics, antidepressants, antianxiety agents, and centrally acting muscle relaxants

Increase metabolic activity of liver enzymes (enzyme induction) and therefore may decrease the effects of drugs biotransformed by those enzymes (eg, acetaminophen, oral anticoagulants, beta-blockers, corticosteroids, oral contraceptives, estrogen, digitalis glycosides, tricyclic antidepressants, and doxycycline)

May inhibit GI absorption of griseofulvin

Effects of barbiturates may be increased by CNS depressants, monoamine oxidase (MAO) inhibitors, chloramphenicol, valproic acid, sulfonamides, acidifying agents, anticholinesterase drugs, and disulfiram

Barbiturates when used with furosemide can produce or aggravate orthostatic hypotension

Chloramphenicol may impair the metabolism of phenobarbital

Nursing Management

Pretherapy Assessment

Assess and record baseline data necessary for detection of adverse effects of barbiturates: General: vital signs (VS), body weight, skin color and temperature, injection site; CNS: orientation, affect, reflexes; GI: liver evaluation, bowel sounds, normal output; Lab: renal and liver function tests, blood and urine glucose, blood urea nitrogen (BUN).

Review medical history and documents for existing or previous conditions that:

a. require cautious use of barbiturates: use in pediatric, elderly, or debilitated patients; presence of fever; hyperthyroidism; diabetes; hepatic, renal, or cardiac impairment; anemia; alcoholism.

b. contraindicate use of barbiturates: allergy to barbiturates; manifest or latent porphyria; marked liver impairment; severe respiratory disease or obstruction; uncontrolled pain; impaired renal function; **pregnancy (Category D)**, lactation (secreted in breast milk; causes drowsiness in nursing infants)

Nursing Interventions

Medication Administration

Observe intravenous injection site for evidence of extravasation (swelling, pain), which may cause tissue necrosis.

Be prepared to deal with an initial period of excitement or confusion in the patient given barbiturates, especially the very young or elderly. Attempt to calm patient and prevent injury.

Always give in combination with an analgesic when pain is present. Given to a patient with severe pain, barbiturates may produce anxiety, restlessness, and an intensified reaction to the pain.

Administer intravenous doses slowly and intramuscular doses deep in a muscle mass.

Do not use a parenteral dosage form if solution is discolored or contains a precipitate.

Ensure ready access to bathroom facilities if GI effects occur.

Surveillance During Therapy

Monitor for toxicity.

Carefully monitor laboratory studies and patient for indications of adverse reactions.

Interpret results of diagnostic tests and contact practitioner as appropriate.

Monitor vital signs continuously when drug is given intravenously. The drug should be administered *slowly* to prevent respiratory depression, laryngospasm, and hypotension, and resuscitative equipment and other supportive measures (eg, IV fluids, vasopressors) should be on hand in case respiratory or circulatory depression occurs.

Maintain appropriate perspective toward administration: Use of barbiturates for prolonged periods, even at therapeutic levels, is associated with a high incidence of dependence and abuse. Barbiturates with the shortest onset of action are most often abused. Discourage long-term use of any barbiturate for daytime sedation.

Monitor patient for signs of excessive dosage (eg, mental clouding, impaired coordination). If these occur, dosage should be reduced accordingly.

Observe patient for signs of developing tolerance (eg, more frequent usage, requests for larger doses, decreased drug effects). Advise practitioner if signs appear, because *gradual* drug withdrawal should be considered.

Carefully evaluate patient response when drugs are used as hypnotics. Barbiturates generally lose effectiveness as hypnotics within 2 weeks of continued usage. Dosage should *not* be increased in an attempt to regain effectiveness.

Assess patient for signs of decreased response when used with other drugs. Because barbiturates enhance the activity of hepatic enzymes, they may diminish effects of drugs metabolized by those enzymes (see **Interactions**). Dosages of such drugs may need to be increased.

Follow regulations for handling and dispensing agents in different schedules because all barbiturates are controlled substances (see also Chapters 10 and 82).

Monitor for possible drug–drug and drug–nutrient interactions: potentiates CNS depression—including respiratory—produced by other sedative-hypnotics, alcohol, narcotics, phenothiazine and other antipsychotic drugs, antihistamines, general anesthetics, antidepressants, antianxiety agents, and centrally acting muscle relaxants; increase metabolic activity of liver enzymes (enzyme induction) and therefore may decrease the effects of drugs biotransformed by those enzymes (eg, acetaminophen, oral anticoagulants, beta-blockers, corticosteroids, oral contraceptives, estrogen, digitalis glycosides, tricyclic antidepressants, and doxycycline); may inhibit GI absorption of griseofulvin; effects of barbiturates may be increased by CNS depressants, MAO inhibitors, chloramphenicol, valproic acid, sulfonamides, acidifying agents, anticholinesterase drugs, and disulfiram; barbiturates when used with furosemide can produce or aggravate orthostatic hypotension; chloramphenicol may impair the metabolism of phenobarbital.

Patient Teaching

Instruct patient to avoid hazardous activities during therapy because drowsiness and impaired motor coordination are often present.

Inform patient that "hangover" effects are common. Suggest rising slowly from bed and walking cautiously until equilibrium is established.

Inform patient of dangers of additive CNS depression if combined with alcohol, antihistamines, tranquilizers, and other central depressants.

Explain potential consequences of abrupt discontinuation of therapy after prolonged use. Withdrawal symptoms, which can be quite serious (eg, tremors, convulsions, delirium), may occur.

Instruct long-term user to note and report the appearance of sore throat, fever, superficial bleeding, bruising, rash, and jaundice, signs of possible hematologic toxicity.

Advise patient *not* to keep more than one night's supply by the bed at night. Drowsiness may cause patient to forget that a dose was taken, and mistaken repeated dosage may result in accidental overdose if large quantities of medication are readily available at the bedside.

Inform patient using oral contraceptives that their efficacy may be reduced by prolonged use of barbiturates.

Discuss adjunctive interventions (eg, warm bath, back rub, quiet atmosphere, mild analgesic, avoidance of coffee at night) that aid in sleep induction.

Selected Bibliography

Gotman J, Bouwer MS, Jones-Gotman M: Intracranial EEG study of brain structures affected by internal carotid injection of amobarbital. Neurology 42:2136, 1992

Hawthorne JL, Maier RC: Drug abuse in an obstetric population of a midsized city. Southern Med J 86(12), 1993

Kitahata LM, Saberski L: Are barbiturates hyperalgesic? Anesthesiology 77(6):1059, 1992

Marx CM et al: Optimal sedation of mechanically ventilated pediatric critical care patients. Crit Care Med 22(1):163, 1994

Smith MC, Riskin BJ: The clinical use of barbiturates in neurological disorders. Drugs 42(3):365, 1991

Sullivan JT, Jasinski DR, Johnson RE: Single dose pharmacodynamics of diazepam and pentobarbital in substance abusers. Clin Pharmacol Ther 54:645, 1993

Zsigmond EK, Flynn K: Effect of secobarbital and morphine on arterial blood gases in healthy human volunteers. J Clin Pharmacol 33:453, 1993

Nursing Bibliography

Carroll K, Magruder C: The role of analgesics and sedatives in the management of pain and agitation during weaning from mechanical ventilation. Critical Care Nursing Quarterly 15(4):68–77, 1993

Vitale R: Pharmacology of conscious sedation. Images 12(1):7-9, 1993

23

Nonbarbiturate Sedative-Hypnotics

Acetylcarbromal

Benzodiazepine hypnotics

Estazolam
Flurazepam
Quazepam
Temazepam
Triazolam

Chloral hydrate
Ethchlorvynol
Glutethimide
Methyprylon
Paraldehyde
Propiomazine
Zolpidem

Nonbarbiturate sedative-hypnotics were developed in an attempt to reduce—or eliminate—the undesirable properties of barbiturates (eg, respiratory depression, enzyme induction, addiction). These attempts have been largely unsuccessful, and most clinically available nonbarbiturate sedative-hypnotics share many common properties with barbiturates. However, one group, the benzodiazepine hypnotics, have several advantages over barbiturates (eg, absence of enzyme induction, little effect on rapid eye movement [REM] sleep, and reduced abuse potential) and are the most widely prescribed hypnotics in clinical medicine.

In general, nonbarbiturate sedative-hypnotics produce significant drowsiness and motor retardation in small doses and induce sleep in therapeutic doses. The dosage difference between the sedative and hypnotic effects is usually small; therefore, most of these drugs (*except* for the benzodiazepines) offer little advantage over the barbiturates in terms of either efficacy or safety. Tolerance develops after approximately 2 weeks of nightly use; adverse reactions, including convulsive seizures, can occur when a physically dependent user is withdrawn from these drugs. Addiction is also similar to that observed during barbiturate use.

Classification of nonbarbiturate sedative-hypnotics is difficult because these agents have different types of molecular structures. However, they all share a common action: the ability to depress the central nervous system (CNS) in a dose-related fashion. The mechanism of this action, however, is not completely understood.

Two antihistamines, found in various over-the-counter (OTC) sleep aids, produce a degree of drowsiness to help a person fall asleep. The recommended doses are 25 to 50 mg diphenhydramine (eg, Compoz, Nytol, Sleep-Eze, Sominex, Twilite), and 25 mg doxylamine (eg, Unisom). Maximum recommended dosages are 100 mg/24 hours. Use of antihistamine-containing sleep aids is recommended for short periods only (7–10 days). These preparations should not be given to children, pregnant women, or patients with asthma, prostate enlargement, or glaucoma (see Chapter 16).

- ***Acetylcarbromal***

Paxarel

A derivative of urea with short-acting sedative-hypnotic properties, acetylcarbromal acts by releasing free bromide ion; it can cause bromide intoxication. Acetylcarbromal is largely an obsolete drug that provides no advantage over most other sedative-hypnotics. Large doses may cause excessive drowsiness, narcosis, and respiratory depression. Prolonged use may cause decreased reflexes, stupor, skin rash, joint pain, and psychotic behavior. Toxicity is best treated by intake of large amounts of sodium chloride and water to promote bromide excretion. The drug is habit forming and should not be used for long-term administration.

Benzodiazepine Hypnotics

- ***Estazolam***
- ***Flurazepam***
- ***Quazepam***
- ***Temazepam***
- ***Triazolam***

Although most benzodiazepine drugs are used for the relief of simple anxiety (see Chapter 25), a few (estazolam, flurazepam, quazepam, temazepam, triazolam) are intended primarily for the short-term management of insomnia and should not be given during the day to control anxiety states. These drugs are Class IV controlled substances (C-IV). They are discussed as a group below, then listed individually in Table 23-1.

Benzodiazepine and barbiturate hypnotics are probably equally effective for the short-term treatment of insomnia. However, the benzodiazepines are safer, do not significantly reduce REM sleep time, and do not cause enzyme induction; thus, they are preferred for acute pharmacological treatment of insomnia.

Mechanism

The primary mechanism of action of benzodiazepines is to enhance gamma-aminobutyric acid (GABA)-induced depression of CNS neurons (benzodiazepines increase the **frequency** of the opening of the $GABA_A$-activated Cl^- channel; more Cl^- flows inside the cell, causing hyperpolarization—and stabilization—of the cell membrane); principal loci of action in the CNS appear to be the limbic system, thalamus, and midbrain reticular formation; unlike the barbiturates, benzodiazepines do not exert a significant effect on higher cortical centers; they possess hypnotic and anticonvulsant actions; minimal suppression of

Table 23-1. **Benzodiazepine Hypnotics**

Drug	*Usual Dosage Range*	*Nursing Considerations*
Estazolam (C-IV) *ProSom*	1 mg at bedtime (0.5 mg in elderly or debilitated patients)	Intermediate-acting (plasma half-life of 10–24 h); no active metabolites; do not use in children younger than 18 y of age
Flurazepam (C-IV) *Dalmane, Durepam (CAN) Apo-Flurazepam, Novoflupam, Somnol*	15–30 mg at bedtime (15 mg in elderly or debilitated patients)	Longest acting benzodiazepine hypnotic; major metabolite is *N*-desalkyl-flurazepam, which is an active hypnotic with prolonged half-life (50–100 h); daytime carryover effects may include decreased alertness, impaired coordination, confusion, and subtle personality changes; maximum hypnotic effectiveness may not be achieved for several nights; residual effects can persist for days after discontinuation of therapy; not recommended for children younger than 15
Quazepam (C-IV) *Doral*	7.5–15 mg at bedtime	Long-acting (plasma half-life of 39 h); biotransformed to several active metabolites; daytime carryover effects can occur, including decreased alertness and coordination
Temazepam (C-IV) *Razepam, Restoril, Temaz*	15–30 mg at bedtime (15 mg in elderly or debilitated patients)	Intermediate acting benzodiazepine (plasma half-life of 9–12 h); no accumulation of metabolites; hangover effects are minimal and early morning wakening is reduced; use in children younger than 18 is not recommended; transient sleep disturbances can occur for several nights after discontinuation of therapy.
Triazolam *Halcion (CAN) Apo-Triazo, Novo-Triolam, Nu-Triazo*	0.25–0.5 mg at bedtime (0.125–0.25 mg in elderly or debilitated patients)	Short-acting hypnotic; plasma half-life is 2–4 h; metabolites are inactive; elicits few daytime hangover effects but may lead to increased wakefulness during the last third of the night; not recommended for children younger than 18; "anterograde amnesia" has occurred, especially if a full night's sleep is not attained, eg, during travel through different time zones.

REM sleep; no enzyme induction; hangover effects can occur, especially with flurazepam.

Uses

Short-term relief of insomnia

Dosage

See Table 23-1

Fate

Oral absorption is good; sleep usually occurs within 15 to 45 minutes with all drugs; peak plasma levels: estazolam at 2 hours, flurazepam at 0.5 to 1 hour, quazepam at 2 hours, temazepam at 2 to 4 hours, and triazolam at 0.5 to 2 hours; flurazepam is converted to an active metabolite with a half-life ($T_{1/2}$) of 50 to 100 hours; thus it has the longest duration of action and can elicit a prolonged hangover effect. Quazepam, with a $T_{1/2}$ of 39 hours, is biotransformed to several active metabolites. Estazolam ($T_{1/2}$ of 10–24 hours), temazepam ($T_{1/2}$ of 9 to 12 hours, and triazolam ($T_{1/2}$ of 1.5–3 hours) are converted to inactive metabolites. Triazolam is very short acting; early morning awakening occurs.

Common Side Effects

Occasional drowsiness, dizziness, headache (especially triazolam), ataxia, lightheadedness (more common in older adults)

Significant Adverse Reactions

(Rare at normal dosage levels)

Lethargy, disorientation, slurred speech, faintness, confusion, anorexia, nervousness, apprehension, weakness, irritability, palpitation, joint pain, nausea, vomiting, diarrhea, heartburn, abdominal and urinary discomfort, short-term memory impairment, depression

Contraindications

Pregnancy. *Cautious use* in patients with renal or hepatic disease, depression, or a history of drug abuse and in elderly or debilitated persons

Interactions

See *also* **Chapter 25**.

Additive CNS depression occurs when benzodiazepines are used with other CNS depressants (eg, alcohol, barbiturates, antihistamines)

Concurrent use of antacids may delay oral absorption of benzodiazepines

Nursing Management

Pretherapy Assessment

Assess and record baseline data necessary for detection of adverse effects of benzodiazepines: General: vital signs (VS), body weight, skin color and temperature; CNS: orientation, affect, reflexes; gastrointestinal (GI): liver evaluation, bowel sounds, normal output; Lab: renal and liver function tests, complete blood count (CBC).

Review medical history and documents for existing or previous conditions that:

a. require cautious use of benzodiazepines: impaired liver or kidney function; debilitation; depression; suicidal tendencies

b. contraindicate use of benzodiazepines: allergy to benzodiazepines; **pregnancy (Category X)**, labor and delivery ("floppy infant" syndrome when mothers are given benzodiazepines during labor), lactation (secreted in breast milk; causes drowsiness, lethargy, and weight loss in nursing infants).

Nursing Interventions

Medication Administration

Assure ready access to bathroom facilities and provide small frequent meals if GI effects occur.

Surveillance During Therapy

Monitor for toxicity.
Carefully monitor laboratory studies and patient for indications of adverse reactions.
Interpret results of diagnostic tests and contact practitioner as appropriate.
Monitor results of laboratory studies. Periodic blood counts and liver and kidney function tests should be performed during prolonged therapy.
Observe patient for indications of habituation with repeated use, especially of larger doses. Although abuse liability is lower than with most similar drugs, dependence may occur. Drugs are classified in Schedule IV.
Monitor for possible drug–drug and drug–nutrient interactions: potentiates CNS depression—including respiratory—produced by other sedative-hypnotics, alcohol, narcotics, phenothiazine and other antipsychotic drugs, antihistamines, general anesthetics, antidepressants, antianxiety agents, and centrally acting muscle relaxants; antacids may delay oral absorption of benzodiazepines.
Provide for patient safety needs if CNS changes occur.

Patient Teaching

Instruct patient to avoid hazardous activities during therapy because drowsiness and impaired motor coordination are often present.
Teach patient that sedative effects of long-acting drugs may persist for several days after termination of use, and that daytime carryover effects are enhanced by alcohol, antianxiety drugs, and other CNS depressants.
Inform patient of dangers of additive CNS depression if combined with alcohol, antihistamines, tranquilizers, and other central depressants.

• Chloral hydrate (C-IV)

Aquachloral Supprettes, Noctec

(CAN) Novochlorhydrate

Mechanism

Depressant effect on cerebral cortex, with minimal involvement of lower brain centers regulating respiration and blood pressure; metabolized quickly to trichloroethanol, considered to be the active metabolite; few hangover or depressant after-effects, and good safety margin; no suppression of REM sleep.

Uses

Temporary relief of insomnia
Preoperative and postoperative sedation

Dosage

Adults:
Hypnosis: 500 to 1,000 mg at bedtime
Sedation: 250 mg 3 times/day
Children:
Hypnosis: 50 mg/kg (maximum, 1,000 mg)
Sedation: 25 mg/kg/day in divided doses

Fate

Quickly absorbed orally or rectally and converted to trichloroethanol, an active metabolite; onset of effect in 30 to 60 minutes; duration is 4 to 8 hours.

Common Side Effects

Unpleasant taste, gastric distress, lightheadedness

Significant Adverse Reactions

Drowsiness, vertigo, motor incoordination, allergic reactions (erythema, urticaria, dermatitis), nightmares, paradoxical excitement and delirium, reduction in white cell count
Prolonged use:
Gastritis, skin eruptions, renal damage, addiction and physical dependence (convulsive seizures may develop during withdrawal from chronic use)

Contraindications

Hepatic or renal impairment, gastritis, severe cardiac disease, history of allergic reactions, and nursing mothers. *Cautious use* in patients with cardiac arrhythmias, asthma, history of drug dependence, and during pregnancy.

Interactions

Effects of other CNS depressants may be potentiated by chloral hydrate
May potentiate the action of acidic protein-bound drugs (eg, anticoagulants, salicylates, oral hypoglycemics) by displacing them from binding sites on plasma proteins
Effects of chloral hydrate can be potentiated by monoamine oxidase (MAO) inhibitors and phenothiazines.
Use of intravenous furosemide with chloral hydrate may cause sweating, tachycardia, and hypertension caused by displacement of thyroid hormone from its bound state.

Nursing Management

Pretherapy Assessment

Assess and record baseline data necessary for detection of adverse effects of chloral hydrate: General: VS, body weight, skin color and temperature; CNS: orientation, affect, reflexes; GI: liver evaluation, bowel sounds, normal output; Lab: renal and liver function tests, CBC with differential, stool guaiac.
Review medical history and documents for existing or previous conditions that:

a. require cautious use of chloral hydrate: cardiac arrhythmias; asthma; history of drug dependence
b. contraindicate use of chloral hydrate: allergy to chloral derivatives; hepatic or renal impairment; gastritis; severe cardiac disease; history of allergic reactions; **pregnancy (Category C)**, lactation (secreted in breast milk; causes drowsiness, lethargy, and weight loss in nursing infants)

Nursing Interventions

Medication Administration

Administer only after pain is controlled with analgesics in patient with severe pain. Otherwise, delirium and excitement may occur.
Administer drug in capsules or well-diluted liquid form with meals to minimize GI irritation.
Follow proper procedures for handling a Schedule IV drug.
Assure ready access to bathroom facilities and provide small frequent meals if GI effects occur.

Surveillance During Therapy

Observe for signs of chronic intoxication (eg, gastritis, skin eruptions); if present, supervised *gradual* withdrawal should be started. Supportive treatment should be available (eg, respiratory aids, pressor agents).
Monitor for toxicity.
Carefully monitor laboratory studies and patient for indications of adverse reactions.
Interpret results of diagnostic tests and contact practitioner as appropriate.
Monitor results of laboratory studies. Periodic blood counts and liver and kidney function tests should be performed during prolonged therapy.
Monitor for possible drug–drug and drug–nutrient interactions: potentiates effects of other CNS depressants; potentiates effects of other acidic, protein-bound drugs; effects of chloral hydrate can be potentiated by MAO inhibitors and phenothiazines.
Provide for patient safety needs if CNS changes occur.

Patient Teaching

Instruct patient to avoid hazardous activities during therapy because drowsiness and impaired motor coordination are often present.
Caution patient to avoid alcohol while taking drug because combination can induce flushing, tachycardia, hypotension, headache, and loss of consciousness.
Warn patient about possible consequences of prolonged use. Chronic users may suddenly exhibit intolerance resulting in hypotension, respiratory depression, and possibly death.
Inform patient of dangers of additive CNS depression if combined with alcohol, antihistamines, tranquilizers, and other central depressants.

• Ethchlorvynol (C-IV)

Placidyl

Mechanism

Not established; short-acting hypnotic with anticonvulsant and muscle-relaxing effects; shortens sleep latency and decreases REM sleep time; dependence is common with prolonged therapy; safety margin is narrow (comparable to that of barbiturates); not widely used.

Uses

Short-term treatment of insomnia (most effective in patients having difficulty falling asleep rather than having frequent awakenings)

Dosage

500 to 1,000 mg at bedtime; a single 200-mg supplement may be given if awakening occurs (not recommended for children)

Fate

Rapidly absorbed orally; onset in 20 to 30 minutes; duration usually 4 to 5 hours; widely distributed and localized in body lipids; less than 0.1% of the dose excreted in the urine within the first 24 hours; extensively metabolized by the liver and slowly excreted

Common Side Effects

Dizziness, blurred vision, facial numbness, unpleasant aftertaste, mild hangover

Significant Adverse Reactions

Nausea, hypotension, skin rash, urticaria, jaundice (rare), ataxia, giddiness if absorption is rapid
Idiosyncratic reactions:
Excitement, hysteria, prolonged hypnosis, muscle weakness, syncope
Prolonged use:
Tremors, incoordination, confusion, slurred speech, hyperreflexia, diplopia, muscle weakness

Contraindications

Porphyria, early pregnancy (first 6 months), and in children. *Cautious use* in depressed patients and those with a history of or potential for drug abuse.

Interactions

Additive depressant effects may occur if used with other CNS depressants or MAO inhibitors
Drug may reduce the effects of oral anticoagulants by decreasing prothrombin time
Delirium can occur if used in combination with tricyclic antidepressants

Nursing Management

Pretherapy Assessment

Assess and record baseline data necessary for detection of adverse effects of ethchlorvynol: General: VS, body weight, skin color and temperature; CNS: orientation, affect, reflexes; GI: liver evaluation, bowel sounds, normal output; Lab: renal and liver function tests, CBC with differential.
Review medical history and documents for existing or previous conditions that:
a. require cautious use of ethchlorvynol: history of drug dependence; depression; impaired hepatic or renal function
b. contraindicate use of ethchlorvynol: allergy to ethchlorvynol, tartrazine; porphyria; use in children;

pregnancy (Category C), lactation (secreted in breast milk; either discontinue drug or nursing the infant)

Nursing Interventions

Medication Administration

Administer only after pain is controlled with analgesics in patient with severe pain.
Administer drug with meals, to minimize GI irritation.
Follow proper procedures for handling a Schedule IV drug.
Assure ready access to bathroom facilities and provide small frequent meals if GI effects occur.

Surveillance During Therapy

Monitor for toxicity.
Monitor for signs of dependence. Drug should be *slowly* discontinued in patient on prolonged therapy. Abrupt withdrawal may precipitate barbiturate-like withdrawal symptoms.
Carefully monitor laboratory studies and patient for indications of adverse reactions.
Interpret results of diagnostic tests and contact practitioner as appropriate.
Monitor results of laboratory studies. Periodic blood counts and liver and kidney function tests should be performed during prolonged therapy.
Monitor for possible drug–drug and drug–nutrient interactions: additive depressant effects if used with other CNS depressants or MAO inhibitors; may reduce effects of oral anticoagulants; may cause delirium if used with tricyclic antidepressants.
Provide for patient safety needs if CNS changes occur.

Patient Teaching

Instruct patient to avoid hazardous activities during therapy because drowsiness and impaired motor coordination are often present.
Caution patient to avoid alcohol while taking drug because combination can induce flushing, tachycardia, hypotension, headache, and loss of consciousness.
Teach patient that the following side effects are common: drowsiness, dizziness, blurred vision, GI upset.
Teach patient to report if the following symptoms occur to their practitioner: skin rash; yellowing of the skin or eyes; bruising.

• Glutethimide (C-II)

Mechanism

Depressive effects are similar to those of the barbiturates, including decreased REM sleep; has no analgesic or anticonvulsant actions; possesses significant anticholinergic activity, most pronounced in the iris (mydriasis) but also affecting the GI tract (decreased motility) and salivary glands (reduced secretions); little respiratory depression in normal doses; stimulates hepatic microsomal enzymes; high degree of psychological and physical dependence; popular drug of abuse.

Uses

Short-term relief of insomnia (essentially obsolete)

Dosage

Insomnia: 250 to 500 mg at bedtime; may repeat once if necessary; maximum dose is 1 g/night

Fate

Erratically absorbed orally because of poor water solubility; onset usually within 30 minutes; duration is 4 to 8 hours; approximately 50% is bound to plasma proteins; quickly distributed to fatty tissues; less than 2% excreted unchanged; most is metabolized by the liver, where it is conjugated and then slowly excreted in the urine; plasma $T_{1/2}$ is approximately 10 hours

Common Side Effects

Skin rash, hangover, dizziness, ataxia, blurred vision, osteomalacia with long-term use

Significant Adverse Reactions

Anorexia, nausea, vomiting, urticaria, exfoliative dermatitis, hypotension, hypersensitivity reactions, blood dyscrasias, peripheral neuropathy, porphyria
Acute overdose: CNS depression (possibly coma), shock, hypothermia (may be followed by fever), depressed reflexes, bladder atony, cyanosis, tachycardia, and sudden apnea; requires immediate treatment. Perform gastric lavage (1:1 mixture of castor oil and water) immediately in cases of overdose. Forced diuresis and urinary alkalinization are *not* recommended. Have adjunctive measures at hand, including vasopressors and mechanical respiratory aids. Do *not* use analeptic drugs to treat overdose.
Chronic intoxication: ataxia, tremors, irritability, slurred speech, hyporeflexia, memory impairment, confusion, delirium. *Withdraw drug slowly.*

Contraindications

Intermittent porphyria, pregnancy, and in children younger than 12. *Cautious use* in patients with glaucoma, prostatic hypertrophy, stenosing peptic ulcer, bladder obstruction, and arrhythmias and in elderly or debilitated persons (danger of paradoxical excitation).

Interactions

Effects of other CNS depressants (eg, alcohol, barbiturates) may be enhanced.
Drug induces liver microsomal enzyme activity so that effects of anticoagulants, antihistamines, corticosteroids, griseofulvin, meprobamate, phenytoin, and other drugs metabolized by these enzymes may be reduced.
May exert an additive anticholinergic effect with tricyclic antidepressants and other anticholinergic drugs

Nursing Management

See **Ethchlorvynol**. In addition:

Medication Administration

Follow proper procedures for handling a Schedule II drug.

Surveillance During Therapy

Monitor patient for prolonged or recurrent signs of overdosage after treatment for overdose. A lethal dose in some individuals is as low as 5 g. The drug is highly lipid soluble and can persist in the body for long periods. As drug is removed from the bloodstream (eg, dialysis), more is gradually released from fat storage back into the bloodstream. This phenomenon can prolong symptoms of overdosage or cause them to recur after dialysis is terminated.

Observe for appearance of skin rash. If one occurs, the drug should be discontinued.

Monitor bowel regularity and urinary output because drug may reduce intestinal motility and cause urinary retention. Provide fluids and roughage as needed.

Patient Teaching

Warn patient that the danger of psychological and physical dependence is high with prolonged or excessive usage.

Advise patient to take glutethimide no later than 4 hours before expected arising because residual effects may persist during the day.

• Methyprylon (C-III)

Mechanism

Largely speculative; may increase brain stem firing threshold; similar to glutethimide in many aspects; suppresses REM sleep and induces hepatic microsomal enzymes.

Uses

Short-term treatment of insomnia (essentially obsolete)

Dosage

Adults: 200 to 400 mg at bedtime

Children: (older than 12 years): 50 to 200 mg at bedtime

Fate

Onset of action is 30 to 45 minutes, and duration lasts 5 to 8 hours; almost completely metabolized in the liver and 60% excreted in the urine, mostly as conjugated metabolites

Common Side Effects

Hangover, GI upset, dizziness

Significant Adverse Reactions

Vomiting, diarrhea, skin rash, paradoxical excitation, esophagitis, neutropenia, thrombocytopenia

Overdose: confusion, somnolence, hypotension, pulmonary edema, respiratory depression, miosis, elevated body temperature, shock, and coma. Treat overdose with gastric lavage, assisted respiration, intravenous fluids, and pressor agents. If excitement is present, a rapid-acting barbiturate can be given. Closely monitor vital signs and urinary output. Hemodialysis may be performed if necessary.

Contraindications

Porphyria, or in children younger than 3 months

Cautious use in the presence of renal or hepatic dysfunction, severe pain, and in pregnant or nursing women or drug abusers

Interactions

See **glutethimide**

Nursing Management

See **Ethchlorvynol**. In addition:

Medication Administration

Follow proper procedures for handling a Schedule III drug.

Patient Teaching

Instruct patient to notify drug prescriber if fever, rash, sore throat, or petechiae (early indications of possible blood dyscrasias) occur.

Prepare patient for the possibility of REM rebound (nightmares, insomnia, hallucinations) if drug is discontinued after prolonged use.

Inform patient that periodic blood counts are advisable with prolonged use.

• Paraldehyde (C-IV)

Paral

Mechanism

Nonspecific CNS depression; therapeutic doses produce minimal effects on respiration and blood pressure; large doses can abolish convulsions and delirium but also produce respiratory depression and hypotension; not widely used.

Uses

General sedative and hypnotic

Production of quietude and sleep in delirium tremens

Dosage

(1 mL liquid equals 1 g paraldehyde)

Oral: (adults): 4 to 8 mL in milk or fruit juice to mask taste and odor

Rectal: (adults): 10 to 20 mL with one to two parts of olive oil or isotonic sodium chloride to minimize rectal irritation

Fate

Well absorbed orally; onset of sleep is within 10 to 15 minutes; duration is 8 to 10 hours; largely metabolized by the liver (70%–80%) or exhaled unchanged through the lungs (11%–28%); rectal administration provides less consistent absorption and onset of action.

Common Side Effects

Oral or rectal mucosal irritation, unpleasant taste and odor on breath

Significant Adverse Reactions

Metabolic acidosis, GI irritation, skin rash

Overdose: Respiratory difficulty, pulmonary edema, marked hypotension, gastritis, renal and hepatic damage (albuminuria, oliguria, nephrosis, azotemia, toxic hepatitis, fatty liver), right-side heart dilatation, and cardiovascular collapse.

Contraindications

Bronchopulmonary disease, GI ulceration, and hepatic insufficiency. *Cautious use* in the presence of severe pain or cough, in pregnant or nursing women, and in persons with a history of drug abuse

Interactions

Effects of other CNS depressants may be potentiated by paraldehyde.
Paraldehyde may antagonize the antibacterial activity of sulfonamides by increasing their rate of metabolism, possibly causing crystalluria.
Tolbutamide (Orinase) may potentiate the hypnotic action of paraldehyde.
Disulfiram (Antabuse) used with paraldehyde may cause a toxic reaction because of excessive blood levels of acetaldehyde.

Nursing Management

Pretherapy Assessment

Assess and record baseline data necessary for detection of adverse effects of paraldehyde: General: VS, body weight, skin color, and temperature; CNS: orientation, affect, reflexes; Lab: renal and liver function tests.
Review medical history and documents for existing or previous conditions that:
a. require cautious use of paraldehyde: history of drug dependence; depression; severe pain or cough
b. contraindicate use of paraldehyde: allergy to paraldehyde; bronchopulmonary disease; GI ulceration; hepatic insufficiency; **pregnancy (Category C)**, lactation (secreted in breast milk; either discontinue drug or nursing the infant)

Nursing Interventions

Medication Administration

Expect drug to be discontinued gradually after prolonged use because delirium, hallucinations, and tremors can occur with rapid withdrawal.
Do not administer paraldehyde if pain is present because it may induce delirium or excitement.
Discard solution if it has a brownish color or an odor of acetic acid; these are indications of decomposition. Fatal poisoning or extreme tissue damage can result from administration of decomposed solution. Discard unused contents of container within 24 hours.
Give oral drug well chilled in fruit juice or milk to mask objectionable odor and taste and to reduce GI irritation.
Dilute drug to be administered rectally in 2 volumes of olive or cottonseed oil (retention enema) or in normal saline to reduce mucosal irritation.
Keep room well ventilated to minimize odor. Inform patient that breath will have a characteristic odor for several hours after administration.

Surveillance During Therapy

Interpret results of certain laboratory tests cautiously. Paraldehyde may produce false-positive plasma and urinary ketone findings and can interfere with urinary steroid measurements.
Follow proper procedures for handling a Schedule IV drug.
Monitor for toxicity.
Carefully monitor laboratory studies and patient for indications of adverse reactions.
Interpret results of diagnostic tests and contact practitioner as appropriate.
Monitor for possible drug–drug and drug–nutrient interactions: additive depressant effects if used with other CNS depressants or MAO inhibitors; may reduce effects of oral anticoagulants; may cause a toxic reaction if used with disulfiram (antabuse).
Provide for patient safety needs if CNS changes occur.

Patient Teaching

Instruct patient to avoid hazardous activities during therapy because drowsiness and impaired motor coordination are often present.
Caution patient to avoid alcohol while taking drug because combination can induce flushing, tachycardia, hypotension, headache, and loss of consciousness.
Teach patient that the following side effects are common: drowsiness, dizziness, blurred vision, GI upset.
Teach patient to report the following symptoms to their practitioner: skin rash; yellowing of the skin or eyes; bruising.

• Propiomazine

Largon

Propiomazine is a phenothiazine derivative possessing sedative, antihistaminic, and antiemetic effects. It is occasionally used IV or IM in a hospital setting as a sedative for the relief of apprehension either before or during surgery, and as an adjunct to analgesics during labor. Peak effects occur within 15 to 30 minutes after intravenous injection, and within 30 to 60 minutes with intramuscular administration. Effects persist 4 to 6 hours with a single injection. Mild elevations in blood pressure and heart rate have been noted, and dizziness, confusion, and restlessness have occurred.

Intravenous injection can cause thrombophlebitis, and therefore drug should be injected only into undamaged vessels, with care being taken to avoid extravasation. Subcutaneous injection is likely to cause tissue irritation, and intra-arterial administration may cause vascular spasm. Because propiomazine can markedly enhance the action of other CNS depressants (eg, barbiturates, narcotics), their dosage should be reduced by approximately 50% when used with propiomazine. Dosage generally ranges from 20 to 40 mg and is frequently combined with 50 mg of meperidine. For sedation during surgery with local or spinal anesthetics, a dosage of 10 to 20 mg is sufficient. For presurgical or postsurgical sedation, children weighing less than 27 kg can be given 0.55 mg/kg; 1.2 mg/kg has been used for children who exhibit a high degree of anxiety

Nursing Management

Medication Administration

Discard solution if it is cloudy or contains a precipitate.
Observe elderly patient carefully after administration, and assist ambulation as necessary because dizziness and confusion may occur.
Expect norepinephrine to be used if a pressor agent is required because of excessive hypotension. Epinephrine

should *not* be used, because hypotension (epinephrine reversal) can occur.

• Zolpidem (C-IV)

Ambien

A new sedative-hypnotic, zolpidem has a molecular structure that is neither a barbiturate nor a benzodiazepine. However, it interacts with the GABA receptor site and has some pharmacological effects similar to those of the benzodiazepines.

Mechanism

Selectively binds to $omega_1$ subtype of the GABA receptor (benzodiazepines bind nonselectively to **all** omega subtypes); the selective binding of zolpidem eliminates the muscle relaxant and anticonvulsant actions characteristic of the benzodiazepines

Uses

Short-term (7–10 days) treatment of insomnia

Dosage

Ten milligrams taken immediately at bedtime; 5 mg is recommended initially in presence of hepatic disease or in debilitated or elderly patients

Fate

Rapid absorption from GI tract; $T_{1/2}$ approximately 2.5 hours; converted to inactive metabolites, which are eliminated by renal excretion; bioavailability and $T_{1/2}$ are increased in patients with hepatic dysfunction ($T_{1/2}$ = 10 hours in presence of cirrhosis) and in geriatric patients; highly protein bound.

Common Side Effects

Drowsiness, dizziness, headache, nausea

Significant Adverse Reactions

CV: tachycardia, hypertension
GI: diarrhea, dry mouth, constipation
GU: urinary incontinence
CNS:lethargy, lightheadedness, depression, confusion, vertigo
Respiratory: sinusitis, pharyngitis, upper respiratory infections
Dermatologic: rash
Other: myalgia, arthralgia, back pain

Contraindications

No absolute contraindications. *Cautious use* in patients with depression, decreased respiratory function, renal or hepatic impairment, and in pregnant or nursing mothers. *Rapid* withdrawal from prolonged use may cause tremors and convulsions.

Interactions

Bioavailability of zolpidem may be decreased by food.
Other CNS depressants (eg, alcohol, benzodiazepines) may enhance the depressive actions of zolpidem.

Nursing Management

See Nursing Management for Benzodiazepine Hypnotics

Note: Unlike benzodiazepine hypnotics, Zolpidem is pregnancy category B.

Selected Bibliography

Biban P et al: Adverse effect of chloral hydrate in two young children with obstructive sleep apnea. Pediatrics 92(3):461, 1993

Hoehns JD, Perry PJ: Zolpidem: A nonbenzodiazepine hypnotic for treatment of insomnia. Clin Pharm 12:814, 1993

Kauffman RE et al: Use of chloral hydrate for sedation in children. Pediatrics 92(3):471, 1993

Morgan K: Hypnotics in the elderly: What cause for concern? Drugs 40(5):688, 1990

Pollak CP, Perlick D, Linsner JP: Sleep and motor activity of community elderly who frequently use bedtime medications. Biol Psychiatry 35:73, 1994

Robin DW, Lee M-H, Hasan SS, Wood AJJ: Triazolam in cirrhosis: Pharmacokinetics and pharmacodynamics. Clin Pharmacol Ther 54:630, 1993

Ronchera CL et al: Administration of oral chloral hydrate to paediatric patients undergoing magnetic resonance imaging. Pharm Weekbl [Sci] 14(6):349, 1992

Steinberg AD: Should chloral hydrate be banned? Pediatrics 92(3):442, 1993

Nursing Bibliography

Blevins S, et al.: Pediatric sedation: When it's time to sleep. Images 11(4): 1–13, 1992

Carroll K, et al.: The use of analgesics and sedatives in the management of pain and agitation during weaning from mechanical ventilation. Critical Care Nursing Quarterly 15(4):68-77, 1993

Cooper J: Use of anxiolytics and hypnotic drugs. Nursing Homes 42(6): 37–39, 1993

Johanson G: Midazolam in terminal care. American Journal of Hospice and Palliative Care 10(1):13–14, 1993

Spitzer L: Sedation and analgesia techniques for regional anesthesia. Current Reviews for Nurse Anesthetists 3(4):190–194, 1992

24

Antipsychotic Drugs

Benzisoxazole
- Risperidone

Butyrophenones
- Droperidol
- Haloperidol

Dibenzoxazepine
- Loxapine

Dibenzodiazepine
- Clozapine

Diphenylbutylpiperidine
- Pimozide

Indolone
- Molindone

Phenothiazines

Aliphatics
- Chlorpromazine
- Methotrimeprazine
- Promazine
- Triflupromazine

Piperazines
- Acetophenazine
- Fluphenazine
- Perphenazine
- Prochlorperazine
- Trifluoperazine

Piperidines
- Mesoridazine
- Thioridazine

Thioxanthenes
- Chlorprothixene
- Thiothixene

Other
- Lithium (antimanic drug)

Antipsychotic drugs reduce the disturbed behavior of psychotic patients without causing significant sedation. They appear to act principally at lower brain centers (eg, mesolimbic area) to improve the distorted thought processes of the psychotic individual; this creates a more favorable mental state for the patient to accept other forms of psychotherapy. The development of effective antipsychotic drugs revolutionized psychiatry and saved thousands of patients from permanent confinement in locked psychiatric wards.

Distinction must be made between antipsychotic drugs, used to treat acute and chronic psychoses, and antianxiety drugs (see Chapter 25) indicated primarily for the relief of anxiety and tension associated with neurotic or psychosomatic disorders. Antipsychotic drugs have more powerful actions on the central nervous system (CNS)—and are more toxic—than antianxiety agents. Unlike the antianxiety agents, however, chronic use of antipsychotic drugs is not associated with development of addiction.

Based on their molecular structures, antipsychotic drugs are divided into many different classifications (Table 24-1).

Several antipsychotic-related drugs (eg, droperidol, lithium, methotrimeprazine, pimozide) with different indications are considered later in this chapter.

The *phenothiazines* constitute the largest and most widely used group of antipsychotic drugs. Based on their structural configuration, they are divided into three groups: 1) aliphatics; 2) piperazines; and 3) piperidines. These groups differ in certain respects, outlined in Table 24-1. **Piperazines** are the most potent derivatives and have the highest incidence of extrapyramidal side effects. **Aliphatics** and **piperidines** are less potent and have a lower rate of extrapyramidal reactions; however, they produce more sedative and hypotensive actions. Generally, antiemetic potency also parallels antipsychotic potency; the only major exception is thioridazine (potent antipsychotic with little or no antiemetic activity). The aliphatics exhibit the greatest anticholinergic activity of the phenothiazines, whereas the piperazines are only weak anticholinergics. Anticholinergic activity leads to a wide range of side effects (xerostomia, blurred vision, urinary hesitancy), but also may reduce the incidence of extrapyramidal reactions.

Thioxanthene derivatives are chemically and pharmacologically similar to the phenothiazines, so the two classes can be used interchangeably. Clinical evidence of an antidepressant action for the thioxanthenes suggests that these agents might be more beneficial than phenothiazines in certain types of withdrawn, retarded, or apathetic psychotic states.

Haloperidol, a butyrophenone derivative, is a potent antipsychotic agent providing an alternative to the phenothiazines in psychotic states characterized by agitation, aggressiveness, or hostility. Its toxicity is quite high (comparable to that of the piperazine group of phenothiazines) but it is only a weak anticholinergic and generally does not cause significant hypotension.

Other drugs used to control psychotic symptoms are chemically unrelated to phenothiazines and butyrophenones but are pharmacologically and toxicologically similar. *Molindone* and *loxapine* are alternative agents to other antipsychotics in unresponsive or intolerant patients; they have no advantages over older compounds except for a lower incidence of certain side effects. *Clozapine* and *risperidone*, two newer drugs, are reputed to be somewhat more effective in many patients than the older drugs; clozapine produces fewer extrapyramidal reactions as well.

A comparison of the potencies and incidence of common side effects among the various classes of antipsychotic drugs is also presented in Table 24-1. Although there are distinct differences in milligram potency and toxicity among the different groups, **no** significant differences exist in the clinical effectiveness of most drugs (ie, when antipsychotic agents are used in therapeutically equivalent doses, their clinical efficacy is essentially equal). However, as indicated above, newer antipsychotic agents, such as clozapine and risperidone, appear to provide clinical improvement in some patients previously unresponsive to the older drugs. The long-term effects of these newer antipsychotic agents, however, remain to be determined.

The pharmacologic actions of the antipsychotic agents are quite complex. In addition to their behavior-modifying effects, these drugs have a wide range of other central and peripheral effects. An outline of the principal pharmacologic actions of the antipsychotics is presented in Table 24-2. Specific information pertaining to individual drugs appears in Table 24-3.

Table 24-1. **Antipsychotic Drugs—Comparison of Effects**

	Approximate Potency Relative to Chlorpromazine	***Relative Incidence of Side Effects***			
		Extrapyramidal Symptoms	*Sedation*	*Hypo-tension*	*Anti-cholinergic*
Phenothiazines					
Aliphatics					
Chlorpromazine	1	++	+++	+++	++
Promazine	0.5	++	++	++	+++
Triflupromazine	4	++	+++	++	+++
Piperazines					
Acetophenazine	5	+++	++	+	++
Fluphenazine	50	+++	+	+	+
Perphenazine	12	+++	+	+	++
Prochlorperazine	10	+++	++	+	+
Trifluoperazine	25	+++	+	+	+
Piperidines					
Mesoridazine	2	+	+++	++	++
Thioridazine	1	+	+++	+++	+++
Thioxanthenes					
Chlorprothixene	1	++	+++	+++	++
Thiothixene	25	+++	+	++	+
Butyrophenone					
Haloperidol	50	+++	+	+	+
Dibenzoxazepine					
Loxapine	5	+++	++	++	+
Dibenzodiazepine					
Clozapine	0.2	+	+++	+++	+++
Indolone					
Molindone	5	+++	++	++	++
Benzisoxazole					
Risperidone	50	+	+	+	+

+++, frequent.
++, occasional.
+, infrequent.

Mechanism

Complex and not completely understood; act primarily at several subcortical brain sites, including the limbic system, hypothalamus, and brain stem; among the known effects of the drugs are reduction of intraneuronal levels of cyclic adenosine monophosphate (cAMP) in brain regions associated with emotion and behavior, and decreased cortical sensory input from ascending spinal tracts by way of collateral nerves to the reticular formation. The major mechanism of action appears to be blockade of dopamine receptors, specifically the D_2 subtype; some agents (eg, clozapine, thioridazine) also block the D_1 subtype. Recent **clinical** evidence (positron emission tomography [PET] scans of human brain in living patients) indicates that—for most agents—significant antipsychotic effects do not occur until 70% to 80% of D_2 receptors are occupied; this level of occupancy is also associated with the appearance of extrapyramidal reactions.

In addition to the antipsychotic activity, these drugs produce other CNS effects including sedation, antiemesis, hypothermia, and altered pituitary hormone release. Peripheral actions responsible for many of the observed side effects include antiadrenergic (alpha$_1$-adrenergic blockade), anticholinergic, antiserotonergic, local anesthetic, and quinidine-like cardiac depressant effects.

Uses

(See Table 24-3 for specific indications of each drug)

- Management of acute and chronic psychoses, either organic or drug induced
- Control of the manic phase of manic-depressive psychoses (lithium)
- Relief of severe nausea and vomiting
- Control of intractable hiccups
- Relief of anxiety, apprehension, and agitation associated with a variety of somatic disorders, or before surgery
- Facilitation of alcohol withdrawal
- Adjunctive treatment of tetanus and acute intermittent porphyria
- Control of aggressiveness in disturbed children
- Control of tics and vocal utterances of Gilles de la Tourette's disease (haloperidol, pimozide)

Table 24-2. **Antipsychotic Drugs—Pharmacologic Effects**

Central Nervous System

Antipsychotic effect: reduced agitation, emotional quieting, decreased paranoid ideation, and lessening of hallucinations and disturbed thought processes.

Antiemetic effect: decreased sensitivity of chemoreceptor trigger zone (CTZ) in medulla to activation by drugs or toxins and direct depression of brain stem vomiting center in large doses

Impaired temperature regulation: hypothermia caused by increased heat loss and decreased compensatory heat production

Endocrine effects: inhibition of FSH and LH release, and increased release of LTH (prolactin), resulting in abnormal lactation. Hormonal effects are due to the blocking action of antipsychotic drugs on dopamine receptors either in the hypothalamic–pituitary pathway or on anterior pituitary cells themselves.

Motor effects: increased involuntary muscle activity (eg, tremors, dyskinesias, akathisias) caused by dopamine blockade in motor-integrating areas of the CNS

Peripheral Nervous System

Antiadrenergic effects: blockade of central and peripheral α-receptors, and possibly inhibition of catecholamine uptake by nerve endings, leading to orthostatic hypotension and reflex tachycardia

Anticholinergic/antihistamine effects: blockade of cholinergic (largely muscarinic) and histaminergic activity

Other

Antiarrhythmic effects: quinidine-like depressant action on the myocardium, and local anesthetic action

Diuretic effect: depression of ADH release and inhibition of water and electrolyte reabsorption (weak effect)

Relief of pain (methotrimeprazine; droperidol [in combination with narcotics])

Dosage

See Table 24-3

Fate

Adequately absorbed orally and well absorbed parenterally; widely distributed to most body tissues and found in high concentrations in the brain; onset and duration of action largely dependent on dosage form and route of administration; clinical effects may not be attained for several weeks after initiation of therapy; most drugs are significantly protein bound, and metabolism and excretion are generally slow; metabolized by the liver and excreted in both the urine and feces; many metabolites are biologically active and contribute to the prolonged effects of some drugs. Enzyme inducers (eg, barbiturates, meprobamate) can accelerate phenothiazine metabolism. Excretion is by way of the kidneys and the enterohepatic circulation.

Common Side Effects

(Most common in early stages of therapy)

Drowsiness, orthostatic hypotension (dizziness, weakness), dry mouth, blurred vision, constipation, nasal stuffiness, palpitations

Significant Adverse Reactions

(Incidence varies among different drugs)

CNS: neuroleptic malignant syndrome (high fever, sweating, muscle rigidity, tachycardia, confusion, delirium), lowering of convulsive threshold, hyperactivity, bizarre dreams, insomnia, depression, cerebral edema

Neuromuscular: extrapyramidal reactions occur within days to weeks of initiation of therapy and include:

- **Akathisia** (motor restlessness)
- **Dystonia** (muscle spasms of face or throat, difficulty in speech or swallowing, extensor rigidity of back muscles, upward rotation of eyeballs)
- **Pseudoparkinsonism**
- Tardive dyskinesias develop slowly during 6 to 24 months of therapy and include
  - Involuntary movements of orofacial area (eg, chewing; protrusion of tongue; puffing of cheeks; puckering of mouth) and possibly of neck and trunk
  - Hyperreflexia

Cardiovascular

Tachycardia, fainting, electrocardiogram (ECG) changes, cardiac arrest (rare)

Hematologic

Blood dyscrasias (agranulocytosis, leukopenia, leukocytosis, anemias, thrombocytopenic purpura, pancytopenia)

Higher frequency of agranulocytosis with clozapine—weekly complete blood count (CBC) *must* be performed with immediate termination of clozapine therapy if $<3{,}000$ white blood cells (WBC)/mm^3 or $<1{,}500$ granulocytes/mm^3!

Any patient who develops agranulocytosis can NOT receive clozapine again.

Hypersensitivity: urticaria, itching, eczema, photosensitivity, contact dermatitis, angioneurotic edema, anaphylactic reaction, exfoliative dermatitis, cholestatic jaundice

Endocrine: abnormal lactation, breast engorgement, gynecomastia, changes in libido, amenorrhea, glycosuria and hyperglycemia, increased appetite

Autonomic: fecal impaction, adynamic ileus, urinary retention, enuresis, incontinence, impotence

Ocular: ptosis, photophobia, pigmentary retinopathy, lens opacities

Respiratory: laryngospasm, bronchospasm, dyspnea

Other: skin pigmentation, polydipsia, aggravation of peptic ulcers, fever, systemic lupus–like reaction, psychotic flare-up

Contraindications

Bone marrow depression, blood dyscrasias, parkinsonism, jaundice, liver damage, renal insufficiency, cerebral arteriosclerosis, coronary disease, circulatory collapse, mitral insufficiency, severe hypotension, chronic alcoholism, comatose states, and subcortical brain damage. *Cautious use* in the presence of glaucoma, prostatic hypertrophy, epilepsy, diabetes, severe hypertension, ulcers, cardiovascular disease, chronic respiratory disorders, liver impairment, in pregnant or lactating women, in children younger than 6 months of age, and in persons exposed to extreme heat, phosphorus insecticides, or pesticides.

(text continues on page 227)

Table 24-3. **Antipsychotic Drugs**

Drug	*Usual Dosage Range*	*Nursing Considerations*
BENZISOXAZOLE		
Resperidone *Risperdal*	Oral: 3 mg 2 times/day	Orthostatic hypotension may occur, especially upon initiation of therapy; low incidence of sedation and anticholinergic effects
BUTYROPHENONES		
Haloperidol *Haldol* *(CAN) Apo-Haloperidol, Novoperidol, Peridol*	*Adults* Oral: 0.5–5 mg 2–3 times/day depending on symptoms (maximum 100 mg/day) IM: 2–5 mg (up to 30 mg if necessary); repeat at 4–8-h intervals as needed Depot injection: 10–15× daily oral dose IM every 4 weeks *Children* (3–12 y) 0.5 mg/day initially in 2–3 divided doses; increase at 0.5-mg increments every 5–7 days until desired effect (range is 0.05–0.15 mg/kg/day)	Indicated in psychotic disorders, manic phase of manic–depressive psychoses, and for management of tics and vocal utterances of Gilles de la Tourette's disease; very potent antipsychotic with high incidence of extrapyramidal reactions; strong antiemetic; less sedation and hypotension than many other similar drugs; do *not* use in children younger than 3 or in parkinsonian patients (drug is a potent dopamine-blocking agent); use cautiously in epileptic individuals because drug may lower convulsive threshold; when used for manic episodes, be alert for reversal to severe depression, which may invite suicidal attempts; concomitant use with lithium may elicit dyskinesias, parkinsonian-like symptoms, or dementia; observe patients closely, and provide emotional support as necessary; perform periodic liver function and blood studies; depot injection is for *chronic* psychoses only
DIBENZOXAZEPINE		
Loxapine *Loxitane* *(CAN) Loxapac*	Initially 10 mg orally twice a day; increase to optimal levels (usually 60–100 mg/day; maximum 250 mg/day) IM: 12.5–50 mg every 4–6 h to control acutely agitated patients	Indicated for manifestations of schizophrenia; elicits strong sedation in early therapy, lowers convulsive threshold, produces hypotension, and is an anticholinergic of moderate potency; has antiemetic activity and may produce ocular toxicity; not recommended in children younger than 16; produces frequent extrapyramidal reactions, usually parkinsonian-like in nature; no endocrine abnormalities have been reported; concentrate should be mixed with orange or grapefruit juice before administration
DIBENZODIAZEPINE		
Clozapine *Clozaril*	Initially: 25 mg 1–2 times/day; target dose of 300–450 mg/day; (maximum, 900 mg/day)	Occasionally effective where other antipsychotics are not; however, significant risk of agranulocytosis; white blood cell count *must* be performed *weekly*; be alert for early signs (fever, sore throat, weakness, lethargy, mucosal ulcers); discontinue drug if WBC count <3,000/mm³; drowsiness, salivation and tachycardia are very common; tardive dyskinesias are *rare*
INDOLONE		
Molindone *Moban*	Initially: 50–75 mg/day Maintenance: 5–25 mg 3–4 times a day depending on symptoms (maximum, 225 mg/day)	Used for control of schizophrenia; not recommended in children younger than 12; provides an alternative drug to the phenothiazines and thioxanthenes in unresponsive patients, although actions are essentially identical to those of other classes of antipsychotics; high degree of initial drowsiness; resumption of menses in previously amenorrheal women has been reported; no ophthalmologic complications have occurred; tablet contains calcium, which may interfere with GI absorption of phenytoin and tetracyclines
PHENOTHIAZINES		
Aliphatics		
Chlorpromazine *Thorazine and several other manufacturers* *(CAN) Largactil, Novochlorpromazine*	Adults *Psychoses* Oral: Initially 50–100 mg/day; increase until desired effect occurs; usual maintenance range is 300–400 mg/day IM: Initially 25 mg; increase gradually up to 400 mg every 4–6 h until patient is quiet and cooperative; substitute oral dosage when possible	Used in acute and chronic psychoses, manic phase of manic–depressive psychoses, for pre- and postoperative sedation, intractable hiccups, acute intermittent porphyria, tetanus, and control of severe nausea and vomiting resulting from drugs, surgery, or toxins; plasma levels after IM injection are several times higher than after oral administration; duration of action ranges from 3–6 h; high incidence of drowsiness, dizziness, and hypotension, especially during first few weeks of therapy and in older

(continued)

Table 24-3. **Antipsychotic Drugs (Continued)**

Drug	Usual Dosage Range	Nursing Considerations
	Nausea/vomiting Oral: 10–25 mg every 4–6 h IM: 25–50 mg every 3–4 h Rectal: 50–100 mg every 6–8 h *Preoperative sedation* Oral: 25–50 mg IM: 12.5–25 mg *Porphyria* Oral: 25–50 mg 3–4 times/day IM: 25 mg 3–4 times/day Children Oral: 0.25 mg/lb 2–4 times/day Rectal: 0.5 mg/lb every 6–8 h IM: 0.125–0.25 mg/lb every 6–8 h IV: 0.25 mg/lb	patients; IV solution should be diluted to 1 mg/mL in saline and administered at a rate of 1 mg/min; doses in excess of 1,000 mg/day for prolonged periods are *not* recommended
Promazine *Sparine, Prozine*	*Adults* Initially: 50–150 mg IM Maintenance: 10–200 mg every 4–6 h orally *or* IM as required *Children* (older than 12): 10–25 mg every 4–6 h	Used primarily for management of psychotic disorders; the preferred parenteral route is IM; IV administration is recommended only in hospitalized patients; when used IV, injections should be given slowly in diluted solutions (25 mg/mL or less); concentrate for oral use should be diluted in fruit juice or other flavored vehicle (2 tsp of diluent for every 25 mg drug); less potent and equally toxic compared with chlorpromazine
Triflupromazine *Vesprin*	Adults *Psychoses* IM: 60–150 mg/day *Nausea/vomiting* IM: 5–15 mg every 4 h IV: 1–3 mg Children (older than 2 y) *Psychoses* IM: 0.2–0.25 mg/kg (maximum, 10 mg) *Nausea/vomiting* IM: 0.2–0.25 mg/kg (maximum, 10 mg)	Effective in psychotic disorders (other than psychotic depression) and for control of nausea and vomiting; sedation and extrapyramidal reactions are common, especially in the elderly and debilitated; has been used as an adjunct for pre- and postoperative management
Piperazines		
Acetophenazine *Tindal*	*Adults:* 20 mg 3 times/day (80–120 mg/day in hospitalized patients) *Children:* 0.8–1.6 mg/kg/day	Used for management of psychotic disorders. In patients with insomnia, last tablet should be taken 1 h before bedtime; infrequently used
Fluphenazine *Permitil, Prolixin* *(CAN) Apo-Fluphenazine, Modecate, Moditen*	*Oral* Initially: 2.5–10 mg/day; (maximum, 20 mg) Maintenance: 1–5 mg/day *IM* HCl: 1.25 mg 2–4 times/day (range 2.5–10 mg/day in divided doses) Enanthate/decanoate (esters in a sesame oil vehicle): 12.5–25 mg every 2–3 wk (may also be given SC); range, 12.5–100 mg at 1–3-wk intervals	Used for control of psychotic manifestations; oral dosage forms and HCl injection are rapid acting and can be used initially to stabilize patient; enanthate and decanoate salts are released slowly from tissue sites and thus have a prolonged effect (1–4 wk); indicated for maintenance therapy in patients who cannot be relied on to follow a regular oral dosage schedule; if given cautiously in *low doses,* may be useful in patients who are hypersensitive to other phenothiazines; very potent drug with high incidence of extrapyramidal reactions and mental depression; decanoate may have a lower incidence of extrapyramidal side effects than other dosage forms; monitor renal function and blood picture periodically in patients on long-term therapy; protect solutions from light and use dry syringe and needle for injection because moisture may cloud the solution; avoid use of antacids with oral dosage forms, because GI absorption is impaired; owing to prolonged effects of enanthate and decanoate salts, advise patients to report appearance of side effects *immediately;* not indicated in children
Perphenazine *Trilafon* *(CAN) Apo-Perphenazine,*	*Oral* Psychoses: 8–16 mg 2–4 times/day (maximum, 64 mg/day) initially; reduce to 4–8 mg 3 times/day for maintenance	Effective in psychoses and in the control of severe nausea and vomiting due to surgery or other acute situations; may also be effective in the management of anxiety and tension due to severe neurosis; *do not use* in children younger

(*continued*)

Table 24-3. **Antipsychotic Drugs (Continued)**

Drug	*Usual Dosage Range*	*Nursing Considerations*
PMS Levazine	Anxiety and tension states: 2–4 mg 3 times/day Nausea and vomiting: 8–16 mg/day in divided doses IM: Initially 5–10 mg; repeat every 6 h (maximum, 30 mg/day); switch to oral therapy as soon as possible IV (severe vomiting only): 1 mg/min infusion of a 0.5 mg/mL dilution (maximum, 5 mg)	than 12; high incidence of extrapyramidal reactions; transient hypotension can occur, especially IV; keep patient recumbent and monitor pulse and pressure; oral concentrate should be diluted (2 oz diluent/5 mL concentrate) with fruit juice, milk, carbonated beverage, or other liquid (tea is *not* recommended)
Prochlorperazine *Chlorpazine, Compazine* *(CAN) PMS-Prochlorperazine, Stemetil*	Adults *Psychoses* Oral: 10 mg 3–4 times/day, increased gradually until maximum effect (usually 100–150 mg/day) IM: 10–20 mg initially; repeat in 2–4 h; switch to oral form as soon as possible *Nausea/vomiting* Oral: 5–10 mg 3–4 times/day Rectal: 25 mg 2 times/day IM: 5–10 mg; repeat every 3–4 h to a maximum of 40 mg/day IV (severe vomiting): 5–10 mg IV injection or 20 mg added to 1 L IV infusion 15–30 min before induction of anesthesia Children (older than 2 y and more than 20 lb) *Psychoses* Oral/rectal: 2.5 mg 2–3 times/day IM: 0.06 mg/lb *Nausea/vomiting* Oral/rectal: 2.5–5 mg 1–2 times/day based on weight IM: 0.06 mg/lb	Used for control of psychotic manifestations in adults and children older than 2 years and for relief of nausea and vomiting; widely used pre- and postoperatively; do not use in short-term vomiting in children or for vomiting of unknown cause; discontinue if signs of restlessness or excitement occur; inject deeply IM (avoid SC use) and do not mix solution with other agents in same syringe; do not confuse *2.5-mg* child suppository with *25-mg* adult suppository; use cautiously in the elderly or debiliated patients and in children who are dehydrated or who have an acute illness because extrapyramidal reactions are common; monitor blood pressure during IV use because hypotension is likely to occur; supervise ambulation after parenteral use
Trifluoperazine *Stelazine* *(CAN) Apo-Trifluoperazine*	*Adults* Oral: Initially 2–5 mg twice a day (maximum, 40 mg/day); maintenance: 1–2 mg twice a day IM: 1–2 mg every 4–6 h (maximum, 10 mg/day) *Children* (older than 6 y) Oral: 1 mg 1–2 times/day (maximum, 15 mg/day in older children) IM: 1 mg 1–2 times/day	Indicated for treatment of psychotic disorders and for controlling manifestations of severe psychoneuroses; very potent agent with high incidence of extrapyramidal reactions; maximum response may be delayed 2–3 weeks; increase dosage very slowly in elderly or debilitated patients; prolonged action of the drug allows once-a-day dosing in many less severe cases; dilute concentrate in 60 mL of appropriate vehicle (liquid or semisolid) to aid palatability; do not give IM injections more frequently than every 4 h because of danger of cumulation
Piperidines		
Mesoridazine *Serentil*	*Psychoses* Oral: Initially 25–50 mg 3 times/day (range, 100–400 mg/day) IM: 25 mg; repeat in 30–60 min if necessary (range, 25–200 mg/day) *Neuroses* Oral: 10 mg 3 times/day (range, 30–150 mg/day) *Alcoholism* 25 mg twice a day (range, 50–200 mg/day)	Used for treatment of schizophrenia, chronic brain syndrome, and psychoneuroses, and as adjunctive therapy in acute and chronic alcoholism; weak antiemetic; low incidence of extrapyramidal reactions but very sedating; may reduce hyperactive behavior associated with mentally deficient states; *not recommended in children younger than 12;* concentrate should be diluted before use
Thioridazine *Mellaril* *(CAN) Apo-Thioridazine, Novoridazine, PMS Thioridazine*	Adults *Psychoses* Initially: 50–100 mg 3 times/day; maintenance 200–800 mg/day in 2–4 divided doses *Depressive neuroses* Initially: 25 mg 3 times/day Maintenance: 20–200 mg/day in 3–4 divided doses *Children* (older than 2 y): 0.5–3.0 mg/kg/day depending on severity of condition	Indicated for psychotic disorders and short-term treatment of depressive neuroses; possibly useful in hyperactive or aggressive children, alcohol withdrawal, intractable pain, and senility; low incidence of extrapyramidal reactions and no antiemetic action, but strong anticholinergic effect and highly sedating; abnormal ECG readings have occurred, especially at high doses; may be potentially cardiotoxic; frequently produces dryness of the mouth, constipation, urinary retention, and impotence in early stages of therapy; discontinue drug or reduce dosage if visual changes (reduced or brownish vision, impaired night vision) occur; periodic blood and liver function tests should be performed during prolonged therapy; dilute oral concentrate immediately before use with fruit juice or water

(*continued*)

Table 24-3. **Antipsychotic Drugs (Continued)**

Drug	*Usual Dosage Range*	*Nursing Considerations*
THIOXANTHENES		
Chlorprothixene *Taractan* *(CAN) Tarasan*	*Adults* Oral: Initially 25–50 mg 3–4 times/day; increase to optimal level (maximum, 600 mg/day) IM: 25–50 mg 3–4 times/day; substitute oral therapy as soon as possible *Children* Oral: 10–25 mg 3–4 times/day IM: Age more than 12 y, same as adult dose	Effective in acute and chronic schizophrenia; produces significant sedation and orthostatic hypotension; when used IM, keep patient recumbent during administration; do *not* give IM in children younger than 12, or orally in children younger than 6; anticholinergic side effects are prominent
Thiothixene *Navane*	Oral: Initially 2–5 mg 2–3 times/day; maintenance 20–60 mg/day in divided doses IM: 4 mg 2–4 times/day (usual range, 16–20 mg/day)	Used for management of acute and chronic schizophrenia; *not* for use in children younger than 12; high incidence of extrapyramidal reactions and drowsiness in early stages of therapy; therapeutic effects may take several weeks to develop with oral administration; do not withdraw drug abruptly because delirium can occur; dosage may need to be adjusted when switching from IM to oral administration

Interactions

Antipsychotic drugs potentiate effects of other CNS depressants (eg, alcohol, barbiturates, general anesthetics, antianxiety agents, narcotic analgesics).

Additive anticholinergic effects may be observed with concomitant use of antipsychotic drugs and other agents having anticholinergic activity (eg, antihistamines, tricyclic antidepressants, antiparkinsonian drugs).

Effects of antipsychotics may be enhanced by estrogens, progestins, anticholinesterases, furazolidone, and monoamine oxidase (MAO) inhibitors.

Hypotensive action of antipsychotic drugs can be increased by antihypertensives, epinephrine, thiazide diuretics, and tricyclic antidepressants.

Antipsychotic drugs may decrease the effectiveness of amphetamines, oral anticoagulants, heparin, anticonvulsants (lowering of seizure threshold), oral hypoglycemics, levodopa, and other antiparkinsonian drugs.

The hypoglycemic effect of insulin may be potentiated by antipsychotics.

Absorption of antipsychotic agents can be impaired by antacids and antidiarrheal preparations.

Lithium and other antipsychotic drugs may exert additive hyperglycemic effects.

The combination of antipsychotic drugs and griseofulvin may precipitate acute porphyria.

Narcotic analgesics may increase the respiratory-depressant action of the antipsychotics.

Antipsychotics can reduce the effectiveness of guanethidine by interfering with its neuronal uptake.

Antipsychotic drugs can potentiate muscle relaxants, possibly resulting in prolonged apnea.

Additive cardiac depressant effects may occur with quinidine and antipsychotic drugs.

Antipsychotic-induced extrapyramidal effects can be reduced by anticholinergic antiparkinsonian drugs, piperazine, and diphenhydramine.

Nursing Management

Pretherapy Assessment

Assess and record baseline data necessary for detection of adverse effects of antipsychotic drugs: General: vital signs (VS), body weight, skin color and temperature; CNS: orientation, affect, reflexes, intraocular pressure (IOP); Cardiovascular system (CVS): orthostatic blood pressure (BP), ECG; GI: liver evaluation, bowel sounds, normal output; Genitourinary (GU): prostate palpation, normal output; Lab: renal, thyroid, and liver function tests, CBC, electroencephalogram (EEG).

Review medical history and documents for existing or previous conditions that:

a. require cautious use of antipsychotic drugs: glaucoma; prostatic hypertrophy; epilepsy; diabetes; chronic respiratory disorders; liver impairment; children younger than 6 years; exposure to extreme heat or organophosphate insecticides.
b. contraindicate use of antipsychotic drugs: allergy to individual drugs; bone marrow depression; blood dyscrasias; parkinsonism; jaundice; liver damage; renal insufficiency; cerebral arteriosclerosis; coronary disease; mitral insufficiency; severe hypertension; chronic alcoholism; coma; subcortical brain damage; thyrotoxicosis; breast cancer; **pregnancy (Category C)**, lactation (secreted in breast milk; discontinue either drug or nursing the infant).

Nursing Interventions

Medication Administration

Keep patient flat for at least 1 hour after parenteral administration of nondepot form, and monitor blood pressure often. Marked hypotension can be treated by placing patient in head-low position and, if necessary, using volume expanders and pressor agents such as levarterenol or dopamine. Epinephrine is *contraindicated*: it can have a reverse effect and aggravate hypotension.

Avoid drug contact with skin or mucous membranes because contact dermatitis can occur.

Discard discolored injectable solutions. Do not mix other solutions in same syringe. Give deep intramuscular injection.

Do not change brands of oral dosage forms or rectal suppositories because bioavailability differences have been documented.

Do not allow patient to chew or crush sustained-release capsules.

Always dilute drug for intravenous injection to a concentration of 1 mg/mL or less.

Supervise emotionally disturbed patient to ascertain that medication is swallowed. Syrup, injection, or depot injection forms may help ensure that patient receives prescribed dose.

Implement measures to prevent constipation (increased intake of fluid and dietary roughage), and monitor bowel and bladder function during prolonged therapy because constipation and urinary retention can occur. A dosage reduction should be considered if these conditions become problematic.

Arrange to discontinue drug gradually after high-dose therapy; gastritis, nausea, dizziness, headache, tachycardia, and insomnia have occurred after abrupt withdrawal.

Protect oral concentrate from light.

Surveillance During Therapy

Monitor for toxicity.

Monitor patient frequently for appearance of fine, wormlike movements of the tongue, an early sign of tardive dyskinesia, which usually develops only during long-term (6–24 months) treatment. Symptoms (see **Significant Adverse Reactions**) may be irreversible; prompt cessation of therapy at onset of the developing syndrome can minimize severity. Antiparkinsonian drugs do *not* alleviate these symptoms and may aggravate them.

Be alert for onset of acute dystonic reactions (ie, neck spasms, eye rolling, dysphagia, convulsions), especially in children with acute illnesses (eg, mumps, measles, severe infections) or who are dehydrated, because they are more susceptible than adults. These reactions are very frightening to most patients. If one occurs, advise practitioner, remain with patient to provide reassurance, and be prepared to discontinue drug.

Assist with periodic evaluation of patient on long-term therapy. Dosage should be kept as low as possible, and drug-free intervals should be employed where possible to minimize incidence of untoward reactions, particularly extrapyramidal syndromes. Antiparkinsonian medication should not be used to *prevent* extrapyramidal reactions. If symptoms appear during therapy, an attempt should be made to eliminate them by reducing the dose of the antipsychotic drug. If symptoms persist, the antiparkinsonian drug should be carefully titrated so that the smallest dose that relieves the symptoms is used (see Chapter 28).

Monitor blood pressure of hospitalized patient before each dose during initial treatment period. Employ appropriate interventions to protect patient from injury caused by orthostatic hypotension.

If patient is on long-term therapy, monitor results of renal function tests. If serum creatinine is elevated, drug dosage may need to be reduced.

Monitor diabetic patient for signs of altered carbohydrate metabolism such as glycosuria, weight loss, and polyphagia. Dosage alterations or dietary changes may be warranted.

Carefully monitor laboratory studies and patient for indications of adverse reactions.

Interpret results of diagnostic tests and contact practitioner as appropriate.

Cautiously interpret results of laboratory tests for pregnancy, iodine-131 uptake, urinary catecholamines, urinary ketones, bilirubin, and steroids, because phenothiazines may interfere with these tests.

Monitor for possible drug–drug and drug–nutrient interactions: See **interactions**.

Provide for patient safety needs if CNS changes occur.

Patient Teaching

Discuss the importance of maintaining a regular dosing schedule, especially during initial stages, because it sometimes takes several weeks for beneficial effects to become manifest. Stress the need for regular follow-up care.

Encourage patient to continue long-term therapy. Another person may need to assume responsibility for ensuring that patient takes medication. *Abrupt* stoppage, particularly if dosage is high, could cause gastritis, vomiting, dizziness, tremors, insomnia, and psychotic behavior. The drug should be withdrawn gradually over several weeks (eg, 10%–25% reduction in dosage every 2 weeks).

Reassure patient that many side effects (drowsiness, dry mouth) are common early in therapy but usually disappear. Others, such as orthostatic hypotension, extrapyramidal reactions, and sedation, may be minimized by selection of proper agent.

Inform patient that no other drugs, including over-the-counter (OTC) preparations, should be taken without consulting the healthcare provider or pharmacist.

Teach patient early signs of blood dyscrasia (fever, sore throat, mucosal irritation, fatigue, upper respiratory infection) that need to be reported to practitioner immediately.

Caution patient not to operate dangerous machinery during initial stages of therapy because drowsiness is common.

Teach patient measures that help control orthostatic hypotension.

Instruct patient to inform practitioner if fever, abdominal pain, rash, itching, diarrhea, or yellowing of skin (signs of developing jaundice) appear.

Suggest interventions to alleviate mouth dryness. Stress meticulous oral hygiene to prevent development of oral candidiasis, especially if oral concentrate is used.

Explain endocrine disturbances that could occur: menstrual irregularities, gynecomastia, breast engorgement, impotence, and altered libido. Reassure patient that it may be possible for practitioners to minimize such changes by adjusting the dosage or substituting another drug.

Instruct patient to be alert for indications of decreased visual acuity, photophobia, and brownish discoloration of objects in visual field, symptoms that call for immediate ophthalmologic examination.

Advise patient to avoid direct sunlight and to use sunscreen lotion because photosensitivity reactions can occur.

Inform patient that drug may discolor the urine (pink to red–brown). Explain that this is not serious and does not necessitate interruption of therapy.

• **Lithium** *(Pregnancy Category D)*

Cibalith-S, Eskalith, Lithane, Lithonate, Lithotabs

(CAN) Carbolith, Duralith, Lithizine

An alkali metal ion effective in the control of the manic phase of manic-depressive psychoses, lithium calms the agitated patient, smoothing out the wide swings in mood between mania and depression. Toxic effects are closely related to serum levels; in many cases, the effective therapeutic level is very near the toxic concentration. Therefore, repeated serum levels should be determined in all patients taking the drug (see **Dosage**).

Mechanism

Specific mechanism for control of mania is unknown. Lithium decreases the release of second messengers in cell membranes by blocking the recycling of inositol substrates, possibly reducing excitatory cholinergic activity; the drug can also alter sodium transport at the nerve ending, thereby changing the electrophysiologic characteristics of nerve cells; decreased norepinephrine turnover and increased serotonin-receptor sensitivity may also play a role in its antimanic action.

Uses

Control of manic symptoms (ie, motor hyperactivity, talkativeness, restlessness, poor judgment, grandiose ideation, aggressiveness, and possibly hostility)

Prophylaxis of recurrent manic-depressive episodes in patients with classic bipolar affective disorder

Adjunctive therapy of psychoses associated with excitement

Investigational uses include management of violent, aggressive behavior in prisoners; prophylaxis of cluster headache and frequent, cyclic migraine attacks; and improvement of the neutrophil count in patients with chronic neutropenia or cancer chemotherapy–induced neutropenia

Dosage

Acute mania: 600 mg 3 times/day (desired serum level is 1.0–1.5 mEq/L); adjust oral dosage to optimal clinical response as well as desired serum level; clinical effects begin to appear within 4 to 7 days.

Prophylaxis: 300 mg 3 to 4 times/day (serum levels 0.6–1.2 mEq/L)

NOTE: Blood samples for determination of serum lithium levels should be taken 12 hours after the night (PM) dose

Fate

Rapidly absorbed orally; peak serum levels in 1 to 2 hours, although optimal clinical response may take a week or more to develop; widely distributed in the body; very little is protein bound; crosses blood–brain barrier; excreted through the kidneys (half-life [$T_{1/2}$] approximately 24 hours), the rate being directly proportional to its plasma concentration; excretion is reduced by low sodium levels (eg, during a low-sodium diet and when diuretic drugs are taken)

Common Side Effects

Fine hand tremors, nausea, thirst, polyuria, fatigue, mild muscle weakness (usually subside with continued therapy)

Significant Adverse Reactions

Usually observed at serum levels above 1.5 mEq/L but can occur at lower concentrations; moderate to severe toxic reactions may develop at levels equal to—or above—2.0 mEq/L.

Neuromuscular: lack of coordination, ataxia, muscle hyperirritability and twitching, choreiform movements, extrapyramidal-like symptoms, coarse hand tremor

CNS: drowsiness, dizziness, restlessness, confusion, slurred speech, tinnitus, incontinence, psychomotor retardation, epileptic-like seizures, stupor, coma

Autonomic: dry mouth, blurred vision

CV: hypotension, arrhythmias, bradycardia, edema, circulatory collapse

GI: anorexia, vomiting, diarrhea, abdominal pain

Urinary: albuminuria, glycosuria, oliguria

Dermatologic: rash, pruritus, thinning of hair, folliculitis, topical anesthesia, acneiform eruptions, cutaneous ulceration

Other: hypothyroidism, transient hyperglycemia, excessive weight gain, leukocytosis, scotomas, flattening and inversion of the T wave, worsening of psoriasis

Contraindications

Severe renal or cardiovascular disease, organic brain syndrome, sodium depletion (low-salt diet, diuretic therapy, dehydration), early pregnancy, and in children younger than 12. *Cautious use* in elderly, debilitated, or dehydrated persons and in the presence of epilepsy or thyroid disease.

Interactions

Effects of lithium may be decreased by acetazolamide, alkalinizing agents (eg, sodium bicarbonate, antacids), aminophylline, caffeine, excess sodium chloride, and urea, all substances that increase its excretion.

Toxic effects of lithium may be intensified by use of diuretics (sodium loss), methyldopa, antipsychotic drugs, phenytoin, carbamazepine, mazindol, and indomethacin.

Combinations of lithium and haloperidol may produce severe encephalopathic symptoms such as parkinsonism, dyskinesias, and dementia.

Profound hypothermia may occur with simultaneous use of benzodiazepines.

Lithium may reduce the pressor effects of sympathomimetic drugs.

Lithium may prolong the effects of neuromuscular blocking agents.

Nursing Management

Pretherapy Assessment

Assess and record baseline data necessary for detection of adverse effects of lithium: General: VS, body weight, skin color, and temperature; CNS: orientation, affect, reflexes, ophthalmologic examination; GI: bowel sounds, normal output; GU: normal output; Lab: renal, thyroid, and liver function tests, CBC with differential, ECG.

Review medical history and documents for existing or previous conditions that:

a. require cautious use of lithium: use in the elderly; dehydration; epilepsy; thyroid disease

b. contraindicate use of lithium: allergy to tartrazine; severe renal or cardiovascular disease; organic brain syndrome; sodium depletion; children younger than 12 years; **pregnancy (Category D)**, lactation (secreted in breast milk; discontinue either drug or nursing the infant).

Nursing Interventions

Medication Administration

Administer drug with food or milk or after meal.

Decrease dose after acute manic symptoms subside.

Provide small, frequent meals and mouth care if GI effects occur.

Consult with prescriber if GI irritation occurs. Administration with meals or use of sustained-release forms or smaller, more frequent doses may help. Monitor results of serum level determinations to ensure that they remain consistent.

Surveillance During Therapy

Monitor serum levels, which should be obtained at least monthly in stabilized outpatient but as frequently as every other day during initial dosing phase. Toxic effects frequently develop when serum level exceeds 1.5 mEq/L.

Expect dosages to be much higher during the acute phase of treatment. To minimize toxicity, dosage should be reduced proportionately as therapeutic effects become evident.

Evaluate patient's response to drug. Optimum therapeutic effects usually occur 7 to 14 days after initiation of treatment. Therapy should *not* be continued beyond 4 weeks if no response is evident.

Test urine periodically for specific gravity, and note signs of polydipsia and polyuria. These are common in the elderly and do not seem to be dose related; if these symptoms are severe, therapy may need to be discontinued.

Observe for signs of developing hypothyroidism (eg, fatigue, weight gain, cold intolerance, puffy face). Symptoms are reversible on cessation of therapy but may be controlled by supplemental thyroxine without discontinuing lithium therapy.

Provide supplemental fluid and salt in cases of prolonged sweating or diarrhea.

Carefully monitor laboratory studies and patient for indications of adverse reactions.

Interpret results of diagnostic tests and contact practitioner as appropriate.

Cautiously interpret results of laboratory tests for pregnancy, ^{131}I uptake, urinary catecholamines, urinary ketones, bilirubin, and steroids because phenothiazines may interfere with these tests.

Monitor for possible drug–drug and drug–nutrient interactions: See **Interactions**.

Patient Teaching

Instruct patient to consult practitioner immediately if signs of toxicity appear, such as diarrhea, vomiting, drowsiness, muscle weakness, ataxia, or tremor.

Stress the importance of adequate intake of salt and 2,500 to 3,000 mL fluid per day. Reduced fluid intake can slow lithium excretion, resulting in increased toxicity.

Caution patient about engaging in activities requiring alertness until reaction to lithium has been established. The drug may cause significant drowsiness and impaired coordination.

Teach patient to check for ankle or wrist edema and to record weekly weight. Sudden changes should be reported to drug prescriber.

• Pimozide

Orap

Pimozide is a centrally acting dopamine receptor antagonist used to suppress severe motor and phonic tics in patients with Gilles de la Tourette's syndrome (disorder characterized by unpredictable and spontaneous outbursts of foul language or barking sounds and other motor abnormalities). Some cases have been successfully managed by haloperidol, another dopamine antagonist, but pimozide appears to be most effective in treating resistant cases.

Prolonged use of pimozide is associated with a high frequency of tardive dyskinesias (as discussed earlier in this chapter with other antipsychotic agents), and dosage must be kept as low as possible to minimize the likelihood of tardive dyskinesias developing. Extrapyramidal reactions occur frequently, often during the first few days of treatment. Their severity and frequency are dose related and are usually reversible with dosage reduction. Many other untoward reactions have occurred in patients receiving pimozide, most of which are also seen with antipsychotic drug use. Refer to earlier **Significant Adverse Reactions** section (ie, other antipsychotics) for a complete listing of potential adverse effects.

Pimozide is *contraindicated* in persons with a history of cardiac arrhythmias or QT interval disturbances, because sudden death has occurred because of ventricular arrhythmias. The drug must be given *with caution* to patients with impaired renal or hepatic function and during pregnancy and nursing. Pimozide may lower the convulsive threshold and may therefore interfere with the action of anticonvulsants, and it can potentiate the effects of other CNS depressants.

The initial dose of pimozide (tablets) is 1 to 2 mg daily in divided doses. Dosage may be gradually increased every other day until an optimal effect is noted. Usual maintenance doses are 10 mg/day or less. Periodic attempts should be made to reduce the dose to see if the tics persist.

Nursing Management

Refer to **Phenothiazines**. In addition:

Patient Teaching

Explain that a baseline ECG is usually prescribed before initiation of therapy. An ECG should also be obtained periodically throughout therapy, especially during periods of dosage adjustment, because cardiotoxicity can occur.

Warn patient to use caution in driving a car or engaging in potentially hazardous activities because hand tremors, drowsiness, and blurred vision may occur.

Teach patient and family how to recognize and report symptoms of extrapyramidal reactions. If dosage reduction fails to alleviate symptoms of a reaction, drug should be discontinued.

Inform patient that concomitant use of other CNS depressant drugs, including alcohol, augment CNS depressant effects of pimozide.

Discuss interventions to help alleviate dry mouth.

Discuss measures to minimize constipation (eg, increased intake of fluid and dietary fiber).

Instruct patient to report other symptoms of anticholinergic effects (eg, urinary retention, ataxia, dizziness). These may necessitate dosage reduction.

• Droperidol

Inapsine

Droperidol is a butyrophenone producing tranquilization, sedation, and mild peripheral vascular dilation. It has a strong antiemetic effect and can potentiate the action of other CNS depressants. Droperidol is principally used in combination with a narcotic analgesic (fentanyl) as Innovar (see Chapter 19) to induce neuroleptanalgesia (condition of tranquility, reduced motor activity, and indifference to pain. Alone, droperidol is given to provide tranquilization, to reduce nausea and vomiting during surgical and diagnostic procedures, and as an adjunct to regional or general anesthesia.

The onset of action with intramuscular or intravenous use is 3 to 10 minutes; the duration is 2 to 4 hours, although altered consciousness may persist up to 12 hours.

Mild hypotension and tachycardia are common side effects and usually subside spontaneously. Postsurgical drowsiness is also a frequent occurrence with use of droperidol, especially when it is given as an adjunct to general anesthesia. Extrapyramidal reactions occur in approximately 1% of patients. Other untoward reactions reported include dizziness, shivering, bronchospasm, and postoperative hallucinations. When used in combination with fentanyl, respiratory depression, muscle rigidity, and elevated blood pressure have been noted.

Droperidol should be used *cautiously* in elderly, debilitated, and other poor-risk patients; during pregnancy; in children younger than 2 years; and in the presence of liver, kidney, or cardiac dysfunction.

Recommended dosage for the indications for droperidol are as follows:

Adults

Premedication: 2.5 to 10 mg IM 30 to 60 minutes preoperatively

Adjunct to general anesthesia: 2.5 mg/9.1 kg to 11.4 kg IV during induction

Maintenance: 1.25 to 2.5 mg IV

Diagnostic procedures: 2.5 to 10 mg IM 30 to 60 minutes before procedure, then 1.25 to 2.5 mg IV as needed

Children (2–12 years of age)

1 to 1.5 mg/9.1kg to 11.4 kg for premedication or induction of anesthesia

Nursing Management

Refer to **Phenothiazines**. In addition:

Nursing Interventions

Surveillance During Therapy

Monitor vital signs closely during use. Have fluids, vasopressors, and other necessary measures at hand to manage hypotension should it occur. Do *not* use epinephrine because reversal of pressor effect can occur, worsening the hypotension.

Observe for additive depressant effects when narcotics or other CNS depressants are used. Dosage of other CNS depressants should be reduced in the presence of droperidol.

Assess for early signs of respiratory depression such as dyspnea, restlessness, and rigidity when used with fentanyl (as Innovar), especially if rapid intravenous injection is given. Be prepared to provide respiratory assistance, and have necessary resuscitative equipment available (eg, endotracheal tube, oxygen, suction apparatus).

Exercise care in moving and positioning patient after administration of droperidol because orthostatic hypotension may develop.

Observe for development of extrapyramidal reactions, which may occur up to 1 to 2 days after administration. They can usually be controlled with an antiparkinsonian agent.

Assist patient with ambulation and other activities postoperatively until drowsiness disappears.

Carefully evaluate reaction of elderly or debilitated patient to initial dose, which should be small. Incremental doses should be based on response.

• Methotrimeprazine

Levoprome

(CAN) Nozinan

A phenothiazine derivative having a profound CNS-depressant effect, methotrimeprazine produces sedation, reduced motor activity, amnesia, and analgesia (comparable to morphine) but rarely produces respiratory depression. There is a high incidence of orthostatic hypotension and sedation, but most other phenothiazine-related side effects (eg, extrapyramidal symptoms, anticholinergic effects) occur less frequently than with other antipsychotic drugs; it has no antitussive action.

The principal indication for use of methotrimeprazine is for relief of moderate to severe pain in nonambulatory patients. Additional uses include obstetrical analgesia when respiratory depression is to be avoided, and as a preanesthetic agent to produce somnolence and reduce anxiety and fear.

The principal side effect of methotrimeprazine is orthostatic hypotension, accompanied by weakness and fainting. This effect can be avoided by keeping the patient supine for at least 6 hours after the injection. The orthostatic hypotensive effect generally diminishes with continued administration. Other adverse effects include nausea and vomiting, abdominal discomfort, disorientation, weakness, urinary hesitancy, xerostomia, nasal congestion, pain and inflammation at the injection site, and agranulocytosis and jaundice with prolonged high-dose therapy.

Use of methotrimeprazine is *contraindicated* in the presence of severe myocardial, renal, or hepatic disease; significant hypotension; and in patients receiving antihypertensive drugs or CNS depressants, because additive effects can occur. The drug should not be used longer than 30 days, except where narcotics are contraindicated or in terminal illnesses. When used for prolonged periods, regular liver function tests and blood studies should be performed.

Methotrimeprazine is given by deep intramuscular injection into a large muscle mass. Intravenous and subcutaneous administration should be avoided. Usual dosage ranges are as follows:

Analgesia: 10 to 20 mg IM every 4 to 6 hours (5–10 mg in elderly patients)

Obstetrical analgesia: 15 to 20 mg IM; repeat as needed

Preanesthetic sedation: 10 to 20 mg IM 1 to 3 hours before surgery, often with atropine or scopolamine in reduced doses

Postoperative analgesia: 2.5 to 7.5 mg IM every 4 to 6 hours as needed

Because methotrimeprazine is a phenothiazine derivative, refer to the discussion of antipsychotic drugs earlier in the chapter for additional information on potential adverse effects as well as drug interactions.

Nursing Management

Refer to **Phenothiazines**. In addition:

Nursing Interventions

Medication Administration

Keep patient recumbent for at least 6 hours after administration to avoid orthostatic hypotension. Supervise ambulation and provide assistance as needed.

Monitor blood pressure and pulse frequently until response stabilizes. If vasopressors are needed to combat hypotension, methoxamine or phenylephrine should be used. Epinephrine is *contraindicated* because reversal can occur.

Administer only by deep intramuscular injection and in a syringe separate from other drugs (except atropine or scopolamine), because incompatibility can result.

Clarify appropriateness of long-term administration, because drug should not be used longer than 30 days, except where narcotics are contraindicated or in terminal illness. When used for prolonged periods, liver function tests and blood studies should be performed regularly.

Selected Bibliography

Ananth J, Johnson K: Psychotropic and medical drug interactions. Psychother Psychosom 58:178, 1992

Balant-Gorgia AE, Balant LP, Andreoli A: Pharmacokinetic optimisation of the treatment of psychosis. Clin Pharmacokinet 25(3):217, 1993

Baldessarini RJ, Frankenburg FR: Clozapine: A novel antipsychotic drug. N Engl J Med 324:746, 1991

Bergen J, Kitchin R, Berry G: Predictors of the course of tardive dyskinesia in patients receiving neuroleptics. Biol Psychiatry 32:580, 1992

Breier A et al: Effects of clozapine on positive and negative symptoms in outpatients with schizophrenia. Am J Psychiatry 151:20, 1994

Farde L et al: Positron emission tomographic analysis of central D_1 and D_2 dopamine receptor occupancy in patients treated with classical neuroleptics and clozapine. Arch Gen Psychiatry 49:538, 1992

Gerner RH: Treatment of acute mania. Psychiatr Clin North Am 16:443, 1993

Green AI et al: Clozapine response and plasma catecholamines and their metabolites. Psychiatry Res 46:39, 1993

Greenblatt DJ: Basic pharmacokinetic principles and their application to psychotropic drugs. J Clin Psychiatry 54(9, suppl):8, 1993

Hamner MB, Diamond BI: Elevated plasma dopamine in post-traumatic stress disorder: A preliminary report. Biol Psychiatry 33:304, 1993

Khot V et al: The assessment and clinical implications of haloperidol acute-dose, steady-state, and withdrawal pharmacokinetics. J Clin Psychopharmacol 13:120, 1993

Koreen AR et al: Relation of plasma fluphenazine levels to treatment response and extrapyramidal side effects in first-episode schizophrenic patients. Am J Psychiatry 151:35, 1994

Levinson DF: Pharmacologic treatment of schizophrenia. Clin Ther 13:326, 1991

Nordstrom A-L et al: Central D_2-dopamine receptor occupancy in relation to antipsychotic drug effects: A double-blind PET study of schizophrenic patients. Biol Psychiatry 33:227, 1993

Reynolds GP: Developments in the drug treatment of schizophrenia. Trends Pharmacol Sci 13:116, 1992

Seeman P: Dopamine receptor sequences: Therapeutic levels of neuroleptics occupy D_2 receptors; clozapine occupies D_4 Neuropsychopharmacology 7:261, 1992

Schou M: Is there a lithium withdrawal syndrome? An examination of the evidence. Br J Psychiatry 163:514, 1993

Schwartz JT, Brotman AW: A clinical guide to antipsychotic drugs. Drugs 44(6):981, 1992

Nursing Bibliography

Foley J: Consideration in the use of benzodiazepine and antipsychotics in the emergency department. Journal of Emergency Nursing 19(5): 448–450, 1993

Forman L: Medication: Reasons and intervention for non-compliance. Journal of Psychosocial Nursing and Mental Health Services 31(10): 23–25, 1993

Glod C: Psychopharmacology and clinical practice. Nursing Clinics of North America 26(2):375–400, 1991

Johnston B: Let's talk about drugs. Psychotropic Medications Home Health Care Nurse 11(3):42–49, 1993

25
Antianxiety Drugs

Benzodiazepines
- Alprazolam
- Chlordiazepoxide
- Clorazepate
- Diazepam
- Halazepam
- Lorazepam
- Midazolam
- Oxazepam
- Prazepam

Benzodiazepine Antagonist
- Flumazenil

Miscellaneous
- Buspirone
- Chlormezanone
- Hydroxyzine
- Meprobamate

Drugs classified as *antianxiety agents* reduce anxiety and tension in doses that, generally, do not impair mental alertness or psychomotor performance; however, sedation can occur within the therapeutic range. Unfortunately, antianxiety agents are often abused.

Pharmacologically, antianxiety drugs are similar to barbiturates in many ways; however, their principal advantage is a significantly higher **hypnotic dose: sedative dose ratio** than that of barbiturates. In other words, the margin between the hypnotic (sleep-inducing) dose and the calming (tension-relieving) dose is much greater with most antianxiety agents than with the barbiturates. Likewise, their safety margin (toxic dose: therapeutic dose ratio) is wider than that of barbiturates. The primary use is to provide a degree of relief from emotional symptoms (such as agitation, anxiety, muscle tension, and motor hyperactivity) associated with neurotic and psychosomatic disorders. However, antianxiety drugs are rarely effective when used **alone** to control severely disturbed psychotic patients; they have been successfully employed when combined with antipsychotic drugs for treatment of acute psychotic episodes.

In contrast to the antipsychotic drugs, however, antianxiety agents have a low incidence of adverse reactions when administered in normal therapeutic doses. Moreover, their central skeletal muscle-relaxant action may contribute to their effectiveness in treating emotional disorders compounded by excessive muscular tension or spasm. Prolonged use of antianxiety agents produces tolerance and physical dependence. In addition, psychological dependence (addiction) is more likely to occur than with the antipsychotic drugs.

Most antianxiety agents also have clinically significant anticonvulsant activity when administered intravenously and can effectively control acute convulsive states such as status epilepticus or those associated with acute alcohol withdrawal. Their use is not accompanied by extrapyramidal reactions or autonomic nervous system side effects.

The currently available antianxiety agents can be conveniently classified as either "benzodiazepines" (eg, alprazolam, chlordiazepoxide, and diazepam) or "miscellaneous" (eg, buspirone, hydroxyzine, meprobamate).

Benzodiazepines

The benzodiazepines are the most widely used antianxiety agents. Much of their popularity derives from their demonstrated effectiveness at dosage levels that are not associated with the high risk of untoward reactions, such as respiratory depression that is characteristic of prolonged barbiturate consumption. The benzodiazepines discussed in this chapter are indicated primarily for the relief of situational anxiety. Other benzodiazepines have somewhat different indications and are found elsewhere in this book. Midazolam, a short-acting agent used IM or IV as an adjunct in minor surgical procedures, is reviewed after the general discussion of the benzodiazepines. Estazolam, flurazepam, quazepam, temazepam, and triazolam are effective nonbarbiturate hypnotics used to relieve insomnia; they are reviewed in Chapter 23. Clonazepam is used to treat epilepsy and bipolar affective disorders and is discussed in Chapter 27.

The effectiveness of benzodiazepines in relieving symptoms of anxiety over prolonged periods has not been conclusively established; these drugs should not be used for longer than 3 to 4 months unless careful patient reassessment establishes a definite need for continued treatment.

Although all clinically useful benzodiazepines share many common pharmacologic properties (mild sedation, skeletal muscle relaxation, anticonvulsant action) and are similar in clinical effectiveness, they differ significantly in their duration of action, which is largely dependent on whether they are converted to active or inactive metabolites. Table 25-1 lists usual doses, onset of action, metabolic activity, and elimination half-lives ($T_{1/2}$) of the benzodiazepine antianxiety drugs. The benzodiazepines are first discussed as a group; characteristics of each individual agent are then outlined in Table 25-2.

Mechanism

Act at several subcortical brain sites such as the limbic system and the midbrain reticular formation; higher cortical function is largely unaffected. Primary mechanism of action is to enhance activity of gamma-aminobutyric acid (GABA), an inhibitory neurotransmitter in the central nervous system (CNS); benzodiazepines increase the **frequency** of the opening of the $GABA_A$-activated Cl^- channel; more Cl^- flows inside the cell, causing hyperpolarization—and stabilization—of the cell membrane; enhancement of GABA activity in the spinal cord decreases activity in motor reflex pathways, resulting in skeletal muscle relaxation; the seizure threshold is elevated, resulting in a clinically significant anticonvulsant action for certain derivatives; unlike barbiturates, the benzodiazepines do not significantly depress the respiratory or vasomotor centers and do not cause enzyme induction.

Table 25-1. **Oral Benzodiazepine Metabolism**

Drug	Usual Daily Dosage Range (mg)	Onset of Action	Activity of Metabolites	Elimination Half-Life (h)
Alprazolam *Xanax*	0.75–1.5	Moderate	Inactive*	10–15
Chlordiazepoxide *Librium*	15–100	Moderate	Active	5–30
Clorazepate *Tranxene*	15–60	Fast	Active	30–90
Diazepam *Valium*	4–40	Very fast	Active	20–80
Halazepam *Paxipam*	80–160	Slow	Active	12–15
Lorazepam *Ativan*	2–8	Moderate	Inactive	10–20
Oxazepam *Serax*	30–120	Slow	Inactive	5–15
Prazepam *Centrax*	20–60	Slow	Active	30–100

* One metabolite is inactive and another shows weak activity.

Uses

Symptomatic relief of anxiety, tension, and irritability associated with neuroses, depression, psychoneuroses, and psychosomatic disorders (short-term use only [maximum, 4 months])

Symptomatic relief of the symptoms of acute alcohol withdrawal (chlordiazepoxide, clorazepate, diazepam, lorazepam, oxazepam)

Preoperative sedation

Relief of muscle hypertonicity associated with anxiety or tension states

Adjunctive therapy in the management of epileptic states (clorazepate, diazepam)

Control of acute (eg, status epilepticus) or severe recurrent convulsive seizure states (diazepam or lorazepam, administered intravenously)

Adjunctive treatment before cardioversion or endoscopic procedures to lessen anxiety and reduce recall (diazepam or lorazepam; intravenous, intramuscular)

Control of nocturnal enuresis and night terrors (experimental use only)

Dosage

See Table 25-2

Fate

Generally well absorbed orally, although rates differ widely; intramuscular absorption of midazolam is rapid and complete, but that of chlordiazepoxide and diazepam is erratic; onset of action ranges from 30 to 60 minutes orally (diazepam has quickest onset of action) and 15 to 30 minutes IM; most drugs have long $T_{1/2}$s, and metabolites may be clinically active as well (see Table 25-1); drugs are lipid soluble and distribute widely throughout the body; protein binding is high (70%–99%); most drugs (except oxazepam and lorazepam) have long elimination $T_{1/2}$s, because their metabolites are also clinically active (see Table 25-1); prazepam and clorazepate are inactive as parent compounds but are metabolized to desmethyldiazepam, an active metabolite; excreted as both unchanged drug and metabolites, largely through the kidneys; elimination may occur in two stages; a rapid (within several hours) phase followed by a slower (within days) phase; danger of accumulation exists with prolonged use

Common Side Effects

Drowsiness, fatigue, lethargy, ataxia (most common during early stages of therapy)

Significant Adverse Reactions

(Not all reactions observed with every drug)

Table 25-2. **Benzodiazepine Antianxiety Drugs**

Drug	Usual Dosage Range	Nursing Considerations
Alprazolam (C-IV) *Xanax* *(CAN)* *Apo-Alpraz,* *Novo-Alprazol,* *Nu-Alpraz*	Initially, 0.25–0.5 mg times/day; maximum total dose, 4 mg/day Elderly persons: 0.25 mg 2–3 times/day	Metabolized to benzophenone which is inactive, and alpha hydroxyalprazolam, which is approximately one-half as active as alprazolam; has a short $T_{1/2}$ (12–15 h) and relatively brief duration of action; possesses antidepressant activity at higher doses; drowsiness and lightheadedness are common during early stages of therapy
Chlordiazepoxide (C-IV) *Libritabs, Librium, Mitran, Reposans-10* *(CAN) Apo-Chlordiazepoxide, Medilium, Novopoxide Solium*	**Oral** *Adults*: Anxiety—5–10 mg 3–4 times/day up to 25 mg 4 times/day Alcohol withdrawal—50–100 mg up to 300 mg/day *Children* (older than 6 y): 5–10 mg 2–4 times/day as needed **Parenteral** Adults: 50–100 mg IM or IV Children (older than 12 y): 25–50 mg IM or IV	Less potent than diazepam and has less anticonvulsive activity; excreted slowly by the kidneys, so danger of accumulation exists; prepare IM solution immediately before administration and discard unused portion; do not use IM diluent if hazy or opalescent; IM solution should *not* be given IV because of air bubbles that form in solution; inject slowly and deeply IM; IV solution can be prepared with sterile water or saline; give IV injection slowly over 1 minute; do *not* inject IV solution IM because pain is common; do *not* add to IV infusion because solution is unstable and quickly deteriorates; sterilization by heating should *not* be attempted; available in combination with amitriptyline as Limbitrol for treatment of anxious depressions
Clorazepate (C-IV) *Gen-Xene, Tranxene* *(CAN) Apo-Clorazepate, Novoclopate, Nu-Clopate*	*Anxiety*: 15–60 mg daily in divided doses *or* 11.25–22.5 mg once a day; elderly persons: 7.5–15 mg/day *Adjunct to anticonvulsants*: Adults: 7.5 mg 3 times/day initially; increase gradually Children: 7.5 mg twice a day; increase gradually *Alcohol withdrawal* Day 1: 30 mg initially, then 30–60 mg in divided doses Day 2: 45–90 mg in divided doses Day 3: 22.5–45 mg in divided doses Day 4: 15–30 mg in divided doses	Slow onset (about 60 min) and fairly long duration (up to 24 h) of action: active metabolite is desmethyldiazepam; single daily dose is usually given at bedtime; recommended in children *only* as adjunct to other anticonvulsant drugs; effects parallel those of diazepam see also Chap. 27.
Diazepam (C-IV) *Valium, Zetran, and several other manufacturers* *(CAN) Apo-Diazepam, Diazemuls, E-PAM, Novodipam, Rival, Vivol*	**Oral** *Adults* Anxiety: 2–10 mg 2–4 times/day *or* 15–30 mg/day sustained-release capsules Alcohol withdrawal: 10 mg 3–4 times/day initially, followed by 5 mg 3–4 times/day Adjunct in muscle spasm and convulsive states; 2–10 mg 2–4 times/day *or* 15–30 mg once daily *Children* (older than 6 mo): 1–2.5 mg 3–4 times/day; may increase gradually as required **Parenteral** *Adults* Psychoneuroses: 2–10 mg IM or IV every 3–4 h as necessary, depending on severity of symptoms Alcohol withdrawal: 5–10 mg IM or IV; repeat every 3–4 h Preoperative and minor surgical procedures (eg, endoscopy): 5–10 mg IM *or* IV before procedure *Status epilepticus*: 5–10 mg IV: repeat at 10–15 min intervals to a maximum of 30 mg Cardioversion: 5–15 mg IV 5–10 min before procedure *Children*: Tetanus: 2–10 mg, IM *or* slow IV every 3–4 h Status epilepticus: younger than 5 y: 0.2–0.5 mg by slow IV every 2–5 min; older than 5 y: 1 mg every 2–5 min	Effects occur within 20–30 min with oral administration, 15–30 min IM, and immediately IV; when using IV, inject slowly (5 mg/min) and avoid small veins to reduce danger of thrombophlebitis and local swelling and irritation; do *not* mix or dilute with other solutions or add to IV fluids; IM injection should be made deeply and slowly into a large muscle such as the gluteus; when used to control convulsions, be prepared to readminister drug if seizures recur, because duration of action with IV use is rather short; use cautiously in patients with chronic lung disease or unstable cardiovascular status; facilities for respiratory assistance should be present when drug is given parenterally; use of diazepam for endoscopic procedures has been associated with coughing, dyspnea, hyperventilation, laryngospasm, and pain in the throat and chest; use a topical anesthetic and have countermeasures available (eg, respiratory assistance); reduce dose of narcotic analgesic by one-third when used with diazepam
Halazepam (C-IV) *Paxipam*	20–40 mg 3 or 4 times/day; elderly persons: 20 mg 1–2 times/day	Long-acting benzodiazepine; maximum plasma levels are attained in 1–3 h; highly protein-bound; do *not* use in children younger than 18

(continued)

Table 25-2. **Benzodiazepine Antianxiety Drugs (Continued)**

Drug	Usual Dosage Range	Nursing Considerations
Lorazepam *Ativan* *(CAN) Apo-Lorazepam, Novolorazem, Nu-Loraz*	**Oral** Anxiety: 1–2 mg 2–3 times/day Insomnia: 2–4 mg at bedtime **IM** Preoperative medication: 0.05 mg/kg 2 h before procedure (maximum, 4 mg) **IV** Acute anxiety: 2–4 mg	Short-acting drug used for anxiety, preanesthetic medication and temporary relief of insomnia; *not* recommended in children younger than 12 y; dosage must be individually titrated; increase dosage gradually to minimize adverse effects; elderly or debilitated persons should receive an initial dose of 1–2 mg/day; less danger of accumulation than with other derivatives because no active metabolites are formed; may be more likely to impair short-term memory than other benzodiazepines; inject IM deep into muscle mass; dilute in appropriate diluent for IV administration; do not use if discolored
Oxazepam (C-IV) *Serax* *(CAN) Apo-Oxazepam, Novoxapam, Ox-Pam, Zapex*	Adults 10–30 mg 3–4 times/day Elderly or debilitated persons: 10 mg 3–4 times/day	Has shorter duration of action than diazepam and produces a lower incidence of "hangover" effects; *not* recommended in children younger than 6 y of age; paradoxical excitation may occur in first 2 wk of therapy; reduce dosage until symptoms subside
Prazepam (C-IV) *Centrax*	Adults: 20–60 mg/day in divided doses Elderly persons: 10–15 mg/day	Slow onset and prolonged duration of action; not indicated in patients younger than 18 y of age; can be used as a single daily dose (20–40 mg) at bedtime; similar to diazepam in actions and toxicity

CNS: confusion, disorientation, memory impairment, agitation, slurred speech, headache, syncope, vertigo, depression, hyporeactivity, stupor, tremor; paradoxical excitement (hostility, rage, muscle spasticity, irritability, vivid dreams, euphoria, insomnia, hallucinations) can occur, especially in psychotic patients

Autonomic: dry mouth, constipation, urinary retention, blurred vision, diplopia

CV: bradycardia, hypotension, edema and weight gain, cardiovascular collapse

Hematologic: agranulocytosis, neutropenia

Hypersensitivity: skin rash, urticaria, fever, angioneurotic edema, bronchial spasm

Other: changes in libido, menstrual irregularities, nasal congestion, salivation, hiccups, difficulty swallowing, hepatic dysfunction (jaundice), pain or thrombophlebitis on intravenous injection

Overdosage with benzodiazepines alone is seldom fatal; most fatalities result from multiple drug ingestion. Symptoms of overdosage include drowsiness, confusion, ataxia, and hypotension, but significant circulatory or respiratory depression is rare. An antagonist (ie, flumazenil) is available for treatment.

Contraindications

Severe psychoses, narrow-angle glaucoma, shock, in children younger than 6 years (except diazepam [children younger than 6 months]). *Cautious use* in addiction-prone persons, in pregnant or nursing women, in elderly or debilitated persons, and in the presence of liver or kidney disease, severe muscle weakness. Injectable benzodiazepines must be given with caution to persons in shock, in acute alcohol intoxication, and those with limited pulmonary reserve

Interactions

Benzodiazepines may enhance the CNS-depressant effects of alcohol, barbiturates, antihistamines, phenothiazines, opiates, and other CNS-depressant drugs.

Effects of phenytoin may be potentiated by benzodiazepines.

An increased muscle-relaxant effect can occur with combinations of benzodiazepines and other centrally and peripherally acting muscle relaxants.

Actions of levodopa may be antagonized by benzodiazepines.

Effects of benzodiazepines may be lessened in individuals who smoke.

Antacids or food may slow oral absorption of some benzodiazepines.

The half-life of some benzodiazepines—but *not* lorazepam or oxazepam—can be prolonged by cimetidine.

Nursing Management

Pretherapy Assessment

Assess and record baseline data necessary for detection of adverse effects of benzodiazepines: General: vital signs (VS), body weight, skin color and temperature; CNS: orientation, affect, reflexes; gastrointestinal (GI): liver evaluation, bowel sounds, normal output; Lab: renal and liver function tests, complete blood count (CBC).

Review medical history and documents for existing or previous conditions that:

a. require cautious use of benzodiazepines: impaired liver or kidney function; debilitation; depression; suicidal tendencies

b. contraindicate use of benzodiazepines: allergy to benzodiazepines; **pregnancy (Category D)**, labor and delivery ("floppy infant" syndrome when mothers given benzodiazepines during labor), lactation (secreted in breast milk; causes drowsiness, lethargy, and weight loss in nursing infants).

Nursing Interventions

Medication Administration

Assure ready access to bathroom facilities and provide small frequent meals if GI effects occur.

Follow proper procedures for handling schedule IV drugs.

Surveillance During Therapy

Monitor for toxicity.

Carefully monitor laboratory studies and patient for indications of adverse reactions.

Interpret results of diagnostic tests and contact practitioner as appropriate.

Monitor results of laboratory studies. Periodic blood counts and liver and kidney function tests should be performed during prolonged therapy.

Observe patient for indications of habituation with repeated use, especially of larger doses. Although abuse liability is lower than with most similar drugs, dependence may occur. Drugs are classified in schedule IV.

Monitor for possible drug–drug and drug–nutrient interactions: See **Interactions**.

Provide for patient safety needs if CNS changes occur.

Patient Teaching

Instruct patient to avoid hazardous activities during therapy because drowsiness and impaired motor coordination are often present.

Teach patient that sedative effects of long-acting drugs may persist for several days after termination of use, and that daytime carryover effects are enhanced by alcohol, antianxiety drugs, and other CNS depressants.

Inform patient of dangers of additive CNS depression if combined with alcohol, antihistamines, tranquilizers, and other central depressants.

Teach patient and family how to identify paradoxical excitatory effects. If they occur, the drug should be discontinued, and appropriate supportive care should be provided.

Instruct patient to report early signs of developing jaundice (nausea, diarrhea, abdominal pain, rash) or blood dyscrasias (sore throat, fever, weakness, mucosal ulceration), which are indications for discontinuing the drug.

Instruct patient not to abruptly discontinue therapy after long-term treatment because withdrawal symptoms (eg, vomiting, cramping, sweating, tremor, convulsions) can occur and may persist for several days. If withdrawal symptoms occur, they should be treated symptomatically as needed.

Inform woman with childbearing potential that congenital malformations can occur if drug is taken during early pregnancy. Discourage use during this period.

• Midazolam

Versed

Midazolam is a short-acting benzodiazepine used parenterally for preoperative and perioperative sedation and as a supplement to nitrous oxide anesthesia for short surgical procedures. Its actions resemble those of the other benzodiazepines with a very rapid onset of sedative action after injection. Midazolam induces a slight to moderate decrease in mean arterial pressure, cardiac output, stroke volume, and systemic vascular resistance.

Mechanism

See general discussion of the benzodiazepines earlier in the chapter.

Uses

Preoperative sedation and reduced recall of perioperative events (intramuscular)

Production of sedation before short diagnostic or endoscopic procedures (alone or with a narcotic drug; intravenous)

Induction of general anesthesia, before administration of other anesthetic agents (intravenous)

Supplementation of nitrous oxide-oxygen anesthesia for short surgical procedures (intravenous)

Dosage

Preoperative/perioperative sedation: 0.07 to 0.08 mg/kg IM 1 hour before surgery

Endoscopic or cardiovascular procedures: 0.1 to 0.15 mg/kg IV (up to 0.2 mg/kg); dosage should be reduced if narcotic premedication is used or if given to patients older than 60 years of age

Induction of general anesthesia: 0.3 to 0.35 mg/kg initially (IV); increments of 25% of the initial dose may be given if needed after 2 to 3 minutes. If patient has received narcotic premedication, the recommended dose is 0.15 to 0.3 mg/kg IV

Fate

Onset of sedation is within 15 minutes after intramuscular injection and 2 to 3 minutes after intravenous administration; anesthesia occurs within 2 minutes after intravenous injection; elimination half-life is variable (1–12 hours); awakening from general anesthesia usually occurs within 2 hours

Common Side Effects

Memory impairment of subsequent events is noted in 80% to 90% of patients. Also, nausea, hiccups, decreased respiratory rate and tidal volume, pain and tenderness on intramuscular injection, headache, muscle stiffness

Significant Adverse Reactions

CAUTION

Midazolam administered IV has been associated with severe respiratory depression and respiratory arrest, resulting in hypoxic encephalopathy or death. Continuous monitoring of respiratory and cardiac function is essential.

CNS: sedation, headache, confusion, dizziness, amnesia, nervousness, agitation, anxiety, delirium, insomnia, nightmares, tremor, involuntary movements, ataxia, paresthesias, slurred speech, blurred vision, and tonic/clonic movements
CV: premature ventricular contractions, tachycardia, bigeminy, hematoma at intramuscular injection site
Respiratory: bronchospasm, laryngospasm, dyspnea, hyperventilation, wheezing, tachypnea
Dermatologic: swelling or feeling of burning or warmth at injection site, rash, pruritus, urticaria
Other: salivation, retching, yawning, lethargy, weakness, chills, toothache
Symptoms of overdosage are characteristic of other benzodiazepines and include somnolence, sedation, confusion, impaired coordination, reduced reflexes, and respiratory distress. Flumazenil, a benzodiazepine antagonist, is available.

Contraindications

Acute narrow-angle glaucoma, acute alcohol intoxication, significantly depressed vital signs, pregnancy. *Cautious use* in persons with respiratory disease, hypotension, congestive heart failure, or renal dysfunction and in elderly or debilitated persons.

Interactions

The duration or degree of respiratory depression may be enhanced by concurrent use of other respiratory depressants, such as barbiturates, narcotics, alcohol, and so on
The dosage of induction or inhalational anesthetics may need to be reduced if midazolam is used preoperatively
The hypnotic effects of midazolam may be accentuated by preanesthetic use of narcotics, barbiturates, or other sedative agents

Nursing Management

Refer to *benzodiazepines*. However, because midazolam use is limited principally to singular occasions, risks associated with ongoing benzodiazepine therapy are negligible. See Caution, above, for risks associated with acute administration.

Benzodiazepine Antagonist

- ***Flumazenil***

Romazicon

Flumazenil is a benzodiazepine antagonist; it reverses benzodiazepine-induced sedation, psychomotor impairment and, **only to some degree**, amnesia and respiratory depression.

Mechanism

Flumazenil displaces benzodiazepines from their binding sites on the GABA–benzodiazepine receptor complex.

Uses

Reversal of CNS depression produced by benzodiazepines when employed in conscious sedation or general anesthesia, or in cases of benzodiazepine overdose

Dosage

Reversal of conscious sedation or in general anesthesia: initial intravenous dose of 0.2 mg over 15 seconds; this dose can be repeated every 60 seconds for a *total* dose of 1 mg. If resedation occurs, this regimen can be repeated at 20-minute intervals as needed with a *limit* of 3 mg/hour.
Management of suspected benzodiazepine overdose: initial intravenous dose of 0.2 mg over 30 seconds; after a 30-second interval, a 0.3-mg dose can be given over the next 30 seconds. Additional doses of 0.5 mg can be given over 30 seconds at 1-minute intervals for a *total* dose of 3 mg. If a patient does not respond to a total dose of 5 mg over 5 minutes, the CNS depression probably was *not* caused by a benzodiazepine.

Fate

Reversal of benzodiazepine-induced CNS depression usually begins within 1 to 2 minutes after completion of the intravenous dose; the elimination half-life ranges from 40 to 80 minutes. It is extensively biotransformed (99%), and elimination is complete within 72 hours.

Common Side Effects

Headache, sweating, pain at injection site, nausea, dizziness

Significant Adverse Reactions

CV: cutaneous vasodilation, arrhythmias
GI: dry mouth, vomiting
CNS: double vision, agitation, anxiety, abnormal vision, paresthesias, paranoia, emotional lability, confusion, convulsions (result of rapid benzodiazepine reversal)

CAUTION

Flumazenil may precipitate seizures in patients who have been using benzodiazepines for prolonged intervals or who have taken overdoses of cyclic antidepressants.

Contraindications

Patients taking benzodiazepines for life-threatening conditions (eg, status epilepticus); antidepressant overdose. *Cautious use* in patients with head injuries, psychiatric disorders, drug or alcohol dependence, liver impairment, and in pregnant or nursing mothers.

Interactions

Use of flumazenil may result in emergence of toxic effects of other drugs taken in overdose together with benzodiazepines.

Nursing Management

Pretherapy Assessment

Assess and record important baseline data necessary for detection of adverse effects of flumazenil: VS (T, P, R, BP); CNS: orientation, reflexes; CVS: peripheral perfusion; GI: liver function, output; GU: renal function; Laboratory: renal function tests, CBC.
Review past medical history and documents for evidence of existing or previous medical history related to conditions that:

a. require caution with flumazenil: pregnancy, breast feeding, use in the elderly, head injuries, psychiatric disorders, drug or alcohol dependence, liver impairment.
b. contraindicate use of flumazenil: allergy to flumazenil or to benzodiazepines, trycyclic antidepressant overdosage, **pregnancy (Category C)**.

Nursing Interventions

Medication Administration

Assure that the patient has a secure airway and intravenous access prior to administration of the drug.
Administer **intravenously through a freely running infusion set; initial recommended dose is 0.2 mg; maximum cumulative dose is 3 mg**.
Be prepared with emergency medications in the event that the patient responds to flumazenil with seizures.

Surveillance During Therapy

Monitor patient for therapeutic effect of flumazenil therapy.
Compare current status with previous status to detect improvements or deterioration in the patient's condition.
Monitor for adverse effects, toxicity, and interactions.
Monitor for signs of hypersensitivity that may require discontinuation of the drug.
Monitor patient for signs of benzodiazepine withdrawal, including hot flashes, agitation and tremors; severe signs of withdrawal include seizures.
Facilitate acquisition of diagnostic tests ordered for ongoing assessment of drug response.
Interpret results of diagnostic tests and contact practitioner/prescriber as appropriate.
Monitor for possible drug–laboratory test interactions.

Patient Teaching

Because this is an emergency medication, patient teaching will typically occur after the patient has received the medication.
If the drug is to be used to reverse conscious sedation and the amnesic effects of benzodiazepines, inform the patient (in writing) that:
their memory and judgment may continue to be impaired despite the use of the drug.
they should not use or operate hazardous machinery or motor vehicles for at least 18 to 24 hours after discharge.
they should not take any alcohol or nonprescription drugs for at least 18 to 24 hours after discharge.

Miscellaneous Antianxiety Agents

• Buspirone

BuSpar

Buspirone is a chemically and pharmacologically unique antianxiety agent that appears to be as effective as the benzodiazepines in treating general anxiety in many patients but does not possess the muscle-relaxant, anticonvulsant, sedative, or alcohol-potentiating actions of the benzodiazepines. In addition, there is no evidence that buspirone use leads to dependence or habituation, and it is *not* a controlled substance.

Mechanism

Interacts with serotonin$_{1A}$ receptor sites in several brain regions; may also function as a dopamine agonist; decreases anxiety without producing significant sedation or muscle relaxation; does *not* interact with GABA as do the benzodiazepines; no anticonvulsant activity; drug has not been shown to increase alcohol-induced CNS depression or motor impairment; tolerance and habituation have not been demonstrated on continual therapy.

Uses

Short-term management of anxiety disorders (efficacy for longer than 3 to 4 weeks has not been conclusively demonstrated, although patients have been given the drug for several months with no obvious untoward effect).

Dosage

Initially, 5 mg 3 times a day
Increase by 5-mg increments at 2- or 3-day intervals as needed
Usual maintenance range is 20 to 30 mg/day in divided doses (maximum, 60 mg/day)

Fate

Oral absorption is rapid, and peak plasma levels occur within 45 to 90 minutes; first-pass hepatic metabolism is extensive; approximately 95% of buspirone is protein bound in the plasma; drug is metabolized by the liver, mainly to inactive hydroxylated metabolites, which are excreted largely in the urine (30%–65%) with lesser amounts in the feces (20%–40%); elimination $T_{1/2}$ is 2 to 3 hours.

Common Side Effects

Nausea, headache, dizziness, lightheadedness, nervousness

Significant Adverse Reactions

CNS: dysphoria, loss of interest, akathisia, fearfulness, hallucinations, seizures, impaired concentration, confusion, depression, paresthesias, tremor, incoordination, slurred speech, cold intolerance, and suicidal ideation
GI: anorexia, dry mouth, diarrhea, salivation, irritable colon, rectal bleeding
Genitourinary: urinary hesitancy, menstrual irregularities, dysuria
Dermatologic: rash, edema, pruritus, flushing, easy bruising, dry skin, hair loss
Musculoskeletal: muscle cramps, arthralgia, muscle spasm
Respiratory: hyperventilation, dyspnea, chest congestion
Neurologic: involuntary movements, slowed reaction time
Other: altered taste or smell sensation, nasal congestion, muscle aching, tinnitus, blurred vision, conjunctivitis, itching of the eyes, altered libido, increased aspartate aminotransferase (AST) (serum glutamic-oxaloacetic transaminase [SGOT]) and alanine aminotransferase (ALT) (serum glutamic-pyruvic transaminase [SGPT]), weight gain, fever

Overdosage can cause vomiting, drowsiness, dizziness, gastric distress, and miosis. No deaths have occurred with doses as high as 375 mg. Treatment is supportive.

Contraindications

No absolute contraindications. *Cautious use* in persons with liver or kidney impairment, parkinsonism, in pregnant or nursing women, and in children younger than 18

Interactions

Buspirone may increase the serum level of haloperidol if administered together.

Buspirone may have additional CNS-depressive effects when given together with other depressants, such as hypnotics, narcotics, and alcohol, although the likelihood of a clinically significant interaction is minimal.

Concurrent use of buspirone and a monoamine oxidase (MAO) inhibitor can result in a hypertensive reaction.

Nursing Management

Pretherapy Assessment

Assess and record baseline data necessary for detection of adverse effects of buspirone: General: VS, body weight, skin color and temperature; CNS: orientation, affect, reflexes; GI: liver evaluation, bowel sounds, normal output; genitourinary (GU): normal output, voiding pattern; Lab: renal and liver function tests, CBC with differential

Review medical history and documents for existing or previous conditions that:

a. require cautious use of buspirone: impaired liver or kidney function; debilitation; parkinsonism; children younger than 18 years
b. contraindicate use of buspirone: allergy to buspirone; **pregnancy (Category B)**, lactation (secreted in breast milk; avoid use in nursing mothers)

Nursing Interventions

Medication Administration

Assure ready access to bathroom facilities and provide small frequent meals if GI effects occur.

Advocate use of a different anxiolytic agent if patient needs either immediate relief from anxiety or an intermittent drug regimen for episodic anxiety, because the antianxiety effects of buspirone are not evident until after 1 or 2 weeks of use.

Surveillance During Therapy

Monitor for toxicity.

Carefully monitor laboratory studies and patient for indications of adverse reactions.

Interpret results of diagnostic tests and contact practitioner as appropriate.

Monitor for possible drug–drug and drug–nutrient interactions: See **Interactions**.

Provide for patient safety needs if CNS changes occur.

Patient Teaching

Instruct patient to avoid hazardous activities during therapy because drowsiness and impaired motor coordination are often present.

Inform patient of dangers of additive CNS depression if combined with alcohol, antihistamines, tranquilizers, and other central depressants.

Inform patient that anxiolytic effects may not be apparent until after 1 or 2 weeks of use.

Instruct patient to be alert for and to immediately report any abnormal involuntary movements (eg, dystonias, facial movements), which can occur because of the drug's dopamine-agonistic activity.

• Chlormezanone

Trancopal

An infrequently used antianxiety drug for the treatment of mild anxiety and tension states, chlormezanone has a usual dosage range of 100 to 200 mg, 3 to 4 times/day for adults, and 50 to 100 mg 3 or 4 times/day in children 5 to 12 years of age. Its onset of action is 15 to 30 minutes, and effects persist for up to 6 hours. Adverse reactions can include dizziness, rash, drowsiness, dryness of the mouth, muscle weakness, edema, and depression.

The warnings, precautions, and nursing considerations discussed previously in connection with the benzodiazepines generally pertain to the use of chlormezanone as well. The drug has no particular advantage over the other antianxiety agents and is largely obsolete.

• Hydroxyzine

Atarax, Vistaril, and several other manufacturers

(CAN) Apo-Hydroxyzine, Multipax, Novo-Hydroxyzine, PMS-Hydroxyzine

Hydroxyzine is a diphenylmethane derivative having a mild CNS-depressant action, together with anticholinergic, antihistaminic, local anesthetic, antiemetic, antispasmodic, antisecretory, and skeletal muscle-relaxant effects. It has a good safety margin, and adverse reactions are minimal at recommended doses; it is frequently used in children as a mild sedative.

Mechanism

Not completely established; may suppress activity in subcortical brain areas but appears to have little effect on the cortex; blocks action of histamine and exerts both a direct and an indirect (through its sedative action) skeletal muscle-relaxant effect; also possesses an antiemetic effect

Uses

Symptomatic treatment of psychoneurotic states characterized by anxiety, tension, hostility, and motor hyperactivity

Adjunctive preoperative and prepartum therapy to help reduce anxiety and lessen narcotic analgesic requirements

Relief of anxiety symptoms associated with organic disturbances such as digestive disorders, allergic conditions, organic brain syndrome, menopause, alcoholism, and behavioral problems, especially in children

Relief of pruritus associated with urticaria, dermatoses, and other histamine-mediated conditions

Adjunctive treatment of alcohol withdrawal or delirium tremens (intramuscular)

Dosage

Oral

Relief of anxiety: adults: 50 to 100 mg 4 times/day; children: 50 to 100 mg/day in divided doses

Relief of pruritus: adults: 25 mg 3 to 4 times/day; children: 50 to 100 mg/day in divided doses

Preoperative sedation: adults: 50 to 100 mg; children: 0.6 mg/kg

Intramuscular

Acute alcoholism: 50 to 100 mg every 4 to 6 hours as needed

Nausea/vomiting: adults: 25 to 100 mg; children: 1.1 mg/kg

Preoperative/postoperative: adults: 25 to 100 mg; children: 1.1 mg/kg

Fate

Rapidly absorbed orally and parenterally; onset of action within 15 to 30 minutes; effects last for up to 6 hours; metabolized primarily in the liver and largely excreted through the bile in the feces; some drug appears in the urine

Common Side Effects

Transitory drowsiness, dry mouth

Significant Adverse Reactions

Involuntary motor activity, dizziness

Rarely, hypersensitivity reactions (urticaria, skin eruptions, erythema multiforme)

Contraindications

Early pregnancy (fetal abnormalities can occur)

Interactions

May exert additive effects with other CNS depressants (eg, alcohol, hypnotics, narcotics)

Nursing Management

Pretherapy Assessment

Assess and record baseline data necessary for detection of adverse effects of hydroxyzine: General: VS, body weight, skin color and temperature; CNS: orientation, affect, reflexes

Review medical history and documents for existing or previous conditions that:

a. require cautious use of hydroxyzine: no significant cautions to use

b. contraindicate use of hydroxyzine: allergy to hydroxyzine; **pregnancy (Category C)**, lactation (secreted in breast milk; safety not established, avoid use in nursing mothers)

Nursing Interventions

Medication Administration

Attempt to determine and arrange treatment for the underlying cause of vomiting because drug may mask signs and symptoms of serious underlying disease.

Inject deeply into large muscle mass when giving intramuscularly. Do not administer by other parenteral routes because risk of adverse effects such as tissue necrosis and hemolysis are great.

Provide frequent mouth care if dry mouth occurs.

Surveillance During Therapy

Monitor for toxicity.

Carefully monitor laboratory studies and patient for indications of adverse reactions.

Interpret results of diagnostic tests and contact practitioner as appropriate.

Monitor for possible drug–drug and drug–nutrient interactions: exerts an additive effect with other CNS depressants (alcohol, hypnotics, narcotics).

Patient Teaching

Instruct patient to avoid hazardous activities during therapy because drowsiness and impaired motor coordination are often present.

Inform patient of dangers of additive CNS depression if combined with alcohol, antihistamines, tranquilizers, and other central depressants.

Teach patient to avoid use of OTC preparations while taking this drug.

Teach patient to inform practitioner if the following adverse effects occur: difficulty breathing; tremors; loss of coordination; sore muscles or muscle spasms.

• Meprobamate

Equanil, Miltown, and several other manufacturers

(CAN) Apo Meprobamate

Meprobamate is an antianxiety agent that more closely resembles a barbiturate than a benzodiazepine. Its CNS depressant actions are similar to those of the barbiturates but are generally shorter in duration. Other effects produced by meprobamate include skeletal muscle relaxation and, in large doses, an anticonvulsant action. It also reduces rapid eye movement (REM) sleep time. Prolonged use can result in habituation and dependence, and meprobamate is somewhat more dangerous in this regard than the benzodiazepines.

Mechanism

Not well established; appears to act at several subcortical loci, including the limbic system and thalamus; no specific depressant effects on the reticular activating system or the autonomic nervous system; suppresses REM sleep and exerts a skeletal muscle-relaxing effect, probably resulting in part from its sedative action

Uses

Short-term relief of anxiety and tension associated with various disease states (alternative drug *only* to the benzodiazepines or buspirone)

Dosage

Adults: 1,200 to 1,600 mg/day in three or four divided doses

Children: (6–12 y): 100 to 200 mg 2 to 3 times/day

Fate

Well absorbed orally; onset of effect within 1 hour; plasma half-life is 6 to 18 hours but is prolonged with long-term use; uniformly distributed in the body; minimal protein binding; metabolized in the liver and largely excreted in the urine mainly as inactive metabolites; meprobamate induces liver microsomal enzymes and readily crosses placental barrier

Common Side Effects

Drowsiness, ataxia, rash

Significant Adverse Reactions

CNS: dizziness, vertigo, slurred speech, weakness, paresthesias, headache, depression, confusion, paradoxical excitation, euphoria, hyperactivity

Hypersensitivity: pruritus, urticaria, fever, edema, petechiae, ecchymoses, adenopathy, bronchospasm, anaphylaxis, exfoliative dermatitis

Hematologic: leukopenia, agranulocytosis, thrombocytopenic purpura, aplastic anemia, pancytopenia

CV: hypotension, flushing, syncope, palpitations, tachycardia, arrhythmias

GI: nausea, vomiting, diarrhea, dry mouth, glossitis

Other: exacerbation of porphyria, increased incidence of grand mal attacks, pain at intramuscular injection site

Contraindications

Acute intermittent porphyria, renal insufficiency (intramuscular use), and children younger than 6. *Cautious use* in epileptics, persons with liver or kidney impairment, addiction-prone persons, and in elderly or debilitated patients.

Interactions

Additive depressant effects can occur between meprobamate and other CNS depressants (eg, alcohol, barbiturates, phenothiazines).

Meprobamate may augment the metabolism of oral anticoagulants and steroid hormones, thereby reducing their pharmacologic effects.

Nursing Management

See Nursing Management for Barbiturates (Chapter 22) and Benzodiazepines.

Selected Bibliography

Greenblatt DJ, Wright CE: Clinical pharmacokinetics of alprazolam: Therapeutic implications. Clin Pharmacokinet 24(6):453, 1993

Labelle A, Lapierre YD: Anxiety disorders—Part 2: Pharmacotherapy with benzodiazepines. Can Fam Physician 39:2205, 1993

Lader M, Russell J: Guidelines for the prevention and treatment of benzodiazepine dependence: Summary of a report from the Mental Health Foundation. Addiction 88:1707, 1993

Laegreid L: Clinical observations in children after prenatal benzodiazepine exposure. Dev Pharmacol Ther 15:186, 1990

McMillan CO et al: Premedication of children with oral midazolam. Can J Anaesth 39(6):545, 1992

Otto MW et al: Discontinuation of benzodiazepine treatment: Efficacy for cognitive-behavioral therapy for patients with panic disorder. Am J Psychiatry 150(10):1485, 1993

Piekarski JM, Rossmann JA, Putman J: Benzodiazepine reversal with flumazenil: A review of the literature. J Can Dent Assoc 58:307, 1992

Pollak CP, Perlick D, Linsner JP: Sleep and motor activity of community elderly who frequently use bedtime medications. Biol Psychiatry 35:73, 1994

Seivewright N, Dougal W: Withdrawal symptoms from high dose benzodiazepines in poly-drug users. Drugs Alcohol Depend 32:15, 1993

Sheikh JI: Anxiety disorders and their treatment. Clin Geriatric Med 8:411, 1992

Tiller JWG, Schweitzer I: Benzodiazepines: Depressants or antidepressants? Drugs 44(2):165, 1992

Van Laar MW, Volkerts ER, Van Willigenburg APP: Therapeutic effects and effects on actual driving performance of chronically administered buspirone and diazepam in anxious outpatients. J Clin Psychopharmacol 12(2):86, 1992

Nursing Bibliography

Aker J: Review of current research on midazolam and diazepam for endoscopic premedication. Gastroenterology Nursing 13(2):245–285, 1990

Alprazolam in PMS: Nurses Drug Alert 17(8):61, 1993

Diazepam for recurring febrile seizures. Nurses Drug Alert 17(9):68–69, 1993

Simms S, et al.: Comparison of prochlorperazine and lorazepam antiemetic regimen in the control of post chemotherapy symptoms. Nursing Research 42(4): 234–239, 1993

26 Antidepressants

Blockade of Neurotransmitter Uptake
- *Tricyclic Antidepressants*
  - *Tertiary*
    - Amitriptyline
    - Clomipramine
    - Doxepin
    - Imipramine
    - Trimipramine
  - *Secondary*
    - Amoxapine
    - Desipramine
    - Nortriptyline
    - Protriptyline
- *Tetracyclic Antidepressant*
  - Maprotiline
- *Atypical Antidepressants*
  - *Serotonin-Selective Inhibitors*
    - Fluoxetine
    - Paroxetine
    - Sertraline
  - *Other*
    - Bupropion
    - Trazodone
    - Venlafaxine

Inhibition of Monoamine Oxidase (MAO Inhibitors)
- *Hydrazines*
  - Isocarboxazid
  - Phenelzine
- *Nonhydrazine*
  - Tranylcypromine

Antidepressants are drugs that alleviate a variety of symptoms (eg, sleep problems, loss of interest in sex, loss of appetite) found in persons presenting with *"depression,"* a condition of significantly lowered mood for a prolonged period. Drug therapy is one approach to treatment of depression; others include psychotherapy and electroconvulsive therapy (ECT).

In general, the various types of depression can be classified as **reactive depression** ("exogenous" or "secondary"; occurs *after* some traumatic event [eg, diagnosis of terminal cancer; stress caused by death of a child]), **major depressive disorder** ("endogenous" or "primary"; no clear identifiable cause; occurs at any age; possibly caused by genetic factors), and **bipolar** ("manic-depression").

To be more specific, "depression" is classified as a condition with a very noticeable and constant reduced mood that has lasted at least 2 weeks and prevents the person from functioning normally every day. In some types of depression, significant therapeutic benefit has been obtained with use of antidepressant drugs. It is recommended that **before** antidepressants are given, a patient should exhibit four—or more—of the following symptoms: change in appetite; increase in fatigue; feelings of guilt or worthlessness; loss of interest in usual activities (eg, decreased sex drive); change in sleep patterns; psychomotor agitation or retardation; impaired concentration (slowed thinking); suicidal thoughts or attempts.

Concurrent use of antidepressants during ECT may increase the hazards, and such therapy should be avoided. Patients receiving tricyclic antidepressants who are to undergo ECT should have the drugs discontinued for 24 to 48 hours before the ECT.

Classification of Antidepressant Drugs

The clinically useful antidepressant drugs can be categorized according to their respective mechanism of action as follows:

I. *Blockade of neurotransmitter uptake*
   A. *Tricyclic antidepressants* (eg, imipramine, amitriptyline)
   B. *Tetracyclic antidepressant* (eg, maprotiline)
   C. *Atypical antidepressants* (eg, bupropion, fluoxetine, trazodone)

II. *Inhibitors of monoamine oxidase (MAO inhibitors)* (eg, isocarboxazid, tranylcypromine)

Antidepressants that block neurotransmitter uptake are the most widely used drugs for the treatment of endogenous depression. The *tricyclic antidepressants* (TCAs) are the largest group of such drugs; differing in molecular structure from the tricyclic drugs—but similar in pharmacological actions—are drugs such as trazodone and bupropion, sometimes referred to as "second-generation" antidepressants because they were developed *after* the TCAs. The newest group of antidepressants, typified by drugs such as fluoxetine and sertraline, are the *selective serotonin uptake inhibitors*, which exhibit a lower incidence of side effects compared with many of the older antidepressants. Monoamine oxidase (MAO) inhibitors are more toxic agents and are reserved for treating severe depressions not managed successfully by other antidepressants. Several central nervous system (CNS) stimulants such as amphetamine derivatives and methylphenidate have been used for short periods in treatment of mild depressive states; they are not "true" antidepressants because they elevate **all** moods, ie, depressed or not (in contrast, "true" antidepressants will increase only a mood that is below normal; they have no clinical effect on normal moods). Central nervous system stimulants also have a high abuse potential. They have other recognized indications, however, and are reviewed in Chapter 29.

Blockade of Neurotransmitter Uptake

Tricyclic Antidepressants

Tricyclic antidepressants (TCAs) are so named because of their characteristic three-ring molecular structure; they are further differentiated into secondary or tertiary amines based on the configuration of their side chain (Table 26-1).

The currently available TCAs are structurally similar to the phenothiazine antipsychotic agents; they share many of the same pharmacologic and toxicologic actions (eg, sedation, anticholinergic activity, orthostatic hypotension). TCAs are characterized by their *specific* blocking action on the uptake of biogenic amines at the nerve ending (presynaptic membrane).

Table 26-1. **Pharmacologic Properties and Side Effects of Antidepressants that Block Neurotransmitter Uptake**

	Reuptake Blocking Activity		*Side Effects*		
	NE	*5-HT*	*Anticholinergic*	*Sedative*	*Orthostatic Hypotension*
Tricyclics					
Tertiary Amines					
Amitriptyline Elavil	+	+++	+++	+++	++
Clomipramine Anafranil	+	++++	+++	+++	++
Doxepin Sinequan, Adapin	+	+	++	+++	++
Imipramine Tofranil	++	+++	++	++	+++
Trimipramine Surmontil	+	+	+++	+++	++
Secondary Amines					
Amoxapine Asendin	++	++	++	++	+
Desipramine Norpramin, Pertofrane	+++	+	+	+	+
Nortriptyline Aventyl, Pamelor	++	++	+	++	+
Protriptyline Vivactil	+++	+	+++	0(+)	+
Tetracyclic					
Maprotiline Ludiomil	++	0(+)	+	++	+
Atypical					
Serotonin Selective					
Fluoxetine Prozac	0(+)	++++	0(+)	0(+)	0(+)
Paroxetine Paxil	0(+)	++++	+	+	0(+)
Sertraline Zoloft	0(+)	++++	0(+)	0(+)	+
Other					
Bupropion Wellbutrin	+	+	++	+	0(+)
Trazodone Desyrel	0(+)	+++	+	++	++
Venlafaxine Effexor	+++	+++	+	++	0*

++++ = Highest effect.
+++ = Strong effect.
++ = Moderate effect.
+ = Slight effect.
0(+) = Little or no effect.
* May cause sustained hypertension.

Because presynaptic uptake of biogenic amines is the primary process by which their activity is terminated, blockade of this process by TCAs prolongs and increases the action of these amines at postsynaptic receptors.

It is important to realize that blockade of biogenic amine uptake into nerve endings is **not** the **only** mechanism produced by these antidepressants.

In fact, clinical observations suggest that it just may be the **initial** event in a series of reactions. It is well known that the therapeutic benefit of antidepressants—relief of depressive symptoms—is observed only after one or more weeks of daily therapy, whereas the blocking effect on amine uptake occurs almost immediately. The current theory to explain this is that inhibition of presynaptic uptake produces increased levels of neurotransmitters in the synapse. This causes increased stimulation of *postsynaptic receptor sites, which then become fewer in number and hypo*sensitive. Loss of postsynaptic receptors or sensitivity is termed *"down-regulation"*; it develops slowly when a patient is started on a tricyclic antidepressant. Of importance is the fact that the time required for down-regulation of postsynaptic receptors corresponds **very closely** to the onset of antidepressant activity. Therefore, down-regulation of postsynaptic receptors appears to play a major role in the therapeutic efficacy of the tricyclic antidepressants.

Selective differences exist among the different tricyclic drugs in their relative potency for blocking norepinephrine versus serotonin uptake. These differences, outlined in Table 26-1, may explain the varying degrees of effectiveness among tricyclics observed in different depressed populations.

Most tricyclic compounds have a sedative action in addition to their antidepressant effect; all derivatives have both central and peripheral anticholinergic actions and can induce orthostatic hypotension, especially in geriatric patients. The frequency of occurrence and degree of severity vary considerably among the different drugs, as outlined in Table 26-1.

Mechanism

Inhibit neuronal uptake of biogenic amines (norepinephrine, serotonin) into presynaptic endings, blocking a major process for inactivation of these amines, which increases their effects; may also exert a blocking effect at presynaptic alpha$_2$ receptor sites, which allows greater release of norepinephrine and possibly serotonin; increased postsynaptic receptor activation causes a gradual decrease in the number and sensitivity of these receptors; the clinical efficacy of these agents is thought to be the result of *down-regulation* of β-adrenergic and serotonergic receptors; TCAs also possess anticholinergic, antihistaminic, and quinidine-like action, and produce peripheral vasodilation and mild hypotension.

Uses

Relief of the symptoms of depression (especially **endogenous** type)
Control of anxiety associated with depressive states
Treatment of depression in patients with manic-depressive disorders
Treatment of obsessive-compulsive disorder (clomipramine)
Investigational uses include enhanced control of acute pain (in combination with narcotic analgesics), prevention of migraine and cluster headaches (especially amitriptyline), treatment of obstructive sleep apnea (protriptyline), symptomatic management of peptic ulcer disease (doxepin, trimipramine), and treatment of attention-deficit disorders (desipramine)

Dosage

See Table 26-2

Dosage should be tailored to patient's needs: Use lowest effective dose for maintenance therapy, and observe patient carefully for continued clinical progress. Gradually taper dosage after symptoms have been controlled for some time (at least 3–6 months), but be alert for possible relapse. Not recommended for use in children younger than 12 years.

Fate

Well absorbed from the gastrointestinal (GI) tract, but undergo extensive first-pass hepatic inactivation; peak plasma concentrations attained within 2 to 4 hours; widely distributed in the body and highly bound to plasma proteins (75%–95%); wide individual variation in plasma levels and plasma half-life (eg, 8–60 hours) caused by variability in liver metabolic activity; metabolized in the liver, often to therapeutically active compounds (eg, imipramine to desipramine; amitriptyline to nortriptyline); hydroxylated metabolites excreted in the urine, along with small amounts of unchanged drug

Common Side Effects

Sedation, anticholinergic effects (dryness of the mouth, blurred vision, tachycardia, constipation, urinary hesitancy), headache, muscle twitching, weight gain
In children (when used for *enuresis*, an *unapproved* indication):
Nervousness, insomnia, lethargy, GI disturbances

Significant Adverse Reactions

CNS: anxiety, restlessness, agitation, irritability, fever, insomnia, nightmares, disorientation, confusion, delusions, hypomania, hallucinations, dizziness, tinnitus, numbness and tingling in extremities, ataxia, tremors, extrapyramidal symptoms, paresthesias, seizures
CV: orthostatic hypotension, arrhythmias, palpitations, congestive heart failure, infarction, heart block, stroke; electrocardiographic (ECG) changes include prolongation of the PR and QT intervals, reduction of the T wave, and formation of a prominent U wave (*caution* in persons with cardiovascular disorders)
Allergic: skin rash, pruritus, urticaria, petechiae, photosensitization, edema, fever
GI: nausea, anorexia, vomiting, diarrhea, cramping, epigastric distress, stomatitis
Endocrine: galactorrhea, gynecomastia, testicular and breast swelling, altered libido, delayed ejaculation or impotence, altered blood sugar levels
Hematologic: blood dyscrasias (agranulocytosis, eosinophilia, leukopenia, thrombocytopenia), bone marrow depression
Other: altered liver function (including jaundice), alopecia, parotid gland enlargement, flushing, sweating, chills, nocturia, nasal congestion, lacrimation
Overdosage is characterized by CNS signs, such as confusion, agitation, hyperreflexia, seizures, and hallucinations; autonomic effects such as dilated pupils, flushing, and hyperpyrexia; and cardiovascular complications such as tachycardia, arrhythmias, pulmonary edema, hypotension, and possibly ventricular fibrillation

Contraindications

Acute recovery phase of myocardial infarction, severe renal or hepatic impairment, **simultaneous** use of MAO inhibitors, narrow-angle glaucoma. *Cautious use* in patients with a history of

Table 26-2. **Antidepressants that Block Neurotransmitter Uptake**

Drug	Usual Dosage Range	Nursing Considerations
Amitriptyline *Elavil, Endep, Enovil* *(CAN) Apo-Amitriptyline, Levate, Novotriptyn*	*Oral* Initially: 75–150 mg/day Maintenance: 50–100 mg/day in divided doses or at bedtime *IM* 20–30 mg 4 times/day initially; replace with oral form as soon as possible	Most effective in endogenous depressions, especially those accompanied by anxiety, or in patients older than 50 y of age; investigational uses include prevention of migraine headaches and control of acute pain, especially in combination with potent narcotics; sedative effect is prominent, especially early in therapy; give drug at bedtime to minimize daytime drowsiness; plasma half-life is 30–40 h
Amoxapine *Asendin*	Initially: 50 mg 2–3 times/day; increase to 100 mg 2–3 times/day on the third day Once effective dose is established, may be given in a single bedtime dose not to exceed 300 mg	Used in a wide range of depressions; exhibits a moderate sedative action; clinical effects are usually observed within 7 days; may be used on a once daily basis at bedtime; highly bound (90%) to plasma proteins, so interactions with other protein-bound drugs can occur; increased risk of seizures; has been associated with development of neuroleptic malignant syndrome (NMS); serum half-life is 8 h, but converted to an active metabolite with a half-life of 30 h; *do not* use in children younger than 16 y; most frequent adverse reactions (10%–15%) are sedation, dry mouth, and constipation
Bupropion *Wellbutrin*	Initially, 100 mg twice daily; may increase to 100 mg 3 times/day after 3 days. Maximum dose is 450 mg/day in 3 divided doses	Increased risk of seizures, especially at high doses; use with caution in patients with history of seizure disorders
Clomipramine *Anafranil*	Initially, 25 mg daily; may increase to 100 mg/day during first 2 weeks. Maximum dose, 250 mg/day	Effective in treating obsessive-compulsive disorder (OCD); may increase risk of seizures; produces sexual dysfunction in males; may also be useful in treating panic attacks
Desipramine *Norpramin, Pertofrane*	Adults: 25–50 mg 3–4 times/day (maximum, 300 mg/day) Geriatric patients: 25–100 mg/day	Active metabolite of imipramine with essentially the same uses and adverse effects; *not* recommended in children; slightly lower incidence of sedation and anticholinergic action than imipramine; increased psychomotor activity may occur in first few weeks of therapy; orthostatic hypotension is common early in treatment—caution against rapid position changes; improvement is usually apparent within 1–2 wks
Doxepin *Adapin, Sinequan* *(CAN) Tridapin*	10–50 mg 3 times/day (maximum, 300 mg/day) *or* 150 mg once daily at bedtime *Do not* use in children younger than 12 y	Indicated for relief of depression and anxiety associated with psychotic or psychoneurotic disorders; antianxiety effects occur within several days, but antidepressant action requires several weeks; sedation is marked during initial stage of treatment; effects of alcohol may be enhanced; dilute oral concentrate with 4 oz water, juice, or milk before administration
Fluoxetine *Prozac*	Initially, 20-mg once daily; increase in 20-mg increments; maximum, 80 mg/day	Used for depression, obsessive-compulsive disorder, and panic attacks; low incidence of sedation and anticholinergic effects; may cause anxiety and insomnia; anorexia can lead to weight loss
Imipramine *Janimine, Tofranil* *(CAN) Apo-Imipramine, Novopramine*	**Depression** *Oral* Initially: 75–150 mg/day in divided doses Maintenance: 50–150 mg/day *IM* 100 mg/day in divided doses **Enuresis** Initially: 25–50 mg/night, orally *or* 25 mg in midafternoon and 25 mg at bedtime	Used for relief of symptoms of endogenous depressions and for reducing enuresis in children 6 y and older; decreases time spent in deep phases of sleep associated with bedwetting but serious side effects have occurred; may be administered in a single nightly dose (Tofranil-PM) for depression; do *not* use the PM (pamoate salt) dosage form in enuresis; plasma half-life is 10–25 h
Maprotiline *Ludiomil*	Initially: 75 mg/day in single or divided doses; adjust to desired maintenance range, usually 75–225 mg/day (maximum, 300 mg/day) Elderly: 50–75 mg/day	A *tetracyclic* antidepressant with a slightly lower incidence of cardiovascular reactions and fewer anticholinergic side effects than most tricyclic compounds; may have a rapid response (within 1 wk) in some patients; used in manic-depressive disorders; most common side effects are dry mouth and drowsiness; *not* indicated in children younger than 18 y; reduce dosage in elderly patient, and during prolonged maintenance therapy
Nortriptyline *Aventyl, Pamelor*	25 mg 3–4 times/day (maximum, 150 mg/day) *Geriatric patients*: 30–50 mg/day	Primarily effective in endogenous depressions; not recommended in children younger than 12 y; drug is a metabolite of amitriptyline and is similar to imipramine in most of its pharmacologic effects

(continued)

Table 26-2. **Antidepressants that Block Neurotransmitter Uptake (Continued)**

Drug	Usual Dosage Range	Nursing Considerations
Paroxetine *Paxil*	Initially: 20 mg daily (maximum, 50 mg/day)	Selective serotonin reuptake inhibitor; shares many properties with fluoxetine (see above); reduce dose in patients with hepatic or renal impairment or in debilitated patients
Protriptyline *Vivactil* *(CAN) Triptil*	5–10 mg 3–4 times/day (maximum, 60 mg/day) Geriatric patients: 5 mg 3 times/day	Most effective in endogenous depressions in withdrawn and anergic patients; use is associated with less sedation, but drug has more CNS-stimulatory, cardiovascular, and anticholinergic action than other tricyclics; *caution* in cardiac patients or in those with insomnia; *not* recommended in children younger than 12 y; last dose should be taken not later than midafternoon to avoid excessive stimulation at bedtime
Sertraline *Zoloft*	50 mg daily (maximum, 200 mg/day)	Selective serotonin reuptake inhibitor (see fluoxetine); long half-life (24 h); may be useful in obsessive-compulsive disorder; weight loss can occur
Trazodone *Desyrel*	Initially, 150 mg/day in divided doses; increase in 50 mg increments; maximum, 600 mg/day in patients	Priapism can occur and may require surgical intervention; sedation is common; may induce arrhythmias in patients with pre-existing heart disease
Trimipramine *Surmontil* *(CAN) Apo-Trimip, Novo-Tripramine, Rhotrimune*	Initially: 75–150 mg/day in divided doses Maintenance: 50–150 mg/day at bedtime Geriatric patients: 50–100 mg/day	Possesses significant sedative action; similar to amitriptyline in most respects; *not* recommended in children
Venlafaxine *Effexor*	Initially: 75 mg/day in divided doses; increase up to 150–225 mg/day if necessary	Elimination $T_{1/2}$ increased in both hepatic and renal disease; dosage reduction is necessary; may cause dose-dependent increase in blood pressure (sustained hypertension)

seizure disorders, cardiovascular disease, urinary dysfunction, or narrow-angle glaucoma. Also in the presence of pregnancy, lactation, hepatic or renal impairment, prostatic hypertrophy, hyperthryoidism, schizophrenia, or other psychoses.

Interactions

Tricyclics may enhance the effects of other CNS depressants (eg, alcohol, barbiturates, benzodiazepines, hypnotics, phenothiazines); catecholamines; other adrenergic drugs (eg, ephedrine, amphetamine); anticholinergics; narcotic analgesics; thyroid drugs; disulfiram; anticoagulants; vasodilators; and centrally acting muscle relaxants.

Tricyclics may antagonize the action of antihypertensives (eg, guanethidine, clonidine); beta-blockers; anticonvulsants (increase incidence of seizures); phenylbutazone; and cholinergic drugs.

Effects of TCAs may be potentiated by phenothiazines, methylphenidate, amphetamines, cimetidine, furazolidone, acetazolamide, MAO inhibitors, and urinary alkalinizers (eg, sodium bicarbonate).

Tricyclics should not be administered within 14 days of MAO inhibitors because hypertension, hyperpyresis, and convulsions can occur.

Reserpine and TCAs can result in a stimulating effect, possibly leading to mania.

Therapeutic effects of TCAs may be reduced by barbiturates (enzyme induction), urinary acidifiers such as ammonium chloride and ascorbic acid (decreased renal tubular reabsorption), and oral contraceptives.

Increased cardiovascular toxic effects may be seen with thyroid drugs, quinidine, or procainamide in combination with TCAs.

Tetracyclic Antidepressant

• Maprotiline

Ludiomil

Maprotiline possess a four-ring nuclear structure; it has a greater effect on blockade of norepinephrine uptake than on serotonin. This agent is similar in most respects to the tricyclic drugs, but may have a lower incidence of some undesirable side effects.

Nursing Management

Pretherapy Assessment

Assess and record baseline data necessary for detection of adverse effects of cyclic antidepressants: General: vital signs (VS), body weight, skin color and temperature; CNS: orientation, affect, reflexes, vision and hearing; cardiovascular (CV): orthostatic blood pressure (BP), perfusion; GI: bowel sounds, normal output, liver evaluation; genitourinary (GU): normal output; Endocrine: usual sexual function, frequency of menses, breast and scrotal examination; Lab: liver function, urinalysis, complete blood count (CBC), ECG.

Review medical history and documents for existing or previous conditions that:

a. require cautious use of cyclic antidepressants: history of seizure disorders; cardiovascular disease; urinary dysfunction; narrow-angle glaucoma; hepatic or renal impairment; prostatic hypertrophy; hyperthyroidism; schizophrenia; other psychoses
b. contraindicate use of cyclic antidepressants: allergy to any cyclic antidepressant or to tartrazine; acute recovery phase of myocardial infarction (MI); severe renal or hepatic impairment; MAO inhibitors; **pregnancy (Category B or C)**, lactation (secreted in breast milk; safety not established, avoid use in nursing mothers).

Nursing Interventions

Medication Administration

Ensure that depressed and potentially suicidal patients have access to only a limited supply of these drugs.

Administer intramuscularly only when oral therapy is impossible; do not administer intravenously.

Administer major portion of daily dose at bedtime if drowsiness or severe anticholinergic effects occur.

Surveillance During Therapy

Carefully assess severely depressed patient during initial improvement phase. Suicidal tendency may be increased as depression and psychomotor retardation are lessened.

Monitor blood pressure and pulse at least twice a day until stable because hypotension, several types of arrhythmias, and other cardiovascular side effects may occur, especially in patients receiving high doses.

Provide emotional support during drug therapy. Encourage patient to engage regularly in physical and social activities. Significant others may need to help motivate patient to participate.

Ensure that baseline blood and liver function studies and ECG have been completed before initiating drug administration.

Assist in evaluating patient's response to drug. The lowest effective dosage should be used for maintenance therapy, and the patient should be carefully observed for continued clinical progress. After symptoms have been controlled for some time (at least 3 months), dosage should be gradually tapered, but patient should be monitored for possible relapse. If no improvement is observed within 8 weeks, the drug should be discontinued and alternative therapy instituted.

Monitor for toxicity.

Carefully monitor laboratory studies and patient for indications of adverse reactions.

Interpret results of diagnostic tests and contact practitioner as appropriate.

Monitor for possible drug–drug and drug–nutrient interactions: See Interactions.

Patient Teaching

Encourage patient to maintain prescribed regimen. Beneficial effects may not become manifest for several weeks, although some drugs (eg, maprotiline) claim a more rapid onset of action (5–7 days).

Explain that abrupt discontinuation of therapy could result in nausea, muscle aching, insomnia, and irritability. The drug should be withdrawn gradually under supervision of the prescriber.

Reassure patient that many side effects common early in therapy disappear or diminish with continued use; others may remain. The patient should inform prescriber if side effects appear or persist, as dosage adjustment or change to another agent may help minimize them.

Warn patient that no other drugs, including over-the-counter (OTC) preparations, should be taken without consulting the healthcare provider.

Explain that tricyclic antidepressants augment the effects of alcohol and other CNS depressants. Motor coordination may be impaired if they are used in combination.

Caution patient not to operate dangerous machinery until response to drug is known because marked sedation is common during early stages of treatment.

Teach patient measures that help control orthostatic hypotension.

Teach patient early signs of blood dyscrasia (fever, sore throat, mucosal irritation, fatigue) that need to be reported to practitioner immediately.

Instruct patient to inform practitioner immediately if fever, nausea, abdominal pain, or rash (early signs of cholestatic jaundice) appear.

Suggest interventions to alleviate mouth dryness, which is common in early therapy.

Teach patient interventions to prevent constipation (increased intake of fluid and dietary roughage), and advise patient to monitor bowel and bladder function because constipation and urinary retention can occur. Dosage adjustment or adjunctive therapy (eg, stool softener, laxative) may be necessary.

Teach diabetic patient how to assess need for adjustment in antidiabetes regimen because both hypoglycemia and hyperglycemia have been reported.

Advise patient to avoid excessive exposure to sunlight because photosensitivity reactions may occur.

Instruct patient to notify practitioner in charge of tricyclic antidepressant use before elective surgery. To reduce operative risks (eg, excessive hypotension or respiratory depression), the drug should be discontinued several days before surgery.

Atypical Antidepressants

Serotonin-Selective Inhibitors

Several newer antidepressants appear to have greater efficacy in treating certain forms of depression, and may be particularly effective in obsessive-compulsive disorders. These agents, which include fluoxetine, paroxetine, and sertraline, have a more *selective* effect on blockade of serotonin uptake than on norepinephrine (see Table 26-1).

Serotonin-selective inhibitors are chemically dissimilar to other available antidepressants but comparable in clinical efficacy. The incidence of anticholinergic, sedative, and hypotensive effects compared with the tricyclics is somewhat reduced, although certain CNS (eg, headache, nervousness) and GI (eg, nausea, diarrhea) side effects appear to occur more often than with other antidepressants

Mechanism

Significantly inhibit neuronal uptake of serotonin, with minimal effects on norepinephrine uptake; antagonism of cholinergic, histaminergic, and α-adrenergic receptors is weak; may slightly reduce heart rate, but no ECG changes have occurred; exhibit weak anorexigenic action and can lead to slight weight loss

Uses

Symptomatic treatment of endogenous depression
Symptomatic treatment of obsessive-compulsive disorder (OCD).

Dosage

See Table 26-2.

Fate

Oral absorption is good and not appreciably decreased by food (food may increase absorption of sertraline); long elimination half-lives ($T_{1/2}$) (**fluoxetine**, 2–3 days [norfluoxetine, *active* metabolite, 7–9 days]; **paroxetine**, 21 hours [biotransformational enzyme can be saturated, causing higher than expected plasma levels during multiple dosing]; **sertraline**, 26 hours); highly bound to plasma proteins.

Common Side Effects

Nausea, vomiting, anorexia, anxiety, nervousness, insomnia, headache, sweating, mild tremor, lightheadedness

Significant Adverse Reactions

Listed in order of approximate decreasing frequency within each organ system

CNS: drowsiness, anxiety, tremor, dizziness, fatigue, decreased libido, abnormal dreams, agitation
GI: diarrhea, dry mouth, constipation, abdominal pain, vomiting, altered taste, flatulence, increased appetite
Dermatologic: rash, pruritus, alopecia, acneiform eruptions, contact dermatitis, urticaria, herpes simplex infection
Respiratory: upper respiratory infection, pharyngitis, flu-like syndrome, nasal congestion, sinusitis, cough, dyspnea, rhinitis, bronchitis
CV: palpitations, hot flashes, migraine, tachycardia
Musculoskeletal: back, joint, or muscle pain
Urogenital: frequent urination, painful menstruation, urinary tract infection
Miscellaneous: fever, asthenia, allergic reactions, visual disturbances, weight loss, chest pain, chills

Contraindications

Patients taking MAO inhibitors. *Cautious use* in persons with a history of seizures, impaired renal or hepatic function, anorexia, mania or hypomania, in pregnant or nursing women, and in the elderly.

Interactions

These agents may interact with other highly protein-bound drugs, resulting in an increased effect of both drugs
The $T_{1/2}$ of diazepam may be prolonged by concomitant administration of fluoxetine
Concurrent use of an MAO inhibitor may lead to increased adverse effects

Nursing Management

Refer to **Tricyclic Antidepressants**. In addition:

Surveillance During Therapy

Carefully evaluate drug effects in patient with liver or kidney disease. Because drug is metabolized primarily in liver, dosage should be lower or another drug should be used if liver function is impaired. Dosage should also be decreased if kidney disease is present.

Patient Teaching

Inform patient that antidepressant effect may not be evident until after 4 weeks or longer of use.
Emphasize importance of promptly reporting any adverse reactions. Drug withdrawal can be problematic because long $T_{1/2}$s of drug and metabolite cause active drug substance to persist weeks after drug is discontinued.

Other Atypical Antidepressants

• Bupropion

Wellbutrin

Bupropion is an aminoketone antidepressant unrelated to any other antidepressant. It is an alternative to the tricyclics for treating endogenous depression not responding to more conventional therapy.

Mechanism

Not established. Blocks dopamine reuptake; weakly inhibits norepinephrine and serotonin uptake; no effect on MAO; possesses CNS stimulating action

Uses

Short-term treatment of depression (effectiveness longer than 6 weeks has not been established)

Dosage

Initially, 100 mg twice a day; may increase to 100 mg 3 times/day after 3 days if necessary; maximum, 450 mg/day in three divided doses

Fate

Well absorbed orally; peak plasma levels occur within 2 hours; average $T_{1/2}$ is 12 to 16 hours; protein binding is approximately 80%; metabolites are eliminated in both urine and feces

Common Side Effects

Dry mouth, insomnia, headache, agitation, nausea/vomiting, constipation, tremor

Significant Adverse Reactions

CAUTION

A risk of seizures is closely associated with use of bupropion. At doses up to 450 mg/day, the risk is about 4 times that seen with other antidepressants. Seizure incidence increases almost 10-fold at doses between 450 and 600 mg/day. The total daily dose should not exceed 450 mg in three equally divided doses, and the drug should be used with extreme caution in persons with a history of seizures, cranial trauma, or other predisposition toward seizures.

CNS: sedation, insomnia, akinesia, confusion, hostility, impaired concentration, decreased libido, anxiety, blurred vision, auditory disturbances
CV: dizziness, tachycardia, hypertension, arrhythmias, palpitation
GI: weight loss, anorexia, diarrhea, dyspepsia
Other: menstrual irregularities, impotence, urinary frequency, rash, pruritus, fatigue, arthritic-like symptoms, fever, chills

Contraindications

Patients with a seizure disorder, anorexia, or bulimia, or those being treated with a MAO inhibitor. *Cautious use* in persons with psychoses, mania, unstable heart disease, impaired liver or kidney function, and in pregnant or nursing women

Interactions

Bupropion is an enzyme inducer in the liver and may increase the metabolism of other drugs metabolized by the hepatic microsomal enzyme system.
Concurrent use of bupropion and levodopa may increase the risk of adverse reactions to levodopa.
The toxicity of bupropion may be enhanced by MAO inhibitors.
Drugs that lower the seizure threshold increase the risk of seizures with bupropion.

Nursing Management

Refer to **Tricyclic Antidepressants**. In addition:

Nursing Interventions

Medication Administration

Use extreme caution when administering bupropion to persons with increased risk of seizures (eg, alcoholics, epileptics, patients with CNS tumors or trauma). Begin at low doses, make dosage changes gradually, and closely monitor patients. Question patient about any prior seizure episodes and be aware of the danger of seizures in persons with a history of seizure activity.

Surveillance During Therapy

Monitor weight during therapy with bupropion. Weight loss occurs commonly and may be excessive.

Patient Teaching

Inform patients that drug may impair the ability to perform tasks requiring judgment or motor skills. Advise caution during early stages of therapy.
Impress patients with the importance of adhering to prescribed dosage schedule to minimize the risk of seizures and other adverse reactions.
Caution against taking any other medication during therapy with bupropion unless approved by healthcare provider.

• Trazodone

Desyrel

Trazodone is an effective antidepressant chemically unrelated to tricyclics, tetracyclics, or MAO inhibitors. Its use is associated with minimal anticholinergic and cardiac conductive effects, although arrhythmogenic incidences have occurred with trazodone, particularly at high doses. Symptomatic improvement is often noted within 1 week.

Mechanism

Selectively inhibits serotonin uptake in the brain but, *unlike* all other antidepressants, *strongly* blocks 5-HT_{1A} and 5-HT_2 receptors; does not elicit CNS stimulation

Uses

Treatment of depression, with or without accompanying anxiety

Dosage

Initially, 150 mg/day in divided doses; increase by 50-mg/day increments every 3 or 4 days until optimal effect is attained.
Maximum dose is 400 mg/day in outpatients and 600 mg/day in inpatients.

Fate

Well absorbed orally; peak plasma levels occur in 1 hour if taken on an empty stomach and within 2 hours if taken with food. Clinically significant therapeutic response is seen within 2 weeks in 75% of responders; metabolized in the liver; elimination $T_{1/2}$ is 4 to 8 hours.

Common Side Effects

Drowsiness, dizziness, lightheadedness, fatigue, dry mouth, constipation, nasal congestion

Significant Adverse Reactions

(See also general discussion of tricyclic antidepressants)

CV: hypotension, syncope, tachycardia, chest pain
CNS: confusion, headache, insomnia, nervousness, disorientation, reduced concentration, malaise
Autonomic: blurred vision, constipation
GI: nausea, vomiting, salivation
Neurologic: incoordination, paresthesias, tremors
Other: allergic skin conditions; myalgia; sinus congestion; tinnitus; weight gain; tired, itching eyes; sweating; dyspnea; decreased libido; altered menses; anemia, leukopenia

Contraindications

No absolute contraindications. *Cautious use* in patients with arrhythmias, hypotension, in pregnant or nursing mothers, and in persons receiving MAO inhibitors. Drug should not be administered concurrently with ECT or during initial recovery phase after myocardial infarction.

Interactions

See general discussion of tricyclic antidepressants. In addition:

Increased serum levels of digoxin and phenytoin have been reported with trazodone therapy.

Increased CNS depression can occur with concurrent use of trazodone and alcohol, barbiturates, and other CNS depressants.

Trazodone may enhance the hypotensive effects of most antihypertensive drugs; however, the effects of clonidine may be inhibited by trazodone.

Nursing Management

Refer to **Tricyclic Antidepressants**.

Patient Teaching

Instruct patient to take drug during or shortly after a meal or snack because absorption is enhanced by the presence of food in the stomach.

Inhibition of Monoamine Oxidase

Drugs that can form stable complexes with—and inhibit the action of—the enzyme MAO have been employed for decades as antidepressants. Currently available drugs include isocarboxazid, phenelzine, and tranylcypromine. MAO is an enzyme system that catalyzes the deamination (inactivation) of several naturally occurring biogenic amines (especially norepinephrine, epinephrine, and serotonin) in numerous body tissues, particularly nerve endings and the liver, kidney, and intestines. MAO is found within the mitochondria of cells of these tissues; its principal role in neuronal transmission is to regulate *intra*cellular neurotransmitter levels. Inhibition of MAO in nerve endings increases the amount of neurotransmitter available for release (*after* arrival of a nerve impulse). By blocking a major process for metabolism of intraneuronal catecholamines and serotonin, MAO inhibitors increase the synaptic level of these amine neurotransmitters, consequently enhancing activation of postsynaptic receptors. As discussed previously under Tricyclic Antidepressants, increased stimulation of postsynaptic receptors reduces the sensitivity—and amount—of these receptor sites; this process is termed *receptor "down-regulation."* The successful reduction of depressive symptoms appears to be the result of such down-regulation.

Although MAO inhibitors were the first clinically effective antidepressants to be introduced, their relatively high toxicity has restricted their usefulness to serving as alternatives to the more effective and less toxic tricyclic antidepressants. MAO inhibitors are frequently employed in a hospital setting in patients not responding to other antidepressants. Their use in outpatients must be **carefully** and **continually** monitored—and necessary precautions taken—to avoid the occurrence of serious adverse reactions and drug interactions.

Because MAO inhibitors interfere with the activity of enzymes responsible for inactivating many endogenous and exogenous amines, the effects of aminergic substances contained in several foods may be markedly enhanced in the presence of an MAO inhibitor. Certain sympathomimetic amines such as tyramine, which is found in many foods, can exert a potent pressor effect. Normally, tyramine is efficiently metabolized by MAO; however, in the presence of an MAO inhibitor, the pressor action of tyramine can be substantially potentiated, and hypertensive crises have occurred with ingestion of tyramine-containing foods (eg, sausages, aged cheeses, smoked fish, chianti wine, caviar) as well as foods containing other pressor substances normally metabolized by MAO.

Mechanism

Inhibit the MAO enzyme system by forming a stable complex with the enzyme (isocarboxazid and phenelzine form irreversible bonds); consequently, intraneuronal breakdown of catecholamines and serotonin is inhibited, and their concentration increases in several body tissues including the CNS, heart, blood, and intestine. Increased intraneuronal concentrations of these amine neurohormones result in a larger pool of neurohormone available for release and thus an enhanced postsynaptic action. The increased activity of norepinephrine, serotonin, and possibly other neurohormones at postjunctional receptor sites in the CNS is believed to underlie the effectiveness of MAO inhibitors in relieving depression. Likewise, increased neurohormone availability in other body tissues is thought to underlie many of the toxic reactions elicited by these agents. These drugs also inhibit hepatic microsomal drug-metabolizing enzymes, thereby prolonging the action of many other drugs.

Uses

Management of severe endogenous, exogenous (atypical), or reactive depressions resistant to treatment with tricyclic antidepressants, ECT, or other adjunctive psychotherapy

Dosage

See Table 26-3

Fate

Readily absorbed orally; enzyme inhibition occurs rapidly, but clinical effects take several weeks to develop, except with tranylcypromine (10–14 days); termination of drug effect after administration of irreversible inhibitors (isocarboxazid, phenelzine) depends largely on regeneration of MAO enzyme, a process taking several weeks; tranylcypromine effects decline within 3 to 5 days after discontinuation of therapy; drugs are metabolized in the liver and excreted in the urine as metabolites and some unchanged drug

Common Side Effects

Orthostatic hypotension, dizziness, weakness, fatigue, jitteriness, hyperactivity, insomnia, GI disturbances, headache, disturbances in cardiac rate and rhythm, dry mouth, blurred vision, hyperhidrosis

Significant Adverse Reactions

CNS: vertigo, tremors, hypomania, euphoria, confusion, memory impairment, drowsiness, ataxia, excessive sweating, delirium, hallucinations, convulsions

Autonomic/cardiovascular: dysuria, incontinence, impotence, palpitations, edema, weight gain

Hematologic/dermatologic: leukopenia, hypochromic anemia, skin rash, hepatocellular jaundice

Other: anorexia, peripheral neuritis, photosensitivity reactions, nystagmus, sodium retention, hypoglycemia, galactorrhea, glaucoma, optic damage

Overdose: restlessness, tachycardia, hypotension, respiratory depression, confusion, incoherence, convulsions, shock

Table 26-3. Monoamine Oxidase Inhibitor Antidepressants

Drug	*Usual Dosage Range*	*Nursing Considerations*
Isocarboxazid *Marplan*	*Initially:* 30 mg/day; reduce to maintenance levels (usually 10–20 mg/day) as soon as possible	Administer with meals to reduce gastric upset; adjust dosage critically, on basis of patient observation; note that although therapeutic effects may take several weeks to develop, toxic interactions can occur within hours; may be administered either as a single dose or in divided doses
Phenelzine *Nardil*	*Initially:* 15 mg 3 times/day; reduce slowly to maintenance levels, usually 15 mg every 1–2 days	Effective in moderate to severe depressive states, especially accompanied by anxiety and agitation; do not exceed 75 mg/day
Tranylcypromine *Parnate*	*Initially:* 20–30 mg/day; reduce to 10–20 mg/day as needed *With concurrent ECT:* 10 mg 1–2 times/day	Incidence of hypertensive reactions is higher than with other MAO inhibitors; latency of therapeutic effect is generally shorter (3–5 days) than with other similar drugs; it is a structural analog of amphetamine and probably exerts a direct receptor activation, as well as MAO inhibition

Contraindications

In children younger than 16 years of age, congestive heart failure, liver disease, pheochromocytoma, hyperthyroidism, hypertension, cardiovascular or cerebrovascular disease, and elderly or debilitated patients. *Cautious use* in patients with epilepsy, diabetes, depression accompanying drug or alcohol addiction, chronic brain syndromes, history of anginal attacks, impaired renal function, and during pregnancy and lactation.

Interactions

Effects of sympathomimetic drugs (eg, amphetamines, catecholamines, L-dopa, ephedrine, phenylephrine, methylphenidate) may be potentiated, resulting in severe hypertension, headache, and possibly cerebrovascular hemorrhage.

Hypertensive reactions can occur in patients taking MAO inhibitors who ingest foods containing tyramine, a pressor substance (eg, cheeses, sour cream, beer, red wines, yeasts, yogurt, pickled herring, chicken livers, aged meats, fermented sausages) as well as caffeine, chocolate, and licorice.

Concurrent use of MAO inhibitors and tricyclic antidepressants (or within 10 days of each other) can result in severe hypertension, convulsions, fever, sweating, delirium, tremor, circulatory collapse, and coma, although some tricyclic antidepressants have been employed safely in conjunction with MAO inhibitors.

MAO inhibitors may increase the toxic effects of barbiturates and phenothiazines by decreasing their metabolism in the liver.

Effects of antihypertensive drugs may be potentiated by MAO inhibitors (increased orthostatic *hypo*tension); however, severe *hypertension* can occur with parenteral use of reserpine or guanethidine, because of release of large amounts of catecholamines.

Hypotension, respiratory arrest, shock, and coma can occur if MAO inhibitors are used in combination with CNS depressants such as alcohol, anesthetics, narcotics (especially meperidine), and sedative–hypnotics.

Increased hypoglycemic effects have occurred with combined use of MAO inhibitors and either insulin or oral hypoglycemics.

Muscle-relaxing action of succinylcholine may be increased because MAO inhibitors interfere with plasma pseudocholinesterase, the enzyme that inactivates succinylcholine.

MAO inhibitors reduce convulsive seizure threshold and may reduce the efficacy of antiepileptic drugs.

Effects of anticholinergic, antihistaminic, and antiparkinsonian drugs may be potentiated by MAO inhibitors, which decrease their rate of metabolism.

Nursing Management

Pretherapy Assessment

Assess and record baseline data necessary for detection of adverse effects of MAO inhibitors: General: VS, body weight, skin color and temperature; CNS: orientation, affect, reflexes, vision; CVS: orthostatic BP, perfusion; GI: bowel sounds, normal output, liver evaluation; GU: normal output; Endocrine: thyroid palpation; Lab: liver, kidney, and thyroid function, urinalysis, CBC, ECG.

Review medical history and documents for existing or previous conditions that:

a. require cautious use of MAO inhibitors: seizure disorders; drug/alcohol dependence; chronic brain syndromes; history of anginal attacks; impaired renal and hepatic dysfunction
b. contraindicate use of MAO inhibitors: allergy to any MAO inhibitor; congestive heart failure; pheochromocytoma; hypertension; use in children or the elderly; **pregnancy (Category C)**, lactation (secreted in breast milk; safety not established, avoid use in nursing mothers)

Nursing Interventions

Medication Administration

Ensure that depressed and potentially suicidal patients have access to only a limited supply of these drugs.

Arrange to discontinue drug and monitor BP carefully if patient reports unusual or severe headache.
Provide phentolamine or other α-adrenergic blocker on standby in case hypertensive crisis occurs.
Establish baseline blood pressure before therapy is initiated and monitor frequently during therapy.

Surveillance During Therapy

Monitor indicators of fluid retention (intake and output, edema, weight gain) until dosage is stabilized. Advise primary care provider of any changes because renal impairment may result in greatly increased toxicity.
Monitor results of liver function studies and blood cell counts, which should be performed before initiation of therapy and at regular intervals thereafter.
Assist with evaluation of patient's response to therapy. If no significant clinical response occurs within 4 weeks, the patient should be reevaluated, and an alternative form of treatment should be considered.
Carefully assess severely depressed patient during initial improvement phase. Suicidal tendency may be increased as depression and psychomotor retardation are lessened.
Monitor for toxicity.
Carefully monitor laboratory studies and patient for indications of adverse reactions.
Interpret results of diagnostic tests and contact practitioner.
Monitor for possible drug–drug and drug–nutrient interactions: See interactions.

Patient Teaching

Encourage patient to maintain prescribed regimen. Beneficial effects may not become manifest for several weeks.
Carefully explain the untoward reactions associated with use of MAO inhibitors, especially the possibility of hypertensive crisis.
Emphasize the need to *closely* follow prescribed drug regimen and diet to minimize the danger of untoward reactions.
Ensure that patient and family have a list of, and fully understand, tyramine-containing foods that should not be eaten. Consumption of such foods could precipitate a hypertensive crisis. Aged cheese, sour cream, imported beer and ale, red wine (especially chianti), yogurt, yeast, pickled herring, aged meat and meat tenderizer, and chicken liver are among the foods that should be avoided. Chocolate and caffeine have also been implicated in blood pressure elevations with MAO inhibitors.
Urge patient not to take any other drugs, including OTC preparations, without consulting the healthcare provider who prescribed the MAO inhibitor, because numerous serious drug interactions can occur.
Stress the importance of noting and reporting early signs of an impending hypertensive reaction (headache, palpitations, neck stiffness, sweating, nausea, photophobia).
Instruct patient not to discontinue drug without supervision. Rapid withdrawal may induce excitability, hallucinations, and possibly severe depression, especially after prolonged use or high dosage.
Warn patient to avoid all foods and drugs that may be hazardous for at least several weeks after the last dose of MAO inhibitor has been taken.
Teach patient interventions to help minimize orthostatic hypotension.
Advise patient and family to be alert for and to report the development of hypomania, which occurs most often when hyperkinetic symptoms have been masked by concurrent depression. Relief of depression by MAO inhibitors can precipitate agitation, delusion, and exaggeration of feelings. Use of sedatives is indicated.
Teach patient how to recognize and report the development of hepatic complications, marked by jaundicelike reactions (eg, rash, abdominal pain, pruritus, yellowing of skin). If they occur, drug may need to be discontinued.
Instruct patient to report immediately any visual disturbances, especially changes in red-green color vision, because these are often the initial signs of drug-induced ocular change.
Suggest interventions to relieve mouth dryness.
Instruct patient to inform practitioner of MAO inhibitor use before surgery. MAO inhibitors should be discontinued at least 1 week before elective surgery to reduce the danger of interaction with anesthetic agents and postoperative narcotics.
Caution patient, especially one with a history of heart disease, to avoid overexertion. MAO inhibitors suppress anginal pain and therefore may mask the warning signs of an ischemic attack.
Teach diabetic patient how to carefully observe for signs of hypoglycemia, and inform patient that the dosage of antidiabetic agent may need to be adjusted.
Explain that abrupt discontinuation of therapy could result in nausea, muscle aching, insomnia, and irritability. The drug should be withdrawn gradually under supervision of the prescriber.
Reassure patient that many side effects common early in therapy disappear or diminish with continued use; others may remain. The patient should inform prescriber if side effects appear or persist, because dosage adjustment or change to another agent may help minimize them.

Selected Bibliography

Ananth J, Johnson K: Psychotropic and medical drug interactions. Psychother Psychosom 58:178, 1992
Greden JF: Antidepressant maintenance medications: When to discontinue and how to stop. J Clin Psychiatry 54(8, suppl):39, 1993
Greenblatt DJ: Basic pharmacokinetic principles and their application to psychotropic drugs. J Clin Psychiatry 54(9, suppl):8, 1993
Henry JA: The safety of antidepressants. Br J Psychiatry 160:439, 1992
Hollister LE, Claghorn JL: New antidepressants. Annu Rev Pharmacol 33:165, 1993
Karson CN et al: Human brain fluoxetine concentrations. J Neuropsychiatry Clin Neurosci 5(3):322, 1993
Kerrick JM, Fine PG, Lipman AG, Love G: Low-dose amitriptyline as an adjunct to opioids for postoperative orthopedic pain: A placebo-controlled trial. Pain 52:325, 1993

Otton SV, et al: Inhibition by fluoxetine of cytochrome P450 2D6 activity. Clin Pharmacol Ther 53:401, 1993

Rasmussen SA, Eisen JL, Pato MT: Current issues in the, pharmacologic management of obsessive compulsive disorder. J Clin Psychiatry 54(6, suppl):4, 1993

Richelson E: Treatment of acute depression. Psychiatry Clin North Am 16(3):461, 1993

Ritch R, Krupin T, Henry C, Kurata F: Oral imipramine and acute angle closure glaucoma. Arch Ophthalmol 112:67, 1994

Stahl SM: Serotonergic mechanisms and antidepressants. Psychol Med 23:281, 1993

Stewart RB: Advances in pharmacotherapy: depression in the elderly—issues and advances in treatment. J Clin Pharm Ther 18:243, 1993

Nursing Bibliography

Gomez G, Gomez E: Depression in the elderly. Journal of Psychosocial Nursing and Mental Health Services 31(5):23–33, 1993

Neese J: Depression in general hospitals. The Nursing Clinics of North America 26(3):613-622, 1991

Steiner D, Marcopulos B: Depression in the elderly: Characteristics and clinical management. Nursing Clinics of North America 26(3): 585–600, 1991

U.S. Department of Health & Human Services: Depression in primary care: Detection, diagnosis and treatment. Journal Psychosocial Nursing and Mental Health Services 31(6):19-28, 1993

27

Anticonvulsants

Barbiturates

Mephobarbital
Phenobarbital

Deoxybarbiturate

Primidone

Hydantoins

Ethotoin
Mephenytoin
Phenytoin

Oxazolidinediones

Paramethadione
Trimethadione

Succinimides

Ethosuximide
Methsuximide
Phensuximide

Benzodiazepines

Clonazepam
Clorazepate
Diazepam

Other

Acetazolamide
Carbamazepine
Felbamate
Gabapentin
Magnesium Sulfate
Phenacemide
Valproic Acid

Anticonvulsant drugs are usually effective in controlling those seizures occurring in patients with epilepsy. Careful regulation of dosage to maintain blood levels of anticonvulsants in the therapeutic range is extremely important for maximum efficacy. Both the drugs used **and** their respective doses must be individualized according to each patient's needs, which can change over time (eg, increased seizures when a patient is going through a stressful condition). Because some anticonvulsant drugs may actually **worsen** certain types of seizure disorders, successful therapy depends on accurate diagnosis, careful selection of each agent, and critical adjustment of dosage. Anticonvulsants are also used in treatment of seizures caused by other conditions such as high fever (in children), head trauma, and brain tumors.

Epilepsy is a chronic central nervous system (CNS) disorder estimated to afflict between 0.5% and 1.5% of the population. Although there are various ways to classify the types of epilepsy, certain characteristics (eg, electroencephalographic [EEG] alterations; muscular hyperactivity [localized or generalized]) can aid in differentiation of the major types of epilepsies; these are outlined in Table 27-1.

Seizures can be broadly categorized as being *generalized* or *partial* (ie, localized). "Generalized seizures" include tonic, clonic, tonic-clonic (grand mal), simple absence (petit mal), atypical absence, myoclonic jerking and atonic-akinetic. In contrast, "partial seizures" may be subdivided according to the degree of total body involvement. Simple partial (focal) seizures are characterized by minimal spread of the discharge, and limited involvement of the extremities. In complex partial seizures, the discharge becomes more widespread, and complex motor or behavioral aberrations are noted. Complex seizures arise primarily in the temporal lobe (therefore sometimes referred to as *temporal lobe* or *psychomotor* epilepsy), spread more widely, and affect more areas of the body.

Therapy usually is initiated with a single agent, but complete control of most seizure types generally requires addition of a second—and often a third—drug. Frequent dosage alterations or too-rapid shifting among anticonvulsant drugs should be avoided. The major requirements of an antiepileptic drug is that it control seizures with little or no sedation or other adverse drug effects. Many currently employed anticonvulsants do provide adequate control of seizures without subjecting the patient to frequent and debilitating adverse reactions. Although these drugs do not *cure* the affliction, they do allow the epileptic patient to function productively.

Stabilization of epileptic patients is a difficult task in most cases. Patients should be advised of the dangers involved if they—without consulting their doctor—change the amount and/or frequency of their drug doses; such **unauthorized** changes can cause blood levels to *increase* into the toxic range or decrease *below* the therapeutic level (Table 27-2). Because physical and emotional stresses can disrupt stable conditions, patients should be taught to carefully monitor themselves and report any unusual symptoms that occur during therapy; such symptoms may indicate early warnings of serious toxicity. Drugs should be discontinued *gradually* whenever necessary, and changes in medication should be accomplished slowly over several weeks. Abrupt discontinuance—or alteration—of drug therapy can precipitate *status epilepticus*, a series of rapid, repetitive seizures that may be fatal unless terminated quickly.

Several agents (including phenobarbital and diazepam) that are employed in the emergency control of acute convulsive states resulting from trauma, hyperthermia of infection, or drug overdosage have already been reviewed in previous chapters. The drugs considered here are used primarily to treat the various forms of epilepsy and therefore may be regarded as specific antiepileptic agents.

Barbiturates

Although all barbiturates can abolish seizure activity at doses sufficient to produce anesthesia, only two barbiturates—phenobarbital and mephobarbital—are useful for treatment of epilepsy. They are usually effective at nonsedating doses, exert a prolonged action, and tend to be well tolerated during extended drug therapy.

Mechanism

Reduce excitability of nerve cells; facilitate gamma aminobutyric acid (GABA) activity, ie, increase *duration* of opening of $GABA_A$-activated Cl^- channel, allowing more Cl^- to flow in, causing **hyper**polarization and stabilization of the cell membrane

Table 27-1. **Classification and Management of Seizures**

Seizure	*Characteristics*	*Useful Drugs*
Partial		
Simple partial	Manifestations differ according to site of the lesion; convulsions may be confined to a single limb or muscle group (Jacksonian seizures); no impairment of consciousness; sensory disturbances also noted; EEG shows spiking at site of focus	Carbamazepine, felbamate, gabapentin, phenobarbital, primidone, valproic acid.
Complex, partial seizures (psychomotor epilepsy)	Confused behavior, with involuntary, purposeless, repetitive motor activity; usually accompanied by autonomic manifestations and loss of consciousness; seizures last several minutes, but patients have no recall of the attack; bizarre actions are sometimes seen; EEG spiking is present in the temporal lobe; control is difficult	Carbamazepine, felbamate, gabapentin, hydantoins, phenobarbital, primidone, valproic acid, phenacemide (?), clonazepam (?)
Generalized		
Tonic Seizures	Opisthotonus; rigidity; loss of consciousness; autonomic manifestations	Carbamazepine, phenytoin, valproic acid
Clonic seizures	Rhythmic alternating contractions of all muscles; loss of consciousness; autonomic manifestations	Carbamazepine, phenytoin, valproic acid
Tonic–clonic seizures (grand mal)	Tonic rigidity of extremities, followed by massive, synchronous clonic jerking for several minutes; urinary incontinence is common; lassitude and stupor ensue	Barbiturates, carbamazepine, hydantoins, primidone, valproic acid
Simple absence seizures (petit mal)	Sudden loss of consciousness lasting up to 30 sec but usually of much shorter duration; can occur hundreds of times a day; characteristic 3/sec spike-wave EEG patterns; may be accompanied by some clonic jerking of the eyelids or extremities and autonomic manifestations but frequently no motor activity is evident; rare in the adult	Carbamazepine, clonazepam, oxazolidinediones, succinimides, valproic acid
Atypical absence seizures	Similar to simple absence seizures but with slower onset and longer duration; EEG pattern is often more heterogenous	Carbamazepine, valproic acid
Myoclonic jerking	Sudden, violent contractions of the extremities, with or without loss of consciousness; occur most often after awakening or before retiring, often in combination with other seizure types; multiple EEG spikes	Carbamazepine, phenytoin, valproic acid
Atonic–akinetic seizures	Sudden loss of muscle tone, usually lasting 10–60 sec; sagging of head and dropping to ground are noted; EEG shows a slow spike-wave pattern; most often due to an organic brain abnormality	Carbamazepine, phenytoin, valproic acid
Infantile spasms (hypsarrhythmia)	Brief, recurrent myoclonic jerks with abrupt flexion or extension of the limbs or whole body; most patients are mentally retarded; high-voltage, slow waves are predominant in the EEG.	Corticosteroids, benzodiazepines

Uses

Generalized tonic-clonic seizures (grand mal); used alone in infants and young children, and most often in combination with phenytoin in adults

Generalized myoclonic jerks

Complex absence seizures with autonomic manifestations

Status epilepticus

Infantile spasms (effectiveness not conclusively demonstrated)

Dosage

See Table 27-3

Fate

Well absorbed orally; onset after oral administration ranges from 30 to 60 minutes; effects are evident in 10 to 15 minutes with intravenous injection of phenobarbital; duration lasts from 8 to 12 hours; partly metabolized in the liver and excreted both as metabolites and unchanged drug in the urine.

Common Side Effects

Lethargy, dizziness, irritability

Significant Adverse Reactions

Nausea, vomiting, diarrhea, skin rash (2% of patients), urticaria, angioedema, muscle and joint pain, bradycardia, hypoventilation, laryngospasm, respiratory depression, paradoxical excitation (especially in children and elderly), megaloblastic anemia, insomnia, nightmares, altered behavior, blood dyscrasias (rare)

Contraindications

Latent or manifest porphyria, respiratory obstruction. *Cautious use* in patients with pulmonary, hepatic, or renal disease, status

Table 27-2. **Therapeutic Serum Levels of Selected Anticonvulsants**

	*Effective Serum Level** (μg/mL)
Carbamazepine	4–12
Clonazepam	0.02–0.08
Ethosuximide	40–100
Phenobarbital	10–40
Phenytoin	10–20†
Primidone	5–15
Valproic Acid	50–100

* Although total (free + bound) serum levels are currently used clinically, the best correlation with therapeutic effectiveness is the *free* [unbound] serum level
† At levels of approximately 20 μg/mL, the biotransformation of phenytoin becomes zero order; a small increase in dose will produce a much larger (very disproportionate) elevation of plasma level
Note: Chronic administration of several anticonvulsants (eg, carbamazepine, phenobarbital, phenytoin, primidone) usually produces enzyme induction; plasma levels decrease and the patient experiences increased frequency of seizures; a small increase in daily dosage will often reestablish the desired therapeutic level.

asthmaticus, hyperthyroidism, diabetes, and in elderly or debilitated patients. Too-rapid intravenous injection can result in hypotension, laryngospasm, respiratory depression, and apnea.

Interactions

See Chapter 22.

Nursing Management

See Chapter 22. In addition:

Nursing Interventions

Medication Administration

Ensure that adequate resuscitative measures are immediately at hand, and monitor vital signs closely when administering drugs intravenously in acute convulsive states. Drugs should be given slowly.

Be prepared to administer vitamin K prophylactically at birth to infants born to mothers receiving the drug. Drugs may cause neonatal hemorrhage by reducing levels of vitamin K–dependent clotting factors produced in the liver.

Follow proper procedures for handling Schedule IV controlled substances.

Patient Teaching

Warn patient that drug may impair mental and physical abilities required for performance of many tasks such as driving.

Prepare patient and family for the possibility of paradoxical excitatory and other unusual affective reactions, which are particularly likely to occur in the elderly and in young children.

Explain that prolonged use, even in rather low doses, can lead to tolerance and habituation. Teach patient to

Table 27-3. **Antiepileptic Barbiturates**

Drug	*Usual Dosage Range*	*Nursing Considerations*
BARBITURATES		
Mephobarbital (C-IV) *Mebaral*	Adults: 400–600 mg/day Children (older than 5 y): 32–64 mg 3–4 times/day; (younger than 5 y) 16–32 mg 3–4 times/day	Similar to phenobarbital in most respects, producing somewhat less sedation; largely converted to phenobarbital within 24 h; used as a single daily dose at bedtime for nocturnal seizures; withdraw slowly when necessary, and reduce dose of other antiepileptics when added to the regimen
Phenobarbital (C-IV) *Various manufacturers*	*Oral* Adults: 50–100 mg 2–3 times/day Children: Initially, 3–5 mg/kg/day for 7–10 days; adjust to blood level of 10 μg/mL to 15 μg/mL IM, IV Adults: 200–300 mg; repeat in 6 h if needed *or* 300–600 mg initially, then 120–240 mg every 20 min as needed Children (IV): 20 mg/kg initially, then 6 mg/kg every 20 min as needed	Very effective alone for treatment of grand mal (especially in children) and as part of the drug regimen in most other forms of epilepsy; also used IV or IM for status epilepticus and other acute convulsive states; after IV injection, 15 min or more may be required to attain peak CNS concentration; thus, give drug *intermittently*, even though convulsions persist; continuous injection can result in excessive CNS levels of drug after convulsions have ceased, possibly leading to respiratory depression; solutions should be prepared in sterile water for injection and should not be used if not completely clear after 5 min of mixing; inject drug within 30 min after preparation of solution; drowsiness is common in early stages of therapy but diminishes with continued use; frequency of IV administration is determined by patient's response; discontinue drug as soon as desired response is obtained
DEOXYBARBITURATE		
Primidone *Mysoline* *(CAN) Apo-Primidone, PMS-Primidone*	*Adults*: Initially 100–125 mg/day for 3 days Usual maintenance range: 250 mg 3–4 times/day *Children*: Initially; 50 mg/day Usual maintenance range: 125–250 mg 3 times/day	Similar to phenobarbital (one of its active metabolites is phenobarbital); may cause blood dyscrasias; monitor hematological changes; clinical effects may take several weeks to become evident; do not discontinue abruptly

recognize signs of tolerance and inform patient that, if drug must be withdrawn, it should be discontinued *slowly* to avoid possibility of delirium, tremors, and convulsions.
Instruct patient to increase intake of vitamin D, because drugs may increase vitamin D requirements by stepping up its metabolism, occasionally leading to rickets or osteomalacia with prolonged use.

Deoxybarbiturate

- ***Primidone*** *(Pregnancy Category D)*

Mysoline

(CAN) Apo-Primidone, PMS-Primidone

Although not a true barbiturate, primidone is structurally related to phenobarbital and has a similar profile of action. Of importance is the fact that primidone is **biotransformed** to two **active** metabolites: phenobarbital and phenylethylmalonamide.

Mechanism

Probably similar to phenobarbital

Uses

Grand mal seizures
Psychomotor seizures
Simple partial seizures (Jacksonian)
Benign familial (essential) tremor (investigational use)

Dosage

See Table 27-3.

Fate

Slowly but well absorbed orally; peak serum levels attained in 3 to 4 hours; prolonged action caused by conversion to active metabolites with half-lives ($T_{1/2}$) of 2 to 4 days; excreted through kidneys, approximately one-fourth as unchanged drug

Common Side Effects

Lethargy, ataxia, vertigo, irritability

Significant Adverse Reactions

Nausea, anorexia, vomiting, fatigue, allergic reactions, severe skin rash (macropapular and morbilliform), lymph gland enlargement, megaloblastic anemia (rare), visual disturbances, impotence, personality disorders, drowsiness, blood dyscrasias (leukopenia, thrombocytopenia), systemic lupus–like reaction

Contraindications

Latent or manifest porphyria.
Cautious use in pregnant or nursing women and in persons who must drive or operate heavy machinery

Interactions

See Barbiturates. In addition:

Concurrent administration of phenytoin may increase the toxic effects of primidone by altering its metabolism
Primidone can decrease plasma levels of carbamazepine
Isoniazid may inhibit the metabolism of primidone to active metabolites

Nursing Management

See **Barbiturates**. In addition:

Nursing Interventions

Monitor for early signs of lymph node enlargement, fever, sore throat, bruising, and weakness, possible indications of blood dyscrasias.
Assess for signs of folic acid deficiency (drug may impair folate absorption), such as anemia, mental dysfunction, neuropathy, and psychiatric disturbances. Use of folic acid (15 mg/day) or vitamin B_6 may be necessary to prevent megaloblastic anemia.
Review patient's medication history for evidence of allergy to barbiturates before initiating administration. A patient allergic to barbiturates is probably allergic to primidone.
Observe for early signs of overdosage (eg, incoordination, slurred speech, blurred vision). If they occur, dosage should be gradually decreased.
Expect dosage adjustments to be made gradually and dosage of other antiepileptics to be readjusted if primidone is added to the regimen.

Patient Teaching

Inform patient that a complete blood count (CBC) is recommended at 6-month intervals with prolonged therapy.

Hydantoins *(Pregnancy Category D)*

- ***Ethotoin***
- ***Mephenytoin***
- ***Phenytoin***

The hydantoin group of antiepileptic agents is effective for the treatment of grand mal seizures; they can also be used to control psychomotor epilepsy. Unlike barbiturates, hydantoins are not strong CNS depressants and, usually, in therapeutic doses, do not reduce normal sensory function. Phenytoin is the most frequently prescribed of the three currently marketed hydantoins; ethotoin and mephenytoin are the others (Table 27-4)

Mechanism

Inhibit spread of seizure activity to neurons surrounding seizure focus in the motor cortex by raising the threshold of excitability of these neurons; block Na^+ and Ca^{2+} channels.

Uses

Grand mal seizures (may be combined with primidone or carbamazepine)
Focal, Jacksonian, or psychomotor seizures, either alone or in combination with primidone
Alcohol withdrawal syndrome
Trigeminal neuralgia
Cardiac arrhythmias (especially ventricular arrhythmias caused by digitalis intoxication [see Chapter 32])

Table 27-4. **Hydantoins**

Drug	Usual Dosage Range	Nursing Considerations
Ethotoin *Peganone*	Adults: 250 mg 4 times/day initially; increase to optimal levels (Usually 2–3 g/day) Children: 750 mg/day initially; maintenance 500–1000 mg/day based on age and weight	Administer with food, and begin therapy at small dose levels; compatible with most other anticonvulsants (dosage must be adjusted) except phenacemide (danger of paranoid reactions); less effective than phenytoin; but somewhat less toxic as well; *not* used as an antiarrhythmic
Mephenytoin *Mesantoin*	Adults: Initial dose 50–100 mg/day; increase gradually to optimal levels (Usual range, 200–600 mg/day) Children: 100–400 mg/day based on age, weight, and severity of seizures	Most toxic of the hydantoins; reserved for patients refractory to less toxic anticonvulsants; may be useful in Jacksonian seizures; possesses a strong sedative action; blood counts should be performed every 2–4 wk; more rapidly absorbed than other hydantoins with an onset of action in 30 minutes
Phenytoin *Dilantin Infatab,* *Dilantin-30 Pediatric,* *Dilantin-125* **Phenytoin Sodium, Extended** *Dilantin Kapseals* **Phenytoin Sodium, Prompt** **Phenytoin Sodium Parenteral** *Dilantin*	*Oral* Adults: Initially, 100 mg 3 times/day; usual range is 300–400 mg/day Children: Initially 5 mg/kg/day in 2 or 3 divided doses; usual maintenance range is 4–8 mg/kg/day in children under 6 IV Status epilepticus Adults: 150–250 mg; repeat in 30 min with 100–150 mg if necessary Children: 250 mg/m^2 body surface area *Arrhythmias* 100 mg every 5 min until arrhythmia is abolished (maximum, 1,000 mg) *IM* *Neurosurgery* 100–200 mg/4 h during surgery and postoperative period (maximum, 1,000 mg/day)	Owing to their slower dissolution rate, *extended* phenytoin sodium capsules (Dilantin) can be used on a more convenient once-daily basis when seizure control has been established with divided doses initially; *do not* administer IM in status epilepticus, because erratic absorption prevents attaining sufficient plasma levels; an IM dose 50% greater than the oral dose is necessary to maintain stable plasma levels; margin between the effective and toxic IV doses is very small; administer slowly and carefully monitor vital signs; do *not* exceed IV infusion rate of 50 mg/min and avoid *continuous* infusion; effective against digitalis-induced arrhythmias (see Chapter 31); phenytoin is also available in combination with phenobarbital (Dilantin-Pb capsules)

Status epilepticus and seizures during neurosurgery (intravenous phenytoin)

Dosage

See Table 27-4

Fate

(Discussion applies to phenytoin, the only hydantoin whose pharmacokinetics has been extensively studied)

Generally slowly absorbed orally; rate and extent of phenytoin absorption vary widely among the different available preparations, the sodium salt being the best absorbed; bioavailability also differs markedly (20%–90%) among products from different manufacturers; oral phenytoin sodium *extended* (Dilantin) attains peak plasma levels in 4 to 12 hours; phenytoin sodium *prompt* achieves peak serum levels in 2 to 3 hours; erratically absorbed after intramuscular injection; peak blood levels occur at varying times up to 24 hours and are significantly lower than blood levels obtained with oral or intravenous administration; highly bound (85%–95%) to plasma proteins; metabolized in the liver and excreted largely as conjugated metabolites in the urine; elimination $T_{1/2}$ ranges from 8 to 60 hours (average, 20–30 hours)

Common Side Effects

Sluggishness, ataxia, nystagmus, confusion, slurred speech

Less commonly—dizziness, insomnia, nervousness, fatigue, irritability

Significant Adverse Reactions

GI: nausea, vomiting, diarrhea, abdominal pain, dysphagia
CNS: headache, depression, tremors, behavioral disturbances
Dermatologic: skin rashes (morbilliform, maculopapular, scarlatiniform), urticaria, keratosis, hirsutism, lupus erythematosus, exfoliative dermatitis (rare)
Hematopoietic: blood dyscrasias, anemias, lymphadenopathy, bone marrow depression
Other: gingival hyperplasia (20%–30% incidence, especially children), periodontal infection, polyarthropathy, hepatitis, liver damage, alopecia, hyperglycemia, edema, chest pain, numbness, photophobia, pulmonary fibrosis, osteomalacia

Intravenous administration has resulted in hypotension, cardiac arrhythmias, hyperkinesis, and cardiovascular collapse.

Contraindications

CAUTION

Consider benefit versus risk ratio in pregnant women. Although fetal damage has been reported (cleft palate), discontinuance of therapy may precipitate status epilepticus with resulting hypoxia to the fetus. Carefully weigh all factors when using these drugs during pregnancy.

Hematologic disorders, severe hepatic dysfunction, incomplete heart block; intravenous phenytoin is contraindicated in sinus bradycardia, sinoatrial block, second- and third-degree atrioventricular (AV) block, and Adams-Stokes syndrome. *Cautious use* in persons with hypotension, myocardial insufficiency, hyperglycemia, anemia, osteoporosis, or acute intermittent porphyria, and in pregnant or nursing mothers. Abrupt withdrawal of the drug may result in status epilepticus.

Interactions

Phenytoin may increase the effects of oral anticoagulants, antihypertensives, thyroid hormones, sedatives and hypnotics, propranolol, and methotrexate.

Phenytoin may diminish the effects of corticosteroids, oral contraceptives, disopyramide, quinidine, digitalis glycosides, and tetracyclines (by increasing their liver metabolism).

The effects of phenytoin can be increased by drugs that 1) *inhibit its metabolism* (eg, allopurinol, cimetidine, diazepam, disulfiram, acute ethanol ingestion, isoniazid, phenacemide, phenylbutazone, succinimides, sulfonamides, trimethoprim, and valproic acid) or 2) *displace the drug from protein-binding sites* (eg, salicylates and anti-inflammatory drugs, valproic acid).

The effects of phenytoin can be reduced by drugs that 1) *increase its metabolism* (eg, barbiturates, carbamazepine, diazoxide, chronic ethanol ingestion, folic acid, and theophylline), 2) *retard its oral absorption* (eg, antacids, antineoplastics, calcium, charcoal) and 3) by several other drugs such as influenza virus vaccine, loxapine, nitrofurantoin, and pyridoxine.

Tricyclic antidepressants may precipitate seizures, so phenytoin dosage should be adjusted accordingly. Valproic acid and phenytoin may result in breakthrough seizures.

Phenytoin can impair the absorption of furosemide.

Concomitant administration of phenytoin and dopamine may lead to hypotension and bradycardia.

Nursing Management

Pretherapy Assessment

Assess and record baseline data necessary for detection of adverse effects of hydantoins: General: vital signs (VS), body weight, skin color and temperature, lymph node palpation; CNS: orientation, affect, reflexes; gastrointestinal (GI): normal output, bowel sounds, liver evaluation, periodontal examination; Lab: liver function, urinalysis, CBC with differential, blood proteins, blood and urine glucose, EEG, electrocardiogram (ECG).

Review medical history and documents for existing or previous conditions that:

a. require cautious use of hydantoins: hypotension; myocardial insufficiency; hyperglycemia; anemia; osteoporosis

b. contraindicate use of hydantoins: allergy to hydantoins; hematologic disorders; severe hepatic dysfunction; intravenous use in sinus bradycardia, sinoatrial block, second- and third-degree AV block and Adams-Stokes syndrome; **pregnancy (Category D)**, lactation (effects not known, use caution in nursing mothers).

Nursing Interventions

Medication Administration

Monitor blood pressure, ECG, and respiration, and ensure that appropriate antidotal measures (eg, vasopressors, oxygen, respiratory aids) are on hand when administering drug intravenously. Hydantoins should be given *slowly* (50 mg/min into running intravenous line) to avoid bradycardia and hypotension, and sterile saline should be injected through the needle or catheter after each injection to avoid local venous irritation caused by alkalinity of the drug solution.

Collaborate with healthcare team to individually adjust dosage to minimize toxicity. In some patients, peak blood levels after full dosage may be associated with transient signs of CNS toxicity, and these adverse effects may be reduced by using multiple smaller doses.

Ensure that brand of phenytoin administered is not changed after therapy is initiated unless serum concentrations are carefully monitored, because bioavailability differs significantly among preparations (see Fate). Note that *only Dilantin products* are approved for once-daily use because of prolonged absorption. All other phenytoin products are classified as *prompt* acting and are used 2 to 4 times a day.

Use parenteral solutions immediately after mixing, and do not add to any intravenous infusion because solubility may be altered by pH differences. Shake suspension thoroughly to obtain correct dosage. Continuous infusions should be avoided.

Administer oral drug with food to enhance absorption and reduce GI upset.

Assure ready access to bathroom facilities if GI effects occur.

Provide small, frequent meals if GI effects occur.

Surveillance During Therapy

Monitor patient for early signs of developing blood dyscrasias (eg, fever, sore throat, mucosal ulceration, malaise) or hepatic dysfunction (dark urine, abdominal cramps, jaundice), and check results of periodic blood counts and urinalyses.

Assess for nystagmus, confusion, ataxia, dysarthria, and unresponsive pupils, which are signs of overdosage. If these occur, dosage should be carefully readjusted.

Observe for signs of folic acid deficiency (anemia, neuropathy, psychiatric disorders, mental dysfunction) because hydantoins may interfere with folic acid availability. Supplemental folic acid should be given as needed. Additional folic acid can, however, increase phenytoin metabolism and may increase seizure frequency. Dosage should be adjusted accordingly.

Monitor patient's blood sugar levels because hydantoins may inhibit insulin release, leading to hyperglycemia. Dosage should be carefully adjusted in the diabetic patient.

Be prepared to administer vitamin K prophylactically during latter stages of pregnancy because hydantoins can reduce levels of vitamin K–dependent clotting factors produced by the liver.

Refer patient for dietary consultation to ensure that intake of vitamin D–containing foods is adequate to prevent hypocalcemia; hydantoins can accelerate vitamin D metabolism.

Question administration to patient with petit mal seizures because hydantoins may worsen the symptoms. Combined drug therapy is indicated when mixed seizure types are present.

Carefully monitor laboratory studies and patient for indications of adverse reactions.

Interpret results of diagnostic tests and contact practitioner as appropriate.

Monitor for possible drug–drug and drug–nutrient interactions: See Interactions.

Patient Teaching

Advise patient to take oral drug with meals, if possible, to minimize gastric irritation; drug is strongly alkaline.

Discuss the importance of proper diet, avoidance of fatigue, stress, or illness, and maintenance of prescribed dosage regimen for good seizure control.

Warn patient that convulsions may occur if dosage is altered or medication is abruptly discontinued.

Advise patient not to take any other drugs, including over-the-counter (OTC) preparations, unless specifically prescribed because hydantoins interact with many drugs. Excessive use of alcohol or other CNS depressants, for example, may reduce the efficacy of hydantoins.

Stress the importance of oral hygiene, regular gum massage, and frequent brushing of the teeth to minimize the severity of gingival hyperplasia, especially in children, in whom the incidence is much higher than in adults.

Inform patient that hydantoins may harmlessly color urine pink to reddish-brown.

Teach significant others proper methods for dealing with a seizure episode.

Urge patient to carry an identification card with pertinent medical information.

Oxazolidinediones *(Pregnancy Category D)*

- ***Paramethadione***
- ***Trimethadione***

The oxazolidinediones are effective drugs for control of simple absence (petit mal) seizures, but cause a high incidence of toxic reactions. They are largely reserved for patients who are intolerant of—or unresponsive to—other less toxic agents. The two currently available drugs, trimethadione and paramethadione, differ only slightly in their pharmacologic properties; thus, they are reviewed together (listed separately in Table 27-5).

Mechanism

Complex and incompletely understood; prolong the recovery period of postsynaptic neurons in those CNS systems (primarily thalamocortical) where repetitive discharges produce absence attacks through a negative feedback mechanism; other central effects include elevating the threshold for seizure discharge in the thalamus and interference with the propagation of seizure activity from a cortical focus to the thalamus; possess little sedative or hypnotic action but may exert an analgesic effect

Uses

Simple absence (petit mal) seizures refractory to other drugs

Dosage

See Table 27-5

Fate

Readily absorbed from GI tract; peak plasma concentrations in 30 to 60 minutes; uniformly distributed and not bound to plasma proteins; metabolized in liver to an active metabolite with an extended $T_{1/2}$; slowly excreted in the urine

Common Side Effects

Drowsiness, GI distress, hiccups, photophobia

Significant Adverse Reactions

CAUTION

Fetal malformations and other serious side effects have occurred during therapy with oxazolidinediones. Use only where other less toxic drugs are ineffective.

GI: nausea, vomiting, abdominal pain, anorexia

CNS: vertigo, irritability, personality changes, headache, paresthesias, precipitation of grand mal seizures

Ocular: diplopia, scotomata, hemeralopia (day blindness), retinal hemorrhage

Hematologic: epistaxis, mucosal bleeding (eg, gums, vagina), blood dyscrasias (especially neutropenia), changes in blood pressure

Dermatologic: skin rash (acneiform, morbilliform), exfoliative dermatitis, erythema multiforme

Other: albuminuria, alopecia, lymphadenopathy, systemic lupus–like reaction, myasthenia gravis–like reaction, nephrosis, hepatitis

Contraindications

Hepatic and renal disease, blood dyscrasias, diseases of the retina or optic nerve, myasthenia gravis, pregnancy. *Cautious use* in nursing mothers and in persons with acute intermittent porphyria. Do not use alone in mixed seizure forms because oxazolidinediones can worsen grand mal symptoms.

Interactions

Central nervous system depression induced by oxazolidinediones may be augmented by other depressants, oral anticoagulants, and *p*-aminosalicylic acid

Nursing Management

Pretherapy Assessment

Assess and record important baseline data necessary for detection of adverse effects of oxazolidinediones: General: VS, body weight, skin color and temperature; CNS: orientation, affect, reflexes; GI: normal output,

Table 27-5. **Oxazolidinediones**

Drug	*Usual Dosage Range*	*Nursing Considerations*
Paramethadione *Paradione*	Adults: 300–600 mg 3–4 times/day (initial dose, 900 mg/day; increase by 300 mg/wk to above range) Children: 300–900 mg/day in 3–4 divided doses	Less effective but slightly less toxic than trimethadione; no myasthenic-like reactions have occurred, but sedation is common; oral solution contains 65% alcohol and should be diluted with water before administration to children
Trimethadione *Tridione*	Adults: Initially, 300 mg 3 times/day; usual maintenance dose 900–2,400 mg/day in divided doses Children: 300–900 mg/day in 3–4 divided doses	Plasma level of dimethadione the active metabolite of trimethadione, may be used as a dosage guide; this level should be maintained about 700 μg/mL for optimal control of petit mal attacks in patients receiving trimethadione; alkalinization of the urine will increase excretion of this metabolite

bowel sounds, liver evaluation, periodontal examination; Lab: liver function, urinalysis, CBC with differential, blood proteins, blood and urine glucose, EEG, ECG.

Review medical history and documents for existing or previous conditions that:

a. require cautious use of oxazolidinediones: acute intermittent porphyria

b. contraindicate use of oxazolidinediones: allergy to oxazolidinediones; hematologic disorders; severe hepatic dysfunction; disease of the retina or optic nerve; myasthenia gravis; **pregnancy (Category D)**, lactation (effects not known, use caution in nursing mothers)

Nursing Interventions

Medication Administration

Administer oral drug with food to enhance absorption and reduce GI upset.

Assure ready access to bathroom facilities if GI effects occur.

Provide small, frequent meals if GI effects occur.

Surveillance During Therapy

Observe closely for early signs of hematologic toxicity (eg, sore throat, mucosal ulceration, fever, malaise, petechiae). If noted, withhold drug and notify practitioner.

Withhold drug and inform practitioner if skin rash, neutrophil depression (see next item), jaundice, albuminuria, scotomas, lymph node enlargement, or myasthenia symptoms occur, because severe toxicity can ensue.

Monitor results of CBCs, liver function tests, and urinalyses, which should be performed before and at regular intervals during therapy. Therapy should be discontinued if neutrophil count decreases to below 2,500/mm^3.

Carefully monitor laboratory studies and patient for indications of adverse reactions.

Interpret results of diagnostic tests and contact practitioner as appropriate.

Monitor for possible drug–drug and drug–nutrient interactions: See interactions.

Patient Teaching

Advise patient to take oral drug with meals, if possible, to minimize gastric irritation; drug is strongly alkaline.

Discuss the importance of proper diet, avoidance of fatigue, stress, or illness, and maintenance of prescribed dosage regimen for good seizure control.

Stress the importance of rigid adherence to prescribed regimen to minimize untoward reactions.

Advise patient to report immediately any development of ocular side effects (eg, glaring, dark spots, blurring), which necessitate dosage reduction. Retinal damage may occur if dosage is too high.

Inform patient that the incidence of petit mal attacks may *increase* during first few days of therapy. Reassure patient that clinical benefit will occur within several days.

Inform patient that drowsiness will diminish with continued use. A mild stimulant such as caffeine may be employed in early stages of therapy to reduce excessive drowsiness.

Inform patient that therapy should be discontinued only under the supervision of a health care provider. The drug should be withdrawn gradually to prevent development of simple absence attacks, which can occur with abrupt discontinuation.

Teach significant others proper methods for dealing with a seizure episode.

Urge patient to carry an identification card with pertinent medical information.

Succinimides

- ***Ethosuximide***
- ***Methsuximide***
- ***Phensuximide***

Although no more effective than the oxazolidinediones in the treatment of simple absence (petit mal) seizures, succinimides remain the drugs of choice primarily because they have a lower toxicity. Because they may increase the frequency of grand mal attacks, their use in patients with mixed seizure patterns **must** be accompanied by other antiepileptics that can control tonic-clonic seizures. Three succinimides are currently available (ethosuximide, methsuximide, and phensuximide) and do not differ significantly. They are discussed as a group, but listed individually in Table 27-6.

Mechanism

Remains to be definitively established; effects generally similar to oxazolidinediones; suppress the three-per-second spike-wave EEG pattern characteristic of absence seizures; evidence suggests a depressant effect on the motor cortex and possible elevation of the firing threshold of cortical neurons; block Ca^{2+} channel.

Uses

Simple absence (petit mal) seizures
Adjunctive treatment of psychomotor and other minor motor seizures (methsuximide *only*)

Dosage

See Table 27-6.

Fate

Well absorbed orally; peak serum levels in 2 to 4 hours; not bound to plasma proteins; short $T_{1/2}$ (2–4 hours) except ethosuximide (30–60 hours); metabolized by the liver and excreted primarily in the urine as both active and inactive metabolites

Common Side Effects

GI distress (nausea, upset, cramping, pain, diarrhea), drowsiness, ataxia, dizziness

Significant Adverse Reactions

CNS: irritability, nervousness, euphoria, aggressiveness, hyperactivity, confusion, lethargy, fatigue, depression, sleep disturbances, night terrors, inability to concentrate, hiccups, insomnia
Ocular: blurred vision, myopia, photophobia, periorbital edema
Hematologic: blood dyscrasias
Dermatologic: urticaria, erythematous rashes, erythema multiforme, systemic lupus erythematosus, Stevens-Johnson syndrome (see Chapter 5)
Genitourinary: urinary frequency, hematuria, albuminuria, renal damage (rare)
Other: alopecia, vaginal bleeding, hyperemia, swelling of the tongue, muscular weakness, hirsutism

Contraindications

Severe liver or renal damage. *Cautious use* in persons with reduced liver function, mixed seizures, behavioral disturbances, and ulcers.

Interactions

Increased libido may result if ethosuximide is combined with other anticonvulsants.

Nursing Management

Pretherapy Assessment

Assess and record baseline data necessary for detection of adverse effects of succinimides: General: VS, body weight, skin color and temperature; CNS: orientation, affect, reflexes, bilateral grip strength, vision examination; GI: normal output, bowel sounds, liver evaluation; Lab: liver function, urinalysis, CBC with differential, blood proteins, blood and urine glucose, EEG.

Review medical history and documents for existing or previous conditions that:

a. require cautious use of succinimides: reduced liver function; mixed seizures; behavioral disturbances; peptic ulcer
b. contraindicate use of succinimides: allergy to succinimides; severe renal or hepatic damage; **pregnancy (Category C)**, lactation (effects not known, use caution in nursing mothers)

Nursing Interventions

Medication Administration

Administer oral drug with food to enhance absorption and reduce GI upset.

Table 27-6. **Succinimides**

Drug	Usual Dosage Range	Nursing Considerations
Ethosuximide *Zarontin*	Adults: Initially 500 mg/day; increase by 250 mg every 4–7 days until control is achieved (maximum, 1,500 mg/day) Children: 250 mg/day increased slowly to optimal level	Inform patient that drug may color urine pink to reddish-brown; appearance of frequent GI distress, dizziness, ataxia, or other neurologic disorders signifies need for dosage adjustment; administer with meals to reduce GI upset; long half-life, therefore do not exceed recommended dosage because danger of accumulation exists
Methsuximide *Celontin*	Initially 300 mg/day for 1 wk; may increase by 300 mg weekly to a maximum of 1,200 mg	Equally effective in petit mal as ethosuximide but somewhat more toxic, especially to the CNS (eg, severe depression, confusion); may be useful in certain cases of psychomotor epilepsy
Phensuximide *Milontin*	Adults: 500–1,000 mg 2–3 times/day (range, 1–3 g/day) Children: 600–1,200 mg 2 or 3 times/day	Slightly less effective and less toxic than other succinimides; may color urine reddish-brown

Assure ready access to bathroom facilities if GI effects occur.
Provide small, frequent meals if GI effects occur.

Surveillance During Therapy

Observe closely for early signs of hematologic toxicity (eg, sore throat, mucosal ulceration, fever, malaise, petechiae). If noted, withhold drug and notify practitioner.
Withhold drug and inform practitioner if skin rash, neutrophil depression (see next item), jaundice, albuminuria, scotomas, lymph node enlargement, or myasthenia symptoms occur because severe toxicity can ensue.
Monitor results of compete blood counts, liver function tests, and urinalyses, which should be performed before and at regular intervals during therapy. Therapy should be discontinued if neutrophil count decreases to below 2,500/mm^3.
Carefully monitor laboratory studies and patient for indications of adverse reactions.
Interpret results of diagnostic tests and contact practitioner as appropriate.
Monitor for possible drug–drug and drug–nutrient interactions: See Interactions.

Patient Teaching

Advise patient to take oral drug with meals.
Discuss the importance of proper diet, avoidance of fatigue, stress, or illness, and maintenance of prescribed dosage regimen for good seizure control.
Caution against engaging in any hazardous activity during initial stages of therapy because drowsiness is common.
Explain the significance of adhering to prescribed dosing schedule. Dosage adjustments should always be made gradually because abrupt changes may precipitate increased seizure activity.
Stress the importance of carefully noting and reporting the development of untoward reactions. Most adverse effects can be minimized or eliminated by a dosage adjustment if detected early.
Instruct patient and family to be alert for and to report development of behavior changes (eg, depression, aggressiveness). Drug should be withdrawn slowly if these occur.
Instruct patient to inform practitioner if rash, dizziness, fever, blurred vision, joint pain, bruising, or bleeding occur, because these may indicate developing toxicity.
Encourage patient to obtain all laboratory studies requested. Periodic blood counts should be performed because several blood dyscrasias have been reported.
Urge patient to carry an identification card with pertinent medical information.

Benzodiazepines

Several benzodiazepines are employed in the treatment of epilepsy, namely clonazepam, clorazepate, and diazepam. Because this drug group has been extensively reviewed (see Chapters 23 and 25), only a few of the factors relevant to their use as anticonvulsants are presented here.

Mechanism

Suppress polysynaptic neuronal activity in spinal cord and mesencephalic reticular formation; suppresses spike-wave discharge characteristic of absence seizures and decreases frequency, duration, amplitude, and spread of minor motor seizure discharges; facilitates the action of GABA, an inhibitory neurotransmitter in the CNS, which increases *frequency* of opening of GABA$_A$-activated Cl^- channel, which then enhances inflow of Cl^- causing *hyper*polarization and membrane stability.

• Clonazepam

Klonopin

(CAN) Rivotril

Clonazepam is used primarily in absence seizures, especially the akinetic and myoclonic variants. Its use is associated with a significant degree of CNS depression and can result in psychological dependence. As many as 50% of users develop tolerance, usually within 3 to 6 months, necessitating a dosage adjustment.

Uses

Petit mal variant (Lennox-Gastaut syndrome)
Myoclonic and akinetic seizures
Simple absence seizures refractory to succinimides (may be used alone or as an adjunct; some evidence of benefit in psychomotor and focal seizures in combination with other drugs)
Investigational uses include treatment of acute manic episodes of bipolar affective disorders, leg movements during sleep, multifocal tic disorders, neuralgias, as adjunctive therapy in schizophrenia, and simple anxiety states.

Dosage

Adults: Initially 0.5 mg 3 times/day; increase by 0.5 to 1.0 mg every 3 days until optimal effect is achieved (maximum, 20 mg/day)
Children: Initially 0.01 to 0.03 mg/kg/day; increase by 0.25 to 0.5 mg every 3 days (usual range, 0.1–0.2 mg/kg/day)

Fate

Onset after oral administration in 30 to 60 minutes; maximum plasma levels occur in 1 to 2 hours; duration, 6 to 12 hours; $T_{1/2}$ varies from 20 to 40 hours; metabolized in the liver and primarily excreted in the urine

Common Side Effects

Drowsiness, ataxia, abnormal behavior

Significant Adverse Reactions

CNS: confusion, insomnia, depression, hysteria, headache, hypotonia, involuntary movements, slurred speech, tremor, vertigo, nystagmus, hallucinations, psychosis

GI: anorexia, constipation, dry mouth, gastritis, nausea, sore gums, hepatomegaly, coated tongue
Respiratory: rhinorrhea, shortness of breath, hypersecretion
Dermatologic: rash, ankle edema, hirsutism
Urinary: dysuria, enuresis, nocturia
Other: palpitations, muscle weakness, fever, lymphadenopathy, dehydration, blood dyscrasias (rare), diplopia, abnormal eye movements, increased salivation

Contraindications

Severe liver disease, narrow-angle glaucoma. *Cautious use* in behaviorally disturbed or drug-addicted persons, persons with renal dysfunction or chronic respiratory diseases, and in pregnant or nursing mothers. Drug should *not* be given alone in the presence of mixed seizures, because it may worsen tonic-clonic seizures.

Interactions

Central nervous system depressive effects may be enhanced by other drugs having a depressant action (eg, alcohol, narcotics, sedatives, phenothiazines, barbiturates).
Phenytoin and phenobarbital can reduce serum clonazepam levels.
Combined use of clonazepam and valproic acid may elicit absence seizures.

Nursing Management

Refer to **Benzodiazepines** (Chap. 25). In addition:

Nursing Interventions

Surveillance During Therapy

Monitor results of complete blood counts and liver function tests, which should be performed periodically during prolonged therapy.
Assist with evaluation of patient response to drug. Dosage should be periodically reviewed and adjusted as necessary. Signs of dependence should be noted and, if drug needs to be discontinued, it should be discontinued slowly to avoid withdrawal symptoms.

Patient Teaching

Caution patient against performing hazardous tasks because incidence of drowsiness is quite high.
Inform patient that drug may induce paradoxical increases in seizure activity. If this occurs, the practitioner should be notified. The drug should not be discontinued abruptly because marked exacerbation of seizures or status epilepticus can result.

• Clorazepate

Tranxene

(CAN) Apo-Clorazepate, Novo-Clopate, Nu-Clopate

This benzodiazepine is used as an adjunct in management of partial seizures. It is not recommended for children younger than 9 years of age. The initial dose is 7.5 mg, given 3 times a day in adults and twice a day in children. Dosage is increased gradually at weekly intervals. Maximum daily doses are 60 mg in children and 90 mg in adults. See also Chapter 25.

• Diazepam

Valium, Val-release, Zetran

(CAN) Apo-Diazepam, Diazemuls, E-PAM, Novodipam, Rival, Vivol

Diazepam is primarily used for control of anxiety states. It may be useful orally as an adjunct in the management of convulsive disorders but is rarely effective alone. Its principal indication is parenterally (intravenously) for the treatment of status epilepticus and other severe recurrent convulsive seizures. Diazepam may also be used for convulsions accompanying acute alcohol withdrawal. The drug is discussed fully in Chapter 25; thus only those aspects relating to its use as an antiepileptic are reviewed here.

Oral adult dosage ranges from 2 to 10 mg 2 to 4 times a day, whereas children may be given 1 to 2.5 mg 3 to 4 times a day. Adult intravenous doses are 5 to 10 mg, to be repeated as needed at 10- to 15-minute intervals to a maximum of 30 mg. Children receive 0.2 to 1 mg every 2 to 5 minutes, depending on age and body weight.

Nursing Management

(See also Chapter 25)

Nursing Interventions

Medication Administration

Observe patient carefully after intravenous administration to control an acute seizure episode. Readministration may be necessary because drug effects are short-lived, and many patients experience recurrent seizure episodes.
Question intravenous administration to patient with petit mal or petit mal variants because status epilepticus can be *precipitated* in such a patient.
Inject intravenous diazepam very slowly (5 mg/min) and do not use small veins (eg, wrist or dorsum of the hand) to help prevent venous thrombosis, swelling, or phlebitis.
Inject deep into large muscle mass when giving intramuscularly. Although the intravenous route is preferred for treating convulsive disorders, the drug may be given intramuscularly if severe convulsions preclude intravenous use.

Other Anticonvulsants

• Acetazolamide

Diamox

(CAN) Apo-Acetazolamide

Acetazolamide is a carbonic anhydrase inhibitor used primarily as an *adjunct* in the control of petit mal and other absence or nonlocalized seizures. This drug has also been employed as a mild diuretic, for relief of migraine headaches, and for treatment of chronic open-angle glaucoma (reduces formation of aqueous humor).

Acetazolamide reduces abnormal discharges from central neurons, although the mechanism of this effect is not well understood. It inhibits the enzyme carbonic anhydrase, reducing formation of H^+ and HCO_3^-; the therapeutic effects may be due to the slight acidosis produced by this agent.

The usefulness of acetazolamide in treating epileptic seizures is greatly limited by the rapid onset of tolerance; seizure activity often returns within a few weeks. The starting dose is 250 mg/day; the usual maintenance dosage range is 375 to 1,000 mg a day, generally in combination with another antiepileptic agent.

The most frequently encountered side effects are paresthesias of the face and extremities. Other untoward reactions observed with acetazolamide include polyuria, glycosuria, drowsiness, confusion, myopia, urticaria, rash, hepatic dysfunction, and flaccid paralysis. Because acetazolamide is a sulfonamide derivative, it is contraindicated in patients with sulfonamide allergy; it is also contraindicated in the presence of acidosis, hypokalemia, kidney or liver dysfunction, adrenal insufficiency, and early pregnancy. The drug should be used with *caution* in diabetic patients because it may increase blood glucose levels and, consequently, the need to increase doses of insulin or oral hypoglycemic drugs.

Nursing Management

Pretherapy Assessment

Assess and record baseline data necessary for detection of adverse effects of acetazolamide: General: VS, body weight, skin color and temperature, edema; CNS: orientation, affect, reflexes, bilateral grip strength, intraocular pressure (IOP); GI: normal output, bowel sounds, liver evaluation; Lab: liver function, urinalysis, CBC with differential, serum electrolytes.

Review medical history and documents for existing or previous conditions that:

a. require cautious use of acetazolamide: diabetes
b. contraindicate use of acetazolamide: allergy to acetazolamide, sulfonamides; hypokalemia; kidney or liver dysfunction; adrenal insufficiency; **pregnancy (Category C)**, lactation (effects not known, use caution in nursing mothers)

Nursing Interventions

Medication Administration

Administer oral drug with food to enhance absorption and reduce GI upset.

Assure ready access to bathroom facilities if GI effects occur.

Provide small, frequent meals if GI effects occur.

Surveillance During Therapy

Monitor for toxicity.

Assess diabetic patient carefully because acetazolamide may alter antidiabetic drug requirements by increasing blood glucose levels.

Use parenteral solution within 24 hours after reconstitution because it contains no preservative.

Carefully monitor laboratory studies and patient for indications of adverse reactions.

Interpret results of diagnostic tests and contact practitioner as appropriate.

Monitor for possible drug–drug and drug–nutrient interactions.

Patient Teaching

Advise patient to take oral drug with meals.

Discuss the importance of proper diet, avoidance of fatigue, stress, or illness, and maintenance of prescribed dosage regimen for good seizure control.

Instruct patient to report signs of hypokalemia (muscle weakness, cramping, cardiac irregularities) and metabolic acidosis (nausea, weakness, malaise, vomiting, abdominal pain, dehydration), which indicate the need for dosage adjustment.

• Carbamazepine

Epitol, Tegretol

(CAN) Apo-Carbamazepine, Novo-Carbamaz

Carbamazepine is structurally related to the tricyclic antidepressants and has a spectrum of action similar to phenytoin. In addition to its use in a variety of epilepsies, it has been employed successfully to treat the pain of trigeminal neuralgia (tic dooloureux), and neuropathic pain in cancer patients.

Mechanism

Increases latency, decreases responsivity, and suppresses afterdischarges in polysynaptic pathways associated with cortical and limbic function; may reduce post-tetanic potentiation; blocks Na^+ channel; has anticholinergic, antidepressant, and muscle-relaxing action (interferes with neuromuscular transmission)

Uses

Psychomotor seizures (alone or with primidone or phenytoin)

Grand mal (with phenytoin)

Adjunctive treatment of mixed seizures or complex partial seizures

Relief of pain associated with trigeminal neuralgia

Neuropathic pain in cancer patients

Experimental uses include treatment of neurogenic diabetes insipidus, alcohol withdrawal syndrome, and certain psychiatric disorders such as bipolar depressive illness and resistant schizoaffective disorders

Dosage

Epilepsy

Adults and children older than 12: Initially 200 mg twice a day; increase by 200 mg/day in divided doses until optimal response is achieved; maximum, 1,200 mg/day; usual maintenance range is 800 to 1200 mg/day

Children aged 6 to 12 years: Initially, 100 mg twice a day; increase by 100 mg/day until optimal response is achieved; usual maintenance level is 400 to 800 mg daily

Trigeminal Neuralgia

Initially 100 mg twice a day; increase by 100 mg/12 hours; usual maintenance range is 400 to 800 mg/day

Fate

Oral absorption is slow but complete; peak plasma levels in 4 to 6 hours; widely distributed and highly (75%) protein-bound;

serum $T_{1/2}$ is 12 to 20 hours on repeated dosing; metabolized in the liver (epoxide metabolite has anticonvulsant activity) and excreted as several metabolites and some unchanged drug through the kidneys

Common Side Effects

Drowsiness, dizziness, ataxia, nausea, blurred vision, diplopia

Significant Adverse Reactions

CAUTION

Serious and sometime fatal blood dyscrasias have occurred with carbamazepine. Early detection is vital, because in some patients aplastic anemia is irreversible. See Nursing Management.

CNS: confusion, incoordination, speech disturbances, involuntary movements, dysphasia, visual hallucinations, tinnitus, depression, peripheral neuritis, paresthesias, nystagmus

Dermatologic: rash, sweating, urticaria, photosensitivity reactions, alopecia, exfoliative dermatitis, erythema multiforme, abnormal pigmentation

Hematologic: blood dyscrasias, (aplastic anemia, leukopenia, agranulocytosis, eosinophilia, leukocytosis, thrombocytopenia)

Genitourinary: urinary frequency, albuminuria, glycosuria, urinary retention, oliguria, impotence

GI: diarrhea, vomiting, abdominal pain, anorexia, xerostomia, glossitis

CV: hypotension, syncope, arrhythmias, aggravation of coronary artery disease and hypertension, thrombophlebitis, AV block, congestive heart failure

Other: abnormal liver function, osteomalacia, hepatitis, jaundice, muscle aching, fever, chills, lenticular opacities, adenopathy

Contraindications

History of bone marrow depression, severe hypertension, and concomitant use of monoamine oxidase (MAO) inhibitors. *Cautious use* in patients with renal, hepatic, or cardiac disease, hypertension, glaucoma, and in elderly, pregnant, or nursing patients.

Interactions

Carbamazepine may accelerate the metabolism and therefore decrease the effects of other anticonvulsants (phenobarbital, phenytoin, primidone), oral anticoagulants, and tetracyclines.

Concurrent use of carbamazepine with MAO inhibitors or tricyclic antidepressants is not recommended because toxicity may be increased.

Carbamazepine is highly protein bound and therefore may potentiate other protein-bound drugs (eg, salicylates, oral hypoglycemics, anticoagulants, anti-inflammatory agents) by displacing them from protein-binding sites.

Cimetidine, isoniazid, erythromycin, and propoxyphene can elevate serum levels of carbamazepine, leading to increased toxicity.

Carbamazepine can result in breakthrough bleeding in women taking oral contraceptives.

Increased CNS toxicity can occur if carbamazepine is used concurrently with lithium.

Nursing Management

Pretherapy Assessment

Assess and record baseline data necessary for detection of adverse effects of carbamazepine: General: VS, body weight, skin color and temperature, lymph node palpation; CNS: orientation, affect, reflexes, bilateral grip strength, ophthalmic examination; GI: normal output, bowel sounds, oral mucous membranes; Lab: liver function, urinalysis, CBC with differential, serum (electrolytes, iron, blood urea nitrogen [BUN], thyroid hormones).

Review medical history and documents for existing or previous conditions that:

a. require cautious use of carbamazepine: renal, hepatic or cardiac disease; hypertension; glaucoma; use in the elderly.
b. contraindicate use of carbamazepine: allergy to carbamazepine or tricyclic antidepressants; bone marrow suppression; severe hypertension; MAO inhibitors; **pregnancy (Category C)**, lactation (effects not known, use caution in nursing mothers)

Nursing Interventions

Medication Administration

Administer oral drug with food to enhance absorption and reduce GI upset.

Assure ready access to bathroom facilities if GI effects occur.

Provide small, frequent meals if GI effects occur.

Surveillance During Therapy

Monitor for toxicity.

Monitor results of complete blood counts, liver function tests, urinalyses, and BUN tests, which should be performed before initiating therapy and at regular intervals thereafter. The drug should be discontinued if findings are abnormal or if any evidence of bone marrow depression develops.

Implement interventions to protect elderly patients from injury, because confusion, agitation, and behavioral disturbances occur more commonly in the elderly.

Carefully monitor laboratory studies and patient for indications of adverse reactions.

Interpret results of diagnostic tests and contact practitioner as appropriate.

Monitor for possible drug–drug and drug–nutrient interactions: See Interactions.

Patient Teaching

Advise patient to take oral drug with meals.

Discuss the importance of proper diet, avoidance of fatigue, stress, or illness, and maintenance of prescribed dosage regimen for good seizure control.

Warn patient to avoid hazardous tasks until reaction to drug has been determined. Drowsiness and dizziness are common in initial stages of therapy.

Explain the importance of adhering to prescribed dosage schedule. Drug withdrawal or dosage adjustments should be implemented slowly. Abrupt changes may provoke seizures or status epilepticus.

Teach patient how to recognize early signs of hematologic toxicity (sore throat, mucosal ulceration, petechiae, bruising, malaise). If any occur, the practitioner should be notified immediately.

Encourage patient to obtain periodic ophthalmologic examinations because drug can cause ocular damage.

• Felbamate

Felbatol

Felbatol is a relatively new agent that is effective in partial seizures, whether they occur alone or with other types of seizures in a particularly severe type of epilepsy known as Lennox-Gastaut syndrome (occurs in childhood; composed of multiple seizure types; associated with mental retardation; refractory to standard anticonvulsant drugs).

Mechanism

Reduces spread of seizures; possible antagonist of NMDA (*N*-methyl-D,L-aspartic acid) receptor; blocks Na^+ channel

Uses

Alone and combined with other anticonvulsants in partial seizures

Adjunctive therapy in treatment of partial seizures occurring in Lennox-Gastaut syndrome in children

Dosage

Adults: initially, 1,200 mg daily in three or four divided doses (provides plasma level of approximately 30 μg/mL); can increase by 600 mg/day every 2 weeks until maximum of 3,600 mg/day (provides plasma level of approximately 83 μg/mL)

Children: as adjunct in Lennox-Gastaut—add at rate of 15 mg/kg/day in divided doses while lowering dose of other anticonvulsant(s); maximum, 45 mg/kg/day

Fate

Good absorption after oral administration; largely unaffected by food; elimination $T_{1/2}$ is approximately 22 hours; approximately 50% of absorbed dose appears unchanged in the urine; only slightly protein bound

Common Side Effects

Nausea, headache, fatigue, anorexia, drowsiness

Significant Adverse Reactions

CV: tachycardia
GI: vomiting, diarrhea, constipation,
GU: intramenstrual bleeding, urinary tract infection
CNS: insomnia, anxiety
Respiratory: upper respiratory tract infection
Hematologic: purpura, leukopenia, aplastic anemia
Dermatologic: photosensitization, acne, rash, pruritus
Other: increased alanine transaminase (ALT)

Interactions

Felbamate can **lower** plasma levels of carbamazepine and **elevate** those of phenytoin and valproic acid.

When added to felbamate therapy, both carbamazepine and phenytoin **decrease** plasma levels of felbamate.

Nursing Management

Pretherapy Assessment

Assess and record important baseline data necessary for detection of adverse effects of felbamate: VS (T, P, R, BP); CNS: orientation, reflexes; GI: output, liver function; GU: menstrual function, renal function; Laboratory: liver function tests, CBC, assessment of serum concentrations of other antiepileptic agents being taken.

Review past medical history and documents for evidence of existing or previous medical history related to conditions that:

a. require caution with felbamate: allergy to carbamates.
b. contraindicate use of felbamate: allergy to felbamate or its ingredients, **pregnancy (Category C)**.

Nursing Interventions

Medication Administration

Administer oral form of drug **with meals**.

Initiate a meal schedule that provides small, frequent meals if GI upset occurs.

Provide ready access to bathrooms and interventions directed at symptom relief if diarrhea occurs.

If the oral suspension is used, shake well before using.

If being used as adjunctive therapy, add felbamate at 1200 mg/d TID while reducing other anticonvulsant medication doses by 20%. Further reduction in primary anticonvulsant doses may be necessary as felbamate dose is increased.

Surveillance During Therapy

Monitor patient for therapeutic effects of felbamate therapy.

Compare current status with previous status to detect improvements or deterioration in the patient's condition.

Monitor for adverse effects, toxicity, and interactions.

Monitor for signs of hypersensitivity (**including photosensitivity**) that may require discontinuation of drug.

Facilitate acquisition of diagnostic tests ordered for ongoing assessment of drug response.

Monitor CBC, urinalysis, and liver and kidney function test results obtained over the course of therapy.

Interpret results of diagnostic tests and contact practitioner/prescriber as appropriate.

Monitor for possible drug–laboratory test interactions.

Patient Teaching

Instruct patient that the prescribed drug is to be taken for the condition for which it is prescribed.

Instruct the patient to keep these drugs and all medications out of the reach of children.

• Gabapentin

Neurontin

A relatively new antiepileptic, gabapentin is structurally related to the neurotransmitter GABA, but does *not* appear to interact with GABA receptors nor is it converted into a GABA-like compound.

Mechanism

Not completely understood; exhibits antiseizure activity in common with other anticonvulsants

Uses

Adjunctive therapy for treatment of partial seizures, with or without generalized seizures

Dosage

Dosage is 900 to 1,800 mg/day in three divided doses; maximum, 3,600 mg/day

Fate

Absorption is good and unaffected by food; plasma protein binding is minimal; not appreciably metabolized but excreted by the kidney as unchanged drug; elimination $T_{1/2}$ is 5 to 7 hours.

Common Side Effects

Somnolence, dizziness, ataxia, nystagmus

Significant Adverse Reactions

CNS: tremor, amnesia, depression
GI: dyspepsia, constipation, dry mouth, nausea, vomiting
Respiratory: rhinitis, pharyngitis, cough
Other: myalgia, pruritus, impotence, diplopia, fatigue, weight gain, back pain
Many other adverse effects have occurred when gabapentin has been used in combination with other antiepileptic drugs; the incidence is less than 1% in most cases.

Contraindications

No absolute contraindications. *Cautious use* in elderly patients, and in pregant or nursing mothers.

Interactions

Antacids can reduce the effectiveness of gabapentin by decreasing its availability.
Cimetidine may reduce clearance of gabapentin.

Nursing Management

Pretherapy Assessment

Assess and record important baseline data necessary for detection of adverse effects of gabapentin: VS (T, P, R, BP); CNS: orientation, reflexes; GI: output; GU: renal function; Laboratory: renal function tests, CBC, assessment of serum concentrations of other antiepileptic agents being taken.
Review past medical history and documents for evidence of existing or previous medical history related to conditions that:
a. require caution with gabapentin: pregnancy, breast feeding, use in the elderly.
b. contraindicate use of gabapentin: allergy to gabapentin or its ingredients, **pregnancy (Category C)**.

Nursing Interventions

Medication Administration

Administer oral form of drug **with meals**.
Compare current status with previous status to detect improvements or deterioration in the patient's condition.
Monitor for adverse effects, toxicity, and interactions.
Monitor for signs of hypersensitivity that may require discontinuation of drug.
Facilitate acquisition of diagnostic tests ordered for ongoing assessment of drug response.
Monitor CBC, urinalysis, and kidney function test results obtained over the course of therapy.
Interpret results of diagnostic tests and contact practitioner/prescriber as appropriate.
Monitor for possible drug–laboratory test interactions.

Patient Teaching

Instruct patient that the prescribed drug is to be taken for the condition for which it is prescribed.
Instruct patient to keep these drugs and all medications out of the reach of children.

• Magnesium Sulfate

Magnesium, in the form of magnesium sulfate, is an effective anticonvulsant to control seizures caused by toxemia of pregnancy and other conditions of abnormally low levels of plasma magnesium. Depending on the speed of action desired, magnesium sulfate may be used IV or IM, although intravenous use is *significantly more hazardous*. Other clinical applications for magnesium sulfate are: oral—cathartic; topical—antipruritic; parenteral—control of uterine tetany, paroxysmal atrial tachycardia, hypertension, and cerebral edema. It has also been employed as an adjunct in hyperalimentation, and for replacement therapy in acute magnesium deficiency.

Magnesium controls convulsions by interfering with neuromuscular transmission, possibly by blocking release of acetylcholine from motor nerve endings. It also exerts a depressant effect on the CNS.

Adult intramuscular doses range from 1 to 5 g of a 25% to 50% solution, up to 5 times a day as necessary. With intravenous injection, 1 to 4 g of a 10% to 20% solution may be given at a rate not exceeding 1.5 mL/min; alternately, 4 g in 250 mL 5% dextrose solution may be infused at a rate not to exceed 3 mL/min. Pediatric intramuscular doses range from 20 to 40 mg/kg in a 20% solution. With repeated administration, knee–jerk reflexes should be tested before every dose; if the reflex is absent, magnesium should *not* be administered. The onset of action is immediate with intravenous injection and within 1 hour with intramuscular administration.

Side effects include flushing (common), sweating, hypotension, sedation, confusion, hypothermia, flaccid paralysis, depressed reflexes, cardiac and respiratory depression, and circulatory collapse. Hypocalcemia with tetany has been reported secondary to magnesium sulfate administration. The drug must be given *cautiously* to persons with renal impairment and is *contraindicated* in the presence of heart block and myocardial insufficiency. Additive CNS-depressant effects can occur when magnesium is given together with narcotics, barbiturates, anesthetics, and other sedative-hypnotic drugs. Magnesium may potentiate the muscle-relaxing action of neuromuscular blocking agents.

Nursing Management

Nursing Interventions

Medication Administration

Ensure that intravenous calcium is on hand as an antidote, along with appropriate respiratory equipment, when magnesium is administered parenterally.

Surveillance During Therapy

Monitor blood pressure and pulse repeatedly during intravenous therapy.
Observe patient for appearance of early signs of magnesium toxicity (thirst, feeling of warmth, confusion, depressed tendon reflexes, muscle weakness), which require discontinuation of the drug.
Monitor intake and output during extended use. The drug should be discontinued if output decreases to below 100 mL during the 4 hours before administration of each dose.
Monitor results of plasma magnesium level determinations during parenteral treatment. Plasma levels above 4 mEq/L are usually associated with untoward reactions.

• Phenacemide

Phenurone

A structural analog of the hydantoins, phenacemide is useful in severe epileptic states, especially mixed forms of psychomotor seizures refractory to other medications. It is generally employed as a last resort, however, because of its extreme toxicity. The exact mechanism of action of phenacemide is unknown.

Recommended doses in adults are 250 to 500 mg orally 3 times a day, initially. The usual maintenance range is 2 to 3 g a day. Children (5–10 years of age) should receive only **50%** of the adult dose.

Phenacemide can produce serious untoward reactions. Most frequently encountered adverse effects are psychic changes (eg, psychosis, depression), gastrointestinal disturbances, skin rash, drowsiness, dizziness, weakness, and headache. In addition, phenacemide administration has been associated with insomnia, paresthesias, fatigue, fever, muscle pain, palpitations, increased serum creatinine, hepatitis (occasionally fatal), blood dyscrasias (eg, leukopenia, aplastic anemia), and bone marrow depression. The drug is contraindicated in persons with personality disorders and in pregnant women. *Cautious use* is warranted in patients with a history of allergy or renal dysfunction, and in nursing mothers. Concomitant use of other antiepileptics, especially ethotoin, can increase the incidence of untoward reactions.

Nursing Management

Nursing Interventions

Surveillance During Therapy

Monitor results of CBCs and liver function tests, which should be performed before initiating therapy and at regular intervals thereafter. The drug should be discontinued if symptoms of jaundice or hepatitis appear or if blood picture is abnormal.

Patient Teaching

Suggest taking drug with food or milk to minimize GI irritation.
Teach patient how to recognize and report early signs of hematologic toxicity (eg, sore throat, fever, mucosal ulceration, malaise) or liver damage (eg, pruritus, yellow skin, frothy amber urine, petechiae). If these occur, the drug should be withdrawn slowly.
Stress the potential toxicity of the drug and the importance of immediately reporting *any* untoward reaction.

• Valproic Acid *(Pregnancy Category D)*

Depakene, Depakote

(CAN) Epival

Although chemically unrelated to other anticonvulsants, valproic acid, its sodium salt, and a stable compound composed of equal parts valproic acid and sodium valproate (ie, divalproex sodium [Depakote]) generally provide improved seizure control when added to the drug regimen of patients with multiple seizure types whose condition is refractory to treatment. They are most effective against simple and complex absence seizures. Divalproex is an enteric-coated dosage form and has a slightly lower incidence of GI side effects than the other dosage forms.

Mechanism

Increases synaptic levels of GABA in CNS, possibly by inhibiting the enzyme responsible for its catabolism; blocks Na^+ channel and may exert a direct membrane stabilizing action

Uses

Simple and complex absence seizures, including petit mal (alone or in combination with other anticonvulsants)
Adjunct in the treatment of multiple-seizure types
Unlabeled uses include treatment of grand mal seizures, myoclonic seizures, infantile spasms, complex and elementary partial seizures, prevention of recurrent febrile seizures, and treatment of bipolar affective disorder

Dosage

(Dosage is expressed in valproic acid equivalents.)
Initially, 15 mg/kg/day; increase by 5 mg/kg to 10 mg/kg weekly until seizures are controlled (maximum, 60 mg/kg/day)

Fate

Valproic acid and sodium valproate are rapidly absorbed orally; divalproex is enteric coated and absorption is delayed but uniform and consistent; peak serum levels occur within 30 to 60 minutes with sodium valproate and within 1 to 4 hours with the other dosage forms; widely distributed and highly (90%) protein bound; drug is metabolized primarily in the liver and is excreted in the urine, almost entirely as conjugated metabolites.

Common Side Effects

Nausea, vomiting, indigestion, sedation, elevated serum transaminases

Significant Adverse Reactions

CAUTION

Fatal hepatic failure has occurred in patients receiving valproic acid, particularly in children younger than 2 years of age; usually occurs during the first 6 months of treatment. *Frequent liver function tests are required, especially during the initial months of therapy.*

Diarrhea, abdominal cramps, lenticular opacities, nystagmus, visual disturbances, diplopia, dizziness, incoordination, tremor, dysarthria, skin rash, petechiae, alopecia, depression, aggression, hyperactivity, behavioral disturbances, altered bleeding time (drug inhibits platelet aggregation), muscle weakness, blood dyscrasias (rare), hepatotoxicity

Note: Because the drug has been used in combination with other antiepileptic medication, it is difficult to ascribe the above adverse effects solely to valproic acid.

Contraindications

Hepatic disease or dysfunction. *Cautious use* in persons with bleeding disorders or renal dysfunction and in pregnant or nursing women.

Interactions

Valproic acid may potentiate the depressant effects of other CNS depressant drugs (eg, barbiturates, narcotics, alcohol).

Serum phenobarbital levels may be elevated by valproic acid.

Simultaneous use of valproic acid and clonazepam may *induce* absence seizures.

Valproic acid interferes with platelet aggregation and therefore may enhance the action of anticoagulants, dipyridamole, and salicylates.

Breakthrough seizures have occurred with use of valproic acid and phenytoin.

Nursing Management

Pretherapy Assessment

Assess and record baseline data necessary for detection of adverse effects of valproic acid: General: VS, body weight, skin color and temperature; CNS: orientation, affect, reflexes; GI: normal output, bowel sounds; Lab: liver function, urinalysis, CBC with differential, serum (ammonia, electrolytes, iron, BUN, thyroid hormones), EEG.

Review medical history and documents for existing or previous conditions that:

a. require cautious use of valproic acid: bleeding disorders; renal dysfunction.
b. contraindicate use of valproic acid: allergy to valproic acid; hepatic disease or dysfunction; **pregnancy (Category D)**, lactation (effects not known, use caution in nursing mothers).

Nursing Interventions

Medication Administration

Administer oral drug with food to enhance absorption and reduce GI upset.

Assure ready access to bathroom facilities if GI effects occur.

Provide small, frequent meals if GI effects occur.

Surveillance During Therapy

Monitor for toxicity.

Monitor results of liver function tests, which should be performed before and at frequent intervals during therapy, because hepatic failure has occurred. The drug should be discontinued at the first sign of hepatic dysfunction as indicated by either serum biochemistry or clinical evaluation.

Interpret urine tests for ketone bodies cautiously. The drug is excreted in part as a ketone-containing metabolite, which can interfere with these tests.

Carefully monitor laboratory studies and patient for indications of adverse reactions.

Interpret results of diagnostic tests and contact practitioner as appropriate.

Monitor for possible drug–drug and drug–nutrient interactions: See Interactions.

Patient Teaching

Advise patient to take oral drug with meals.

Discuss the importance of proper diet, avoidance of fatigue, stress, or illness, and maintenance of prescribed dosage regimen for good seizure control.

Instruct patient to swallow capsule whole to avoid local mouth and throat irritation and to take with food to minimize GI irritation.

Warn patient not to use alcohol or other CNS depressants with valproic acid because additive CNS depression can occur.

Advise patient not to engage in hazardous activities because drowsiness and dizziness can occur.

Instruct patient to report any visual disturbances immediately because ocular toxicity has been noted.

Inform patient that periodic blood counts are advisable during therapy because platelet dysfunction and blood dyscrasias have been reported.

Selected Bibliography

Bellver MJG et al: Plasma protein binding kinetics of valproic acid over a broad dosage range: Therapeutic implications. J Clin Pharm Ther 18:191, 1993

Brodie MJ, Porter RJ: New and potential anticonvulsants. Lancet 336: 425, 1990

Dodson WE et al: Treatment of convulsive status epilepticus. JAMA 270:854, 1993

Faingold CL, Fromm GH (eds): Drugs for Control of Epilepsy: Actions on Neuronal Networks involved in Seizure Disorders. Boca Raton, Fla, CRC Press, 1992

Gomez Bellver MJ et al: Plasma protein binding kinetics of valproic acid over a broad dosage range: therapeutic implications. J Clin Pharm Ther 18:191, 1993

Halman MH et al: Anticonvulsant use in the treatment of manic syndromes in patients with HIV-1 infection. J Neuropsychiatry Clin Neurosci 5:430, 1993

Kaneko S et al: Teratogenicity of antiepileptic drugs and drug specific malformations. Japan J Psychiat Neurol 47(2):306, 1993

Kodama Y et al: Effect of unbound clearance on binding parameters of valproic acid to serum proteins. J Clin Pharm 33:130, 1993

Lenn NJ, Robertson M: Clinical utility of unbound antiepileptic drug blood levels in the management of epilepsy. Neurology 42:988, 1992

Lifshitz M et al: Monitoring phenytoin therapy using citric acid-stimulated saliva in infants and children. Ther Drug Monit 12:334, 1990

Morse TG, Zeigler V: Phenytoin: It's not just for seizures anymore. Am J Matern/Child Nurs 19(1):33, 1994

Privitera MD: Clinical rules for phenytoin dosing. Ann Pharmacother 27:1169, 1993

Scholtes FB, Renier WO, Meinardi H: Generalized convulsive status epilepticus: Pathophysiology and treatment. Pharm World Sci 15(1): 17, 1993

VanValkenburg C, Kluznik JC, Merrill R: New uses of anticonvulsant drugs in psychosis. Drugs 44(3):326, 1992

Yajnik S, Singh GP, Singh G, Kumar M: Phenytoin as a coanalgesic in cancer pain. J Pain Symptom Manage 7:209, 1992

Nursing Bibliography

Dichter M: Deciding to discontinue anti-epileptic medication. Hospital Practice 27(10A):16, 21–22, 1992

Gold C, Mathew J: Expanding uses of anticonvulsants in the treatment of bipolar disorders. Journal of Psychosocial Nursing and Mental Health Services 31(5):37–39, 1993

Neurologic therapies in critical care. Critical Care Nursing Clinics of North American 5(2):L237–246, 1993

Shantz D, Spitz M: What you need to know about seizures. Nursing '93 23(11):34–40, 1993

28
Antiparkinsonian Drugs

Dopaminergic Agents
- ***Dopamine precursor***
  - Levodopa
  - Carbidopa/levodopa
- ***Dopamine releaser***
  - Amantadine
- ***Dopamine receptor agonists***
  - Bromocriptine
  - Pergolide
- ***Inhibitor of dopamine inactivation***
  - Selegiline

Anticholinergic/ Antihistaminergic Agents
- Benztropine
- Biperiden
- Diphenhydramine
- Ethopropazine
- L-Hyoscyamine
- Procyclidine
- Trihexyphenidyl

Parkinson's disease, or *paralysis agitans*, is a chronic progressive disorder of the CNS. Although a significant degree of research is currently devoted to Parkinson's disease , the cause(s) remain largely unknown. *"Parkinsonism"* is the term used to describe the condition that occurs either from the disease itself or as a toxic effect produced by certain drugs (eg, phenothiazines [see Chapter 24]). Although the appearance of signs and symptoms depend on the stage of this disease—which becomes more disabling as it progresses—the three primary manifestations are the following:

- *Akinesia (bradykinesia)*: a lack of or difficulty in initiating voluntary muscle movement; advanced disease states are characterized by "frozen" muscles, resulting in an unchanging (masklike) facial expression, impairment of postural reflexes, and inability to adequately care for oneself
- *Rigidity*: usually of the "plastic" or "cogwheel" type; the affected area usually can be moved without great difficulty but often remains fixed once again in its new position
- *Tremor*: coarse (3 to 7 cycles/second), repetitive muscle activity, usually worse when the person is at rest; commonly manifested as a "pill-rolling" motion of the hands and a bobbing of the head

Besides these principal signs, affected patients may show disturbances in gait or posture, impaired speech, muscular weakness, and autonomic *hyper*activity (eg, increased saliva formation; seborrhea). In contrast, advanced stages are frequently characterized by autonomic *insufficiency*, resulting in severe orthostatic hypotension; these effects can be exacerbated by anticholinergic drugs used in treatment.

Onset usually occurs in middle age; during early stages, the signs are frequently much worse on one side of the body, and a diagnosis is usually made from these signs. Definite biochemical changes are present in the central nervous system (CNS), the most characteristic being a degeneration of those dopaminergic neurons with cell bodies in the substantia nigra. Because motor regulatory areas such as the corpus striatum receive their dopamine supply from the substantia nigra, degeneration of these nigral-striatal neurons decreases the functional amount of dopamine available to nuclei of the corpus striatum (ie, caudate nucleus, putamen). This upsets the normal balance between the inhibitory transmitter dopamine and the excitatory transmitter acetylcholine in these brain regions; that is, the intact cholinergic pathways now become predominant.

Although striatal dopamine deficiency provides a common basis for the various signs of parkinsonism, the only *true* abnormality resulting from low striatal dopamine is akinesia. Therefore, akinesia is the motor defect most responsive to dopamine-replacement therapy. Tremor and rigidity occur because of the *imbalance* between low dopaminergic activity and a *compensatory* high cholinergic action; thus, they are more effectively controlled by both dopamine replacement *and* cholinergic antagonism.

Drug therapy of parkinsonism is directed either toward augmentation of central dopaminergic function or reduction of central cholinergic activity. Drugs effective in the control of Parkinson's disease may be grouped as follows:

I. Dopaminergic agents
   A. Dopamine precursor (eg, levodopa)
   B. Dopamine-releasing agent (eg, amantadine)
   C. Dopamine receptor agonist (eg, bromocriptine)
   D. Inhibitor of dopamine inactivation (eg, selegiline)
II. *Anticholinergic/antihistaminergic agents* (eg, benztropine, diphenhydramine)

In addition to proper drug treatment—which is not curative but simply palliative—adjunctive therapy for parkinsonism should include physical therapy and emotional support; both will reduce the feelings of helplessness and inadequacy as the disease progresses and limits the patient's activities.

New approaches to the treatment of Parkinson's disease have emerged in recent years, although they are still in the experimental stages. Among the more promising is implantation—into the brain—of adrenal medullary tissue or fetal nigral tissue to replace the deficient dopamine-producing cells of the substantia nigra.

A somewhat different type of drug-induced parkinsonism has been reported among drug abusers. Attempts by certain illegal laboratories to synthesize a meperidine-like narcotic drug have resulted in the formation of certain by-products, one of which is l-methyl-4-phenyl-1,2,5,6-tetrahydropyridine (MPTP). When this substance was accidentally injected, these relatively young persons developed severe parkinsonism within 2 weeks; they were actually "frozen" in position. Subsequent investigations proved that MPTP is a neurotoxin that can selectively destroy dopaminergic neurons in the substantia nigra, leading

Malseed, RT; Goldstein, FJ; and Balkon, N: PHARMACOLOGY: DRUG THERAPY AND NURSING CONSIDERATIONS, Fourth Edition.

to the development of classic parkinsonism that is *irreversible* and requires antiparkinsonian drug therapy. MPTP is now being evaluated in the preclinical laboratory as a model for Parkinson's disease.

Dopaminergic Agents

Four types of drugs are available that can enhance dopaminergic functioning in the motor regulatory centers of the CNS. *Levodopa* (L-dopa) is the metabolic precursor of dopamine, and its use results in increased concentrations of dopamine in the corpus striatum. It is given rather than dopamine itself because L-dopa readily passes the blood–brain barrier; dopamine does not and, therefore, will not accumulate in sufficient amounts in the brain after systemic administration. Levodopa is now used almost exclusively in a fixed-ratio combination with carbidopa, the latter being an inhibitor of peripheral dopa decarboxylase, which biotransforms dopa to dopamine. (see following discussion of carbidopa/levodopa).

Another drug employed to enhance the effects of dopamine in the CNS is *amantadine*. Originally developed as an antiviral agent against the Asian (A) influenza strain, amantadine was observed to have a beneficial action in those parkinsonian patients to whom it was administered for the flu. Because amantadine appears to increase release of dopamine from presynaptic nerve endings, its effectiveness is most apparent in those patients having sufficient stores of dopamine available in striatal brain areas. Such patients are likely to be in the early stages of the disease.

A third type of dopaminergic drug is typified by *bromocriptine* and *pergolide*, dopamine receptor agonists principally used in parkinsonism patients with a poor response to conventional therapy; they are employed as adjuncts to levodopa/carbidopa treatment. These drugs can provide additional therapeutic benefit in those patients whose condition has begun to deteriorate, in other words, they may allow a reduction in levodopa dosage, which reduces adverse reactions associated with levodopa therapy. However, patients whose condition does not respond to levodopa are not likely to benefit from bromocriptine or pergolide.

Finally, *selegiline*, an inhibitor of monoamine oxidase B (MAO-B; enzyme that inactivates dopamine in presynaptic nerve endings), is employed; it blocks conversion of environmental toxins into free radicals that can destroy nigral neurons and cause Parkinson's disease.

Dopamine Precursor

- ***Levodopa***

  Dopar, Larodopa

- ***Carbidopa/levodopa***

  Sinemet

Although levodopa is the active pharmacologic agent in treating the symptoms of Parkinson's disease, it is seldom used alone but rather as a fixed combination of carbidopa: L-dopa (either 1:4 or 1:10). Carbidopa competes for the enzyme dopa decarboxylase, thereby reducing *peripheral* biotransformation of L-dopa. This enzyme inhibition allows more of the L-dopa dose to pass through the blood–brain barrier, resulting in higher dopamine levels in central motor regulatory centers. Carbidopa itself does not cross the blood–brain barrier and therefore does not interfere with conversion of L-dopa to dopamine in the CNS. Because its half-life ($T_{1/2}$) and, consequently, plasma levels are increased, levodopa dosage requirements are reduced by approximately 75% when combined with carbidopa. Because less dopamine is formed peripherally (compared with the use of L-dopa alone), there is a lower incidence of many systemic side effects, especially nausea, vomiting, and cardiovascular disturbances. However, adverse *CNS* effects (eg, dyskinesias) may occur sooner and at lower doses of L-dopa when combined with carbidopa (than when given alone) because more levodopa is reaching the brain to be converted there to dopamine.

Although most parkinsonian patients can be managed adequately with the carbidopa/levodopa combination (Sinemet), certain patients may require **individual titration** of each drug, especially when nausea and vomiting are prominent. Therefore, carbidopa is also available **alone** in 25-mg tablets (Lodosyn); this allows the practitioner to more carefully titrate the dosage ratio to obtain better symptom control. Individual dosing of the two drugs (ie, levodopa and carbidopa) allows separate titration of each agent; this method may provide better control of the disease and fewer side effects than use of the fixed-dosage combinations.

The pharmacologic and toxicologic properties of carbidopa/levodopa are similar to those of levodopa in most respects. However, the fixed ratio combinations allow use of lower doses of L-dopa, provide a smoother response, and permit more rapid dosage adjustments than can be obtained with L-dopa alone. Untoward reactions, contraindications, and drug interactions observed with carbidopa/levodopa are essentially the same as those noted with levodopa itself, although blood levels of urea nitrogen, uric acid, and creatinine are lower during carbidopa/levodopa administration than during treatment with levodopa alone.

Levodopa must be discontinued at least 8 hours before initiating therapy with carbidopa/levodopa, which should be substituted at a dosage level that will provide approximately 25% of the previous levodopa dose. The combination is *not* recommended in patients younger than 18.

Mechanism

Levodopa is a precursor of dopamine that readily passes the blood–brain barrier and is then decarboxylated to dopamine. Increased formation of dopamine in motor-regulatory areas of the CNS restores the depleted dopamine levels and improves the symptoms of Parkinson's disease; levodopa is most effective in relieving akinesia and bradykinesia, somewhat less efficacious in controlling rigidity, and seldom of significant benefit in reducing tremor; response to levodopa is greatest at the outset of therapy but diminishes gradually over 2 to 5 years, at which time it is usually necessary to initiate therapy with other antiparkinsonian drugs, such as anticholinergics, amantadine, or bromocriptine

Uses

Treatment of parkinsonism, whether idiopathic, postencephalitic, or secondary to injury or cerebral arteriosclerosis

Control of drug-induced extrapyramidal symptoms

Dosage

Levodopa alone

Highly individualized; initially 0.5 to 1 g/day in two or more divided doses; increase gradually in increments of 0.75 g every 3 to 7 days; maximum dose is 8 g/day

Carbidopa/levodopa

The dosage of carbidopa/levodopa, like that of levodopa itself, is highly individualized. Tablets are available in a fixed ratio of either 10 mg carbidopa/100 mg levodopa, 25 mg carbidopa/100 mg levodopa, or 25 mg carbidopa/250 mg levodopa. Dosage schedules are as follows:

Patients not receiving levodopa: Initially, 1 tablet (10/100 or 25/100) 3 times/day; increase by 1 tablet daily until 6 tablets/day; if more L-dopa is necessary, substitute 1 tablet (25/250) 3 or 4 times/day; increase by ½ to 1 tablet/day to a maximum of 8 tablets (25/250) per day

Patients receiving levodopa: (Discontinue L-dopa for at least 8 hours); initially, 1 tablet (25/250) 3 or 4 times/day in patient previously requiring 1,500 mg or more of levodopa alone per day; *otherwise*, 1 tablet (10/100) 3 or 4 times/day; adjust by ½ to 1 tablet a day until control is obtained

Fate

Levodopa is well absorbed from GI tract; peak plasma levels occur in 1 to 2 hours; significant amounts are metabolized to dopamine in the stomach, intestines, and liver; a relatively small fraction of administered dose reaches CNS unchanged as levodopa (1%–2%); dopamine metabolites are rapidly and almost completely excreted in the urine. Carbidopa inhibits the decarboxylation of peripheral levodopa but does not cross the blood–brain barrier and therefore does not interfere with the conversion of dopa to dopamine in the CNS. Concurrent use of carbidopa with levodopa reduces the required dose of levodopa by 70% to 80% and increases its plasma $T_{1/2}$.

Common Side Effects

Nausea, vomiting, anorexia, orthostatic hypotension, salivation, dry mouth, dysphagia, ataxia, headache, confusion, dizziness, weakness, fatigue, hand tremor, insomnia, anxiety, euphoria, choreiform and other involuntary movements, nightmares, agitation

Use of carbidopa with levodopa may reduce the incidence of peripheral side effects but can exacerbate the centrally mediated side effects. Dyskinesias occur in most patients receiving long-term therapy and tend to develop with smaller doses as treatment continues.

Significant Adverse Reactions

GI: diarrhea, GI bleeding, ulceration

CV: palpitations, tachycardia, arrhythmias, phlebitis, hemolytic anemia

Neurologic/psychiatric: bradykinetic episodes (on/off phenomena—see Patient Teaching), muscle twitching, grinding of the teeth, convulsions, paranoid ideation, psychotic reactions, depression, dementia

Ocular: spasmodic winking (blepharospasm), diplopia, blurred vision

Other: urinary retention, bitter taste, skin rash, sweating, hot flashes, edema, alopecia, leukopenia

Drug may elevate blood urea nitrogen (BUN), aspartate aminotransferase (AST), alanine aminotransferase (ALT), lactate dehydrogenase (LDH), bilirubin, alkaline phosphatase, and protein-bound iodine (PBI); may also reduce white blood cells (WBC), hemoglobin, and hematocrit.

Contraindications

Narrow-angle glaucoma, undiagnosed skin lesions or history of melanoma (Levodopa can activate malignant melanoma.), acute psychoses, and in patients on MAO inhibitor therapy. *Cautious use* in patients with severe cardiovascular, pulmonary, renal, hepatic, or endocrine disease; peptic ulcer; chronic wide-angle glaucoma; diabetes; psychiatric disturbances (including depression); a history of myocardial infarction with residual arrhythmias; and in pregnant or nursing women.

Interactions

Effects of L-dopa may be *decreased* by antipsychotics, phenytoin, papaverine, pyridoxine, reserpine, phenylbutazone, benzodiazepines (eg, diazepam), and tricyclic antidepressants.

L-Dopa may enhance the hypotensive effect of methyldopa, guanethidine, diuretics, and possibly other antihypertensive drugs.

Therapeutic effects of L-dopa may be potentiated by propranolol, methyldopa, and anticholinergics.

Cardiovascular effects of sympathomimetic drugs such as amphetamines, ephedrine, and epinephrine can be increased by L-dopa.

Diabetic control with oral hypoglycemic drugs may be adversely affected by L-dopa.

Concurrent use of L-dopa and either tricyclic antidepressants or MAO inhibitors can result in tachycardia and hypertension.

Nursing Management

Pretherapy Assessment

Assess and record baseline data necessary for detection of adverse effects of levodopa: General: VS, body weight, skin color and temperature; CNS: orientation, affect, reflexes, bilateral grip strength; CVS: orthostatic BP, perfusion; GI: bowel sounds, normal output, liver evaluation; GU: normal output, voiding pattern, prostate palpation; Endocrine: thyroid palpation; Lab: liver, kidney and thyroid function, urinalysis, CBC with differential.

Review medical history and documents for existing or previous conditions that:

a. require cautious use of levodopa: severe cardiovascular, pulmonary, renal, hepatic or endocrine disease; peptic ulcer; chronic wide angle glaucoma; diabetes; history of myocardial infarction (MI) with residual arrhythmias
b. contraindicate use of levodopa: allergy to levodopa; narrow-angle glaucoma; undiagnosed skin lesions or history of melanoma; acute psychoses; MAO inhibitor use; **pregnancy (Category C)**, lactation (secreted in breast milk; safety not established, avoid use in nursing mothers)

Nursing Interventions

Medication Administration

Administer with meals if GI upset occurs.
Observe all patients for development of suicidal tendencies.
Provide small, frequent meals and frequent mouth care if GI effects occur.
Ensure that patient voids before receiving each dose of drug if urinary retention is a problem.

Surveillance During Therapy

Monitor vital signs during early dosage regulation.
Check results of tests of hepatic, renal, and cardiovascular function, which should be performed periodically during prolonged therapy.
Monitor for toxicity.
Carefully monitor laboratory studies and patient for indications of adverse reactions.
Interpret results of diagnostic tests and contact practitioner as appropriate.
Monitor for possible drug–drug and drug–nutrient interactions: See Interactions.
Provide for patient safety needs if CNS, visual, or hypotensive effects occur.

Patient Teaching

Advise taking drug with food to lessen GI irritation.
Instruct patient to promptly report appearance of muscle twitching and blepharospasm (intermittent winking), early signs of overdosage.
Teach patient measures to help minimize orthostatic hypotension, which is common during early months of therapy.
Explain that prolonged use often leads to development of abnormal involuntary movements, especially of the face, mouth, tongue, and head, in which case an attempt should be made to reduce the dosage to the lowest effective level to minimize these effects.
Prepare patient for the possibility of a *sudden* worsening of symptoms (eg, extreme weakness, bradykinesia) during prolonged high-dosage therapy, the so-called *on/off phenomenon*. This condition, which usually lasts several hours, is apparently caused by temporarily excessive L-dopa levels, perhaps resulting from altered metabolism.
Advise patient to avoid multiple-vitamin preparations containing vitamin B_6 (pyridoxine) because it will reduce the effects of L-dopa by increasing its *peripheral* conversion to dopamine.
Inform patient that some improvement generally occurs within 2 to 3 weeks, but in some cases it may be several months before benefits are evident.
Advise diabetic patient to monitor condition closely for possible loss of control. Blood sugar should be checked frequently during therapy. Inform patient that drug can cause false-negative urine test with Clinistix and false-positive with Clinitest.
Inform patient that drug may cause urine and sweat to darken.

Dopamine Releaser

• Amantadine

Symadine, Symmetrel

A synthetic antiviral agent originally used for prophylaxis against the Asian strain of influenza, amantadine can also effectively relieve symptoms of parkinsonism (especially akinesia and rigidity). It is effective in up to 40% of patients initially, but its efficacy tends to diminish within 1 to 2 years. Amantadine may be used as initial therapy in milder forms of Parkinson's disease and in conjunction with levodopa in more advanced stages.

Mechanism

Not completely understood; may enhance release of dopamine from presynaptic nerve endings, and block presynaptic reuptake of dopamine; effectiveness is greatly reduced in the absence of functional dopamine stores in the corpus striatum; no anticholinergic activity

Antiviral action has been attributed to prevention of the release of viral nucleic acid into host cells; does not interfere with the influenza A viral vaccine (see Chapter 73).

Uses

Symptomatic treatment of parkinsonism and drug-induced extrapyramidal reactions
Prophylaxis against Asian influenza virus strains, especially in high-risk patients (see Chapter 73)
Symptomatic management of respiratory disease caused by Asian influenza virus (see Chapter 73)

Dosage

Parkinsonism: 100 mg 1 or 2 times/day (maximum, 400 mg/day)
Drug-Induced extrapyramidal reactions: 100 mg twice a day (maximum, 300 mg/day)

Fate

Well absorbed orally; peak plasma levels in 2 to 4 hours; long duration of action ($T_{1/2}$ 18–24 hours); not metabolized to any extent and excreted almost entirely intact through the kidneys; excretion is enhanced in an acid urine

Common Side Effects

Irritability, nausea, dizziness, insomnia

Significant Adverse Reactions

Orthostatic hypotension, vomiting, headache, weakness, fatigue, ataxia, confusion, mild depression, constipation, urinary retention, peripheral edema, livedo reticularis (skin mottling), dyspnea, anxiety, tremors, visual disturbances, skin rash, dermatitis, ankle edema, congestive heart failure, psychotic reactions, leukopenia, neutropenia

Contraindications

No absolute contraindications. *Cautious use* in patients with a history or evidence of epilepsy, congestive heart failure, or peripheral edema; also in patients with dermatitis, hypotension, psychotic disturbances, liver or kidney disease, and in elderly patients.

Interactions

Amantadine may worsen the side effects of anticholinergics (eg, hallucinations, confusion).
Excessive CNS stimulation may occur when given with other stimulants.

Nursing Management

Pretherapy Assessment

Assess and record baseline data necessary for detection of adverse effects of amantadine: General: VS, body weight, skin color and temperature; CNS: orientation, affect, reflexes, vision, speech; cardiovascular system (CVS): orthstatic blood pressure (BP), perfusion, edema; genitourinary (GU): normal output; Lab: BUN, creatinine clearance.
Review medical history and documents for existing or previous conditions that:
a. require cautious use of amantadine: history or evidence of epilepsy; congestive heart failure; peripheral edema; dermatitis; hypotension; psychotic disturbances; liver or kidney disease; use in the elderly
b. contraindicate use of amantadine: allergy to amantadine; **pregnancy (Category C)**, lactation (secreted in breast milk; safety not established, avoid use in nursing mothers)

Nursing Interventions

Medication Administration

Administer with meals if GI upset occurs.
Provide small, frequent meals and frequent mouth care if GI effects occur.

Surveillance During Therapy

Monitor for toxicity.
Carefully monitor laboratory studies and patient for indications of adverse reactions.
Interpret results of diagnostic tests and contact practitioner as appropriate.
Monitor for possible drug–drug and drug–nutrient interactions: See Interactions.
Provide for patient safety needs if CNS, visual, or hypotensive effects occur.

Patient Teaching

Advise taking drug with food to lessen GI irritation.
Suggest that patient avoid taking last dose close to bedtime because insomnia can result.
Inform patient that *abrupt* discontinuation of drug can markedly worsen symptoms. Dosage should be tapered gradually.
Warn patient that dizziness, drowsiness, and blurred vision may impair ability to drive a car or operate machinery.
Instruct patient to make position changes slowly, especially when arising from bed, because orthostatic hypotension may occur.
Explain that livedo reticularis (skin mottling, usually of lower extremities) may occur, particularly if patient is exposed to cold. Effect generally appears early in therapy and will subside once drug is discontinued or possibly when dose is reduced.

Dopamine Receptor Agonists

• Bromocriptine

Parlodel

Bromocriptine is primarily used orally as adjunctive therapy to provide additional therapeutic benefits in patients currently maintained on L-dopa who are beginning to show signs of deterioration in their condition. Because of the progressive degenerative nature of parkinsonism, even persons receiving maximum doses of L-dopa in combination with carbidopa are eventually susceptible to breakthrough effects. These are sometimes referred to as "late L-dopa failures." Examples of such conditions are return of tremor or rigidity, "end-of-dose" failure (appearance of akinesia between dosing), and "on/off" phenomena (abrupt loss of mobility). Bromocriptine may delay the onset of late L-dopa failure and may also ameliorate the symptoms (eg, dyskinesias) associated with excessive L-dopa levels by allowing a dosage reduction.

Mechanism

Functions as a direct receptor agonist at dopaminergic sites in the CNS, resulting in increased dopamine receptor activation in the corpus striatum; may provide increased control of parkinsonian symptoms in patients whose condition has begun to deteriorate after prolonged L-dopa therapy; also activates dopamine receptors in the tuberoinfundibular dopaminergic system of the pituitary, resulting in secretion of prolactin inhibitory factor (PIF) from the hypothalamus; secretion of PIF blocks release of prolactin from the anterior pituitary

Uses

Adjunctive treatment of Parkinson's disease (usually in combination with levodopa/carbidopa) or drug-induced parkinsonian-like symptoms (may provide increased symptom control and reduce the incidence of levodopa-induced side effects by permitting use of a smaller dose)
Treatment of amenorrhea/galactorrhea associated with hyperprolactinemia (*not* indicated in patients with normal prolactin levels)
Treatment of female infertility associated with hyperprolactinemia
Prevention of postpartum lactation
Reduction of plasma growth hormone levels in patients with acromegaly

Dosage

Parkinson's disease: 1.25 to 2.5 mg twice daily initially; increase by 2.5-mg increments every 2 to 4 weeks until optimal response occurs
Amenorrhea/galactorrhea: 2.5 mg 2 to 3 times a day; not to exceed 6 months
Prevention of lactation: 2.5 mg 2 to 3 times a day for 14 to 21 days
Treatment of infertility: initially 2.5 mg once daily; increase to 2 or 3 times a day within the first week

Acromegaly: 1.25 to 2.5 mg daily for 3 days; increased slowly every 3 to 7 days as tolerated; usual therapeutic range is 20 to 30 mg daily to a maximum of 100 mg daily

Fate

Approximately one-fourth of an oral dose is absorbed from the gastrointestinal tract; drug is highly protein bound (90%–95%); metabolized in the liver and excreted almost entirely through the bile into the feces; less than 5% of the dose is eliminated in the urine.

Common Side Effects

Nausea, vomiting, headache, dizziness, drowsiness, lightheadedness, confusion, visual disturbances, nasal congestion, shortness of breath, abdominal discomfort, diarrhea, insomnia, hypotension

Significant Adverse Reactions

Nightmares, anxiety, anorexia, dysphagia, foot and ankle edema, skin mottling, paresthesia, skin rash, urinary frequency, and epileptiform seizures. In addition, signs and symptoms of ergotism have occurred, such as numbness and tingling in the extremities, cold feet, muscle cramping, and Raynaud's syndrome.

Elevations in BUN, ALT, AST, creatine phosphokinase (CPK), alkaline phosphatase, and serum uric acid have been noted, but are usually of a transient nature.

Contraindications

Severe ischemic heart disease, peripheral vascular disease, sensitivity to ergot alkaloids, and in pregnant or nursing women. *Cautious use* in the presence of severe hypotension, epilepsy, psychoses, cardiac arrhythmias, and impaired hepatic or renal function; safety and efficacy of bromocriptine in children younger than 15 years of age have not been established.

Interactions

Bromocriptine can potentiate the hypotensive action of other blood pressure–lowering drugs.

Antipsychotic drugs that are dopamine blockers may antagonize the action of bromocriptine.

Nursing Management

Pretherapy Assessment

Assess and record baseline data necessary for detection of adverse effects of bromocriptine: General: VS, body weight, skin color and temperature (especially fingers), lesions, nasal mucous membranes; CNS: orientation, affect, reflexes, vision, speech, bilateral grip strength; CVS: orthostatic BP; GI: normal output, bowel sounds, liver evaluation; Lab: liver and kidney function tests, CBC with differential.

Review medical history and documents for existing or previous conditions that:

a. require cautious use of bromocriptine: severe hypotension; epilepsy; psychoses; cardiac arrhythmias; impaired renal or hepatic dysfunction; peptic ulcer; history of MI with residual arrhythmias
b. contraindicate use of bromocriptine: allergy to bromocriptine or any ergot alkaloid; severe ischemic heart disease; peripheral vascular disease; **pregnancy (Category C)**, lactation (Do not use in women who elect to breast feed, because drug inhibits lactation.)

Nursing Interventions

Medication Administration

Carefully evaluate patients with amenorrhea/galactorrhea before drug therapy begins to assure that syndrome does not result from a pituitary adenoma that requires surgical or radiologic intervention.

Administer with meals if GI upset occurs.

Provide small, frequent meals and frequent mouth care if GI effects occur.

Surveillance During Therapy

Provide for patient safety needs if CNS, visual, or hypotensive effects occur.

Collaborate with patient, significant others, and health-care team to ensure that adequate provision is made for patient's safety in home environment because side effects such as dizziness and hypotension may limit ability to manage self-care, especially early in therapy.

Arrange to taper dosage in patients with Parkinson's disease if drug must be discontinued.

Monitor for toxicity.

Carefully monitor laboratory studies and patient for indications of adverse reactions.

Interpret results of diagnostic tests and contact practitioner as appropriate.

Monitor for possible drug–drug and drug–nutrient interactions: See Interactions.

Patient Teaching

Advise taking drug with food to lessen GI irritation.

Inform amenorrheic woman that treatment with bromocriptine may restore fertility. Encourage use of effective contraceptive measures.

Inform woman with childbearing potential that periodic pregnancy tests are recommended during therapy. Treatment should be discontinued immediately if pregnancy occurs.

Warn patient to use caution in operating machinery or engaging in other potentially hazardous activities because dizziness and fainting may occur.

• Pergolide

Permax

Pergolide is a dopamine receptor agonist that directly stimulates dopamine receptors in the nigrostriatal system. It is similar to bromocriptine but is about 100 times more potent on a milligram basis. It is used as adjunctive therapy to L-dopa in Parkinson's disease, allowing for a 5% to 30% reduction in the dose of L-dopa. Most frequently encountered side effects are dyskinesia, nausea, dizziness, hallucinations, rhinitis, somnolence, and confusion. Orthostatic hypotension may also occur frequently, especially during the initial stages of treatment. Cardiac arrhythmias have been reported. The clinical efficacy of pergolide may be decreased by concurrent use of dopamine antagonists such as phenothiazine antipsychotics or metoclopramide. Initial dose is 0.05 mg/day for the first 2 days. Dosage is then increased by 0.1 mg or 0.15 mg/day every third day for 2 weeks, then by 0.25 mg/day until an optimal therapeutic dosage is achieved. The drug is usually administered in three divided doses. The usual daily dose is 3 mg/day; efficacy of doses above 5 mg/day has not been determined.

Nursing Management

See **Bromocriptine**.

Inhibitor of Dopamine Inactivation

• Selegiline

Eldepryl

Mechanism

Irreversibly inhibits MAO-B enzyme in nerve endings in the brain, thereby increasing the intraneuronal levels of dopamine; as a result, more dopamine is available for release; also interferes with dopamine reuptake into nerve endings; may delay progression of symptoms by protecting against nerve cell damage resulting from formation of free radicals in the CNS; does not appear to interfere with activity of MAO-A, the enzyme found in the liver and intestines

Uses

Adjunctive treatment of Parkinson's disease in patients being treated with L-dopa when the response begins to deteriorate

Delay need for treatment with L-dopa in Parkinson's disease (investigational use)

Dosage

Dosage is 5 mg twice a day, at breakfast and lunch. After 2 or 3 days of treatment, attempt to reduce dose of L-dopa by 10% to 30%. Further reductions may be possible with continued selegiline use.

Fate

Rapidly absorbed orally; peak plasma levels are attained in 1 to 2 hours; quickly metabolized to at least three metabolites, which are excreted largely in the urine

Common Side Effects

Nausea, dizziness, lightheadedness

Significant Adverse Reactions

CNS: confusion, vivid dreams, headache, anxiety, insomnia, depression, hallucinations, delusions, tremor, involuntary motor movements, personality changes, dyskinesias

CV: palpitations, orthostatic hypotension, tachycardia, arrhythmias, sinus bradycardia, peripheral edema

GI: vomiting, diarrhea, anorexia, weight loss, heartburn, dysphagia

Urinary: urinary retention, nocturia, prostatic hypertrophy

Dermatologic: sweating, hair loss, rash, photosensitivity

Other: dry mouth, acne, leg pain, back pain, diplopia, blurred vision, asthma, tinnitus, migraine, chills, altered taste, numbness of fingers and toes

Contraindications

No absolute contraindications. *Cautious use* in persons in whom dizziness and drowsiness may prove hazardous and in pregnant or nursing women. Doses exceeding 10 mg/day should not be used, because nonselective inhibition of MAO-A may occur, leading to the possibility of hypertensive reactions with tyramine-containing foods (see Chapter 26).

Interactions

Concurrent use of meperidine and MAO inhibitors may result in severe and sometimes fatal interactions.

Nursing Management

Pretherapy Assessment

Assess and record baseline data necessary for detection of adverse effects of selegiline: General: VS, body weight, skin color and temperature; CNS: orientation, affect, reflexes; GI: normal output, bowel sounds, liver evaluation.

Review medical history and documents for existing or previous conditions that:

a. require cautious use of selegiline: use in persons whom dizziness or drowsiness may prove hazardous
b. contraindicate use of selegiline: allergy to selegiline; **pregnancy (Category C)**, lactation (effects not known, use caution in nursing mothers)

Nursing Interventions

Medication Administration

Administer only as adjunct with levodopa/carbidopa therapy in patients whose symptoms are deteriorating.

Administer twice a day with breakfast and with lunch.

Ensure that dosage does not exceed 10 mg/day, because MAO-B selectivity may be lost and patient will be at risk for severe hypertensive reactions.

Surveillance During Therapy

Provide for patient safety needs if CNS, visual, or hypotensive effects occur.

Collaborate with patient, significant others, and health-care team to ensure that adequate provision is made for patient's safety in home environment because side effects such as dizziness and hypotension may limit ability to manage self-care, especially early in therapy.

Arrange to taper dosage in patients with Parkinson's disease if drug must be discontinued.

Monitor for toxicity.

Carefully monitor laboratory studies and patient for indications of adverse reactions.

Interpret results of diagnostic tests and contact practitioner as appropriate.

Monitor for possible drug–drug and drug–nutrient interactions: See Interactions.

Patient Teaching

Advise taking drug with food to lessen GI irritation.

Caution patients not to exceed the recommended dose (10 mg/day), because higher doses inhibit MAO-A and may result in a hypertensive reaction to many foods containing tyramine, a potent pressor agent (see Chapter 26).

Inform patients of the signs of an MAO-inhibitor hypertensive reaction, such as severe headache, sweating, or flushing.

Anticholinergic/Antihistaminergic Agents

The first drugs used for the treatment of Parkinson's disease were the belladonna alkaloids atropine and scopolamine. For many years they were the only effective drugs available for this disease but now are only occasionally employed; they have been replaced by synthetic drugs having central anticholinergic—and in some instances antihistaminergic—activity (eg, benztropine, diphenhydramine, trihexyphenidyl).

Anticholinergics, useful in patients with mild symptoms, are effective in relieving rigidity and occasional tremor. They are often prescribed *in combination* with levodopa to obtain better control of the condition than either drug alone. Their usefulness is limited by their side effects, such as blurred vision, dizziness, and dysuria. Moreover, large doses may cause adverse CNS effects such as confusion, ataxia, delirium, and hallucinations, *especially in geriatric patients*.

In addition to their use in parkinsonism, these drugs are employed to control the extrapyramidal manifestations (akinesia, dystonias, akathisia, tremor) characteristic of treatment with antipsychotic agents.

Because the anticholinergic/antihistaminergic drugs used in Parkinson's disease are pharmacologically and toxicologically similar, they are reviewed as a group. Most of the individual drugs have been mentioned previously, either in Chapter 13 (anticholinergics) or Chapter 16 (antihistamines). They are listed again here in Table 28-1, where specific information is provided relating to their use in parkinsonism and extrapyramidal disorders.

Mechanism

Block central cholinergic pathways that have become too powerful as dopamine—which normally counterbalances acetylcholine—decreases in Parkinson's disease; may also reduce the storage and presynaptic reuptake of dopamine

Uses

Sole or adjunctive treatment of parkinsonian symptoms

Prevention and relief of extrapyramidal reactions resulting from antipsychotic drug therapy

Dosage

See Table 28-1

Fate

Generally well absorbed orally; onset usually in 30 to 60 minutes; duration of action is variable (average, 4–6 hours), except for sustained-release preparations (8–12 hours); excreted primarily by the kidney, both as metabolites and intact drug.

Common Side Effects

Dryness of mouth, blurred vision, dizziness, nausea, nervousness, drowsiness, urinary hesitancy

Significant Adverse Reactions

(Usually due to excessive dosage)

Confusion, agitation, delirium, hallucinations, depression, memory loss, vomiting, constipation, paralytic ileus, dilatation of the colon, skin rash, flushing, decreased sweating, tachycardia, palpitation, weakness, mild orthostatic hypotension, paresthesias, numbness in extremities, muscle cramping, elevated temperature, mydriasis, diplopia, headache, increased intraocular pressure

Contraindications

Acute narrow-angle glaucoma, pyloric or duodenal obstruction, peptic ulcer, prostatic hypertrophy, myasthenia gravis. *Cautious use* in patients with open-angle glaucoma; cardiac, liver, or kidney disorders; and in small children, elderly or debilitated patients; alcoholics, and pregnant or nursing women.

Interactions

Combined use with other drugs having an anticholinergic action (eg, phenothiazines, tricyclic antidepressants) may result in increased toxicity

May potentiate the sedative action of other CNS depressants (eg, alcohol, barbiturates, narcotics)

Certain centrally acting anticholinergic drugs can impair the antipsychotic effectiveness of phenothiazines and haloperidol by increasing their rate of GI metabolism.

Oral absorption of levodopa can be reduced by anticholinergic drugs because they delay gastric emptying, thus increasing the gastric degradation of levodopa. However, the reduced gastrointestinal motility may increase absorption of slowly dissolving preparations such as digoxin.

Nursing Management

Pretherapy Assessment

Assess and record baseline data necessary for detection of adverse effects of anticholinergic/antihistaminics: General: VS, body weight, skin color and temperature; CNS: orientation, reflexes, vision; GI: bowel sounds, normal output; GU: prostate palpation; Lab: CBC with differential.

Review medical history and documents for existing or previous conditions that:

a. require cautious use of anticholinergic/antihistaminics: cardiovascular disease; convulsive disorders; renal or hepatic impairment; hypertension; urinary retention; glaucoma; diabetes; asthma; or other chronic lower respiratory disease; and hyperthyroidism, and in young children, elderly, or debilitated patients

b. contraindicate use of anticholinergic/antihistaminics: allergy to antihistamines, narrow-angle glaucoma; peptic ulcer; prostatic hypertrophy; GI or bladder obstruction; patients on MAO inhibitor therapy; **pregnancy (Category C)**, lactation (secreted in breast milk, contraindicated in nursing mothers because of possible adverse effects to the neonate; may inhibit lactation, nursing mothers should avoid this drug)

Table 28-1. **Anticholinergic/Antihistaminergic Drugs Used in Parkinson's Disease**

Drug	Usual Dosage Range	Nursing Considerations
Benztropine *Cogentin* *(CAN) ApoBenzotropine, Bensylate, PMS Benztropine*	*Parkinsonism*: 1–2 mg/day (range, 0.5–6 mg) *Extrapyrmidal reactions* 1–4 mg 1–2 times/day	IM injection used for rapid response in acute dystonic reactions (onset 15 min); do *not* use in children younger than 3; effects are cumulative and may take several days to develop; usually not effective against tremors
Biperiden *Akineton*	*Parkinsonism* 2 mg 3 or 4 times/day *Extrapyrmidal reactions* Oral: 2 mg 1–3 times/day IM, IV: 2 mg; may repeat every 30 min to a total of 4 doses	Most effective against akinesia and rigidity; effectively reduces salivation and seborrhea; may produce mood elevation or temporary euphoria, especially parenterally; IV injection can cause hypotension and incoordination
Diphenhydramine *Benadryl and others; see also* Chapter 16	Oral: 25–50 mg 3–4 times/day IV, IM: 10–50 mg (maximum, 400 mg/day)	Effective in mild parkinsonism and extrapyramidal reactions (especially dystonias); often combined with other anticholinergics or L-dopa; see Chapter 16 for adverse effects, contraindications, and interactions
Ethopropazine *Parsidol* *(CAN) Parsitan*	Initially 50 mg 1–2 times/day Increase gradually to a maximum of 600 mg/day in severe cases	A phenothiazine derivative with significant anticholinergic activity; effectively controls most symptoms, including tremor; does *not* potentiate other CNS depressants; high incidence of side effects and poorly tolerated by many older patients; used for treatment of extrapyramidal reactions, even though it is a phenothiazine itself
L-Hyoscyamine *Levsin*	0.125–0.25 mg every 4 h as needed	Used to decrease excessive salivation and sweating; may also reduce tremor and improve rigidity; use with caution in patients exposed to high temperatures—may cause heat stroke (see also Chapter 13)
Procyclidine *Kemadrin* *(CAN) PMS Procyclidine, Procyclid*	*Parkinsonism*: Initially 2.5 mg 3 times/day; increase gradually to a maximum of 20 mg/day *Extrapyramidal reactions*: 2.5 mg 3 times/day (usual range, 10–20 mg/day)	Anticholinergic and smooth muscle antispasmodic; most effective against rigidity; controls excessive salivation as well; may temporarily worsen tremor as rigidity is relieved; be alert for confusion, agitation, and behavioral changes, which are common in elderly persons with hypotension; similar to trihexyphenidyl
Trihexyphenidyl *Artane, Trihexy* *(CAN) Aparkane, Apo-Trihex, Novohexidyl*	*Parkinsonism* Initially 1–2 mg; increase by 2-mg increments every 3–5 days to a maximum of 15 mg/day Usual range: 6–10 mg/day, in 3–4 divided doses or 5 mg sustained-release once or twice a day *Extrapyramidal reactions* Initially 1 mg; increase by 1 mg every few hours until control is obtained Usual range: 5–15 mg/day in divided doses	Anticholinergic and smooth muscle relaxant; do *not* use sustained-release capsules for initial therapy because they do not allow enough flexibility in dosage regulation; major effect is on rigidity; although most symptoms improve to some extent; effects may be potentiated by MAO inhibitors

Nursing Interventions

Medication Administration

Determine whether patient has any contraindicated condition before initiating administration.

Oral drug may be administered with food to facilitate absorption.

Administer syrup form if patient is unable to take tablets.

Give intramuscular antihistamine deep into large muscle mass to reduce tissue irritation. Subcutaneous injection should not be used.

Withhold drug and seek clarification if prescribed for patient who received an MAO inhibitor drug within past 2 weeks.

Provide small frequent meals if GI upset occurs.

Surveillance During Therapy

Monitor urinary output and bowel function during prolonged therapy.

Be alert for possible early signs of paralytic ileus (eg, abdominal pain, distention, constipation). Alert practitioner if these occur.

Monitor for toxicity.

Observe patient closely during parenteral use. Hypersensitivity reactions are more likely to occur with parenteral rather than with oral administration. Inform patient that brief stinging sensation may occur.

Interpret results of diagnostic tests and contact practitioner as appropriate.

Monitor for possible drug–drug and drug–nutrient interactions: See Interactions.

Provide for patient safety needs if CNS effects or hypotension occur.

Patient Teaching

Instruct the patient to avoid over-the-counter (OTC) preparations.

Suggest taking drug with meals to minimize GI irritation.

Stress the importance of adhering to prescribed dosage levels. Clinical improvement may not occur for several days or even weeks.

Warn patient to exercise caution in driving a car or operating machinery because physical and mental abilities may be impaired, especially during early therapy.

Explain that the ability to sweat may be hampered, which may interfere with maintenance of heat equilibrium. If a problem occurs, a dosage reduction should be considered, and patient should be instructed to avoid exertion as much as possible.

Suggest interventions to alleviate dry mouth.

Emphasize the importance of periodic ophthalmic examinations for patient on prolonged therapy.

Advise patient that if drugs are used for prolonged periods, tests may be performed periodically to assess blood, kidney, and liver function.

Instruct patient to notify practitioner promptly at first sign of: skin rash; difficulty breathing, night cough; hallucinations, tremors, loss of coordination; unusual bleeding or bruising; visual disturbances; irregular heartbeat.

Teach patient about the types of side effects expected with therapy: dizziness; drowsiness; epigastric distress, diarrhea, or constipation; dry mouth, thickening of bronchial secretions, dryness of nasal mucosa.

Selected Bibliography

Contin M et al: No effect of chronic bromocriptine therapy on levodopa pharmacokinetics in patients with Parkinson's disease. Clin Neuropharmacol 15(6):505, 1992

Good PF, Olanow CW, Perl DP: Neuromelanin-containing neurons of the substantia nigra accumulate iron and aluminum in Parkinson's disease: A LAMMA study. Brain Res 593:343, 1992

Hubble JP, Koller WC, Waters C: Effects of seligiline dosing on motor fluctuations in Parkinson's disease. 16(1):83, 1993

Hutton JT, Morris JL: Long-acting carbidopa-levodopa in the management of moderate and advanced Parkinson's disease. Neurology 42(suppl 1):51, 1992

Koller WC: Initiating treatment of Parkinson's disease. Neurology 42 (suppl 1):39, 1992

Kopin IJ: Pharmacology of Parkinson's disease therapy: An update. Annu Rev Pharmacol 33:467, 1993

Kulkarni J et al: Psychotic symptoms resulting from intraventricular infusion of dopamine in Parkinson's disease. Biol Psychiatry 31: 1225, 1992

Montastruc JL, Rascol O, Senard JM: Current status of dopamine agonists in Parkinson's disease management. Drugs 46(3):384, 1993

Peter SA, Autz A, Jean-Simon ML: Bromocriptine-induced schizophrenia. J Natl Med Assoc 85(9):700, 1993

Pleet AB: Newly-diagnosed Parkinson's disease: A therapeutic update. Geriatrics 47:24, 1992

Wessel K, Szelenyi I: Selegiline: An overview of its role in the treatment of Parkinson's disease. Clin Invest 70:459, 1992

Ziv I et al: Short-term beneficial effect of deprenyl monotherapy in early Parkinson's disease. Clin Neuropharmacol 16(1):54, 1993

Nursing Bibliography

Goetz C, Jarkovic J, Paulson G: Update on Parkinson's disease. Patient Care: 172–208, 1992

McPherson M: Management of Parkinson's disease. Journal of Home Health Care Practice 4(4):31–35, 1992

Paulson G: Management of the patient with newly diagnosed Parkinson's disease. Geriatrics 48(2):38–34, 39–40, 1993

Sprinzeles L: Decreasing hallucinations in residents with Parkinson's disease. Provider 19(2):41, 1992

29
Central Nervous System Stimulants

Respiratory Stimulant (Analeptic)
- Doxapram

Caffeine

Amphetamines
- Amphetamine
- Dextroamphetamine
- Methamphetamine

Anorexiants
- Benzphetamine
- Diethylpropion
- Fenfluramine
- Mazindol
- Phendimetrazine
- Phentermine
- Phenylpropanolamine

Methylphenidate

Pemoline

Although many therapeutic agents have a stimulating effect on the central nervous system (CNS), the number of drugs actually used clinically for this purpose is small. A useful classification of therapeutically effective CNS stimulants is as follows:

I. Respiratory stimulant (analeptic; eg, doxapram)
II. Caffeine
III. Amphetamines (eg, dextroamphetamine, methamphetamine)
IV. Anorexiants (eg, phentermine, diethylpropion)
V. Methylphenidate
VI. Pemoline

Analeptics are used to antagonize respiratory depression caused by overdosage with CNS depressants; the only currently available analeptic is doxapram.

Caffeine is the most widely used CNS stimulant, largely because it is consumed in coffee, tea, soda, and many over-the-counter (OTC) drug combinations. In small amounts it is a relatively weak stimulant that aids in maintaining mental alertness. Caffeine can relieve the pain of vascular headaches by constricting cerebral blood vessels, and is also employed parenterally as a respiratory stimulant. *Amphetamines* are powerful CNS stimulants with a high potential for abuse. They have been used to treat obesity but are effective for only a few weeks. Other approved indications for amphetamines are in treatment of narcolepsy and of attention deficit disorder (ADD). *Anorexiants* are drugs related to amphetamines; they are used in the therapy of obesity and have most of the same limitations as amphetamine.

The remaining CNS stimulants (ie, methylphenidate and pemoline) are primarily employed for treatment of ADD in children.

Respiratory Stimulants (Analeptics)

Analeptics act at the level of the respiratory center in the brain stem—as well as on peripheral carotid chemoreceptors—to increase the depth and, frequently, the rate of respiration. Analeptics are used mainly to overcome respiratory depression caused by drug overdosage with several classes of CNS depressants (eg, sedative-hypnotics, narcotics) or overdosage resulting from general anesthesia. However, their clinical effectiveness in treating drug-induced respiratory depression has been questioned, and their potential for producing additional adverse reactions is high.

A primary disadvantage is that CNS areas other than the respiratory center (eg, vasomotor center, vomiting center, brain stem reticular formation) are also stimulated; this causes many undesirable effects ranging from mild cardiovascular stimulation to marked central activation leading to vomiting, hyperreflexia, and convulsions. Because respiratory stimulants have a narrow safety margin, they must be administered cautiously by trained personnel and only in conjunction with appropriate adjunctive measures (eg, mechanical assistance, oxygen, suction, anticonvulsants, muscle relaxants and, where appropriate, narcotic antagonists or cholinergic drugs). Obviously, maintenance of an open airway is essential with use of respiratory stimulants.

• Doxapram

Dopram

Mechanism

Enhances depth and rate of respiration by direct stimulation of peripheral carotid chemoreceptors and—in large doses—the medullary respiratory center; large doses also stimulate the vasomotor center (increase blood pressure and cardiac output) and may cause convulsions; little direct action on cerebral cortex

Uses

Reversal of postanesthetic respiratory depression or apnea (except due to muscle relaxants)

Adjunctive treatment of drug-induced CNS and respiratory depression, to hasten arousal and facilitate return of laryngopharyngeal reflexes (*Note*: respiratory depression due to CNS-depressant overdosage is *best* managed by mechanical ventilation.)

Prevention of elevated arterial CO_2 tension during O_2 administration in patients with chronic obstructive pulmonary disease (COPD) who are having acute respiratory insufficiency

Dosage

Postanesthesia: 0.5 to 1 mg/kg intravenous injection (maximum 2 mg/kg) or 5 mg/min by intravenous infusion until satisfactory response, then 1 to 3 mg/min to maintain respiration

Drug-induced respiratory depression: 2 mg/kg intravenous injection; repeat in 5 minutes, then at 1- to 2-hour intervals until arousal is sustained (total maximum dose

is 3 g); alternatively, 1 mg to 3 mg/min by intravenous infusion after initial priming dose given above (total maximum dose is 3 g)
Chronic obstructive pulmonary disease: 1 mg to 3 mg/min by intravenous infusion (2 mg/mL solution) for a maximum of 2 hours

Fate

Onset of action is 20 to 40 seconds and peak effect occurs within 1 to 2 minutes; duration ranges from 5 to 12 minutes

Common Side Effects

Mild hypertension, variations in heart rate

Significant Adverse Reactions

CNS: headache, dizziness, disorientation, convulsions
Autonomic: flushing, sweating, pruritus, paresthesias, mydriasis, tremors, involuntary movements, muscle spasticity, increased deep tendon reflexes
Respiratory: cough, dyspnea, bronchospasm, laryngospasm, hiccups, rebound hypoventilation
CV: chest pain and tightness, phlebitis, depressed T waves, arrhythmias
GI: nausea, vomiting, diarrhea
Other: urinary retention, incontinence, proteinuria, decreased hemoglobin or hematocrit

Contraindications

Epilepsy or other convulsive states, airway obstruction, incompetence of the ventilatory mechanism, pneumothorax, extreme dyspnea, acute bronchial asthma, suggested or confirmed pulmonary embolism, respiratory failure caused by neuromuscular disorders, pulmonary fibrosis, severe hypertension, head injury, coronary artery disease, and uncompensated heart failure. *Cautious use* in the presence of cerebral edema, severe tachycardia, arrhythmias, cardiac disease, pheochromocytoma, history of bronchial asthma, hyperthyroidism, peptic ulcer, acute agitation; in pregnant women and in children younger than 12 years.

Interactions

Additive pressor effects may occur if doxapram is combined with sympathomimetics or monoamine oxidase (MAO) inhibitors.

Doxapram releases epinephrine and thus may increase the incidence of arrhythmias with those general anesthetics that sensitize the myocardium (eg, halothane, enflurane, cyclopropane).

Doxapram may enhance the CNS effects of amantadine (see Chapter 28).

Nursing Management

Pretherapy Assessment

Assess and record baseline data necessary for detection of adverse effects of doxapram: General: VS, body weight, skin color and temperature; CNS: orientation, affect, reflexes; GI: normal output, bowel sounds, liver evaluation.

Review medical history and documents for existing or previous conditions that:

a. require cautious use of doxapram: cerebral edema; severe tachycardia; arrhythmias; cardiac disease; pheochromocytoma; bronchial asthma; hyperthyroidism; peptic ulcer; children younger than 12 years
b. contraindicate use of doxapram: allergy to doxapram; epilepsy; airway obstruction; pneumothorax; mechanical disorders of respiration; severe hypertension; uncompensated heart failure; **pregnancy (Category B)**, lactation (effects not known, use caution in nursing mothers)

Nursing Interventions

Medication Administration

Ensure that airway is patent and oxygenation is adequate before drug is administered.

Use intravenous infusion control pump to regulate flow rate of infusion, and have proper measures and drugs available (eg, oxygen, resuscitative equipment, anticonvulsants, antiarrhythmics) to treat possible doxapram overdosage.

Delay administration of doxapram for 10 to 15 minutes after anesthetics (eg, halothane, enflurane) have been discontinued because doxapram-induced release of epinephrine may elicit arrhythmias.

Immediately notify practitioner if sudden dyspnea or hypotension occurs because the drug should be discontinued.

Carefully avoid extravasation of solution because thrombophlebitis can result.

Ensure that arterial blood gas levels have been determined before doxapram is administered in patient with obstructive pulmonary disease. Blood gases should then be monitored at least every 30 minutes during infusion. Drug should not be infused for more than 2 hours. Supplemental oxygen should be provided as needed.

Continue to observe patient closely for at least 1 hour after injection or until patient is fully alert and pharyngeal and laryngeal reflexes are restored.

Expect subsequent doses of doxapram to be readministered only to patient who has responded to initial dose.

Do not mix doxapram injection with alkaline solutions because precipitation will result. Injection is compatible with normal saline or dextrose in water.

Surveillance During Therapy

Monitor blood pressure, pulse, and deep tendon reflexes during administration to prevent overdosage. If signs of toxicity (tachycardia, hyperactive reflexes, hypertension) occur, the infusion rate should be reduced or the drug should be discontinued.

Carefully monitor laboratory studies and patient for indications of adverse reactions.

Interpret results of diagnostic tests and contact practitioner as appropriate.

Monitor for possible drug–drug and drug–nutrient interactions: See Interactions.

Patient Teaching

Because drug is an emergency medication, opportunity for patient teaching is focused on teaching family members about clinical aspects of emergency patient care.

Caffeine

• Caffeine

Cafedrine, No Doz, Quick Pep, Tirend, Vivarin

• Caffeine and Sodium Benzoate

Caffeine is a xanthine derivative possessing weak CNS-stimulant, smooth-muscle relaxant, vasodilatory, diuretic, and myocardial stimulant actions. However, it constricts cerebral arteries and enhances the contraction of skeletal muscles. CNS stimulant effects are exerted mainly on the cortex in small doses, relieving fatigue and improving sensory awareness. Larger doses can further excite lower brain centers (eg, vasomotor, respiratory, vagal). The drug is used orally, as tablets or capsules containing dextrose or sucrose, and parenterally combined with sodium benzoate.

Mechanism

Competitively blocks receptors for adenosine (substance that depresses CNS neurons) which increases neuronal firing; also increases concentration of cyclic adenosine monophosphate (cAMP) in tissues by inhibiting phosphodiesterase (enzyme that inactivates cAMP); can increase release of calcium from sarcoplasmic reticulum, improving skeletal muscle tone; stimulates all levels of CNS when used in sufficient amounts

Uses

Reduces fatigue and increases sensory awareness (orally)
Treatment of mild to moderate respiratory depression caused by overdosage with CNS depressants such as morphine or alcohol (parenterally)
Relieves pain associated with vascular headaches or spinal puncture (orally or parenterally, often with ergotamine)

Dosage

Oral: 100 to 200 mg every 4 hours *or* 200 mg sustained-release capsules every 3 to 4 hours. Oral administration of caffeine is not recommended in children
Parenteral: 500 mg intramuscularly or slow intravenous injection; maximum, 2.5 g/24 hours

Fate

Readily absorbed after injection; well absorbed orally, peak plasma levels occur within 30 to 45 minutes; readily crosses the blood–brain barrier; half-life ($T_{1/2}$) is 3 to 6 hours; minimally protein bound; partially demethylated and oxidized in the liver; excreted largely through the kidney, 10% as unchanged drug

Common Side Effects

Nervousness, insomnia, gastric irritation

Significant Adverse Reactions

(Usually with large doses)

Nausea, vomiting, hematemesis, restlessness, irritability, excitement, tinnitus, scotomas, tremors, flushing, palpitation, tachycardia, extrasystoles, diuresis, hypotension, delirium, respiratory distress

Contraindications

No absolute contraindications. *Cautious use* in patients with diabetes (may produce *hyperglycemia*), gastric ulcers, myocardial infarction, and respiratory depression.

Interactions

Caffeine may cause hypertensive reactions in combination with MAO inhibitors.
Caffeine can increase CNS stimulation caused by propoxyphene overdosage, resulting in convulsions.
Increased effects of caffeine can occur when combined with oral contraceptives, fluoroquinolone antibiotics, or cimetidine (These drugs inhibit caffeine metabolism.).
Smoking may increase elimination of caffeine.

Nursing Management

Pretherapy Assessment

Assess and record baseline data necessary for detection of adverse effects of caffeine: General: vital signs (VS), body weight, skin color and temperature; CNS: orientation, affect, reflexes; gastrointestinal (GI): normal output, bowel sounds, liver evaluation.
Review medical history and documents for existing or previous conditions that:
a. require cautious use of caffeine: gastric ulcers; myocardial infarction; respiratory depression; diabetes
b. contraindicate use of caffeine: allergy to methylxanthines; **pregnancy (Category B)**, lactation (effects not known, use caution in nursing mothers)

Nursing Interventions

Medication Administration

Administer caffeine and sodium benzoate slowly. Do not exceed 1,000 mg per dose because increased respiratory depression may result.
Have a short-acting barbiturate on hand when drug is given intramuscularly or intravenously to counteract excessive CNS stimulation.

Surveillance During Therapy

Monitor blood pressure, pulse, and deep tendon reflexes during administration to prevent overdosage. If signs of toxicity (tachycardia, hyperactive reflexes, hypertension) occur, the infusion rate should be reduced or the drug should be discontinued.
Carefully monitor laboratory studies and patient for indications of adverse reactions.
Interpret results of diagnostic tests and contact practitioner as appropriate.
Monitor for possible drug–drug and drug–nutrient interactions: See Interactions.

Patient Teaching

Inform patient with diabetes that regular use of caffeine may alter insulin and/or dietary requirements.

Amphetamines

- **Amphetamine**
- **Dextroamphetamine**
- **Methamphetamine**

The amphetamines are synthetic sympathomimetic amines with marked CNS-stimulatory action. They increase alertness and concentration, temporarily elevate mood, and stimulate motor activity. Depending on both the dose and personality of the user, amphetamines can induce varying degrees of euphoria. Major peripheral effects of these compounds include elevation of blood pressure, relaxation of bronchiolar smooth muscle, contraction of the urinary sphincter, and mydriasis.

Prolonged oral use of amphetamines can cause insomnia, dizziness, and irritability. The stimulation resulting from amphetamine usage is followed by an equally intense depression, fatigue, and listlessness. The desire to overcome this post-stimulatory depression often leads to repetitive amphetamine dosing; this process may cause amphetamine addiction in the susceptible person. The acute behavioral changes that can develop include disorientation, hallucinations, and paranoid ideation; users are given to violent outbursts that can endanger themselves and others. Chronic abuse of amphetamines can produce a behavioral state of paranoia that is difficult to distinguish from paranoid schizophrenia. Obviously, the danger is greatly increased when these agents are abused parenterally (especially intravenously); see Chapter 82 for a discussion of amphetamine abuse.

Approved clinical indications for amphetamines are few; use of these drugs must be undertaken cautiously with close monitoring of patients. The amphetamines are discussed as a group (listed individually in Table 29-1).

Mechanism

Promote release of catecholamines from—and reduce reuptake into—presynaptic nerve terminals; net effect is potentiation of endogenous catecholamine activity; may directly activate adrenergic receptor sites and inhibit MAO (enzyme that biotransforms amines such as norepinephrine, dopamine, and serotonin); stimulant effect thought to be caused by activation of cerebral cortex and possibly reticular formation; anorexiant action may be caused by stimulation of β-receptor–mediated satiety center in lateral hypothalamus; usefulness in attention deficit disorder has been related to potentiation of dopamine action in CNS (and possibly to enhanced stimulus discrimination related to increased activity of the reticular activating system)

Uses

Short-term (ie, 4–8 weeks) adjunct in the treatment of obesity, as an aid to a total weight control program (potential benefit does *not* outweigh inherent risks—see below)

Treatment of narcolepsy

Treatment of attention deficit disorder (ADD) in children

Dosage

See Table 29-1.

Fate

Rapidly absorbed from GI tract and widely distributed in the body; high concentrations are found in the brain and cere-

Table 29-1. **Amphetamines**

Drug	***Usual Dosage Range***	***Nursing Considerations***
Amphetamine Sulfate (C-II)	*Narcolepsy* 5–60 mg/day in divided doses *Attention deficit disorder* 3–5 y; 2.5 mg/day; increase by 2.5 mg/wk if necessary Older than 6 y: 5 mg 1–2 times/day; increase by 5 mg/wk of necessary *Obesity* 5–30 mg/day in divided doses 30–60 min before meals	Note development of insomnia or anorexia and reduce dose; give first dose on awakening and last dose 4–6 h before bedtime if possible; attempt to provide drug-free periods in children with attention deficit disorder, especially during periods of reduced stress (eg, summer vacation, holidays); be aware that response is more variable in children than in adults, and observe more closely
Dextroamphetamine Sulfate (C-II) *Dexedrine*	*Narcolepsy* 5–60 mg/day in divided doses *Obesity* 2.5–10 mg 1–3 times/day *Attention deficit disorder* Older than 3 y: 2.5–5 mg/day; increase gradually to optimal effect (maximum, 40 mg/day)	More potent CNS stimulant than amphetamine but less of an effect on the cardiovascular and peripheral nervous systems; give last dose at least 6 h before bedtime; tolerance usually develops within several weeks; possesses the same pharmacologic properties and hazards as amphetamine, and should be used sparingly and cautiously
Methamphetamine (C-II) *Desoxyn*	*Obesity* 5 mg 3 times/day (long-acting—1 tablet daily) *Attention deficit disorder* Older than 6 y: initially, 5 mg 1 or 2 times/day; increase by 5 mg/week to optimal level (usual range, 20–25 mg/day)	CNS effect slightly greater than amphetamine; do *not* use long-acting tablets to initiate dosage; give 30 min before meals and last dose at least 6 h before bedtime; large doses may result in cardiac stimulation; tolerance develops quickly; so drug has high abuse potential; commonly called *speed* among abusers; has caused severe psychotic reactions following repeated injections of dissolved tablets

brospinal fluid; onset of action is usually in 30 to 60 minutes; plasma $T_{1/2}$ is approximately 4 to 6 hours, but effects may persist for up to 24 hours; partially metabolized in the liver; metabolites may lead to development of amphetamine psychosis with prolonged use; some unchanged drug is eliminated in the urine

Common Side Effects

Nervousness, palpitations, insomnia, tachycardia, unpleasant taste

Significant Adverse Reactions

CNS: dizziness, euphoria or dysphoria, headache, chills, tremor; large doses may cause confusion, hallucinations, panic, aggressiveness, and psychotic episodes

CV: hypertension, arrhythmias

GI: nausea, vomiting, diarrhea, anorexia and weight loss, cramping

Other: impotence, urticaria, delayed or difficult urination; large doses can cause dyspnea, anginal pain, syncope, convulsions, and coma

Overdosage: restlessness, irritability, tremor, sweating, hyperreflexia, confusion, hypertension, delirium, arrhythmias, convulsions

Contraindications

Cardiovascular disease, hypertension, hyperthyroidism, arteriosclerosis, glaucoma, agitated states, severe endogenous depression, history of drug abuse, within 14 days of MAO-inhibitor administration; in children younger than 3 years, and in pregnancy. *Cautious use* in emotionally disturbed persons, in the presence of cardiac arrhythmias, and in nursing mothers.

Interactions

Amphetamines can reduce the antihypertensive effects of guanethidine, methyldopa, hydralazine, and possibly other antihypertensive drugs.

Effects of amphetamines can be potentiated by acetazolamide, cocaine, furazolidone, propoxyphene, tricyclic antidepressants, MAO inhibitors, and by sodium bicarbonate and other substances that alkalinize the urine.

Amphetamines may be antagonized by urinary acidifying agents (ascorbic acid, methenamine, glutamic acid, fruit juices), which increase renal excretion, and by lithium, haloperidol, and phenothiazines.

Amphetamines may delay the effects of phenytoin, ethosuximide, and related anticonvulsants by impairing their GI absorption.

Amphetamines, when used with general anesthetics, may increase the risk of cardiac arrhythmias.

Nursing Management

Pretherapy Assessment

Assess and record baseline data necessary for detection of adverse effects of amphetamines: General: VS, body weight, skin color and temperature; CNS: orientation, affect, reflexes; GI: normal output, bowel sounds, liver evaluation; Lab: thyroid function, blood and urine glucose, baseline electrocardiogram (ECG).

Review medical history and documents for existing or previous conditions that:

a. require cautious use of amphetamine: emotionally disturbed; cardiac arrhythmias
b. contraindicate use of amphetamine: allergy to sympathomimetic amines, tartrazine; cardiovascular disease; hypertension; hyperthyroidism; glaucoma; severe endogenous depression; drug abuse; within 14 days of MAO inhibitor therapy; **pregnancy (Category C)**, lactation (effects not known, use caution in nursing mothers)

Nursing Interventions

Medication Administration

Observe patient closely for signs of tolerance when administering an amphetamine for weight control. If tolerance develops, the drug should be discontinued rather than increasing the dose.

Assist with efforts to determine the *lowest* effective dose for each patient to minimize dangers of adverse effects and habituation.

Collaborate with healthcare team to plan for provision of appropriate educational, psychological, and social interventions, along with drug therapy, when used for attention deficit disorder in children.

Follow proper procedures for handling schedule II substances (see Chapter 10).

Surveillance During Therapy

Monitor for toxicity.

Carefully monitor laboratory studies and patient for indications of adverse reactions.

Interpret results of diagnostic tests and contact practitioner as appropriate.

Monitor for possible drug–drug and drug–nutrient interactions: See Interactions.

Patient Teaching

CAUTION

The risk of both psychological and physcial dependence with amphetamines is considerable. Therefore, they should be used for weight control *only* after other programs have failed, and they should be given for no more than a few weeks.

Suggest taking last dose at least 6 hours before bedtime, if possible, to minimize insomnia.

Caution patient that ability to drive or operate machinery may be impaired.

Warn patient that post-stimulatory depression may occur. Emphasize the need for proper rest and avoidance of hazardous activities during this period.

Explain that abrupt discontinuation of drug after prolonged therapy can cause extreme fatigue, depression, and even psychotic behavior.

Inform diabetic patient that amphetamines may alter insulin or dietary requirements. Urge patient to report any symptomatic changes.

Instruct patient to avoid excessive intake of foods high in tyramine (eg, aged cheese, beer, red wine, liver, broad beans, soy sauce) because they can cause an excessive increase in blood pressure when amphetamines are being taken.

Stress the importance of adhering to dietary program to obtain maximal benefit if patient is using drug for weight reduction.

Anorexiants

A group of drugs related structurally to amphetamine have been used in treating obesity. These agents, termed *anorexiants, anorectics*, or *anorexigenics*, possess essentially the same pharmacologic and toxicologic actions as amphetamine. With the exception of fenfluramine, which depresses the CNS, all these drugs are stimulants, an action largely responsible for their anorectic effect. They are primarily indicated for the *temporary* (ie, few weeks) adjunctive management of obesity in conjunction with a carefully supervised program of caloric restriction *and* proper exercise. Although none of these agents is superior to amphetamine in effectiveness, some have less potential for addiction than amphetamines and may be preferable for short-term therapy. It is important to recognize, however, that *all* of these drugs can produce both psychological **and** physical dependence with continued use.

All of these anorexiants are available only by prescription except for the decongestant *phenylpropanolamine*, an adrenergic compound available as an OTC diet aid either alone or in combination with vitamins or grapefruit extract. A weak CNS stimulant, phenylpropanolamine has been recommended for the short-term management of obesity despite its very questionable efficacy. Moreover, because phenylpropanolamine stimulates α-adrenergic receptors and releases norepinephrine, it can significantly elevate blood pressure and should not be taken by anyone with even mild hypertension. Severe hypertensive episodes have occurred during administration of phenylpropanolamine combined with propranolol or indomethacin. Contraindications to phenylpropanolamine include hypertension, diabetes, kidney disease, arteriosclerosis, symptomatic cardiovascular disease, and hyperthyroidism. Recommended dosages of phenylpropanolamine are 25 mg 3 times/day or 75 mg (sustained-release) once daily. Strict supervision is necessary whenever these nonprescription diet aids are used.

The anorexigenic drugs are discussed as a group, followed by a tabular listing of the agents indicating significant differences in their actions (Table 29-2). As with amphetamines, the chance of suffering serious adverse reactions from anorexigenic drugs is *greater* than their therapeutic benefit.

Mechanism

Probably similar to amphetamine; exert a CNS-stimulant effect on the cortex and may activate hypothalamic satiety center regulating food intake to decrease appetite; most drugs (except

Table 29-2. **Anorexiant Drugs**

Drug	*Usual Dosage Range*	*Nursing Considerations*
Benzphetamine (C-III) *Didrex*	Initially 25–50 mg/day; increase as necessary (usual range 50–150 mg/day)	Usually given as a single daily dose, midmorning or midafternoon
Diethylpropion (C-IV) *Tenuate, Tepanil* *(CAN) Nobesine*	25 mg 3 times/day 1 h before meals and in midevening if needed *or* 75 mg daily in the morning	Less effective but somewhat less hazardous than amphetamines; caution in epileptics because drug has been shown to increase convulsions; may alter ECG (T-wave changes)
Fenfluramine (C-IV) *Pondimin* *(CAN) Ponderal*	Initially 20 mg 3 times/day before meals; increase by 20 mg/week to a maximum of 120 mg/day	Differs from other anorexiants because it often produces CNS *depression*; may enhance glucose uptake by skeletal muscles; *use cautiously* in depression and diabetes; diarrhea is often noted early in therapy; reduce dosage or discontinue if severe; do not discontinue abruptly because severe depression can ensue; avoid use in alcoholics, because psychiatric symptoms can develop; may potentiate effects of both CNS stimulants and CNS depressants
Mazindol (C-IV) *Mazanor, Sanorex*	1 mg 3 times/day before meals *or* 2 mg daily before lunch	Take with food if necessary to reduce GI discomfort; may alter drug requirements by lowering blood glucose levels; elicits CNS and cardiovascular stimulation, and appears to alter mood by action on the limbic system
Phendimetrazine (C-III) *Several manufacturers*	35 mg 2–3 times/day 1 h before meals *or* 105 mg once a day	Similar to amphetamine in action but somewhat less potent
Phetermine (C-IV) *Ionamin and several other manufacturers*	8 mg 3 times/day before meals *or* 15–37.5 mg daily in the morning	Less potent stimulant of CNS and cardiovascular activity than amphetamine; available as a resin-complex capsule (15 mg, 30 mg) providing prolonged action (1–15 h); do *not* use resin complex if patient has diarrhea because effectiveness is lost
Phenylpropanolamine *Acutrim, Dexatrim, and several other manufacturers*	25 mg 3 times/day *or* 50–75 mg once daily in the morning	Over-the-counter diet aid possessing weak central stimulatory action; can activate peripheral α and β receptors, resulting in vasoconstriction and cardiac stimulation; also used as a nasal decongestant (see Chapter 14); use must be closely supervised because blood pressure elevations have occurred; discontinue drug if tachycardia, dizziness, nervousness, or insomnia occur; do *not* exceed recommended dose

fenfluramine) possess a central excitatory action and can elevate blood pressure

Uses

Short-term (8–12 weeks) adjunctive management of exogenous obesity in conjunction with caloric restriction
Fenfluramine has been used investigationally in treating autistic children with elevated serotonin levels.

Dosage

See Table 29-2

Fate

Most drugs are quickly and completely absorbed orally; onset of action occurs within 1 hour, and effects generally persist 4 to 6 hours; sustained-release formulations may have prolonged action (12–18 hours). Tolerance develops within several weeks; metabolized by the liver and excreted both as unchanged drug and metabolites by the kidney

Common Side Effects

Nervousness, irritability, insomnia, tachycardia, palpitations

Significant Adverse Reactions

CV: hypertension, precordial pain, arrhythmias, syncope
CNS: anxiety, dizziness, headache, euphoria, tremors, confusion, incoordination; occasionally depression, (especially fenfluramine), dysphoria, dysarthria; also, drowsiness and impotence with fenfluramine
GI: nausea, vomiting, unpleasant taste, cramping, constipation, glossitis, stomatitis
Genitourinary: dysuria, polyuria, diuresis, cystitis, impotence, menstrual irregularities, changes in libido, gynecomastia
Other: rash, urticaria, erythema, mydriasis, blurred vision, muscle pain, chills, flushing, fever, sweating, alopecia, blood dyscrasias (rare)

Contraindications

See Amphetamines. *Cautious use* in pregnant or nursing women, and in persons with glaucoma, diabetes, epilepsy, or anxiety neuroses.

Interactions

See Amphetamines. In addition:
Fenfluramine may augment the effects of other CNS depressants (eg, alcohol, narcotics, barbiturates) and may potentiate the action of antihypertensive drugs.
Mazindol may potentiate the pressor effects of exogenous catecholamines and increase the risk of lithium toxicity.
Anorexiants may reduce diabetic drug requirements by increasing glucose uptake by skeletal muscle cells, necessitating dosage adjustment.

Nursing Management

Refer to **Amphetamines**. In addition:

Nursing Interventions

Medication Administration

Expect therapy to be discontinued after several weeks to avoid development of tolerance and possible habituation. The recommended dose should not be exceeded in an attempt to increase anorectic effect.
Monitor for signs of excessive stimulation (tachycardia, dizziness, restlessness, hypertension), and notify practitioner immediately if any occur.
Follow proper procedures for handling controlled substances. Individual drugs are classified in schedules III and IV (see Chapter 10).

Patient Teaching

Instruct patient to swallow the delayed or sustained-action dosage forms whole. Chewing or crushing the tablets may release large quantities of medication too quickly.
Suggest taking last dose at least 6 hours before bedtime to minimize insomnia. Because much overeating occurs at night, advantages and disadvantages of an evening dose should be considered.
Caution patient to avoid activities requiring mental alertness and coordination because dizziness and confusion may occur.
Explain that extreme fatigue and depression may ensue if drug is abruptly discontinued after use for a prolonged period.
Emphasize the importance of careful adherence to the *total* treatment regimen (ie, drugs, diet, exercise) if weight control is to be successful. Clarify the danger of overreliance on the drug as the answer to an obesity problem.
Ensure that patient understands dietary restrictions that must accompany drug therapy to obtain maximal benefit.
Advise patient to avoid excessive consumption of foods high in tyramine content (eg, aged cheese, broad beans, red wine, beer, liver, soy sauce) because they can cause hypertensive reactions in persons taking amphetamine-like drugs.

• Methylphenidate (C-II)

Ritalin

A CNS stimulant with a pharmacologic profile of action similar to that of amphetamine, but having a more marked effect on mental rather than physical or motor activities at normal doses, methylphenidate shares the potential for habituation and psychological addiction possessed by the amphetamines. However, its central excitatory effects are weaker. In usual therapeutic dosage, it does not elevate the blood pressure, heart rate, or respiratory rate; however, with large doses, signs of generalized CNS excitation can occur (eg, tremors, tachycardia, hyperpyrexia, confusion). It is most widely used as an adjunct in the therapy of ADD in children, where its effectiveness equals that of the amphetamines.

Mechanism

Not definitively established, but probably similar to amphetamine; major action appears to be on the cerebral cortex; increases release of catecholamines from presynaptic nerve endings

Uses

Adjunctive therapy of attention deficit disorder in children
Treatment of narcolepsy
Investigational uses include treatment of depression in elderly, cancer or post-stroke patients

Dosage

Adults: Initially 10 mg 2 or 3 times/day (maximum, 60 mg/day)
Children: (older than 6 years): Initially 5 mg 2 times/day; increase by 5 to 10 mg/week to optimal dose (maximum, 60 mg/day)

During prolonged therapy in children, periodic discontinuation of therapy should be attempted to assess the patient's condition. Drug treatment is not intended to be indefinite.

Fate

Absorbed well from GI tract; distributed throughout the body, including CNS; onset of action occurs in 30 to 60 minutes, and peak blood levels are achieved in 1 hour to 3 hours; effects persist up to 6 hours with oral administration; excreted through the kidneys, largely as metabolites

Common Side Effects

Nervousness, insomnia
In children: anorexia, mild weight loss, and tachycardia are also frequent

Significant Adverse Reactions

CNS: nausea, dizziness, drowsiness, headache, dyskinesia, agitation, toxic psychoses
CV: palpitations, blood pressure changes, tachycardia, anginal attacks, arrhythmias
Allergic: skin rash, fever, urticaria, arthralgia, erythema multiforme, necrotizing vasculitis, exfoliative dermatitis
Other: visual disturbances, alopecia, abdominal pain, anemia

Contraindications

Marked tension, anxiety or agitated states, glaucoma, seizure disorders, and *severe* depression. *Cautious use* in patients with hypertension, in patients with a history of drug dependence or alcoholism, and during pregnancy.

Interactions

Methylphenidate may increase the effects of oral anticoagulants, anticonvulsants, tricyclic antidepressants, and phenylbutazone by inhibiting their metabolism.
Hypertensive reactions may occur with vasopressors, MAO inhibitors, and furazolidone.
Methylphenidate decreases the antihypertensive action of guanethidine.
Effects of methylphenidate can be antagonized by phenothiazines and propoxyphene.

Nursing Management

Refer to **Amphetamines**. In addition:

Nursing Interventions

Medication Administration

Collaborate with healthcare team to plan for provision of appropriate educational, psychological, and social intervention, along with drug therapy, when used for attention deficit disorder in children.
Follow proper procedures for handling a Schedule II drug (see Chapter 10).

Surveillance During Therapy

Carefully evaluate drug-taking patterns, especially in emotionally unstable person, because chronic abuse can occur.
Monitor blood pressure, weight, and results of blood counts, which should be performed periodically during extended periods of treatment.

Patient Teaching

Suggest taking last dose no later than 4 or 5 hours before bedtime to minimize insomnia.
Advise patient that nervousness and insomnia may occur early in therapy but generally lessen with time. Dosage reduction may be required.
Explain that drug should be withdrawn gradually to avoid precipitation of severe depressive episodes or psychotic behavior. The drug should *not* be prescribed for a severely depressed patient.

• Pemoline (C-IV)

Cylert

Pemoline is a CNS stimulant that is pharmacologically similar to amphetamine and methylphenidate but has minimal sympathomimetic effects. It appears to have a lower abuse potential than most other CNS stimulants.

Mechanism

Not established; increases alertness and motor activity and induces a mild euphoria, probably by an action on the cerebral cortex; may increase dopaminergic transmission in CNS structures

Uses

Treatment of attention deficit disorder in children
Treatment of narcolepsy and excessive sleepiness

Dosage

Initially 37.5 mg/day as single morning dose; increase by 18.75 mg/week until optimal effects are noted; maximum dose, 112.5 mg/day

Fate

Absorbed from GI tract, with peak blood levels in 2 to 4 hours; onset of action is gradual over 3 to 4 weeks; plasma $T_{1/2}$ approximately 12 hours; metabolized by the liver and excreted in the urine both as unchanged drug (45%) and as several conjugated metabolites

Common Side Effects

Insomnia, anorexia

Significant Adverse Reactions

Nausea, diarrhea, dizziness, headache, drowsiness, irritability, nystagmus, dyskinesias, abdominal pain, skin rash, jaundice, convulsive movements, hallucinations

Contraindications

Children younger than 6. *Cautious use* in patients with impaired renal or hepatic function, in those with a history of drug abuse, and in pregnant or lactating women.

Interactions

May enhance the effects of other CNS stimulants (eg, caffeine, amphetamines)

Nursing Management

Refer to **Amphetamines**. In addition:

Nursing Interventions

Medication Administration

Collaborate with healthcare team to plan for provision of appropriate educational, psychological, and social intervention, along with drug therapy, when used for ADD in children.

Follow proper procedures for handling a schedule IV drug (see Chapter 10).

Surveillance During Therapy

Monitor results of liver function tests, which should be performed periodically during prolonged therapy. Drug should be discontinued if aspartate aminotransferase (AST), alanine aminotransferase (ALT), or serum lactate dehydrogenase (LDH) levels are significantly elevated.

Monitor weight of children on prolonged therapy because growth suppression and weight loss can occur.

Patient Teaching

Suggest that drug be taken once a day in the morning to minimize insomnia.

Selected Bibliography

Bruera E, Fainsinger R, MacEachern T, Hanson J: The use of methylphenidate in patients with incident cancer pain receiving regular opiates: A preliminary report. Pain 50:75, 1992

Elia J: Drug treatment for hyperactive children: Therapeutic Guidelines. Drugs 46(5):863, 1993

Fine S: Drug and placebo side effects in methylphenidate-placebo trial for attention deficit hyperactivity disorder. Child Psychiat Hum Dev 24(1):25, 1993

Fox AM, Rieder MJ: Risks and benefits of drugs used in the management of the hyperactive child. Drug Safety 9(1):38, 1993

Goldberg TE et al: Cognitive and behavioral effects of the coadministration of dextroamphetamine and haloperidol in schizophrenia. Am J Psychiatry 148(1):78, 1991

Hando J, Hall W: HIV risk-taking behaviour among amphetamine users in Sydney, Australia. Addiction 89:79, 1994

Patt RB: An evolving role for the psychostimulants in pain management. Am Pain Soc Bull 3(4):1, 1993

Schteingart DE: Effectiveness of phenylpropanolamine in the management of moderate obesity. Int J Obesity 16:487, 1992

Seiden LS, Sabol KE, Ricaurte GA: Amphetamine: Effects on catecholamine systems and behavior. Annu Rev Pharmacol 33:639, 1993

Silverstone T: Appetite suppressants: A review. Drugs 43:820, 1992

Simeon JG, Wiggins DM: Pharmacotherapy of attention-deficit hyperactivity disorder. Can J Psychiatry 38:443, 1993

Stallone DD, Stunkard AJ: Long-term use of appetite suppressant medication: Rationale and recommendations. Drug Dev Res 26:1, 1992

Nursing Bibliography

Funk J: Attention deficit hyperactivity disorder, creativity and the effects of methylphenidate. Pediatrics 91(4):816–819, 1993

Selvaggi L: Caffeine consumption and fibrocystic breast disease. Florida Nurse 40(10):11–12, 1992

III

Drugs Acting on the Cardiovascular System

30
Cardiovascular Physiology: A Review

The cardiovascular system functions as a highly integrated unit to establish and maintain, within a wide range of conditions, the hemodynamic state necessary to meet the moment-to-moment needs of each body tissue.

The rhythmic pumping action of the heart establishes blood flow at an adequate level of pressure. The elastic recoil of the aorta and large arteries transforms the intermittent output of the heart into a relatively steady peripheral flow of blood. Unidirectional flow of blood is maintained by suitable pressure gradients and is aided by strategically placed valves. Blood pressure is maintained by delicate reflex mechanisms, and blood flow to individual body tissues is controlled by local metabolic needs as well as by central integrating mechanisms.

The Heart

The human heart is a four-chambered, highly muscular organ lying within the mediastinum enclosed by a double-layered pericardium (Fig. 30-1). The heart wall is composed of three layers: an outer thin transparent *epicardium* (visceral pericardium); a thick middle muscular *myocardium;* and an inner serous lining, or *endocardium*. In addition to lining the chambers of the heart, the endocardium covers the valves of the heart and is continuous with the endothelium of the blood vessels.

The thin-walled superior chambers, or *atria*, function primarily as reservoirs for blood returning to the heart. The right atrium receives systemic venous blood from the superior and inferior venae cavae and coronary venous blood chiefly through the coronary sinus. The left atrium receives oxygenated blood from the lungs by way of four pulmonary veins. Because no true valves separate the great veins near the heart from the atrial chambers, elevations in right atrial pressure are reflected backward into the systemic venous circulation, whereas elevations in left atrial pressure lead to pulmonary congestion.

The inferior chambers or *ventricles* are thick walled, being formed by three indistinct layers of muscle arranged in a complex spiral fashion. During contraction, the myocardium of each ventricle generates a force sufficient to overcome the existing pressure in the receiving artery. The right ventricle ejects its contents into the pulmonary artery, while the left ventricle pumps oxygenated blood into the aorta. Because the pulmonary circulation is maintained at a considerably lower pressure than the systemic circulation, the thickness of the right ventricular wall is approximately one-third that of the left, reflecting the lighter workload of the right ventricle.

Unidirectional blood flow through the heart is maintained by two types of valves: the *atrioventricular* (AV) valves and the *semilunar* valves. The AV valves separate the atria from the ventricles. Each valve is composed of leaflets or cusps that attach to the papillary muscles of the ventricles by way of chordae tendineae. A *tricuspid* valve separates the right atrium from the right ventricle, and a *bicuspid* or mitral valve is found between the left atrium and left ventricle.

The semilunar valves consist of three symmetrical cuplike cusps secured onto a fibrous ring. The *pulmonic* valve is situated between the right ventricle and the pulmonary artery, and the *aortic* valve is located between the left ventricle and the aorta. Immediately above the free margins of the aortic valve are the sinuses of Valsalva and the openings of the coronary arteries.

The Coronary Circulation

The myocardium is richly vascularized, its blood supply coming by way of the coronary circulation. The coronary vessels course around the heart in two external anatomic grooves: the atrioventricular groove and the interventricular groove.

The coronary arteries arise from the ascending aorta immediately above the free margins of the aortic semilunar valve. They form a crown around the heart and provide branches to supply the atrial and ventricular myocardium.

The right coronary artery, with its marginal and posterior interventricular branches, supplies the right atrium, right ventricle, and a portion of the left ventricle. The left coronary artery and its major branches, the circumflex and anterior interventricular arteries, supply the left atrium, left ventricle, and part of the right ventricle. Anastomoses between arterial branches exist and serve as potential routes for collateral circulation if gradual occlusion of a vessel occurs. Coronary veins accompany the coronary arteries. The most significant myocardial venous return occurs by way of the coronary sinus, which opens into the right atrium near the orifice of the inferior vena cava.

Blood flow through the coronary arteries occurs primarily during ventricular relaxation (*diastole*) because ventricular contraction (*systole*) compresses the arteries and impedes arterial flow. The reduced time in diastole that occurs at rapid heart rates can markedly decrease coronary arterial perfusion, a potentially critical situation in patients with coronary artery or cardiac disease.

Coronary perfusion is intrinsically autoregulated, although it may also be affected by autonomic nerve activity. Coronary arteries dilate in response to oxygen lack and to elevated local concentrations of CO_2, H^+, K^+, and adenosine.

If vascular spasm restricts coronary blood flow or if a coronary artery is partially occluded by a plaque or thrombus, the vasodilation that automatically occurs distal to the block may provide sufficient blood flow to meet the needs of a resting heart. During exercise or emotional stress, however, such vasodilation may not be sufficient to meet the increased demand on the heart, and ischemia may result. Moderate inadequacy of coronary perfusion is associated with a characteristic substernal thoracic pain that occasionally radiates along the medial

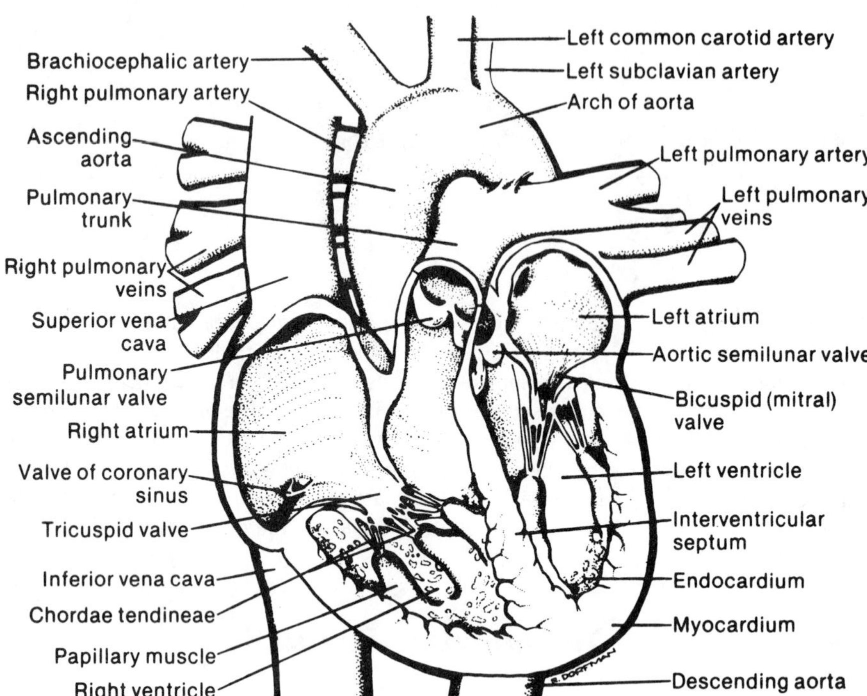

Figure 30-1 The human heart contains four chambers and is enclosed by a double-layered pericardium.

aspect of the left arm and is termed *angina pectoris*. Angina pectoris is usually relieved by rest and vasodilators such as nitroglycerin. Severe and prolonged ischemia of the myocardium causes irreversible damage to the heart. This state, termed *myocardial infarction*, is characterized by severe substernal oppression and may lead to shock, arrhythmias, cardiac dysfunction, or sudden death.

The Conduction System

The heart muscle, or *myocardium*, exhibits the physiologic properties of excitability, conductivity, contractility, and autorhythmicity. The heart spontaneously and rhythmically generates electrical impulses (action potentials) that are distributed along specialized conduction pathways to all parts of the myocardium, permitting synchronous contraction of the ventricular myocardium. Like all excitable tissues, the myocardium exhibits refractory periods. During such times of decreased reactivity, the myocardium is unresponsive to a second stimulus.

The rhythmic synchronized activity of the heart is maintained by a spontaneously active, highly specialized conduction system illustrated in Figure 30-2.

The cardiac impulse normally originates in the *sinoatrial (SA) node*, a small mass of modified myocardial tissue located in the posterior wall of the right atrium, below the opening of the superior vena cava.

A second specialized mass of conduction tissue, the *AV node*, lies in the posterior right side of the interatrial septum near the opening of the coronary sinus. The AV node is continuous with a tract of conducting tissue termed the *AV bundle* or the *bundle of His*. Descending along the interventricular septum, the AV bundle divides into right and left bundle branches that descend along opposite sides of the interventricular septum and ultimately terminate in an extensive network of fine branches known as *Purkinje fibers*.

The spread of the cardiac impulse over the Purkinje fibers is extremely rapid, thereby ensuring virtually simultaneous excitation of the entire ventricular myocardium. Adjacent myocardial cells approximate at specialized junctions of low resistance, called *intercalated discs*. These intercalated discs contain gap junctions that facilitate the rapid spread of excitation from cell to cell, thereby allowing the heart to function as a *syncytium*.

The SA node initiates a wave of depolarization that spreads rapidly throughout the atria. On reaching the AV node, the impulse is delayed briefly (0.08–0.12 seconds) to allow completion of atrial contraction. Excessive delay or failure of impulse conduction at the AV node results in heart block. After the normally brief delay at the AV node, the cardiac impulse then proceeds along the bundle of His and its right and left bundle branches to the rapidly depolarizing fibers of the Purkinje network. The impulse sweeps through the ventricular myocardium from the endocardial (inner) to the epicardial (outer) surface.

Although all parts of the conduction system can rhythmically discharge cardiac action potentials, the cells of the SA node intrinsically depolarize at the highest frequency (60–100 times/minute), thereby setting the pace or rhythm of the heart. Hence the SA node is commonly termed the cardiac *pacemaker*. The discharge rate of the SA node may be affected extrinsically by the autonomic nervous system, as well as by certain hormones, drugs, and even temperature changes. If the SA node fails to generate rhythmic cardiac impulses, other sites, such as the AV node or AV bundle, may assume a pacemaker role.

Disturbances of normal cardiac rhythm, or *arrhythmias*, are caused by altered myocardial electrophysiology. Cardiac arrhythmias may result from abnormal sites of impulse formation (ectopic foci), abnormal rates of impulse formation, or abnormal rates or routes of impulse conduction (see Chapter 32). A shortened myocardial refractory period may also contribute to the development of cardiac arrhythmias. Other predisposing factors include cardiac ischemia, electrolyte imbalance, excessive autonomic stimulation, and drug toxicity.

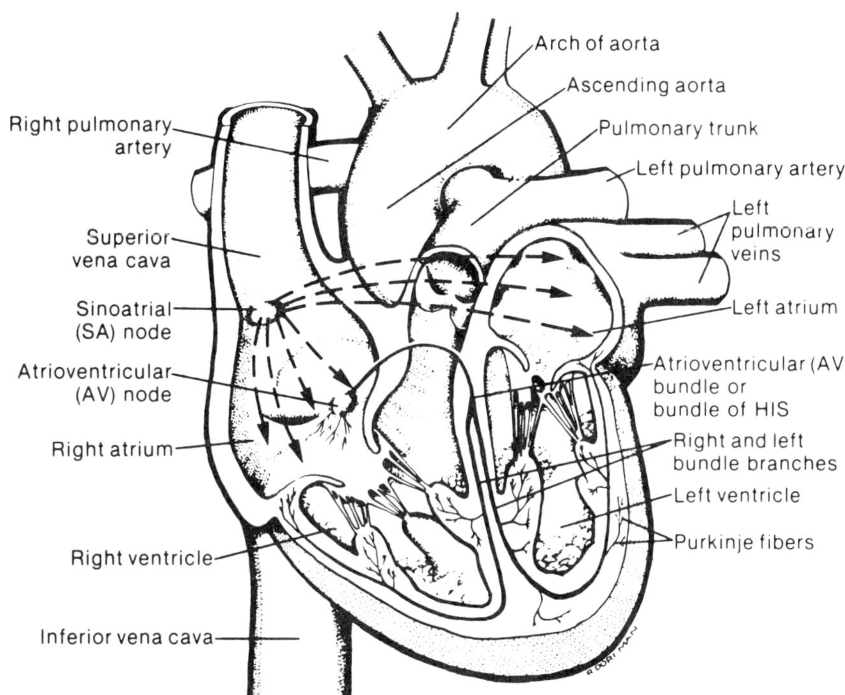

Figure 30-2 A highly specialized conduction system maintains the rhythmic synchronized activity of the heart.

The Electrocardiogram

The *electrocardiogram* (ECG) is a graphic record of the electrical activity of the heart. A typical ECG (lead II tracing) is shown in Figure 30-3. The *P wave* depicts atrial depolarization, the *QRS complex* depicts ventricular depolarization, and the *T wave* depicts ventricular repolarization.

The PR interval (normally 0.12–0.20 seconds) indicates conduction time through the atria and includes the delay at the AV node. Abnormal prolongation of the PR interval indicates first-degree heart block.

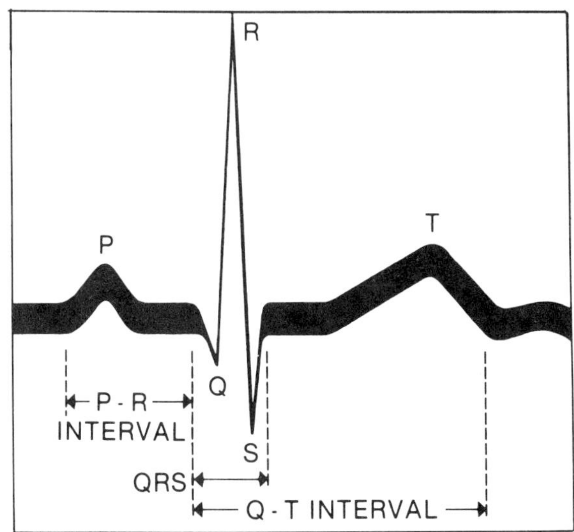

Figure 30-3 A typical electrocardiogram includes the following features: the P wave (depicting atrial depolarization), the QRS complex (depicting ventricular depolarization), and the T wave (depicting ventricular repolarization).

The QT interval encompasses both ventricular depolarization and repolarization. The QT interval may be prolonged by some antiarrhythmic drugs such as quinidine.

The T wave may be flattened or inverted by digitalis overdosage. Hyperkalemia causes peaking and elevation of the T wave. To a skilled reader, the ECG offers valuable information about cardiac rhythm (atrial and ventricular rates), conduction rate, chamber hypertrophy, ischemia, presence of infarction, ionic imbalance, and drug effects.

The Cardiac Cycle

The *cardiac cycle* consists of an orderly sequence of interdependent electrical and mechanical events associated with one complete cycle of contraction (systole) and relaxation (diastole) of the heart. Electrical excitation of the heart precedes contraction.

During diastole, the atrial and ventricular chambers are relaxed and the semilunar valves are closed. Blood that has entered the atria through the great veins flows passively from the atria to the ventricles through the open AV valves. The initial rapid ventricular filling is followed by a slow ventricular filling, termed *diastasis*, which occurs in mid-diastole. During late diastole, a wave of depolarization (P wave) sweeps through the atria, leading to contraction of the atrial musculature. Atrial contraction (atrial systole) contributes approximately 30% to the ventricular blood volume.

Ventricular contraction follows the wave of depolarization through the ventricular conduction system and myocardium (QRS complex). When the ventricular pressures exceed the atrial pressures, the AV valves close, generating the first heart sound. During this phase of ventricular systole, the arterial pressures within the aorta and pulmonary artery exceed the ventricular pressures, thereby keeping the semilunar valves closed and maintaining the ventricular volumes constant (period of isovolumetric contraction). Eventually the sustained ventricular contraction generates sufficient ventricular pressure to exceed the arterial pressure. At this point the semilunar valves open, and the ventricles eject the blood into the pulmonary artery and aorta.

A wave of repolarization (T wave) sweeps through the ventricles, causing the ventricular myocardium to relax. As the ventricles relax, the ventricular pressures fall below the arterial pressures of the pulmonary artery and aorta, causing the semilunar valves to close and generating the second heart sound.

The initial part of ventricular diastole is the period of isovolumetric relaxation. With continued ventricular relaxation, the ventricular pressures fall below the atrial pressures, causing the AV valves to open. The venous blood that has been accumulating in the atria during ventricular systole now rapidly flows through the open AV valves into the ventricles. At rest, approximately 70% of ventricular filling takes place before atrial systole.

Cardiac Output

The work of the heart may be expressed in terms of *cardiac output*, that is, the volume of blood ejected from each ventricle in 1 minute. Cardiac output represents the product of *stroke volume* and *heart rate*. The cardiac output of an adult at rest averages 5 L/minute; however, during exercise, it may approach 20 to 25 L/minute. Many factors contribute to the control of cardiac output through an effect on stroke volume and/or heart rate.

The *stroke volume* (the volume of blood ejected from a ventricle during a single contraction) is equal to the difference between the end-diastolic volume (EDV) and end-systolic volume (ESV). The EDV represents the degree of ventricular filling, and it is determined by factors such as ventricular filling time, atrial contraction, myocardial distensibility, and the effective filling pressure. Normally, the bulk of ventricular filling occurs during early diastole, so that ventricular filling time is inversely related to the heart rate. At very rapid heart rates, the shortened time spent in diastole may reduce passive ventricular filling, in which case atrial contraction may contribute significantly to the ventricular volume.

The effective filling pressure is directly related to the venous return, which is determined largely by the circulating blood volume and venous tone. Venous return to the heart is enhanced by sympathetically mediated venoconstriction and by skeletal muscle contraction, which increases venous pressure through external compression of the veins. Venous return is also facilitated by the thoracicoabdominal pump. The pressure within the thorax is negative with respect to atmospheric pressure, whereas the pressure within the abdominal cavity is slightly positive. The pressure gradient, which becomes even greater during inspiration, thus favors the return of blood from the abdomen to the thorax.

According to the *Frank-Starling Law of the Heart*, there is, within physiologic limits, a direct relationship between myocardial fiber length and the force of ventricular contraction. The degree of stretch of myocardial fibers before contraction is termed *preload*, and it is determined largely by the EDV. Increased preload will, within physiologic limits, increase the force of ventricular contraction and thereby increase the stroke volume.

The end-systolic volume is primarily determined by the afterload and the contractility of the myocardium. *Afterload* determines the amount of tension that a ventricle must develop during systole in order to open the semilunar valve and to eject blood into the receiving artery. Afterload is a function of arterial pressure and ventricular size. As the size of a ventricle increases, the ventricle must develop a greater tension in order to generate a given pressure. Therefore, a dilated ventricle would have to develop a greater tension than a normal ventricle to generate the same systolic pressure.

Elevations in arterial pressure and stenosis of a semilunar valve also increase resistance to the outflow of blood from a ventricle, thereby necessitating an increase in ventricular tension. Chronic or excessive increases in afterload adversely affect the cardiac output and lead to pathologic changes in the heart that may result in eventual cardiac failure.

The contractility of the myocardium is affected by a multitude of factors, including the metabolic state of the myocardium, physical and mechanical factors (Frank-Starling's Law of the Heart), nervous activity, hormones, and pharmacologic agents.

Factors that enhance the contractility of the myocardium are said to have a positive inotropic effect on the heart. Physiologically, sympathetic stimulation and epinephrine enhance the contractile force of the myocardium and thereby increase stroke volume and cardiac output. Other positive inotropic agents include glucagon, caffeine, theophylline, and digitalis. Hypoxia, hypercapnia, acidosis, and certain drugs (eg, disopyramide, verapamil) decrease myocardial contractility.

Cardiac output may also be altered by changes in heart rate. Heart rate is responsive to extrinsic control by the autonomic nervous system. The SA and AV nodes are richly innervated by sympathetic and parasympathetic nerve fibers. The atria receive some innervation from each division of the autonomic nervous system, whereas the ventricles are innervated principally by sympathetic fibers. Sympathetic stimulation, through the release of norepinephrine from adrenergic nerve terminals, accelerates the heart rate and the speed of cardiac impulse conduction. Sympathetic activation also can markedly enhance the force of myocardial contractility.

Parasympathetic nerves to the heart are anatomically vagal and functionally cardioinhibitory. Vagal stimulation, through mediation of the neurotransmitter acetylcholine, produces a notable decrease in the heart rate and the speed of impulse conduction and a slight reduction of cardiac contractility. At rest, the dominant nervous influence on cardiac activity is parasympathetic.

Blood Flow: Hemodynamics

The cardiovascular system forms a continuous closed circuit for the distribution of blood to all body tissues. With each contraction, the left ventricle ejects the blood with a force sufficient to propel it through the entire systemic circuit. The elasticity of the aorta and large arteries transforms the intermittent output of the heart into a relatively steady peripheral blood flow. Blood flows through the arteries, arterioles, capillaries, venules, and veins according to existing pressure gradients, the progressive decrease in pressure across the systemic circuit promoting undirectional forward flow.

According to Poiseuille's law, blood flow is directly proportional to the driving pressure and inversely proportional to the resistance. Resistance to blood flow is directly related to the viscosity of blood and is inversely related to the vascular radius. The viscosity of blood depends on the hematocrit, the rate of flow, and the diameter of the vessel. With a constant hematocrit, the viscosity changes over normal ranges of flow are insignificant. The variable resistance to blood flow is determined largely by the radius of the blood vessels, notably the small muscular arteries and arterioles (resistance vessels). Because the vascular resistance to flow varies inversely as the fourth power of the vascular radius, even a small change in the caliber of a blood vessel can produce a pronounced change in blood flow.

Blood flow varies widely among the different organs and tissues of the body. The brain and kidneys, which represent only a small fraction of the total body mass, receive a generous blood supply; skeletal muscle, despite its large mass, receives only a small percentage of the cardiac output at rest.

Distribution of the cardiac output among the organs and tissues is determined by individual metabolic requirements of the tissue as well as by neural and humoral factors. Because the needs of individual body tissues are continually changing, blood flow must continually be adjusted. Blood flow to a given organ may be enhanced by increasing the cardiac output or by shunting blood from other body tissues. Distribution of the cardiac output is controlled by intrinsic as well as extrinsic mechanisms, which will now be examined in greater detail.

Intrinsic Control of Blood Flow

Local metabolic conditions and individual tissue requirements play an important role in the regulation of regional blood flow. Factors involved in the intrinsic control of blood flow include tissue oxygen requirements and availability, rate of tissue metabolism, and presence of certain tissue metabolites. The vascular smooth muscle of the microcirculation (arterioles, precapillaries, and precapillary sphincters) is highly sensitive to lack of oxygen. The vessels respond to tissue ischemia by vasodilation. Local increases in carbon dioxide and hydrogen ions also produce vasodilation and increased blood flow independently of nervous reflexes. Local control of perfusion is particularly evident in the heart, brain, and skeletal muscle.

In addition to changes in pH and gas tension, endogenous vasodilators such as adenosine, potassium ions, and histamine may act locally to increase blood flow, the latter being especially involved during times of tissue injury or inflammation. *Endothelial-derived relaxing factor (EDRF)*, now known to be *nitric oxide*, produces vasodilation, and the *endothelins* induce vasoconstriction.

Autoregulation of blood flow assumes the inherent ability of a vascular bed to maintain a relatively constant flow rate despite fluctuations in arterial pressure. Central to the mechanism of autoregulation is the ability of vascular smooth muscle to respond to distention caused by increased intraluminal pressure with appropriately graded contraction.

Extrinsic Control of Blood Flow

The walls of small arteries and arterioles are abundantly innervated by autonomic vasomotor fibers, most of which are sympathetic. Sympathetic vasoconstrictor nerves are important in the regulation of peripheral resistance. Arteriolar vasomotor tone changes in accordance with the level of sympathetic activity. Increased sympathetic discharge of vasoconstrictor fibers leads to a reduction in vascular caliber and thereby to an increase in peripheral resistance to blood flow. All vasoconstrictor fibers are adrenergic.

Vasodilator nerves are of minor functional significance in most vascular beds, with the exception of skeletal muscle. In addition to possessing sympathetic adrenergic vasoconstrictor fibers, the vasculature of skeletal muscle is uniquely equipped with sympathetic cholinergic vasodilator nerves that elicit vasodilation in response to stress or exercise. Parasympathetic vasodilator nerves (also cholinergic) innervate only certain organs such as the salivary glands, bladder, and external genitalia. These vasodilator fibers do not significantly influence peripheral vascular resistance. Rather, their specific and limited distribution suggests a more specialized physiologic role.

In addition to neural regulation, humoral agents extrinsically influence peripheral vascular resistance and blood flow. Circulating vasoconstrictors include the catecholamines (epinephrine and norepinephrine), angiotensin II, and vasopressin. Vasodilators include bradykinin, atrial natriuretic hormone, and vasoactive intestinal peptide.

Arterial Blood Pressure

The arterial blood pressure serves as the driving force for blood flow through the vascular system. The magnitude of arterial blood pressure changes throughout the cardiac cycle. The maximum pressure (*systolic pressure*) occurs at the peak of ventricular contraction or systole. The magnitude of systolic pressure may be altered by changes in cardiac output or arterial distensibility. An increase in stroke volume, and hence cardiac output, elevates systolic pressure, as does a reduction in arterial distensibility such as that occurring in arteriosclerosis.

The lowest pressure (*diastolic pressure*) occurs during diastole, just before ventricular contraction. Changes in peripheral resistance alter the level of diastolic pressure. The difference between the systolic and diastolic pressures is termed *pulse pressure*.

The mean arterial pressure is generally assumed to equal the diastolic pressure plus one-third of the pulse pressure. At rapid heart rates, the times spent in systole and diastole are more nearly equal, and mean arterial pressure equals approximately one-half the sum of systolic and diastolic pressures.

The mean arterial pressure equals the product of cardiac output and peripheral resistance. Any factor or condition that alters either or both of these variables therefore affects the blood pressure.

The arterial blood pressure must be constantly and carefully regulated to provide a driving force sufficient to distribute blood to all body tissues without imposing an excessive load on the heart and blood vessels. Several control mechanisms exist for the continuous and precise regulation and integration of cardiovascular functions.

Within the medulla of the brain stem are cardiovascular (cardiac and vasomotor) control centers that receive and integrate input from numerous sensory receptors. Homeostatically, the most important of these are the pressure-sensitive baroreceptors located in the carotid sinus and aortic arch. Associated with the baroreceptors are branches of the glossopharyngeal (IX) and vagus (X) nerves, which serve as "buffer" nerves for the physiologic regulation and maintenance of systemic arterial pressure.

In response to blood pressure changes detected by the

baroreceptors, afferent (sensory) impulses travel along the glossopharyngeal (sinus) and vagus (aortic) nerves to the cardiovascular integrating centers of the medulla. Activation of autonomic sympathetic and parasympathetic efferent nerves to the heart and blood vessels produces appropriate changes in cardiac output and peripheral resistance for the homeostatic restoration of blood pressure.

Efferent responses to an elevated blood pressure include the following: 1) a slowing of the heart (bradycardia) induced by increased parasympathetic and decreased sympathetic activity; 2) reduced myocardial contractility caused by decreased sympathetic discharge; and 3) vasodilation resulting from decreased sympathetic tone. The reduction in cardiac output (resulting from a decreased heart rate and stroke volume) and the decreased peripheral vascular resistance restore the blood pressure toward normal.

The activity of the medullary cardiovascular integrating centers may also be influenced by afferent impulses from higher brain centers such as the hypothalamus and cerebral cortex. It is through such afferent input that emotional responses, for example, fear or rage, alter blood pressure.

A peripheral mechanism operative in the control of blood pressure is the renin–angiotensin–aldosterone system, which is outlined in Figure 30-4. Renin is released from renal juxtaglomerular cells (see Fig. 38-3) in response to a number of stimuli, including hypotension, hyponatremia, hypovolemia, reduced renal perfusion pressure, and β-adrenergic stimulation. Renin acts on the plasma protein angiotensinogen to form the decapeptide angiotensin I, which is then converted by endothelial cell and plasma enzymes into the physiologically active angiotensin II. Angiotensin II is a potent vasopressor that acts through several mechanisms, but primarily by direct stimulation of vascular smooth muscle, to produce intense vasoconstriction and increased peripheral resistance. Angiotensin II also stimulates release of aldosterone from the adrenal cortex. Aldosterone stimulates renal tubular reabsorption of sodium, thereby promoting water reabsorption and increasing blood volume. The increased blood volume and the increased

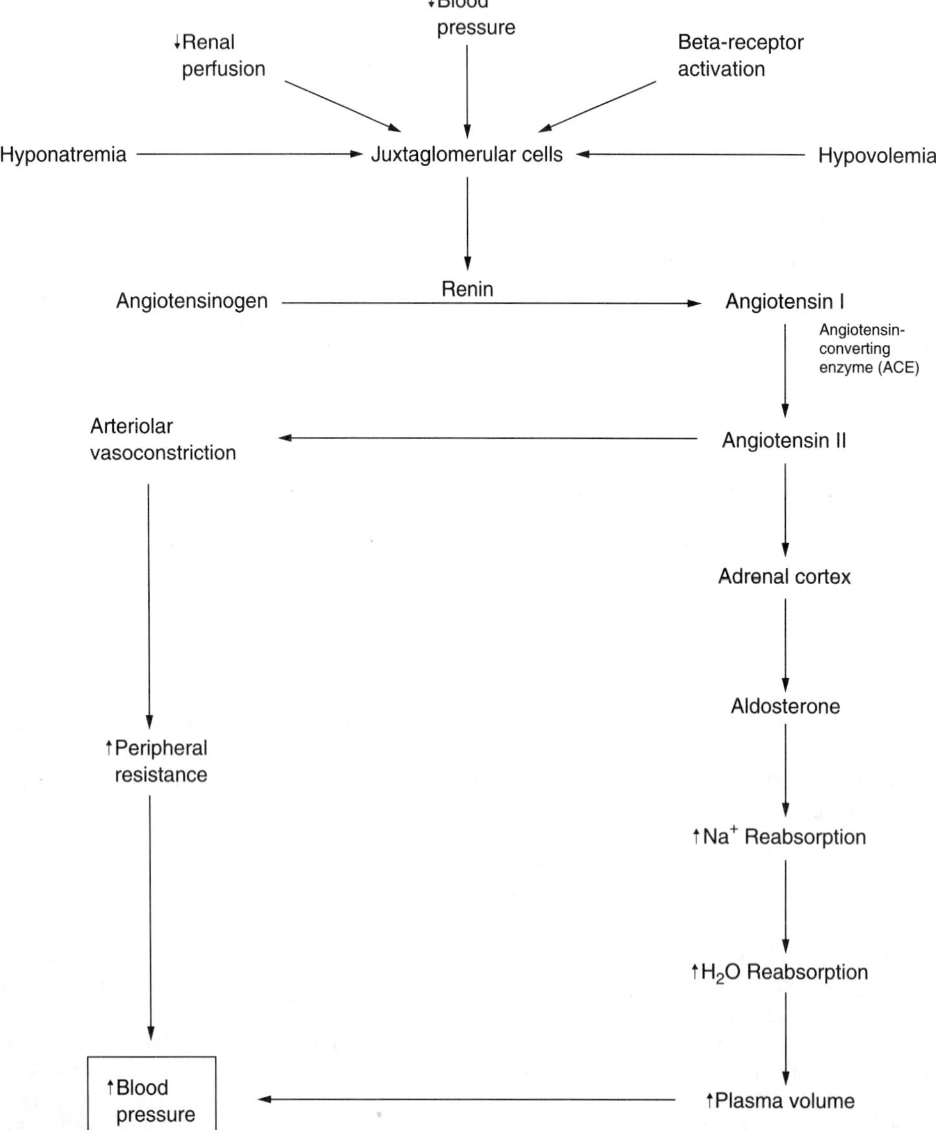

Figure 30-4 Renin-angiotensin-aldosterone mechanism for blood pressure regulation.

peripheral resistance both contribute to the elevation of blood pressure.

The renin–angiotensin–aldosterone system can be affected by a number of drugs, such as angiotensin converting enzyme (ACE) inhibitors and drugs that decrease renin secretion (eg, β-adrenergic blockers. These drugs are useful in treating hypertensive states and in the case of the ACE inhibitors, are also effective in treating congestive heart failure (see Chapter 33).

31
Cardiotonic Drugs

Digitalis Glycosides
- Digoxin
- Digitoxin

Digoxin Immune Fab

Positive Inotropic Agents
- Amrinone
- Milrinone

Drugs that have a cardiotonic action are capable of increasing the force of contraction of cardiac muscle, thus improving its functional capability. The term has traditionally been applied to a group of drugs known as the digitalis glycosides, although newer drugs that exhibit similar properties are now available and are termed positive inotropic agents. Cardiotonic drugs are primarily indicated for the treatment of congestive heart failure because of their ability to improve the force of contraction of the failing heart. In addition to the digitalis glycosides and the positive inotropic agents discussed in this chapter, other drugs are used in managing the symptoms of congestive heart failure. Thus, diuretics (see Chapter 39) and vasodilators (see Chapters 33 and 34) also are of great use in treating certain types of congestive heart failure. Optimal therapy often includes two or more of these drugs.

Cardioactive (Digitalis) Glycosides

The cardioactive glycosides are two semisynthetic steroidal compounds having qualitatively similar effects on cardiac function. These drugs are derived from the leaves of either *Digitalis purpurea* or *Digitalis lanata*, both species of the foxglove plant. Because "digitalis" is the name of the principal botanical source of these agents, they also are referred to collectively as the digitalis glycosides.

Although the digitalis glycosides have similar pharmacologic effects on the heart, they differ with respect to onset and duration of action (owing to differences in absorption, biotransformation, and extent of protein binding) as well as mode of administration. The major characteristics of the available cardioactive glycosides, grouped according to their methods of administration, are listed in Table 31-1.

The digitalis glycosides increase myocardial contractility in both healthy and failing hearts. Consequently, there is significant improvement in cardiovascular performance and an associated decrease in the size of the ventricles. Although there is some increase in oxygen demand because of increased contractility, this is more than compensated for by the reduced oxygen demand that occurs as ventricular size is reduced. Therefore, in the failing heart, there is an overall increase in efficiency (work performed in relation to energy required).

The overall cardiodynamic effects of the digitalis agents are quite complex, being a combination of direct actions on the myocardium and indirect actions that alter the normal electrophysiologic properties of the heart (automaticity, conductivity, refractoriness). Moreover, the benefits of the digitalis drugs are significantly greater in the failing heart than in the healthy heart, a further indication that the drugs act to correct the hemodynamic imbalances associated with heart failure.

The direct action of the digitalis glycosides on the myocardium is largely responsible for the increased force of contraction (positive inotropic effect) noted with these drugs. Conversely, their effects on the heart's electrical properties play an essential role in their ability to alter the rate and rhythm of the heartbeat. This latter action is responsible for both the therapeutic effect of the drugs in managing certain supraventricular arrhythmias, and their toxic effects on the heart, namely the development of other types of arrhythmias. Table 31-2 provides a review of the major cardiovascular actions of the digitalis glycosides.

The progressive atrioventricular (AV) block seen with increasing dosage can lead to a major manifestation of digitalis toxicity—disturbances in cardiac rhythm. The arrhythmias that develop after administration of these drugs also are attributable to a shortened AV refractory period, suppression of normal pacemaker activity, and increased ventricular automaticity. Many factors can predispose the heart to digitalis toxicity, the most important being hypokalemia (reduced serum potassium levels), hypercalcemia (elevated serum calcium levels), catecholamine depletion, concurrent use of quinidine, systemic alkalosis, and renal or hepatic impairment. These drugs display a rather narrow safety margin, and signs of toxicity develop in between 10% and 20% of patients receiving them.

After administration, digitalis glycosides are distributed widely in the body, into both inactive reservoir (binding) sites and active receptor sites in the myocardium. Therefore, to achieve the desired effect at the active myocardial receptor sites, it is necessary to administer sufficient drug to saturate the reservoir of nonspecific binding sites. In *acute* congestive failure, large loading doses of drug may be administered rapidly to achieve the desired effect quickly. This process, termed *digitalization*, carries the risk of serious toxicity if the loading dose is excessive. Therefore, in less acute conditions, the patient should be loaded (digitalized) more slowly to reduce the risk of potential toxicity. Such slow loading often can be effectively accomplished simply by administering the small recommended maintenance doses from the beginning of therapy.

The *maintenance* dose is the amount of drug sufficient to replace the amount of drug eliminated between dosings, and thereby maintain a steady-state plasma level of the drug. Maintenance doses therefore are smaller than rapid loading doses and must be individually adjusted according to the patient's condition and the type of digitalis preparation used (long or short acting). Periodic clinical assessment is necessary to ensure that the optimal maintenance dose of the cardiac glycoside is being used and that adverse reactions are kept at a minimum. Because there is a substantial difference between the digitalizing and

Table 31-1. **Characteristics of Digitalis Glycosides**

	Onset		*Peak Effect*		*Plasma Half-Life*	*Extent of GI Absorption*	*Protein Binding*
	IV	*PO*	*IV*	*PO*			
Oral/Parenteral							
Digoxin	5–30 min	1–2 h	2–4 h	2–6 h	30–40 h	60%–90%	20%–30%
Oral							
Digitoxin		1–4 h		6–12 h	5–7 d	90%–98%	90%–100%

maintenance doses of some agents, both dosage ranges are given for each drug throughout this chapter.

The digitalis glycosides are reviewed as a group because they have similar pharmacologic properties; characteristics of individual drugs are given in Table 31-3.

- **Digoxin**
- **Digitoxin**

Mechanism

Inhibit sodium–potassium (Na^+–K^+) membrane adenosine triphosphatase (ATPase), the enzyme responsible for breakdown of ATP to supply energy for the cellular Na^+–K^+ pump; therefore, electrical properties of the myocardium are altered, and intracellular sodium and extracellular potassium concentrations are elevated; subsequently, calcium exchange occurs across the sarcolemmal membrane and additional calcium is liberated from binding sites on the sarcoplasmic reticulum; elevated free intracellular calcium levels facilitate the interaction of actin and myosin by removing the inhibitory effect of the troponin–tropomyosin complex; therefore, cardiac contraction is enhanced and cardiac output is increased. Heart rate is slowed by both vagal and extravagal mechanisms. Vagally, the drugs stimulate medullary vagal nuclei and increase sensitivity of pacemaker cells to the action of acetylcholine; extravagally, the drugs decrease AV conduction and increase the AV refractory period. Diuretic effect is primarily caused by increases in renal blood flow and glomerular filtration rate secondary to higher cardiac output, but also may involve a reduction in aldosterone release and possibly direct interference with sodium reabsorption in renal tubules.

Table 31-2. **Cardiovascular Actions: Digitalis Glycosides**

Excitability of myocardium
  Small doses 0 (↑)
  Large doses ↓
Conduction velocity
  AV conduction system ↓ (dose-dependent)
  Cardiac muscle 0 (↑)
Refractory period
  AV conduction system ↑ (dose-dependent)
  Cardiac muscle ↓
Heart rate ↓
Force of contraction ↑
Cardiac output ↑
Blood pressure
  Venous ↓
  Systolic slight ↑
  Diastolic slight ↓
ECG
  P–R interval prolonged
  Q–T interval shortened
  S–T segment depressed
  T wave decreased *or* inverted
Diuretic action
  Renal blood flow and glomerular filtration ↑
  Aldosterone release ↓
  (deactivation of renin–angiotensin mechanism)
  Sodium reabsorption in renal tubules ↓

0, no effect; ↑, increased or prolonged; ↓, decreased or shortened; AV, atrioventricular; ECG, electrocardiogram.

Uses

Treatment of congestive heart failure, especially low-output failure associated with depressed left ventricular function.
NOTE: Drugs are of little value in "high-output" congestive heart failure or in patients with mitral stenosis and normal sinus rhythm.
Treatment of certain cardiac arrhythmias, including atrial fibrillation, atrial flutter, and paroxysmal atrial tachycardia, in which ventricular rate is elevated
Treatment of cardiogenic shock accompanied by pulmonary edema

Dosage

See Table 31-3.

Fate

Different rates of absorption, onset of action, and duration of effect are observed between the two digitalis glycosides (see Table 31-1). Digitoxin is highly lipid soluble and extensively absorbed orally. Digoxin is somewhat less well absorbed (60%–90%). The digitalis glycosides are widely distributed in peripheral tissues; preparations are bound to different degrees by plasma proteins (see Table 31-1) and are excreted through the kidneys, either as unchanged drug (eg, digoxin,) or as hepatic metabolites (eg, digitoxin).

Common Side Effects

Anorexia, nausea, slow or irregular pulse, altered color perception (yellow or green vision).

Significant Adverse Reactions

More common at large doses.

GI: vomiting, diarrhea, abdominal pain
CNS: weakness, lethargy, disorientation, headache, confu-

Table 31-3. Cardioactive Glycosides

Drug	Usual Dosage Range: Digitalizing	Usual Dosage Range: Maintenance	Nursing Considerations
Digitoxin *Crystodigin*	*Rapid:* 0.6 mg initially, followed by 0.4 mg, then 0.2 mg at intervals of 4–6 h *Slow:* 0.2 mg twice a day for 4 days *Children* <1 y: 0.045 mg/kg 1–2 y: 0.04 mg/kg 2–12 y: 0.03 mg/kg	*Adults:* 0.05–0.3 mg/day (usual—0.1 mg/day) Children: one tenth of digitalizing dose	Long-acting, potent glycoside mainly used for maintenance rather than digitalizing therapy; slow onset and extremely long half-life makes digitalization difficult; danger of accumulation toxicity is high with this drug; do *not* give full digitalizing doses to patients receiving other digitalis glycosides within the preceding 3 wk
Digoxin *Lanoxin, Lanoxicaps (CAN) Novodigoxin*	**Oral** *Adults* Rapid: 0.5–0.75 mg initially, followed by 0.25–0.5 mg every 6–8 h to a total of 1–1.5 mg Slow: 0.125–0.25 mg daily for 7 days *Children* Newborn: 25–35 μg/kg 1 mo–2 y: 35–60 μg/kg 2–5 y: 30–40 μg/kg 5–10 y: 20–35 μg/kg >10 y: 10–15 μg/kg **IV** *Adults:* 0.25–0.5 mg initially, then 0.25 mg every 4–6 h to a total of 1 mg *Children* Newborn: 20–30 μg/kg 1–24 m: 30–50 μg/kg 2–5 y: 25–35 μg/kg 5–10 y: 15–30 μg/kg >10 y: 8–12 μg/kg	**Oral/IV** *Adults:* 0.125–0.5 mg/ day (average 0.25 mg/ day) *Children:* 20%–30% of the total digitalizing dose daily	Widely used for both rapid digitalization and maintenance therapy; little danger of accumulation because drug is rapidly excreted; capsules have greater bioavailability than tablets; therefore 0.2-mg capsule is equivalent to 0.25-mg tablet and 0.1-mg capsule is equivalent to 0.125-mg tablet; drug can be given IM but absorption is erratic; administration with food slows rate of absorption but does not affect the total amount absorbed; closely monitor patients with renal insufficiency because drug is primarily excreted unchanged through the kidney; dosage may need to be decreased in patients receiving quinidine (see Interactions)

sion, depression, paresthesias, amblyopia, diplopia, visual disturbances (eg, flashes, halos, white dots, "snowflakes"), neuralgia-like pain, delirium

Cardiac: arrhythmias (all types are possible); most common are ventricular premature beats and paroxysmal atrial tachycardia

Other: thromboembolism, pruritus, urticaria, fever, facial edema, joint pain, gynecomastia

Contraindications

Ventricular tachycardia or fibrillation, severe myocarditis. *Cautious use* in patients with Adams-Stokes syndrome, acute myocardial infarction, severe pulmonary disease, advanced heart failure, myxedema, incomplete AV block, chronic constrictive pericarditis, or hypertrophic subaortic stenosis; also in the presence of hypoxia, hypomagnesemia, hypokalemia, hypercalcemia, renal or hepatic insufficiency, and in elderly, debilitated, pregnant, or nursing patients.

Interactions

Absorption of digitalis drugs may be reduced by antacids, cholestyramine resin, colestipol, laxatives, metoclopramide, neomycin, and possibly other oral aminoglycosides.

Effects of digitoxin can be reduced by agents that increase their metabolism, such as anticonvulsants, barbiturates, and rifampin.

Toxic effects of cardiac glycosides (especially arrhythmias) may be increased by adrenergics, amphotericin, calcium salts, corticosteroids, diuretics (except potassium-sparing drugs), glucose, insulin, magnesium, reserpine, succinylcholine, thyroid preparations, and nondepolarizing muscle relaxants.

Marked bradycardia may develop if digitalis drugs are given in combination with carbamazepine, guanethidine, phenytoin, beta-blockers, and reserpine.

Amiodarone, quinidine, nifedipine, verapamil, bepridil, diltiazem, and propafenone can increase serum levels of digoxin, possibly by displacement from tissue-binding sites or reduced renal clearance.

Increased plasma levels of digitalis drugs can result from combined use with spironolactone or anticholinergics.

Nursing Management

Pretherapy Assessment

Assess and record baseline data necessary for detection of adverse effects of digitalis: General: vital signs (VS), body weight, skin color and temperature; CNS: orientation, affect, reflexes, vision; Cardiovascular system (CVS): baseline electrocardiogram (ECG), peripheral pulses and perfusion, edema; GI: normal output, bowel sounds, liver evaluation; Laboratory: liver function, urinalysis, serum electrolytes.

Review medical history and documents for existing or previous conditions that:

a. require cautious use of digitalis drugs: Adams-Stokes syndrome; acute myocardial infarction; severe pulmonary disease; advanced heart failure; myxedema; incomplete AV block; chronic constrictive pericarditis; hypertrophic subaortic stenosis; hypoxia; hypomagnesemia; hypokalemia; hypercalcemia; renal or hepatic insufficiency; in the elderly or debilitated.

b. contraindicate use of digitalis drugs: allergy to digitalis preparations; ventricular tachycardia; myocarditis; **pregnancy (Category C)**; lactation (effects not known, use with caution in nursing mothers).

Nursing Interventions

Medication Administration

Check dosage and preparation carefully.

Avoid administering oral dosage form with food.

Ensure that baseline data (ie, clinical symptoms, serum electrolytes, vital signs) have been obtained before initiating administration.

Expect to give drug parenterally only when oral administration is not feasible (eg, need for *rapid* digitalization, severe vomiting, unconsciousness).

Take apical pulse for 1 minute immediately before giving drug. Determine pulse deficit (apical minus radial pulse) in patient with atrial fibrillation. Check with practitioner to determine limits (both high and low) for withholding drug.

The practitioner should be notified immediately if nausea and vomiting develop while the patient is receiving digitalis glycosides, because they may indicate onset of digitalis toxicity.

Surveillance During Therapy

Closely monitor patient for early symptoms of impending toxicity (weakness, nausea, vomiting, diarrhea, blurred vision, diplopia, halo vision, dizziness, precordial pain, palpitations, anxiety, and facial pain) because the margin between the therapeutic and toxic doses of cardiac glycosides is extremely narrow. Many symptoms of digitalis intoxication are, however, the same as those associated with conditions for which digitalis is used (eg, nausea and vomiting due to heart failure, arrhythmias). Careful determination of cause (ie, disease versus digitalis overdose) is essential to proper management.

Monitor for early indications of potassium deficiency (eg, drowsiness, paresthesias, muscle weakness, anorexia, depressed reflexes, orthostatic hypotension, polyuria), especially if patient is receiving potassium-wasting diuretics, because hypokalemia greatly increases the incidence of digitalis toxicity. Potassium supplementation (KCl liquid, orange juice, bananas) should be considered.

Monitor for changes in pulse rate (eg, sudden increase above 120 when rate has been slowing or a fall below 60/minute) or rhythm, possible signs of overdosage. Ventricular arrhythmias may occur even when other signs of digitalis toxicity are absent, especially in the patient with advanced heart failure, severe pulmonary disease, rheumatic carditis, or Wolff-Parkinson-White syndrome.

Carefully assess for presence of atrial arrhythmias if the patient is a child. Atrial arrhythmias are often the most reliable indication of developing toxicity because nausea, vomiting, and neurologic and visual disturbances rarely occur in children. Premature, immature, and newborn infants arc particularly sensitive to digitalis drugs and should be digitalized very cautiously. Arrhythmias also occur very frequently in children with rheumatic carditis.

Carefully monitor laboratory studies and patient for indications of adverse reactions.

Monitor intake–output and body weight, and check for edema. Dosage adjustments may be necessary to improve renal function if fluid retention occurs.

Monitor results of renal and liver function tests and ECG and serum electrolyte determinations, which should be performed periodically.

Interpret results of diagnostic tests and contact practitioner as appropriate.

Monitor for possible drug–drug and drug–nutrient interactions; see Interactions.

Patient Teaching

Emphasize importance of adhering to prescribed dosage regimen and recommended diet to obtain maximal benefit with minimal toxicity.

Instruct patient not to take an "extra" dose of medication to compensate for a missed dose. The possibility of toxicity is increased if doses are taken too close together because of the danger of accumulation.

Teach patient how to monitor pulse rate, urinary output, and weight to determine if therapy is appropriate.

Instruct patient to report untoward reactions immediately because toxicity can develop rapidly.

Instruct patient to notify practitioner at once if protracted diarrhea or vomiting occur because these conditions can alter electrolyte balance and possibly lead to toxicity.

Advise patient to avoid using over-the-counter drugs high in sodium (eg, Alka Seltzer, Bromo Seltzer, Bisodol).

Refer patient to dietitian for instruction regarding reduction of overall salt intake. High-salt foods as well as addition of table salt to foods generally should be avoided.

Refer to appropriate resource for assistance with a weight reduction program to lessen demands on cardiovascular system if the patient is overweight.

Inform patient that consumption of large quantities of licorice, which contains glycyrrhizic acid, may cause salt and water retention, hypokalemia, and other symptoms of congestive heart failure.

Digoxin Antidote

• Digoxin Immune Fab–Ovine

Digibind

Digoxin immune Fab consists of antigen-binding fragments (Fab) derived from antidigoxin antibodies produced in immunized sheep. The antibodies are papain digested, and digoxin-specific Fab fragments are then isolated and purified. The preparation contains 40 mg/vial of lyophilized powder for reconstitution. Each vial binds approximately 0.6 mg of digoxin (or digitoxin).

Digoxin immune Fab is used to treat potentially life-threatening digoxin (or digitoxin) intoxication. In most instances, amelioration of signs and symptoms of intoxication is noted within 1 hour. The drug is administered intravenously (IV) over 30 minutes, but may be given as a bolus injection if cardiac arrest is imminent. Dosage guidelines are provided with the drug packaging and differ according to the amount of digoxin (or digitoxin) to be neutralized. If this value is not readily obtainable, administration of 20 vials (800 mg) is usually adequate to treat most life-threatening intoxications in adults and children. Larger doses have a more rapid onset of action than smaller doses but are associated with a greater likelihood of febrile or allergic reactions. Hypokalemia also may occur, and withdrawal from the effects of digoxin may result in reduced cardiac output and worsening of congestive heart failure.

Positive Inotropic Agents

The positive inotropic agents amrinone and milrinone are structurally and mechanistically unlike the digitalis glycosides. Amrinone and its close structural analogue milrinone increase myocardial contractility and exert a peripheral vasodilatory action. They can provide additional symptomatic relief of congestive heart failure in patients whose condition is not satisfactorily controlled by conventional therapy (ie, digitalis drugs, diuretics, vasodilators). The drugs are administered IV only in an acute setting; prolonged use of amrinone increases the likelihood of thrombocytopenia and should be avoided.

- ***Amrinone***

  Inocor

- ***Milrinone***

  Primacor

Mechanism

Appear to inhibit myocardial cell phosphodiesterase III (the enzyme responsible for inactivating cyclic AMP), thus increasing cellular levels of cyclic AMP, which facilitates the contractions of myocardial muscle cells; also exhibit a relaxant effect on vascular smooth muscle, thereby reducing both preload and afterload (see review of cardiac physiology in Chapter 30); drugs are *not* beta-adrenergic agonists, nor do they inhibit the activity of Na^+–K^+ ATPase, as do the digitalis glycosides; increased inward calcium flux during the action potential also has been postulated as a contributory mechanism; effects noted after administration include enhanced myocardial contractility *even after full doses of digitalis*, increased cardiac output, reduced ventricular filling pressure and pulmonary capillary wedge pressure, increased left ventricular ejection fraction, and improved exercise capacity; there is little change in heart rate or arterial pressure.

Uses

Short-term management of congestive heart failure in patients who have not responded adequately to digitalis drugs, diuretics, and vasodilators.

Dosage

Amrinone: Initially, 0.75 mg/kg by IV bolus over 2 to 3 minutes, followed by a maintenance infusion of 5 to 10 μg/kg/min to a total daily dose of 10 mg/kg (including bolus); an additional bolus injection may be given 30 minutes after the initial bolus, if needed

Milrinone: Initially, 50 μg/kg over 10 minutes, followed by a maintenance infusion of 0.375 to 0.75 μg/kg/min; dosage must be adjusted for impaired renal function

Fate

Amrinone: Peak effect occurs within 10 minutes; duration of action is dose dependent (range, 30 min–2 h); protein binding is variable (10%–50%); metabolized in the liver; elimination half-life is 3 to 4 hours, although it can range from 3 to 15 hours depending on status of heart function.

Milrinone: Peak effect occurs within 5 to 15 minutes; 83% eliminated unchanged in the urine, elimination half-life is 2.4 hours.

Significant Adverse Reactions

Amrinone: Arrhythmias (3%) and thrombocytopenia (2.5%) can occur, especially with prolonged therapy; other adverse effects associated with amrinone therapy are nausea, vomiting, anorexia, abdominal pain, hepatotoxicity, hypotension, fever, chest pain, burning at injection site; asymptomatic platelet count reductions (less than 150,000/mm^3) may be noted and are usually reversed within 1 week of dosage reduction.

Milrinone: Ventricular arrhythmias (12%); other adverse effects associated with milrinone therapy are hypotension, angina/chest pain, headache, hypokalemia, tremor, and thrombocytopenia (0.4%).

Contraindications

No absolute contraindications. *Cautious use* in patients with aortic or pulmonic valvular disease, hypertrophic subaortic stenosis, arrhythmias, thrombocytopenia, hypotension, and after an acute myocardial infarction or vigorous diuretic therapy. Safety for use in pregnant or nursing women and in children has not been established.

CAUTION

If liver enzymes are elevated or platelet count is reduced *together* with clinical symptoms, amrinone should be discontinued. If these changes occur in the *absence* of clinical symptoms, consider the benefit-to-risk ratio in deciding whether to discontinue therapy.

Interactions

Additive hypotensive effects may occur with concurrent use of disopyramide and amrinone.

Nursing Management

Pretherapy Assessment

Assess and record baseline data necessary for detection of adverse effects of amrinone/milrinone: General: VS, body weight, skin color and temperature; CNS: orientation; CVS: peripheral pulses and perfusion, edema; GI: normal output, bowel sounds, liver evaluation; Laboratory: liver function, urinalysis, serum electrolytes, platelet count.

Review medical history and documents for existing or previous conditions that:

a. require cautious use of amrinone/milrinone: valvular disease; idiopathic hypertrophic subaortic stenosis; arrhythmias; thrombocytopenia; hypotension; acute myocardial infarction.

b. contraindicate use of amrinone/milrinone: allergy to amrinone, bisulfite; **pregnancy (Category C)**; lactation (effects not known, use with caution in nursing mothers).

Nursing Interventions

Medication Administration

Protect drug from light.

Provide access to bathroom facilities.

Dilute with normal saline because drug is extremely irritating if given as a bolus in a peripheral IV. Irritation is not a problem with a central line.

Do not dilute drug with solutions containing dextrose because a chemical interaction occurs with prolonged contact.

Do not administer through an IV line with other drugs because physical incompatibilities are highly likely.

There is an immediate chemical interaction causing precipitation when furosemide is injected into an infusion of milrinone.

Surveillance During Therapy

Assess patient for evidence of unusual bleeding, such as petechiae, purpura, hematuria, or melena.

Monitor results of platelet counts, which should be obtained regularly. Levels below 150,000/mm^3 represent thrombocytopenia.

Assess patient for signs and symptoms of hepatotoxicity.

Monitor results of liver enzyme determinations, which should be performed periodically.

Check results of ECGs, which should be performed periodically to detect arrhythmias.

Carefully monitor laboratory studies and patient for indications of adverse reactions.

Interpret results of diagnostic tests and contact practitioner as appropriate.

Assess patient for presence of GI symptoms (eg, anorexia, nausea, vomiting, abdominal pain). Symptoms can be ameliorated by reducing drug dosage.

Carefully monitor fluid and electrolyte changes and renal function.

Monitor potassium levels and correct hypokalemia as necessary.

Monitor for possible drug–drug and drug–nutrient interactions; see Interactions.

Patient Teaching

Teach patient the reason for frequent blood pressure and pulse monitoring.

Teach the patient to report any of the following: dizziness; weakness or fatigue; numbness or tingling.

Selected Bibliography

DeBono D: Digoxin in eurhythmic heart failure: Proved or "not proven"? Lancet 343:128, 1994

Feldman AM: Can we alter survival in patients with congestive heart failure. JAMA 267:1956, 1992

Honerjayer P, Nawrath H: Pharmacology of bipyridine phosphodiesterase III inhibitors. Eur J Anaesthesiol 5(Suppl):7, 1992

Kelly RA, Smith TW: Digoxin in heart failure: Implications of recent trials. J Am Coll Cardiol 22(4 Suppl A):107A, 1993

Leier CV: Current status of non-digitalis positive inotropic drugs. Am J Cardiol 69:120G, 1992

Om A, Hess ML: Inotropic therapy of the failing myocardium. Clin Cardiol 16:5, 1993

Packer M: The development of positive inotropic agents for chronic heart failure: How have we gone astray? J Am Coll Cardiol 22(4 Suppl A):119A, 1993

Packer M, Gheorghiade M, Young JB: Withdrawal of digoxin from patients with chronic heart failure treated with angiotensin-converting-enzyme inhibitors. N Engl J Med 329:1, 1993

Powers ER, Bergin JD: Recent advances in evaluating and managing congestive heart failure. Modern Medicine 60:54, 1992

Weintraub NL, Chaitman BR: Newer concepts in the medical management of patients with congestive heart failure. Clin Cardiol 16:380, 1993

Nursing Bibliography

Brown K: Boosting the failing heart with inotropic drugs. Nursing '93 23(4):34, 1993

Cross J: Pharmacologic management of heart failure: Positive inotropic agents. Critical Care Nursing Clinics of North America 5:589, 1993

Lasater M: Combining vasoactive infusions for maximal cardiac performance in the postoperative period. Critical Care Nursing Quarterly 16(2):11, 1993

Meissner J, Gever L: Reducing the risks of digitalis toxicity. Nursing '93 23(7):46, 1993

Moser D: Pharmacologic management of heart failure: Neurohormonal agents. Critical Care Nursing Clinics of North America 5:599, 1993

Murphy T: Digoxin toxicity: Ventricular dysrhythmias to watch for. Am J Nurs 12(1):37, 1994

Walthall S, Odtohan B, McCoy M, Fromm B, Frankovich D, Lehmann M: Routine withholding of digitalis for heart rate less than 60 BPM: Widespread nursing misconceptions. Heart Lung 22:472, 1993

Whalen D, Izzi G: Pharmacologic treatment of acute congestive heart failure resulting from left ventricular systolic or diastolic dysfunction. Critical Care Nursing Clinics of North America 5:261, 1993

32

Antiarrhythmic Drugs

Quinidine
Procainamide
Disopyramide
Moricizine
Lidocaine
Tocainide
Phenytoin
Mexiletine
Flecainide
Encainide
Propafenone
Propranolol
Acebutolol
Esmolol
Bretylium
Amiodarone
Sotalol
Verapamil
Diltiazem
Adenosine

Cardiac arrhythmias can be regarded as any deviation from the normal rate and rhythm of contractions of the heart. Depending on the type of arrhythmia present, a number of hemodynamic complications can ensue, cardiac output may be reduced, and serious rhythm alterations may be lethal.

The conductile system of the heart is discussed in detail in Chapter 30 and outlined schematically in Figure 30-2. Deviations from the orderly propagation and conduction of impulses through this cardiac conductile system result in a decrement in cardiac function and reduced flow of oxygenated blood to the body organs. Irregularities in rate and rhythm of the heart markedly impair its ability to function and are a cause of eventual development of cardiac failure.

Cardiac arrhythmias arise from electrophysiologic disturbances of cardiac function. The two principal alterations are:

Disorders of impulse formation: impulses arise in areas of the heart other than the normal sinoatrial (SA) node; these are often termed *ectopic beats*.

Disorders of impulse conduction: impulses spread throughout the heart by abnormal pathways; examples include delayed atrioventricular (AV) conduction (AV block), bundle branch block, and reentry excitation, a complex phenomenon in which impulses reenter an area of the myocardium from a direction opposite to normal flow, reactivating the fibers.

Although certainly serious, *atrial arrhythmias* usually are not life threatening if normal ventricular function is maintained. Conversely, disturbances in *ventricular* rhythm of even a few minutes' duration can be fatal, and therefore require immediate and vigorous therapy. The purposes of antiarrhythmic drug treatment, therefore, are twofold: to restore normal cardiac rhythm, and to prevent recurrence or extension of an existing arrhythmia.

Although the electrophysiologic properties of antiarrhythmic drugs are quite complex, attempts have been made to classify these drugs based on their primary mechanisms of action. Table 32-1 outlines the different groups of antiarrhythmic drugs categorized according to their principal actions on the heart. Drugs within a particular group (eg, group IA) generally share similar electrophysiologic effects but can differ significantly in other respects, such as oral versus parenteral availability and frequency and type of side effects.

Selection of an appropriate antiarrhythmic agent depends on the type of arrhythmia present as well as the characteristics of the drugs themselves—their onset, duration, type, and incidence of side effects, in addition to other factors. The major pharmacokinetic properties as well as the electrophysiologic effects of the principal antiarrhythmic drugs are listed in Table 32-2.

Drugs used in treating arrhythmias alter the heart's basic electrical properties, including excitability, conduction velocity, refractory period, and automaticity. These, then, are potentially dangerous drugs. Because not all arrhythmias require drug therapy, careful diagnosis of the type of disordered rhythm present is essential for effective and safe management of these conditions. Because the overall pharmacology and toxicology vary to a significant degree among the different drugs, they are discussed individually in this chapter.

Group IA Drugs

• Quinidine

Cardioquin, Cin-Quin, Duraquin, Quinaglute Dura-Tabs, Quinatime, Quinidex Extentabs, Quinora, Quin-Release

(CAN) Apo-Quinidine, Biquin Durules, Novoquinidin, Quinate

Mechanism

Complexes with lipoproteins in myocardial cell membrane, thereby decreasing sodium influx during depolarization and potassium efflux during repolarization; depresses cardiac excitability (elevates firing threshold to screen out weak ectopic impulses), slows conduction velocity, and prolongs effective refractory period of the myocardium; slows phase 0 (depolarization) and prolongs phase 4 (diastolic depolarization) of the ventricular action potential; exerts anticholinergic action (decreases vagal tone and prevents cardiac slowing due to vagal activation).

Uses

Treatment of the following arrhythmias:
- Paroxysmal supraventricular tachycardia
- Atrial flutter and fibrillation (after digoxin to prevent excessive rise in ventricular rate)
- Premature atrial and ventricular contractions
- Paroxysmal AV junctional rhythm
- Paroxysmal ventricular tachycardia not associated with complete heart block

Maintenance therapy after electrical conversion of atrial flutter or fibrillation

Dosage

Oral

Usual: 10 to 20 mg/kg/day in 4 to 6 divided doses (200–300 mg 4 times/day) individually adjusted to patient's response

Table 32-1. **Classification of Antiarrhythmic Drugs**

Group	Drugs	Principal Cardiac Actions	Major Indications
IA	Quinidine Procainamide Disopyramide Moricizine*	Slow conduction velocity Prolong myocardial refractory period Prolong action potential duration	Prophylaxis of atrial fibrillation Premature atrial contractions Premature ventricular contractions Ventricular tachycardia
IB	Lidocaine Tocainide Phenytoin† Mexiletine	Enhance conduction Shorten repolarization	Premature ventricular contractions Ventricular tachycardia Digitalis-induced arrhythmias
IC	Flecainide Encainide Propafenone	Decrease conduction (especially His–Purkinje) Prolong ventricular refractory period	Life-threatening ventricular arrhythmias
II	Propranolol Acebutolol Esmolol	Slow AV conduction Prolong AV nodal refractory period Decrease automaticity of SA node	Atrial tachycardia or flutter Supraventricular tachycardia Exercise-induced arrhythmias
III	Bretylium Amiodarone Sotalol	Prolong refractory period Increase action potential duration	Life-threatening ventricular arrhythmias (not responding to other treatment)
IV	Verapamil Diltiazem	Prolong AV nodal refractory period Decrease sinus node automaticity	Supraventricular tachyarrhythmias Control of rapid ventricular rate in atrial fibrillation
—	Adenosine	Decrease automaticity of SA node Decrease AV conduction velocity Prolong AV refractory period	Supraventricular tachyarrhythmias

* Moricizine exhibits properties of group IA, IB, and IC drugs.
† Phenytoin is *not* approved for treatment of arrhythmias but is used for digitalis-induced arrhythmias.

Paroxysmal supraventricular tachycardia: 400 to 600 mg every 2 to 3 hours until paroxysm is terminated
Premature atrial and ventricular contractions: 200 to 300 mg 3 to 4 times/day
Atrial fibrillation: 200 mg every 2 to 3 hours for 5 to 8 doses; increase gradually until sinus rhythm is restored (maximal daily dose is 3–4 g)
Maintenance: 200 to 300 mg 3 to 4 times/day (sustained-release forms: 1–2 tablets 2–3 times/day)
Intramuscular (IM; rarely used): 600 mg gluconate salt initially, then 400 mg every 2 hours as needed
Intravenous (IV; rarely used): 200 to 750 mg gluconate salt or equivalent by slow IV infusion of a dilute (800 mg gluconate/50 mL 5% glucose) solution at a rate of 1 mL (16 mg) per minute

NOTE: Use prolonged-acting forms of quinidine (ie, Quinaglute Dura-Tabs, Quinidex Extentabs) for maintenance therapy only. Make appropriate dosage adjustments when changing preparations (Quinaglute Dura-Tabs are 62% base; quinidine sulfate is 82% base).

Fate

Completely absorbed orally; maximum effects occur in 1 to 3 hours, and action persists for at least 6 to 8 hours (8–12 h with sustained-release forms); widely distributed in the body and significantly bound (70%–90%) to plasma proteins; metabolized in the liver and excreted through the kidneys both as metabolites (80%) and unchanged drug (20%); elimination half-life is 6 hours.

Common Side Effects

Nausea, diarrhea, abdominal distress; large doses can result in *cinchonism*, characterized by headache, tinnitus, dizziness, blurred vision, and mild tremor.

Significant Adverse Reactions

GI: vomiting, cramping
CNS: fever, vertigo, impaired hearing, altered color perception, photophobia, diplopia, scotomas, excitement, confusion, delirium, syncope
CV: ventricular ectopic beats, cardiac asystole, hypotension, severe bradycardia, atrial or ventricular flutter and fibrillation, arterial embolism
Hematologic–dermatologic: acute hemolytic anemia, thrombocytopenic purpura, leukopenia, agranulocytosis (rare), flushing, urticaria, angioedema, pruritus, sweating
Other: arthralgia, dyspnea, respiratory depression, asthmatic episodes
IV use: sweating, nervousness, vomiting, cramping, urge to urinate or defecate

Contraindications

AV conduction defects or complete AV block, ectopic impulses and rhythms due to escape mechanisms, thrombocytopenic purpura, acute rheumatic fever, myasthenia gravis, cardiac enlargement due to congestive heart failure, renal dysfunction with azotemia. *Cautious use* in the presence of incomplete heart block, digitalis intoxication, congestive heart failure, hy-

Table 32-2. **Pharmacokinetic and Electrophysiologic Properties of Antiarrhythmic Drugs**

	Pharmacokinetics				Electrophysiology							
					Automaticity		Conduction Velocity		Refractory Period			Heart Rate
Drugs	Onset (min)	Duration (h)	Plasma Half-life (h)	Protein Binding (%)	SA Node	Ectopic Pacemakers	AV Node	Purkinje Fibers	AV	Purkinje	Ventricle	
Quinidine	30	6–10	6–7	70–90	↑ ↓	↓	↑ ↓	↓	↑	↑	↑	↑ ↓
Procainamide	30	3–5	3–5	15–25	↑ ↓	↓	↑ ↓	↓	↑	↑	↑	↑ ↓
Disopyramide	30	5–7	4–8	30–60	↑ ↓	↓	↑	↓	↑	↑	↑	↑ ↓
Lidocaine	1–3*	0.2	1–2	40–80	0	↓	↑	↑	↑ ↓	↑ ↓	↑ ↓	0
Phenytoin	30–60	24	24–36	90–95	↑ ↓	↓	↑	↑	↑ ↓	↑ ↓	↑ ↓	↑ ↓
Tocainide	30–60	4–8	10–15	10–20	↑ ↓	↓	0	0	↓	↑ ↓	↓	0
Mexiletine	30–60	4–8	10–12	50–60	↓	↓	0	0	↑ ↓	↑	↑	—
Flecainide	30–60	8–12	12–24	40–50	↓	↓	↓	↓	0	↑	↑	0
Encainide	30–60	8–12	1–2	75–85	↑ ↓	↓	↓	↓	↑	↑	↑	0
Propafenone	30–60	8	2–10	97	0	↓	↓	↓	↑	↑	↑	0
Moricizine	120	10–24	2–4	95	0	↓	↓	↓	0	0	0–↑	0–↑
Propranolol	30	3–6	2–4	90–95	↓	↓	↓	↓	↑	0	0	↑
Acebutolol	30	12–16	3–4	25–30	↓	↓	↓	↓	↑	0	0	↓
Esmolol	1–2	0.1	0.2	55	↓	↓	↓	0	↑	0	0	↓
Bretylium	1–3*	6–8	6–10	10	↑	↑	0	↑	↑ ↓	↑	↑	0
Amiodarone	†	†	1–4 days	95	↓	↓	↓	↓	↑	↑	↑	—
Sotalol		8–12	12	0	↓	↓	↓	0	↑	↑ ↑	↑ ↑	↓
Verapamil	30	6–8	4–8	90	↓	↓	↓	0	↑	0	0	↓
Diltiazem	5	1–3	5	70	0–↓	↓	↓	↓	↑	0	0	↓
Adenosine	0.5	0.01	—	—	↓	↓	↓	0	↑	0	0	↑

* Onset reflects time after IV administration.
† Onset may take several weeks and effects persist from weeks to months, even after drug is discontinued.
↑, increase; ↓, decrease; 0, no significant effect; ↑ ↓, variable effect.

potension, respiratory disorders, potassium imbalance (eg, diuretic therapy), and impaired renal or hepatic function.

Interactions

Quinidine may increase the effects of oral anticoagulants, antihypertensives, neuromuscular blocking agents, anticholinergics, digitalis, and other antiarrhythmics.

Blood levels of quinidine can be elevated by substances that alkalinize the urine (eg, sodium bicarbonate, antacids, carbonic anhydrase inhibitors), thereby retarding quinidine excretion.

Effects of cholinergic drugs (eg, neostigmine, edrophonium) may be antagonized by quinidine.

Additive cardiac-depressant effects may occur with use of propranolol or phenothiazines with quinidine.

Administration of phenytoin, rifampin, or barbiturates may reduce the serum half-life of quinidine because of enzyme induction.

Quinidine may elevate blood levels of digoxin by reducing its tissue binding or by retarding its renal clearance.

Cimetidine may enhance the effects of quinidine by slowing its hepatic metabolism.

Concurrent use of nifedipine and quinidine may result in lowered plasma levels of quinidine.

Nursing Management

Pretherapy Assessment

Assess and record baseline data necessary for detection of adverse effects of quinidine: General: vital signs (VS), body weight, skin color and temperature; CNS: cranial nerves, reflexes, orientation, bilateral grip strength; Cardiovascular system (CVS): peripheral pulses and perfusion, edema; GI: normal output, bowel sounds, liver evaluation; Laboratory: liver function, urinalysis, complete blood count (CBC).

Review medical history and documents for existing or previous conditions that:

a. require cautious use of quinidine: incomplete heart block; digitalis intoxication; congestive heart failure; hypotension; respiratory disorders; potassium imbalance; impaired renal or hepatic function.
b. contraindicate use of quinidine: allergy or idiosyncrasy to quinidine or quinine; AV conduction defects or block; thrombocytopenia; acute rheumat-

ic fever; myasthenia gravis; renal dysfunction with azotemia; **pregnancy (Category C)**; lactation (secreted in breast milk; effects not known, use with caution in nursing mothers).

Nursing Interventions

Medication Administration

Provide access to bathroom facilities.
Administer drug with food if GI upset occurs.
Keep patient supine during IV administration, and monitor blood pressure for development of severe hypotension. Monitor results of serum quinidine levels, which should be determined frequently to prevent the cardiac toxicity that often occurs at levels greater than 8 mg/L.
Ensure that patients with atrial flutter or fibrillation have been pretreated with digoxin before administering quinidine to slow AV conduction, reducing the danger of ventricular tachycardia resulting from a progressive reduction in the degree of AV block to a 1 : 1 ratio.
Monitor electrocardiogram (ECG), pulse rate and rhythm, and blood pressure during parenteral therapy. Have sodium lactate, vasopressors, and cardiopulmonary resuscitative equipment available.

Surveillance During Therapy

Assess patient for evidence of unusual bleeding, such as petechiae, purpura, hematuria, or melena.
Monitor results of platelet counts, which should be obtained regularly. Levels below 150,000/mm^3 represent thrombocytopenia.
Carefully monitor laboratory studies and patient for indications of adverse reactions.
Closely monitor patient receiving quinidine (especially parenterally or in large oral doses), and note evidence of developing cardiotoxicity (widening of QRS complex by more than 25%, ventricular extrasystoles, abolition of P waves). Advise practitioner immediately if signs of toxicity appear, because the drug should be discontinued.
Interpret results of diagnostic tests and contact practitioner as appropriate.
Monitor for possible drug–drug and drug–nutrient interactions; see Interactions.

Patient Teaching

Suggest taking drug with food to minimize GI distress.
Inform patient that diarrhea is common early in therapy but should disappear. Advise consulting practitioner if diarrhea persists because dosage adjustment may be required.
Instruct patient to be alert for signs of quinidine overdosage, collectively termed *cinchonism*. If tinnitus, impaired vision, dyspnea, palpitations, nausea, headache, or chest tightness appear, the practitioner should be informed, and the dosage should be reduced.
Instruct patient to report immediately feelings of dizziness or faintness, possible indications of ventricular arrhythmias and depressed cardiac output.
Encourage patient on prolonged therapy to obtain the periodic blood counts, serum electrolyte determinations, and liver and kidney function tests that should be performed.
Advise patient to use moderation in the consumption of caffeine or alcohol and in smoking, which can alter the irritability of the heart.
Instruct patient to avoid consumption of large amounts of citrus fruits because they can alkalinize the urine and reduce excretion of quinidine.

• Procainamide

Procan, Pronestyl, and other products

Mechanism

Essentially identical to quinidine in pharmacologic actions; decreases cardiac excitability (screening out weaker ectopic impulses), slows conduction in the atria, ventricles, and bundle of His, and prolongs the refractory period of the atria; little effect on contractility or cardiac output; may elicit tachycardia because of its anticholinergic (ie, vagal blocking) action; produces peripheral vasodilation (especially IV) and hypotension; large doses can result in progressive AV block and ventricular extrasystoles.

Uses

Treatment of premature ventricular contractions (PVCs), ventricular tachycardia, paroxysmal atrial tachycardia (PAT), and atrial fibrillation
Treatment of arrhythmias associated with surgery, general anesthesia, or myocardial infarction (IV administration)

Dosage

Oral: Less urgent arrhythmias: initially, 1-g loading dose, then 50 mg/kg/day in divided doses every 3 hours (every 6 h with sustained-release tablets)
IM: Initially, 50 mg/kg/day in divided doses every 3 to 6 hours; switch to oral therapy as soon as possible (for arrhythmias during anesthesia or surgery, 0.1–0.5 g IM). *Deep* IM injection is recommended
IV injection: 100 mg every 5 minutes by slow IV injection (25–50 mg/min) to a maximum of 500 mg; usual serum level is 4 to 8 μg/mL; continuous ECG monitoring must be performed
For *life-threatening arrhythmia*: 20 to 30 mg IV per minute until one of the following occurs:
Arrhythmia is suppressed
Hypotension occurs
QRS is greater than 50% of baseline
1000 mg has been given

If suppression of arrhythmia occurs, start a continuous infusion of 1 to 4 mg/min.

Therapeutic plasma levels are 3 to 10 μg/mL.

Fate

Well absorbed orally, except in patients with severely compromised cardiovascular function; onset is 30 minutes with oral use and duration is 3 to 4 hours (up to 6 h with sustained-release preparations); onset after IM or IV administration is rapid; maximum plasma levels in 15 to 30 minutes; minimal protein binding (15%–25%); slowly hydrolyzed by liver esterases, approximately one fourth converted to *N*-acetylprocainamide, an active metabolite with a 6-hour half-life; primarily (60%–70%) excreted by the kidneys, at least half as the unchanged drug; half-lives of procainamide and metabolites are prolonged in patients with congestive heart failure.

Common Side Effects

Anorexia, nausea (orally); hypotension (IV).

Significant Adverse Reactions

Orally: vomiting, diarrhea, urticaria, angioedema, maculopapular rash, weakness, depression, psychotic behavior, agranulocytosis, systemic lupus-like reaction (fever, rashes, muscle and joint pain, pericarditis, skin lesions seen with prolonged use), pleural effusion, hepatomegaly, hemolytic anemia, thrombocytopenia
IV: flushing, ventricular asystole, ventricular fibrillation, hypotension

Contraindications

Myasthenia gravis, second- or third-degree AV block, and hypersensitivity to local anesthetics (drug is a derivative of procaine). *Cautious use* in patients with liver or kidney disease because accumulation can occur; advise patient to report possible signs of renal dysfunction (eg, dysuria, oliguria).

Interactions

Procainamide may potentiate the muscle-relaxing action of neuromuscular blocking agents and those antibiotics (especially aminoglycosides) having a skeletal muscle-relaxant effect.
Additive effects on the heart may occur with combinations of procainamide and other antiarrhythmic or digitalis-like drugs.
Procainamide may increase the hypotensive effects of antihypertensives and diuretics.
Effects of procainamide can be potentiated by agents that alkalinize the urine and reduce urinary excretion, such as acetazolamide, sodium lactate, and sodium bicarbonate.
The action of cholinesterase inhibitors in treating myasthenia gravis can be antagonized by procainamide.
Cimetidine can reduce the renal clearance of procainamide and its metabolite.

Nursing Management

Pretherapy Assessment

Assess and record baseline data necessary for detection of adverse effects of procainamide: General: VS, body weight, skin color and temperature; CNS: reflexes, orientation, bilateral grip strength; CVS: peripheral pulses and perfusion, edema; GI: normal output, bowel sounds, liver evaluation; Laboratory: liver function, urinalysis, CBC.
Review medical history and documents for existing or previous conditions that:
a. require cautious use of procainamide: liver or kidney disease; renal dysfunction (eg, dysuria, oliguria).
b. contraindicate use of procainamide: allergy to procainamide, procaine or similar drugs; myasthenia gravis; second- or third-degree AV block; **pregnancy (Category C)**; lactation (secreted in breast milk; effects not known, use with caution in nursing mothers).

Nursing Interventions

Medication Administration

Provide access to bathroom facilities.
Administer drug with food if GI upset occurs.
Keep patient supine during IV infusion and monitor ECG and blood pressure continually. If blood pressure falls by more than 15 mm Hg or if ventricular rate slows significantly without development of regular AV conduction, infusion should be discontinued. Have pressor agent (eg, levarterenol or dopamine) available to combat extreme hypotension.
Be prepared to stop infusion when arrhythmia is terminated or if excessive widening of QRS complex or prolongation of PR interval occurs. Arrhythmias usually are abolished within minutes after IV infusion.
Be alert for sudden development of ventricular tachycardia when rapid atrial rate is slowed during drug infusion, in the treatment of atrial arrhythmias, allowing 1 : 1 AV conduction. Prior digitalization reduces this danger.
Observe carefully for signs of possible lupus-like reaction (eg, fever, arthralgia, skin lesions, pericarditis, chest pain, coughing, pleural effusion) in patient receiving large oral doses over prolonged periods. Review results of antinuclear antibody titers, which should be measured periodically. The drug should be discontinued if clinical signs of lupus appear or if titer rises (quinidine may be substituted). Steroid therapy should be initiated if symptoms persist or worsen.
Expect dosage of oral anticoagulant to remain unchanged for patient taking an oral anticoagulant simultaneously with procainamide. Procainamide does not appear to increase effects of oral anticoagulants, as does quinidine.

Surveillance During Therapy

Carefully monitor laboratory studies and patient for indications of adverse reactions.
Interpret results of diagnostic tests and contact practitioner as appropriate.
Watch for indications of developing agranulocytosis (fever, sore throat, mucosal ulceration, respiratory tract infection), and check results of leukocyte counts. Medication should be discontinued if values are abnormal.
Monitor results of ECG determinations and blood counts, which should be performed periodically in patients on prolonged therapy.
Monitor for possible drug–drug and drug–nutrient interactions; see Interactions.

Patient Teaching

Suggest taking drug with meals or milk to reduce GI upset.
Inform patient that drug may cause lightheadedness and dizziness owing to hypotensive effect. Advise caution in driving a car or operating machinery.

Advise patient to avoid using other medications, including over-the-counter (OTC) preparations, that can alter cardiac stability (eg, sympathomimetics, anticholinergics) during long-term therapy with procainamide.

Disopyramide

Norpace

(CAN) Rythmodan

Mechanism

Decreases the rate of diastolic depolarization (phase 4) in myocardial cells, and decreases upstroke velocity of the action potential (phase 0); prolongs action potential duration and effective refractory period of the atria and ventricles, thereby decreasing automaticity and conduction velocity; minimal effect on AV conduction or AV nodal refractory period; possesses some anticholinergic activity and exerts a negative inotropic effect (decreased force of contraction), especially in patients with reduced left ventricular function.

Uses

Suppression and prevention of recurrence of the following arrhythmias:

- Unifocal premature (ectopic) ventricular contractions
- Premature (ectopic) ventricular contractions of multifocal origin
- Paired premature ventricular contractions
- Episodes of ventricular tachycardia

Dosage

CAUTION

Patients with atrial flutter or fibrillation should be digitalized before administering disopyramide to ensure that the drug-induced increase in AV conduction does not result in unacceptably rapid ventricular rates.

- Initially, 200 to 300 mg loading dose, followed by 150 mg every 6 hours; controlled-release capsules (Norpace CR) may be given every 8 hours; usual dose is 400 to 800 mg/day
- In patients weighing less than 50 kg, or in those with hepatic or mild renal insufficiency: 200-mg loading dose followed by 100 mg every 6 hours
- In patients with cardiomyopathy or cardiac decompensation: 100 mg every 6 hours with *no* loading dose
- Pediatric dosage (divided doses every 6 h):
  - *1 to 4 years*: 10 to 20 mg/kg/day
  - *4 to 12 years*: 10 to 15 mg/kg/day
  - *12 to 18 years*: 6 to 15 mg/kg/day

Fate

Rapidly and almost completely absorbed; onset within 30 minutes; peak serum levels occur within 2 to 3 hours; duration approximately 4 to 6 hours; plasma half-life 4 to 10 hours; approximately 25% to 30% protein bound; excreted mainly in the urine, one half as unchanged drug; remainder is excreted as metabolites, either through the kidney or in the feces; renal excretion is independent of urinary pH.

Common Side Effects

Dry mouth, urinary hesitancy, nausea, bloating, GI pain, constipation, blurred vision, fatigue, headache, malaise.

Significant Adverse Reactions

CV: Hypotension, congestive heart failure (due to decreased force of contraction), edema, cardiac conduction disturbances, QRS widening, AV block, chest pain, dyspnea
CNS: Dizziness, nervousness, insomnia, depression
Dermatologic–hematologic: Rash, pruritus, dermatoses, decreased hemoglobin, thrombocytopenia, agranulocytosis (rare)
Other: Urinary retention; anorexia; diarrhea; vomiting; elevated liver enzymes; impotence; elevated creatinine; reversible cholestatic jaundice; elevated cholesterol, triglycerides, and blood urea nitrogen; hypokalemia; hypoglycemia; anaphylactoid reaction

Contraindications

Cardiogenic shock, second- or third-degree AV block, uncompensated congestive heart failure or hypotension, and in nursing mothers. *Cautious use* in patients with glaucoma, urinary retention, prostatic hypertrophy, sick sinus syndrome, Wolff-Parkinson-White syndrome, bundle branch block, renal impairment, hepatic dysfunction, and in children and pregnant women.

Interactions

- Effects of disopyramide may be enhanced by concurrent use of other antiarrhythmic drugs, beta-adrenergic blockers, and calcium channel blockers.
- Plasma levels can be increased by the presence of other protein-bound drugs (eg, sulfonamides, antiinflammatory agents, oral anticoagulants, oral hypoglycemics).
- Therapeutic effects may be reduced by the presence of hypokalemia (eg, during diuretic therapy).
- Effects of cholinesterase inhibitors in relieving myasthenia gravis may be impaired by disopyramide.
- Plasma levels of disopyramide may be lowered by the presence of enzyme inducers, such as phenytoin, barbiturates, glutethimide, or primidone.

Nursing Management

See **Procainamide**. In addition:

Nursing Interventions

Medication Administration

Expect dosage to be reduced if first-degree heart block occurs. If block persists, benefits of continuing therapy should be weighed against risk of causing higher degrees of heart block.

Surveillance During Therapy

- Monitor blood pressure and cardiac function closely. Be alert for signs of developing toxicity, such as excessive widening of QRS complex, hypotension, conduction disturbances, bradycardia, and worsening of congestive heart failure. Progressive congestive failure should be treated with cardiac glycosides and diuretics.
- Monitor intake and output because urinary retention can occur.

Patient Teaching

Warn patient not to drive a car until effects of drug are known because lightheadedness and dizziness can occur.
Advise patient to avoid using all drugs, including OTC preparations, that have sympathomimetic effects (eg, cough or cold preparations, nasal decongestants) because they may alter cardiac stability.
Suggest interventions to relieve the mouth dryness that often occurs.

• Moricizine

Ethmozine

Mechanism

Exhibits some properties of groups of IA, IB, and IC drugs. Like the other group IA agents, it decreases sodium influx during depolarization; however, it decreases conduction velocity in the AV node, the duration of the action potential, and effective refractory period.

Uses

Treatment of life-threatening ventricular arrhythmias.

Dosage

Usual: 200 mg orally every 8 hours, adjust dose in increments of 150 mg/day at 3-day intervals, usual range 600 to 900 mg per day.

Fate

Undergoes extensive metabolism by the liver immediately after absorption; peak concentrations within 0.5 to 2 hours; approximately 95% bound to plasma proteins; accelerates its own metabolism; duration of action is 10 to 24 hours.

Common Side Effects

Palpitations, nausea, dizziness, headache, fatigue.

Significant Adverse Reactions

CV: sustained ventricular tachycardia, chest pain, cardiac death, hypotension, bradycardia
CNS: paresthesias, confusion, seizure, coma, nystagmus, ataxia
GI: abdominal pain, bitter taste, anorexia
Respiratory: dyspnea, apnea
Genitourinary: urinary retention
Other: arthralgia, dry mouth, blurred vision, drug fever

Contraindications

Cardiogenic shock, second- or third-degree heart block, right bundle branch block associated with left hemiblock unless a pacemaker is used.

Interactions

Moricizine may have an additive effect with digoxin and propranolol and may prolong the PR interval.
Cimetidine decreases the clearance of moricizine, therefore increasing moricizine plasma levels.
Moricizine may increase the clearance of theophylline.

Nursing Management

Pretherapy Assessment

Assess and record baseline data necessary for detection of adverse effects of moricizine: General: VS, body weight, skin color and temperature; CNS: reflexes, orientation; CVS: ECG, exercise testing; GI: normal output, bowel sounds, liver evaluation; Laboratory: liver function, urinalysis, serum electrolytes.
Review medical history and documents for existing or previous conditions that:
a. require cautious use of moricizine: liver or kidney disease; renal dysfunction (eg, dysuria, oliguria); sick sinus syndrome.
b. contraindicate use of moricizine: allergy to moricizine; second- or third-degree AV block; cardiogenic shock; congestive heart failure; **pregnancy (Category B)**; lactation (secreted in breast milk; serious adverse effects are possible, use with caution in nursing mothers).

Nursing Interventions

Medication Administration

Provide access to bathroom facilities.
Administer drug with food if GI upset occurs.
Administer only to patients with life-threatening arrhythmias who do not respond to conventional therapy.
Patient should be hospitalized and monitored during initiation of therapy.

Surveillance During Therapy

Closely monitor patients receiving digoxin. If second-degree block occurs, notify the practitioner.
Carefully monitor laboratory studies and patient for indications of adverse reactions.
Interpret results of diagnostic tests and contact practitioner as appropriate.
Monitor for possible drug–drug and drug–nutrient interactions; see Interactions.

Patient Teaching

Suggest taking drug with food to minimize GI distress.
Instruct the patient to report any dizziness, chest pain, or palpitations to a practitioner immediately.
Advise the patient not to stop taking this medication abruptly without consulting the practitioner because rebound arrhythmias may occur.

Group IB Drugs

• Lidocaine

Lidopen, Xylocaine

(CAN) Xylocard

Mechanism

Increases the electrical stimulation threshold of the ventricle during diastole; suppresses automaticity of ectopic pacemaker, shortens the refractory period, and decreases the duration of the action potential in Purkinje fibers, thereby slowing spontaneously firing ectopic ventricular rhythms; little effect on atrial muscle, AV conduction, systolic arterial pressure, myocardial contractility, and cardiac output; also has a local anesthetic action (see Chapter 18).

Uses

Management of acute ventricular arrhythmias such as those resulting from myocardial infarction, cardiac surgery, or catheterization, and digitalis intoxication

Emergency control of arrhythmias when IV administration is impractical, such as in a mobile emergency unit (IM administration)

Dosage

Loading dose is given initially, followed by a maintenance infusion to maintain a therapeutic plasma level of 2 to 5 µg/mL.

IV injection: 1 mg/kg at a rate of 25 to 50 mg/min; may repeat at one third to one half initial dose in 5 minutes if necessary; maximum is 300 mg/h

IV infusion: 20 to 50 µg/kg/min (1–4 mg/min) of a 0.1% to 0.2% solution (1–2 g lidocaine in 1 L 5% dextrose in water)

IM: 300 mg in an average 70-kg person (approximately 4.3 mg/kg); may repeat in 60 to 90 minutes; use only 10% solution, or LidoPen Auto-Injector (300 mg/3 mL).

Fate

Onset with IV injection is immediate and duration is 10 to 20 minutes; after IM injection, onset is 5 to 15 minutes and duration is approximately 60 to 120 minutes. Plasma half-life is 1 to 2 hours, although the initial distribution half-life from the plasma is 5 to 10 minutes; widely distributed in the body and significantly bound to plasma proteins (40%–80%); largely (90%) metabolized in the liver and excreted in the urine.

Common Side Effects

Drowsiness; lightheadedness; slurred speech; sensations of heat, cold, or numbness; paresthesias; mild tremor.

Significant Adverse Reactions

CNS: dizziness, impaired hearing or vision, anxiety, apprehension, euphoria, vomiting, muscle twitching, tremors, convulsions, respiratory depression

CV: hypotension, bradycardia, cardiovascular collapse, cardiac arrest (overdosage)

Dermatologic: urticaria, peripheral edema, cutaneous lesions

Other: pain at IM injection site, excessive perspiration, local thrombophlebitis (IV infusion); *rarely*, malignant hyperthermia

Contraindications

Adams-Stokes syndrome; Wolff-Parkinson-White syndrome; severe SA, AV, or intraventricular block; hypersensitivity to local anesthetics. *Cautious use* in the presence of liver or kidney disease, congestive heart failure, severe respiratory depression, hypovolemia, shock, or myasthenia gravis.

CAUTION

In patients with sinus bradycardia or incomplete heart block, acceleration of the heartbeat with isoproterenol or electric pacing should be accomplished before administering lidocaine to avoid precipitation of more frequent or serious ventricular arrhythmias or complete heart block.

Interactions

Cardiac depression may increase if lidocaine is used along with other antiarrhythmic drugs, especially phenytoin or propranolol.

Concurrent administration of procainamide may result in additive neurologic effects.

Muscle-relaxant effects of neuromuscular blocking agents (eg, succinylcholine, aminoglycosides) may be increased by lidocaine.

Lidocaine inhibits the antibacterial action of sulfonamides.

Barbiturates may decrease the action of lidocaine through enzyme induction.

Serum levels of lidocaine can be elevated by concurrent use of cimetidine or beta-blockers.

Nursing Management

Pretherapy Assessment

Assess and record baseline data necessary for detection of adverse effects of lidocaine: General: VS, body weight, skin color and temperature; CNS: reflexes, orientation; CVS: continuous ECG; GI: normal output, bowel sounds, liver evaluation; Laboratory: liver function, urinalysis, serum electrolytes.

Review medical history and documents for existing or previous conditions that:

a. require cautious use of lidocaine: liver or kidney disease; congestive heart failure; severe respiratory depression; hypovolemia; shock; myasthenia gravis.
b. contraindicate use of lidocaine: allergy to lidocaine or amide-type local anesthetics; Adams-Stokes syndrome; Wolff-Parkinson-White syndrome; severe SA, AV, or intraventricular block; **pregnancy (Category B)**; labor and delivery (epidural anesthesia may prolong the second stage of labor. Monitor for fetal and neonatal CVS and CNS toxicity); lactation (secreted in breast milk; serious adverse effects are possible, use with caution in nursing mothers).

Nursing Interventions

Medication Administration

Have resuscitative equipment (eg, respiratory aids) and drugs (eg, IV fluids, vasopressors, muscle relaxants) available to treat adverse reactions involving the CNS or the cardiovascular or respiratory systems.

Use microdrip IV administration set and an infusion control device to ensure accuracy. Monitor flow rate continuously. Adequate plasma levels must be maintained because lidocaine has a short duration of action.

Monitor cardiac function and blood pressure closely. Infusion should be discontinued if signs of cardiac depression (eg, prolonged PR interval, widened QRS complex) or increased arrhythmias develop.

Do *not* add lidocaine to transfusion assemblies.

Do not use lidocaine solutions containing either preservatives or epinephrine for treatment of arrhythmias.

Give IM injections into deltoid muscle because therapeutic blood levels occur sooner, and peak blood level is higher than with other IM injection sites.

Interpret serum creatine phosphokinase (CPK) levels cautiously because levels may be increased if IM route is used. This can interfere with diagnosis of myocardial infarction.

Have IV diazepam available in case convulsions occur.

Surveillance During Therapy

Observe patient carefully for indications of CNS toxicity (eg, confusion, paresthesias, excitement, tremors), particularly during IV infusion. CNS effects are especially problematic in patient with congestive heart failure. Be prepared to terminate IV infusion as soon as cardiac rhythm is stable (or signs of toxicity develop). Patient should be changed to oral antiarrhythmic for maintenance as soon as possible, usually within 24 hours.

Carefully monitor laboratory studies and patient for indications of adverse reactions.

Monitor for malignant hyperthermia (jaw muscle spasm, rigidity); have life support equipment and IV dantrolene ready.

Interpret results of diagnostic tests and contact practitioner as appropriate.

Monitor for possible drug–drug and drug–nutrient interactions; see Interactions.

Provide for patient safety needs if CNS effects occur.

Patient Teaching

Teach patient that drowsiness, dizziness, numbness, and double vision, and nausea and vomiting, can occur as typical side effects of lidocaine therapy.

Reassure patient during frequent IV rate checks when lidocaine is used as an antiarrhythmic.

• Tocainide

Tonocard

Mechanism

Similar to that of lidocaine but effective orally; decreases myocardial cell excitability, reduces automaticity, and decreases the effective refractory period of the Purkinje fibers and ventricular muscle cells; sinus node function is largely unaltered and conduction times are not changed appreciably. No significant changes in heart rate, blood pressure, or myocardial contractility, although a slight degree of depression of left ventricular function is noted, usually without appreciable change in the cardiac output in well compensated patients; a slight increase in vascular resistance and pulmonary arterial pressure may occur.

Uses

Treatment of symptomatic ventricular arrhythmias such as premature ventricular contractions, ventricular tachycardia, and unifocal or multifocal couplets.

Dosage

Initially, 400 mg orally every 8 hours; usual maintenance range is 1200 to 1800 mg/day in divided doses; maximum dose is 2400 mg/day.

Fate

Oral absorption is rapid and complete; peak serum levels are attained in 30 minutes to 3 hours; food delays the rate but not the extent of absorption; only 10% to 20% of a dose is protein bound; drug is inactivated in the liver and is excreted in the urine as metabolites as well as unchanged drug (30%–50%); elimination half-life is approximately 12 to 15 hours and is increased in the presence of severe renal dysfunction; pharmacokinetics of the drug are not appreciably altered in patients with a myocardial infarction.

Common Side Effects

Lightheadedness, dizziness, nausea, paresthesias, numbness, mild tremor, giddiness.

Significant Adverse Reactions

CNS: nervousness, visual disturbances, tinnitus, headache, drowsiness, nystagmus, ataxia, anxiety, incoordination, confusion, disorientation, altered mood, hallucinations

CV: bradycardia, hypotension, palpitations, chest pain, ventricular arrhythmias, congestive heart failure, AV or bundle branch block, cardiomegaly

GI: anorexia, loose stools, diarrhea, vomiting, abdominal pain, dysphagia

Other: sweating, rash, skin lesions, arthralgia; rarely, blood dyscrasias, lupus-like syndrome, pulmonary fibrosis and edema, pneumonia

Contraindications

Second- and third-degree heart block, hypersensitivity to amide-type local anesthetics. *Cautious use* in patients with heart failure, reduced cardiac reserve, conduction disturbances, atrial arrhythmias (ventricular rate may increase), pulmonary dysfunction, hypokalemia, severe liver or kidney disease, and in pregnant or nursing women.

Interactions

Concurrent use of tocainide with other drugs having a negative inotropic action (eg, beta-blockers, verapamil, disopyramide) may further depress left ventricular function.

Nursing Management

See **Lidocaine**. In addition:

Nursing Interventions

Medication Administration

Carefully review patient's past medication history for evidence of allergy to amide-type local anesthetics, a contraindication to tocainide use.

Surveillance During Therapy

Assess patient carefully for indications of CNS toxicity (eg, drowsiness, dizziness, lightheadedness, confusion, headache, visual disturbances, tinnitus, mood alterations, hallucinations). Neurologic side effects usually are early warning signs of toxicity.

Monitor ECG results for manifestations of prodysrhythmic effect (incidence estimated at approximately 1%–2% for tocainide).

Assess patient for evidence of GI symptoms (eg, nausea, vomiting, anorexia, diarrhea). The patient who has GI or CNS side effects on divided doses every 12 hours may tolerate therapy better if drug instead is given every 8 hours and is taken with a meal.

Patient Teaching

Recommend that bedtime doses be taken with snacks.

Inform patient that most side effects are transient. If symptoms persist, however, the practitioner should be notified.

Instruct patient to report any unusual bleeding (eg, petechiae, bruising, hematuria) because thrombocytopenia has occurred in rare instances.

Instruct patient to report signs of infection (eg, sore throat, fever, chills) because leukopenia and agranulocytosis have occurred, although infrequently.

Advise patient to report respiratory problems (eg, exertional dyspnea, cough, wheezing) because pulmonary reactions such as fibrosis, pneumonitis, pneumonia, and edema have occurred on rare occasions.

Phenytoin

Dilantin, Diphenylan

Although this is not an approved indication, phenytoin has been used in treating certain arrhythmias, particularly those resulting from digitalis toxicity.

Mechanism

Depresses ectopic pacemaker activity and shortens action potential duration in isolated Purkinje tissue; improves AV and intraventricular conduction in the digitalis-depressed heart; increases membrane responsiveness in Purkinje fibers; slightly impairs force of contraction and has little effect on arterial pressure; exerts an anticonvulsant activity (see Chapter 27), and is widely used in grand mal seizures.

Uses

Treatment of paroxysmal atrial tachycardia, particularly if associated with digitalis intoxication

Treatment of ventricular ectopic rhythms, especially those resulting from digitalis overdosage

Dosage

IV injection: 100 mg every 5 to 10 minutes until arrhythmia is abolished or toxicity appears (maximum dose is 1000 mg/24 h)

Oral: Initially 1000 mg first day in divided doses, then 500 to 600 mg on second and third days; maintenance is 100 mg 2 to 4 times/day; usual serum level is 10 to 20 μg/mL

Fate

Also see Chapter 27. Onset of action orally is 30 to 60 minutes; plasma half-life is 24 to 36 hours; highly protein bound (85%–95%); metabolized by the liver and excreted largely by the kidneys as conjugated metabolites.

Common Side Effects

Nystagmus, diplopia, nausea, GI upset (also see Chapter 27).

Significant Adverse Reactions

See Chapter 27.

CV: bradycardia, hypotension, cardiac arrest

CNS: confusion, nervousness, ataxia, drowsiness, tremors, visual disturbances

Contraindications

Also see Chapter 27. Severe bradycardia, second-degree or complete heart block.

Interactions

See Chapter 27.

Nursing Management

See Chapter 27. In addition:

Nursing Interventions

Medication Administration

Have atropine available to reverse bradycardia or heart block during IV administration. Inform patient that infusion may be quite painful, and check infusion site frequently for signs of phlebitis. Infusion may be accomplished with a dilute solution (1 g/L of dextrose in water) given over 2 to 4 hours.

Rate of infusion should not exceed 50 mg/min.

Expect to administer large initial doses in some cases. It takes 6 to 12 days to attain steady-state plasma levels with oral administration because of long half-life.

Refer to Chapter 27 for discussion of potential adverse effects when drug is given orally for prolonged periods. Because of these, therapy should be limited to the shortest feasible period of time. Because most arrhythmias respond to phenytoin at plasma concentrations below toxic levels, however, cautious therapy should eliminate most short-term adverse effects.

Mexiletine

Mexitil

Mechanism

Similar to lidocaine and tocainide in its actions; reduces the rate of rise of phase 0 of the action potential, decreases the effective refractory period in Purkinje fibers, and shortens the action potential duration; mexiletine has minimal effects on impulse generation or propagation, cardiac output, force of contraction, pulse rate, blood pressure, and peripheral vascular resistance.

Uses

Management of symptomatic ventricular arrhythmias (eg, premature ventricular contractions, ventricular tachycardia).

Dosage

Initially, 200 mg orally every 8 hours (up to 400 mg initially may be given for rapid control of ventricular arrhythmias); adjust dosage in 50-mg increments to optimal response.

Fate

Oral absorption is good; peak serum levels occur in 2 to 3 hours; the effective plasma range of 0.5 to 2 μg/mL can be maintained with 2-to 3-times-daily dosing; 50% to 60% protein bound, drug is metabolized in the liver and metabolites are excreted in the urine together with approximately 10% unchanged drug; elimination half-life is 10 to 12 hours with normal liver function, but may be prolonged up to 25 to 30 hours in patients with liver impairment.

Common Side Effects

GI distress, lightheadedness, dizziness, impaired coordination, palpitations, nervousness, headache, mild tremor.

Significant Adverse Reactions

CAUTION

Mexiletine can worsen arrhythmias, especially in more seriously ill patients.

GI: diarrhea, loss of appetite, abdominal pain, dysphagia, GI bleeding, peptic ulcer, altered taste, oral mucosal ulceration

CNS: confusion, short-term memory loss, depression, hallucinations, convulsions, psychotic behavior

CV: angina-like pain, premature ventricular contractions, bradycardia, hypotension, syncope, edema, conduction disturbances, atrial arrhythmias

Other: rash, arthralgia, fever, urinary hesitancy, hiccups, dyspnea, sweating, hair loss, decreased libido, impotence, systemic lupus-like syndrome, blood dyscrasias, abnormal liver function tests, positive antinuclear antibody (ANA) titer

Contraindications

Cardiogenic shock, second- and third-degree heart block. *Cautious use* in patients with sinus node dysfunction, conduction abnormalities, hypotension, congestive heart failure, liver or kidney disease, or history of convulsive disorders, and in pregnant or nursing women.

Interactions

Phenytoin, phenobarbital, rifampin, and other hepatic enzyme inducers may lower mexiletine plasma levels.

Mexiletine may increase theophylline levels.

Drugs that alkalinize the urine may slow mexiletine excretion, whereas acidifying agents can enhance its rate of excretion.

Nursing Management

See Tocainide. In addition:

Nursing Interventions

Surveillance During Therapy

Monitor results of liver function studies, which should be performed periodically to detect hepatotoxicity.

Patient Teaching

Recommend that drug be taken with food or antacid to slow absorption time, which may help to reduce side effects. CNS and GI side effects may be quite disabling, can occur with normal doses, and may necessitate dosage reduction.

Warn patient to limit driving or operation of hazardous equipment until response to drug is known because dizziness and drowsiness may occur.

Teach patient interventions to help minimize orthostatic hypotension related to drug's hypotensive effects.

Group IC Drugs

• Flecainide

Tambocor

Mechanism

Possesses membrane-stabilizing activity and has local anesthetic-like properties; decreases conduction in all parts of the heart, with the greatest effect noted in the His–Purkinje system; ventricular refractory period is prolonged; suppresses single and multiple premature ventricular contractions and can decrease the recurrence of ventricular tachycardia; alterations in heart rate and blood pressure are minimal; drug can cause new arrhythmias or worsen existing ones, and its use is associated with a wide range of untoward reactions.

Uses

Treatment of documented life-threatening ventricular arrhythmias (eg, sustained ventricular tachycardia)—*only approved indication*: see CAUTION.

Dosage

Initially, 100 mg every 12 hours; increase in 50-mg increments twice a day every 4 days *only*; most patients are controlled at 300 mg/day; maximum dose 400 mg/day.

Fate

Oral absorption is complete and peak plasma levels are attained in about 3 hours; steady-state plasma levels occur within 3 to 5 days, and the plasma half-life ranges from 12 to 24 hours; accumulation rarely occurs during prolonged therapy; plasma protein binding is approximately 40%; about one third of an oral dose is eliminated unchanged in the urine; the remainder is metabolized in the liver and conjugated metabolites are excreted in the urine; renal impairment lengthens the drug's half-life.

Common Side Effects

Lightheadedness, faintness, visual disturbances, headache, nausea, dizziness, palpitations, dyspnea, constipation.

Significant Adverse Reactions

CAUTION

The National Heart, Lung and Blood Institutes' Cardiac Arrhythmia Suppression Trial (CAST) demonstrated an excessive mortality or nonfatal cardiac arrest rate with flecainide and encainide. Use of these agents is reserved for patients in whom the benefits outweigh the risks. Therapy with flecainide should be initiated in the hospital and patients monitored closely because fatalities have occurred.

The drug also exhibits a negative inotropic effect and may cause or worsen congestive heart failure, particularly in patients with cardiomyopathy, preexisting heart failure, or low ejection fractions.

CV: sinus bradycardia, sinus arrest, second- or third-degree heart block, angina-like symptoms, hypotension

CNS: flushing, sweating, tinnitus, paresthesias, ataxia, somnolence, anxiety, depression, weakness, speech disorders, stupor, amnesia, euphoria, convulsions, morbid dreams

GI: diarrhea, vomiting, anorexia, dyspepsia, dry mouth, altered taste

Ocular: blurred vision, diplopia, photophobia, eye pain, nystagmus

Other: decreased libido, impotence, polyuria, skin rash, urticaria, pruritus, exfoliative dermatitis, fever, swollen lips or tongue, bronchospasm, arthralgia, myalgia, leukopenia, thrombocytopenia

Large doses may significantly lengthen the PR interval; increase the QRS duration, QT interval, and amplitude of the T wave; and reduce heart rate and contractile force. Conduction disturbances, hypotension, respiratory failure, and asystole have resulted from overdosage.

Contraindications

Second- or third-degree heart block, bundle branch block, cardiogenic shock. *Cautious use* in patients with congestive heart failure, myocardial dysfunction, sick sinus syndrome, renal impairment, electrolyte imbalances, liver disease, or implanted pacemakers, and in pregnant or nursing women.

Interactions

Concurrent use of flecainide with propranolol (and probably other beta-blockers), verapamil, or disopyramide can cause additive negative inotropic effects.

Acidification of the urine can increase the renal elimination of flecainide, whereas alkalinization reduces the rate of excretion.

Plasma levels of flecainide and propranolol may both be increased when the two drugs are given together.

Nursing Management

Pretherapy Assessment

Assess and record baseline data necessary for detection of adverse effects of flecainide: General: VS, body weight, skin color and temperature; CNS: reflexes, orientation, vision; CVS: ECG, edema; GI: normal output, bowel sounds, liver evaluation; Laboratory: liver function, CBC, urinalysis, serum electrolytes.

Review medical history and documents for existing or previous conditions that:

a. require cautious use of flecainide: congestive heart failure; myocardial dysfunction; sick sinus syndrome; renal impairment; electrolyte imbalances; liver disease; or implanted pacemakers.

b. contraindicate use of flecainide: allergy to flecainide; second- or third-degree heart block, bundle branch block, cardiogenic shock; **pregnancy (Category C)**; labor and delivery (safety not established); lactation (secreted in breast milk; serious adverse effects are possible, use with caution in nursing mothers).

Nursing Interventions

Medication Administration

Have IV diazepam available in case convulsions occur.

Carefully review patient's medication history for evidence of allergy to amide-type local anesthetics, a contraindication to drug use.

Ensure that baseline assessment of ECG and cardiovascular function is obtained before therapy is initiated because many cardiovascular side effects can occur.

Check serum potassium before administration.

Drug may be administered without regard to meals.

Have life support equipment available in case serious CVS and CNS effects occur.

Surveillance During Therapy

Assess patient for signs of developing congestive heart failure. Most side effects develop within 1 to 2 weeks after initiation of therapy.

Monitor results of serum drug level determinations, which should be obtained periodically. Drug should be administered every 12 hours because effectiveness is enhanced by maintenance of consistent blood levels.

Assess patient for indications of CNS toxicity (eg, drowsiness, dizziness, lightheadedness, confusion, headache, visual disturbances, tinnitus, mood alterations, hallucinations). Neurologic side effects are usually the early warning signs of toxicity.

Carefully monitor laboratory studies and patient for indications of adverse reactions.

Interpret results of diagnostic tests and contact practitioner as appropriate.

Monitor for possible drug–drug and drug–nutrient interactions; see Interactions.

Provide for patient safety needs if CNS effects occur.

Patient Teaching

Instruct patient to report immediately any rapid weight gain, swelling of hands or feet, or difficulty in breathing, possible signs of congestive heart failure.

Instruct patient to report any unusual bleeding (eg, petechiae, bruising, hematuria) because thrombocytopenia has occurred in rare instances.

• Encainide

Enkaid

Encainide has been voluntarily withdrawn from the market by the manufacturer because of continuing uncertainty about the implications of the CAST trial (see flecainide). The drug is available on a limited basis from the manufacturer only.

Mechanism

Similar to flecainide; blocks sodium channel of Purkinje fibers and myocardium and slows phase 0 depolarization; increases the ratio of the effective refractory period : action potential duration; decreases intracardiac conduction in all parts of the heart; blood pressure is unchanged.

Uses

Treatment of documented, life-threatening ventricular arrhythmias.

Dosage

Initially, 25 mg orally every 8 hours; increase to 35 mg every 8 hours after 3 to 5 days, and, if necessary, to 50 mg every 8 hours; maximum dose for life-threatening arrhythmias is 75 mg 4 times daily.

Fate

Oral absorption is complete; peak plasma levels occur within 30 to 90 minutes; plasma protein binding is 75% to 85%; steady-state plasma levels are attained within 3 to 5 days; drug has two active metabolites that are eliminated more slowly than the parent compound (4–8 h vs. 1–2 h); major route of elimination is through the kidneys.

Common Side Effects

Dizziness, blurred vision, headache.

Significant Adverse Reactions

CAUTION

Encainide can initiate or worsen an existing ventricular arrhythmia in approximately 10% of patients, and some fatalities have occurred; these proarrhythmic events occur most often during the first week of therapy and are more common when doses exceed 200 mg/day.

CV: palpitations, tachycardia, syncope, peripheral edema, prolonged QRS interval, congestive heart failure
CNS: nervousness, somnolence, tremor, anorexia, insomnia
GI: abdominal pain, constipation, nausea, vomiting, dry mouth
Other: dyspnea, cough, skin rash, tinnitus, altered taste, paresthesia, lower extremity pain, chest pain

Contraindications

Preexisting second- or third-degree heart block, right bundle branch block (unless a pacemaker is present), cardiogenic shock. *Cautious use* in patients with congestive heart failure, electrolyte disturbances, sick sinus syndrome, or renal or hepatic impairment, and in pregnant or nursing women.

Interactions

Concurrent use of cimetidine may increase the plasma levels of encainide.

Nursing Management

See **Flecainide**.

• Propafenone

Rythmol

Mechanism

Exerts a local anesthetic effect and exhibits membrane-stabilizing activity; reduces upstroke velocity; ventricular refractory period is prolonged; decreases resting heart rate approximately 8%; causes prolongation of AV nodal and His–Purkinje conduction time.

Uses

Treatment of life-threatening ventricular arrhythmias
Investigational uses include treatment of arrhythmias associated with Wolff-Parkinson-White syndrome

Dosage

Initially, 150 mg every 8 hours, titrate the dose at 3- to 4-day intervals to 225 mg every 8 hours, up to a maximum of 300 mg every 8 hours.

Fate

Very well absorbed, peak plasma levels in 3.5 hours, extensive first-pass metabolism in the liver. Increasing the dose may saturate the metabolic systems; therefore, increasing the dose 3-fold may lead to a 10-fold increase in steady-state plasma concentration. Metabolism is complex; 90% of patients have an elimination half-life of 2 to 10 hours, whereas the half-life in remaining patients may be as long as 32 hours.

Common Side Effects

Dizziness, nausea or vomiting, altered taste, constipation, first-degree AV block, intraventricular conduction delays.

Significant Adverse Reactions

CAUTION

The National Heart Lung and Blood Institutes' Cardiac Arrhythmia Suppression Trial (CAST) demonstrated an excessive mortality or nonfatal cardiac arrest rate with encainide and flecainide. The applicability of these results to other group IC agents is unknown; however, use of group IC agents usually is reserved for life-threatening arrhythmias in which the benefits are thought to outweigh the risks.

CV: Proarrhythmic effects, increased premature ventricular contractions, ventricular fibrillation, torsades de pointes.
CNS: confusion, numbness, coma, seizures
GI: elevated liver enzymes, cholestasis, gastroenteritis, hepatitis.
Hematologic: agranulocytosis, anemia, thrombocytopenia
Other: nephrotic syndrome, alopecia, syndrome of inappropriate antidiuretic hormone secretion (SIADH)

Contraindications

Cardiogenic shock, second- or third-degree block, sick sinus syndrome.

Interactions

Serum propafenone levels may be increased by local anesthetics, cimetidine, and quinidine.
Oral anticoagulant effects may be increased by propafenone.
Propafenone may increase serum levels and effects of beta-blockers, digoxin, and cyclosporine.

Nursing Management

See **Flecainide**. In addition:

Nursing Interventions

Medication Administration

Ensure that baseline assessment of ECG and cardiovascular function is obtained before therapy is initiated because many cardiovascular side effects can occur.

Review the patients medications history to screen for potential drug interactions.

Surveillance During Therapy

Monitor ECG for signs of proarrhythmic effects.

Patient Teaching

Assess if the patient adequately understands the importance of reporting adverse effects to a practitioner.
Instruct the patient to report immediately any increased or bothersome chest pain, palpitations, or difficulty breathing.
Instruct the patient to report any unusual bleeding (eg, petechiae, bruising, hematuria) because thrombocytopenia has occurred is rare instances.
Instruct the patient to contact a practitioner if a fever, sore throat, or chills develop, because agranulocytosis has occurred in rare instances.

Group II Drugs (Beta-Adrenergic Blockers)

- **Propranolol**

Inderal

(CAN) Apo-Propranol, Detensol, Novopranol, PMS Propranolol

- **Acebutolol**

Sectral

(CAN) Monitan, Rhotral

- **Esmolol**

Brevibloc

Propranolol and acebutolol are beta-adrenergic blocking agents that have been used in treating a variety of arrhythmias, particularly exercise-induced arrhythmias or those associated with excessive sympathetic stimulation or circulating catecholamine levels. Esmolol is a rapid-acting, parenteral beta-blocker used primarily to control a rapid ventricular response secondary to atrial fibrillation or atrial flutter. Esmolol may also be used for sinus tachycardia. The beta-blockers are used for a number of pathologic conditions, and they are reviewed in detail as a group in Chapter 15. The following discussion is limited to their usefulness in treating arrhythmias.

Mechanism

Competitively antagonize the action of adrenergic agents at beta receptor sites; on the heart, specifically, they reduce rate, force of contraction, irritability, AV conduction, and automaticity of the SA node and ectopic pacemaker activity; large doses exert a direct quinidine-like depressant effect on the myocardium, suppressing overall cardiac function.

Uses

Treatment of the following arrhythmias:

Exercise-induced ventricular tachycardia
Supraventricular tachyarrhythmias
Digitalis-induced arrhythmias
Tachycardia due to thyrotoxicosis or excessive catecholamine activity
Persistent premature ventricular extrasystoles

Dosage

Propranolol
Oral: 10 to 30 mg 3 to 4 times/day
IV (life-threatening arrhythmias *only*): 1 to 3 mg at a rate of 1 mg/min

Acebutolol
Oral: initially, 200 mg twice a day; increase gradually until desired response is achieved; usual range 600 to 1200 mg daily

Esmolol
IV: Initial loading dose of 500 µg/kg/min for 1 minute, followed immediately by a continuous infusion of 50 µg/kg/min for 4 minutes. If the desired response is not achieved, repeat the loading dose and increase the infusion to 100 µg/kg/minute. Repeat the above steps every 5 minutes until desired response or a maximum continuous infusion of 300 µg/kg/min.

Fate

Orally, see Chapter 15. With IV administration of propranolol, onset is 1 to 2 minutes and duration lasts 3 to 6 hours; with esmolol, onset is 1 to 2 minutes, and its elimination half-life is only 9 minutes.

Nursing Management

See Chapter 15. In addition:

Nursing Interventions

Medication Administration

Be alert for development of severe bradycardia and hypotension when propranolol is administered IV, especially in patients with digitalis intoxication. Keep patient supine, closely monitor ECG and blood pressure, and have atropine injection available.

Surveillance During Therapy

Closely monitor patient on propranolol and digitalis therapy because their effects are additive in depressing AV conduction. Use of propranolol in digitalis overdosage may further depress myocardial contractility and can lead to cardiac failure. Propranolol should be withdrawn if signs of cardiac failure persist.

Group III Drugs

- **Bretylium**

Bretylol

(CAN) Bretylate

Mechanism

Complex and incompletely understood; prolongs the effective refractory period of Purkinje fibers and ventricular muscle fibers; increases ventricular fibrillation threshold and action potential duration; initially releases norepinephrine from adrenergic nerve endings, which may result in tachycardia, increased blood pressure, and a transient worsening of arrhythmias; subsequently, release of norepinephrine is reduced in response to nerve stimulation, although stores in the nerve ending are not depleted.

Uses

Treatment of *life-threatening* ventricular arrhythmias that have not responded to lidocaine or procainamide (use is restricted to intensive care or coronary care units with appropriate facilities for continuous monitoring of cardiac function).

Dosage

Acute ventricular fibrillation, IV: 5 mg/kg (undiluted) by rapid injection; may repeat at 10 mg/kg every 15 to 30 minutes to a total dose of 30 mg/kg

Other ventricular arrhythmias, IV: 5 to 10 mg/kg of a diluted solution by IV infusion over 10 to 30 minutes; repeat at 1- to 2-hour intervals

Dilution: 10 mL (500 mg) diluted to a minimum of 50 mL with dextrose or sodium chloride injection

IM (do *not* dilute): 5 to 10 mg/kg; may repeat in 1 to 2 hours, then every 6 to 8 hours thereafter (maximum injection volume is 5 mL)

Maintenance dosage: 5 to 10 mg/kg of diluted solution infused over 8 to 10 minutes every 6 hours or 1 to 2 mg/kg of diluted solution by constant infusion

Fate

Adequately absorbed IM; peak plasma concentrations in 60 to 90 minutes; however, maximum antiarrhythmic effects are not seen for 6 to 9 hours; effects of a single dose persist for 6 to 8 hours; onset after IV injection within minutes; excreted largely unchanged by the kidneys, approximately 70% to 80% of a dose within 24 hours.

Common Side Effects

Hypotension, nausea and vomiting (especially with rapid IV injection), lightheadedness.

Significant Adverse Reactions

Vertigo, syncope, bradycardia, transitory hypertension, increased arrhythmias (initially), anginal attacks, substernal pressure and pain.

Other (cause–effect relationship has not been definitively established): diarrhea, flushing, hyperthermia, dyspnea, anxiety, abdominal pain, erythematous rash, diaphoresis, confusion, nasal congestion, renal dysfunction.

Contraindications

There are no absolute contraindications to use in treating life-threatening ventricular arrhythmias; use in less serious arrhythmias is contraindicated in severe pulmonary hypertension or in aortic stenosis, and in patients with fixed cardiac output. *Cautious use* in pregnant women, in children, and in patients with reduced renal function.

Interactions

May increase digitalis toxicity by releasing norepinephrine.

Peripheral vasodilation occurring in patients already receiving procainamide or quinidine may be increased by bretylium.

Nursing Management

Pretherapy Assessment

Assess and record baseline data necessary for detection of adverse effects of bretylium: General: VS, body weight, skin color and temperature; CNS: reflexes, orientation, speech; CVS: ECG; GI: normal output, bowel sounds, liver evaluation; Laboratory: renal function tests.

Review medical history and documents for existing or previous conditions that:

a. require cautious use of bretylium: reduced renal function.
b. contraindicate use of bretylium: allergy to bretylium; severe pulmonary hypertension; aortic stenosis; patients with fixed cardiac output; **pregnancy (Category C)**; lactation (safety not established).

Note: because bretylium is used in life-threatening situations, the benefits usually outweigh any possible risks of therapy.

Nursing Interventions

Medication Administration

Expect dosage to be reduced in patient with impaired renal function to prevent accumulation toxicity because drug is excreted primarily through the kidneys.

Monitor patient closely and inform practitioner if effects of transient hypertension and arrhythmias are severe or prolonged because they can develop during *early* stages of therapy owing to initial release of catecholamines.

Surveillance During Therapy

Keep patient supine until tolerance to hypotensive action of the drug has developed, which often does not occur for several days. Assist with ambulation as needed.

Monitor cardiac function closely during therapy, and have appropriate equipment and drugs (eg, dopamine) available to treat adverse effects such as hypotension.

Carefully monitor laboratory studies and patient for indications of adverse reactions.

Interpret results of diagnostic tests and contact practitioner as appropriate.

Monitor for possible drug–drug and drug–nutrient interactions; see Interactions.

Provide for patient safety if orthostatic hypotension occurs.

Patient Teaching

Teach patient that blood pressure will fall during drug therapy and it is important for the patient to remain lying down.

Amiodarone

Cordarone

Mechanism

Prolongs myocardial cell action potential duration and refractory period; possesses both an alpha-adrenergic and a beta-adrenergic blocking action; vascular smooth muscle is relaxed and peripheral vascular resistance is reduced; automaticity of cardiac cells is decreased, but amiodarone can cause marked sinus bradycardia and has resulted in heart block and sinus arrest; ECG changes include increased PR and QT intervals, appearance of U waves, and altered T-wave contour.

Uses

Treatment of life-threatening recurrent ventricular arrhythmias (ventricular fibrillation, hemodynamically unstable ventricular tachycardia) that do not respond to other antiarrhythmics.

Dosage

Initially, loading doses of 800 to 1600 mg daily in divided doses; when arrhythmia is controlled, reduce dosage to 600 to 800 mg daily for 1 month, then to 400 mg daily.

Fate

Oral absorption is slow and variable; peak plasma levels occur in 3 to 7 hours, but clinical effects often take days to weeks to become manifest; widely distributed in the body and accumulates in fatty tissue; protein binding is approximately 95%; eliminated largely through the bile after hepatic metabolism; plasma half-life is extremely variable (20–120 days).

Common Side Effects

Nausea, vomiting, corneal microdeposits, photosensitivity, fatigue, tremor, incoordination, paresthesias.

Significant Adverse Reactions

CAUTION

Amiodarone is a highly toxic drug. Fatalities have occurred as a result of pulmonary toxicity (eg, interstitial pneumonitis; alveolitis), liver disease, arrhythmias, heart block, and sinus bradycardia. Owing to its slow onset and very prolonged duration of action, even after drug discontinuation, patients must be monitored very closely during therapy and for several months after termination of therapy. Drug treatment should be initiated in a hospital setting, and prolonged hospitalization may be required in unstable patients.

CNS: insomnia, headache, dizziness, ataxia, anorexia, sleep disturbances, decreased libido, visual disturbances, photophobia

CV: bradycardia, congestive heart failure, SA node dysfunction, hypotension, conduction abnormalities, arrhythmias (most often exacerbation of existing arrhythmias)

Dermatologic: Solar dermatitis, blue skin discoloration, rash, alopecia, spontaneous ecchymoses

Other: Abdominal pain, dryness of the eyes, peripheral neuropathy, hepatic disease, hepatitis, abnormal taste and smell, salivation, edema, altered thyroid function, coagulation abnormalities, pulmonary inflammation

Contraindications

Marked sinus bradycardia, second- or third-degree heart block, syncope due to bradycardia. *Cautious use* in patients with reduced hepatic function, thyroid abnormalities (drug increases levels of thyroxine [T_4] and reduces levels of triiodothyronine [T_3]), electrolyte disturbances, coagulation difficulties, pulmonary disease, and in pregnant or nursing women.

Drug should be discontinued if the following develop: pulmonary infiltrates or fibrosis, paroxysmal ventricular tachycardia, congestive heart failure, or symptoms of hepatic dysfunction.

Interactions

Amiodarone can increase serum levels of digoxin, quinidine, procainamide, and phenytoin if given concurrently. Dosage reductions of one third to one half may be necessary for these drugs.

Beta-blockers and calcium channel blockers (especially verapamil) may result in potentiation of bradycardia and increase the risk of AV block or sinus arrest when given together with amiodarone.

Amiodarone may increase the hypoprothrombinemic effects of warfarin, leading to serious bleeding.

Nursing Management

Pretherapy Assessment

Assess and record baseline data necessary for detection of adverse effects of amiodarone: General: VS, body weight, skin color and temperature; GI: normal output, bowel sounds, liver evaluation; Laboratory: thyroid, liver and kidney function tests, CBC, urinalysis.

Review medical history and documents for existing or previous conditions that:

a. require cautious use of amiodarone: reduced hepatic function; thyroid abnormalities (drug increases levels of T_4 and reduces levels of T_3); electrolyte disturbances; coagulation difficulties; pulmonary disease.
b. contraindicate use of amiodarone: allergy to amiodarone; marked sinus bradycardia; second- or third-degree heart block; syncope due to bradycardia; **pregnancy (Category C)**; lactation (secreted in breast milk, safety not established; if drug is required, do not nurse).

Nursing Interventions

Medication Administration

Weigh patient daily to monitor early development of congestive heart failure.

Measure intake and output to monitor possible fluid retention.

Review results of baseline and periodic determinations of arterial blood gases and hepatic function (hepatotoxicity may also occur).

Administer with food if GI disturbances occur. Because absorption is slow, however, food may merely prolong symptoms.

Implement interventions to prevent constipation (eg, increased intake of fluid and dietary fiber). Laxatives should be avoided if possible because they may impair drug absorption.

Surveillance During Therapy

Monitor patient closely because a wide range of debilitating side effects can occur. The drug usually is used only as a last resort when other drugs have failed. Unfortunately, side effects may not resolve for days to weeks even after cessation of therapy because the drug has a long half-life.

Assess patient for evidence of developing congestive heart failure (eg, dyspnea, rales, edema, lip cyanosis, neck vein distention) or pulmonary fibrosis.

Instill artificial tears 4 to 6 times daily to facilitate excretion of small crystals deposited because some of drug is excreted through lacrimal ducts. Complete ocular examinations should be performed when therapy is initiated and periodically thereafter during therapy because corneal deposits may develop.

Assess patient's neurologic status periodically because headaches and peripheral neuropathies, especially in hands and feet, can occur.

Monitor results of thyroid function studies (T_3, T_4), which should be obtained periodically, because either hyperthyroidism or hypothyroidism (more likely) may occur.

Carefully monitor laboratory studies and patient for indications of adverse reactions.

Interpret results of diagnostic tests and contact practitioner as appropriate.

Monitor for possible drug–drug and drug–nutrient interactions; see Interactions.

Patient Teaching

Warn patient that photophobia is likely to occur. Dark glasses may afford sufficient protection, but some patients are unable to go outdoors at all in the daytime.

Instruct patient to report development of blurred vision, halos around lights (especially at night), or altered visual acuity.

Advise patient to use sunscreens and protective clothing and to limit exposure to direct sunlight because photosensitivity reactions may occur.

Inform patient that a reversible blue-gray skin discoloration may occur, particularly in fair-skinned women.

Instruct patient to report development of symptoms of hyperthyroidism (eg, rapid heart rate, increased perspiration, increased appetite with weight loss, and insomnia) or hypothyroidism (eg, lethargy, puffy hands and feet, periorbital edema, cool skin, vertigo, constipation).

• Sotalol

Betapace

Mechanism

Lengthens cardiac repolarization and effective refractory period in all cardiac tissues; drug is a unique beta-blocker that lacks cardioselectivity, intrinsic sympathomimetic activity, or membrane-stabilizing actions.

Uses

Treatment of life-threatening ventricular arrhythmias.

Dosage

Initially, 80 mg orally twice daily. Allow 2 to 3 days until further titration, usual dosage range 160 to 320 mg/day. Doses as high as 640 mg/day have been used.

Fate

Well absorbed orally; not metabolized or protein bound; excreted unchanged in the urine; elimination half-life is 12 hours in patients with normal renal function.

Common Side Effects

Fatigue, lethargy, decreased libido, dyspnea, bradycardia, dizziness.

Significant Adverse Reactions

Torsades de pointes, ventricular arrhythmias.

Contraindications

Asthma, sinus bradycardia, second- or third-degree AV block, long QT syndromes, cardiogenic shock, uncontrolled congestive heart failure.

Interactions

Group IA antiarrhythmics may prolong the effective refractory period if given with sotalol.

Calcium channel blockers and sotalol may have additive depressant effects on the AV node.

Nursing Management

See Chapter 15 (**beta-blockers**). In addition:

Nursing Interventions

Surveillance During Therapy

Monitor ECG for signs of bradycardia or proarrhythmic effects.

Monitor serum glucose levels, especially in patients with diabetes; dosage of insulin or oral antidiabetic drugs may need to be adjusted.

Monitor renal function and advise practitioner of any changes that may require sotalol dosage adjustment.

Group IV Drugs

• Verapamil

Calan, Isoptin, Verelan

• Diltiazem

Cardizem

Verapamil and diltiazem are calcium channel blockers that, together with other calcium channel blockers, are used orally for the treatment of angina (see Chapter 34). These drugs are also used orally for the control of hypertension (see Chapter 33). In addition, verapamil and diltiazem are indicated for the treatment of supraventricular tachyarrhythmias because of their effects on the SA and AV node. Their use as antiarrhythmics is discussed in the following.

Mechanism

Inhibits influx of calcium ions through slow channels into cells of the cardiac conductile system; AV conduction is slowed and the effective refractory period of the AV node is prolonged, thus reducing elevated ventricular rate, interrupting AV nodal impulse reentry, and restoring normal sinus rhythm in supraventricular tachycardias; decreases myocardial contractility and reduces aortic impedance to left ventricular ejection (ie, afterload); may transiently lower systemic arterial pressure, and raise left ventricular filling pressure.

Uses

Treatment of supraventricular tachyarrhythmias, such as paroxysmal atrial tachycardia
Control of excessive ventricular rate in patients with atrial flutter or atrial fibrillation
Long-term management of angina (see Chapter 34)
Treatment of mild to moderate hypertension (see Chapter 33)

Dosage

Verapamil (given by slow IV injection)
Adults: initially, 5 to 10 mg over 2 to 3 minutes; repeat with 10 mg 30 minutes after first dose if initial response is inadequate
Children: 0 to 1 years, 0.75 to 2 mg over 2 minutes; 1 to 15 years, 2 to 5 mg over 2 minutes; may repeat initial dose in 30 minutes, if necessary
Diltiazem: Initially 0.25 mg/kg over 2 minutes; if after 15 minutes response is inadequate, administer 0.35 mg/kg over 2 minutes. For continued response, start diltiazem infusion at 5 mg/h, may increase to 15 mg/h.

Fate

Effects are usually noted within 2 to 5 minutes of injection. Duration of action of a single injection is 30 to 45 minutes. Elimination half-life is 3 to 8 hours. Verapamil is rapidly metabolized in the liver, and metabolites are excreted in the urine (70%) and feces (15%–20%). It is highly protein bound (90%).

Common Side Effects

Transient hypotension and dizziness, bradycardia.

Significant Adverse Reactions

CV: tachycardia, marked hypotension, asystole, AV block, congestive heart failure
CNS: headache, depression, vertigo, fatigue, nystagmus
GI: nausea, abdominal discomfort
Other: diaphoresis, muscle weakness

Contraindications

Severe hypotension, cardiogenic shock, second- or third-degree AV block, severe congestive heart failure, sick sinus syndrome, concurrent administration of IV beta-blocker or disopyramide. *Cautious use* in patients with hypertrophic cardiomyopathy and renal or hepatic dysfunction.

Interactions

Verapamil may be potentiated by other strongly protein-bound drugs, such as oral anticoagulants, antiinflammatory drugs, and sulfonamides.
The desired effects of calcium channel blockers may be reduced by administration of supplemental calcium.
The depressant action of calcium channel blockers on the myocardium and AV node can be enhanced by simultaneous use of an IV beta-blocking drug or disopyramide.
Excessive bradycardia or AV block can occur if calcium channel blockers are given together with a digitalis drug. Prolonged calcium channel blocker therapy increases serum digoxin levels.
Calcium channel blockers can enhance the blood pressure-lowering action of antihypertensive drugs.

Nursing Management

Pretherapy Assessment

Assess and record baseline data necessary for detection of adverse effects of calcium channel blockers: General: VS, body weight, skin color and temperature; CNS: orientation, reflexes; CVS: baseline ECG, peripheral perfusion; GI: normal output, bowel sounds, liver evaluation; Laboratory: liver and kidney function tests, CBC, urinalysis.
Review medical history and documents for existing or previous conditions that:
a. require cautious use of calcium channel blockers: hypertrophic cardiomyopathy; renal or hepatic dysfunction.
b. contraindicate use of calcium channel blockers: allergy to calcium channel blockers; severe hypotension; cardiogenic shock; second- or third-degree AV block; severe congestive heart failure; sick sinus syndrome; use with administration of IV beta-blocker or disopyramide; **pregnancy (Category C)**; lactation (secreted in breast milk, safety not established; if drug is required, do not nurse).

Nursing Interventions

Medication Administration

Ensure that complete monitoring and proper resuscitative equipment is available when calcium channel blockers are first administered because patient may respond with rapid ventricular rate, or, conversely, with marked hypotension and extreme bradycardia. Cardioversion, lidocaine, or procainamide are effective in treating rapid ventricular rate. Norepinephrine or metaraminol may be used to treat hypotension, and isoproterenol or atropine is indicated to reverse bradycardia or AV block.
Administer verapamil IV injection over at least 3 minutes in older patient to minimize possibility of adverse reactions. Keep patient recumbent for 1 hour after injection to minimize hypotension. Closely monitor patient receiving verapamil along with digitalis drugs, beta-blockers, or other antiarrhythmic drugs because adverse effects can be increased.

Surveillance During Therapy

Monitor urinary output because impaired renal function can prolong duration of action.
Be prepared for possible occurrence of complexes resembling premature ventricular contractions during conversion to normal sinus rhythm. These events have no clinical significance.
Carefully monitor laboratory studies and patient for indications of adverse reactions.
Interpret results of diagnostic tests and contact practitioner as appropriate.
Monitor for possible drug–drug and drug–nutrient interactions; see Interactions.

Patient Teaching

Explain to patient on prolonged therapy that OTC products containing calcium may impair effectiveness of calcium channel blockers.

Miscellaneous Antiarrhythmic Drugs

- **Adenosine**

Adenocard

Mechanism

An endogenous nucleoside that is found in all cells of the body; slows conduction through the AV node; may briefly depress the SA and AV node.

Uses

Conversion of paroxysmal supraventricular tachycardia into sinus rhythm, including that associated with Wolff-Parkinson-White syndrome.

Dosage

Initially, 6 mg rapid (over 1–2 sec) IV bolus; must follow with a rapid saline flush. May repeat in 1 to 2 minutes with a 12-mg rapid IV bolus, again followed by a saline flush. This 12-mg dose may be repeated a second time.

Fate

Adenosine is taken up by erythrocytes and vascular endothelial cells very rapidly; elimination half-life is less than 10 seconds.

Common Side Effects

Flushing, headache, chest pain, shortness of breath, lightheadedness, asystole.

Significant Adverse Effects

Transient heart block, brief asystole, arrhythmias. Owing to short half-life, adverse effects are quickly self-limiting.

Contraindications

Second- or third-degree AV block, atrial flutter or fibrillation, ventricular tachycardia.

Interactions

Methylxanthines, such as theophylline and caffeine, block the effects of adenosine and patients may not respond to usual doses.
Carbamazepine and dipyridamole may increase the effects of adenosine.

Nursing Management

Medication Administration

Proper administration is critical owing to the short elimination half-life of adenosine. A three-way stopcock may be useful. Draw up desired dose of adenosine and 20-mg saline flush. Place each syringe on its own port, open port for adenosine, and inject rapidly (1–2 sec), then run stopcock to saline and flush.

Selected Bibliography

Anderson JL: Reassessment of benefit–risk ratio and treatment algorithms for antiarrhythmic drug therapy after the Cardiac Arrhythmia Suppression Trail. J Clin Pharmacol 30:981, 1990
Baker B, Cacchione J: Dermatologic cross-sensitivity between diltiazem and amlodipine. Ann Pharmacother 28:118, 1994
Camm AJ, Garratt CJ. Adenosine and supraventricular tachycardia. N Engl J Med 325:1621, 1991
Cooper GS, Marinchak RA, Rials SJ, Kowey PR: Cardiac arrhythmias: Recent therapeutic changes. Drug Therapy 22:15, 1992
Freedman MD, Somberg JC: Pharmacology and pharmacokinetics of amiodarone. J Clin Pharmacol 31:1061, 1991
Garrett MM: Practical management of atrial fibrillation. Postgrad Med 87:40, 1990
Leibowitz D: Sotalol: A novel beta-blocker with class III anti-arrhythmic activity. J Clin Pharmacol 33:508, 1993
MacNeil DJ, Davies RO, Deitchman D: Clinical safety profile of sotalol in the treatment of arrhythmias. Am J Cardiol 72:44A, 1993
Mann HJ: Moricizine: A new class I antiarrhythmic. Clin Pharm 9:842, 1990
Nattel S, Bois D: Injectable diltiazem in early intervention against atrial fibrillation and flutter. Hosp Formul 27(Suppl):4, 1992
Pratt CM, Moyle LA: The cardiac arrhythmia suppression trial: Background, interim results and implications. Am J Cardiol 65:20B, 1990
Pritchett ELC: Management of atrial fibrillation. N Engl J Med 326:1264, 1992
Rosen MR, Bigger JT, Breithardt G, Brown AM: The Sicilian gambit: A new approach to the classification of antiarrhythmic drugs based on their actions on arrhythmogenic mechanisms. Circulation 84:1831, 1991

Nursing Bibliography

Benz M: Pharmacologic management of ventricular arrhythmias. Critical Care Nursing Clinics of North America 14(3):8, 1991
Creveling Paul S: New pharmacologic agents for emergency management of supraventricular tachydysrhythmias. Critical Care Nursing Quarterly 16(2):35, 1993
Schoenbaum M, Drew B: Proarrhythmia: Mechanisms, evaluations and treatment. Critical Care Nursing Clinics of North America 14(2):10, 1991
Starks Bledsoe D, Vespe M: Heading off sudden cardiac death. Nursing '92 22(11):52, 1992

33
Antihypertensive Drugs

Diuretics

Beta-Adrenergic Blocking Agents

Labetalol

Angiotensin-Converting Enzyme Inhibitors

- Benazepril
- Captopril
- Fosinopril
- Lisinopril
- Enalapril
- Quinapril
- Ramipril

Alpha$_1$-Adrenergic Blocking Agents

- Doxazosin
- Prazosin
- Terazosin

Calcium Channel Blockers

- Amlodipine
- Diltiazem
- Felodipine
- Isradipine
- Nicardipine
- Nifedipine
- Verapamil

Central Alpha$_2$-Adrenergic Agonists

- Clonidine
- Guanabenz
- Guanfacine
- Methyldopa

***Rauwolfia* Derivatives**

- Rauwolfia Whole Root
- Rescinnamine
- Reserpine

Vascular Smooth Muscle Relaxants

- Hydralazine
- Minoxidil

Peripheral Antiadrenergics

- Guanadrel
- Guanethidine

Drugs for Hypertensive Emergencies

- Diazoxide, Parenteral
- Nitroprusside
- Trimethaphan

Miscellaneous Antihypertensive Drugs

- Mecamylamine
- Metyrosine
- Phenoxybenzamine
- Phentolamine

Drug therapy of hypertension is directed toward reducing elevated arterial pressure, which is believed to be the primary cause of vascular degeneration and other complications that impair health and reduce life expectancy. The etiology of most cases of hypertension is unknown, and thus treatment is essentially palliative—that is, directed at lowering the elevated systolic and diastolic pressures.

Nevertheless, judicious use of one or more of the available antihypertensive agents can provide excellent control of blood pressure for extended periods. Drug therapy has clearly been shown to reduce the cardiovascular morbidity associated with hypertension. *The Fifth Report of the Joint National Committee on the Detection, Evaluation, and the Treatment of High Blood Pressure* (JNC V) has been published; a new classification system for hypertension discourages the terms "mild hypertension" and "moderate hypertension" (Table 33-1). This was done because most people with high blood pressure were labeled as having mild hypertension. This term did not emphasize the seriousness of the condition, even though most of the morbidity and mortality is seen in this group. In addition, the previous steps in the stepped-care approach, as outlined in previous editions, have been changed to reflect the importance of lifestyle modifications in addition to drug therapy in treating milder forms of hypertension. An algorithm that outlines the new approach to stepped-care treatment of hypertension is presented in Figure 33-1. Drug therapy is now only one aspect of a complete therapeutic regimen that also should include proper diet, exercise, and reduced salt intake.

The wide range of antihypertensive medications in clinical use today allows the physician carefully to tailor drug therapy to the needs of each hypertensive patient. Stage 1 hypertension frequently can be controlled by single-drug therapy, whereas more elevated pressures may require one or more additional antihypertensive agents in the regimen. Combination drug therapy enhances the pharmacologic effects of each drug, so that smaller individual doses can be used and the incidence and severity of untoward reactions thereby reduced. Control of all degrees of blood pressure can therefore be attained, in most instances, with minimal untoward effects on the patient.

The treatment goal is a systolic blood pressure below 140 mm Hg and a diastolic blood pressure below 90 mm Hg. In some patients, the goal may be even lower (130/85).

Clinically effective antihypertensive drugs act at many sites in the body and through numerous mechanisms. They have a wide range of potencies, side effects, and potential interactions. Choice of a suitable antihypertensive drug depends on many factors, such as the degree of hypertension being treated, the presence of other disease states (eg, reserpine is contraindicated in active hepatic disease), the presence of other drugs (eg, antidepressants reduce guanethidine's effectiveness), and a patient's acceptance of the mild yet often inescapable side effects of many agents. Although many antihypertensive drugs have more than one site or mechanism of action, they can be conveniently grouped according to their *principal sites* of action, recognizing, however, that these may not be the only active sites for many of the compounds. Such a grouping is presented in Table 33-2.

Diuretics and beta-blockers are the only two classes of antihypertensive agents that have been shown to reduce morbidity and mortality. For this reason, the JNC V recommends these two classes as first-line agents unless they are contraindicated. Alternative agents include angiotensin-converting enzyme (ACE) inhibitors, calcium channel blockers, alpha$_1$ receptor blockers, and labetalol. These drugs may be used when diuretics and beta-blockers are contraindicated or when they can treat a coexisting disease (eg, benign prostatic hypertrophy that can be treated with an alpha$_1$-blocker).

If initial therapy does not produce the desired results, either

Table 33-1. **Classification of Blood Pressure for Adults Aged 18 Years and Older**

Category	*Systolic (mm Hg)*	*Diastolic (mm Hg)*
Normal	<130	<85
High normal	130–139	85–89
Hypertension		
Stage 1 (mild)	140–159	90–99
Stage 2 (moderate)	160–179	100–109
Stage 3 (severe)	180–209	110–119
Stage 4 (very severe)	≥210	≥120

the dose must be increased, another drug substituted, or a second agent from a different class added. When diuretics are not used initially, and when they are not contraindicated, they usually should be the second agent added. The agents mentioned thus far, either as monotherapy or combination therapy, produce effective results in most patients. Other agents, however, such as methyldopa, clonidine, peripheral adrenergic antagonists, or vascular smooth muscle relaxants (hydralazine, minoxidil), may be used in certain clinical settings as supplemental agents.

Hypertensive emergencies are best managed by intravenous (IV) sodium nitroprusside or diazoxide, both vascular smooth muscle relaxants, or by trimethaphan, a ganglionic blocking agent. Pheochromocytoma, a catecholamine-secreting tumor of chromaffin tissue (eg, adrenal medulla), leads to marked elevations in blood pressure. Metyrosine or possibly phentolamine can be used to reduce the excessively high blood pressure seen in pheochromocytoma.

Several classes of antihypertensive agents have been discussed in previous chapters (eg, alpha- and beta-adrenergic blocking agents, ganglionic blocking agents); only those aspects related to their antihypertensive action are mentioned here. Likewise, diuretics are reviewed in detail in Chapter 39, and are not considered in this chapter. Calcium channel blockers also are useful antihypertensive agents because of their peripheral vasodilating action; their antihypertensive action is discussed in this chapter, whereas their other uses are considered in Chapters 32 and 34.

Preferred First-Line Agents

Diuretics are still recognized as initial drugs of choice for stage 1 hypertension *in most patients*, and their overall safety record is quite good, especially when electrolyte levels are controlled. Serious untoward reactions, however, such as arrhythmias (some fatal), and increases in serum triglycerides, blood viscosity, and platelet aggregation have been associated with use of diuretics, particularly in large doses or in patients with cardiac abnormalities. These have prompted a reevaluation of the relative role of diuretics versus beta-blockers as initial therapy in treating mild, uncomplicated hypertension, and have also suggested a possible role for the ACE inhibitors as drugs for treating mild hypertension.

Owing to the concerns about diuretics, there is increasing support for the use of beta-blockers in the initial pharmacologic treatment of mild hypertension, although it must be recognized that these drugs are capable of causing untoward reactions as

Table 33-2. **Antihypertensive Drugs: Principal Sites of Action**

CNS

Cardiovascular centers (hypothalamus, medulla)
- Clonidine/guanabenz/guanfacine
- Methyldopa
- Beta-adrenergic blockers

Sympathetic Ganglia

Ganglionic blocking agents

Adrenergic Nerve Endings

Alpha-adrenergic blockers
Beta-adrenergic blockers
Reserpine and rauwolfia derivatives
Guanethidine/guanadrel
Metyrosine
Pargyline

Vascular Smooth Muscle

Hydralazine
Diazoxide
Minoxidil
Nitroprusside
Diuretics
Calcium channel blockers

Kidney and Afferent Arteriole

Diuretics
Beta-adrenergic blockers

Renin–Angiotensin System

Angiotensin-converting enzyme inhibitors

well, such as bradycardia, congestive heart failure, and bronchoconstriction. Although the choice of a diuretic versus a beta-blocker is still largely a matter of physician preference, there are definite precautions that must be observed when making this choice. Diuretics usually are preferred in patients with congestive heart failure, sinus bradycardia, and asthma, whereas beta-blockers are a logical choice in patients with cardiac arrhythmias, tachycardia, angina, hyperuricemia, and coagulation disorders.

Diuretics

See Chapter 39.

Beta-Adrenergic Blocking Agents

- ***Acebutolol***
- ***Atenolol***
- ***Betaxolol***
- ***Bisoprolol***
- ***Carteolol***
- ***Metoprolol***
- ***Nadolol***
- ***Penbutolol***
- ***Pindolol***
- ***Propranolol***
- ***Timolol***

Beta-blockers have numerous clinical indications, and are considered in detail in Chapter 15. Most of the available beta-

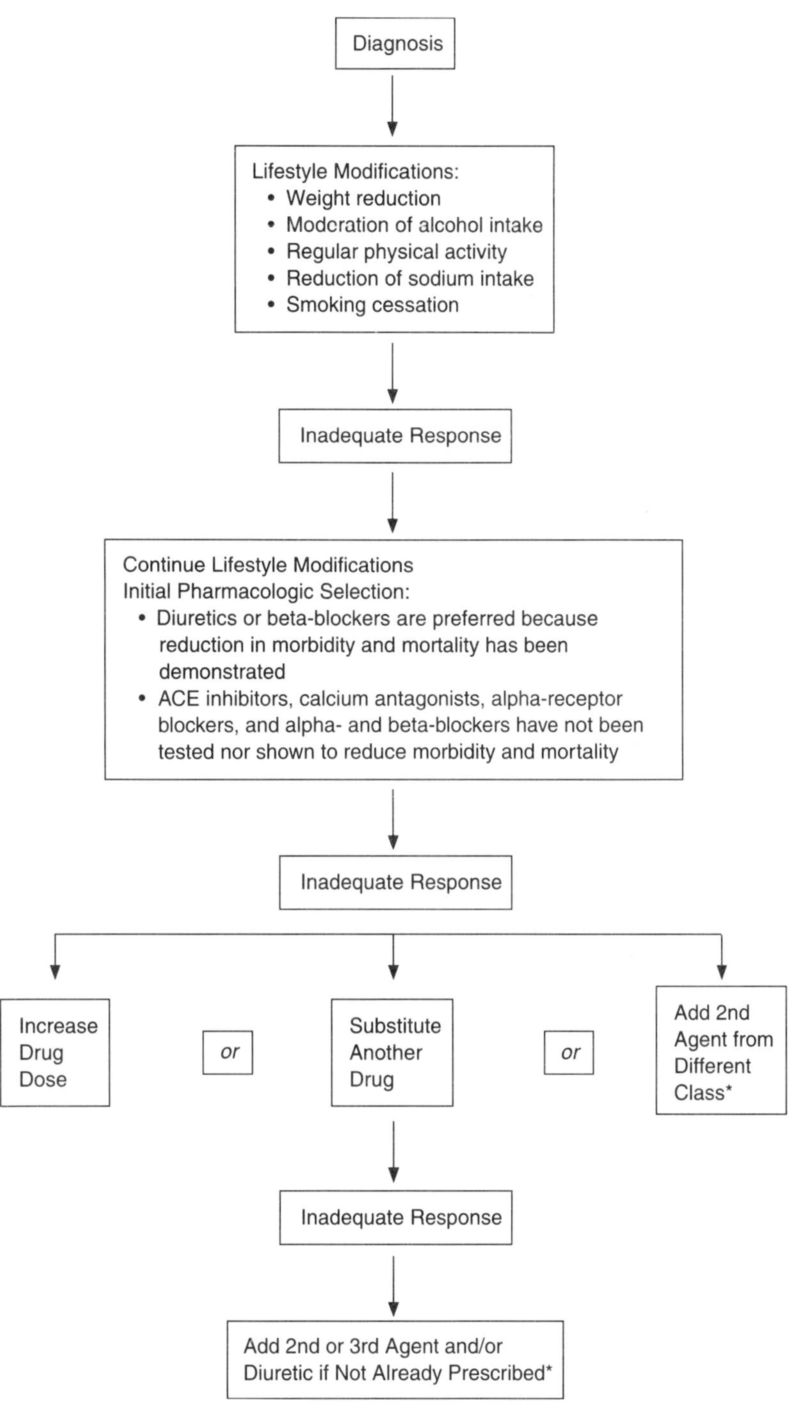

Figure 33-1. Algorithm for treatment of hypertension.

*Other agents include alpha$_2$ agonists, peripherally acting antiadrenergics, vascular smooth muscle relaxants, and rauwolfia derivatives.

blockers are approved for use in treating hypertension, and that particular indication is discussed in the following sections.

Mechanism

Not completely established; these agents can decrease cardiac output, reduce release of renin from the juxtaglomerular cells of the kidney (thus decreasing production of angiotensin and secretion of aldosterone), and impede outflow of sympathetic (ie, vasoconstrictor and cardioaccelerator) impulses from brain stem vasomotor control centers to peripheral organs; in addition, beta-blockers may retard release of norepinephrine from adrenergic nerve endings by blockade of presynaptic beta receptors, thereby reducing the vasoconstrictive action of endogenous norepinephrine.

Dosage

For hypertension only.

Acebutolol (Sectral): Initially, 400 mg in a single or twice-daily dose; usual dosage range is 400 to 800 mg daily, to a maximum of 1200 mg/day

Atenolol (Tenormin; [CAN] Apo-Atenol, Novo-Atenol, Nu-Atenol): Initially, 50 mg as a single daily dose; increase to 100 mg as a single dose if an optimal response is not achieved within 2 weeks; further dosage increases are unlikely to provide additional benefit; available in combination with chlorthalidone (25 mg) as Tenoretic

Betaxolol (Kerlone): Initially, 10 mg once a day, increase the dose to 20 mg once a day if desired effect is not seen within 7 to 14 days; may increase to 40 mg once a day

Bisoprolol (Zebeta): Initially 2.5 to 5 mg, adjust up to a maximum of 20 mg daily if necessary

Carteolol (Cartrol): Initially, 2.5 mg as a single daily dose; may increase up to 10 mg once daily if necessary; usual dosage range 2.5 to 5 mg once daily

Metoprolol (Lopressor; [CAN] Apo-Metoprolol, Betaloc, Novometoprol): Initially 100 mg/day in a single dose or 2 divided doses; increase at weekly intervals until optimal blood pressure reduction is attained; usual maintenance range is 100 to 450 mg/day; once-daily administration with lower doses of immediate-release preparations may not provide 24-hour control, which may require extended-release product; available in combination with hydrochlorothiazide as Lopressor HCT

Nadolol (Corgard; [CAN] Apo-Nadol, Syn-Nadolol): Initially, 40 mg once daily; increase gradually in 40- to 80-mg increments until optimal effect is noted; usual maintenance range is 80 to 320 mg/day in a single dose; also available in fixed combination with bendroflumethiazide (5 mg) as Corzide

Penbutolol (Levatol): 20 mg once daily; may increase to 40 to 80 mg once daily if necessary

Pindolol (Visken; [CAN] Apo-Pindol, Novo-Pindol, Nu-Pindol, Syn-Pindolol): Initially, 5 mg twice a day; adjust dosage in increments of 10 mg/day at 2- to 3-week intervals; maximum dose is 60 mg/day

Propranolol (Inderal; [CAN] Apo-Propranolol, Detensol, Noropranol, PMS Propranolol): Initially, 40 mg twice a day or 80 mg (sustained-release) once daily; adjust gradually to optimal effect; usual dosage ranges are 120 to 240 mg/day in 2 to 3 divided doses or 120 to 160 mg once daily as sustained-release dosage forms; maximum daily dose is 640 mg; available in combination with hydrochlorothiazide as Inderide

Timolol (Blocadren; [CAN] Apo-Timol): Initially, 10 mg twice a day; usual maintenance range is 20 to 40 mg/day in 1 or 2 divided doses; maximum dose is 60 mg/day in 2 divided doses; available in combination with hydrochlorothiazide as Timolide

Alpha/Beta Adrenergic Blocking Agent

• Labetalol

Normodyne, Trandate

Mechanism

A unique adrenergic blocking agent that combines an alpha$_1$ blocking action with a nonspecific beta-blocking action at both beta$_1$ and beta$_2$ receptor sites; ratio of alpha-to-beta blockade with oral administration is approximately 1:3; blood pressure is lowered by labetalol, standing pressure more so than supine (owing to the alpha$_1$ blocking action), but changes in heart rate are minimal; exercise-induced increases in heart rate and blood pressure are blunted, and elevated plasma renin levels are reduced; cardiac output and renal function are relatively unaffected, as are atrioventricular conduction time and refractory period; also appears to possess some intrinsic beta$_2$ agonist activity, although the clinical significance of this action is not known; postural hypotension can occur.

Uses

Treatment of mild to moderate hypertension, either alone or combined with other antihypertensive agents, especially diuretics

Emergency control of blood pressure in severe hypertension (IV administration)

Dosage

Oral: 100 mg twice a day as an initial dose; increased in increments of 100 mg twice a day every 2 to 3 days until the desired effect is obtained; usual oral maintenance dose is 200 to 400 mg twice a day, although up to 2400 mg/day has been used in severe hypertension

IV (hypertensive emergency): 20 mg injected over 2 minutes; additional injections of 40 to 80 mg can be given every 10 minutes thereafter until the desired supine blood pressure is attained or a total of 300 mg has been administered; alternatively, 2 mg/min (2 mL/min of diluted injection solution) can be infused IV until the desired blood pressure response has been attained; usual IV dosage range is 50 to 200 mg. Labetalol is compatible with and stable in 5% dextrose, 0.9% sodium chloride, dextrose and sodium chloride mixtures, Ringer's solution, and lactated Ringer's solution. It is *not* compatible with 5% sodium bicarbonate injection

Fate

Completely absorbed orally; peak plasma levels occur within 1 to 2 hours; maximum effects with a single dose are noted within 2 to 4 hours, and effects persist 8 to 12 hours; undergoes extensive first-pass hepatic metabolism; drug is approximately 50% protein bound.

Maximum effect after IV injection occurs within 5 minutes and persists for up to 12 to 15 hours after discontinuation; drug is partially metabolized in the liver and excreted both in the urine and feces and by way of the bile as conjugated metabolites as well as unchanged drug; elimination half-life after oral and IV administration is 6 hours and 5.5 hours, respectively.

Common Side Effects

Nausea, fatigue, dizziness, rash, tingling of skin and scalp.

Significant Adverse Reactions

Systemic lupus-like reaction; in addition, refer to Chapter 15 for the adverse reactions associated with alpha- and beta-adrenergic blockers, which may also occur with labetalol.

Contraindications

Bronchial asthma, severe bradycardia, second- or third-degree heart block, cardiac failure, cardiogenic shock. *Cautious use* in patients with bronchitis, emphysema, diabetes mellitus, or hepatic dysfunction, and in pregnant or nursing women.

Interactions

Labetalol can reduce the bronchodilator effects of beta-adrenergic agonists.
The incidence of tremor with combined use of labetalol and tricyclic antidepressants is significantly higher than with use of labetalol alone.
Cimetidine can increase the plasma levels of labetalol.
Labetalol reduces the reflex tachycardia seen with direct-acting vasodilators.

In addition, see Chapter 15 for a list of other potential interactions for $alpha_1$ antagonists and beta-adrenergic antagonists.

Nursing Management

Pretherapy Assessment

Assess and record baseline data necessary for detection of adverse effects of labetalol: General: VS, body weight, skin color and temperature; CNS: orientation, reflexes; CVS: baseline ECG, peripheral perfusion; GI: normal output, bowel sounds, liver evaluation; Laboratory: liver and thyroid function tests, blood and urine glucose, urinalysis.
Review medical history and documents for existing or previous conditions that:
a. require cautious use of labetalol: bronchitis, emphysema, diabetes mellitus, or hepatic dysfunction.
b. contraindicate use of labetalol: allergy to beta-blockers; bronchial asthma; severe bradycardia; second- or third-degree heart block; cardiac failure; cardiogenic shock; **pregnancy (Category C)**; lactation (secreted in breast milk, safety not established; if drug is required, do not nurse).

Nursing Interventions

Medication Administration

Take lying and standing blood pressures 1 to 3 hours after an initial oral dose or dose increment to detect postural hypotension.
Prepare patient for prolonged supine positioning before IV administration. During and for up to 3 hours after IV administration, maintain patient in supine position to avoid postural hypotension (high incidence).
Take patient's supine blood pressure (maximum effect usually occurs within 5 minutes after injection) immediately before IV injection and at 5 and 10 minutes after each injection.
Monitor blood pressure every 15 to 30 minutes during IV infusion.
Use microdrip IV administration set and an infusion control device to ensure accuracy. Monitor flow rate continuously.
Administer 1 hour before or 2 hours after meals.
Provide small, frequent meals if GI upset is severe.

Surveillance During Therapy

Review results of antinuclear antibody titers, which should be performed periodically to detect a systemic lupus-like reaction, for patient on long-term therapy.
Recognize that drug has both alpha- and beta-antiadrenergic effects. Unlike drugs with only beta-antiadrenergic effects, labetalol does not require routine monitoring of heart rate and cardiac output.
Carefully monitor laboratory studies and patient for indications of adverse reactions.
Interpret results of diagnostic tests and contact practitioner as appropriate.
Monitor for possible drug–drug and drug–nutrient interactions; see Interactions.

Patient Teaching

Recommend that patient take drug with food if nausea occurs. Nausea is an early, but usually transient, side effect.
Instruct patient on long-term therapy to report any symptoms of a systemic lupus-like reaction, such as joint pain, stiffness, or dyspnea.

Angiotensin-Converting Enzyme (ACE) Inhibitors

- ***Benazepril***
- ***Captopril***
- ***Enalapril***
- ***Fosinopril***
- ***Lisinopril***
- ***Quinapril***
- ***Ramipril***

These drugs are orally effective antihypertensive drugs that are used either alone or in combination with other antihypertensive agents in treating mild to moderate hypertension. These drugs (especially captopril) also may be used at higher doses for controlling more severe, resistant forms of hypertension, although at these elevated dose levels serious toxicity such as blood dyscrasias or renal damage can occur with captopril. They are discussed as a group in the following sections, and listed individually in Table 33-3.

Mechanism

ACE inhibitors inhibit the angiotensin-converting enzyme that hydrolyzes inactive angiotensin I to active angiotensin II in the plasma and lungs (see Fig. 30-4). Inhibition of ACE reduces the formation of the pressor substance angiotensin II and decreases the angiotensin-mediated secretion of aldosterone from the adrenal cortex. Peripheral vascular resistance is lowered, and salt and water retention is reduced. Plasma renin activity increases owing to loss of negative feedback, and serum potassium may rise owing to absence of aldosterone activity. No significant change in cardiac output occurs, but renal blood flow is increased. Both supine and standing blood pressure are lowered to approximately the same extent. Orthostatic hypotension is rare, and reflex tachycardia seldom occurs.

Table 33-3. Angiotensin-Converting Enzyme (ACE) Inhibitors

Drug	*Usual Dosage Range*	*Nursing Considerations*
Captopril *Capoten (CAN) Apo-Captopril, Novo-Capto, Syncaptopril*	*Mild hypertension:* 12.5–25 mg 2–3 times/day; increase gradually as needed *Moderate–severe hypertension:* initially 25 mg 3 times/day; usual dosage range 50–150 mg 2–3 times/day *Congestive heart failure:* Initially 25–50 mg 3 times/day; usual maintenance dose is 50–100 mg 3 times/day	Used alone for mild hypertension and most often together with a diuretic and other antihypertensives for severe hypertension; also used as adjunctive therapy in congestive heart failure (see Chapter 31), because it reduces preload and afterload; rash is a common occurrence; proteinuria and neutropenia can occur at high doses
Enalapril *Vasotec*	*Oral:* initially 5 mg once daily; usual dosage range 10–40 mg daily in a single or 2 divided doses *IV:* 1.25 mg every 6 h given over 5 min; in patients receiving diuretics, 0.625 mg IV over 5 min *Congestive heart failure:* Initially 2.5 mg 1–2 times/day; usual maintenance dose is 5–20 mg/day in two divided doses	After absorption, drug is hydrolyzed to enalaprilat, a more potent ACE inhibitor; also used in congestive heart failure; headache and dizziness are most common side effects; may elevate serum potassium; also available for IV injection as enalaprilat; peak effects may not occur for 4 h, however; has been used up to 7 days IV
Lisinopril *Prinivil, Zestril*	Initially 10 mg once daily; usual dosage range 20–40 mg/day *Congestive heart failure:* 5–20 mg/day as a single dose	Long-acting ACE inhibitor; a diuretic may be added if control with lisinopril alone is inadequate; reduce initial dose in elderly and in patients with impaired renal function
Benazepril *Lotensin*	Initially 10 mg daily; usual range 20–40 mg/day as a single or divided dose	Benazepril, fosinopril, quinapril, and ramipril are all long-acting ACE inhibitors with similar characteristics. The following is applicable to all of them: Serum potassium levels can be elevated by concurrent use of ACE inhibitors and potassium-sparing diuretics or potassium supplements; excessive hypotension has occurred after ACE inhibitor administration, especially in severely salt- or volume-depleted patients, such as those with severe congestive heart failure who are receiving diuretics; excessive perspiration, vomiting, diarrhea, or dehydration may increase the likelihood of extreme hypotension; caution must be used when initiating therapy with these agents in patients who are receiving other blood pressure-lowering drugs such as diuretics or adrenergic inhibitors; drugs frequently produce a dry, hacking cough
Fosinopril *Monopril*	Initially 10 mg once daily; usual dosage range 20–40 mg once, or twice daily	
Quinapril *Accupril*	Initially 10 mg once daily; usual dosage range 20–80 mg/day as a single or divided dose	
Ramipril *Altace*	Initially 1.25–2.5 mg once daily; usual dosage range 2.5–20 mg/day as a single or divided dose	

Inhibition of the converting enzyme by these drugs also appears to *decrease* the inactivation of bradykinin, a potent endogenous vasodilator, an action that may also contribute to the blood pressure-lowering effect. An increased synthesis of prostaglandin E, which may result in peripheral vasodilation, has been proposed as an additional action, possibly resulting from the increased levels of bradykinin.

In patients with congestive heart failure, these agents decrease systemic vascular resistance (ie, afterload) and pulmonary capillary wedge pressure, and increase cardiac output

Uses

Treatment of all degrees of hypertension, either alone or combined with other drugs, especially diuretics, because blood pressure-lowering effects are additive
- *Small doses* may be used in stage 1 hypertension in patients with normal renal function, especially when alternative drugs are inappropriate or ineffective
- *Large doses* may be used in moderate to severe forms of hypertension in patients who fail to respond to or cannot tolerate other multiple-drug regimens (risk of toxicity is significantly increased)

Treatment of refractive congestive heart failure, sometimes combined with digoxin, a diuretic, or both

Treatment of diabetic neuropathy

Symptomatic treatment of rheumatoid arthritis, idiopathic edema and Raynaud's disease (investigational uses for captopril)

Dosage

See Table 33-3.

Fate

ACE inhibitors are adequately absorbed orally, although the presence of food can reduce absorption of captopril by 30% to 40%; maximal blood pressure-lowering effect is achieved within 60 to 90 minutes with captopril and within 4 to 6 hours with enalapril and lisinopril; however, optimal clinical antihypertensive effects may require several weeks to develop. After absorption, enalapril is converted to enalaprilat, a more potent ACE inhibitor. The elimination half-life of captopril is less than 2 hours, but may be up to 12 hours for lisinopril and up to 36 hours for enalaprilat. Approximately 95% of a dose of each drug is eliminated within 24 hours, in both the urine and the feces. Benazepril, fosinopril, quinapril, and ramipril are long-acting drugs, similar to lisinopril.

Common Side Effects

(Incidence varies among individual drugs.) Gastrointestinal (GI) upset, loss of taste sensation, rash, pruritus, headache, dizziness, fatigue, chronic nonproductive cough.

Significant Adverse Reactions

CAUTION

Excessive hypotension has occurred after ACE inhibitor administration, especially in severely salt- or volume-depleted patients, such as those with severe congestive heart failure who are receiving diuretics. Excessive perspiration, vomiting, diarrhea, or dehydration may increase the likelihood of extreme hypotension. Caution must be used when initiating therapy with these agents in patients who are receiving other blood pressure-lowering drugs such as diuretics or adrenergic inhibitors.

NOTE: Not all of the following adverse reactions have been noted with each drug.

CV: tachycardia, chest pain, palpitations, flushing, hypotension, angina, congestive heart failure, myocardial infarction (rare)
GI: nausea, gastric irritation, abdominal pain, diarrhea, vomiting, peptic ulcer,
CNS: malaise, insomnia, headache
Hematologic: neutropenia, agranulocytosis, eosinophilia, hemolytic anemia
Dermatologic: photosensitivity, angioedema, paresthesias, flushing, pallor, alopecia, hyperhidrosis, rash, pruritus
Renal: proteinuria, oliguria, polyuria, urinary frequency, renal insufficiency
Other: dry mouth, dyspnea, lymphadenopathy, Raynaud's disease, laryngeal edema, elevated liver enzymes.

Contraindications

CAUTION

ACE inhibitors can cause fetal and neonatal morbidity and death when administered during pregnancy, especially during the second and third trimesters. When pregnancy is confirmed, ACE inhibitors should be discontinued.

Cautious use in patients with severe renal dysfunction, systemic lupus-like syndrome, reduced white cell counts, valvular stenosis, or diabetes mellitus, and in pregnant or nursing women.

Interactions

The hypotensive effects of ACE inhibitors may be increased by diuretics, adrenergic blocking agents, other antihypertensive drugs, nifedipine, and by severe salt or fluid restriction (see CAUTION under Significant Adverse Reactions).
Serum potassium levels can be elevated by concurrent use of ACE inhibitors and potassium-sparing diuretics or potassium supplements.
Vasodilators (eg, nitrites) may be potentiated by these agents and should be discontinued before beginning therapy with ACE inhibitors.
The antihypertensive efficacy of captopril can be reduced by indomethacin and possibly by aspirin and other salicylates.
Plasma levels of digoxin and lithium may be increased after adding an ACE inhibitor.

Nursing Management

Pretherapy Assessment

Assess and record baseline data necessary for detection of adverse effects of ACE inhibitors: General: vital signs (VS), body weight, skin color and temperature; CNS: orientation, reflexes; Cardiovascular system (CVS): baseline electrocardiogram (ECG), peripheral perfusion; GI: normal output, bowel sounds, liver evaluation; Laboratory: liver and kidney function tests, complete blood count (CBC) with differential, urinalysis.
Review medical history and documents for existing or previous conditions that:
a. require cautious use of ACE inhibitors: severe renal dysfunction; systemic lupus-like syndrome; reduced white cell counts; valvular stenosis; diabetes mellitus.
b. contraindicate use of ACE inhibitors: allergy to captopril or other angiotensin converting enzyme inhibitors; **pregnancy (Category C [first trimester]; Category D [second and third trimester])**; lactation (secreted in breast milk, safety not established; if drug is required, do not nurse).

Nursing Interventions

Medication Administration

Administer 1 hour before or 2 hours after meals.
Arrange for bowel program if constipation occurs.
Provide small, frequent meals if GI upset is severe.

Surveillance During Therapy

Monitor results of urinary protein estimates, which should be performed before therapy and at monthly intervals thereafter. If proteinuria exceeds 1 g/day, drug should be discontinued unless benefits clearly outweigh risks.
Review results of white blood cell and differential counts, which should be obtained before therapy and at 2-week intervals during early months of treatment.
Monitor closely in any situation that may lead to a fall in blood pressure because excessive hypotension may occur.
Carefully monitor laboratory studies and patient for indications of adverse reactions.
Interpret results of diagnostic tests and contact practitioner as appropriate.

Monitor for possible drug–drug and drug–nutrient interactions; see Interactions.

Patient Teaching

Explain that several weeks of careful monitoring may be required to titrate the dosage gradually to achieve full therapeutic benefit.
Instruct patient to take drug with water either 1 hour before or 2 hours after a meal (to enhance absorption).
Advise patient that drug may alter taste perception during therapy.
Stress importance of reporting any signs of infection (fever, sore throat), possible signs of neutropenia, which are indications for withdrawing drug if white cell count is abnormal.
Instruct patient to notify practitioner if mouth sores, swelling of hands or feet, irregular heartbeat, or chest pains occur.
Recommend that patient maintain the same salt intake as before therapy because salt restriction can lead to a precipitous drop in blood pressure with initial doses of these drugs.
Warn patient that excessive perspiration and dehydration (eg, due to diarrhea, vomiting) may lead to drastic reduction in blood pressure.
Consult practitioner or pharmacist before using aspirin or other nonprescription pain relievers.

Alpha$_1$-Adrenergic Blocking Agents

- **Prazosin**

Minipress

(CAN) Apo-Prazo, Novo-Prazin, Nu-Prazo

- **Terazosin**

Hytrin

- **Doxazosin**

Cardura

Mechanism

Selectively block postsynaptic alpha$_1$ receptor sites and dilate both resistance (ie, arterioles) and capacitance (ie, veins) vessels; therefore, little change in cardiac output, heart rate, renal blood flow, or glomerular filtration rate; blood pressure is lowered in both supine and standing positions, and effects are most pronounced on the diastolic pressure; reduce venous return (preload) and aortic impedance to left ventricular ejection (afterload); sodium and water retention can occur.

Uses

Treatment of mild to moderate hypertension, either alone or with a diuretic or other antihypertensive agent
Adjunctive treatment of severe, refractive congestive heart failure
Treatment of benign prostatic hyperplasia (terazosin *only*)

Dosage

Prazosin: Initially 1 mg 2 to 3 times/day; increase slowly to optimal response, up to 20 mg/day; usual maintenance range is 6 to 15 mg/day in 2 or 3 divided doses
Terazosin: Initially, 1 mg at bedtime; increase slowly to optimal response; usual dose range is 1 to 5 mg daily; maximum dose 20 mg/day
Benign prostatic hyperplasia: Initially 1 mg at bedtime; increase stepwise to 10 mg/day, the usual maintenance dose
Doxazosin: Initially 1 mg daily; measure the standing blood pressure 2 to 6 hours after the dose; depending on the response, increase the dose to 2 mg; further titrations to 4, 8, and 16 mg may be necessary

Fate

Oral absorption is not affected by food; peak plasma levels occur within 1 to 3 hours; protein binding is 90% to 98%; elimination half-life for prazosin, terazosin, and doxazosin are 2 to 3 hours, 9 to 12 hours, and 22 hours, respectively; drugs are excreted both in the urine and the bile.

Common Side Effects

Dizziness, headache, malaise, drowsiness, weakness, palpitations, nausea, nasal congestion.

Significant Adverse Reactions

Causal relationships not established in all cases.

GI: vomiting, constipation, abdominal pain
CV: tachycardia, angina, syncope (see Nursing Management regarding first-dose phenomenon) edema, orthostatic hypotension
CNS: nervousness, paresthesias, vertigo, depression
Other: urinary frequency or incontinence, impotence, rash, pruritus, dyspnea, blurred vision, tinnitus, dry mouth, epistaxis, diaphoresis, arthralgia, leukopenia, drug-induced lupus-like syndrome (rare)

Contraindications

No absolute contraindications. *Cautious use* in people who must drive or operate heavy machinery during early stages of therapy.

Interactions

Beta-blockers may increase the risk of postural hypotension after the first dose of prazosin; terazosin and doxazosin have been combined with beta-blockers safely.
Calcium channel blockers such as verapamil and nifedipine may produce significant hypotension when used in combination with prazosin.
Indomethacin can reduce the antihypertensive action of prazosin.
Alpha$_1$-blockers can decrease the antihypertensive effectiveness of clonidine.

Nursing Management

Pretherapy Assessment

Assess and record baseline data necessary for detection of adverse effects of alpha$_1$-blockers: General: VS, body weight, skin color and temperature; CNS: orientation, reflexes, ophthalmologic exam; CVS: orthostatic blood pressure, supine blood pressure, peripheral perfusion, edema; GI: normal output, bowel sounds, liver evaluation; Laboratory: kidney function tests, blood and urine glucose, urinalysis.

Review medical history and documents for existing or previous conditions that:

a. require cautious use of alpha$_1$-blockers: congestive heart failure; renal failure; use in people who must drive or operate equipment during the early phase of therapy.
b. contraindicate use of alpha$_1$-blockers: allergy to the drugs; **pregnancy (Category C)**; lactation (secreted in breast milk, safety not established; if drug is required, do not nurse).

Nursing Interventions

Medication Administration

Arrange to administer first dose of drug (at bedtime) to lessen likelihood of first-dose effect (syncope due to excessive postural hypotension). The initial dose of these drugs should be limited to 1 mg, dosage adjustments should be made gradually, and other antihypertensive medications should be added cautiously to avoid excessive hypotensive reactions.

Administer 1 hour before or 2 hours after meals.

Provide small, frequent meals if GI upset is severe.

Provide ready access to bathroom facilities if GI effects occur.

Monitor blood pressure frequently during changes in drug regimen.

Surveillance During Therapy

Monitor for orthostatic hypotension, which is most marked in the morning and accentuated in hot weather, with exercise, and with the use of alcohol.

Monitor for edema (body weight) in incipient cardiac decompensation; arrange to add a diuretic if sodium and fluid retention occur.

Carefully monitor laboratory studies and patient for indications of adverse reactions.

Interpret results of diagnostic tests and contact practitioner as appropriate.

Monitor for possible drug–drug and drug–nutrient interactions; see Interactions.

Provide for patient safety needs if CNS or hypotensive changes occur.

Patient Teaching

Recommend that patient take drug with food if nausea occurs. Nausea is an early, but usually transient, side effect.

Inform patient that fainting caused by excessive orthostatic hypotension can occur shortly after small, initial doses of alpha$_1$-blockers (first-dose phenomenon).

Teach patient to avoid use of over-the-counter (OTC) preparations, which can cause dangerous effects.

Teach patient that the following effects may occur as a result of therapy: dizziness, weakness; GI upset; impotence; dry mouth; stuffy nose.

Instruct patient to inform the practitioner if frequent dizziness or faintness occur.

Calcium Channel Blockers

Amlodipine (Norvasc)
Diltiazem (Cardizem, Dilacor XR)
Felodipine (Plendil)
Isradipine (DynaCirc)
Nicardipine (Cardene)
Nifedipine (Adalat CC, Procardia XL)
Verapamil (Calan, Isoptin, Verelan)

In addition to their use in treating arrhythmias (see Chapter 32) and for the prophylaxis of angina (see Chapter 34), several calcium channel blockers have been used for the control of mild to moderate hypertension. The drugs relax vascular smooth muscle and elicit peripheral vasodilation, thereby lowering blood pressure. They are well tolerated by most patients, the most frequent side effects being headache, nausea, dizziness, and mild peripheral edema. Adverse effects such as impotence, depression, and elevated serum lipids that have occurred with other agents used in mild hypertension do not seem to occur with calcium channel blockers.

Dosage

(see also Table 34-3)

Amlodipine: Initially, 5 mg daily; for elderly patients or those with hepatic failure, start with 2.5 mg daily; increase the dose after 7 to 14 days up to 10 mg daily if necessary

Diltiazem (sustained release)

Cardizem SR: 60 to 120 mg twice daily; adjust dosage every 2 weeks; usual dosage range is 240 to 360 mg per day

Cardizem CD/Dilacor XR: 180 to 240 mg daily, adjust dosage every 2 weeks, usual dosage range 240 to 360 mg per day for Cardizem CD; 180 to 480 mg per day for Dilacor XR

Felodipine: Initially 5 mg daily; adjust after 14 days; usual dosage range is 5 to 10 mg (maximum 20 mg daily)

Isradipine: Initially, 2.5 mg twice daily; adjust after 2 to 4 weeks; usual dosage range is 5 to 10 mg daily

Nicardipine

Immediate release: initially, 20 mg three times daily; usual range is 20 to 40 mg three times daily

Sustained release: Initially, 30 mg twice daily; usual range is 30 to 60 mg twice daily

Nifedipine (sustained release): Initially, 30 or 60 mg once daily; adjust doses every 7 to 14 days up to 120 mg daily

Verapamil: Initially, 80 mg three times daily; increase gradually as needed up to 360 mg daily. Maintenance with sustained release tablets is usually 240 mg once daily.

Contraindications

Diltiazem, Verapamil: Second- or third-degree heart block, systolic hypotension (<90 mm Hg), sick sinus syndrome

Diltiazem: Acute myocardial infarction and pulmonary congestion

Nicardipine: Advanced aortic stenosis

Verapamil: Severe left ventricular dysfunction, cardiogenic shock, severe congestive heart failure unless secondary to supraventricular tachycardia

Nursing Management

See Chapters 32 and 34 and Table 34-3.

Central Alpha$_2$-Adrenergic Agonists

- **Clonidine**

  Catapres

  (CAN) Dixarit

- **Guanabenz**

  Wytensin

- **Guanfacine**

  Tenex

Clonidine, guanabenz, and guanfacine are similar, orally active antiadrenergic agents that are indicated in the treatment of mild to moderate hypertension. In addition, clonidine is available as a transdermal patch (Clonidine-TTS). They are centrally acting antihypertensive drugs with a very low incidence of serious toxicity; principal side effects are drowsiness and dry mouth.

Mechanism

Activation of presynaptic adrenergic alpha$_2$ receptors in cardiovascular integrating centers in the brain stem, resulting in a decreased outflow of sympathetic vasoconstrictor and cardioaccelerator impulses; moderate reduction in pulse rate and cardiac output; decrease in plasma renin activity; initially, may stimulate peripheral alpha-adrenergic receptors, causing transient vasoconstriction.

Uses

Treatment of mild to moderate degrees of hypertension, either alone or with a diuretic or another antihypertensive drug

Investigational uses for *clonidine* include prophylaxis of migraine, treatment of episodes of menopausal flushing, symptomatic management of opiate detoxification, and treatment of Gilles de la Tourette disease

Dosage

Clonidine (for hypertension): Initially, 0.1 mg twice a day; increase by 0.1 to 0.2 mg/day to desired response; usual range is 0.2 to 0.8 mg/day in divided doses; maximum 2.4 mg/day; may be effective as a single daily dose; transdermal patch, apply 1 patch every 7 days; begin with 0.1-mg system and increase in 0.1-mg increments as needed

Guanabenz: Initially, 4 mg twice a day; increase in increments of 4 to 8 mg/day every 1 to 2 weeks; maximum dose is 32 mg a day in divided doses

Guanfacine: Initially, 1 mg daily at bedtime (usually with a diuretic); may increase up to 3 mg/day if necessary

Fate

Onset for all drugs is 30 to 60 minutes after oral administration; maximum effect in 2 to 4 hours; duration 6 to 8 hours; plasma half-life is 12 to 16 hours for clonidine and guanfacine and 6 to 8 hours for guanabenz; metabolized by the liver and excreted mainly in the urine both as unchanged drug and as metabolites.

Common Side Effects

Dry mouth, drowsiness, sedation, constipation, dizziness, headache, fatigue.

Significant Adverse Reactions

Not all reactions observed with all drugs.

GI: anorexia, nausea, vomiting, parotid pain, liver function test abnormalities

CNS: insomnia, nervousness, anxiety, depression, vivid dreams or nightmares

Dermatologic: rash, angioedema, urticaria, hives, hair loss, pruritus

CV: Raynaud's phenomenon (pallor, cyanosis, pain in extremities), palpitation, flushing, congestive heart failure (rare)

Other: weight gain, hyperglycemia, gynecomastia, urinary retention, impotence, itching or burning of eyes, pallor, dryness of nasal mucosa

Contraindications

No absolute contraindications. *Cautious use* in patients with coronary insufficiency, cerebrovascular disease, chronic renal failure, thromboangiitis obliterans, history of depression or recent myocardial infarction, and in pregnant women.

Interactions

Clonidine, guanabenz, and guanfacine may intensify the CNS-depressant effects of alcohol, barbiturates, narcotics, and other depressants.

Effects of clonidine, guanabenz, and guanfacine may be antagonized by tricyclic antidepressants (except doxepin) and tolazoline.

Excessive bradycardia can occur when clonidine, guanabenz, and guanfacine are used in combination with digitalis agents, propranolol, or guanethidine.

Nursing Management

Pretherapy Assessment

Assess and record baseline data necessary for detection of adverse effects of alpha$_2$ agonists: General: VS, body weight, skin color and temperature; CNS: orientation, reflexes, ophthalmologic examination; CVS: orthostatic blood pressure, supine blood pressure, peripheral perfusion, edema; GI: normal output, bowel sounds, liver evaluation; Laboratory: liver function tests, ECG.

Review medical history and documents for existing or previous conditions that:

a. require cautious use of alpha$_2$ agonists: coronary insufficiency; cerebrovascular disease; chronic renal failure; thromboangiitis obliterans; history of depression; recent myocardial infarction.
b. contraindicate use of alpha$_2$ agonists: allergy to

$alpha_2$ agonists or any component of the clonidine transdermal system; **pregnancy (Category C)**; lactation (concentrated in breast milk, safety not established; if drug is required, do not nurse).

Nursing Interventions

Medication Administration

Administer 1 hour before or 2 hours after meals.
Provide small, frequent meals if GI upset is severe.
Provide ready access to bathroom facilities if GI effects occur.
Use the transdermal system exactly as prescribed.
Do not discontinue therapy abruptly, because agitation, tachycardia, and rebound hypertension can occur. Discontinue therapy gradually over 3 to 4 days. If symptoms occur, be prepared to reinstitute drug or to administer both an alpha- and a beta-adrenergic blocker.

Surveillance During Therapy

Carefully monitor laboratory studies and patient for indications of adverse reactions.
Interpret results of diagnostic tests and contact practitioner as appropriate.
Monitor for possible drug–drug and drug–nutrient interactions; see Interactions.
Provide for patient safety needs if CNS or hypotensive changes occur.

Patient Teaching

Recommend that patient take drug with food if nausea occurs. Nausea is an early, but usually transient, side effect.
Teach patient to avoid use of OTC preparations, which can cause dangerous effects.
Suggest that significant others closely observe patient with a prior history of mental depression because these drugs can evoke depressive episodes.
Instruct patient to report any changes in pattern of urination because urinary hesitancy can occur.
Instruct patient to undergo periodic eye examinations during prolonged therapy because retinal degeneration may occur.
Inform patient that tolerance to drug effects can develop. If tolerance occurs, therapy should be reevaluated, and addition of other antihypertensive medications should be considered.
Inform patient that sensitivity to alcohol may be increased.
Teach patient that the following effects may occur as a result of therapy: dizziness; weakness; GI upset; impotence; dry mouth; stuffy nose; breast enlargement, tenderness.
Instruct patient to inform the practitioner if frequent dizziness, faintness, urinary retention, changes in vision, blanching of fingers, or skin rash occur.

• Methyldopa

Aldomet, Amodopa

(CAN) Apo-Methyldopa, Dopamet, Novomedopa, PMS Dopazide

Mechanism

Inhibits the enzyme aromatic amino acid decarboxylase by competitive antagonism, and is itself converted to alpha-methylnorepinephrine, which functions as an activator of central $alpha_2$-adrenergic receptors. Stimulation of brain stem $alpha_2$ receptors results in a decreased outflow of sympathetic vasoconstrictor and cardioaccelerator impulses, thereby producing vasodilation and bradycardia; may reduce plasma renin activity but does not significantly affect renal blood flow; cardiac output is usually decreased; diurnal blood pressure variations occur rarely; has a sedative action and promotes sodium and water retention.

Uses

Treatment of sustained moderate to moderately severe hypertension, either alone or more commonly with other antihypertensive agents
Treatment of acute hypertensive crises (methyldopate ester, IV); infrequently used owing to slow onset of action

Dosage

Oral
Adults: Initially 250 mg 2 to 3 times/day; adjust dosage by increments at intervals of not less than 2 days until desired response occurs; usual maintenance dosage 500 to 2000 mg/day in 2 to 4 divided doses (maximum 3 g/day)
Children: 10 mg/kg/day in 2 to 4 divided doses adjusted to desired level; maximum dose 65 mg/kg or 3 g daily
IV Infusion
Adults: 250 to 500 mg at 6-hour intervals (dose is added to 100 mL 5% dextrose injection and infused over 30 to 60 min); maximum dose 1 g every 6 hours
Children: 20 to 40 mg/kg in divided doses every 6 hours; maximum dose 3 g/day

Fate

Oral absorption is variable (range, 10%–60%); peak plasma levels occur in 2 to 4 hours, but maximal antihypertensive effect may not occur for several days; duration may persist for 24 hours even though elimination half-life is 2 to 3 hours; after IV infusion, maximal effects are seen in 4 to 8 hours and last 12 to 16 hours; appears rapidly in the urine, predominantly in unaltered form.

Common Side Effects

Sedation, headache, weakness, dry mouth, nasal stuffiness, weight gain, and positive direct Coombs' test (see Nursing Management, Surveillance During Therapy).

Significant Adverse Reactions

CV: bradycardia, anginal pain, orthostatic hypotension, edema, myocarditis, paradoxical pressor response with IV use
CNS: dizziness, paresthesias, Parkinson-like symptoms, choreoathetoid movements, psychoses, depression, nightmares, memory impairment
GI: nausea, vomiting, constipation, "black" tongue, abdominal distention, pancreatitis, sialadenitis

Hematologic: hemolytic anemia, leukopenia, thrombocytopenia, granulocytopenia
Hepatic: jaundice, liver dysfunction
Other: fever, myalgia, arthralgia, dermatoses, rash, nasal congestion, breast enlargement, gynecomastia, lactation, impotence, decreased libido
Laboratory test variations: abnormal liver function tests; positive tests for antinuclear antibody, lupus erythematosus cells, and rheumatoid factor; rise in blood urea nitrogen; falsely high urinary catecholamines

Contraindications

Active hepatic disease, blood dyscrasias. *Cautious use* in patients with chronic liver dysfunction, angina, renal impairment, pheochromocytoma, endocrine disorders, or anemia, and in pregnant or nursing women.

Interactions

Additive hypotensive effects can occur with methyldopa and anesthetics, alcohol, calcium channel blockers, diuretics and other antihypertensive drugs, fenfluramine, narcotics, methotrimeprazine, levodopa, quinidine, vasodilators.
Hypotensive action of methyldopa can be antagonized by amphetamines, catecholamines (except levodopa), tricyclic antidepressants, monoamine oxidase (MAO) inhibitors, phenothiazines, sympathomimetics, and vasopressors.
Methyldopa can potentiate the hypoglycemic action of tolbutamide.
Elevated serum lithium levels can occur with methyldopa.
Psychiatric disturbances can result from combined use of methyldopa and haloperidol.
Phenoxybenzamine and methyldopa together have resulted in reversible urinary incontinence.
Combinations of methyldopa and propranolol have occasionally resulted in paradoxical hypertension.

Nursing Management

Pretherapy Assessment

Assess and record baseline data necessary for detection of adverse effects of methyldopa: General: VS, body weight, skin color and temperature; CNS: orientation, reflexes, ophthalmologic examination; CVS: orthostatic blood pressure, supine blood pressure, peripheral perfusion, edema; GI: normal output, bowel sounds, liver evaluation; Endocrine: breast examination; Laboratory: liver and kidney function tests, urinalysis, CBC with differential, direct Coombs' test.
Review medical history and documents for existing or previous conditions that:

a. require cautious use of methyldopa: chronic liver dysfunction; angina; renal impairment; pheochromocytoma; endocrine disorders; anemia.
b. contraindicate use of methyldopa: allergy to methyldopa; active hepatic disease; blood dyscrasias; **pregnancy (Category C)**; lactation (concentrated in breast milk, safety not established; if drug is required, do not nurse).

Nursing Interventions

Medication Administration

Administer 1 hour before or 2 hours after meals.
Provide small, frequent meals if GI upset is severe.
Provide ready access to bathroom facilities if GI effects occur.
Check blood pressure repeatedly until stabilized and monitor urinary output during IV administration.
Be alert for development of paradoxic pressor response with IV use of methyldopate ester.

Surveillance During Therapy

Monitor results of complete blood counts and direct Coombs' tests, which should be performed before initiating therapy and periodically during drug treatment, because a positive Coombs' test, as well as hemolytic anemia and liver disorders, can occur and can lead to potentially fatal complications. A positive Coombs' test is observed in approximately 20% of patients on chronic therapy. It is dose dependent and may persist for 3 to 18 months after drug is withdrawn. In most cases, it is *not* clinically significant in the absence of other complications (eg, anemia, hepatitis). If a positive test develops, hemolytic anemia needs to be ruled out. Although a positive test is not in itself an indication for stopping therapy, if Coombs'-positive hemolytic anemia, non–dose-dependent drug fever, or hepatitis occur, the drug should be discontinued immediately.
Carefully monitor laboratory studies and patient for indications of adverse reactions.
Interpret results of diagnostic tests and contact practitioner as appropriate.
Monitor for possible drug–drug and drug–nutrient interactions; see Interactions.
Provide for patient safety needs if CNS or hypotensive changes occur.

Patient Teaching

Recommend that patient take drug with food if nausea occurs.
Teach patient to avoid use of OTC preparations, which can cause dangerous effects.
Teach patient to be alert for development of fever, chills, headache, pruritus, rash, arthralgia, and enlarged liver because reversible methyldopa hepatotoxicity occasionally occurs, especially during the first few months of therapy. Patient should notify practitioner if these occur so that liver function tests can be performed. If fever, jaundice, or liver function abnormalities appear, the drug should be discontinued.
Instruct patient to watch for appearance of involuntary movements and to advise practitioner if these occur, because the drug should be discontinued.
Inform patient that a breakdown product of drug may harmlessly darken urine.
Inform patient that tolerance to drug effects can develop. If tolerance occurs, therapy should be reevaluated, and addition of other antihypertensive medications should be considered.

Teach patient that the following effects may occur as a result of therapy: dizziness, weakness, dreams, nightmares, memory impairment, GI upset, impotence, dry mouth, stuffy nose, breast enlargement and tenderness.

Instruct patient to inform the practitioner if unexplained, prolonged general fatigue; yellowing of the skin or eyes; fever; bruising; or skin rash occur.

Rauwolfia Alkaloids

Rauwolfia whole root
Rescinnamine
Reserpine

The rauwolfia derivatives are a group of products derived from the *Rauwolfia* family of plants, comprising whole-root rauwolfia and the refined alkaloids rescinnamine and reserpine. These agents are infrequently used today, because they are no more effective than most other available antihypertensive medications and have the potential to elicit a wide range of troublesome side effects. They deplete central and peripheral neuronal stores of biogenic amines (ie, norepinephrine, serotonin) by blocking amine uptake into vesicular storage sites within the nerve ending, thus decreasing blood pressure, heart rate, and cardiac output. Rauwolfia derivatives are occasionally used in treating mild to moderate essential hypertension, usually in combination with other antihypertensive medications. Their maximum antihypertensive effect requires several weeks to develop and effects persist for weeks after discontinuation of therapy. Common side effects include drowsiness, nasal congestion, diarrhea, and bradycardia. Many other adverse effects have occurred during therapy with these agents, frequently involving the central nervous system. Rauwolfia drugs are contraindicated in mental depression, active peptic ulcer, ulcerative colitis, pheochromocytoma, and in patients receiving MAO inhibitors. *Cautious use* is required in patients with arrhythmias, obesity, epilepsy, bronchitis, gallstones, renal or hepatic dysfunction, and in pregnant women or nursing mothers.

Interactions

Enhanced hypotensive effects may be seen when rauwolfia derivatives are combined with anesthetics, barbiturates, diuretics and other antihypertensive drugs, methotrimeprazine, phenothiazines, quinidine, propranolol, and vasodilators.

Cardiac arrhythmias can occur if reserpine is given with digitalis, quinidine, or theophylline.

CNS-depressant effects of other agents (eg, alcohol, barbiturates, narcotics, antihistamines, phenothiazines) may be enhanced by reserpine.

Rauwolfia derivatives may decrease the effects of anticholinergics (antisecretory action), anticonvulsants, indirect-acting sympathomimetics (eg, ephedrine, amphetamine), levodopa, morphine, salicylates, vasopressors (eg, metaraminol, mephentermine).

If used with tricyclic antidepressants, rauwolfia derivatives may cause excitation and mania.

Excitation and hypertension can initially result from combined use of rauwolfia drugs and MAO inhibitors, but prolonged therapy can lead to severe depression and markedly increased GI activity.

Nursing Management

Pretherapy Assessment

Assess and record baseline data necessary for detection of adverse effects of rauwolfia alkaloids: General: VS, body weight, skin color and temperature; CNS: orientation, reflexes, ophthalmologic examination; CVS: orthostatic blood pressure, peripheral perfusion, edema; GI: normal output, bowel sounds, liver evaluation; Endocrine: breast examination; Laboratory: liver and kidney function tests, urinalysis, CBC with differential, stool guaiac test.

Review medical history and documents for existing or previous conditions that:

a. require cautious use of rauwolfia alkaloids: arrhythmias; obesity; epilepsy; bronchitis; gallstones; renal or hepatic dysfunction.
b. contraindicate use of rauwolfia alkaloids: allergy to rauwolfia derivatives; mental depression; active peptic ulcer; ulcerative colitis; pheochromocytoma; in patients receiving electroconvulsive therapy; therapy with MAO inhibitors; **pregnancy (Category C)**, lactation (secreted in breast milk, safety not established; if drug is required, do not nurse).

Nursing Interventions

Medication Administration

Administer with food or milk to minimize GI distress.

Provide small, frequent meals if GI upset is severe.

Provide ready access to bathroom facilities if GI effects occur.

Surveillance During Therapy

Carefully monitor laboratory studies and patient for indications of adverse reactions.

Interpret results of diagnostic tests and contact practitioner as appropriate.

Monitor for possible drug–drug and drug–nutrient interactions; see Interactions.

Provide for patient safety needs if CNS or hypotensive changes occur.

Patient Teaching

Recommend that drug be taken with food or milk to minimize GI distress.

Teach patient and significant others to report the first signs of drug-induced depression (despondency, insomnia, anorexia, impotence). Depressive effects of drug can, however, persist for months after withdrawal.

Inform patient that, although orthostatic hypotension is uncommon, dizziness and fainting may occur.

Inform patient that alcohol may increase both the hypotensive and CNS-depressant effects of the drug.

Explain that therapeutic effects may persist for up to 1 month after termination of therapy.

Inform patient that after prolonged use of rauwolfia alkaloids, ingestion of agents containing sympathomimetic amines, such as decongestants, cold preparations, or adrenergic bronchodilators, can result in excessive elevation of blood pressure because the receptivity of postsynaptic adrenergic receptors may be increased when presynaptic neurohormonal stores are depleted.

Instruct patient to inform practitioner of drug use before elective surgery because the drug should be discontinued several weeks earlier to avoid severe hypotension during anesthesia.

Teach patient that the following effects may occur as a result of therapy: dizziness, weakness, dreams, nightmares, memory impairment, GI upset, impotence, dry mouth, stuffy nose, breast enlargement or tenderness.

Instruct patient to inform the practitioner if bruising; nose bleeds; skin rash; depression or loss of interest in surroundings; habitual early morning awakening; painful urination; or black, tarry, or bloody stools occur.

Vascular Smooth Muscle Relaxants

• Hydralazine

Alazine, Apresoline

(CAN) Apo-Hydralazine, Novo-Hylazin, Nu-Hydral

Mechanism

Direct relaxation of vascular smooth muscle, primarily arteriolar, leading to decreased peripheral resistance; little effect on venous capacitance vessels; diastolic pressure is usually lowered more than systolic; no change or possibly an increase in renal and cerebral blood flow; reflex increase in heart rate, stroke volume, and cardiac output. In congestive heart failure, drug lowers peripheral arteriolar resistance, thereby improving cardiac output.

Uses

Management of moderate forms of hypertension, sometimes alone but more commonly in combination with other antihypertensive medications

Short-term treatment of severe essential hypertension (IV or IM)

Adjunctive treatment of congestive heart failure and severe aortic insufficiency, and after valve replacement

Dosage

Oral: initially 10 mg 4 times/day for 2 to 4 days; increase to 25 mg 4 times/day for balance of week; for second and subsequent weeks, increase to 50 mg 4 times/day; adjust to lowest effective levels for maintenance; twice-daily dosage may be adequate

IM, IV: initially, 5 to 10 mg; titrate upward slowly as needed and give at 30-minute intervals

Children: 0.1 to 0.2 mg/kg every 4 to 6 hours

Fate

Well absorbed orally; peak plasma levels occur within 2 hours; half-life is 2 to 8 hours; effects last for 6 to 8 hours; highly protein bound (85%–90%); onset after IM injection is 10 to 15 minutes and duration lasts 3 to 4 hours; IV administration results in immediate onset, with maximal response in 1 hour; metabolized by the liver and rapidly excreted, largely in the urine as metabolites.

Common Side Effects

Headache, nausea, vomiting, diarrhea, sweating, palpitations, tachycardia.

Significant Adverse Reactions

Paresthesias, numbness and tingling in extremities, anginal pain, tremors, disorientation, anxiety, depression, flushing, lacrimation, conjunctivitis, urticaria, pruritus, fever, chills, nasal congestion, muscle cramping, arthralgia, eosinophilia, constipation, difficulty in micturition, dyspnea, and paralytic ileus.

Reduced hemoglobin, leukopenia, agranulocytosis, and purpura.

Systemic lupus-like syndrome (doses greater than 400 mg/day) marked by fever, dermatoses, myalgia, arthralgia, anemia, splenomegaly, edema, and lymphadenopathy.

Contraindications

Rheumatic heart disease, coronary artery disease, and systemic lupus erythematosus. *Cautious use* in people with renal impairment, cerebral vascular disease, or peripheral neuritis, and in pregnant or nursing women.

Interactions

Additive hypotensive effects can occur with combined use of hydralazine and other antihypertensives.

Use with caution in patients receiving MAO inhibitors; a synergistic effect may cause excessive hypotension.

Nursing Management

Pretherapy Assessment

Assess and record baseline data necessary for detection of adverse effects of hydralazine: General: VS, body weight, skin color and temperature; CNS: orientation, reflexes, ophthalmologic examination; CVS: orthostatic blood pressure, supine blood pressure, peripheral perfusion, edema; GI: normal output, bowel sounds, liver evaluation; Endocrine: breast examination; Laboratory: liver and kidney function tests, urinalysis, CBC with differential, lupus erythematosus (LE) cell preparations; antinuclear antibody (ANA) preparations.

Review medical history and documents for existing or previous conditions that:

a. require cautious use of hydralazine: renal impairment; cerebral vascular disease; peripheral neuritis.
b. contraindicate use of hydralazine: allergy to hydralazine, tartrazine; rheumatic heart disease; coronary artery disease; systemic lupus erythematosus; **pregnancy (Category C)**; lactation (secreted in breast milk, safety not established; if drug is required, do not nurse).

Nursing Interventions

Medication Administration

Administer with food or milk to increase bioavailability.

Use parenteral hydralazine immediately after opening ampule. Hydralazine changes color after contact with metal; discolored solutions should be discontinued.

Arrange for CBC, LE cell preparations, antinuclear antibody titers before and periodically during therapy. Arrange to discontinue drug if blood dyscrasias occur.
Provide small, frequent meals if GI upset is severe.
Provide ready access to bathroom facilities if GI effects occur.

Surveillance During Therapy

Closely observe patient receiving large amounts (dosage should not exceed 400 mg/day) for signs of lupus-like reaction (eg, fever, myalgia, dermatoses, arthralgia, anemia, skin lesions). Drug should be discontinued and alternative antihypertensive medication used if signs develop. Most symptoms regress when drug is withdrawn, but residual effects may persist for years.
Carefully monitor laboratory studies and patient for indications of adverse reactions.
Interpret results of diagnostic tests and contact practitioner as appropriate.
Monitor for possible drug–drug and drug–nutrient interactions; see Interactions.
Provide for patient safety needs if CNS or hypotensive changes occur.

Patient Teaching

Suggest taking drug with meals because bioavailability is reportedly *enhanced* by ingestion when taken with food, which may decrease first-pass hepatic metabolism.
Inform patient that headache and palpitations may occur during early stages of therapy, but usually disappear.
Teach significant others how to recognize changes in patient's mental acuity because these may indicate cerebral ischemia. The practitioner should be notified if these occur.
Instruct patient to report signs of hydralazine-induced peripheral neuritis (paresthesias, numbness, tingling) to practitioner. Pyridoxine (vitamin B_6) may be used to alleviate these symptoms.
Explain to patient that periodic blood counts, lupus erythematosus cell preparations, and antinuclear antibody titer determinations should be performed during prolonged therapy.
Teach patient that the following effects may occur as a result of therapy: dizziness, weakness, nightmares, memory impairment, GI upset, impotence, dry mouth, stuffy nose.
Instruct patient to inform the practitioner if persistent or severe constipation, unexplained fever or malaise, or muscle or joint ache occur.

• Minoxidil

Loniten

Mechanism

Direct relaxation of arteriolar smooth muscle, possibly secondary to blockade of calcium uptake through the cell membrane, thus decreasing peripheral vascular resistance—little effect on venous tone; microcirculatory blood flow is maintained in all systemic vascular beds; does not enter CNS or interfere with vasomotor reflexes, and therefore does not elicit orthostatic hypotension; reflexly increases heart rate and cardiac output, renin secretion, and salt and water retention; topical application (as Rogaine) may increase hair growth in balding areas but effect lasts only as long as drug is applied.

Uses

Treatment of severe hypertension not manageable by maximum doses of a diuretic plus two other antihypertensive drugs; usually given together with a diuretic or a beta-blocker, or both; methyldopa and clonidine also have been used concurrently
Treatment of male pattern baldness (alopecia areata, androgenic alopecia) based on drug's ability to increase growth of fine body hair (see Common Side Effects)

Dosage

Usually given with a diuretic to minimize fluid retention and with a beta-blocker to reduce reflex bradycardia.

Adults: initially 5 mg/day orally as a single dose; increase stepwise to 40 mg/day in divided doses, or until optimal control is attained; usual range is 10 to 40 mg/day (maximum is 100 mg/day)

Children (<12 y): initially, 0.2 mg/kg/day as a single dose; increase in 50% to 100% increments until optimal control is attained; usual range is 0.25 to 1.0 mg/kg/day (maximum is 50 mg/day)

Fate

Well absorbed from the GI tract; maximum plasma levels occur within 60 minutes, effects are maximal in 2 to 3 hours and persist up to 24 hours; half-life is approximately 4 hours; almost completely metabolized in the liver and excreted principally in the urine; does not bind to plasma proteins.

Common Side Effects

Hypertrichosis (elongation, thickening, and enhanced pigmentation of fine body hair in 80% of patients within 3–6 weeks), temporary edema, ECG (ie, T-wave) changes *not* associated with other symptoms, sweating, headache, temporary edema.

Significant Adverse Reactions

CAUTION

Use only in severe hypertension because serious adverse reactions have occurred. Pericardial effusion, occasionally progressing to tamponade, has been reported, and anginal symptoms may be exacerbated.

Nausea; vomiting; fatigue; pericardial effusion; tamponade; reflex tachycardia; breast tenderness; temporary decreases in hemoglobin, hematocrit, and erythrocytes; increases in alkaline phosphatase and serum creatinine; hypersensitivity reactions.

Contraindications

Pheochromocytoma, acute myocardial infarction, dissecting aortic aneurysm. *Cautious use* in patients with cardiac disease, renal or hepatic insufficiency, in edematous states, and in pregnant or nursing women.

Interactions

Minoxidil may markedly worsen the degree of orthostatic hypotension caused by guanethidine.

Nursing Management

Pretherapy Assessment

Assess and record baseline data necessary for detection of adverse effects of minoxidil: General: VS, body weight, skin color and temperature; CVS: orthostatic blood pressure, supine blood pressure, peripheral perfusion, edema; GI: normal output, bowel sounds, liver evaluation; Endocrine: breast examination; Laboratory: kidney function tests, urinalysis, CBC with differential.

Review medical history and documents for existing or previous conditions that:

a. require cautious use of minoxidil: cardiac disease; renal or hepatic insufficiency; edematous states.

b. contraindicate use of minoxidil: allergy to minoxidil; pheochromocytoma; acute myocardial infarction; dissecting aortic aneurysm; **pregnancy (Category C)**; lactation (secreted in breast milk, safety not established; if drug is required, do not nurse).

Nursing Interventions

Medication Administration

Administer without regard to meals.

Provide small, frequent meals if GI upset is severe.

Provide ready access to bathroom facilities if GI effects occur.

Surveillance During Therapy

Closely monitor laboratory studies and patient for development of adverse reactions. Minoxidil should be administered only under close supervision to patient with severe hypertension who has not responded to maximum doses of a diuretic plus two other antihypertensive drugs.

Carefully assess patient for evidence of a pericardial disorder; if one is suspected, echocardiographic studies should be performed. Pericardial effusion occurs in about 3% of treated patients not on dialysis, especially those with impaired renal function.

Continually monitor blood pressure after minoxidil administration to detect a too-large or too-rapid drop when minoxidil is used in a patient already receiving guanethidine. The patient should be hospitalized.

Monitor fluid and electrolyte balance, intake–output ratio, and body weight.

Help to evaluate patient's response to drug. At least 3 days should elapse between dosage adjustments to permit the full response to a given dose to become manifest.

Interpret results of diagnostic tests and contact practitioner as appropriate.

Monitor for possible drug–drug and drug–nutrient interactions; see Interactions.

Provide for patient safety needs is CNS or hypotensive changes occur.

Patient Teaching

Stress the importance of taking other antihypertensive medications exactly as prescribed along with minoxidil to increase drug's effectiveness and to reduce untoward reactions. Patient should not discontinue any other drugs without consulting drug prescriber.

Teach patient how to detect and report increased pulse rate (20 or more beats/min over normal), rapid weight gain, swelling in the extremities, dyspnea, or chest pain. If these occur, a dosage adjustment is indicated.

Inform patient that fine body hair will probably increase and darken within 3 to 6 weeks (80% incidence). Although bothersome, this is not associated with hormonal changes and is probably not dangerous. It is first noticeable in eyebrows, sideburns, and temple area, later extending to back, arms, and legs. This condition regresses and eventually disappears within 2 to 6 months after treatment is discontinued.

• Guanadrel

Hylorel

• Guanethidine

Ismelin

(CAN) Apo-Guanethidine

Guanadrel and guanethidine are two antihypertensive drugs with similar pharmacologic and toxicologic properties. Both drugs are effective in the treatment of moderate to severe refractive hypertension not responding adequately to diuretics and other antihypertensive agents.

Mechanism

Accumulate in peripheral adrenergic nerve endings, where they inhibit norepinephrine release in response to nerve stimulation; a gradual depletion of norepinephrine stores in the nerve endings ensues, resulting in a prolonged reduction in heart rate and peripheral vascular resistance; venous return is diminished, cardiac output is reduced, and plasma renin activity is decreased; blood pressure reduction is greater in the standing than prone position, and orthostatic effects are common and can result in significant dizziness and weakness; renal blood flow is reduced relative to blood flow to the heart and brain, and thus sodium and water retention is significant; sensitivity of adrenergic receptors to circulating norepinephrine is enhanced owing to impaired neuronal uptake.

Uses

Treatment of moderate to severe hypertension not adequately controlled by other antihypertensive drugs.

Treatment of renal hypertension, including that secondary to renal artery stenosis and pyelonephritis

Dosage

Guanadrel: Initially, 10 mg/day; increase gradually until optimal effect is seen; usual dosage range is 20 to 75 mg in twice daily doses

Guanethidine

Ambulatory patients: initially 10 mg/day; increase gradually every 5 to 7 days to achieve optimal response; usual dose is 25 to 50 mg/day in a single dose

Hospitalized patients: initially 10 to 50 mg, depending on other antihypertensive drugs being used; increase by 10 to 25 mg every 2 to 4 days until desired response is obtained

Children: initially 0.2 mg/kg/day as a single oral dose; increase by 0.2-mg/kg/day increments every 7 to 10 days; maximum dose is 3 mg/kg/day

Fate

Guancthidinc is poorly but consistently absorbed orally; peak effect occurs within 8 hours of a single dose; half-life is 5 days, so drug accumulates slowly; partially metabolized by the liver and excreted as active drug and inactive metabolites primarily by the kidneys.

Guanadrel is rapidly absorbed orally and attains peak plasma concentration in 1.5 to 2 hours; effects are noted within 2 hours and maximal blood pressure decreases occur within 4 to 6 hours; excreted primarily in the urine, approximately 40% as unchanged drug.

Common Side Effects

Fatigue, headache, faintness, drowsiness, nocturia, urinary urgency, increased bowel movements, diarrhea, shortness of breath on exertion, palpitations, bradycardia, fluid retention, ejaculation disturbances.

Significant Adverse Reactions

Nausea, vomiting, paresthesias, incontinence, dermatitis, anorexia, constipation, leg cramps, hair loss, nasal congestion, blurred vision, asthma, chest pains, myalgia, tremor, depression, and cardiac irregularities.

Contraindications

Pheochromocytoma, congestive heart failure not caused by hypertension, and concurrent use with MAO inhibitors. *Cautious use* in patients with fever, bronchial asthma, renal disease, coronary insufficiency, recent myocardial infarction, cerebral vascular disease, colitis, or peptic ulcer, and during pregnancy.

Interactions

The antihypertensive effects of guanethidine and guanadrel may be antagonized by amphetamines, antidepressants, antihistamines, antipsychotics (eg, phenothiazines, thioxanthenes, haloperidol), cocaine, diethylpropion, ephedrine, MAO inhibitors, methylphenidate, oral contraceptives, and sympathomimetic agents.

Enhanced hypotensive effects may be observed when guanethidine or guanadrel is given in combination with alcohol, diuretics, hydralazine, levodopa, methotrimeprazine, propranolol, quinidine, reserpine, or vasodilator drugs.

Excessive bradycardia can occur if guanethidine or guanadrel is used in combination with digitalis drugs.

Guanethidine or guanadrel may impair the hyposecretory effect of anticholinergics.

Guanethidine or guanadrel may exert an additive hypoglycemic effect with insulin or oral antidiabetic drugs.

Increased responses to adrenergic agents (eg, catecholamines, phenylephrine, metaraminol) may occur with guanethidine or guanadrel.

Nursing Management

Pretherapy Assessment

Assess and record baseline data necessary for detection of adverse effects of guanethidine and guanadrel: General: VS, body weight, skin color and temperature; CNS: orientation, reflexes, ophthalmologic examination; CVS: orthostatic blood pressure, supine blood pressure, peripheral perfusion, edema; GI: normal output, bowel sounds, liver evaluation; Endocrine: breast examination; Laboratory: kidney function tests, urinalysis, CBC with differential.

Review medical history and documents for existing or previous conditions that:

a. require cautious use of guanethidine and guanadrel: fever; bronchial asthma; renal disease; coronary insufficiency; recent myocardial infarction; cerebral vascular disease; colitis; or peptic ulcer.

b. contraindicate use of guanethidine and guanadrel: allergy to guanethidine and guanadrel; pheochromocytoma; congestive heart failure not caused by hypertension; MAO inhibitors; **pregnancy (Category C)**; lactation (secreted in breast milk, safety not established; if drug is required, do not nurse).

Nursing Interventions

Medication Administration

Administer without regard to meals.

Provide small, frequent meals if GI upset is severe.

Provide ready access to bathroom facilities if GI effects occur.

Note prominently on patient's chart that patient is receiving drug if emergency surgery is needed because reductions in preanesthetic medications and in anesthetics will be needed.

Surveillance During Therapy

Monitor patient for orthostatic hypotension.

Monitor patient for signs of fluid retention indicative of incipient cardiac decompensation.

Carefully monitor laboratory studies and patient for indications of adverse reactions.

Interpret results of diagnostic tests and contact practitioner as appropriate.

Monitor for possible drug–drug and drug–nutrient interactions; see Interactions.

Provide for patient safety needs if CNS or hypotensive changes occur.

Patient Teaching

Instruct patient to inform practitioner of development of persistent diarrhea, sudden weight gain, or edema. Dosage adjustment or additional medication may be required.

Instruct patient to be alert for development of adverse reactions such as urinary hesitancy or retention, weakness, and bradycardia, and to report these effects promptly.

Inform patient that periodic blood counts and liver and kidney function tests are advisable when therapy is prolonged.

Explain that practitioner in charge should be informed of drug use before surgery. If possible, drugs should be withdrawn 48 to 72 hours before the use of general anesthetics to reduce the possibility of vascular collapse and cardiac arrest.
Explain that drugs have prolonged durations of action. Dosage adjustments should be made carefully, and sufficient time should be allowed between dosage changes (eg, 3–5 days) for effects to become manifest.
Inform patient that a diuretic is often given along with drug to minimize sodium and water retention as well as to enhance hypotensive response.
Encourage patient on antihyperglycemic medication to monitor blood sugar carefully because guanadrel or guanethidine may have additive hypoglycemic effects.
Warn patient that alcohol may intensify the hypotensive reaction.

Drugs for Hypertensive Emergencies

Hypertensive emergencies, or sudden, marked elevations in blood pressure, require immediate treatment to avoid serious and often life-threatening complications. A number of drugs are available to lower blood pressure rapidly, and they are commonly administered IV, frequently with or after a diuretic. Among the drugs indicated for hypertensive emergencies that have been discussed previously are trimethaphan, a ganglionic blocking agent (reviewed in Chapter 13), and methyldopa, hydralazine, and labetalol, three orally effective antihypertensive drugs, discussed in this chapter, that can also be given IV in acute hypertension. The other drugs frequently used in acute hypertensive emergencies are diazoxide parenteral and nitroprusside; these are considered in detail in the following sections.

• Diazoxide, Parenteral

Hyperstat IV

Mechanism

Direct relaxation of arteriolar smooth muscle, resulting in vasodilation; reflexly increases heart rate, stroke volume, and cardiac output; renal blood flow is increased; causes sodium and water retention and inhibits tubular secretion of uric acid; elicits hyperglycemia by inhibiting insulin secretion from the pancreas; elevates serum free fatty acids.

Uses

Acute treatment (IV) of hypertensive emergencies and severe hypertension
Production of controlled hypotension during surgery
Management of hypoglycemia caused by hyperinsulinism (eg, islet cell carcinoma); available in *oral* form as Proglycem—see Chapter 44

Dosage

IV: 1 to 3 mg/kg (maximum 150 mg per injection) by IV push within 30 seconds or less; repeat at intervals of 5 to 15 minutes until a satisfactory response is attained, then at 4- to 24-hour intervals until a regimen of oral antihypertensive drug becomes effective.

NOTE: Do not give for longer than 10 days or by IV *infusion*.

Fate

Onset usually within 1 to 2 minutes, with maximal blood pressure decrease in 5 minutes; pressure then slowly increases over 2 to 12 hours; extensively bound to serum proteins (90%); excreted slowly through the kidneys; plasma half-life is 20 to 36 hours.

Common Side Effects

Nausea, hypotension, dizziness, weakness (most often seen with large doses); repeated injections can result in fluid retention and hyperglycemia.

Significant Adverse Reactions

CV: myocardial and cerebral ischemia, palpitations, arrhythmias, sweating, flushing, supraventricular tachycardia
CNS: (secondary to blood flow changes in the brain) confusion, headache, lightheadedness, somnolence, hearing impairment, euphoria, convulsions, paralysis
GI: abdominal pain, vomiting, anorexia, parotid swelling, salivation, dry mouth, constipation or diarrhea, ileus
Dermatologic–hypersensitivity: rash, fever, leukopenia
Respiratory: cough, dyspnea, choking sensation
Other: pancreatitis, weakness, lacrimation, cellulitis, pain along injected vein, back pain, nocturia, hyperuricemia

Contraindications

Hypersensitivity to thiazide diuretics, coronary artery disease, compensatory hypertension (eg, aortic coarctation, arteriovenous shunt), and dissecting aortic aneurysm. *Cautious use* in the presence of impaired cerebral or coronary circulation, hyperglycemia, or congestive heart failure, and in pregnant or nursing women.

Interactions

Combined use of diuretics with diazoxide may intensify its hyperglycemic, hyperuricemic, and antihypertensive effects.
Diazoxide may potentiate the action of other highly protein-bound drugs (eg, oral anticoagulants, antiinflammatory agents, sulfonamides, phenytoin, quinidine, propranolol) by displacing them from binding sites.
Chlorpromazine and furosemide may potentiate the hyperglycemic effect of diazoxide.
An increased hypotensive response can occur when diazoxide is used along with other antihypertensive drugs such as vasodilators (eg, nitrites, hydralazine), catecholamine-depleting drugs (eg, reserpine), beta-blockers, or centrally acting agents.
Diazoxide can accelerate the hepatic metabolism of phenytoin.
Diazoxide may blunt the effectiveness of oral hypoglycemic agents by impairing insulin secretion.

Nursing Management

Pretherapy Assessment

Assess and record baseline data necessary for detection of adverse effects of diazoxide: General: VS, body weight, skin color and temperature; CVS: peripheral perfusion, edema; GI: normal output, bowel sounds, liver evaluation; Laboratory: liver and kidney function tests, urinalysis, CBC with differential, glucose, electrolytes, uric acid.

Review medical history and documents for existing or previous conditions that:

a. require cautious use of diazoxide: impaired cerebral or coronary circulation; hyperglycemia; congestive heart failure.

b. contraindicate use of diazoxide: allergy to thiazides or other sulfonamides; coronary artery disease; compensatory hypertension (eg, aortic coarctation, arteriovenous shunt); dissecting aortic aneurysm; **pregnancy (Category C)**; lactation (secreted in breast milk, safety not established; if drug is required, do not nurse).

Nursing Interventions

Medication Administration

Administer undiluted IV only in small doses.

Have vasopressors (eg, metaraminol) available to treat marked hypotension when drug is administered. Smaller-than-recommended doses can be given by IV injection with less danger of sharp drop in blood pressure. IV infusion may be effective if patient is also receiving another antihypertensive.

Assist with drug administration as needed. Drug should be given only in a peripheral vein, and extravasation should be avoided because solution is alkaline and very irritating.

Keep patient recumbent during, and for at least 30 minutes after, injection. Monitor blood pressure closely until stabilized, then hourly during expected duration of effect. Check blood pressure with patient in upright position before ending surveillance.

Assess patient for, and inform practitioner of, signs of developing congestive heart failure (cough, dyspnea, edema, distended neck veins, rales) and renal or bowel dysfunction (urinary hesitancy, decreased urine output, constipation, abdominal distention) with repeated injections.

Protect oral drug suspensions from light.

Provide small, frequent meals if anorexia, altered taste occur.

Check urine glucose and ketones daily.

Surveillance During Therapy

Ensure that appropriate blood glucose and electrolyte determinations are obtained (usually at start of therapy and frequently during repeated dosing).

Keep patient supine for 8 to 10 hours because of added hypotensive effect when diuretics are used in conjunction with diazoxide. Concomitant diuretic use prevents sodium and water retention elicited by diazoxide and increases the antihypertensive effect.

Monitor diabetic patient for signs of hyperglycemia. Diazoxide-induced hyperglycemia is usually transient, reversible, and clinically insignificant in the nondiabetic patient, but the dosage of antidiabetic drugs may need to be adjusted in the diabetic patient.

Be prepared to administer a beta-blocker (eg, propranolol) if reflex tachycardia and increased cardiac output become clinically significant.

Carefully monitor laboratory studies and patient for indications of adverse reactions.

Interpret results of diagnostic tests and contact practitioner as appropriate.

Monitor for possible drug–drug and drug–nutrient interactions; see Interactions.

Patient Teaching

Teach patient to check urine daily for glucose and ketones; report elevated levels to practitioner.

Instruct patient to weigh themselves daily at the same time of day.

Instruct patient to report any of the following if they occur to practitioner: weight gain of more than 5 lb (11 kg) in 2 to 3 days; increased thirst; nausea; vomiting; confusion; fruity odor on breath; abdominal pain; swelling of extremities; difficulty breathing; bruising; bleeding.

• Nitroprusside

Nipride, Nitropress

Mechanism

Direct relaxation of arteriolar and venular smooth muscle, resulting in marked reduction of arterial pressure, slight reflex increase in heart rate, and a small decrease in cardiac output; renin activity is markedly increased.

In the presence of left ventricular failure, reduces both afterload (aortic resistance) and preload (ventricular filling pressure), improves cardiac output, and reduces pulmonary capillary wedge pressure. Heart rate is essentially unchanged.

Uses

Emergency treatment of hypertensive crises (NOTE: Oral antihypertensive medication should be initiated while blood pressure is being controlled by IV nitroprusside)

Production of controlled hypotension during surgery or anesthesia

Adjunctive therapy of severe, refractory congestive heart failure, treatment of lactic acidosis secondary to reduced peripheral perfusion, and attenuation of the vasoconstrictor effects of norepinephrine and dopamine

Dosage

Adults and children (by IV infusion only): 3 μg/kg/min (range, 0.5–10 μg/kg/min) of a 50 mg in 250 to 1000 mL of 5% dextrose in water dilution.

Fate

Immediate onset of action (30–60 sec); effects are maximum within 1 to 2 minutes; on termination of the infusion, blood pressure can return to pretreatment levels within several minutes; decomposes to cyanide in the blood, which either reacts with methemoglobin to form cyanmethemoglobin or is converted in the liver and kidneys to thiocyanate, which is slowly cleared by the kidneys; in patients with impaired renal function, prolonged infusion or excessive doses can cause cyanide or thiocyanate toxicity.

Common Side Effects

Usually result of too-rapid infusion—nausea, sweating, headache, restlessness, muscle twitching, palpitations, dizziness, substernal discomfort.

Significant Adverse Reactions

Usually caused by thiocyanate accumulation (see Fate), especially in patients with impaired renal function—blurred vision, tinnitus, dyspnea, ataxia, diminished reflexes, mydriasis, delirium, and convulsions; also, hypothyroidism, methemoglobinemia.

Contraindications

Compensatory hypertension (arteriovenous shunt, aortic coarctation), and inadequate cerebral circulation. *Cautious use* in patients with hypothyroidism, renal or hepatic impairment, anemia, hypovolemia, and in elderly patients or those who are poor surgical risks.

Interactions

Enhanced hypotension can occur if nitroprusside is given to patients receiving other antihypertensive medications, circulatory depressants, and volatile liquid anesthetics.

Tolbutamide may decrease the effects of nitroprusside.

Nursing Management

Pretherapy Assessment

Assess and record baseline data necessary for detection of adverse effects of nitroprusside: General: VS, body weight, skin color and temperature; CVS: peripheral perfusion, edema; GI: normal output, bowel sounds, liver evaluation; Laboratory: liver and kidney function tests, urinalysis, CBC with differential, glucose, electrolytes, uric acid.

Review medical history and documents for existing or previous conditions that:

a. require cautious use of nitroprusside: hypothyroidism; renal or hepatic impairment; anemia; hypovolemia; in elderly patients or those who are poor surgical risks.

b. contraindicate use of nitroprusside: allergy to thiocyanates and ferricyanates; compensatory hypertension (arteriovenous shunt, aortic coarctation); inadequate cerebral circulation; **pregnancy (Category C)**; lactation (safety not established; if drug is required, do not nurse).

Nursing Interventions

Medication Administration

Administer *only* by slow IV infusion. Determine blood pressure frequently, and adjust rate of flow to achieve desired response. Do not allow systolic pressure to go below 70 mm Hg.

Do not exceed infusion rate of 10 μg/kg/min. If blood pressure is not reduced within 10 minutes at this dose, drug should be discontinued. Dosage should be reduced in patient already receiving antihypertensive medication.

Have drugs available to treat cyanide intoxication in case of overdose because nitroprusside is metabolized to cyanide, then to thiocyanate. If treatment is continued longer than 2 to 3 days, thiocyanate blood levels should be determined; drug should be discontinued if levels exceed 10 mg/100 mL. To treat overdosage, 2.5 to 5 mL/minute of 3% sodium nitrite is injected to a total of 15 mL, followed by sodium thiosulfate 12.5 g/50 mL of 5% dextrose over 10 minutes by IV infusion. Treatment is repeated at one half of these doses if signs of overdose reappear.

Discard any solution that is strongly colored (freshly prepared solutions have a faint brownish tinge), and use solutions within 4 hours after preparation. Cover infusion container with opaque material to exclude light, which can increase rate of decomposition to cyanide ion.

Do *not* add other drugs or preservatives to infusion solution.

Check infusion site for indications of extravasation (eg, swelling, pain) because irritation may occur.

Ensure that preexisting anemia or hypovolemia has been corrected before nitroprusside administration when drug is used to produce controlled hypotension during surgery.

Expect patient to be started on oral antihypertensive medication as soon as possible. Oral drug may be started while blood pressure is being brought under control by nitroprusside.

Surveillance During Therapy

Monitor acid–base balance (metabolic acidosis is an early sign of cyanide toxicity) and serum cyanate levels during prolonged therapy, especially in renal impairment.

Carefully monitor laboratory studies and patient for indications of adverse reactions.

Interpret results of diagnostic tests and contact practitioner as appropriate.

Monitor for possible drug–drug and drug–nutrient interactions; see Interactions.

Patient Teaching

Inform patient that frequent monitoring of blood pressure, blood tests, and checks of IV dosage and rate will be required.

• Trimethaphan

Arfonad

Trimethaphan is a ganglionic blocking agent used parenterally for rapid blood pressure reduction. In addition to blocking ganglionic receptor sites, it also may exert a direct relaxant effect on peripheral vascular smooth muscle. Onset of action is rapid, and the effects persist for only a short time after the infusion is terminated. Trimethaphan is discussed in Chapter 13.

Uses

Production of controlled hypotension during surgery
Short-term management of hypertensive emergencies (eg, dissection of the aorta)
Emergency treatment of pulmonary edema in patients with pulmonary hypertension

Dosage

Dilute 500 mg of drug to 500 mL 5% dextrose injection; infuse initially at a rate of 3 to 4 mL/min and adjust to desired blood pressure control; range is 0.3 to 6 mL/min.

Miscellaneous Antihypertensive Drugs

• Mecamylamine

Inversine

Mecamylamine is a potent, orally effective ganglionic blocking agent that exerts a considerable orthostatic hypotensive effect. Owing primarily to its many side effects, it is used only for the control of severe hypertension in patients not responding to a combination of other antihypertensive drugs. The drug is reviewed further in Chapter 13.

Dosage

Initially 2.5 mg twice a day; increase by 2.5 mg every 2 days until desired response is attained; average dose is 25 mg/day in 2 to 4 divided doses; usually given after meals, with the larger fraction of the dose administered later in the day.

• Metyrosine

Demser

Mechanism

Inhibits tyrosine hydroxylase, the enzyme that catalyzes the conversion of tyrosine to dopa, which is the initial reaction in the biosynthesis of the catecholamines dopamine, norepinephrine, and epinephrine. Therefore, catecholamine production is reduced.

Uses

Symptomatic treatment of patients with pheochromocytoma (a tumor of the sympathetic nervous system, usually of the adrenal medulla):
- Preoperative preparation
- Management of patients when surgery is contraindicated
- Chronic therapy of malignant pheochromocytoma

Dosage

Initially, 250 mg 4 times/day; increase by 250 to 500 mg every day as needed to a maximum of 4 g/day in divided doses

Common Side Effects

Sedation, extrapyramidal symptoms (drooling, fine tremor, speech difficulties), diarrhea.

Significant Adverse Reactions

Anxiety, depression, hallucinations, confusion, headache, nasal congestion, decreased salivation, vomiting, dry mouth, abdominal pain, impotence, galactorrhea, breast swelling, crystalluria, dysuria, hematuria, hypersensitivity reactions (urticaria, rash, pharyngeal edema).

Interactions

Extrapyramidal effects may be intensified by concurrent use of phenothiazines or other antipsychotic drugs.
Metyrosine may have additive effects with alcohol or other CNS depressants.

Nursing Management

Nursing Interventions

Medication Administration

Ensure that patient receiving metyrosine maintains adequate postoperative intravascular fluid volume to avoid hypotension and reduced perfusion of vital organs.
Continually monitor blood pressure and ECG during surgery because arrhythmias can occur. Have lidocaine and a beta-adrenergic blocking agent available.
Be prepared to add an alpha-adrenergic blocking agent to drug regimen if patient's blood pressure is not adequately controlled with metyrosine.

Surveillance During Therapy

Observe for, and inform practitioner of, first signs of drooling, speech difficulty, fine tremors, diarrhea, disorientation, or jaw stiffness.
Interpret results of urinary catecholamine measurements cautiously because the drug can interfere with them.

Patient Teaching

Encourage patient to maintain fluid intake sufficient to achieve daily urine volume of 2000 mL or more to minimize danger of drug crystallization in urine.

• Phenoxybenzamine

Dibenzyline

An orally effective, long-acting, nonselective alpha-adrenergic blocking agent indicated for the control of episodes of hypertension and sweating associated with pheochromocytoma. Phenoxybenzamine produces a chemical sympathectomy, interrupting impulse transmission through alpha-adrenergic receptor sites, thereby reducing blood pressure and increasing blood flow to the skin, mucosa, and abdominal organs. In addition to its use in pheochromocytoma, it has been shown effective in disorders of the bladder that cause impaired urination.

Principal adverse reactions with phenoxybenzamine are nasal congestion, orthostatic hypotension, miosis, tachycardia, and impaired ejaculation. These effects are secondary to adrenergic blockade and usually disappear with time. Phenoxybenzamine should be used with *caution* in patients with coronary or cerebral vascular insufficiency or renal damage. Phenoxybenzamine is discussed in detail in Chapter 15.

Dosage

Initially 10 mg/day orally; increase by 10 mg every 4 days until desired response is achieved; usual dosage range is 20 to 60 mg/day.

Note: At least 2 weeks usually are required to attain significant improvement, and possibly several more weeks are required for full benefits.

• Phentolamine

Regitine

(CAN) Rogitine

Phentolamine is a nonselective alpha-adrenergic blocking agent used by injection to control hypertensive episodes that might occur in patients with pheochromocytoma during surgery for removal of the chromaffin tumor. The drug also has been used to prevent the dermal necrosis and sloughing that can occur on extravasation during IV infusion of epinephrine, norepinephrine, or dopamine solutions. Treatment of rebound hypertension during withdrawal of antihypertensive medications has also been accomplished by injection of phentolamine. In addition to its alpha-blocking action, the drug has a direct relaxant effect on vascular smooth muscle.

Tachycardia and cardiac arrhythmias may occur with use of phentolamine. Other adverse effects include weakness, dizziness, flushing, orthostatic hypotension, nasal stuffiness, vomiting, and diarrhea.

Dosage

Hypertension (IV, IM): 5 mg in adults; 1 mg in children
Necrosis/sloughing: 10 mg/L of IV infusion solution, or 5 to 10 mg/10 mL saline injected into area of extravasation

Selected Bibliography

Babamoto KS, Hirokawa WT: Doxazosin: A new alpha$_1$-adrenergic antagonist. Clin Pharm 11:415, 1992

Burnier M, Waeber B, Brunner HR: First-line pharmacological treatment of hypertension. Ann Intern Med 232:381, 1992

Cunningham FG, Lindheimer MD: Hypertension in pregnancy. N Engl J Med 326:927, 1992

Dimsdale JE: Reflections on the impact of antihypertensive medications on mood, sedation, and neuropsychologic functioning. Arch Intern Med 152:35, 1992

Freis ED. Veterans Administration Cooperative Study Group on Hypertensive Agents: Effects of age on treatment results. Am J Med 90 (Suppl):3A20S, 1991

Frishman WH: Comparative pharmacokinetic and clinical profiles of angiotensin-converting enzyme inhibitors and calcium antagonists in systemic hypertension. Am J Cardiol 69:17C, 1992

Frishman WH, Landau A, Cretkovic A: Combination drug therapy with calcium-channel blockers in the treatment of systemic hypertension. J Clin Pharmacol 33:752, 1993

Gifford RW, Alderman MH, Chobanian AV, Cunningham SL: The Fifth Report of the Joint National Committee on Detection, Evaluation, and Treatment of High Blood Pressure. Arch Intern Med 153:154, 1993

Hansson L. Review of state-of-the-art beta-blocker therapy. Am J Cardiol 67:43B, 1991

Harper KJ, Forker AD: Antihypertensive therapy: Current issues and challenges. Postgrad Med 91:163, 1992

Hebert PR, Moser M, Mayer J, Glynn RJ, Hennekens CH: Recent evidence on drug therapy of mild to moderate hypertension and decreased risk of coronary heart disease. Arch Intern Med 153:578, 1993

Houston MC: New insights and approaches to reduce end-organ damage in the treatment of hypertension: Subsets of hypertension approach. Am Heart J 123:1337, 1992

Kaplan NM: Cardiovascular risk reduction: The role of antihypertensive treatment. Am J Med 90(Suppl):2A19S, 1991

Murphy MB: Selecting optimum antihypertensive therapy: Indications for choosing a calcium channel blocker. Am J Med 93(Suppl):2A38S, 1992

Perry MH: Efficacy and safety of atenolol, enalapril, and isradipine in elderly hypertensive women. Am J Med 96:77, 1994

Pool JL: Combination antihypertensive therapy with terazosin and other antihypertensive agents: Results of clinical trails. Am Heart J 122 (Suppl):926, 1991

Prisant LM, Carr AA, Hawkins DW: Treating hypertensive emergencies: Controlled reduction of blood pressure and protection of target organs. Postgrad Med 93:92, 1993

Schnaper HW: Angiotensin-converting enzyme inhibitors for systemic hypertension in young and elderly patients. Am J Cardiol 69:54C, 1992

Studer JA, Piepho RW: Antihypertensive therapy in the geriatric patient. II: A review of the alpha$_1$-adrenergic blocking agents. J Clin Pharmacol 33:2, 1993

Nursing Bibliography

Bridges J, Strong A: Angiotensin converting enzyme inhibition: Pharmacologic management to minimize postinfarction heart failure. Critical Care Nursing Quarterly 16(2):17, 1993

Gullickson C: Client ordered drug choice: An alternative approach in managing hypertension. The Nurse Practitioner 18(2):3, 1993

Hockenberry B: Multiple drug therapy in the treatment of essential hypertension. Nursing Clinics of North America 26:417, 1991

Uber L, Uber W: Hypertensive crisis in the 1990s. Critical Care Nursing Quarterly 16(2):27, 1993

Winer N: Hypertensive crisis. Critical Care Nursing Quarterly 13(3):23, 1990

34

Antianginal Agents and Vasodilators

Nitrates

- Amyl nitrate
- Erythrityl tetranitrate
- Isosorbide dinitrate
- Isosorbide mononitrate
- Nitroglycerin
- Pentaerythritol tetranitrate

Calcium Channel Blockers

- Amlodipine
- Bepridil
- Diltiazem
- Felodipine
- Isradipine
- Nicardipine
- Nifedipine
- Nimodipine
- Verapamil

Beta-Adrenergic Blockers

- Atenolol
- Metoprolol
- Nadolol
- Propranolol

Dipyridamole

Ticlopidine

Peripheral Vasodilators

- Cyclandelate
- Ergoloid mesylates
- Isoxsuprine
- Papaverine
- Ethaverine

Drugs that improve blood flow through circulatory vessels by increasing their diameters are termed *vasodilators*. These agents usually are effective in reducing the incidence and severity of exertional pain in patients with coronary artery disease (eg, angina) but are of limited clinical usefulness for improving circulation in peripheral vascular diseases. The drugs discussed in this chapter are therefore divided into those principally used for the treatment of angina pectoris and those usually indicated for the treatment of peripheral and cerebrovascular insufficiency.

Antianginal Agents

Angina pectoris is a condition characterized by intermittent substernal (chest) pain, often of a "crushing" nature, which may remain localized in the sternal region or may radiate to other areas of the body (eg, the left shoulder or left arm). The pain is the result of ischemia (reduced blood supply) in an area of the myocardium, leading to decreased cardiac oxygenation, especially during periods of exertion or stress.

Angina may be classified on the basis of the etiology of the myocardial ischemia as:

- *Classic, stable angina*: increased oxygen demand resulting from exercise, stress, physical exertion
- *Unstable angina*: pain occurs even at rest; probably owing to significantly compromised coronary blood flow
- *Vasospastic (Prinzmetal) angina*: ischemia results from coronary vasospasm; death can occur from attendant arrhythmias

Acute anginal attacks are triggered when the oxygen demand of the heart exceeds the capacity of the coronary circulation to supply the needed oxygen. Merely increasing myocardial blood flow by coronary artery dilation, however, is not usually beneficial unless the workload on the heart is also reduced. Effective management of the anginal condition requires the use of drugs that can increase *overall* myocardial oxygenation. In fact, the primary effect of the vasodilators such as the nitrates used in the treatment of angina is reduction of *total* peripheral vascular resistance rather than selective dilation of coronary arteries. The resultant decrease in venous return to the heart and in systemic vascular resistance reduces the workload on the anginal heart and hence the oxygen requirement of the myocardium.

Drug therapy of angina is twofold: namely, to provide relief of pain during an acute anginal attack, and to decrease the overall frequency and severity of attacks by improving the oxygen supply : demand ratio. Treatment of an acute anginal attack usually consists of sublingual administration of one of the rapid-acting nitrites or nitrates (eg, nitroglycerin, isosorbide dinitrate), drugs that have a quick onset and a relatively short duration of action. Prophylaxis against anginal episodes can be conferred by use of longer-acting preparations of orally effective nitrates (eg, isosorbide mononitrate), topical nitroglycerin, beta-adrenergic blockers, and calcium channel blockers.

Whereas the efficacy of the rapid-acting agents in aborting an acute anginal attack is unquestioned, controversy surrounds the use of the long-acting nitrates as prophylactic drugs. Although clinical evidence suggests that these long-acting agents may improve exercise tolerance in some patients with angina, there are conflicting data on their efficacy in reducing the incidence and severity of anginal attacks when used repeatedly. Tolerance to the effects of nitrates develops rapidly with continued use, and attempts to maintain stable plasma levels of these drugs with a *regular* dosing schedule invariably lead to loss of effectiveness, sometimes within a matter of days. Similarly, use of nitrates as transdermal patches or topical ointment quickly leads to a loss of improvement in exercise tolerance owing to rapid development of tolerance to the drug. Many clinicians are now advocating "pulse" dosing of nitrates, in which the drugs are given for a portion of each day but the patient remains drug free for a given period each day, such as overnight. This dosing method reportedly results in much less tolerance and increased effectiveness.

A chemically unique type of compound, the calcium channel blocker, is also indicated for *prophylaxis* of anginal attacks. The calcium channel blockers act by reducing the influx of calcium through the so-called slow membrane channels, thus reducing the contractile activity of smooth muscle and cardiac muscle. They are effective in alleviating pain and improving exercise tolerance in many anginal patients while exhibiting a fairly low incidence of side effects. The calcium channel blockers are used orally in chronic, stable angina as well as in the vasospastic (Prinzmetal) variant form. In addition, verapamil (and to a lesser extent, diltiazem) reduce atrioventricular (AV) conduction and sinoatrial nodal automaticity and prevent abnormal impulse reentry at the AV node; they are also used intravenously (IV) in the management of supraventricular tachyarrhythmias, a condition in which they are considered by many to be the drugs of choice. This latter indication is reviewed in detail in Chapter 32. Calcium channel blockers are also useful in treating hypertension, and this aspect of their pharmacology in considered in Chapter 33.

The nitrites and nitrates are discussed as a group because they exhibit qualitatively similar actions; individual drugs are listed in Table 34-1. The calcium channel blockers are likewise considered together, and the individual drugs are detailed in Tables 34-2 and 34-3. Beta-blockers useful in the prophylaxis of angina are reviewed briefly here because they are considered in detail in Chapter 15.

• Nitrites/Nitrates

Amyl nitrite
Erythrityl tetranitrate
Isosorbide mononitrate
Isosorbide dinitrate
Nitroglycerin
Pentaerythritol tetranitrate

Mechanism

Direct relaxing effect on vascular smooth muscle (due to liberation of nitric oxide, which activates the enzyme guanylyl cyclase, increasing synthesis of cyclic guanosine monophosphate [GMP]), resulting in generalized vasodilation; venous effects predominate, leading to pooling of blood in the great veins and reduced venous return, which lowers the left ventricular end-diastolic pressure (LVEDP), also known as the *preload*. Decreased venous return also leads to reduced cardiac output and lowered myocardial oxygen demand. Decline in LVEDP results in improved blood flow to deeper (subendocardial) layers of the myocardium, which may be oxygen starved.

Relaxation of arteriolar smooth muscle occurs to a lesser extent, which lowers systemic vascular resistance and aortic

Table 34-1. **Nitrites and Nitrates**

Drug	*Usual Dosage Range*	*Nursing Considerations*
Amyl nitrite *Aspirols, Vaporole*	0.3 mL inhaled as required	Available as thin ampules in a woven fabric cover; ampule is wrapped in gauze or cloth, crushed between fingers, and contents inhaled; drug has a strong, fruity odor; volatile and highly flammable; tachycardia often occurs for a brief period after inhalation; has been used to relieve renal and gallbladder colic but infrequently used now because of odor, cost, and inconvenience; excessive doses may cause methemoglobinemia, an impaired oxygen-carrying capacity of red blood cells
Erythrityl tetranitrate *Cardilate*	*Sublingual:* 5–10 mg 3 times/day or before stressful episodes *Oral:* 10 mg 3 times/day	Comparable onset but longer duration (4 h) of action than nitroglycerin; used mainly for prophylaxis in patients with frequent, recurrent anginal pain and reduced exercise tolerance; vascular headaches are common early in therapy—less frequent with oral than sublingual administration; gastrointestinal disturbances are noted with high oral doses
Isosorbide dinitrate *Isordil, Sorbitrate, and several other manufacturers* *(CAN) Apo-ISDN, Cedocard-SR, Coradur, Coronex, Novosorbide*	*Sublingual:* 2.5–10 mg as needed for relief of pain *or* every 2–3 h for prophylaxis *Chewable:* 5–10 mg every 2–3 h for prophylaxis *Tablets:* 10–40 mg 3 times a day for prophylaxis *Sustained-release:* 40–80 mg every 8 h twice a day	Sublingual and chewable forms rated "probably effective" for treatment of acute anginal attacks and to prevent attacks in high-risk situations (eg, stress); oral dosage forms rated "possibly effective" for prevention of anginal episodes; should be taken on an empty stomach unless vascular headaches are severe—then drug may be taken with meals; duration after sublingual administration is 1–3 h, and up to 6 h with oral administration (8 h with sustained-release forms); tolerance to these agents may develop; consider administering the short-acting preparations 2 or 3 times a day (last dose no later than 7 PM), and once daily or twice daily at 8 AM and 2 PM for the sustained-release preparations
Isosorbide mononitrate *Imdur, Ismo, Monoket*	20 mg twice daily with the two doses given 7 h apart *or* 60 mg (Imdur) given once daily	Suggested regimen is to give the first dose on awakening and the second dose 7 h apart; this regimen helps prevent the development of nitrate tolerance; alternatively, Imdur (60 mg) may be given once daily
Nitroglycerin, sublingual *Nitrostat*	0.15–0.6 mg under the tongue or in the buccal pouch at first indication of acute anginal	Very effective in relieving pain of acute anginal episodes and for preventing attacks when taken imme-

(*continued*)

Table 34-1. **Nitrites and Nitrates (Continued)**

Drug	*Usual Dosage Range*	*Nursing Considerations*
	attack; repeat approximately every 5 min until relief is obtained; take no more than 3 tablets in 15 min	diately before a stressful event; onset is almost immediate, and effects persist 30–45 min; keep bottles tightly capped, store in cool and dry place
Nitroglycerin, translingual *Nitrolingual*	1–2 sprays onto oral mucosa; no more than 3 sprays within 15 min	Oral spray used for relief of an acute attack of angina *or* prophylactically immediately before engaging in strenuous activities; if chest pain persists after three sprays, prompt medical attention is needed; spray should not be inhaled
Nitroglycerin, transmucosal *Nitrogard*	1 tablet placed in buccal pouch every 3–5 h while awake	Tablets are placed between lip and gum above incisors or between cheek and gum and adhere to mucosa; drug is slowly absorbed over several hours; used for long-term management of angina; caution must be exercised in drinking and eating; if tablet is accidentally swallowed, insert a new tablet because most of the drug that is swallowed is metabolized on first pass through the liver
Nitroglycerin, topical ointment *Nitro-Bid, Nitrol*	Initially, half-inch strip of ointment every 4–8 h; apply by spreading a thin, uniform layer on skin; do *not* rub in; increase by half-inch increments until optimal response is obtained; usual dose is 1–2 in/8 h, although up to 4–5 in have been used every 4 h	Effective prevention of anginal attacks, especially at night; begin with half-inch of ointment/dose, and increase by half-inch every succeeding dose until vascular headache occurs, then decrease slightly; ointment is measured by squeezing a ribbon onto calibrated measuring tapes provided; rotate sites of application to prevent dermal inflammation and sensitization; area may be covered with plastic wrap to protect clothing; equally effective when applied to any skin area; *gradually* reduce dosage and frequency of application on termination of drug to prevent sudden withdrawal reaction; 1 inch ointment equals approximately 15 mg nitroglycerin
Nitroglycerin, sustained release *Nitro-Bid, and several other manufacturers*	Initially 2.5 mg every 6–8 h; increase in 2.5-mg increments 2–4 times/day until side effects limit the dose	Rated "possibly effective" for prophylaxis of anginal attacks; drug should be taken on an empty stomach, and tablets or capsules should be swallowed whole; monitor blood pressure closely
Nitroglycerin, injection *Nitro-Bid IV, Tridil*	Initially 5 μg/min by intravenous infusion; increase gradually in 5-μg/min increments every 3–5 min up to 20 μg/min; if no response, further increases should be made in increments of 10 μg/min, then 20 μg/min until an effect is noted	Used to reduce the incidence of myocardial ischemic injury resulting from an acute myocardial infarction, to control hypertension associated with certain surgical procedures, to provide "controlled hypotension" during surgery, and to treat acute angina pectoris in patients not responding to other means of therapy; dilute and store solutions only in glass containers because nitroglycerin can be absorbed by plastic; use only non-PVC (polyvinyl chloride) tubing to prevent absorption; some preparations contain alcohol; use caution with intracoronary injections; to discontinue, gradually decrease dose 5μg/min every 5 min and monitor blood pressure
Nitroglycerin transdermal systems *Deponit, Minitran, Nitrocine, Nitrodisc, Nitro-Dur, Transderm-Nitro*	Apply one patch to a nonhairy skin area once every 16–18 h (remove patch for 6–8 h overnight)	Transdermal patch system provides for continuous drug absorption, although rates and hence nitroglycerin plasma levels can vary significantly; tolerance develops rapidly if patches are left on 24 h/day; dosage is stated in amount of drug absorbed over 24 h; patch must be in complete contact with skin to be effective; any tears or breaks in the patch system change the rate of absorption; rotate application sites to minimize undue skin irritation; dosage is individualized and titrated to clinical response and tolerance of side effects (eg, headache, hypotension); terminate usage gradually over 4–6 wk to prevent sudden withdrawal reactions; *not* intended for treatment of acute anginal attacks
Pentaerythritol tetranitrate *Peritrate, and other manufacturers*	Initially 10–20 mg 3 times/day; increase gradually to a maximum 40 mg 3 times/day; maintenance 30–80 mg sustained-release forms every 12 h	Rated "possibly effective" for prophylactic treatment of angina; observe for development of skin rash or persistent headaches and caution patient that prolonged use may reduce effectiveness of rapid-acting drugs

impedance to left ventricular ejection (*afterload*), also reducing the workload on the heart. Pulmonary vascular pressures are reduced, and heart size is decreased.

Total coronary blood flow is probably not significantly increased by nitrites/nitrates; however, the drugs may cause a shunting or redistribution of flow to ischemic areas by dilation of collateral channels; most nonvascular smooth muscle is transiently relaxed, and reflex tachycardia due to a drop in blood pressure can occur.

Uses

Relief of pain of acute anginal attacks (rapid-acting dosage forms, eg, sublingual, translingual spray)
Prevention of anginal episodes and reduction in frequency and severity of acute attacks (long-acting or sustained-release forms of nitrates; transdermal nitroglycerin)
Reduction of cardiac workload in patients with myocardial infarction or congestive heart failure
Production of controlled hypotension or control of blood pressure during surgery (IV nitroglycerin)

Dosage

See Table 34-1.

Fate

Onset with sublingual administration is 1 to 2 minutes; duration ranges from 30 to 45 minutes (nitroglycerin) to 2 hours (isosorbide); onset after oral ingestion is 20 to 30 minutes, with a duration of 4 to 6 hours for regular tablets or capsules, and perhaps up to 12 hours with sustained-release dosage forms. Topical administration (ointment, transdermal patch) produces effects within 30 to 60 minutes; initial duration of action is 4 to 6 hours with ointment, and up to 24 hours with transdermal patch; however, rapid tolerance occurs, and duration of action declines quickly with continued use; drugs are rapidly metabolized in the liver. After oral administration, there is extensive first-pass hepatic metabolism, although hepatic enzyme activity can be saturated by large oral doses of these drugs; two metabolites have some vasodilator activity and longer plasma half-life than the parent compounds; metabolites are excreted in the urine.

Common Side Effects

Most frequent with rapid-acting drugs—headache, flushing, dizziness, palpitation, burning sensation in sublingual area. Topical application causes localized irritation.

Significant Adverse Reactions

Orthostatic hypotension, tachycardia, vertigo, confusion, weakness, skin rash, and exfoliative dermatitis (rare).

Occasional hypersensitivity reaction marked by vomiting, profound weakness, restlessness, tachycardia, incontinence, syncope, perspiration, pallor, pronounced hypotension, and collapse.

Contraindications

Severe anemia, marked hypotension, increased intracranial pressure, cerebral hemorrhage, and acute stages of myocardial infarction. *Cautious use* in patients with hypotension, glaucoma, severe hepatic or renal disease, and in pregnant or nursing women.

Interactions

Hypotensive effects of nitrites and nitrates may be enhanced by alcohol, beta-blockers, antihypertensives, narcotics, tricyclic antidepressants.
Nitrates can potentiate the effects of antihistamines, tricyclic antidepressants, and other anticholinergic drugs.
Cross-tolerance can occur between all nitrites and nitrates.
Nitrites and nitrates can antagonize the pressor actions of sympathomimetic drugs.

Nursing Management

Pretherapy Assessment

Assess and record baseline data necessary for detection of adverse effects of nitrates: General: vital signs, body weight, skin color and temperature; Central nervous system (CNS): orientation, reflexes, affect; Cardiovascular system: peripheral perfusion, orthostatic blood pressure, baseline electrocardiogram; Genitourinary (GI): normal output, bowel sounds, liver evaluation; Laboratory: liver and kidney function tests, urinalysis, complete blood count with differential, hemoglobin.
Review medical history and documents for existing or previous conditions that:
a. require cautious use of nitrates: hypotension; glaucoma; severe hepatic or renal disease.
b. contraindicate use of nitrates: allergy to nitrates; severe anemia; marked hypotension; increased intracranial pressure; cerebral hemorrhage; acute stages of myocardial infarction; **pregnancy (Category C)**; lactation (safety not established; if drug is required, do not nurse)

Nursing Interventions

Medication Administration

Administer sublingual preparations under tongue or in buccal pouch. Encourage patient not to swallow. Ask patient if tablet "fizzles" or burns. Discard unused drug 6 months after bottle is opened.
Administer sustained-release preparations with water; advise patient not to chew tablets or capsules.
Administer transdermal systems to skin free of hair and not subject to much movement.
Administer transmucosal tablets by placing them between the lip and gum above the incisors or between cheek and gum.
Administer translingual spray directly into oral mucosa; preparation is not to be inhaled.
Do not give IV push; do not mix with other drugs; use only with glass IV bottles; protect from light and extremes of temperature.

Surveillance During Therapy

Carefully monitor laboratory studies and patient for indications of adverse reactions.
Interpret results of diagnostic tests and contact practitioner as appropriate.
Monitor for possible drug–drug and drug–nutrient interactions; see Interactions.

Patient Teaching

Teach appropriate administration techniques for the various dosage forms of nitroglycerin.
Inform patient that the following side effects may occur with therapy: dizziness, lightheadedness; headache; flushing of the neck or face.
Instruct the patient to inform the practitioner if any other of the following effects occur: blurred vision; persistent or severe headache; skin rash; more frequent or severe angina attacks; fainting.
Encourage patient to avoid situations that might precipitate angina (eg, stress, heavy exercise, smoking, overeating). Recommend, as appropriate, reduction in caloric intake and development of a program of regular exercise.
Recommend using sublingual nitroglycerin in anticipation of situations in which acute anginal episodes have predictably occurred.
Instruct patient to place sublingual tablets under the tongue. Long-acting tablets or capsules should be swallowed whole.
Advise patient to sit or lie down to take medication and to rest for 10 to 15 minutes after taking drug because dizziness, weakness, syncope, and other signs of orthostatic hypotension can occur after administration, especially sublingual.
Instruct patient to take additional sublingual tablets (up to 3) at 5-minute intervals if necessary. If pain is not relieved after 15 minutes, either a practitioner should be contacted immediately or patient should report to a hospital.
Reassure patient that headaches that may occur after drug administration usually disappear within 20 to 30 minutes. Prolonged headache can be relieved with analgesics.
Discuss danger associated with alcohol consumption in conjunction with nitroglycerin therapy: A shock-like syndrome (flushing, pallor, weakness, hypotension, syncope) can occur.
Instruct patient to inform practitioner if skin rash, visual disturbances, dry mouth, or severe or persistent headaches occur because the medication may need to be adjusted.
Warn patient to be alert for development of tolerance to rapid-acting drug (inadequate pain relief after several tablets). Temporary discontinuation (several days) usually is sufficient to restore sensitivity. Tolerance can be minimized by using smallest effective dose.
Assist patient to develop a system for recording frequency of anginal attacks, number of tablets required for relief, and development of side effects.
Instruct patient to store drug (especially sublingual nitroglycerin) in original container. Tablets may rapidly lose potency in metal, plastic, or cardboard containers.
Suggest that patient discard unused sublingual tablets 6 months after original container is opened because potency is probably reduced.
Explain that topical nitroglycerin dosage forms are *not* intended for relief of acute anginal attacks because their onset of action is slower.
Advise patient to check patch to ensure that it is intact after showering, swimming, or heavy perspiration, which may affect drug response.
Explain that increased anginal episodes can result from excessive consumption of caffeine (in coffee, tea, and other foods).

• Calcium Channel Blockers

Amlodipine
Bepridil
Diltiazem
Felodipine
Isradipine
Nicardipine
Nifedipine
Nimodipine
Verapamil

Most types of smooth muscle and cardiac muscle cells depend on transmembrane calcium influx for maintenance of normal resting tone and for activation. This influx occurs subsequent to the rapid influx of sodium noted during the initial depolarization phase and proceeds at a much slower rate by way of membrane channels that are relatively selective for calcium. These *slow membrane channels* are blocked by a group of drugs known as calcium channel blockers. The entry of extracellular calcium into smooth muscle cells and myocardial cells is inhibited by these agents, resulting in vasodilation, bradycardia, decreased force of contraction, and reduced AV nodal conduction. Some of these agents are useful in treating angina, mild hypertension, and certain types of arrhythmias. In addition, nimodipine is indicated as an adjunctive agent in subarachnoid hemorrhage (see Uses). The following discussion pertains to the oral use of these agents in angina. Although all of the calcium blockers except nimodipine, isradipine, and felodipine are approved for the treatment of angina pectoris, significant differences exist among the drugs with regard to their pharmacologic effects on cardiovascular function. Table 34-2 outlines some of the more important differences in the actions of the calcium channel blockers, and Table 34-3 presents dosage ranges and additional information.

Mechanism

Calcium channel blockers inhibit the influx of extracellular calcium ions into cardiac muscle and smooth muscle cells through specific slow calcium channels. Antianginal effects include dilation of coronary arteries and arterioles and prevention of coronary artery spasm. Dilation of peripheral arterioles also occurs, reducing total resistance against which the heart must work; thus, there is a corresponding reduction in myocardial energy consumption and oxygen demand. Verapamil and, to a lesser extent, diltiazem also markedly decrease calcium influx into cardiac contractile and conductile cells of the sinoatrial node and AV node. This latter action slows AV conduction, prolongs effective AV refractory period, and interrupts reentry of impulses at the AV node, thus restoring normal sinus rhythm. Nimodipine appears to have a greater effect on cerebral rather than peripheral arteries and may prevent arterial spasm subsequent to subarachnoid hemorrhage

Table 34-2. **Pharmacokinetic and Pharmacologic Properties of Calcium Channel Blockers**

	Diltiazem	*Nifedipine*	*Verapamil*	*Nicardipine*	*Nimodipine*	*Isradipine*	*Felodipine*	*Amlodipine*	*Bepridil*
Pharmacokinetics									
Onset of action (min)	15–30	20	30 (2–5 IV)	20	—	120	120–300	—	60
Half-life (h)	3–6	2–4	4–8	2–4	1–2	8	11–16	30–50	24
Protein binding (%)	70–80	90–95	85–90	95–98	95–98	95	>99	93	>99
Pharmacologic effects									
Peripheral vasodilation	↑	↑↑↑	↑↑	↑↑↑	—	↑↑↑	↑↑↑	↑↑↑	↑
Heart rate	↓	↑ (reflex)	↑ or ↓	↑	—	0 (↑)	↑	0 ↑	↓
Contractility	0 (↓)	↑ (reflex)	↓↓	0	—	0	↑ (reflex)	↑ (reflex)	↓
AV nodal conduction	↓↓	0 (↓)	↓↓↓	0 (↑)	—	0	0	0	↓
SA nodal automaticity	↓	0	↓↓	0	—	0	0	0	↓

↑↑↑ or ↓↓↓, marked effect; ↑↑ or ↓↓, moderate effect; ↑ or ↓, minimal effect; 0 (↑) or 0 (↓), variable effect; 0, no effect; —, no data.

Table 34-3. **Calcium Channel Blockers**

Drug	*Usual Dosage Ranges*	*Nursing Considerations*
Diltiazem *Cardizem, Cardizem SR, Cardizem CD, Dilacor XR (CAN) Apo-Diltiaz, Novo-Diltiazem, Nu-Diltiaz, Syn-Diltiazem*	*Angina:* Initially 30 mg 4 times/day; increase gradually at 1–2-day intervals to achieve optimal response; maximum dose is 360 mg/day in divided doses *Hypertension:* 60–120 mg sustained-release twice a day; usual dosage range is 240–360 mg/day Cardizem CD: start with 120 or 180 mg once daily; titrate at 7–14 day intervals. Maximum dose is 480 mg once a day. *Arrhythmias:* see Chapter 32	Potent coronary vasodilator with little or no negative inotropic effect; also used in treating mild–moderate hypertension; and IV for supraventricular arrhythmias; heart rate is slightly reduced; slows AV conduction and may have additive bradycardic effects with beta-blockers or digitalis; incidence of adverse reactions is very low; nausea, headache, and peripheral edema are occasionally reported; elevated serum transaminases and hyperbilirubinemia have occurred but are reversible on cessation of therapy; *not* recommended for children
Nicardipine *Cardene, Cardene SR*	*Angina/Hypertension:* Initially 20 mg 3 times/day; usual range is 20–40 mg 3 times/day *Sustained release:* 30 mg twice a day; usual range 30–60 mg twice a day	Potent peripheral vasodilator used for treating angina and mild–moderate hypertension; significantly increases cardiac output; may also be useful in adjunctive treatment of congestive heart failure; decrease dosage in patients with hepatic impairment
Nifedipine *Adalat, Procardia, Procardia XL, Adalat CC (CAN) Apo-Nifed, Gen-Nifedipine, Novo-Nifedin, Nu-Nifed*	Initially 10 mg 3 times/day; increase slowly until optimal effect is noted; usual dosage range is 10–20 mg 3 times/day; maximum recommended dose is 180 mg/day *Sustained release:* 30–60 mg once daily; titrate over 7–14-day period	Orally effective calcium blocker used in chronic, stable angina as well as vasospastic angina; does not alter conduction system of the heart as does verapamil, thus is of no use in arrhythmias; marked reduction in peripheral resistance coupled with minimal increase in heart rate makes drug effective as an antihypertensive; discontinue drug gradually if necessary; decreases platelet aggregation
Nimodipine *Nimotop*	60 mg every 4 h for 21 consecutive days	Orally effective drug used to improve neurologic deficit due to cerebral arterial spasm subsequent to subarachnoid hemorrhage; treatment should be initiated within 96 h of the onset of hemorrhage; may also be effective in treating migraine and cluster headaches.
Verapamil *Calan, Isoptin, Verelan, Calan SR, Isoptin SR (CAN) Apo-Verap, Novo-Veramil, Nu-Verap*	Oral *Angina:* Initially 80 mg 3–4 times/day; increase at daily or weekly intervals until optimal effect is attained; usual dosage range is 300–480 mg daily *Hypertension:* Initially, 4–80 mg 3 times/day; usual dose is 240 mg as a single dose IV See Chapter 32	Orally effective calcium blocker used in angina and for relief of mild to moderate hypertension; also administered IV for treatment of supraventricular tachyarrhythmias (see Chapter 32); significantly reduces SA nodal automaticity and AV conduction and decreases force of contraction; high oral doses are necessary owing to extensive first-pass metabolism; use with *caution* in patients with left ventricular dysfunction
Isradipine *DynaCirc*	Initially, 2.5 mg twice a day; titrate dosage in 5 mg/day increments over 2–4 wk intervals; maximum dose is 20 mg per day	Potent peripheral vasodilator used for treating hypertension; most patients show no additional responses to doses >10 mg/d
Felodipine *Plendil*	Initially, 5 mg once a day; titrate dosage over 2–4 wk to a maximum of 10 mg/d	Potent peripheral vasodilator used for treating hypertension; patient should be told to swallow whole; do not crush or chew; fluid retention may occur but responds to diuretics
Amlodipine *Norvasc*	*Hypertension:* Dosage must be individualized; usual dose is 5 mg/d; maximum dosage is 10 mg; titrate over 2–4 wk *Angina:* 5–10 mg/d; elderly patients and patients with hepatic disease require lower dosage	Potent peripheral vasodilator used for both hypertension and angina; bioavailability is not affected by food; may be taken without regard to meals
Bepridil *Vascor*	*Chronic stable angina:* Usual initial dose is 200 mg/d; after 10 d, adjust dose depending on response; maximum dose is 400 mg/d	Bepridil has caused serious ventricular arrhythmias and also agranulocytosis; therefore, this agent should be reserved for patients who have failed to respond to or are intolerant of other antianginals

Uses

Management of all forms of angina (chronic stable, unstable, or vasospastic)
Treatment of supraventricular tachyarrhythmias and control of rapid ventricular rate in atrial flutter or atrial fibrillation (IV verapamil or diltiazem—see Chapter 32)
Control of mild to moderate hypertension (see Chapter 33)
Improvement of neurologic deficits resulting from cerebral arterial spasm after subarachnoid hemorrhage (nimodipine only)
Investigational uses include treatment of bronchial asthma and Raynaud's phenomenon, and migraine prophylaxis

Dosage

See Table 34-3.

Fate

See Table 34-2. All drugs are well absorbed orally, but undergo extensive first-pass hepatic metabolism (except amlodipine); onset of action and duration of action varies considerably among the products. All drugs are highly protein bound. Hepatic metabolism is extensive and excretion proceeds largely through the kidneys, except for diltiazem, which is eliminated primarily in the feces.

Common Side Effects

Frequency varies among individual drugs—flushing, headache, weakness, dizziness, nausea, lightheadedness, peripheral edema; also, constipation with verapamil and giddiness with nifedipine.

Significant Adverse Reactions

CV: palpitations, hypotension, bradycardia, myocardial infarction, heart failure; in addition, third-degree AV block with verapamil and ventricular tachycardia or arrhythmias with bepridil
Respiratory: dyspnea, cough, wheezing, chest congestion, pulmonary edema
GI: heartburn, diarrhea, cramping, flatulence, sore throat
CNS: fatigue, tremor, nervousness, confusion, mood changes, blurred vision, insomnia
Musculoskeletal: muscle cramping, joint stiffness, inflammation
Other: hair loss, menstrual irregularities, claudication, dermatitis, urticaria, fever, sweating, chills, impotence

Contraindications

Verapamil and diltiazem—severe left ventricular dysfunction, sick sinus syndrome, second- or third-degree heart block, cardiogenic shock, systolic pressure less than 90 mm Hg; *diltiazem* is also contraindicated in acute myocardial infarction and pulmonary congestion; nicardipine is contraindicated in advanced aortic stenosis; *bepridil* is contraindicated in patients with a history of serious ventricular arrhythmias or uncompensated cardiac insufficiency. *Cautious use* in patients with impaired hepatic or renal function, hypotension, reduced left ventricular function, or pulmonary edema, and in pregnant women and nursing mothers.

Interactions

Calcium blockers and beta-blockers together may be beneficial in some patients with chronic, stable angina but can also increase the likelihood of congestive heart failure or severe hypotension and may worsen existing angina, especially when given IV in patients with left ventricular dysfunction or conduction defects.
Verapamil, nifedipine, felodipine, diltiazem, and bepridil can elevate serum levels of digoxin if used concurrently, possibly leading to digitalis toxicity.
Calcium blockers may have an additive antihypertensive effect if administered together with other antihypertensive drugs.
The effectiveness of verapamil may be reduced by combined use with calcium and vitamin D.
Nifedipine may decrease serum quinidine levels in patients with diminished left ventricular function.
Cimetidine may augment the effects of calcium channel blockers by decreasing their hepatic metabolic rate.
Lithium plasma levels may be decreased by verapamil and diltiazem.
Plasma levels of cyclosporine, prazosin, encainide, and carbamazepine can be increased by diltiazem, verapamil, and possibly other calcium channel blockers.
Severe hypotension has been reported with concurrent use of fentanyl and calcium channel blockers.

Nursing Management

See **Calcium Channel Blockers** in Chapter 32. In addition:

Nursing Interventions

Surveillance During Therapy

Carefully monitor blood pressure during initial stages of therapy and whenever dosages are altered because excessive hypotension can occur, especially in patient already receiving beta-blocker or other antihypertensive drug.
Monitor electrocardiogram for development of bradycardia, sometimes accompanied by nodal escape rhythms, because verapamil and, to a lesser extent, diltiazem have significant negative inotropic effects and markedly slow AV conduction (see Table 34-2). First-degree AV block may also occur. If such changes persist or worsen, the dose should be reduced, and preparations should be made to institute appropriate antidotal therapy if necessary. The agent may have to be discontinued.
Assess for signs of developing congestive heart failure, especially if patient is also receiving a beta-blocker. Mild peripheral edema can occur, usually in the legs, especially with nifedipine, and may be treated with diuretics. This must be differentiated from the edema that results from heart failure. If heart failure develops, the drug should be discontinued.
Monitor results of liver enzyme determinations, which should be obtained periodically because occasional elevations of transaminase and alkaline phosphatase have been reported. Although elevations usually are

not associated with clinical symptoms, and their significance is unclear, the potential for hepatic injury exists.

Patient Teaching

Inform patient that sublingual nitroglycerin may be used as needed to control acute anginal attacks while taking a calcium channel blocker.

Beta-Blockers

The beta-adrenergic blocking agents approved for use in the treatment of angina include atenolol, metoprolol, propranolol, and nadolol. They are particularly suited for patients who experience frequent or severe acute attacks at rest because they can markedly reduce the myocardial oxygen demand. The principal hemodynamic actions of the beta-blockers responsible for this effect include a decreased heart rate, blood pressure, and myocardial contractility, all of which reduce cardiac workload. Decreased heart rate may also result in lengthened diastolic perfusion time, leading to increased coronary blood flow. Although beta-blockers may cause a slight increase in the end-diastolic pressure owing to the slowed heart rate, this potentially undesirable action can be offset readily by concurrent use of one of the nitrates. Conversely, the reflex tachycardia frequently seen with nitrates is attenuated by beta-blockers. Therefore, combined nitrate–beta-blocker therapy is frequently more advantageous than use of either drug alone.

The beta-blockers are discussed in detail in Chapter 15, and only those aspects of the use of propranolol, metoprolol, nadolol, and atenolol in the control of angina are considered here.

• Propranolol

Inderal, Inderal LA

(CAN) Apo-Propranolol, Detensol, Novopranol, PMS Propranolol

A nonselective beta-blocker used for management of moderate to severe angina, frequently in combination with nitrates.

Dosage

Initially 10 to 20 mg 3 to 4 times/day; increase gradually at weekly intervals until optimal response is obtained; usual maintenance dosage range is 80 to 160 mg/day in a single (sustained-release) or divided doses.

• Metoprolol

Lopressor, Toprol XL

(CAN) Apo-Metoprolol, Betaloc, Novometoprol

A beta-selective blocker that is well absorbed orally and displays moderate lipid solubility. It is useful for treating angina as well as hypertension and for preventing reinfarction after a myocardial infarction.

Dosage

Initially, 50 mg twice a day, increase gradually at weekly intervals as necessary; usual dosage range is 100 to 400 mg daily in two divided doses.

• Nadolol

Corgard

A nonspecific beta-adrenergic blocking agent indicated for the long-term management of patients with angina; its actions resemble those of propranolol. The long half-life of nadolol (20–24 h) permits once-daily dosing.

Dosage

Initially 40 mg once daily; increase by 40 to 80 mg at 3- to 7-day intervals until optimal clinical response is observed, or until there is pronounced slowing of heart rate; usually maintenance dose is 80 to 240 mg/day.

• Atenolol

Tenormin

A $beta_1$-selective blocker with a long half-life (once-daily dosing) and low lipid solubility, which decreases the incidence of central side effects such as drowsiness.

Dosage

50 mg once daily; may increase to 100 mg once daily.

Nursing Management

See Chapter 15. In addition:

Nursing Interventions

Surveillance During Therapy

Assist with ongoing evaluation of patient's response to drug because dosage requirements may change as condition stabilizes or deteriorates.

• Dipyridamole

Persantine, Pyridamole

(CAN) Apo-Dipyridamole

Dipyridamole is an orally effective coronary vasodilator and inhibitor of platelet aggregation. It has been used to prevent reinfarction and to decrease the incidence of transient ischemic attacks due to platelet hyperaggregation, although these indications are viewed solely as investigational. The drug has been extensively used as an anginal prophylactic agent although, this is no longer an FDA-approved indication.

Mechanism

Inhibits the activity on adenosine deaminase, thereby increasing functional levels of adenosine and other vasodilatory nucleotides; also appears to block the action of phosphodiesterase, resulting in elevated levels of cyclic AMP, another coronary vasodilator; increased cyclic AMP also reduces platelet aggregation; synthesis of prostacyclin is increased by dipyridamole, resulting in further vasodilation and impaired platelet aggregation; blood pressure is relatively unchanged, and systemic blood flow is largely unaffected; a mild positive inotropic action has also been reported.

Uses

Adjunct to coumarin anticoagulants in preventing postoperative thromboembolic complications of cardiac valve replacement

Investigational uses include prevention of thrombotic complications associated with cerebrovascular or ischemic heart diseases, prevention of myocardial reinfarction and mortality after infarction, and prevention of coronary bypass graft occlusion

Dosage

75 to 100 mg 4 times a day as an adjunct to the usual anticoagulant dose (the average for most other nonapproved uses is 50 mg 3 times a day, 1 h before meals; clinical effects may take several months to become evident).

Fate

Oral absorption is good, although bioavailability is variable (25%–75%). Peak plasma concentrations occur within 2 to 3 hours, although, as noted, therapeutic effects may not be evident for weeks to months. Protein binding is extensive (90%–97%). The drug is metabolized in the liver and excreted in the feces by enterohepatic recirculation.

Significant Adverse Reactions

Infrequent—headache, nausea, GI distress, weakness, dizziness, syncope, skin rash; occasionally, aggravation of angina pectoris.

Contraindications

No absolute contraindications. *Cautious use* in the presence of hypotension.

Interactions

Dipyridamole can enhance the effects of oral anticoagulants and heparin.

• Ticlopidine

Ticlid

Mechanism

Decreases platelet aggregation by inhibiting adenosine diphosphate-induced platelet fibrinogen binding; inhibitory effect is irreversible.

Uses

Alternative therapy to reduce risk of thrombotic stroke in patients who are at high risk (*not* a first-line drug owing to danger of blood dyscrasias—see CAUTION under Significant Adverse Reactions)

Unlabeled uses include treatment of intermittent claudication, chronic arterial occlusion, and sickle cell disease; also preoperatively in open heart surgery

Dosage

250 mg twice a day

Fate

Rapidly absorbed orally; peak plasma levels occur within 2 hours; greater than 50% inhibition of platelet aggregation is noted within 4 days, with maximum effects occurring in 8 to 12 days; highly bound to plasma proteins; metabolized extensively in the liver and excreted both in the urine (60%) and feces (35%).

Common Side Effects

GI pain, diarrhea, nausea, rash.

Significant Adverse Reactions

CAUTION

Neutropenia has occurred in 2% to 3% of patients receiving ticlopidine. The onset typically begins within 3 weeks to 3 months of the start of therapy. Complete blood counts and differential white cell counts must be performed at least every 2 weeks beginning from the second week of therapy. If neutropenia is present, discontinue the drug. Neutrophil counts usually return to normal within 1 to 3 weeks.

GI: vomiting, anorexia, GI bleeding, flatulence, abnormal liver function test results

Hematologic: epistaxis, hematuria, ecchymosis, conjunctival hemorrhage

Other: purpura, pruritus, dizziness, tinnitus

Contraindications

Presence of hemostatic disorders or active bleeding, neutropenia (see CAUTION), thrombocytopenia, severe liver impairment. *Cautious use* in patients with peptic ulcer, increased serum lipids, impaired renal function, and in pregnant or nursing mothers.

Interactions

Ticlopidine may increase plasma levels of theophylline.

The antiplatelet effects of aspirin can be enhanced by ticlopidine.

Cimetidine may decrease the clearance of ticlopidine, increasing its effects.

Peripheral Vasodilators

Vasodilator drugs may increase blood flow through circulatory vessels by either a direct action (smooth muscle relaxation) or an indirect action (interference with sympathetic nerve supply). Although these agents may improve blood flow to limbs and body organs in the otherwise *healthy* person, their efficacy in relieving the ischemia of peripheral vascular disease is severely limited. It is unlikely that any peripheral vasodilator can markedly increase blood flow distal to an occlusion. Moreover, regulatory mechanisms in cerebral and skeletal vascular beds elicit compensatory vasodilation in response to ischemia; thus, vasodilator drugs probably increase blood flow primarily to nonischemic areas. Therefore, minimal therapeutic benefit should be expected from the treatment of peripheral vascular disease with the peripheral vasodilators. Despite this fact, they continue to be prescribed for symptomatic treatment of chronic occlusive vascular disease, often at a significant cost to the public. Their use in treating cerebrovascular insufficiency in the elderly patient is particularly hazardous, inasmuch as these drugs can elicit a significant degree of hypotension, which can actually result in *reduced* cerebral perfusion, negating any potential benefit derived from dilation of cerebral vessels. Peripheral circulation should be closely monitored when any of these drugs is used. In addition, reflex tachycardia can occur with use of the peripheral vasodilators, which may prove dangerous in the patient with cardiac disease. Also, increased intraocular pressure may occur. Patients taking these drugs should be warned immediately to report any vision change or eye pain.

• Cyclandelate

Cyclan, Cyclospasmol

Cyclandelate is a direct-acting vascular smooth muscle relaxant with no significant sympathomimetic or adrenergic blocking action. It is rated only "possibly effective" for treatment of ischemic peripheral and cerebrovascular disease (eg, intermittent claudication, arteriosclerosis obliterans, Raynaud's phenomenon, thrombophlebitis, nocturnal leg cramps).

Initial oral dosage is 400 mg 3 to 4 times a day, which is gradually reduced to the usual maintenance dosage of 400 to 800 mg/day in 2 to 4 divided doses. Side effects include flushing, headache, weakness, sweating, dizziness, tachycardia, and GI distress. Most of these are transient; GI distress can be minimized by taking the drug with meals. The drug must be used cautiously in patients with glaucoma, severe coronary artery or cerebrovascular disease, and bleeding tendencies (prolonged bleeding time has been noted at high doses). Clinical benefit, if any, is slow to develop.

• Ergoloid Mesylates

Gerimal, Hydergine

Ergoloid mesylates contain equal parts of three dihydrogenated ergotoxine alkaloids, namely dihydroergocornine, dihydroergocristine, and dihydroergocryptine. The compound is used to provide symptomatic relief of those signs and symptoms associated with a decline in mental acuity and capacity in the elderly, such as confusion and forgetfulness and lessened self-care, sociability, and appetite. A degree of improvement in these conditions is observed within 8 to 12 weeks and may be related to improved cerebral circulation. Although the precise mechanism by which ergoloid mesylates are able to improve mentation is not known, it is believed the drug may increase metabolic activity of the brain, thereby improving cerebral blood flow. Vasodilation of cerebral vessels may also play a role, albeit a minor one, in the action of the drug. Blood pressure may decline, reducing cerebral perfusion, and orthostatic effects have been noted.

The drug is erratically absorbed orally when administered as a tablet, capsule, or liquid, and undergoes extensive first-pass hepatic metabolism. Thus, the preferred route of administration is sublingual, although this may be difficult in elderly or senile patients. Recommended starting dosage is 1 mg 3 times a day. Onset of clinical response is gradual, and results may not be evident for 3 to 4 weeks. Doses up to 12 mg/day have been used for extended periods.

Side effects are generally mild and include GI upset, nausea, sublingual irritation, lightheadedness, nasal stuffiness, blurred vision, skin rash, and orthostatic hypotension. Ergoloid mesylates should not be used in people with acute or chronic psychosis, or in people with a history of acute intermittent porphyria.

• Isoxsuprine

Vasodilan, Voxsuprine

Isoxsuprine is a peripheral vasodilator that can increase resting blood flow in skeletal muscle. The drug possesses a beta-adrenergic agonistic, alpha-adrenergic antagonistic, and direct vascular smooth muscle relaxant effect. Because its vasodilatory actions are *not* blocked by beta-blocking agents, it is doubtful whether its beta-agonistic properties contribute to its vasodilatory action. Isoxsuprine can also increase heart rate, myocardial contractility, and cardiac output, and can relax uterine smooth muscle, probably by means of a beta-activating action. High doses may inhibit platelet aggregation. It is rated only "possibly effective" for the relief of symptoms associated with cerebral and peripheral vascular insufficiency. In addition, isoxsuprine has been used intramuscularly to inhibit premature labor and to prevent threatened abortion, although these latter indications are considered experimental.

Oral dosage is 10 to 20 mg 3 to 4 times a day. When given IM, 5 to 10 mg may be administered 2 to 3 times a day. The drug should not be given IV because the likelihood of side effects is greatly increased. Flushing, palpitations, nausea, dizziness, skin rash, tachycardia, abdominal distress, hypotension, and nervousness have been reported with the use of isoxsuprine. The drug is discussed further in Chapter 14.

• Papaverine

Cerespan, Pavabid, and others

• Ethaverine

Ethaquin, Ethatab, Ethavex-100, Isovex

Papaverine and its closely related analogue, ethaverine, exert a direct, nonspecific relaxant effect on smooth muscle. Vasodilatory effects are noted on the coronary, cerebral, pulmonary, and systemic blood vessels. The drugs may elevate the levels of cyclic AMP in vascular smooth muscle. Cerebral blood flow may be increased by means of decreased cerebral vascular resistance; however, blood pressure may decline, offsetting the beneficial effect of reduced cerebral vascular resistance. Papaverine and ethaverine have been used orally for relieving cerebral, myocardial, and peripheral ischemia resulting from vascular spasm, although their clinical effectiveness has not been conclusively demonstrated. They have also been used as smooth muscle spasmolytics for treatment of a number of spastic states of GI, urinary, ureteral, or biliary smooth muscles.

Oral dosage of *papaverine* is 100 to 300 mg 3 to 5 times a day or 150-mg sustained-release preparation every 12 hours. IV or IM dosage ranges from 30 to 120 mg every 3 hours. For immediate effect, the IV route is recommended, and administration may be by *slow* injection or intermittent infusion. Absorption from sustained-release preparations is highly variable, and plasma levels may be very low after this mode of administration. Recommended dosage for *ethaverine* is 100 to 200 mg 3 times a day.

Side effects associated with these drugs include nausea, abdominal distress, flushing, sweating, headache, fatigue, skin rash, diarrhea, dizziness, tachycardia, and anorexia. Hepatic hypersensitivity also can occur, and may be manifested as eosinophilia, jaundice, and elevated serum transaminases and alkaline phosphatase. IV administration of papaverine can lead to increased blood pressure, respiratory rate, and heart rate, and to profound sedation. Large doses of these agents can suppress AV nodal conduction and may lead to arrhythmias. The drugs are contraindicated in severe liver disease, complete AV block, and serious arrhythmias, and they must be used with caution in patients with glaucoma (increase intraocular pressure), myocardial depression, or impaired liver function.

Intraocular pressure may increase during drug use. The patient should be told immediately to report any change in vision, eye pain, or scleral redness.

Nursing Management

Patient Teaching

Recommend that patient exercise caution in driving and performing other hazardous tasks until effects of drug have been determined because dizziness and drowsiness may occur.

Teach patient interventions to minimize orthostatic hypotension.

Teach patient how to monitor heart rate because abnormalities can occur. Dosage should be reduced or drug should be discontinued if heart rate is significantly altered.

Inform patient that flushing, a sensation of warmth, and headache can occur during initial stages of therapy, but that they usually disappear with slight dosage reduction.

Explain that beneficial effects may occur gradually and that adherence to dosage schedule is important to obtain maximal therapeutic benefit.

Stress the importance of good health practices (eg, proper diet, rest, exercise, cessation of smoking) in the successful management of peripheral vascular disease.

Selected Bibliography

Cruikshank JM, McAinsh J: Beta blockers and quality of life. Br J Clin Pract 46:34, 1992

Katz RJ: Mechanisms of nitrate tolerance: A review. Cardiovasc Drugs Ther 4:427, 1990

Klaus D: The role of calcium antagonists in the treatment of hypertension. J Cardiovasc Pharmacol 20(Suppl 6):S5, 1992

Mark DB: Effects of coronary angioplasty, coronary bypass surgery, and medical therapy on employment in patients with coronary artery disease. Ann Intern Med 120:111, 1994

Rinde-Hoffman D, Glaser SP, Arnett Dk: Update on nitrate therapy. J Clin Pharmacol 31:697, 1991

Triggle DJ: Calcium-channel antagonists: Mechanisms of action, vascular selectivities, and clinical relevance. Cleve Clin J Med 59:617, 1992

Walton T, Symes LR: Felodipine and isradipine: New calcium-channel-blocking agents for the treatment of hypertension. Clin Pharm 12:261, 1993

35

Prophylaxis of Atherosclerosis: Hypolipemic Drugs

Bile Acid-Sequestering Resins
- Cholestyramine
- Colestipol

Clofibrate
Dextrothyroxine
Gemfibrozil

HMG-CoA Reductase Inhibitors
- Fluvastatin
- Lovastatin
- Pravastatin
- Simvastatin

Nicotinic Acid
Probucol

Atherosclerosis is a condition characterized by deposition of lipid (fatty) material within the walls of the arterial system, resulting in a gradual occlusion of blood flow. Clinical consequences of this lipid deposition include the development of ischemic heart disease, cerebrovascular disease (including stroke), peripheral ischemia, and renovascular hypertension. The presence of generalized atherosclerosis greatly increases the risk of mortality from one or more of these conditions.

Although the basic mechanism involved in the development of the atherosclerotic process is still somewhat uncertain, there appears to be a metabolic disturbance in the synthesis, transport, and use of lipids; this, in combination with damage to the vascular endothelial lining, results in the adherence and eventual build-up of fatty deposits within the lining of the vessel walls.

Lipids do not circulate freely in the bloodstream, but rather are bound to plasma proteins (albumin, globulins). These complexes are termed *lipoproteins* and contain varying proportions of high-density proteins and low-density lipids. The following is a list of the four major types of lipoproteins, with a brief description of their characteristics.

Chylomicrons: largest and lightest of the lipoproteins, formed in the intestine during absorption of dietary fat; composed mainly (80%–90%) of triglycerides and impart a cloudiness to plasma; normally cleared rapidly from the blood; their presence in plasma taken from a fasting patient suggests an inability to handle dietary fats

Very–low-density lipoproteins (VLDL): prebeta-lipoproteins containing large amounts (50%–60%) of triglycerides that were synthesized in the liver; major means by which endogenous triglycerides are carried from the liver to the plasma

Low-density lipoproteins (LDL): beta-lipoproteins derived partly from breakdown of VLDL, containing about 50% to 60% cholesterol, 25% protein, and very few triglycerides; most of the circulating serum cholesterol is transported in this form, and elevated plasma levels of LDL indicate excessive cholesterol levels and suggest that the patient is at high risk for development of atherosclerosis

High-density lipoproteins (HDL): alpha-lipoproteins, the smallest and most dense (heaviest) of the lipoproteins, containing approximately 50% protein, 25% cholesterol, and very small amounts of triglycerides; believed to play an important role in clearing cholesterol from body tissues and may protect against development of atherosclerosis by blocking uptake of LDL cholesterol by vascular smooth muscle cells

Approximately one fourth of all adults have elevated levels of one or more of the plasma lipids or lipoproteins, which may reflect improper diet, excessive alcohol consumption, secondary disease (such as hypothyroidism or diabetes), or an inherited trait. Measurements of serum cholesterol and triglycerides can easily be done and are a common component of laboratory blood studies. A more accurate and useful classification of patients with defects in lipid metabolism or transport, however, is based on the types of lipoproteins that are elevated in the plasma. This grouping allows precise diagnosis and treatment of each patient's condition. The term *hyperlipoproteinemia* is used to indicate an increase in one or more of the classes of lipoproteins. Table 35-1 lists the types of hyperlipoproteinemias that are recognized, with a brief description of each type and the most effective treatment of each subgroup.

There is good evidence that lowering serum levels of cholesterol and other lipids reduces the risk of atherosclerosis. It appears that elevated plasma cholesterol or LDL is a major risk factor for development of atherosclerosis, and results of a multicenter, randomized clinical study strongly suggest that reductions in plasma concentrations of LDL cholesterol can significantly reduce the risk of coronary artery disease.

Several therapeutic strategies may be used in the treatment of hyperlipoproteinemias. The cornerstone of therapy remains diet modification and weight reduction. Reduced consumption of cholesterol and saturated animal fats is recommended for all types of hyperlipoproteinemias. Protein intake is either maintained or increased in most instances. Other risk factors should be eliminated as well, through cessation of smoking, curtailment or abstinence from alcohol, treatment of elevated blood pressure, and maintenance of an adequate program of exercise and physical fitness.

Drug therapy of hyperlipoproteinemia involves the use of agents that can lower plasma concentrations of lipoproteins, either by blocking their production or by enhancing their removal from the plasma. These drugs, termed *hypolipemic* or *hypolipidemic* agents, are used in a significant percentage of the population with hyperlipoproteinemia. In view of the potential for many hypolipemic drugs to cause untoward reactions, however, dietary changes are usually undertaken before drug ther-

Table 35-1. **Classification of Hyperlipoproteinemias**

Type	Descriptive Name	Characteristic Features	Treatment: Diet	Treatment: Drugs
I	Fat induced (exogenous)	Relatively rare; increase in plasma chylomicrons containing large amounts of triglycerides of dietary origin; frequently seen in infancy and marked by abdominal pain; does not lead to atherosclerosis	Low fat; no alcohol; no restrictions on proteins, carbohydrates, or cholesterol	None effective
IIa	Familial hypercholesterolemia	High levels of LDL; normal VLDL; slight elevation of triglycerides; fairly common, and a definite risk for development of atherosclerosis and coronary artery disease	Low cholesterol; low saturated fats; increased intake of polyunsaturated fats	Nicotinic acid Cholestyramine Colestipol Dextrothyroxine Lovastatin Simvastatin Pravastatin Probucol
IIb	Combined hyperlipoproteinemia	Elevated LDL and VLDL; presence of hypercholesterolemia and hypertriglyceridemia; lipid deposits occur on feet, elbows, knees	See IIa	Cholestyramine Colestipol Dextrothyroxine Lovastatin Pravastatin Simvastatin Gemfibrozil Nicotinic acid Probucol
III	Broad beta-lipoproteinemia	Elevated LDL and VLDL; cholesterol and triglycerides are elevated; relatively uncommon but associated with atherosclerosis; recessively inherited disorder	Weight reduction; low cholesterol; low saturated fats; maintain high protein	Clofibrate Nicotinic acid
IV	Carbohydrate induced (endogenous)	Marked elevation of VLDL; triglycerides are increased but LDL and cholesterol are normal or slightly elevated; most common type; definite risk for atherosclerosis and coronary artery disease	Weight reduction; low carbohydrate; low cholesterol; low alcohol; maintain protein intake	Clofibrate Gemfibrozil Nicotinic acid
V	Mixed hyperlipemia	Elevated VLDL and triglycerides; chylomicrons are increased; relatively uncommon type not generally associated with atherosclerosis or heart disease; xanthomas, hyperuricemia and pancreatitis can occur	Low fat; high protein, low carbohydrate; low alcohol	Clofibrate Gemfibrozil Nicotinic acid

apy is instituted. If diet alone is ineffective in controlling plasma lipids, drug therapy is then warranted, but only on careful diagnosis of the type of hyperlipoproteinemia present. There is some evidence that therapy with cholesterol-lowering agents may cause regression of atherosclerotic lesions.

Bile Acid-Sequestering Resins

Cholestyramine
Colestipol

These two bile acid-sequestering agents are anion-exchange resins that combine with bile acids in the intestines, preventing their reabsorption and therefore increasing their excretion in the feces. They are effective plasma cholesterol-lowering drugs, and cholestyramine is also used for relieving pruritus associated with partial biliary obstruction. They are discussed together here, and listed individually in Table 35-2.

Mechanism

Form an insoluble complex with bile acids in the intestine, increasing their fecal excretion; this leads to increased oxidation of cholesterol to bile acids, decreased serum cholesterol levels, and reduced beta-lipoprotein (LDL) levels; little effect on serum triglyceride levels; may interfere with absorption of calcium, fats, fat-soluble vitamins (A, D, E, K), and many other drugs (see Interactions).

Uses

Adjunctive treatment of primary type II hyperlipoproteinemia

Relief of pruritus associated with partial biliary obstruction (cholestyramine only)

Investigational uses for cholestyramine include treatment of antibiotic-induced pseudomembranous colitis, treatment of poisoning with the pesticide chlordecone (Kepone), and treatment of digitalis toxicity

Dosage

See Table 35-2.

Fate

Not absorbed from the GI tract nor hydrolyzed by digestive enzymes; excreted in feces as insoluble bile acid complex.

Common Side Effects

Constipation (occasionally severe), abdominal discomfort, flatulence, belching, nausea, anorexia.

Significant Adverse Reactions

Vomiting; steatorrhea; fecal impaction; vitamin K deficiency with bleeding tendencies; vitamin A, D, and E deficiencies; rash

Table 35-2. **Bile Acid-Sequestering Resins**

Drug	Usual Dosage Range	Nursing Considerations
Cholestyramine *Cholybar, Questran, Questran Light*	Initially 4 g resin 1–6 times/d before meals, adjust to patient's needs (range, 16–24 g/d)	Place drug on surface of 4–6 oz liquid; allow to stand 1–2 min without stirring, then gently twirl container or stir slowly to obtain a uniform suspension; rinse glass with fluid to ensure taking entire dose; may also be mixed with soups or pulpy fruits (eg, apple sauce); relief of pruritus may take 1–2 wk to become evident; decline in serum cholesterol is usually apparent by 1 mo
Colestipol *Colestid*	5–30 g/d in divided doses 2–4 times/d	Add prescribed amount of drug to at least 3 oz of liquid and stir until completely mixed (does *not* dissolve); may also be added to cereals, soups, or pulpy fruits; does not have the disagreeable odor or taste of cholestyramine

and irritation of the skin, tongue, and perianal region; osteoporosis.

A wide variety of other adverse reactions has been reported in people taking these drugs, but their relationship to the drugs themselves is unclear.

Contraindications

Complete biliary obstruction. *Cautious use* in patients with constipation, anemia, bleeding tendencies, systemic acidosis, or hypothyroidism, and in pregnant or nursing women.

Interactions

May interfere with oral absorption of acetaminophen, amiodarone, anticoagulants, corticosteroids, digitalis drugs, gemfibrozil, iopanoic acid, iron preparations, phenylbutazone, propranolol, pravastatin, thiazide diuretics, thyroid drugs, trimethoprim, vitamins A, D, E, and K.

Nursing Management

Pretherapy Assessment

Assess and record baseline data necessary for detection of adverse effects of bile acid sequestrants: General: vital signs (VS), body weight, skin color and temperature; Central nervous system (CNS): orientation, affect, reflexes; Cardiovascular system (CVS): baseline electrocardiogram ECG, peripheral perfusion; GI: liver evaluation; Laboratory: liver function tests, lipid profiles, clotting profile.

Review medical history and documents for existing or previous conditions that:

a. require cautious use of bile acid sequestrants: constipation; anemia; bleeding tendencies; systemic acidosis; hypothyroidism.
b. contraindicate use of bile acid sequestrants: allergy to bile acid sequestrants; severe anemia; marked hypotension; increased intracranial pressure; cerebral hemorrhage; acute stages of myocardial infarction; **pregnancy (Category C)**; lactation (safety not established; if drug is required, do not nurse).

Nursing Interventions

Medication Administration

Advocate supplemental therapy with parenteral or water-miscible forms of vitamins A, D, and E in patient on prolonged therapy because deficiencies can occur.

Administer drug before meals.

Establish bowel program to deal with constipation.

Provide small, palatable meals.

Prepare drug as instructed before giving orally (see Table 35-2). Dissolve powder in an appropriate vehicle (eg, flavored liquid, thin soup, juice) to disguise disagreeable taste. Ingestion of powder alone is very irritating and may cause esophageal impaction.

Surveillance During Therapy

Consult with dietitian regarding low-cholesterol meals.

Monitor bowel function for development of constipation, especially when dose is high or patient is elderly. If bowel function is problematic, dosage may be lowered, or a stool softener or laxative may be used.

Observe patient for early symptoms of hypoprothrombinemia related to vitamin K deficiency, such as petechiae, mucosal bleeding, and tarry stools. Parenteral vitamin K_1 is indicated if this occurs. Recurrences can be prevented by oral administration of vitamin K (2.5–10 mg).

Carefully observe infant or child because hypochloremic acidosis has occurred in these patients. Therapy should be initiated with small doses because a dosage schedule has not been established for infants or children.

Monitor results of serum cholesterol and triglyceride levels, which should be determined at start of therapy and at regular intervals thereafter.

Carefully monitor laboratory studies and patient for indications of adverse reactions.

Interpret results of diagnostic tests and contact practitioner as appropriate.

Monitor for possible drug–drug and drug–nutrient interactions; see Interactions.

Provide for patient safety needs if CNS effects occur.

Patient Teaching

Instruct patient to take other oral medications at least 1 hour before or 4 hours after cholestyramine or colestipol administration, if possible, to avoid interference with their absorption.

Instruct patient to eat foods high in bulk (fruit, raw vegetables) and to maintain liberal fluid intake to minimize constipation.

Inform patient that GI side effects usually subside with continued therapy.
Inform patients that the following side effects are likely to occur: constipation; nausea; heartburn; loss of appetite; dizziness, vertigo, fainting; headache; muscle and joint aches.
Report any of the following to practitioner if they occur: unusual bleeding or bruising; severe constipation; severe GI upset; chest pain; difficulty breathing; rash, fever.

• Clofibrate

Atromid-S

(CAN) Claripex, Novofibrate

Mechanism

Not definitively established; lowers elevated triglyceride and VLDL levels, possibly by increasing breakdown of free fatty acids in the liver through action of lipoprotein lipase; also, decreases release of VLDL from liver to plasma and interferes with binding of free fatty acids to albumin; may slightly reduce plasma cholesterol and LDL, presumably by inhibiting cholesterol biosynthesis and increasing biliary and fecal excretion of cholesterol; reduces serum fibrinogen levels and platelet adhesiveness.

Uses

Adjunctive treatment of type III hyperlipoproteinemia that does not respond adequately to diet
Adjunctive treatment of types IV and V hyperlipoproteinemia characterized by very high serum triglyceride levels and a risk of pancreatitis

Dosage

Adults: Initially 2 g/day in divided doses; adjust to desired response
NOTE: Drug should be discontinued after 3 months if response is inadequate

Fate

After administration, drug is hydrolyzed to *p*-chlorophenoxyisobutyric acid (CPIB), the active form of the drug, which is slowly but completely absorbed; peak CPIB plasma levels occur in 3 to 6 hours; plasma half-life ranges from 6 to 24 hours; much longer (up to 100 h) in patients with renal impairment; CPIB is highly protein bound (90%–95%) and is largely metabolized in the liver and excreted in the urine.

Common Side Effects

Nausea, dyspepsia, abdominal distress, flatulence.

Significant Adverse Reactions

CAUTION

Clofibrate has produced benign and malignant tumors in rats at five to eight times the human dose. The drug has the potential to elicit hepatic tumors in humans, produce cholelithiasis (twice the risk of nonusers), and evoke a wide range of other untoward reactions. Because of these characteristics, coupled with the lack of substantial evidence for a beneficial effect for clofibrate on cardiovascular mortality, it should be reserved for those patients with *significant hyperlipidemia* and a high risk of coronary artery disease who have not responded adequately to diet, weight loss, and other less toxic drugs.

GI: diarrhea, vomiting, gastritis, stomatitis, increased gallstones, hepatomegaly
CV: arrhythmias, swelling, and phlebitis at site of xanthoma, angina, thromboembolic complications
Dermatologic: rash, urticaria, pruritus, alopecia, dry skin, dry hair
Hematologic: leukopenia, anemia, eosinophilia
Neurologic: drowsiness, weakness, dizziness, headache
Other: myalgia and flulike symptoms, arthralgia, impotence, decreased libido, dysuria, hematuria, decreased urinary output, weight gain, polyphagia, abnormal liver function test results, hepatic tumors

Contraindications

Hepatic or renal dysfunction, primary biliary cirrhosis, and in pregnant and nursing women. *Cautious use* in the presence of peptic ulcer, cardiac arrhythmias, or gout, and in patients receiving oral anticoagulants or oral hypoglycemic drugs (see Interactions).

Interactions

Clofibrate may enhance the effects of oral anticoagulants, hypoglycemic agents, cholinesterase inhibitors, furosemide, and thyroxine.
Oral contraceptives, other estrogens, and rifampin can antagonize the action of clofibrate.
Probenecid may increase the therapeutic and toxic effects of clofibrate.

Nursing Management

Pretherapy Assessment

Assess and record baseline data necessary for detection of adverse effects of clofibrate: General: VS, body weight, skin color and temperature; CVS: baseline ECG, peripheral perfusion, edema; GI: liver evaluation; Laboratory: liver function tests, lipid profiles, clotting profile.
Review medical history and documents for existing or previous conditions that:
a. require cautious use of clofibrate: peptic ulcer; cardiac arrhythmias; gout; oral anticoagulants; oral hypoglycemic drugs (see Interactions).
b. contraindicate use of clofibrate: allergy to clofibrate; hepatic or renal dysfunction; primary biliary cirrhosis; **pregnancy (Category C)**; lactation (safety not established; if drug is required, do not nurse).

Nursing Interventions

Medication Administration

Administer drug with meals or milk if GI upset occurs.
Establish bowel program to deal with constipation.
Provide small, palatable meals.

Surveillance During Therapy

Consult with dietitian regarding low-cholesterol meals.
Monitor results of liver function tests and blood counts, which should be performed frequently during therapy. Drug should be withdrawn if results are abnormal.
Monitor results of serum cholesterol and triglyceride analyses, which should be performed before initiating therapy and at 2- to 4-week intervals during treatment. A *rebound rise* in lipid levels may occur after 2 to 3 months of therapy, but further decreases will then ensue.
Carefully monitor laboratory studies and patient for indications of adverse reactions.
Interpret results of diagnostic tests and contact practitioner as appropriate.
Monitor for possible drug–drug and drug–nutrient interactions; see Interactions.

Patient Teaching

Instruct patient to notify practitioner immediately if chest pain, dyspnea, irregular heartbeat, stomach pain, vomiting, fever, chills, sore throat, hematuria, oliguria, or swelling of the extremities occur.
Instruct patient to report development of flulike symptoms (muscle aching, weakness, soreness, cramping) because these may indicate a need for dosage reduction.
Encourage woman with childbearing potential to use effective birth control measures because fetal damage can occur. Drug should be withdrawn several months before attempted conception.
Stress the importance of adhering to recommended diet.

• Dextrothyroxine

Choloxin

Mechanism

Synthetic D-isomer of thyroxine, possessing much less metabolic stimulating action than the naturally occurring L-isomer (L-thyroxine); reduces serum cholesterol and LDL levels but has no *consistent* effect on triglycerides or VLDL; accelerates breakdown of cholesterol in the liver, resulting in increased biliary excretion; may also increase number of LDL receptors on all membranes.

Uses

Adjunctive treatment for reduction of elevated cholesterol and LDL levels in type II euthyroid patients with no evidence of organic heart disease.

Dosage

Adults: initially 1 to 2 mg/day; increase by 1- to 2-mg increments at monthly intervals to a maintenance range of 4 to 8 mg/day
Children: initially 0.05 mg/kg/day; increase by 0.05-mg/kg/month increments to a maximum of 0.4 mg/kg or 4 mg; maintenance dose 0.1 mg/kg/day

Fate

Adequately absorbed from GI tract; minimal protein binding metabolized by the liver and rapidly excreted in the urine.

Common Side Effects

Nervousness, sweating, flushing, palpitations, dyspepsia.

Significant Adverse Reactions

Most common in hypothyroid patients or patients with organic heart disease.

CV: angina, arrhythmias, myocardial damage, increased heart size
CNS: insomnia, tremors, headache, hyperthermia, dizziness, visual disturbances, tinnitus, paresthesias, psychic changes
GI: vomiting, diarrhea, anorexia
Other: hair loss, weight loss, diuresis, menstrual irregularities, altered libido, hoarseness, muscle pain, skin rash, gallstones, hyperglycemia, elevated protein-bound iodine levels, worsening of peripheral vascular disease

Contraindications

Organic heart disease (angina, arrhythmias, myocardial infarction, congestive heart failure, rheumatic heart disease), hypertension (other than mild, labile forms), liver or kidney disease, pregnancy, and lactation. *Cautious use* in patients with diabetes mellitus.

Interactions

Dextrothyroxine may potentiate the effects of oral anticoagulants.
Therapeutic effect of digitalis preparations may be decreased.
Dextrothyroxine can antagonize the effects of oral hypoglycemics and insulin by increasing blood sugar levels.
Increased response to injections of epinephrine or norepinephrine (eg, episodes of coronary insufficiency) may occur in the presence of dextrothyroxine.
Concurrent use of dextrothyroxine and other CNS stimulants (tricyclic antidepressants, amphetamines, caffeine) may result in increased CNS excitation and tachycardia.

Nursing Management

Pretherapy Assessment

Assess and record baseline data necessary for detection of adverse effects of dextrothyroxine: General: VS, body weight, skin color and temperature; CVS: baseline ECG, peripheral perfusion, edema; GI: liver evaluation; Laboratory: liver function tests, lipid profiles, clotting profile.
Review medical history and documents for existing or previous conditions that:
a. require cautious use of dextrothyroxine: peptic ulcer; cardiac arrhythmias; gout; oral anticoagulants; oral hypoglycemic drugs (see Interactions).
b. contraindicate use of dextrothyroxine: allergy to thyroid agents; hepatic or renal dysfunction; primary biliary cirrhosis; **pregnancy (Category C)**; lactation (safety not established; if drug is required, do not nurse).

Nursing Interventions

Medication Administration

Administer drug with meals or milk if GI upset occurs.
Establish bowel program to deal with constipation.
Provide small, palatable meals.

Surveillance During Therapy

Consult with dietitian regarding low-cholesterol meals.
Monitor results of liver function tests and blood counts, which should be performed frequently during therapy. Drug should be withdrawn if results are abnormal.
Monitor results of serum cholesterol and triglyceride analyses, which should be performed before initiating therapy and at 2- to 4-week intervals during treatment. A *rebound rise* in lipid levels may occur after 2 to 3 months of therapy, but further decreases will then ensue.
Carefully assess patient with known or suspected cardiac disease for signs of increasing cardiac decompensation (eg, dyspnea, nocturnal coughing, pain on exertion, palpitations, edema). If signs appear, inform practitioner immediately; dosage reduction or discontinuation of drug is warranted.
Question prescription of more than 4 mg dextrothyroxine/day because myocardial oxygen requirements may be dangerously elevated in a patient with organic heart disease.
Interpret results of serum protein-bound iodine levels appropriately. Increased levels occur in patient taking dextrothyroxine, but they indicate drug absorption and transport rather than a hypermetabolic state. Levels in the range of 10 to 25 μg/dL are common and do not necessitate dosage adjustment.
Carefully monitor laboratory studies and patient for indications of adverse reactions.
Interpret results of diagnostic tests and contact practitioner as appropriate.
Monitor for possible drug–drug and drug–nutrient interactions; see Interactions.

Patient Teaching

Advise patient promptly to report symptoms of iodism (excessive use of iodine-containing compounds) such as acneiform rash, itching, coryza, conjunctivitis. Drug may have to be withdrawn if these occur.
Encourage woman of childbearing potential to use effective birth control measures because fetal damage can occur.
Teach diabetic patient to carefully assess blood glucose control. Loss of control (eg, glycosuria, polyuria, polydipsia) may require dosage adjustments (increase antidiabetic drugs or decrease dextrothyroxine).
Encourage patient to obtain all blood tests requested. Serum lipids should be determined before therapy and monthly during therapy.
Inform patient that decreased cholesterol levels may not occur for several weeks after initiation of therapy and that maximal response may require 2 to 3 months.

• Gemfibrozil

Lopid

Mechanism

Not completely established; lowers elevated serum triglycerides, primarily the VLDL fraction and less frequently the LDL fraction; also increases the high-density lipoprotein fraction, an action considered to be beneficial in atherosclerosis; biochemical mechanisms of action may include inhibition of peripheral lipolysis, reduction of liver triglyceride production, and impairment in the synthesis of VLDL carrier apoprotein; may also reduce incorporation of long-chain fatty acids into newly formed triglycerides and accelerate removal of cholesterol from the liver.

Uses

Treatment of type IV and V hyperlipoproteinemia associated with high serum triglyceride levels and a definite risk of pancreatitis in patients who do not respond adequately to dietary therapy
Treatment of type IIB hyperlipoproteinemia in patients who have low HDL levels and elevated LDL and triglyceride levels and who have not responded to other measures

Dosage

600 mg twice a day, 30 minutes before the morning and evening meals.

Fate

Well absorbed from the GI tract; peak serum levels occur in 1 to 2 hours; plasma half-life is 1 to 2 hours but elimination half-life is considerably longer owing to enterohepatic circulation; excreted in the urine largely as unchanged drug (70%) and some metabolites; small amounts are also eliminated in the feces.

Common Side Effects

Abdominal pain, diarrhea, nausea.

Significant Adverse Reactions

CAUTION

Because of pharmacologic similarities between gemfibrozil and clofibrate, the serious adverse effects reported in patients receiving clofibrate must be considered a possibility in patients receiving gemfibrozil as well. Refer to the discussion of clofibrate for details.

GI: vomiting, constipation, dry mouth, gas pain, anorexia
CNS: headache, dizziness, blurred vision, vertigo, insomnia, tinnitus, paresthesias
Musculoskeletal: arthralgia, back pain, myalgia, muscle cramping, swollen joints
Dermatologic: rash, dermatitis, pruritus, urticaria
Hepatic: liver function abnormalities (increased serum transaminases, lactate dehydrogenase, creatine phosphokinase, alkaline phosphatase)
Other: anemia, eosinophilia, leukopenia, malaise, syncope, cholelithiasis

Contraindications

Hepatic or severe renal dysfunction, gallbladder disease, biliary cirrhosis. *Cautious use* in patients with diabetes mellitus, cardiac arrhythmias, or altered liver function values, and in pregnant or nursing women.

Interactions

Gemfibrozil may potentiate the effects of oral anticoagulants.
An increased incidence of myositis and elevated creatine kinase, possibly leading to acute renal failure, can occur when combined with lovastatin and possibly also simvastatin, pravastatin, or fluvastatin.

Nursing Management

Pretherapy Assessment

Assess and record baseline data necessary for detection of adverse effects of gemfibrozil: General: VS, body weight, skin color and temperature, gait, range of motion; GI: liver evaluation; Laboratory: liver and renal function tests, complete blood count (CBC), lipid profiles, clotting profile, blood glucose.
Review medical history and documents for existing or previous conditions that:
a. require cautious use of gemfibrozil: diabetes mellitus; cardiac arrhythmias; altered liver function values.
b. contraindicate use of gemfibrozil: allergy to gemfibrozil; hepatic or severe renal dysfunction; gallbladder disease; biliary cirrhosis; **pregnancy (Category B)**, lactation (safety not established; if drug is required, do not nurse).

Nursing Interventions

Medication Administration

Administer drug with meals or milk if GI upset occurs.
Establish bowel program to deal with constipation.
Provide small, palatable meals.

Surveillance During Therapy

Consult with dietitian regarding low-cholesterol meals.
Monitor results of liver function tests and blood counts, which should be performed periodically during therapy. Drug should be discontinued if abnormalities persist for any length of time or worsen.
Assist with evaluation of patient's response to drug. If lipid response is still inadequate after 3 months as determined by serum lipid levels, drug should be withdrawn.
Carefully monitor laboratory studies and patient for indications of adverse reactions.
Interpret results of diagnostic tests and contact practitioner as appropriate.
Monitor for possible drug–drug and drug–nutrient interactions; see Interactions.

Patient Teaching

Instruct patient to notify practitioner if GI symptoms (abdominal pain, nausea, vomiting, diarrhea) persist or worsen. Dosage may have to be reduced or drug discontinued.
Instruct patient to notify practitioner if symptoms of gallbladder disease occur (eg, upper abdominal discomfort, bloating, belching, fried-food intolerance). Appropriate diagnostic studies should be performed. Drug should be discontinued if gallstones are found.
Carefully explain that adherence to prescribed diet and restricted intake of sugars, cholesterol, saturated fats, and alcohol are very important to successful control of hyperlipidemia.

HMG-CoA Reductase Inhibitors (*Pregnancy Category X*)

- ***Fluvastatin***

Lescol

- ***Lovastatin***

Mevacor

- ***Pravastatin***

Pravachol

- ***Simvastatin***

Zocor

Mechanism

Hydrolyzed to a beta-hydroxy acid form, which is a potent inhibitor of HMG-CoA reductase, an enzyme that catalyzes the conversion of HMG-CoA to mevalonate, an early and *rate-limiting* step in the biosynthesis of cholesterol; lowers both normal and elevated LDL cholesterol levels; reduces the concentration of circulating LDL particles, increases HDL cholesterol levels, and reduces VLDL cholesterol and plasma triglycerides; does not appear to affect steroidogenesis adversely.

Uses

Adjunct to diet for reducing elevated total and LDL cholesterol levels in patients with primary hypercholesterolemia (types IIa and IIb)
Reduction of elevated LDL cholesterol levels in patients with combined hypercholesterolemia and hypertriglyceridemia

Dosage

Lovastatin: Initially, 20 mg once daily; usual dosage range 20 to 80 mg daily in a single or divided doses
Pravastatin: Initially, 10 to 20 mg daily at bedtime; initial dose for elderly patients is 10 mg daily at bedtime; usual dose range: 10 to 40 mg daily at bedtime
Simvastatin: Initially, 5 to 10 mg daily in evening; initial dose for elderly patients is 5 mg daily at bedtime; usual dose range: 5 to 40 mg daily; adjust dose at intervals of at least 4 weeks

Fluvastatin: Initially, 20 mg once daily at bedtime; usual dosage range is 20–40 mg as a single evening dose

Fate

Lovastatin: Less than one third of an oral dose is absorbed, and the drug undergoes extensive first-pass hepatic metabolism such that less than 5% of an oral dose reaches the systemic circulation as active drug or metabolite; maximum therapeutic response occurs within 4 to 6 weeks and is maintained by single daily dosing in the evening; both lovastatin and its beta-hydroxy acid metabolite are highly protein bound in the plasma (95%); excretion is largely in the feces by way of the bile (about 85%), with some drug and metabolite (10%–15%) appearing in the urine.
Pravastatin: Approximately 34% of a dose is absorbed. The drug undergoes extensive first-pass hepatic metabolism such that 17% of an oral dose reaches the systemic circulation. Pravastatin is 50% protein bound, with 20% excreted in the urine and 70% in the feces.
Simvastatin: Approximately 85% of a dose is absorbed. The drug undergoes extensive first-pass metabolism such that less than 5% of an oral dose reaches the systemic circulation. Simvastatin is 95% protein bound, with 13% excreted in the urine and 60% in the feces.
Fluvastatin: Almost completely absorbed orally; undergoes extensive first-pass metabolism; highly protein bound; primarily excreted in the feces as several metabolites.

Common Side Effects

Headache, abdominal discomfort, flatulence, diarrhea, nausea, rash, pruritus, elevated creatine phosphokinase.

Significant Adverse Reactions

Dizziness, insomnia, blurred vision, peripheral neuropathy, increased serum transaminases with prolonged therapy, myalgia, muscle tenderness.

Contraindications

Acute liver disease, persistent elevation of serum transaminases, pregnancy, or lactation. *Cautious use* in patients at risk for development of renal failure (such as those with severe acute infections, hypotension, trauma, or severe metabolic, endocrine, or electrolyte disturbances), and in those with uncontrolled seizures, chronic liver dysfunction, or skeletal muscle disorders.

Interactions

HMG-CoA reductase inhibitors can increase the anticoagulant effect of warfarin.
Bile acid sequestrants can decrease the bioavailability of pravastatin by 40% to 50%.
Severe myopathy or rhabdomyolysis may occur when these drugs are used in combination with cyclosporine, erythromycin, gemfibrozil, and niacin.

Nursing Management

Pretherapy Assessment

Assess and record baseline data necessary for detection of adverse effects of HMG-CoA reductase inhibitors: General: VS, body weight, skin color and temperature, gait, range of motion; CNS: orientation, affect, ophthalmic examination; GI: liver evaluation; Laboratory: liver and renal function tests, CBC, lipid profiles, clotting profile, blood glucose.
Review medical history and documents for existing or previous conditions that:
a. require cautious use of HMG-CoA reductase inhibitors: renal failure (such as those with severe acute infections, hypotension, trauma, or severe metabolic, endocrine, or electrolyte disturbances); uncontrolled seizures; chronic liver dysfunction; skeletal muscle disorders.
b. contraindicate use of HMG-CoA reductase inhibitors: allergy to HMG-CoA reductase inhibitors, fungal by-products; acute liver disease; persistent elevation of serum transaminases; **pregnancy (Category X)**; lactation (safety not established; if drug is required, do not nurse).

Nursing Interventions

Medication Administration

Administer drug in the evening, when cholesterol synthesis rates are highest.
Establish bowel program to deal with constipation.
Provide small, palatable meals.

Surveillance During Therapy

Consult with dietitian regarding low-cholesterol meals.
Monitor results of serum cholesterol determinations, which should be obtained periodically throughout therapy to guide dosage adjustments.
Monitor results of liver function tests, which the manufacturer recommends be obtained every 4 to 6 weeks for the first 15 months of therapy and periodically thereafter, because unexplained elevations of serum transaminases may occur. The patient who consumes large amounts of alcohol or has a history of liver disease should be monitored especially carefully.
Carefully monitor laboratory studies and patient for indications of adverse reactions.
Interpret results of diagnostic tests and contact practitioner as appropriate.
Monitor for possible drug–drug and drug–nutrient interactions; see Interactions.

Patient Teaching

Emphasize that drug acts in conjunction with reductions in dietary fat and cholesterol.
Refer patient to dietitian for instruction regarding low-fat, low-cholesterol diet.
Instruct patient to take once daily with evening meal (lovastatin) or at bedtime (other drugs); evening doses appear to be more effective than morning doses.
Advise patient to use caution in performing hazardous activities until drug effects have been determined, because dizziness and blurred vision may occur.
Report unexplained muscle pain, tenderness, or weakness, especially if accompanied by fever or malaise.

• Nicotinic Acid—Niacin

Nicotinic acid (vitamin B_3) is a water-soluble vitamin that is discussed in Chapter 75. In large doses, it can lower elevated plasma lipid levels and has been used as adjunctive therapy in certain types of hyperlipoproteinemias.

Mechanism

Not completely established; reduces lipolysis and release of free fatty acids from adipose tissue and decreases hepatic synthesis of VLDL and triglycerides; LDL formation is also reduced; increases activity of lipoprotein lipase and accelerates removal of chylomicron triglycerides; hepatic cholesterol synthesis may also be inhibited.

Uses

Adjunctive therapy in patients with elevated cholesterol or triglycerides who do not respond adequately to diet and weight loss.

Dosage

1 to 2 g three times/day; increase slowly, first to 4.5 g then to 6 g/day after several weeks if necessary. Lower starting doses may be used in an effort to increase patient tolerance.

Fate

Readily absorbed orally; peak serum levels occur within 1 hour; elimination half-life is 45 to 60 minutes; partially metabolized by the liver and excreted as both metabolites and unchanged drug by the kidneys.

Common Side Effects

GI distress, flushing, feeling of warmth, pruritus, paresthesias.

Significant Adverse Reactions

Headache, dizziness, palpitations, diarrhea, hypotension, hyperuricemia, gouty arthritis, skin rash, dermatoses, epigastric pain, jaundice, decreased glucose tolerance, activation of peptic ulcer, increased sebaceous gland activity, toxic amblyopia, and impaired liver function.

Contraindications

Hepatic dysfunction, active peptic ulcer, severe hypotension, hemorrhaging, and gastritis. *Cautious use* in patients with allergic disorders, glaucoma, gallbladder disease, diabetes, or gout, and in pregnant or lactating women.

Interactions

Nicotinic acid may enhance the blood pressure-lowering effects of antihypertensive medications.

Nicotinic acid may antagonize the effects of hypoglycemic agents by elevating blood glucose levels.

HMG-CoA reductase inhibitors can increase the incidence of myopathy.

Nursing Management

Pretherapy Assessment

Assess and record baseline data necessary for detection of adverse effects of nicotinic acid: General: VS, body weight, skin color and temperature, gait, range of motion; GI: liver evaluation; Laboratory: liver and renal function tests, serum uric acid, glucose tolerance test.

Review medical history and documents for existing or previous conditions that:

a. require cautious use of nicotinic acid: allergic disorders; glaucoma; gallbladder disease; diabetes; gout.
b. contraindicate use of nicotinic acid: allergy to nicotinic acid, nicotinamide, aspirin, tartrazine; hepatic dysfunction; active peptic ulcer; severe hypotension; hemorrhaging; gastritis; **pregnancy (Category C)**; lactation (safety not established; if drug is required, do not exceed nutritional requirements during lactation).

Nursing Interventions

Medication Administration

Administer drug in the evening, when cholesterol synthesis rates are highest.

Establish bowel program to deal with constipation.

Provide small, palatable meals.

Surveillance During Therapy

Consult with dietitian regarding low-cholesterol meals.

Monitor results of serum cholesterol determinations, which should be obtained periodically throughout therapy to guide dosage adjustments.

Carefully monitor laboratory studies and patient for indications of adverse reactions.

Interpret results of diagnostic tests and contact practitioner as appropriate.

Monitor for possible drug–drug and drug–nutrient interactions; see Interactions.

Patient Teaching

Instruct patient to take drug with food to minimize GI distress and with cold water, not hot beverages, to facilitate swallowing. Reduction in serum lipids may be enhanced if tablets are chewed, rather than swallowed whole, and ingested with large amounts of water.

Inform patient that liver function tests and blood glucose determinations usually are performed frequently during early stages of therapy to determine if adverse effects are occurring.

Warn patient that hypotension with accompanying dizziness or weakness can occur after ingestion of nicotinic acid. If this occurs, practitioner should be informed because dosage may need to be reduced.

Pretreatment with 325 mg of aspirin given 30 minutes before niacin may help reduce flushing.

• Probucol

Lorelco

Mechanism

Not determined; may inhibit hepatic synthesis of cholesterol at an early stage; does not affect later stages; increased excretion of fecal bile acids occurs, and absorption of dietary cholesterol may be impaired.

Uses

Treatment of elevated serum cholesterol in patients with primary hypercholesterolemia (type II hyperlipoproteinemia) who have not responded to diet and weight reduction (*not* indicated where hypertriglyceridemia is the predominant factor).

Dosage

500 mg twice a day with meals.

Fate

Variable GI absorption; peak blood levels are higher and less variable when taken with food; accumulates in fatty tissues and is very slowly eliminated in the feces by way of the bile.

Common Side Effects

Diarrhea, flatulence, abdominal pain, nausea.

Significant Adverse Reactions

Headache, dizziness, paresthesias, vomiting, decreased hemoglobin, rash, pruritus, insomnia, impotence, blurred vision, tinnitus, impaired taste, anorexia, indigestion, GI bleeding, petechiae, nocturia, angioedema, palpitations, syncope, chest pain, eosinophilia, thrombocytopenia, peripheral neuritis, and elevated levels of serum transaminases, bilirubin, alkaline phosphatase, uric acid, glucose, and creatine phosphokinase.

Contraindications

Patients with cardiac arrhythmias or prolongation of the QT interval, pregnant or nursing women.

Nursing Management

Pretherapy Assessment

Assess and record baseline data necessary for detection of adverse effects of probucol: General: VS, body weight, skin color and temperature, gait, range of motion; CNS: orientation, affect, reflexes; CVS: baseline ECG, peripheral perfusion; GI: bowel sounds, normal output; Laboratory: lipid profiles, CBC, clotting profiles.

Review medical history and documents for existing or previous conditions that:

a. require cautious use of probucol: hypokalemia; hypomagnesemia; severe bradycardia; atrioventricular block; recent or acute myocardial infarction; myocardial inflammation.

b. contraindicate use of probucol: allergy to probucol; **pregnancy (Category B)**; lactation (safety not established, secreted in breast milk).

Nursing Interventions

Medication Administration

Administer drug with meals.

Provide small, palatable meals.

Surveillance During Therapy

Consult with dietitian regarding low-cholesterol meals.

Monitor results of serum triglyceride analyses, which should be performed during therapy. If levels are elevated and remain so, probucol therapy should be discontinued, and another drug that reduces both cholesterol and triglycerides should be prescribed.

Carefully monitor laboratory studies and patient for indications of adverse reactions.

Interpret results of diagnostic tests and contact practitioner as appropriate.

Monitor for possible drug–drug and drug–nutrient interactions; see Interactions.

Patient Teaching

Instruct patient to take drug with food to minimize GI upset and to provide more consistent blood levels.

Inform patient that serum cholesterol levels are usually determined before initiation of therapy and frequently during initial months of therapy. Reductions should occur within first 2 months of therapy. Drug may be continued as long as favorable trend continues.

Encourage woman with childbearing potential to use effective birth control measures during therapy and for several months thereafter.

Selected Bibliography

Arca M, Vega GL, Grundy SM: Hypercholesterolemia in postmenopausal women: Metabolic defects and response to low-dose lovastatin. JAMA 271:453, 1994

Burris JF: Beta-blockers, dyslipidemia, and coronary artery disease. Arch Intern Med 153:2085, 1993

Expert Panel on Detection, Evaluation and Treatment of High Blood Cholesterol in Adults: Summary of the second report of the National Cholesterol Education Program (NCEP) expert panel on detection, evaluation, and treatment of high blood cholesterol in adults (Adult Treatment Panel II). JAMA 269:3015, 1993

Franceschini G, Paoletti R: Pharmacological control of hypertriglyceridemia. Cardiovasc Drugs Ther 7:297, 1993

Gotto AM Jr: Dyslipidemia and atherosclerosis: A forecast of pharmacological approaches. Circulation 87(4 Suppl):III54, 1993

Kichura GM, Cohen JD: Guidelines for the use of cholesterol-lowering drugs. Drug Ther 21:17, 1991

Pravastatin, simvastatin, and lovastatin for lowering serum cholesterol concentrations. Med Lett Drugs Ther 57:34, 1992

Smith GD, Song F, Sheldon TA: Cholesterol lowering and mortality: The importance of considering initial level of risk. Br Med J 306: 1367, 1993

Nursing Bibliography

Glueck C, Oakes N, Speirs J, et al: Gemfibrozil–lovastatin therapy for primary hyperlipoproteinemias. Am J Cardiol 70:1, 1992

36
Antianemic Drugs

Oral Iron Preparations

Ferrous Fumarate
Ferrous Gluconate
Ferrous Sulfate
Polysaccharide–Iron Complex

Parenteral Iron Preparation

Iron Dextran

Vitamin B_{12} and Folic Acid

Cyanocobalamin, Crystalline
Hydroxocobalamin, Crystalline
Folic Acid
Leucovorin Calcium

The term *anemia* describes a group of clinical conditions characterized by a reduction in the number of erythrocytes or in the hemoglobin concentration within erythrocytes, or both. Because oxygen is transported in the bloodstream primarily in combination with hemoglobin contained within red blood cells, either condition will impair the oxygen-carrying capacity of the blood, thereby leading to inadequate tissue oxygenation.

Red cells are formed continually in the bone marrow, with their synthesis requiring many nutrients, of which the most important are iron, folic acid, and vitamin B_{12} (cyanocobalamin). These substances usually are present in sufficient amounts in the diet; if they are adequately absorbed from the GI tract, erythrocyte formation and hemoglobin synthesis proceed normally. If, however, the diet is deficient in any of these nutrients, or if their GI absorption is impaired, symptoms of anemia develop. Anemia may also result from extreme loss or destruction of red blood cells (eg, trauma, hemorrhage, excessive menstruation), thereby increasing the nutritional requirements above the level that can be supplied by diet alone.

Although anemias can occur in a number of ways (eg, deficiency or impaired availability of dietary factors, excessive destruction or loss of red blood cells, loss of bone marrow cells), most anemias are the result of inadequate amounts of iron, folic acid, or vitamin B_{12}, and so they are considered *deficiency* anemias. Correction of the deficiency has proved highly successful in treating these conditions, if an accurate diagnosis of the type of anemia as well as any underlying causative factor, such as ulcers or malignancy, has been made.

Of the deficiency anemias, those that result from lack of iron are characterized by fewer-than-normal erythrocytes, which are frequently smaller (microcytic) and paler (hypochromic) than usual, because they contain less hemoglobin. These anemias are referred to as *microcytic* or *hypochromic*. Other hypochromic microcytic anemias result from failure to incorporate adequate iron into the developing cells, although an actual nutritional deficiency mav not be present.

Anemias that occur because of insufficient levels of folic acid or vitamin B_{12} (ie, dietary deficiency, reduced absorption) are characterized by the presence of large, immature red cells (megaloblasts) in the bone marrow and blood, as well as enlarged erythrocytes (macrocytes) that may contain abnormally high levels of hemoglobin. These anemias are labeled *megaloblastic, macrocytic*, or *hyperchromic*.

Other types of anemias include *acute hemorrhagic anemia*; *aplastic anemia*, which is caused by bone marrow damage; and *hemolytic anemia*, which is secondary to destruction of circulating red cells. The latter two anemias usually are the result of drug toxicity, and are discussed in Chapter 5.

Because hypochromic and hyperchromic anemias seldom occur together, the importance of accurate diagnosis for proper replacement therapy is obvious. Likewise, carefully differentiating those anemias caused by nutritional iron deficiency from those caused by failure of iron incorporation into red blood cells is essential, because supplemental iron in the latter case is not only ineffective but can result in iron overload (hemochromatosis) and subsequent toxicity. The "shotgun" approach of combining many factors (eg, iron, vitamin B_{12}, folic acid) in treating anemias has no place in clinical medicine and should never be used in lieu of careful diagnosis and *selective* replacement of the deficient factor, as well as correction of any underlying pathologic disorder.

The antianemic drugs discussed in this chapter include the iron preparations, folic acid, and vitamin B_{12}. In addition to these agents, therapy also may include other drugs and measures to correct any underlying abnormality that may be responsible for the anemia. Self-medication with any of the antianemic drugs should be strongly discouraged, because the apparent beneficial effects gained by treating oneself often may mask the symptoms of a more serious underlying disorder (eg, internal bleeding, neurologic dysfunction).

Oral Iron Preparations

Ferrous fumarate
Ferrous gluconate
Ferrous sulfate
Polysaccharide–iron complex

The primary use of supplemental iron is the prevention or treatment of iron-deficiency anemia. The most common cause of iron deficiency in adults is blood loss, which can result from heavy or frequent menstruation, as well as from GI bleeding, especially if it goes unrecognized for extended periods. GI bleeding must always be considered as a cause of unexplained iron-deficiency anemia, and careful evaluation is necessary to rule out a more serious underlying disorder, such as GI carcinoma or peptic ulcers.

Iron-deficiency states also can occur in infants (especially premature infants), in young children during periods of rapid growth, and in pregnant and lactating women. Supplemental iron is frequently given during these periods in the growth and reproductive cycle to meet the increased need.

Several types of preparations containing iron (capsules, tablets, liquids, injections) are used as replacement therapy in iron-deficiency anemias. The oral forms of therapy are preferred; parenteral administration of iron is largely restricted to those people who cannot tolerate oral iron because of its gastric irritative action, those who do not absorb sufficient iron from the GI tract, or those who are unable to comply with an oral regimen. Oral iron is available in either the bivalent (ferrous) or trivalent (ferric) forms; bivalent iron is more widely used because it is better absorbed and somewhat less irritating than the trivalent form. An acid environment favors reduction of trivalent to bivalent iron, which increases absorption. GI distress can be reduced by using one of the iron complexes or sustained-release forms, but the absorption of elemental iron may be retarded with use of these specialized dosage forms, because much of their iron content may be released beyond the major iron absorptive sites in the duodenum and jejunum.

The oral iron preparations are essentially alike in terms of their pharmacologic action, because they all release elemental iron, and therefore they are reviewed as a group. Individual salts and dosage forms are listed in Table 36-1. The parenteral iron preparation, iron dextran, is discussed in detail in a subsequent section.

Mechanism

Provide replacement for insufficient iron, thereby correcting the hemoglobin and tissue iron deficiency; iron is an essential component of hemoglobin because transport of oxygen by hemoglobin requires molecular iron in the bivalent state; corrects the abnormal red blood cell condition.

Uses

Prevention and treatment of iron-deficiency anemias
Prophylactic therapy during periods of increased iron requirements (eg, pregnancy, rapid growth, and sustained hemorrhaging)

Dosage

See Table 36-1.

Fate

Absorption occurs primarily from the duodenum and jejunum; only 5% to 10% of dose is absorbed in otherwise healthy people, and up to 20% in iron-deficient patients. Ferrous iron (ie, Fe^{+2}) is much more efficiently absorbed than ferric iron (ie, Fe^{+3}). Bivalent iron is converted to trivalent iron in gastric mucosal cells and then either combined with transferrin for transport to bone marrow cells or converted to ferritin or hemosiderin and stored in gastric mucosal cells, liver, spleen, or bone marrow. Excretion of iron is minimal (generally less than 1 mg/day) and occurs mainly in feces through sloughing of iron-containing intestinal mucosal cells. Very small amounts of iron may also be eliminated in the urine and sweat.

Common Side Effects

GI irritation, nausea, constipation, darkened stools.

Significant Adverse Reactions

Usually occur with large doses—vomiting, diarrhea, allergic reactions, drowsiness, abdominal pain, stomach and intestinal erosion, hypotension, weak pulse, shock, convulsions.

Contraindications

Peptic ulcer, ulcerative colitis, regional enteritis, hemochromatosis, hemosiderosis, hemolytic anemia. *Cautious use* in hepatic cirrhosis.

Interactions

Absorption of iron may be impaired by antacids (especially those containing magnesium trisilicate), cholestyramine, colestipol and pancreatic extracts, as well as by ingestion of eggs or milk.

Table 36-1. **Oral Iron Preparations**

Drug	***Usual Dosage Range***	***Nursing Considerations***
Ferrous Fumarate *Femiron, Feostat, Fumasorb, Fumerin, Hemocyte, Ircon, Span-FF* *(CAN) Neo-Fer-50, Novofumar, Palafer*	*Adults:* 200–300 mg 1–3 times/d *Children (<6 y):* 100 mg–300 mg/day in divided doses	Contains 33% elemental iron; essentially similar to ferrous sulfate in most respects, with slightly lower incidence of some GI side effects; available in combination with docusate as timed-release capsules (Ferocyl, Ferro-Sequels)
Ferrous Gluconate *Fergon, Ferralet, Simron* *(CAN) Apo-Ferrous Gluconate, Fertinic, Novoferrogluc*	*Adults:* 300–650 mg 3 times/d *Children (6–12 y):* 300 mg 1–3 times/d *Children (<6 y):* 100–300 mg/d in divided doses	Contains 11.6% elemental iron; somewhat better tolerated and better used than other forms of iron; lower incidence of GI distress
Ferrous Sulfate *Feosol, Fer-In-Sol, Fer-Iron, Ferralyn, Ferra-TD, Fero-Gradumet, Fero-space, Mol-Iron, Slow FE* *(CAN) Apo-Ferrous sulfate, Novoferrosulfa, PMS Ferrous sulfate*	*Adults:* 300–1200 mg/d in divided doses *Children (6–12 y):* 120–600 mg/d in divided doses *Children (<6 y):* 300 mg/d in divided doses	Contains 20% elemental iron; most widely used form of oral iron; best absorbed and least expensive; high degree of GI irritation that can be minimized by using sustained-release forms
Polysaccharide–Iron Complex *Hytinic, Niferex, Nu-Iron*	*Adults:* 50–300 mg/d in divided doses as required *Children:* 50–100 mg/d	Water-soluble complex of elemental iron and a low-molecular-weight polysaccharide; fewer GI side effects than with other forms of iron, no teeth staining, and no metallic aftertaste; fairly expensive

Oral iron retards absorption of tetracyclines, penicillamine, and quinolones.
Vitamin C may facilitate iron absorption by maintaining it in the ferrous state.
Chloramphenicol can delay clearance of iron from the plasma and its incorporation into red blood cells.

Nursing Management

Pretherapy Assessment

Assess and record baseline data necessary for detection of adverse effects of oral iron preparations: General: vital signs (VS), body weight, skin color and temperature; Laboratory: complete blood count (CBC), hemoglobin (Hgb), hematocrit (Hct), serum ferritin.
Review medical history and documents for existing or previous conditions that:
a. require cautious use of oral iron preparations: hepatic cirrhosis.
b. contraindicate use of oral iron preparations: allergy to any ingredient in preparations; tartrazine; peptic ulcer; ulcerative colitis; regional enteritis; hemochromatosis; hemosiderosis; hemolytic anemia. NOTE: **pregnancy (Category A)**; lactation (no evidence of risk).

Nursing Interventions

Medication Administration

Administer drug with meals (avoiding milk, eggs, coffee, and tea) if GI discomfort is severe.
Provide small, palatable meals.
Establish bowel program if constipation becomes a problem.
Provide small, frequent meals if GI upset is severe.

Surveillance During Therapy

Refer patient to dietitian for assessment of dietary iron intake, if possible, and note other drugs patient is taking that may contribute to anemia (eg, quinidine, anti-inflammatory drugs, sulfonamides). Blood counts and hemoglobin values should be obtained before iron is prescribed.
Note that oral iron preparations are available in combination with many other drugs (eg, B and C vitamins, folic acid, desiccated liver, antacids, stool softeners).
Carefully monitor laboratory studies and patient for indications of adverse reactions.
Interpret results of diagnostic tests and contact practitioner as appropriate.
Monitor for possible drug–drug and drug–nutrient interactions; see Interactions.

Patient Teaching

Warn patient that self-medication with iron preparations may mask symptoms of a more severe underlying disease.
Inform patient that GI disturbances (irritation, cramping, constipation) are common in initial stages of therapy but usually can be minimized by reducing the dose, taking the drug with food, or changing the type of preparation taken.
Suggest taking drug with food if GI irritation occurs, although this may reduce absorption. Milk or antacids should be avoided because they may further impair absorption.
Instruct patient using liquid form to take drug through a straw and to rinse mouth immediately after ingestion because preparation can stain teeth.
Inform patient that oral iron preparations can cause black or dark green stools, which are *not* usually a sign of GI bleeding.
Inform patient that hemoglobin and reticulocyte values will probably be checked periodically during therapy. Improvement should be noted within 2 to 4 weeks. If not, reassessment is warranted.

Parenteral Iron Preparation

• Iron Dextran

InFeD

Iron dextran is a complex of ferric hydroxide with dextran in physiologic saline used either IV or IM for treating iron-deficiency anemias in patients intolerant of or resistant to oral iron preparations.

Mechanism

Hydrolysis of the iron–dextran complex by reticuloendothelial cells of liver, spleen, and bone marrow releases ferric iron, which combines with transferrin and is transported to the bone marrow to be used in the synthesis of hemoglobin, as it is gradually converted to a usable form of iron.

Uses

Treatment of iron-deficiency anemias in patients in whom oral iron administration is ineffective or poorly tolerated.

Dosage

1 mL iron dextran complex equals 50 mg elemental iron; to determine quantity of iron needed, the following formula may be used:

$$0.3 \times \text{weight (lbs)} \times \left[100 - \frac{\text{hemoglobin (g/dL)} \times 100}{14.8}\right]$$

A more practical rule is 250 mg iron for each gram of hemoglobin below normal.

Recommended dosing procedures are:

IM: Test dose of 25 mg (ie, 0.5 mL) on first day to test for allergic reactions—if no evidence of hypersensitivity within 1 to 2 hours, the remainder of the first day's dose can be given; each day's dose should not exceed 25 mg iron for infants weighing less than 4.5 kg (10 lb), 50 mg iron for children less than 9 kg (20 lb), 100 mg iron for other patients, until the calculated total dose has been given

IV infusion: Dilute the calculated iron dose in 250 to 1000 mL of normal saline; administer a test dose of 25 mg over 5 minutes; if no adverse effects occur, infuse the rest of the dose over 1 to 6 hours

NOTE: IV infusion of iron dextran is not a labeled indication, but it is widely used because it eliminates the need for multiple IM injections, pain and skin staining at the IM injection site, danger of abscess formation, and the possibility of poor absorption from muscle. It is used in patients who have poor IM absorptive capacity or uncontrolled bleeding, or in whom prolonged therapy is indicated.

Fate

Slowly but well absorbed from IM injection sites (60% within 2–3 days and 90% within 1–2 wk); distributed through the reticuloendothelial system; excreted in urine, bile, and feces.

Common Side Effects

Flushing, dizziness (especially with too-rapid IV administration).

Significant Adverse Reactions

Anaphylactic reactions, other hypersensitivity reactions (rash, pruritus, urticaria, dyspnea, arthralgia, fever, chills, sweating, myalgia), soreness and inflammation at injection site, brown discoloration and sterile abscesses at IM injection sites, headache, vomiting, shivering, hypotension, lymphadenopathy, local phlebitis (IV injection), chest pain, tachycardia, arrhythmias, and convulsions.

Contraindications

Anemias other than iron-deficiency anemias and marked liver impairment. *Cautious use* in patients with asthma or a history of allergies, rheumatoid arthritis, liver impairment, or ankylosing spondylitis, during pregnancy, and in women of childbearing potential.

Nursing Management

Pretherapy Assessment

Assess and record baseline data necessary for detection of adverse effects of parenteral iron preparations: General: VS, body weight, skin color and temperature; Neuromuscular: range of motions, joints; GI: liver evaluation; Laboratory: CBC, Hgb, Hct, serum ferritin, liver function.

Review medical history and documents for existing or previous conditions that:

a. require cautious use of parenteral iron preparations: hepatic cirrhosis.

b. contraindicate use of parenteral iron preparations: allergy to iron dextran; anemias other than iron-deficiency anemias; marked liver impairment; **Pregnancy (Category B)**; lactation (safety not established).

Nursing Interventions

Medication Administration

Have epinephrine (1 : 1000) solution available to treat acute hypersensitivity because fatal anaphylactic-type reactions have occurred. A small initial test dose should always be administered to determine patient's sensitivity, and patient should be carefully observed for signs of hypersensitivity.

Keep patient recumbent for 30 to 60 minutes after IV administration to minimize orthostatic hypotension. Drug should be used IV only in patient with insufficient muscle mass, impaired IM absorptive capacity (eg, edema), or uncontrolled bleeding, or for whom massive or prolonged therapy is indicated.

Administer IM injections into upper, outer quadrant of buttock using a large (19- or 20-gauge, 2–3 in) needle. Use Z-track technique to avoid leakage into and staining of overlying subcutaneous tissue (see Chapter 2).

Have patient bear weight on leg opposite injection site when giving IM to patient who is standing. Place supine patient in lateral position with injection site uppermost.

Do not use multiple-dose vials for IV administration because they contain a preservative (phenol).

Do not mix other drugs in solution with iron dextran.

Surveillance During Therapy

Refer patient to dietitian for assessment of dietary iron intake, if possible, and note other drugs patient is taking that may contribute to anemia (eg, quinidine, antiinflammatory drugs, sulfonamides). Blood counts and hemoglobin values should be obtained before iron is prescribed.

Monitor results of hemoglobin, hematocrit, and reticulocyte analyses, which should be obtained periodically during therapy. *Oral* iron therapy should be initiated as soon as feasible.

Assess degree of pain and swelling experienced by patient with rheumatoid arthritis periodically because iron–dextran may cause an increase.

Carefully monitor laboratory studies and patient for indications of adverse reactions.

Interpret results of diagnostic tests and contact practitioner as appropriate.

Monitor for possible drug–drug and drug–nutrient interactions; see Interactions.

Patient Teaching

Teach patient that the following side effects may occur with therapy: pain at injection site; headache; joint and muscle aches; GI upset.

Instruct patient to report to practitioner if any of the following effects occur: difficulty breathing; pain at the injection site; rash; itching.

Vitamin B_{12} and Folic Acid

Vitamin B_{12} and folic acid are two vitamins essential for normal DNA synthesis. A deficiency of either can result in impaired DNA synthesis, inhibition of normal cell division, and anemia.

• Cyanocobalamin, Crystalline

Betalin 12, Redisol, and other manufacturers

(CAN) Anacobin, Rubion and other manufacturers

Cyanocobalamin (vitamin B_{12}) is a cobalt-containing substance essential for normal growth, cell reproduction, hematopoiesis, and nucleoprotein synthesis. It is a biologically potent compound, so only minute amounts (1–2 μg) are necessary in the daily diet to supply the normal body needs. The most common cause of vitamin B_{12} deficiency is insufficient GI absorption, due primarily to reduced availability of the *intrinsic factor*, a glycoprotein secreted by the gastric mucosal cells that is necessary for adequate absorption of B_{12}. This condition is referred to as *pernicious anemia* and is characterized hematologically by megaloblasts in the bone marrow and macrocytes in the plasma. The patient feels fatigued, and frequently there are GI and neurologic complications. Symptoms are usually readily reversed by supplemental injections of cyanocobalamin, crystalline.

Cyanocobalamin is available as an over-the-counter tablet preparation for oral use, and by prescription for IM or SC injection. Tablets containing less than 500 μg are *not* intended for treatment of pernicious anemia but should only be used as nutritional supplements (see Chapter 76).

Mechanism

Activate folic acid coenzymes necessary for the synthesis of red blood cells, and facilitate the maturation of megaloblasts into normal erythrocytes; in vitamin B_{12} deficiency states, cyanocobalamin improves GI function; relieves neurologic symptoms such as numbness, tingling, and incoordination; and arrests further neurologic damage.

Uses

Treatment of vitamin B_{12} deficiency states caused by impaired GI absorption (eg, pernicious anemia, GI dysfunction or surgery, tapeworm infestation, sprue)

Prevention of vitamin B_{12} deficiency resulting from increased requirements (eg, pregnancy; hemorrhage; malignancy; thyroid, liver, or renal disease) or inadequate dietary intake (eg, poverty, famine, alcoholism, vegetarian diet)

Performance of the vitamin B_{12} absorption test (Schilling test)

Treatment of nutritional vitamin B_{12} deficiency (see Chapter 76)

Dosage

Dependent on extent of vitamin B_{12} deficiency:

Initially: 30 to 100 μg IM or SC daily for 5 to 10 days, then on alternate days for 2 weeks, then every third or fourth day for 2 to 3 weeks, then 100 to 200 μg once a month (up to 1000 μg/day has been used in seriously ill patients); may be given orally if GI absorptive mechanisms are *not* impaired

Children: 100 μg/dose to a total of 1 to 5 mg over 2 weeks, then 30 to 60 μg monthly

Schilling test: 1000 μg IM 2 hours after an oral dose of radioactive cobalt–B_{12} (0.5–1 μg); urine is collected for 24 hours and radioactivity is measured; impaired absorption indicated by less than 5% urinary excretion of vitamin B_{12} (normal is 10%–30%)

Fate

Intestinal absorption depends on the availability of sufficient intrinsic factor and calcium; vitamin B_{12}–intrinsic factor complex is transported through cells of the distal ileum by a specific receptor-mediated transport system; absorption from IM or SC sites is rapid and the plasma level peaks within 1 hour; stored mainly in the liver and slowly released as needed for cellular metabolism; deficiency states develop only after considerable time in the absence of supplemental B_{12}; trace amounts (2–5 μg) are normally lost in the urine and feces; however, when administered in large doses, 50% to 98% of the dose appears in the urine within 48 hours, mostly within the first 8 hours.

Common Side Effects

Usually with parenteral therapy—transient diarrhea, itching, flushing.

Significant Adverse Reactions

Urticaria, pain at injection site, hypokalemia, peripheral vascular thrombosis, pulmonary edema, congestive heart failure, polycythemia vera, optic nerve atrophy, and anaphylactic shock.

Contraindications

Cobalt hypersensitivity, optic nerve damage. *Cautious use* in patients with infections, uremia, bone marrow depression, pulmonary edema, hypokalemia, neurologic disorders.

Interactions

GI absorption of cyanocobalamin may be impaired by alcohol, *p*-aminosalicylic acid, colchicine, neomycin, and potassium chloride.

Chloramphenicol may antagonize the beneficial therapeutic response to vitamin B_{12}.

Nursing Management

Pretherapy Assessment

Assess and record baseline data necessary for detection of adverse effects of cyanocobalamin: General: VS, body weight, skin color and temperature; Central nervous system: ophthalmic examination; Cardiovascular system: peripheral perfusion; GI: liver evaluation; Laboratory: CBC, Hgb, Hct, vitamin B_{12}, folic acid levels.

Review medical history and documents for existing or previous conditions that:

a. require cautious use of cyanocobalamin: infections; uremia; bone marrow depression; pulmonary edema; hypokalemia; neurologic disorders.

b. contraindicate use of cyanocobalamin: allergy to cobalt, vitamin B_{12}, or any component of these medications; optic nerve damage; Leber disease; **pregnancy (Category C)**; lactation (secreted in breast milk; required nutrient during lactation [4 μg/d]).

Nursing Interventions

Medication Administration

Expect to administer vitamin B_{12} parenterally in cases of pernicious anemia because oral administration is unreliable, and prolonged oral therapy may therefore result in permanent neurologic complications.

Surveillance During Therapy

Monitor results of serum potassium tests, which should be performed before treatment and regularly during initial days of therapy. Improvement of condition increases erythrocyte potassium requirements and may result in severe hypokalemia, with a possibly fatal outcome.

Assess patient for indications of pulmonary edema (eg, dyspnea, night cough), which can occur early in therapy.

Refer patient to dietitian for a dietary history. If possible, dietary deficiencies should be corrected. Strict vegetarian diets can lead to vitamin B_{12} deficiency. Good sources of vitamin B_{12} are red meats, liver, egg yolk, dairy products, clams, oysters, and sardines. Because single vitamin B_{12} deficiency is rare, multiple-vitamin supplementation is often indicated.

Interpret results of vitamin B_{12} or folic acid blood assays cautiously if patient is taking an antibiotic or methotrexate.

Assist with evaluation of drug therapy. Therapeutic response is usually rapid (within 48 h), as measured by improved hematologic status, lessened GI and neurologic symptoms, and decreased fatigue. Reticulocyte counts rise in 3 to 4 days, peak in 7 to 8 days, then gradually decline as erythrocyte counts and hemoglobin rise.

Carefully monitor laboratory studies and patient for indications of adverse reactions.

Interpret results of diagnostic tests and contact practitioner as appropriate.

Monitor for possible drug–drug and drug–nutrient interactions; see Interactions.

Patient Teaching

Instruct patient to take oral vitamin B_{12} with meals to increase absorption (food stimulates production of intrinsic factor) and to avoid mixing drug with citrus juices because ascorbic acid may adversely affect its stability.

Stress the importance of *continual* vitamin B_{12} therapy in patient with pernicious anemia. Interruption of treatment can result in progressive neurologic damage.

Explain that excessive consumption of alcohol may cause malabsorption of vitamin B_{12}.

Instruct patient to report the development of an infection because decreased vitamin B_{12} effectiveness can result. Dosage may have to be temporarily increased.

Instruct patient to check with practitioner before using multiple B vitamin preparations because doses of vitamin B_{12} greater than 10 μg/day may mask symptoms of folate deficiency.

• Hydroxocobalamin, Crystalline

AlphaRedisol and several other manufacturers

(CAN) Acti-B_{12}

Hydroxocobalamin is a source of vitamin B_{12} similar to cyanocobalamin in its actions, indications, and untoward reactions. It is more slowly absorbed than cyanocobalamin, resulting in a more sustained rise in serum cobalamin levels and less urinary excretion of cobalamin after each injection, and may be taken up by the liver in larger quantities than cyanocobalamin.

Hydroxocobalamin is used for the same indications as cyanocobalamin and is preferred by some because it remains in the circulation longer. In addition, hydroxocobalamin has been used to treat cyanide toxicity, such as that associated with excessive doses of sodium nitroprusside (see Chapter 33). It can combine with cyanide to yield cyanocobalamin, which is nontoxic and readily excreted in the urine. IM dosage is 30 μg/day for 5 to 10 days, then 100 to 200 μg/month as maintenance. Mild pain and irritation at injection site has been reported.

• Folic Acid

Folvite

(CAN) Apo-Folic, Novofolacid

Folic acid, also known as folate or vitamin B_9, is a member of the B-complex vitamin group essential for synthesis of nucleoproteins and maintenance of normal erythrocyte production. Folic acid stimulates production of red and white blood cells as well as platelets in megaloblastic anemias. Dietary folate is ultimately converted in the body to tetrahydrofolic acid, which functions as a coenzyme in may reactions, especially the synthesis of purine and pyrimidine precursors of nucleic acids. Folate is available in many different foods (eg, vegetables, milk, eggs, liver), so deficiencies rarely occur. Most likely causes are malnutrition, greatly increased demands (eg, repeated pregnancy), and malabsorption syndromes such as sprue or celiac disease. Patients lacking sufficient folic acid usually manifest a megaloblastic anemia similar to that observed in pernicious anemia, although the incidence of neurologic damage is much less than that observed in cases of vitamin B_{12} deficiency. Oral or parenteral administration of folic acid readily corrects the anemia, both symptomatically and hematologically, and improvement can be maintained by very small daily doses of folic acid.

Mechanism

Converted to tetrahydrofolic acid, which is essential for proper synthesis of purines and pyrimidines, and ultimately nucleic acids; deficiency of folic acid impairs production of bone marrow blood cell precursors.

Uses

Treatment of megaloblastic anemias caused by deficiency of folic acid, as seen in malnutrition, alcoholism, pregnancy, infancy, sprue or celiac disease.

Dosage

Initially up to 1.0 mg daily until clinical symptoms have subsided; maintenance is 0.1 to 0.4 mg daily depending on age; 0.8 mg daily for pregnant or lactating women.

Fate

Well absorbed from GI tract and widely distributed; highly bound to plasma proteins; in the liver; excreted in the urine, feces, and breast milk.

Common Side Effects

Rare—flushing after IV injection.

Significant Adverse Reactions

Rare—allergic reactions (rash, itching, bronchospasm), GI distress, irritability, confusion, and depression.

Contraindications

Pernicious, aplastic, and normocytic anemias.

Interactions

Effects of folic acid may be decreased by barbiturates, chloramphenicol, oral contraceptives, phenytoin, and primidone.

Folic acid may reduce phenytoin blood levels, requiring an increase in dosage.

Trimethoprim, triamterene, and pyrimethamine may interfere with utilization of folic acid.

Nursing Management

Nursing Interventions

Medication Administration

Expect to administer drug orally, although it can be given IM, IV, or SC in severe diseases or if GI absorption is impaired, and to use higher-than-normal dosages in the presence of alcoholism, hemolytic anemia, chronic infection, and anticonvulsant therapy (especially with hydantoins).

Surveillance During Therapy

Assist with evaluation of drug therapy. Beneficial effects may appear within 24 hours (decreased malaise, improved outlook), although it may take 3 to 5 days for hematologic studies to improve.

Patient Teaching

Caution patient against self-medication with folic acid because this may delay recognition of other types of anemia.

Inform patient that foods high in folates include green vegetables, fruits, liver, and yeasts, and that much of the folate content is destroyed by prolonged cooking or canning.

• Leucovorin Calcium—Folinic Acid

Wellcovorin

Leucovorin is a metabolite of folic acid that is used IM to treat folate-deficient megaloblastic anemia when oral folic acid therapy is not feasible. The drug is also indicated for "leucovorin rescue," that is, to minimize the cellular toxicity resulting from large doses of methotrexate used in certain neoplastic diseases. Leucovorin prevents severe methotrexate-induced toxicity by preferentially protecting or "rescuing" normal cells from the action of folic acid antagonists such as methotrexate without interfering with the desired oncolytic action of the drug. This cellular protective function is considered further in Chapter 74.

In treating megaloblastic anemia, leucovorin is administered IM in a dose of 1 mg/day. It should not be used in anemias secondary to a vitamin B_{12} deficiency, because the hematologic picture may improve while the neurologic deficit continues to accrue. Allergic reactions comprise the principal group of adverse reactions.

Selected Bibliography

Bushnell FK: A guide to primary care of iron-deficiency anemia. Nurse Pract 17(11):68, 1992

Hibbard BM: Folates and fetal development. Br J Obstet Gynaecol 100: 307, 1993

Marcuard SP, Albernaz L, Khazanic PG: Omeprazole therapy causes malabsorption of cyanocobalamin (vitamin B_{12}). Ann Intern Med 120:211, 1994

Oski FA: Iron deficiency in infancy and childhood. N Engl J Med 329:190, 1993

Streiff RR: Anemia and nutritional deficiency in the acutely hospitalized patients. Med Clin North Am 77:911, 1993

Nursing Bibliography

Brigden M: Iron deficiency anemia: Every case is instructive. Postgrad Med 93:181, 1993

Brown S: Recombinant human erythropoietin and renal failure. Care of the Critically Ill 8(1):12, 1992

Hoffman J: Iron deficiency anemia: An update. Journal of Perinatal and Neonatal Nursing 6(4):192, 1993

37

Anticoagulant, Thrombolytic, and Hemostatic Drugs

Anticoagulant Drugs

Parenteral anticoagulants

Heparin
Enoxaparin

Heparin antagonist

Protamine sulfate

Oral anticoagulants

Dicumarol
Warfarin
Anisindione

Oral anticoagulant antagonist

Phytonadione

Hemorheologic agent

Pentoxifylline

Thrombolytic Agents

Alteplase, recombinant
Anistreplase
Streptokinase
Urokinase

Hemostatic Drugs

Systemic hemostatics

Aminocaproic acid
Tranexamic acid
Antihemophilic factor, human
Antiinhibitor coagulant complex
Factor IX complex, human
Antithrombin III, human

Topical hemostatics

The process of blood clot formation, and subsequent clot resolution, or lysis, is characterized by a chemically complex series of events that involves the interaction of a large number of substances (coagulation factors) present in blood plasma, blood cells (especially platelets), and, to a lesser extent, in body tissues.

The *coagulation factors*, which are listed in Table 37-1, function in either of two distinct pathways, the intrinsic clotting pathway and the extrinsic clotting pathway. The *intrinsic pathway* is so named because all of the coagulation proteins are present in the blood itself. The reactions are relatively slow, and several minutes are required to produce a clot. The *extrinsic pathway* is triggered by clotting factors derived from injured cells in tissues. It is a much more rapidly acting system: It can cause a blood clot to form within seconds. The interaction of the intrinsic and extrinsic pathways to produce a fibrin clot is shown schematically in Figure 37-1.

Drugs capable of affecting the coagulation process generally act on one or more of the stages shown in Figure 37-1. Agents preventing the formation of new clots are termed *anticoagulants*. Drugs increasing the rate of resolution (or lysis) of preformed clots are referred to as *thrombolytic agents*. Compounds enhancing blood clot formation, thereby reducing bleeding, are characterized as *hemostatic drugs*.

Anticoagulant Drugs

Therapy with anticoagulant drugs is directed primarily toward preventing development of intravascular thromboses, a major cause of death in thromboembolic disorders. Although these compounds are widely used, therapy with them is often empirical (ie, based on clinical experience), and their efficacy in treating some conditions for which they are used has been questioned. Moreover, they are potentially dangerous drugs, capable of causing severe, possibly fatal hemorrhaging, and therefore must be carefully prescribed and closely monitored. *Long-term* therapy with anticoagulant drugs remains a controversial area; nevertheless, when judiciously selected and properly used, the several anticoagulant agents have an important place in clinical therapy and can markedly reduce the likelihood of vascular clotting, thus improving the quality of life and preventing mortality.

There are two classes of therapeutically useful anticoagulant drugs, the parenteral and oral agents. Heparin and enoxaparin are the parenteral agents, whereas the oral anticoagulant group encompasses several drugs characterized as either coumarin or indandione derivatives. After separate discussions of heparin and enoxaparin, the oral anticoagulants are discussed as a group, followed by a listing of individual drugs. Mention is also made under this heading of both protamine sulfate, a heparin antagonist, and vitamin K and its derivatives, which are antagonists of the oral anticoagulant drugs. Finally, pentoxifylline, a drug that decreases blood viscosity and improves vascular flow, is considered under anticoagulants in this chapter.

Parenteral Anticoagulants

- ***Heparin Sodium***

Liquaemin

(CAN) Hepalean, Heparin Leo

- ***Heparin Calcium***

Calciparine

(CAN) Calcilean, Minihep

Heparin is a mucopolysaccharide extracted from bovine lung or porcine intestinal tissue. Its potency is standardized by a biologic assay and is expressed in units. The compound is a strong organic acid, possessing an electronegative charge that is essential for its anticoagulant activity. Blood clotting is inhibited in vivo as well as in vitro, and the effects of heparin are noted immediately on administration. Heparin is usually given as the sodium salt but is also available as heparin calcium, which is equally effective.

Mechanism

Accelerates the rate at which antithrombin III, an alpha$_2$-globulin produced by the liver, inactivates factors IX, X, XI, and XII, as

Table 37-1. **Blood Coagulation Factors**

Factor	*Name*	*Function*
I	Fibrinogen	Precursor of fibrin
II	Prothrombin	Precursor of thrombin
III	Tissue Thromboplastin	Triggers extrinsic coagulation pathway
IV	Calcium	Essential for several reactions in coagulation pathways
V	Proaccelerin (Labile factor)	Accelerates conversion of prothrombin to thrombin
VII	Proconvertin	Accelerates the extrinsic coagulation pathway
VIII	Antihemophilic factor	Accelerates activation of factor X
IX	Christmas factor (plasma thromboplastin component; PTC)	Accelerates activation of factor X
X	Stuart-Prower factor	Accelerates conversion of prothrombin to thrombin
XI	Plasma thromboplastin antecedent (PTA)	Accelerates activation of factor IX
XII	Hageman factor	Triggers intrinsic coagulation pathway—activates factor XI
XIII	Fibrin stabilizing factor	Strengthens fibrin clot when activated by thrombin and calcium

well as thrombin; thus, conversion of fibrinogen to fibrin is blocked, and activation of the fibrin-stabilizing factor (XIII) is also impaired; the rate-limiting step in the coagulation cascade is activation of factor X, which is inhibited by lower doses of heparin than those needed to neutralize thrombin; thus, prophylactic therapy is accomplished with much lower doses than those necessary once the coagulation process has begun; may also reduce platelet adhesiveness; no fibrinolytic activity, but may exert a diuretic and hypolipemic action, although the latter two actions are of no clinical value.

Uses

- Prophylaxis and treatment of venous thromboses, pulmonary embolism, and atrial fibrillation with embolization
- Prevention of postoperative deep venous thrombosis and pulmonary embolism in patients undergoing major (abdominothoracic, cardiac, arterial) surgery (low-dose regimen)
- Prevention of cerebral thrombosis in evolving stroke
- Diagnosis and treatment of acute and chronic consumption coagulopathies (disseminated intravascular coagulation)
- Prevention of peripheral venous thrombosis after acute myocardial infarction
- Anticoagulant in blood transfusion, dialysis procedures, blood samples for laboratory procedures, and extracorporeal circulation

Dosage

The dosage depends on the patient's coagulation tests. Dosage is adequate when whole blood clotting time is 2.5 to 3 times the control value *or* the partial thromboplastin time (PTT) is 1.5 to 2 times the control value. *Recommended dosage guidelines for average-size patients*:

Anticoagulation

Subcutaneous (SC): 10,000 to 20,000 units initially, then 8000 to 10,000 units every 8 hours or 15,000 to 20,000 units every 12 hours

Intravenous (IV) injection: 10,000 units initially, then 5000 to 10,000 units every 4 to 6 hours

IV infusion: 20,000 to 40,000 units/day in 1000 mL of isotonic sodium chloride solution, preceded by a 5000-unit IV loading dose

Children: 50 units/kg bolus initially, followed by 100 units/kg IV infusion every 4 hours *or* 20,000 units/m^2/24 hours by continuous infusion

Postoperative prophylaxis: SC: 5000 units 2 hours before surgery and 5000 units every 8 to 12 hours for 7 days after surgery

Heart/blood vessel surgery: IV: 150 to 400 units/kg depending on length of surgery

Blood transfusion: 7500 units/100 mL sterile sodium chloride injection; 6 to 8 mL of dilution is added per 100 mL whole blood

Laboratory samples: 70 to 150 units/10 to 20 mL whole sample

Fate

Not active orally; immediate onset IV, with peak effect in 5 to 10 minutes and duration of 2 to 6 hours; gradually absorbed SC, with onset of 30 to 60 minutes and duration of 8 to 12 hours; highly bound to plasma proteins; plasma half-life averages 60 to 90 minutes but is prolonged at high doses; partially metabolized by the liver, and excreted in the urine as metabolites and unchanged drug; not found in appreciable amounts in the fetus or in breast milk.

Common Side Effects

Spontaneous bleeding, local irritation at SC and intramuscular (IM) injection sites (avoid IM injection routes).

Significant Adverse Reactions

CAUTION

Thrombocytopenia may occur in up to one third of patients receiving heparin and is of two types. *Early* thrombocytopenia develops within 2 to 3 days after initiating therapy, is

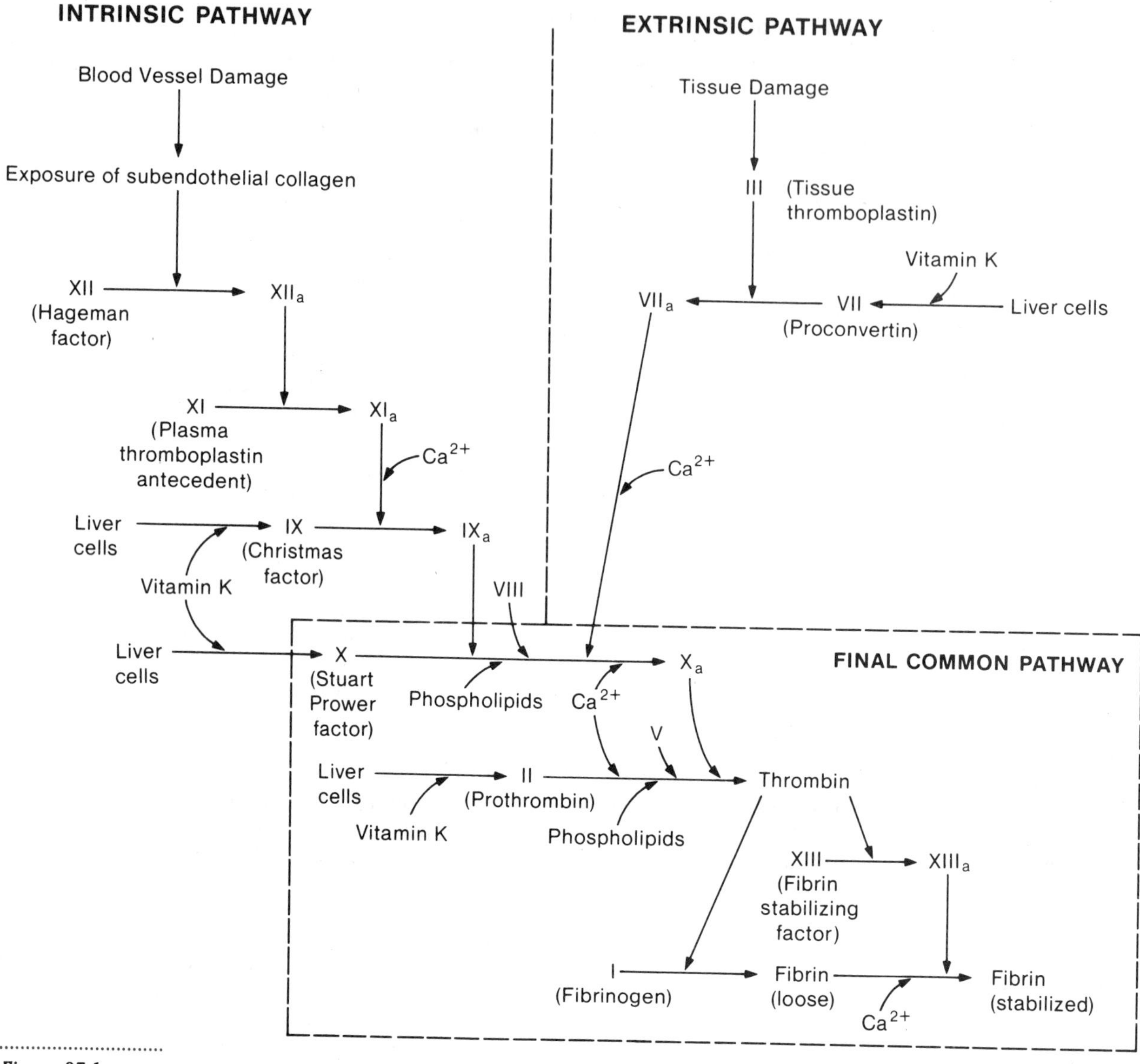

Figure 37-1. Coagulation pathways involved in hemostasis.

usually mild, and is seldom of clinical consequence. It appears to be the result of a direct action of heparin on platelets and may remain stable or even reverse, even if heparin is continued. *Delayed* thrombocytopenia occurs 6 to 12 days after initiation of therapy, probably reflects the presence of an immunoglobulin that induces platelet aggregation, and may be associated with hemorrhage and paradoxic thromboembolic episodes due to irreversible aggregation of platelets, the so-called white clot syndrome. This condition may lead to skin necrosis, gangrene, pulmonary embolism, myocardial infarction, or stroke. If significant thrombocytopenia develops during heparin therapy, the drug should be discontinued and oral anticoagulants substituted. Most instances of delayed thrombocytopenia are attributable to heparin prepared from bovine lung rather than porcine intestine.

Hemorrhaging, hypersensitivity (chills, urticaria, fever, rhinitis, asthma-like reaction, lacrimation, diarrhea, anaphylactic reaction), vasospastic reaction, increased serum transaminases, elevated blood pressure, chest pain, alopecia, osteoporosis, and impaired renal function.

Contraindications

Active bleeding or significant bleeding tendencies (eg, hemophilia, purpura, thrombocytopenia), presence of a drainage tube, and threatened abortion. *Cautious use* in patients with a history of allergy (heparin is derived from animal tissue), renal or hepatic disease or alcoholism; during menstruation, pregnancy, or the immediate postpartum period; when administering acid citrate dextrose (ACD)–converted blood, because heparin activity persists for several weeks after conversion of such blood; and in any condition in which there is increased risk of hemorrhage (eg, after surgery of the brain, eye, or spinal cord); shock; severe hypertension; jaundice; ulcerative lesions; and in patients with indwelling catheters.

Interactions

An increased risk of bleeding is present when heparin is used in combination with other drugs that can interfere with platelet aggregation or cause coagulopathies, such as salicylates, nonsteroidal antiinflammatory drugs, dipyridamole, valproic acid, dextran, ticlopidine, penicillins, cephalosporins, and pentoxifylline.

The action of heparin may be partially reduced by nitroglycerin (IV) and streptokinase.

Nursing Management

Pretherapy Assessment

Assess and record baseline data necessary for detection of adverse effects of heparin: General: vital signs (VS), body weight, skin color and temperature; Cardiovascular system (CVS): baseline electrocardiogram (ECG), peripheral perfusion; Gastrointestinal (GI): liver evaluation; Laboratory: complete blood count (CBC), hemoglobin, hematocrit (Hct), platelet count, PTT.

Review medical history and documents for existing or previous conditions that:

a. require cautious use of heparin: renal or hepatic disease; alcoholism; menstruation; the immediate postpartum period; when administering ACD-converted blood; after surgery of the brain, eye, or spinal cord; shock; severe hypertension; jaundice; ulcerative lesions; and in patients with indwelling catheters.
b. contraindicate use of heparin: allergy to heparin, to pork or beef products; active bleeding or significant bleeding tendencies (eg, hemophilia, purpura, thrombocytopenia), presence of a drainage tube, and threatened abortion; **pregnancy (Category C)**. NOTE: lactation (not secreted in breast milk).

Nursing Interventions

Medication Administration

Have protamine sulfate available, a specific heparin antagonist (see section on protamine sulfate), as well as whole blood or plasma, in case of heparin overdosage. Monitor vital signs during therapy.

Check results of most recent clotting test, such as activated partial thromboplastin time (APTT), before each SC or IV injection. During early stages of IV infusion, tests should be performed every 4 hours. Careful titration of dosage based on test results is critical for safe, effective therapy. Heparin should not be administered to any patient who cannot be kept under careful observation with periodic coagulation tests.

Adjust dose according to results of coagulation test results determined before injection.

Administer SC or IV only because hematoma can occur with IM administration.

Give SC injection deep into fatty layers of abdomen or above iliac crest to minimize local irritation. Alternate injection sites, and observe for hematoma. Do not aspirate syringe. Use "bunching" technique or Z-track method (see Chapter 2).

Ensure that at least 5 hours elapse after the last IV dose and 24 hours after the last SC dose before blood is drawn for a prothrombin time when administering heparin with oral anticoagulants. Heparin may be withdrawn when prothrombin activity is in the desired range. Oral anticoagulant and heparin therapy usually overlap for 3 to 5 days.

Note that solutions of heparin diluted in saline (10 or 100 units/mL) are available for use as an IV flush (Heparin Sodium Lock Flush Solution) to maintain the patency of indwelling IV catheters. These solutions are *not* intended for therapeutic use.

Surveillance During Therapy

Monitor results of platelet counts, which should be performed before initiating therapy and regularly thereafter to detect thrombocytopenia (see Common Side Effects).

Assess patient frequently for signs of unusual bleeding (eg, discoloration of urine or feces, bruising, petechiae, or low back pain, which may indicate abdominal bleeding).

Observe for early signs of an allergic reaction (chills, fever, itching, dyspnea).

Inform practitioner if fever or other symptoms of infection develop, because the patient with an infection, as well as the postoperative patient or one with thrombophlebitis, thrombosis, myocardial infarction, or cancer, may be resistant to heparin.

Carefully monitor laboratory studies and patient for indications of adverse reactions.

Interpret results of diagnostic tests and contact practitioner as appropriate.

Monitor for possible drug–drug and drug–nutrient interactions; see Interactions.

Patient Teaching

Warn patient that indiscriminate use of alcohol or over-the-counter preparations containing aspirin or ibuprofen may alter response to heparin.

Reassure patient that alopecia, if it occurs, is temporary.

Instruct patient to inform all health-care providers that they are taking this medication.

Instruct patient to report any of the following to his or her practitioner: nosebleed, bleeding of gums, unusual bleeding; black or tarry stools; cloudy or dark urine; abdominal or lower back pain; severe headache.

• Enoxaparin

Lovenox

Mechanism

Enoxaparin is a low–molecular-weight heparin obtained from unfractionated porcine heparin. At recommended doses there is no significant effect on prothrombin time, APTT, platelet function, or bleeding time. It has a higher ratio of anti-factor Xa to anti-factor IIa activity than unfractionated heparin.

Uses

Prevention of deep vein thrombosis after hip replacement

Investigational use for prevention of deep vein thrombosis after knee replacement

Dosage

30 mg twice a day subcutaneously with the first dose as soon as possible after the surgery. Continue until risk of deep vein thrombosis has diminished. The average duration is 7 to 10 days.

Fate

Enoxaparin is completely absorbed after subcutaneous injection. The onset of anticoagulant activity as measured by antifactor Xa activity is approximately 3 hours. Enoxaparin is mainly eliminated by the kidney.

Common Side Effects

Spontaneous bleeding, local irritation at subcutaneous injection sites.

Significant Adverse Reactions

Hemorrhaging, thrombocytopenia.

Contraindications

Active major bleeding; thrombocytopenia and a positive antiplatelet antibody test in the presence of enoxaparin; hypersensitivity to enoxaparin, heparin, or pork products.

Interactions

Enoxaparin may result in increased bleeding tendencies in combination with oral anticoagulants or platelet inhibitors.

Nursing Management

See **Heparin**.

Heparin Antagonist

• Protamine Sulfate

Protamine sulfate is a mixture of proteins exhibiting a strongly positive charge that is capable of chemically combining with heparin, producing a stable salt and thereby neutralizing the anticoagulant action of heparin; however, it may exert an anticoagulant effect when administered alone or when dosage exceeds that required to neutralize heparin.

Uses

Treatment of heparin overdosage.

Dosage

Each milligram of protamine sulfate neutralizes approximately 90 units of heparin activity derived from lung tissue and 115 units of heparin activity derived from intestinal mucosa; administer slowly IV over 10 minutes; do not exceed a dose of 50 mg.

Fate

Onset of action within 5 minutes; duration lasts 1 to 2 hours.

Common Side Effects

Flushing, feeling of warmth.

Significant Adverse Reactions

Especially with too-rapid injection—sudden hypotension, bradycardia, dyspnea, and allergic reactions.

Contraindications

No absolute contraindications. *Cautious use* in patients with cardiovascular disease or fish allergies (protamine is derived from fish sources); have facilities available to treat shock.

Nursing Management

Pretherapy Assessment

Assess and record baseline data necessary for detection of adverse effects of protamine: General: VS, body weight, skin color and temperature; Central nervous system (CNS): orientation, reflexes; CVS: baseline ECG, peripheral perfusion; Laboratory: plasma prothrombin time.

Review medical history and documents for existing or previous conditions that:

a. require cautious use of protamine: cardiovascular disease.
b. contraindicate use of protamine: allergy to protamine, fish products; **pregnancy (Category C)**; lactation (effects not known).

Nursing Interventions

Medication Administration

Administer IV, very slowly.

Do not exceed 50 mg per 10-minute period.

Do not mix in lines with incompatible antibiotics (penicillins, cephalosporins).

Surveillance During Therapy

Monitor vital signs during administration and for at least 3 to 4 hours afterward.

Observe patient for signs of increased bleeding if very large doses are used because protamine itself has weak anticoagulant properties. It should not be used to treat hemorrhage resulting from any condition other than heparin overdosage.

Monitor results of blood coagulation studies (eg, heparin titration test, plasma thrombin time), which should be performed to determine the need for repeat doses.

Carefully monitor laboratory studies and patient for indications of adverse reactions.

Interpret results of diagnostic tests and contact practitioner as appropriate.

Monitor for possible drug–drug and drug–nutrient interactions; see Interactions.

Patient Teaching

This drug is used in emergency situations; patient teaching is therefore restricted to informing the patient as to what is being given and why. The patient should be instructed to report any of the following: flushing; dizziness; lack of orientation; shortness of breath and difficulty breathing.

Oral Anticoagulants (*Pregnancy Category D*)

Dicumarol
Warfarin
Anisindione

Mechanism

Depress the hepatic synthesis of vitamin K-dependent clotting factors II, VII, IX, and X by inhibiting vitamin K_2, 3-epoxide reductase enzymes; factor VII is the first to be depleted (because it has the shortest half-life), followed sequentially by factors IX,

X, and II, which have longer half-lives. Thus, initial prolongation of prothrombin time occurs within 8 to 12 hours, but maximal anticoagulant activity requires several days to develop. These drugs exert no effect on established thrombus but may prevent further extension of the formed clot, thereby preventing secondary thromboembolic complications

Uses

Prophylaxis and treatment of venous thrombosis and its extension
Treatment of atrial fibrillation with embolism
Prophylaxis and treatment of pulmonary embolism
Adjunctive treatment of coronary occlusion
Prophylaxis in patients with prosthetic valves
Investigational uses include prevention of recurrent transient ischemic attacks and reduction of risk of recurrence after myocardial infarction

Dosage

See Table 37-2.

Fate

See Table 37-2 for individual drug properties. Most are almost completely absorbed orally, although absorption rates vary widely; peak activity usually occurs within 2 to 3 days; effects persist 2 to 5 days with warfarin, 2 to 10 days with dicumarol, and 1 to 3 days with anisindione; all drugs are highly but weakly bound to plasma proteins; metabolized by hepatic microsomal enzymes, and excreted primarily in the urine as inactive metabolites.

Common Side Effects

Hemorrhagic episodes (nosebleed, petechiae, bleeding gums, hematuria, bleeding from wounds).

Significant Adverse Reactions

Coumarins: nausea, anorexia, severe bleeding, adrenal hemorrhage, vomiting, abdominal cramping, diarrhea, urticaria, dermatitis, alopecia, fever, agranulocytosis, leukopenia, mucosal ulceration, nephropathy
Indandione: dermatitis, urticaria, fever, diarrhea, jaundice, nephropathy, agranulocytosis

Contraindications

Hemorrhagic tendencies; hemophilia; thrombocytopenic purpura; recent or contemplated surgery (especially eye or CNS surgery); active bleeding; ulcerative, traumatic, or surgical wounds; visceral carcinoma; diverticulitis; colitis; aneurysm; acute nephritis; suspicion of cerebrovascular hemorrhage; eclampsia or preeclampsia; threatened abortion; uncontrolled hypertension; hepatic insufficiency; polyarthritis; polycythemia vera; subacute bacterial endocarditis; ascorbic acid (vitamin C) deficiency; spinal puncture; continuous GI drainage; and regional block anesthesia. *Cautious use* in the presence of congestive heart failure, mild liver or kidney dysfunction, alcoholism, tuberculosis, history of ulcerative disease, diabetes, allergic disorders, poor nutritional states, collagen disease, pancreatic disorders, vitamin K deficiency, hypothyroidism, radiation therapy, edema, and hyperlipidemia.

Interactions

The hypoprothrombinemic effect of oral anticoagulants may be enhanced by drugs that decrease vitamin K levels (aminoglycosides, cholestyramine, mineral oil, tetracycline, vitamin E); drugs that displace the anticoagulants from their protein binding sites (clofibrate, chloral hydrate, diazoxide, miconazole, nalidixic acid, phenylbutazone, salicylates, sulfonamides, oral hypoglycemics); drugs that inhibit the metabolism of anticoagulants (alcohol, allopurinol, amiodarone, chloramphenicol, cimetidine, co-trimoxazole, disulfiram, ifosfamide, lovastatin, methylphenidate, metronidazole, omeprazole, phenylbutazone, propafenone, propoxyphene, sulfinpyrazone, tricyclic antidepressants); and also by anabolic steroids, erythromycin, gemfibrozil, glucagon, sulindac, danazol, ketoconazole, propranolol, and thyroid drugs.
Increased incidence of hemorrhage can occur with combined use of oral anticoagulants and inhibitors of platelet aggregation (cephalosporins, dipyridamole,

Table 37-2. **Oral Anticoagulants**

Drug	*Usual Dosage Range*	*Nursing Considerations*
COUMARINS		
Dicumarol *Dicumarol*	200–300 mg first day; 25–200 mg/day thereafter, depending on PT	Slowly and incompletely absorbed orally; peak effect in 3–5 days; be alert for accumulation toxicity (especially bleeding), because drug is long acting; poorly water soluble; half-life increases with increasing dose
Warfarin Sodium *Coumadin, Panwarfin, Sofarin* *(CAN) Warfilone*	Initially 10 mg daily for 2–4 days; thereafter, adjust based on PT Usual maintenance— 2–10 mg/day based on PT	Well absorbed orally; peak effect in 1–3 days, and duration of 3–5 days; most widely used oral anticoagulant, giving most uniform response; reduce dose by half in elderly or debilitated patients
INDANDIONE		
Anisindione *Miradon*	300 mg first day, 200 mg second day, 100 mg third day; then 25–250 mg daily for maintenance	Indandione derivative infrequently used as oral anticoagulant; peak effects occur with 2–3 days and persist for 1–3 days; dermatitis is the most common side effect; may turn urine red–orange

PT, prothrombin time.

indomethacin, penicillins, pyrazolones, salicylates, ticlopidine), inhibitors of procoagulant factors (antimetabolites, alkylating agents, quinidine, salicylates), or ulcerogenic drugs (corticosteroids, indomethacin, pyrazolones, potassium salts, salicylates).

A decreased anticoagulant effect may be observed if oral anticoagulants are used in the presence of enzyme inducers (barbiturates, carbamazepine, ethchlorvynol, glutethimide, griseofulvin, phenytoin, rifampin); activators of procoagulant factors (estrogens, oral contraceptives, vitamin K); and drugs that can decrease GI absorption (cholestyramine, colestipol).

Oral anticoagulants may potentiate the action of phenytoin and the oral hypoglycemic drugs by inhibiting their liver metabolism.

Oral anticoagulants, when used with thrombolytic agents (see discussion later in this chapter), can increase the risk of bleeding.

Nursing Management

Pretherapy Assessment

Assess and record baseline data necessary for detection of adverse effects of oral anticoagulants: General: VS, body weight, skin color and temperature; CNS: orientation, reflexes; CVS: baseline ECG, peripheral perfusion; Laboratory: CBC, urinalysis, guaiac stools, prothrombin time, renal and hepatic function tests.

Review medical history and documents for existing or previous conditions that:

a. require cautious use of oral anticoagulants: congestive heart failure; mild liver or kidney dysfunction; alcoholism; tuberculosis; ulcerative disease; diabetes; allergic disorders; poor nutritional states; collagen disease; pancreatic disorders; vitamin K deficiency; hypothyroidism; radiation therapy; edema; hyperlipidemia.

b. contraindicate use of oral anticoagulants: allergy to oral anticoagulants, tartrazine; hemorrhagic tendencies; hemophilia; thrombocytopenic purpura; recent or contemplated surgery (especially eye or CNS surgery); active bleeding; ulcerative, traumatic, or surgical wounds; visceral carcinoma; diverticulitis; colitis; aneurysm; acute nephritis; suspicion of cerebrovascular hemorrhage; eclampsia or preeclampsia; threatened abortion; uncontrolled hypertension; hepatic insufficiency; polyarthritis; polycythemia vera; subacute bacterial endocarditis; ascorbic acid (vitamin C) deficiency; spinal puncture; continuous GI drainage; and regional block anesthesia; **pregnancy (Category D)**; lactation (secreted in breast milk; use heparin if anticoagulant effect is required).

Nursing Interventions

Medication Administration

Obtain careful drug history before initiation of therapy.

Expect dosages to be prescribed daily after results of prothrombin times are available. Initial doses are based on anticipated maintenance levels. Excessive loading doses have been associated with increased bleeding complications. Heparin is preferred if rapid anticoagulation is desired.

Do not administer IM injections while patient is on oral anticoagulant therapy.

Double-check any other drug that is ordered for potential drug–drug interaction: dosage of both drugs may need to be adjusted.

Have vitamin K available in case of overdosage.

Surveillance During Therapy

Monitor results of prothrombin determinations, which should be obtained daily during initial stages of therapy and during periods of dosage adjustment or addition of other drugs. International normalized ratios (INRs) should be maintained in the range of 2 to 3 for most conditions. An INR of 2 to 3 corresponds to a prothrombin time ratio of 1.3 to 1.5 for a thromboplastin with an ISI of 2.8. INR is calculated as follows: INR = (observed PT ratio)^{ISI}, where ISI (International Sensitivity Index) is the calibration factor and is available from the manufacturer for each batch of thromboplastin. The PT ratio is prothrombin time (observed)/prothrombin time (control).

Observe for signs of overdosage during early stages of therapy because onset of clinical effects is delayed several days, during which time the drug may accumulate.

Ensure that prothrombin time is determined at 1- to 4-week intervals depending on drug response during maintenance therapy. Periodic blood counts, urinalyses, and liver function tests should also be obtained.

Expect therapy to be withdrawn gradually over 3 to 4 weeks. It should not be terminated abruptly. Prothrombin activity returns to normal within 2 to 10 days after cessation of therapy.

Carefully monitor laboratory studies and patient for indications of adverse reactions.

Interpret results of diagnostic tests and contact practitioner as appropriate.

Monitor for possible drug–drug and drug–nutrient interactions; see Interactions.

Provide for patient safety needs to protect from injury.

Patient Teaching

Stress the importance of strict compliance with the prescribed dosage schedule (see Plan of Nursing Care 1-2). Compliance is poorest in elderly, alcoholic, and emotionally unstable patients. Their drug-taking practices should be closely monitored.

Caution patient to avoid starting or discontinuing any other medications without professional guidance.

Ensure that patient understands the need to observe for signs of abnormal bleeding (eg, hematuria, tarry stools, hematemesis, petechiae, ecchymoses, bleeding gums, nosebleed, excessive menses). Bleeding should be immediately reported to health care provider because dosage adjustment is indicated.

Inform patient that minor overdosage, which is characterized by petechiae, oozing from cuts, or bleeding of gums after brushing, can be treated by omitting one or more doses until prothrombin time returns to therapeutic range. More severe bleeding can be treated with oral (2.5–10 mg) or parenteral (5–25 mg) vitamin K (phytonadione), depending on severity. Occasionally, transfusions with fresh whole blood or fresh-frozen plasma may be required.

Warn patient to note development of early signs of agranulocytosis (fever, chills, sore throat, malaise, mucosal ulceration) or hepatitis (itching, dark urine, jaundice) and report at once. Discontinuation of medication is advisable.

Advise patient that many factors may affect anticoagulant response, including maintenance of a well balanced diet and avoidance of excessive alcohol consumption.

Encourage patient to carry some form of identification at all times stating the type of medication taken and health-care provider's name.

Instruct patient to restrict intake of foods rich in vitamin K (see Chapter 75) because they may reduce the effectiveness of oral anticoagulants.

Advise patient to consult with his or her practitioner before undergoing dental work or elective surgery.

Oral Anticoagulant Antagonist

Vitamin K is effective as an antidote to overdosage with the oral anticoagulant drugs. Two forms of vitamin K are available: phytonadione (vitamin K_1), a fat-soluble derivative resembling naturally occurring vitamin K; and menadiol (vitamin K_4), a synthetic, water-soluble analogue that is converted to menadione (vitamin K_3) in vivo. Phytonadione is the preferred drug for treatment of anticoagulant-induced prothrombin deficiency because menadiol is less potent, less dependable, less rapid acting, and shorter acting than K_1.

The complete pharmacology of the vitamin K preparations is reviewed in detail in Chapter 75. The present discussion is limited to the use of phytonadione (vitamin K_1), the preferred antidote, for the treatment of oral anticoagulant overdosage.

• Phytonadione (Vitamin K_1)

AquaMEPHYTON, Konakion, Mephyton

Mechanism

Promotes hepatic synthesis of blood clotting factors II, VII, IX, and X, thereby reversing oral anticoagulant-induced prothrombin depression; no antidotal effects against heparin.

Uses

Treatment of anticoagulant-induced prothrombin deficiency (oral or parenteral K_1)

Treatment of hypoprothrombinemia secondary to antibacterial therapy, obstructive jaundice, biliary fistulas, or salicylate administration (oral or parenteral K_1)

Prophylaxis and therapy of newborn hemorrhagic disease (parenteral K_1)

Treatment of hypoprothrombinemia secondary to malabsorption or impaired synthesis of vitamin K such as can occur in ulcerative colitis, obstructive jaundice, celiac disease, intestinal resection, or regional enteritis (parenteral K_1)

Dosage

Use smallest effective dose. Anticoagulant overdosage:

Oral: 2.5 to 10 mg (maximum 50 mg) initially; repeat in 12 to 48 hours as needed

SC, IM: 2.5 to 10 mg (maximum 50 mg) initially; repeat in 6 to 8 hours as needed

IV (emergency only—see Significant Adverse Reactions): 0.5 to 10 mg at a rate of 1 mg/min

Fate

Effects appear in 6 to 10 hours with oral use and 1 to 2 hours with parenteral use (15 min after IV injection); oral absorption requires presence of bile in the GI tract; normal prothrombin level usually is obtained within 12 to 16 hours.

Common Side Effects

Flushing, GI upset.

Significant Adverse Reactions

CAUTION

Severe anaphylactic reactions have occurred after IV injection of AquaMEPHYTON (an aqueous colloidal solution of vitamin K_1), resulting in shock, cardiac arrest, and respiratory arrest. Therefore, the IV route should be used *only* when other routes are not feasible, and with full consideration of all risks.

Pain, swelling, and tenderness at injection site, allergic reactions (bronchospasm, dyspnea, anaphylaxis), cramping, chills, fever, weakness, dizziness, chest constriction, profuse sweating, erythema, cyanosis.

Contraindications

No absolute contraindications. *Cautious use* during pregnancy and in the presence of severe liver disease.

Interactions

Concurrent administration of phytonadione with mineral oil or bile acid-binding resins may result in impaired vitamin K absorption.

When large doses of phytonadione are used, temporary resistance to oral anticoagulants may be encountered; if anticoagulant therapy becomes necessary, heparin may be required.

Oral antibiotics, quinidine, and salicylates may interfere with vitamin K activity.

Nursing Management

Pretherapy Assessment

Assess and record baseline data necessary for detection of adverse effects of phytonadione: General: VS, body weight, skin color and temperature; CVS: peripheral perfusion; Laboratory: prothrombin time, renal and hepatic function tests.

Review medical history and documents for existing or previous conditions that:

a. require cautious use of phytonadione: severe liver disease.

b. contraindicate use of phytonadione: allergy to any component of the preparation; **pregnancy (Category C)**; lactation (secreted in breast milk).

Nursing Interventions

Medication Administration

Be prepared to administer whole blood or plasma transfusions in cases of severe hemorrhage because it takes several hours for vitamin K to enhance prothrombin synthesis.
Use IV dilution immediately, and discard unused portion. Protect from light by wrapping container during use.
Dilute IV injection with sodium chloride or dextrose solution, and administer very slowly. Severe reactions, including fatal anaphylaxis, have occurred after IV injection (see Significant Adverse Reactions).
Expect to administer the smallest dose that is effective in restoring normal prothrombin time. Overzealous use may promote return of thromboembolic complications and can interfere with action of oral anticoagulants for an extended period (2–3 wk). If patient who has received large doses of phytonadione exhibits resistance to subsequent oral anticoagulant therapy, larger-than-normal doses of the oral drugs or use of heparin may be required.

Surveillance During Therapy

Monitor results of prothrombin times or INRs, which should be performed frequently during therapy to aid in determining dosage and frequency of administration.
Question the use of drugs that can interfere with vitamin K activity (eg, oral antibiotics, quinidine, salicylates) during phytonadione therapy.
Carefully monitor laboratory studies and patient for indications of adverse reactions.
Interpret results of diagnostic tests and contact practitioner as appropriate.
Monitor for possible drug–drug and drug–nutrient interactions; see Interactions.

Patient Teaching

Instruct patient to restrict intake of foods rich in vitamin K (see Chapter 75) during therapy.
Instruct the patient to report to the practitioner any of the following: rash; pain at injection site; difficulty breathing; nausea, vomiting.

Hemorheologic Agent

• Pentoxifylline

Trental

Pentoxifylline is a xanthine derivative, structurally related to caffeine and theophylline. It is termed a hemorheologic agent, inasmuch as it lowers blood viscosity and improves the flexibility of red blood cells. Therefore, in patients with impaired blood flow in microcirculatory areas, pentoxifylline can increase oxygenation of tissues supplied by these occluded vessels by improving microcirculatory blood flow. It is used principally in the treatment of intermittent claudication resulting from chronic occlusive arterial disease of the limbs.

Mechanism

Improves regional blood flow by reducing blood viscosity and improving red blood cell flexibility; increases cellular adenosine triphosphate content, thereby decreasing tendency of red cells to aggregate; may also stimulate release of prostacyclin and impair formation of thromboxane A_2, which also decreases likelihood of platelet aggregation and promotes vasodilation.

Uses

Symptomatic treatment of intermittent claudication due to chronic occlusive arterial disease
Symptomatic treatment of cerebrovascular insufficiency (investigational use)

Dosage

400 mg three times daily with meals for at least 8 weeks. If gastrointestinal or central nervous system side effects are bothersome, dosage may be decreased to 400 mg twice a day.

Fate

After oral administration, peak plasma levels occur within 2 to 4 hours and remain constant thereafter; plasma half-life ranges from 30 to 90 minutes, but therapeutic effects generally are not seen for 4 to 8 weeks; the drug is metabolized in the liver and excreted primarily in the urine.

Common Side Effects

Nausea, dyspepsia, dizziness.

Significant Adverse Reactions

Vomiting, dry mouth, anorexia, constipation, headache, anxiety, mild tremor, nasal congestion, epistaxis, flulike symptoms, pruritus, rash, urticaria, brittle fingernails, blurred vision, conjunctivitis, scotomata, bad taste in mouth, earache, salivation, malaise, sore throat, dyspnea, hypotension, edema, swollen glands, and leukopenia.

Contraindications

Sensitivity to methylxanthines, such as caffeine. *Cautious use* in patients with angina, arrhythmias, or severe hypotension, and in pregnant or nursing women.

Nursing Management

Pretherapy Assessment

Assess and record baseline data necessary for detection of adverse effects of pentoxifylline: General: VS, body weight, skin color and temperature; CNS: orientation, reflexes; CVS: peripheral perfusion; Laboratory: CBC.
Review medical history and documents for existing or previous conditions that:

a. require cautious use of pentoxifylline: angina; arrhythmias; severe hypotension.
b. contraindicate use of pentoxifylline: allergy to any methylxanthine (caffeine, theophylline, dyphylline); **pregnancy (Category C)**; lactation (secreted in breast milk).

Nursing Interventions

Medication Administration

Provide small, frequent meals if GI upset occurs.
Administer drug with meals.
Provide comfort measures for headache.

Surveillance During Therapy

Monitor for angina; chest pain; hypotension; dyspnea; dyspepsia; nausea; dizziness; headache.
Carefully monitor laboratory studies and patient for indications of adverse reactions.
Interpret results of diagnostic tests and contact practitioner as appropriate.
Monitor for possible drug–drug and drug–nutrient interactions; see Interactions.

Patient Teaching

Instruct patient to take drug with meals to minimize GI side effects.
Caution patient to notify drug prescriber if persistent nausea, dyspepsia, dizziness, or headache occur because dosage reduction may be indicated.
Explain that beneficial effects of drug may not be apparent for 2 to 4 weeks. Results are often manifested by gradual increase in ability to walk longer distances without experiencing pain (claudication).
Inform patient that treatment will probably continue for at least 8 weeks.

Thrombolytic Drugs

Alteplase, recombinant
Anistreplase
Streptokinase
Urokinase

Thrombolytic (or fibrinolytic) drugs facilitate the dissolution of blood clots by activating the fibrinolytic enzyme plasmin (fibrinolysin). They are used in the treatment of several thromboembolic disorders and have become widely used in the early stages of a myocardial infarction to effect recanalization of an occluded coronary artery. Most evidence indicates that thrombolytic drugs are most effective when administered within 2 to 4 hours of the *onset* of symptoms of a myocardial infarction; more delayed administration is much less successful in promoting reperfusion of occluded vessels.

The available thrombolytic drugs are enzymes, one derived from beta-hemolytic streptococci (streptokinase), another from human kidney cells (urokinase), a third produced in tissue culture by recombinant DNA techniques (alteplase), and a streptokinase–plasminogen activator complex (anistreplase). These drugs are associated with a definite risk of bleeding, especially from sites of invasive procedures; such procedures should be limited within the first 48 hours after administration. Streptokinase and urokinase can produce a *generalized* lytic state, in which normally protective hemostatic thrombi are lysed as well as the intracoronary thrombi. This condition can lead to internal bleeding and represents a potentially serious complication of thrombolytic therapy. Alteplase appears to be more *clot specific*, inasmuch as it produces only limited amounts of plasmin in the absence of fibrin. The reduced systemic lytic potential of alteplase brought about its increasing use in myocardial infarction.

Because these four drugs are quite similar in their actions, they are reviewed as a group; individual agents are listed in Table 37-3.

Mechanism

Convert plasminogen (profibrinolysin), an inactive plasma protein, to plasmin (fibrinolysin), an active fibrinolytic enzyme, which degrades fibrin clots, fibrinogen, and other plasma proteins. Streptokinase first combines with plasminogen to form an activator complex, resulting in cleavage of peptide bonds on plasminogen to form plasmin; *urokinase* activates plasminogen directly; *alteplase* binds to fibrin and converts the enmeshed plasminogen to plasmin, with only limited conversion to plasmin in the systemic circulation. Increased formation of fibrin degradation products provides for additional anticoagulant activity. Anistreplase is inactive until injected into human blood; when activated, it results in cleavage of peptide bonds on plasminogen to form plasmin.

Uses

Lysis of coronary artery thrombi associated with an evolving myocardial infarction, as an aid to reperfusion of the blocked vessel (most effective if given within 4 hours of onset of symptoms)
Lysis of acute, massive pulmonary emboli (urokinase, alteplase)
Lysis of acute, extensive deep vein thromboses (streptokinase)
Clearance of occluded arteriovenous cannulae (streptokinase)
Restoration of patency of IV and central venous catheters obstructed by clotted blood (urokinase)

Dosage

See Table 37-3.

Fate

Plasminogen is activated almost immediately on IV infusion of these drugs; their metabolism is poorly understood; plasma half-life of streptokinase is 15 to 20 minutes initially, while antistreptokinase antibodies are present; after saturation of antibodies with a loading dose, half-life is prolonged up to 90 minutes; serum half-life of urokinase is less than 20 minutes but is prolonged in the presence of impaired liver function; alteplase is cleared quickly from the plasma, more than one half the dose within 5 minutes; excretion is by way of the urine and bile; anistreplase has a plasma half-life of 70 to 120 minutes.

Common Side Effects

Minor bleeding episodes (especially at sites of invasive procedures), bruising. Mild allergic reactions, fever, headache and muscle pain are common with *streptokinase*.

Significant Adverse Reactions

Severe hemorrhage (cerebral, GI, retroperitoneal); allergic reactions (dyspnea, angioedema, periorbital swelling, bronchospasm, anaphylactic reaction); blood pressure alterations, and phlebitis at site of IV injection.

Contraindications

Active internal bleeding, intracranial or intraspinal surgery, intracranial neoplasm, and recent cerebrovascular accident. *Cautious use* in the following situations: recent or imminent surgery, ulcerative wounds, trauma with internal injuries, malignancies,

Table 37-3. **Thrombolytic Agents**

Drug	*Usual Dosage Range*	*Nursing Considerations*
Alteplase, recombinant *Activase*	*Myocardial infarction* 10 mg IV bolus, followed by 90 mg given over 90 min *Pulmonary embolism* 100 mg by IV infusion over 2 h	Thrombolytic prepared by recombinant DNA technique using a human melanoma cell line; relatively clot specific—requires fibrin as a cofactor, therefore is less likely to produce systemic lysis than other thrombolytics; heparin is given concurrently for at least 48 h; aspirin or dipyridamole may be given either during or after heparin; doses of 150 mg have been associated with increased intracranial bleeding; reconstitute *only* with sterile water for injection and use within 8 h; do *not* add other medications to infusion solution
Anistreplase *Eminase*	*Myocardial infarction* 30 units by IV injection over 2–5 min	May not be effective if given between 5 days and 6 months of prior streptokinase or anistreplase injection or streptococcal infections owing to the presence of antistreptokinase antibodies; reconstitute vial with 5 mL of sterile water, directing stream to side of vial rather than directly into the powder; vial is rolled or tilted gently to reconstitute the drug, but should *not* be shaken; the medication must be used within 30 min of reconstitution
Streptokinase *Kabikinase, Streptase*	*Myocardial infarction* IV: 1,500,000 U in a single IV infusion over 1 h *Intracoronary*: 20,000 U by bolus initially, followed by 2000 U/min for 1 h *Venous thrombosis and pulmonary or arterial embolism* Initially: 250,000 U IV over 30 min, *then*: 100,000 U/h over 72 h for venous thrombosis *or* 100,000 U/h over 24–72 h for pulmonary embolism or arterial thrombosis *Arteriovenous cannula occlusion* Infuse by pump at a constant rate, 250,000 U/2 mL IV solution, into each occluded limb of cannula over 30 min, then clamp off for 2 h; aspirate contents of infusion cannula, flush with saline, and reconnect cannula	Used by either IV (preferred) or intracoronary route of administration; fever is common and is treated symptomatically; may not be effective if given between 5 days and 6 months of prior streptokinase or anistreplase injection or streptococcal infections owing to the presence of antistreptokinase antibodies; reconstitute contents of each vial with 5 mL sodium chloride injection or 5% dextrose injection directed to the side of the vial rather than directly into the powder; vial is rolled or tilted gently to reconstitute the drug but should *not* be shaken; contents are then diluted further to total volume as recommended for the specific indication; refer to package instructions for additional diluting information
Urokinase *Abbokinase*	Initial priming dose of 4400 U/kg is given over 10 min at a rate of 1.5 mL/min, followed by continuous infusion of 4400 U/kg/h at rate of 15 mL/h for 12 h; tubing is then flushed with normal saline injection or 5% dextrose injection at same rate; approximately 3–4 h after urokinase therapy, a continuous heparin IV infusion should be initiated *Lysis of coronary artery thrombi*: After a bolus dose of heparin (2500–10,000 U), urokinase infused into occluded artery at rate of 4 mL/min (6000 U/min) for up to 2 h; therapy should be continued until artery is maximally opened	Used for treating coronary artery thrombosis and pulmonary emboli and for restoring patency to IV catheters; does not result in antibody formation as does streptokinase; powder is reconstituted by adding 5.2 mL of sterile water for injection to the vial, rolling it gently to aid mixing (*do not shake*), then diluting with either normal saline or 5% dextrose injection to the desired concentration before infusing; drug should be mixed immediately before infusing because the solution contains no preservatives; do *not* add other medications to the solution

urinary or GI lesions (eg, colitis, diverticulitis), severe hypertension, diabetic retinopathy, hepatic or renal disease, hemorrhagic disorders, chronic lung disease, rheumatic heart disease, subacute bacterial endocarditis, history of allergic reactions, pregnancy, immediate postpartum period, and in children.

Interactions

Drugs that alter platelet function (eg, salicylates, dipyridamole, indomethacin, phenylbutazone, ticlopidine) or coagulation (eg, heparin, warfarin) may increase the risk of hemorrhage.

Nursing Management

Pretherapy Assessment

Assess and record baseline data necessary for detection of adverse effects of thrombolytic agents: General: VS, body weight, skin color and temperature; CNS: orientation, reflexes; CVS: baseline ECG, peripheral perfusion; Laboratory: CBC, Hct, platelet count, thrombin time, APTT, prothrombin time.

Review medical history and documents for existing or previous conditions that:

a. require cautious use of thrombolytic agents: ulcerative wounds; trauma with internal injuries; malignancies; urinary or GI lesions (eg, colitis, diverticulitis); severe hypertension; diabetic retinopathy; hepatic or renal disease; hemorrhagic disorders; chronic lung disease; rheumatic heart disease; subacute bacterial endocarditis; history of allergic reactions.
b. contraindicate use of thrombolytic agents: allergy to the thrombolytic agent; active internal bleeding; intracranial or intraspinal surgery; intracranial neo-

plasm; recent cerebrovascular accident; **pregnancy (Category C)**; lactation (safety not established).

Nursing Interventions

Medication Administration

Avoid unnecessary delays in initiating thrombolytic therapy for myocardial infarction. The sooner a thrombolytic drug is given after symptoms of myocardial infarction are first noted, the more likely it is that the drug will limit damage to the heart muscle. Treatment should begin within 4 to 6 hours of the onset of symptoms.

Ensure that a blood sample is drawn to determine thrombin time before initiating therapy.

Surveillance During Therapy

Monitor patient for signs of potentially serious internal or external bleeding (hematuria, ecchymoses, epistaxis, bleeding from sites of recent invasive procedures).

Discontinue infusion if serious bleeding occurs and cannot be controlled adequately by local application of pressure or if thrombin time is less than half normal. Whole fresh blood, packed red cells, or fresh-frozen plasma may be administered. Aminocaproic acid may be given if hemorrhage is unresponsive to blood replacement. Therapy should be reinstituted only if signs of bleeding cease.

Avoid arterial invasive procedures before and during treatment. If an arterial puncture is performed, apply manual pressure to the site for 30 minutes, then apply a pressure dressing. Perform venipuncture as carefully and infrequently as possible, and apply prolonged manual pressure to site afterward. Avoid IM injections because hematomas are likely to form.

Monitor patient very carefully during first few hours of infusion for signs of serious allergic reactions (eg, wheezing, hypotension). Discontinue infusion, and prepare to assist with symptomatic treatment (eg, epinephrine, antihistamines, corticosteroids) if allergic manifestations occur.

Check results of streptokinase resistance levels when streptokinase or anistreplase is used, which should be measured before instituting therapy. Although recent streptococcal infection may require use of higher loading doses, streptokinase should not be given if resistance levels exceed 1,000,000 units.

Maintain patient on bed rest during entire course of therapy and avoid handling patient unnecessarily because bruising occurs readily.

Begin continuous IV heparin infusion after completion of therapy with streptokinase or urokinase; or when used with alteplase, begin continuous IV heparin infusion when initiating alteplase therapy. Heparin therapy is followed by oral anticoagulant therapy. Heparin should be discontinued when prothrombin time reaches two to three times the normal control value.

Carefully monitor laboratory studies and patient for indications of adverse reactions.

Interpret results of diagnostic tests and contact practitioner as appropriate.

Monitor for possible drug–drug and drug–nutrient interactions; see Interactions.

Patient Teaching

Teach the patient about the disease being treated, the reasons for the frequent blood tests, and why IV injections are being used.

Hemostatic Drugs

Hemostatic drugs may be used to control bleeding in a variety of situations. Systemically administered agents are used to elevate or replenish one or more coagulation factors that may be deficient because of a hereditary or acquired defect, and to treat excessive systemic bleeding resulting from surgical complications, hematologic disorders, or neoplastic disease. Topically applied hemostatics are primarily used to control continual oozing or mild bleeding from capillaries and other small blood vessels (eg, after surgery), or in the treatment of decubitus or chronic leg ulcers.

Systemic Hemostatics

• *Aminocaproic Acid*

Amicar

Mechanism

Inhibits plasminogen activators and interferes with binding of plasmin to fibrin, thereby retarding clot breakdown.

Uses

Treatment of severe bleeding resulting from systemic hyperfibrinolysis, such as that associated with heart surgery, hematologic disorders, abruptio placentae, cirrhosis of the liver, or neoplastic disorders

Treatment of urinary hyperfibrinolysis, such as that associated with severe trauma, shock, prostatectomy, nephrectomy, or renal malignancies

Treatment of overdosage with fibrinolytic drugs (eg, alteplase, anistreplase, streptokinase, urokinase; investigational use)

Preventing recurrence of subarachnoid hemorrhage, aborting or preventing attacks of hereditary angioneurotic edema, and decreasing need for platelet transfusion in cases of amegakaryocytic thrombocytopenia (investigational uses only)

Dosage

Oral: 5 g initially, followed by 1 to 1.25 g/h for 8 hours or until bleeding has ceased; maximum dose 30 g/day

IV infusion: 4 to 5 g in 250 mL diluent during first hour, followed by continuous infusion at a rate of 1 g/h in 50 mL diluent for 8 hours or until bleeding ceases

Fate

Rapidly absorbed orally; peak plasma levels occur in 1 to 2 hours; widely distributed; rapidly excreted, largely in the form of unmetabolized drug.

Common Side Effects

Nausea, cramping, diarrhea, malaise.

Significant Adverse Reactions

Dizziness, tinnitus, weakness, fatigue, pruritus, headache, hypotension, delirium, nasal congestion, skin rash, menstrual cramping, reversible acute renal failure, thrombophlebitis, and auditory and visual hallucinations.

Contraindications

Active intravascular clotting, hematuria of upper urinary tract origin. *Cautious use* in people with cardiac, renal, or hepatic disease, in pregnant women, and in children.

Interactions

Oral contraceptives may increase the danger of increased coagulation.

Serum potassium levels can be elevated by aminocaproic acid.

Nursing Management

Pretherapy Assessment

Assess and record baseline data necessary for detection of adverse effects of aminocaproic acid: General: VS, body weight, skin color and temperature; CNS: orientation, reflexes; CVS: baseline ECG, peripheral perfusion; Laboratory: CBC, Hct, platelet count, thrombin time, APTT, prothrombin time.

Review medical history and documents for existing or previous conditions that:

a. require cautious use of aminocaproic acid: cardiac, renal, or hepatic disease.

b. contraindicate use of aminocaproic acid: allergy to the aminocaproic acid; active intravascular clotting; hematuria of upper urinary tract; **pregnancy (Category C)**; lactation (safety not established).

Nursing Interventions

Medication Administration

Provide ready access to bathroom facilities if diarrhea occurs.

Provide small, frequent meals if GI upset occurs.

Be prepared to administer emergency treatment in life-threatening bleeding situations, such as fresh whole blood transfusions or fibrinogen infusions.

Surveillance During Therapy

Be alert for signs of possible thromboembolic complications (eg, chest or leg pain, dyspnea).

Monitor results of plasma levels, which should be 0.13 mg/mL or higher to inhibit systemic hyperfibrinolysis.

Carefully monitor laboratory studies and patient for indications of adverse reactions.

Interpret results of diagnostic tests and contact practitioner as appropriate.

Monitor for possible drug–drug and drug–nutrient interactions; see Interactions.

Provide for patient safety needs if CNS changes occur.

Patient Teaching

Inform the patient that the following side effects may occur with this treatment; dizziness; weakness; headache; hallucinations; nausea; diarrhea; cramps; infertility problems; malaise; fatigue.

Instruct the patient to inform the practitioner if any of the following occur: severe headache; restlessness; muscle pain or weakness; blood in the urine.

• Tranexamic Acid

Cyklokapron

Mechanism

Competitively inhibits plasminogen activation; may also directly interfere with action of plasmin at high concentrations; prolongs thrombin time but does not alter platelet aggregation or coagulation time.

Uses

Reduction or prevention of hemorrhage during and after tooth extraction in patients with hemophilia (short-term use, 2–8 days).

Dosage

Oral: 25 mg/kg 3 to 4 times/day 1 day before dental surgery, then 25 mg/kg 3 to 4 times/day for up to 8 days after surgery

IV: 10 mg/kg immediately before surgery then 10 mg/kg 3 to 4 times a day if unable to take oral medications; adjust for renal dysfunction

Fate

Oral absorption is 25% to 50% of administered dose; peak plasma levels occur in 2 to 3 hours; plasma protein binding is minimal; effective plasma concentrations persist for up to 8 hours; more than 95% of a dose is eliminated unchanged in the urine.

Common Side Effects

Nausea, diarrhea with oral use; hypotension with too-rapid IV injection.

Significant Adverse Reactions

Vomiting, visual disturbances (eg, altered color vision).

Contraindications

Subarachnoid hemorrhage, acquired defective color vision. *Cautious use* in people with renal insufficiency and in pregnant or nursing women.

Nursing Management

Pretherapy Assessment

Assess and record baseline data necessary for detection of adverse effects of tranexamic acid: General: VS, body weight, skin color and temperature; CNS: orientation, reflexes; CVS: baseline ECG, peripheral perfusion; Laboratory: CBC, Hct, platelet count, thrombin time, APTT, prothrombin time.

Review medical history and documents for existing or previous conditions that:

a. require cautious use of tranexamic acid: renal insufficiency.

b. contraindicate use of tranexamic acid: allergy to

tranexamic acid; subarachnoid hemorrhage; acquired defective color vision (prevents assessment of toxicity); **pregnancy (Category B)**; lactation (secreted in breast milk; safety not established).

Nursing Interventions

Medication Administration

Provide ready access to bathroom facilities if diarrhea occurs.
Provide small, frequent meals if GI upset occurs.
Do not mix solution with blood or with solutions that contain penicillin.
Administer solution at rate of 1 mL/min with IV injection. If drug is injected too rapidly, hypotension may occur.

Surveillance During Therapy

Monitor patient taking drug for more than several days for changes in visual acuity, color vision, visual fields, or visual fundus. If changes are found, drug should be discontinued.
Carefully monitor laboratory studies and patient for indications of adverse reactions.
Interpret results of diagnostic tests and contact practitioner as appropriate.
Monitor for possible drug–drug and drug–nutrient interactions; see Interactions.
Provide for patient safety needs if CNS changes occur.

Patient Teaching

Inform the patient that the following side effects may occur with this treatment: nausea, diarrhea, cramps.
Instruct the patient to inform the practitioner if any of the following occur: persistent nausea, vomiting, or diarrhea; any visual changes; pain in calves.

• Antihemophilic Factor, Human (AHF)

Hemofil M, Koate-HS, Monoclate

(CAN) Kryobulin VH

Mechanism

A plasma protein (factor VIII) that is essential for the conversion of prothrombin to thrombin; replaces deficient endogenous factor VIII in cases of classic hemophilia, thereby decreasing bleeding tendency.

Uses

Treatment of classic hemophilia A, in which there is a demonstrated deficiency of clotting factor VIII, to control bleeding episodes or perform surgical procedures.

Dosage

Administered IV. Dosage expressed in AHF units; one AHF unit (U) equals the activity present in 1 mL of human plasma pooled from at least 10 donors and tested within 1 hour of collection.

Dose is individually adjusted on the basis of patient's weight, severity of bleeding, presence of factor VIII inhibitors, and the desired level of factor VIII. Therapy should be based on factor VIII level assays. The following average doses are recommended:

Prophylaxis of spontaneous hemorrhage: 10 U/kg as a single dose; do not repeat in mild cases unless further bleeding occurs
Moderate hemorrhage/minor surgery: 15 to 25 U/kg initially, followed by 10 to 15 U/kg every 8 to 12 hours as needed
Severe hemorrhage: 40 to 50 U/kg initially, followed by 20 U/kg every 8 to 12 hours

Doses less than 34 U/mL may be given at a rate of 10 to 20 mL over 3 minutes; doses greater than 34 U/mL should be given at a maximum rate of 2 mL/min. If a significant increase in pulse rate occurs, the rate of administration should be decreased.

Fate

Coagulant levels rise rapidly after administration, then quickly decrease. Plasma half-life after the initial dose ranges from 8 to 24 hours and increases with subsequent doses.

Common Side Effects

Mild allergic reactions, headache, flushing.

Significant Adverse Reactions

Nausea, vomiting, chills, erythema, hives, fever, tachycardia, hypotension, backache, visual disturbances, clouded consciousness; massive doses may cause hemolytic anemia, increased bleeding tendency, and hyperfibrinogenemia.

CAUTION

Because this product is prepared from human plasma, the risk of transmitting viral hepatitis and the human immunodeficiency virus (HIV) exists, and although minimal, must be recognized.

Contraindications

Approximately 5% to 10% of patients with hemophilia A have inhibitors to factor VIII. In these patients, the response to AHF may be markedly reduced or absent; such patients may be candidates for antiinhibitor coagulant complex (see following section). Large or frequent doses of AHF in patients with blood types A, B, or AB may result in intravascular hemolysis and anemia; appropriate blood monitoring is necessary during extended or high-dosage therapy.

Nursing Management

Pretherapy Assessment

Assess and record baseline data necessary for detection of adverse effects of AHF: General: VS, body weight, skin color and temperature; CNS: orientation, reflexes; CVS: baseline ECG, peripheral perfusion; Laboratory: factor VIII levels, Hct, direct Coombs' test, HIV screening, hepatitis screening.
Review medical history and documents for existing or previous conditions that:

a. require cautious use of AHF: large or frequent doses of AHF in patients with blood types A, B, or AB.
b. contraindicate use of AHF: allergy to mouse proteins; inhibitors to factor VIII; **pregnancy (Category C)**; lactation (safety not established).

Nursing Interventions

Medication Administration

Question administration if diagnosis of factor VIII deficiency has not been made. Drug is of no benefit in other bleeding disorders.

Administer at a rate no greater than 10 mL/min because vasomotor reactions can occur.

Be prepared to administer much larger than normal doses of antihemophilic factor or antiinhibitor coagulation complex (see following discussion) to the patient who is one of a small percentage in whom inhibitors to factor VIII develop (incidence is about 10%).

Store drug vials between 2°C and 8°C until reconstituted. Warm concentrate and diluent to room temperature before mixing.

Rotate vial gently but do not shake during reconstitution. Do not use if gel formation occurs.

Do *not* refrigerate after reconstitution because precipitation can occur.

Administer within 3 hours after reconstitution to avoid possible untoward effects caused by bacterial contamination during mixing. Use plastic syringe because solution may adhere to surface of glass syringes.

Surveillance During Therapy

Carefully monitor laboratory studies and patient for indications of adverse reactions.

Interpret results of diagnostic tests and contact practitioner as appropriate.

Monitor for possible drug–drug and drug–nutrient interactions; see Interactions.

Patient Teaching

Inform the patient that the following side effects may occur with this treatment: headache; rash; itching; backache; difficulty breathing.

Instruct the patient to inform the practitioner if any of the following occur: headache; rash; itching; backache; difficulty breathing.

• Antiinhibitor Coagulant Complex

Autoplex, Feiba VH Immuno

Mechanism

Concentrate of activated and precursor clotting factors and factors of the kinin-generating system prepared from pooled human plasma; reduces level of factor VIII inhibitory activity in patients with hemophilia, thus decreasing bleeding episodes.

Uses

Treatment of symptoms of hemophilia in patients with significant levels of factor VIII inhibitors who are bleeding or about to undergo surgery.

Dosage

IV only: 25 to 100 factor VIII correctional units/kg depending on severity of bleeding at a rate of 2 to 10 mL infusion solution/min; repeat in 6 hours if necessary (1 unit of factor VIII correctional activity is that amount of activated prothrombin complex which, on addition to an equal amount of factor VIII-deficient plasma, will correct the clotting time to 35 sec).

Significant Adverse Reactions

CAUTION

This product is prepared from large pools of human plasma and the risk of transmission of viral diseases such as hepatitis or acquired immunodeficiency syndrome (AIDS) exists and, although minimal, must be recognized.

Hypersensitivity reactions (fever, chills, alterations in blood pressure); headache, flushing, tachycardia, hypercoagulability (dyspnea, chest pain, cough, changes in pulse rate).

Contraindications

Fibrinolysis, disseminated intravascular coagulation. *Cautious use* in patients with liver disease or a history of allergies, and in small children.

Interactions

The possibility of hypercoagulability states is increased with concomitant use of antiinhibitor coagulant complex and aminocaproic acid.

Nursing Management

Pretherapy Assessment

Assess and record baseline data necessary for detection of adverse effects of antiinhibitor coagulant complex: General: VS, body weight, skin color and temperature; CNS: orientation, reflexes; CVS: baseline ECG, peripheral perfusion; Laboratory: clotting factor levels, fibrinogen levels, liver function tests.

Review medical history and documents for existing or previous conditions that:

a. require cautious use of antiinhibitor coagulant complex: liver disease; history of allergies; use in small children.
b. contraindicate use of antiinhibitor coagulant complex: fibrinolysis; disseminated intravascular coagulation; **pregnancy (Category C)**; lactation (safety not established).

Nursing Interventions

Medication Administration

Ensure that appropriate medications (eg, epinephrine, corticosteroids, antihistamines) are available to manage any hypersensitivity reactions that may develop.

Avoid rapid infusion rates (eg, 5–10 mL/min) because incidence of side effects is much higher.

Store unreconstituted product under refrigeration. Use diluent provided to prepare infusion solution according to package directions. Each bottle is labeled with units of factor VIII correctional activity that it contains.

Complete infusion in 1 hour for Autoplex and in 3 hours for Feibo VH Immuno.

Surveillance During Therapy

Provide patient with appropriate reassurance and emotional support with regard to the risk of contracting

viral hepatitis and possibly other diseases (eg, AIDS) with administration of product.
Observe closely for indications of intravascular coagulation (eg, dyspnea, coughing, chest or leg pain). Infusion should be terminated if these occur.
Carefully monitor laboratory studies and patient for indications of adverse reactions.
Interpret results of diagnostic tests and contact practitioner as appropriate.
Monitor for possible drug–drug and drug–nutrient interactions; see Interactions.

Patient Teaching

Instruct the patient to inform the practitioner if any of the following side effects occur: headache; rash; itching; backache; difficulty breathing.

• Factor IX Complex, Human

Konyne-HT, Profilnine Heat-Treated, Proplex T

Mechanism

Concentrate of dried plasma fractions of human coagulation factors II, VII, IX, and X with small amounts of other plasma proteins; provides replacement therapy for a congenital or acquired deficiency of one or more factors that can result in increased bleeding tendencies.

Uses

Treatment of factor IX deficiency (hemophilia B or Christmas disease) to prevent or control bleeding episodes (*not* a substitute for fresh-frozen plasma in patients with *mild* factor IX deficiency)
Control of bleeding episodes in patients with factor VIII inhibitors (Proplex T)
Reversal of oral anticoagulant-induced hemorrhaging
Prevention or control of bleeding episodes in patients with factor VII deficiency (Proplex T *only*)

Dosage

Highly individual, depending on patient status, severity of bleeding, and degree of factor deficiency as determined by coagulation assays before treatment; dosage measured in units (1 unit is the activity present in 1 mL of normal plasma less than 1 h old). Potency is adjusted based on factor IX, because the other factors (II, VII, X) are present in approximately the same amount.

Recommended IV dosage guidelines are as follows:

Treatment of bleeding in hemophilia A patients with inhibitors to factor VIII: 75 U/kg; repeat in 12 hours if needed
Reversal of Coumarin effect: 15 U/kg
Hemarthroses in hemophiliacs with factor VIII inhibitors: 75 U/kg; repeat in 12 hours if necessary
Prophylaxis in patients with congenital deficiency of procoagulant factors: 10 to 20 U/kg once or twice a week to prevent spontaneous bleeding

The infusion rate should not exceed 3 mL/min.

Common Side Effects

Flushing, tingling (especially with too-rapid infusion).

Significant Adverse Reactions

CAUTION

This product is obtained from pooled human plasma and therefore is associated with the risk of transmission of viral diseases such as hepatitis or AIDS; although minimal, this risk must be recognized.

Chills, fever, headache, tachycardia, hypotension, viral hepatitis, and intravascular hemolysis.

Contraindications

Liver disease with signs of intravascular coagulation or fibrinolysis.

Not for use in the treatment of factor VII deficiency (except for Proplex T).

Nursing Management

Pretherapy Assessment

Assess and record baseline data necessary for detection of adverse effects of factor IX complex: General: VS, body weight, skin color and temperature; CNS: orientation, reflexes; CVS: baseline ECG, peripheral perfusion; Laboratory: clotting factor levels, fibrinogen levels, liver function tests.
Review medical history and documents for existing or previous conditions that:
a. require cautious use of factor IX complex: none.
b. contraindicate use of factor IX complex; liver disease; signs of intravascular coagulation or fibrinolysis; **pregnancy (Category C)**; lactation (safety not established).

Nursing Interventions

Medication Administration

Infuse *slowly* IV. Rapid infusion (more than 3 mL/min) can produce vasomotor symptoms (eg, tachycardia, hypotension). If chills, fever, tingling, flushing, or headache occur during infusion, dosage reduction (slower infusion rate) is indicated.
Store product under normal refrigeration until reconstituted, but do not freeze. Warm to room temperature just before mixing. Do *not* use if gel forms.
Administer within 3 hours after reconstitution, and do *not* refrigerate reconstituted solution because precipitation can occur.

Surveillance During Therapy

Provide patient with appropriate reassurance and emotional support with regard to the risk of contracting viral hepatitis and possibly other diseases (eg, AIDS) with administration of product.
Monitor infusion rate constantly, and note development of symptoms (eg, cough, chest pain, respiratory distress, altered pulse and blood pressure) that signify increased intravascular coagulation. If these occur, infusion should be stopped immediately. To minimize risk of intravascular coagulation, no attempt should be made to raise factor IX level to more than 50% of normal.

Monitor results of coagulation assays, which should be performed before initiation of treatment and regularly thereafter. Dosage is adjusted on the basis of assay results.
Monitor levels of coagulation factors, which should be checked repeatedly during infusion because excessive levels increase the risk of intravascular coagulation.
Carefully monitor laboratory studies and patient for indications of adverse reactions.
Monitor results of prothrombin times. Drug should not be reinfused unless *post*infusion prothrombin time is at least two thirds of the *pre*infusion value.
Interpret results of diagnostic tests and contact practitioner as appropriate.
Monitor for possible drug–drug and drug–nutrient interactions; see Interactions.

Patient Teaching

Instruct the patient to inform the practitioner if any of the following side effects occur: headache; rash; itching; backache; difficulty breathing; unusual bleeding or bruising.

• Antithrombin III (Human)

ATnativ

Mechanism

Antithrombin III is produced from pooled human plasma from healthy donors. Antithrombin III inactivates thrombin and activated forms of factors IX, X, XI, and XII.

Uses

Treatment of patients who have hereditary antithrombin III deficiency in connection with surgical or obstetric procedures, or when they experience thromboembolism.

Dosage

The dosage is based on antithrombin III levels. They will increase 1% to 2.1% with administration of 1 IU/kg by IV infusion. Levels should be maintained at 75% to 120% of normal. Do not exceed an infusion rate of 2 mL/min; 1 mL/min is recommended.

Significant Adverse Reactions

Adverse effects have been strikingly absent. Rapid administration may cause dyspnea and increased blood pressure.

Interactions

The anticoagulant effect of heparin is increased by concomitant antithrombin III administration.

Nursing Management

Nursing Interventions

Medication Administration

Do not shake when reconstituting.
Use within 3 hours after reconstitution.
Avoid rapid infusion rates (eg, 2 mL/min or more) because of possible dyspnea.

Surveillance During Therapy

Provide patient with appropriate reassurance and emotional support with regard to the risk of contracting viral hepatitis and possibly other diseases (eg AIDS) with administration of product.

Topical Hemostatics

A variety of substances are applied topically to control minor bleeding episodes and to reduce oozing and leakage from small blood vessels that may occur as a result of trauma or surgery. These topical hemostatics rarely are effective in controlling extensive hemorrhaging. Many of these products are used during or after surgery to retard blood loss through capillary and small vessel leakage. Most of the products are slowly absorbable and therefore provide a temporary framework on which platelets can adhere. Others are composed of gelatin, which can absorb many times its weight in blood and which adheres to the damaged site, slowing further blood loss. The clinically available topical hemostatic products are discussed briefly in the following.

• Gelatin Film, Absorbable

Gelfilm, Gelfilm Ophthalmic

Mechanism

Nonantigenic, absorbable gelatin film with the consistency of cellophane; moistened and cut to desired size and shape, and applied to tissue to reduce bleeding; absorbed completely within 1 to 6 months.

Uses

Reduce local bleeding in thoracic, ocular, or neurosurgery.

Dosage

Immerse in sterile saline, and allow to soak until pliable; fit to desired size and shape, and apply to surface of tissue.

Nursing Management

Nursing Interventions

Medication Administration

Do not use in grossly contaminated or infected surgical wounds, because rate of absorption is markedly increased.
Use immediately after opening package envelope to minimize contamination.

• Gelatin Sponge, Absorbable

Gelfoam

Mechanism

A pliable, nonantigenic sponge capable of absorbing many times its weight in whole blood; prepared from specially treated, purified gelatin solution; completely absorbed in 4 to 6 weeks when implanted into tissues; presence of anticoagulants does not interfere with its effectiveness; liquefies within several days when applied to actively bleeding areas.

Uses

Providing control of capillary and small blood vessel bleeding in many forms of surgery

Enhancing wound healing by providing a framework for granulation tissue

Dosage

Use sterile technique. Cut to desired size, and apply either dry or saturated with sodium chloride injection or thrombin solution to desired area. Hold in place with moderate pressure for 10 to 15 seconds, then allow to remain in contact with bleeding site. Wound may be closed over sponge.

Decubitus ulcers may be packed with sponge and a dressing applied.

Contraindications

Presence of infection, postpartum bleeding, menorrhagia, bleeding due to blood dyscrasias, and closure of skin incisions.

Nursing Management

Nursing Interventions

Medication Administration

Compress sponge before inserting into cavities or closed tissue spaces to reduce expansion and possible disturbances of surrounding structures. Do *not* overpack a particular area, because sponge may expand excessively, interfering with function of surrounding structures.

Note that effectiveness can be enhanced by soaking in a thrombin solution.

Use sponges as soon as possible after opening package to minimize bacterial contamination.

Do not resterilize by heating (changes absorption time) or with ethylene oxide (irritating to tissues).

• Gelatin powder, absorbable

Gelfoam

Mechanism

Acts as a hemostatic when applied locally; promotes growth of granulation tissue and facilitates healing of ulcerated areas.

Uses

Control of bleeding from cancellous bone when other conventional procedures are ineffective or impractical

Stimulation of granulation tissue in treating leg ulcers, decubitus ulcers, and other oozing lesions (unlabeled use)

Dosage

Contents of jar (1 g) are poured into a beaker and 3 to 4 mL of sterile saline is added to prepare a paste, which is smeared onto cut surface of bone. Excess is removed when bleeding stops.

Contraindications

Closure of skin incisions, postpartum bleeding or menorrhagia, presence of infection, or use as the sole hemostatic agent in patients with blood dyscrasias.

• Microfibrillar Collagen Hemostat

Avitene

Mechanism

A dry, fibrous, water-insoluble preparation of purified bovine corium collagen; when applied to the source of bleeding, it attracts platelets, which adhere to the fibrils of the preparation, triggering further platelet aggregation into thrombi; stimulates a mild, chronic inflammatory response; response is not inhibited by heparin; does not interfere with bone regeneration or healing.

Uses

Adjunct to hemostasis in surgical procedures when control of bleeding by conventional procedures (eg, ligation) is ineffective or impractical.

Dosage

Compress surface to be treated with a dry sponge before applying dry hemostat preparation, then apply pressure over the hemostat for several minutes. The amount of product required depends on size of area and severity of bleeding. Remove excess material after several minutes. Do *not* handle with wet instruments or gloves.

Significant Adverse Reactions

Potentiation of infection, hematomas (sealing over of exit site for deeper hemorrhage), adhesion formation, and allergic reactions.

Contraindications

Closure of skin incisions, use on bone surfaces to which prosthetic materials are to be attached.

Nursing Management

Nursing Interventions

Medication Administration

Do not sterilize product because it is inactivated by autoclaving. Avoid wetting product because its hemostatic efficacy is impaired.

Avoid spilling product on nonbleeding surfaces (especially abdominal or thoracic viscera) because it will adhere to any moist surface, possibly resulting in adhesions.

Remove excess material after several minutes by gentle teasing or irrigation. If breakthrough bleeding occurs, apply additional hemostat.

Do not use gloved fingers to apply pressure; a dry sponge is preferred.

• Oxidized Cellulose

Oxycel, Surgicel

Mechanism

On saturation with blood, cellulose material swells into a gelatinous, tenacious mass that serves as a clot nucleus; slowly absorbed from sites of implantation with minimal tissue reaction; does not alter normal blood clotting mechanism.

Uses

Adjunctive control of minor hemorrhage (capillary, venous, small arterial) in cases in which conventional methods (eg, ligation) are inappropriate
Production of hemostasis in oral and dental surgery

Dosage

Place pad, strip, or pellet of material of desired size on bleeding site; usually removed after development of hemostasis by irrigation with sterile water or saline.

Significant Adverse Reactions

Stinging, burning, headache, sneezing (nasal application), foreign body reactions, encapsulation of fluid, obstruction (eg, urinary, intestinal) caused by adhesion formation, necrosis of nasal membranes.

Contraindications

Implantation in bone defects (eg, fractures), use as packing or wadding (must be removed after hemostasis), hemorrhage from large arteries, and control of nonhemorrhagic oozing.

Nursing Management

Nursing Interventions

Medication Administration

Do not enclose oxidized cellulose in contaminated wounds without drainage.
Always remove after development of hemostasis in laminectomy procedures (may cause nerve damage), from foramina of bone, and from large open wounds.
Do not apply silver nitrate or other similar materials before using oxidized cellulose because absorption may be impaired.
Avoid wadding or packing the cellulose material, especially within rigid cavities, because swelling may cause obstruction or necrosis.
Ensure that none of the material is aspirated by the patient, as when it is used to control bleeding after tonsillectomy or to reduce epistaxis.
Avoid adding antiinfective agents, buffers, or other hemostatics to oxidized cellulose. The low pH of the product destroys these other additives.
Always irrigate before removal of oxidized cellulose to avoid tearing tissues and reinstituting bleeding.
Do not moisten before application because hemostatic effect is greater when dry.
Do not resterilize because autoclaving causes physical breakdown. Discard opened, unused product.
Use least amount necessary to produce hemostasis. Remove any excess before surgical closure.

• Thrombin, Topical

Thrombinar, Thrombostat

Mechanism

Catalyzes the conversion of fibrinogen to fibrin.

Uses

Reduce oozing and minor bleeding from capillaries and small venules (eg, laryngeal or nasal surgery, plastic surgery, bleeding from cancellous bone, dental extractions).

Dosage

Prepare solutions in sterile distilled water or saline; intended use determines concentration of solution, which may range from 100 to 2000 units/mL, depending on extent and severity of bleeding.

Spray or flood area (using syringe and fine-gauge needle) with solution; alternatively, dried powder from vial may be placed directly on area *or* absorbable gelatin sponge may be soaked in thrombin solution and then placed on area of bleeding.

Significant Adverse Reactions

Allergic reactions, fever.

Nursing Management

Nursing Interventions

Medication Administration

Never administer thrombin parenterally or allow it to enter large blood vessels because extensive intravascular clotting and death can result.
Use solutions the day they are prepared. Refrigerate solutions if several hours are to elapse between preparation and use.
Be aware that acids, alkalis, heat, and heavy metal salts reduce thrombin activity.
Do not sponge-treat surfaces because clot may be dislodged.
Ensure that wound is relatively free from blood before application of drug.

Selected Bibliography

Anderson HV, Willerson JT: Thrombolysis in acute myocardial infarction. N Engl J Med 329:703, 1993
Bruno A: Ischemic stroke: Part 2. Optimal treatment and prevention. Geriatrics 48(3):37, 1993
Cairns JA, et al: Antithrombotic agents in coronary artery disease. Chest 102:456, 1992
Leach RA: A tPA ninety-minute protocol. Journal of Emergency Nursing 19:338, 1993
Phillips DE, Payne K, Mills GM: Heparin-induced thrombotic thrombocytopenia. Ann Pharmacother 28:43, 1994
Pratt CW, Church FC: Antithrombin: Structure and function. Semin Hematol 28:3, 1991
Shammas NW, Zeitler R, Fitzpatrick P: Intravenous thrombolytic therapy in myocardial infarction: An analytical review. Clin Cardiol 16:282, 1993
Sila CA: Prophylaxis and treatment of stroke: The state of the art in 1993. Drugs 45:329, 1993
Simonneau G, Charbonnier, Decousus H: Subcutaneous low-molecular weight heparin compared with continuous intravenous unfractionated heparin in the treatment of proximal deep vein thrombosis. Arch Intern Med 153:1541, 1993
Verstraete M: Advances in thrombolytic therapy. Cardiovasc Drugs Ther 6:111, 1992

Nursing Bibliography

Aragon D, Martin M: What you should know about thrombolytic therapy for acute MI. Am J Nurs 9(1):24, 1993

Burns D: Review of thrombolytic use in acute myocardial infarction, pulmonary embolism, and cerebral thrombosis. Critical Care Nursing Quarterly 15(4):1, 1993

Deutsche J, Green D: Deep vein thrombosis in the critically ill patient. Critical Care Nursing 13(2):29, 1990

Dunn S, Senerchia C: Bleeding complications in the patient with cardiac disease following thrombolytic and anticoagulant therapies. Critical Care Nursing Clinics of North America 5:511, 1993

Majoros K: Comparisons and controversies in clot buster drugs. Critical Care Nursing Quarterly 16(2):46, 1993

Moseley M: Thrombolytic therapy: A case study. Critical Care Nurse 12(3):62, 1992

Pickett S: Women, thrombolytic treatment and the gender gap: Recommendations for practice. Journal of Emergency Nursing 19:491, 1993

Qureshi W, et al: Acute bleeding from peptic ulcers: How to restore hemostasis and prevent reoccurrence. Postgrad Med 93:167, 1993

Weiner B: Thrombolytic agents in critical care. Critical Care Nursing Clinics of North America 5:355, 1993

IV

Drugs Acting on the Renal System

38
Renal Physiology: A Review

The kidneys play a major role in the maintenance of homeostasis by regulating the volume and composition of the extracellular fluid that serves as the internal environment for each cell. In addition to controlling the water, electrolyte, and solute concentrations of the extracellular fluid, the kidneys selectively excrete drugs, hormones, and by-products of metabolism. The kidneys also participate in the maintenance of acid–base balance, renin secretion, erythropoietin production, and vitamin D metabolism.

Gross Anatomy of the Kidney

General Remarks

The kidneys are paired, bean-shaped organs located retroperitoneally on each side of the vertebral column at the level of T12 to L3. The right kidney is slightly lower than the left because of displacement by the liver.

Each kidney is invested by a fibrous capsule that is interrupted medially at the *hilus* for passage of blood vessels, lymphatics, nerves, and a ureter.

A frontal section of the kidney reveals an outer granular *cortex* located deep to the capsule and an inner *medulla* composed of several striated *pyramids* (Fig. 38-1). Interspersed among the pyramids are columns of cortical tissues known as the renal columns of Bertin.

The apex of each renal pyramid forms a *papilla*, which projects into a cup-like minor *calyx*. Several minor calyces unite to form major calyces, and the latter merge to form the *renal pelvis*. The renal pelvis is continuous with the *ureter*, which drains its contents into the *urinary bladder*.

Renal Blood Supply

Paired *renal arteries* arise from the abdominal aorta, branching as they enter the hilus. These branches divide into *interlobar arteries*, which pass between the medullary pyramids. At the corticomedullary junction the vessels form the *arcuate arteries*, which arch over the bases of the pyramids. Branching from the arcuate arteries are numerous *interlobular arteries*, which penetrate the cortical substance and give rise to *afferent arterioles* supplying individual nephron units.

Each afferent arteriole terminates in a tuft of capillaries, the *glomerulus*; these capillaries rejoin to form the *efferent arteriole*. Efferent arterioles terminate in *peritubular capillaries*, which surround the renal tubules. The peritubular capillaries eventually converge into venules that carry the blood into a series of veins corresponding in name and in course to the arteries described above.

A series of long, straight, peritubular capillaries termed *vasa recta* course through the medulla, turning sharply at various levels. The vasa recta participate in countercurrent exchange of substances between the renal tubules and vascular bed, as detailed later in this chapter.

Microscopic Anatomy of the Kidney

General Remarks

The basic anatomic and functional unit of the kidney is the *nephron* (Fig. 38-2). There are approximately 1 million nephrons in each human kidney. A nephron consists of a renal corpuscle and a long, often tortuously coiled renal tubule composed of the following anatomically modified and functionally distinct segments: the proximal convoluted tubule, the loop of Henle, and the distal convoluted tubule, which empties into a confluent collecting tubule.

Each nephron originates as a double-walled cup, the *Bowman capsule*, which encloses the glomerular capillaries. Collectively, the Bowman capsule and the glomerulus are termed the *renal (malpighian) corpuscle*. The epithelium of the Bowman capsule is of the simple squamous type, with the inner (visceral) layer containing modified cells called *podocytes*. The podocytes exhibit numerous, foot-like extensions called *pedicels*, which contact the basement membrane of the glomerular capillaries, except at narrow spaces called *filtration slits*.

The podocyte layer (visceral epithelium) of the Bowman capsule, together with the basement membrane and fenestrated endothelium of the glomerulus, forms a functional filtration membrane.

The outer (parietal) layer of the Bowman capsule becomes continuous with the epithelium of the *proximal convoluted tubule*. The proximal convoluted tubule then straightens and plunges toward the medulla, forming the thick descending segment (pars recta) of the *loop of Henle*.

The loop of Henle is a U-shaped structure composed of a thick descending segment (pars recta), a thin segment, and a thick ascending segment. The thick ascending segment becomes continuous with the *distal convoluted tubule* at a modified site, the *macula densa*, where the tubular cells and their prominent nuclei are densely crowded.

The distal tubule coils in the area of the renal cortex before joining a collecting duct. The latter descends into the medulla as part of a renal pyramid and empties through the papilla into a minor calyx.

The epithelium of the collecting ducts contains two types of cells: *principal cells* and *intercalated cells*. The water permeability and sodium transport of the principal cells are controlled by *antidiuretic hormone* (ADH; vasopressin) and *aldosterone*, respectively. The intercalated cells secrete hydrogen ions by primary active transport.

Histologically, the proximal and distal segments of the tubule differ somewhat, reflecting differences in function. The epithelium of the proximal segments (proximal convoluted

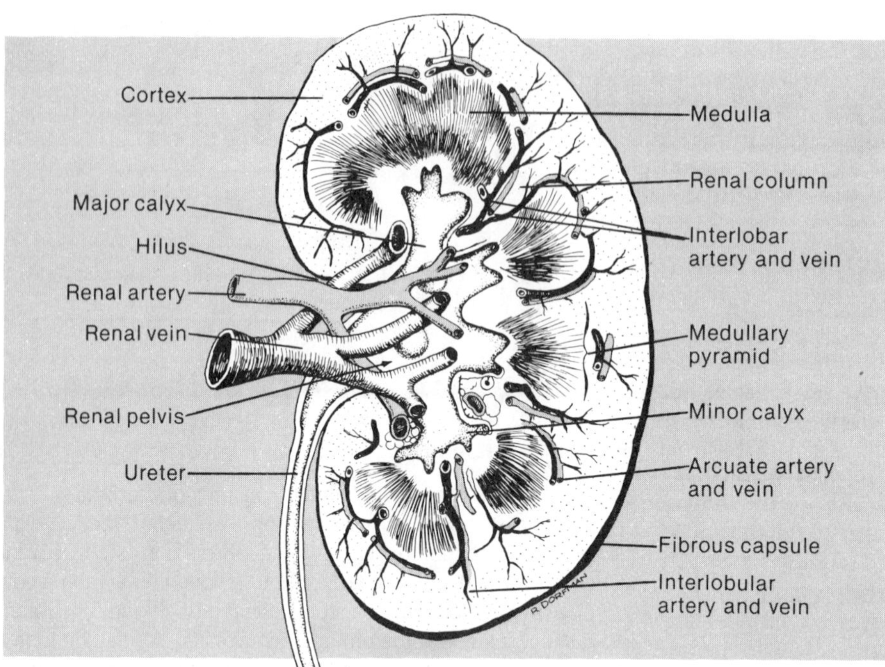

Figure 38-1. Frontal section of a human kidney.

tubule and pars recta) is characterized by a luminal "brush border" of extensive microvilli that greatly increase the free surface area available for reabsorption of filtered substances. By contrast, the epithelia of the thick ascending limb of the loop of Henle and the distal tubule are flatter, with few microvilli. The epithelium of the thin segment of the loop of Henle is simple squamous and lacks microvilli.

Two types of nephrons exist: *cortical nephrons* and *juxtamedullary nephrons*. These differ primarily in the lengths and placement of their loops of Henle and the associated arrangement of the peritubular capillaries. Cortical nephrons have relatively short loops of Henle that extend only slightly into the renal medulla. The juxtamedullary nephrons, however, have long loops of Henle that descend into the depths of the medulla. Hairpin loops of peritubular capillaries, the *vasa recta*, parallel the passage of these long loops of Henle through the medulla. The functional significance of this anatomic arrangement is discussed later in this chapter, in the section on the Countercurrent Mechanism.

Juxtaglomerular Apparatus

At its origin, the distal convoluted tubule lies close to the afferent and efferent arterioles. Here the distal tubular epithelial cells with their prominent nuclei are densely crowded, forming a discrete area termed the *macula densa*. Adjacent to the macula densa are modified afferent arteriolar cells called *juxtaglomerular cells*, which contain granules of the proteolytic enzyme *renin*. Collectively, the juxtaglomerular cells and the macula densa are termed the *juxtaglomerular apparatus* (Fig. 38-3).

The juxtaglomerular cells secrete renin in response to reduced renal perfusion (renal ischemia), hypotension, hyponatremia, hypovolemia, and beta-adrenergic receptor stimulation.

By way of the macula densa, the nature of the tubular fluid in the distal tubule can also influence secretion of renin by the juxtaglomerular cells.

On entering the blood, renin converts the plasma protein *angiotensinogen* into the decapeptide *angiotensin I*. Angiotensin-converting enzymes, found largely in the lungs, split a dipeptide from angiotensin I to form the physiologically active *angiotensin II*. Angiotensin II is a potent vasopressor substance that elevates blood pressure by promoting intense peripheral vasoconstriction and by stimulating secretion of the sodium-retaining hormone aldosterone, as outlined in Figure 30-4 (Chapter 30).

Control of Renal Blood Flow

Sympathetic vasoconstrictor nerve fibers arising from thoracolumbar segments of the spinal cord innervate the kidneys. In an average adult at rest the kidneys receive 20% to 25% of the cardiac output. Pain, cold, fright, strenuous exercise, hemorrhage, deep anesthesia, and other stressors reduce renal blood flow by activating sympathetic mechanisms for constriction of renal blood vessels.

Renal Physiology

The formation of urine by the nephrons involves three basic processes: glomerular filtration, renal tubular reabsorption, and renal tubular secretion.

Glomerular Filtration

Glomerular filtration is a process whereby approximately one fifth of the plasma flowing through each glomerulus is passively transferred into the Bowman capsule. The glomerular filtration membrane acts as a sieve, allowing passage of small molecules while restricting transfer of high–molecular-weight substances such as proteins.

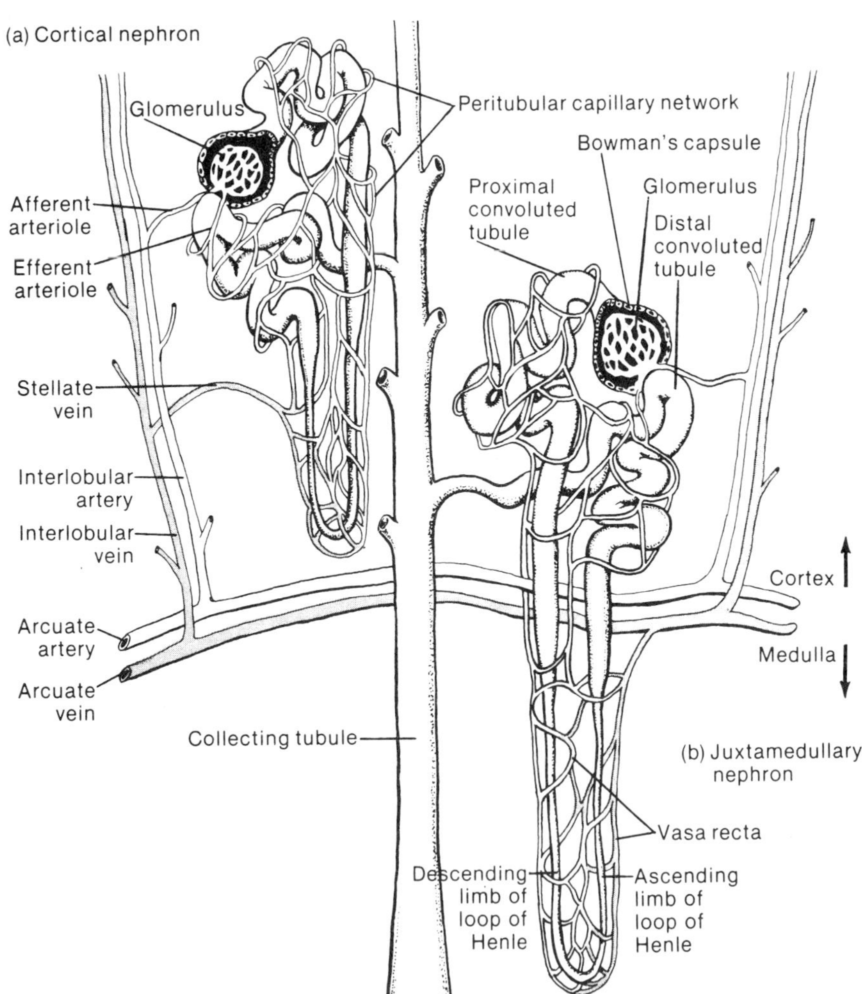

Figure 38-2. Diagram of two nephrons and their blood supply. One nephron (*left*) has a short loop of Henle; the other nephron (*right*) has a long loop of Henle and a more extensive blood supply. (After Chaffee EE, Lytle IM: Basic Physiology and Anatomy, 4th ed. Philadelphia, JB Lippincott, 1980.)

The driving force for filtration is the hydrostatic pressure within the glomerular capillaries, which is ultimately derived from the work of the heart. The hydrostatic pressure in the glomerular capillaries is notably higher than that in other capillaries because each glomerulus is interposed between two arterioles.

Forces opposing filtration include the colloidal osmotic pressure of the plasma and the hydrostatic pressure of the Bowman capsule. The colloidal osmotic pressure of the Bowman capsule is close to zero because the glomerular filtrate is essentially protein free.

Net filtration pressure (NFP) is equal to glomerular capillary hydrostatic pressure (GCHP) *minus* the sum of the plasma colloidal osmotic pressure (PCOP) and the capsular hydrostatic pressure (CHP). This rule can be expressed as a formula: $NFP = GCHP - [PCOP + CHP]$.

For example, with a glomerular capillary hydrostatic pressure of 50 mm Hg, a plasma colloidal osmotic pressure of 30 mm Hg, and a capsular hydrostatic pressure of 10 mm Hg, the net filtration pressure would be: (50 mm Hg) − (30 mm Hg + 10 mm Hg) = 10 mm Hg *NFP*.

Glomerular filtration may be affected by changes in plasma colloidal osmotic pressure, a force that opposes glomerular filtration. Decreases in plasma colloidal osmotic pressure enhance filtration, and vice versa. Elevations in capsular hydrostatic pressure resulting from urinary tract obstructions (eg, urinary stones, prostatic enlargement) may lead to a reduction in glomerular filtration.

In an adult, the average glomerular filtration rate is 125 mL/min. Intrinsic mechanisms of autoregulation keep the glomerular filtration rate remarkably stable within a rather wide range of arterial blood pressure variations. A *myogenic* mechanism inherent in the vascular smooth muscle of the arterioles, and a *tubuloglomerular feedback* mechanism involving the juxtaglomerular apparatus, operate jointly to maintain a constant flow of blood to the glomerular capillaries despite fluctuations in arterial blood pressure.

The high rate of glomerular filtration (125 mL/min) yields a total of 180 L of plasma filtered in 1 day, yet the average volume of urine excreted in 1 day is less than 2 L. Hence, over 99% of the glomerular filtrate is reabsorbed during passage through the renal tubules.

Renal Tubular Reabsorption and Secretion

Renal tubular reabsorption involves the transport of filtered substances across the renal tubular epithelium from the tubular lumen to the blood of the peritubular capillaries.

In contrast, renal tubular secretion involves transtubular movement of substances from the blood of the peritubular capillaries to the tubular lumen.

Substances may be reabsorbed or secreted passively by

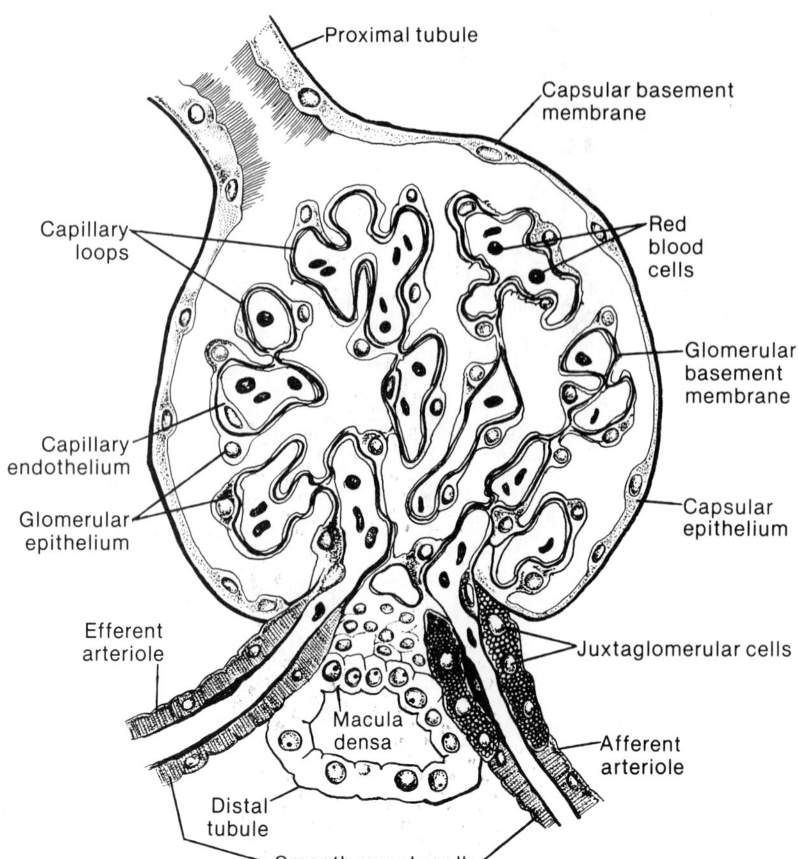

Figure 38-3. Semidiagrammatic drawing of a renal corpuscle. Note that the distal tubule appears to be attached to the afferent arteriole. Also depicted are the macula densa and the juxtaglomerular cells. The combined structure at the point of attachment is called the juxtaglomerular apparatus.

diffusion along existing chemical, electrical, or osmotic gradients. They also may be actively transported against electrical or chemical gradients into or out of the tubular lumen by selective, carrier-mediated, and energy-requiring transport systems. Each active renal transport system exhibits a *transport maximum* (T_m), which is the maximal rate at which a given substance can be carried across the renal tubular epithelium. For actively reabsorbed substances such as glucose, the plasma concentration of the substance that causes its transport maximum to be exceeded is termed the *renal threshold*.

Filtered nutrients such as glucose and amino acids are normally 100% reabsorbed from the proximal tubule by a sodium-dependent, secondary active transport (symport) mechanism. Uric acid, an end product of purine metabolism, is actively reabsorbed and actively secreted in the proximal tubule. Urea, the major end product of nitrogen metabolism, is formed chiefly in the liver in accordance with the rate of protein catabolism. Filtered urea is passively reabsorbed by the renal tubules to an extent determined by the rate of urine flow and degree of water reabsorption.

Creatinine, a product of muscle metabolism, and histamine are actively secreted in the proximal tubule.

Many organic compounds of medical importance are also actively secreted in the proximal tubule. Because renal tubular secretion supplements glomerular filtration and enhances the removal of substances from the blood, impaired renal function may interfere with the excretion of therapeutic agents and may therefore require an adjustment (reduction) in drug dosage.

Renal Handling of Ions and Water

Renal handling of sodium is of singular importance to the maintenance of extracellular fluid volume, because renal tubular reabsorption of sodium is the major driving force for the passive reabsorption of water. Also linked to the active reabsorption of sodium are the reabsorption of glucose, amino acids, chloride, and bicarbonate, as well as the secretion of hydrogen and potassium in certain tubular segments.

Sodium is actively reabsorbed throughout most of the nephron, with approximately two thirds of the filtered sodium being reabsorbed from the proximal tubule. In the proximal tubule, the active reabsorption of sodium creates an electrical gradient that favors the passive reabsorption of anions, such as chloride and bicarbonate. The resulting osmotic gradient promotes the passive reabsorption of water. Thus, the tubular fluid (filtrate) remains isoosmotic with the plasma during its passage through the proximal tubule.

In the thick ascending loop of Henle, sodium is carried out of the tubular lumen by a Na^+-K^+-$2Cl^-$ cotransporter. Because the ascending limb of the loop of Henle is essentially impermeable to water, this outward transport of sodium contributes to the hyperosmolarity of the renal medullary interstitium (see the section on the Countercurrent Mechanism).

Sodium is actively reabsorbed in the distal tubules and collecting ducts. Although much of the reabsorbed sodium is accompanied by chloride, some of the reabsorbed sodium may be exchanged for secreted potassium or hydrogen. The prin-

Table 38-1. **Summary of Renal Reabsorption and Secretion by Nephron Segments**

Nephron Segment	*Activity*
Proximal tubule	Reabsorption of filtered Na^+, Cl^-, K^+, Ca^{2+}, HCO_3^-, HPO_4^{3-}, urea, uric acid, glucose, amino acids, water Secretion of H^+, NH_4^+, organic acids, and bases
Loop of Henle (descending limb)	Reabsorption of water
Loop of Henle (ascending limb)	Reabsorption of Na^+, K^+, Cl^-, Ca^{2+}
Distal tubule	Reabsorption of Na^+, Cl^-, HCO_3^-, Ca^{2+}, HPO_4^{3-}, water Secretion of H^+, NH_4^+, K^+
Collecting duct	Reabsorption of Na^+, Cl^-, HCO_3^-, urea, water Secretion of H^+, NH_4^+, K^+

cipal cells in the cortical collecting ducts are sensitive to aldosterone, which stimulates sodium reabsorption and potassium secretion.

Water reabsorption in the loop of Henle is limited to the descending limb. In the late distal tubules and collecting ducts, the passive reabsorption of water is controlled by ADH (vasopressin), as detailed later in this chapter.

The renal handling of electrolytes, water, nutrients, and metabolic products is summarized in Table 38-1. Several hormones affect renal function: aldosterone promotes sodium reabsorption by the cortical collecting ducts, and ADH allows water reabsorption to occur in the late distal tubules and collecting ducts. Parathyroid hormone increases calcium reabsorption in the distal tubule, and it inhibits phosphate reabsorption in the proximal tubule.

Countercurrent Mechanism

The conservation of water and concentration of urine by the kidneys is made possible by the operation of a countercurrent mechanism within the renal medulla. In this mechanism, the loops of Henle act as countercurrent multipliers that establish an osmotic gradient in the renal medulla, whereas the vasa recta serve as countercurrent exchangers to maintain this gradient.

The unique permeability and transport characteristics of the loop of Henle are essential to the operation of the countercurrent multiplication mechanism. The epithelium of the descending limb of the loop of Henle is freely permeable to water, yet it does not extrude sodium, and is the only nephron segment that does not actively transport sodium. The epithelium of the ascending limb of the loop of Henle actively extrudes NaCl from the tubular lumen; however, it is essentially impermeable to water. Thus, a vertical osmotic gradient is established in the renal medullary interstitium through the active outward transport of NaCl from the tubular lumen of the water-impermeable ascending limb of the loop of Henle. The recycling of urea between the collecting ducts and the loops of Henle in the inner medulla also contributes to the hyperosmolarity of the medullary interstitium.

The hyperosmolar renal medullary interstitium provides an osmotic gradient favoring water reabsorption from the collecting ducts passing through the renal pyramids. The actual amount of water reabsorption from the late distal tubules and the collecting ducts is controlled by ADH which, operating through a cyclic adenosine monophosphate second messenger mechanism, increases the water permeability of the epithelial cells in these segments.

In the presence of ADH, the kidneys excrete a highly concentrated urine owing to the greater degree of water reabsorption from the late distal tubules and collecting ducts. In the absence of ADH, a dilute urine is excreted because the epithelium of these nephron segments is virtually impermeable to water. Factors that control ADH secretion are discussed in Chapter 40, the review of endocrine physiology.

Renal Function in Acid–Base Regulation

The kidneys participate in acid–base regulation by replenishing plasma levels of sodium bicarbonate through the reabsorption of filtered bicarbonate (HCO_3^-) as well as through addition of new bicarbonate, and by secreting H^+ and ammonia. For every H^+ secreted, one Na^+ and one HCO_3^- are added to the plasma. The H^+ ions are derived from the dissociation of carbonic acid (H_2CO_3), which forms when CO_2 and H_2O combine inside renal tubular cells in the presence of the enzyme *carbonic anhydrase*.

The secreted H^+ may combine with filtered HCO_3^- present in the tubular lumen to form CO_2 and H_2O. This is the mechanism involved in the reabsorption of *filtered* bicarbonate, which occurs mainly in the proximal tubules.

Some H^+ secreted into the tubular lumen may combine chemically with phosphate buffers present in the tubular fluid to form monosodium phosphate (NaH_2PO_4).

Secreted hydrogen ions also may combine with the ammonia produced by the renal tubular epithelium from the deamination of amino acids such as glutamine. The secreted hydrogen ions and ammonia combine to form the ammonium ion (NH_4^+), which is excreted together with tubular anions such as chloride (Cl^-).

In the proximal tubule, the secretion of H^+ occurs through the secondary active transport mechanism of Na^+,H^+ antiport. In the late distal tubules and collecting ducts, intercalated cells secrete H^+ through primary active transport.

39

Diuretics

Carbonic Anhydrase Inhibitors

Loop (High-Ceiling) Diuretics

Osmotic Diuretics

Potassium-Sparing Diuretics

Thiazides and Related Diuretics

A *diuretic* is an agent capable of increasing the volume of urine and promoting a net loss of body water. The retention of excess fluid by the body depends in large measure on the retention of sodium. Therefore, the effectiveness of a diuretic is primarily related to its ability to increase the excretion of sodium, which is accomplished in most cases by interfering with the reabsorption of sodium ions in the tubules of the kidney. Loss of sodium is accompanied by excretion of an osmotically equivalent quantity of water, which is derived from body fluids removed from the tissues.

The handling of electrolytes by the kidney involves a complex series of interrelated mechanisms. Drugs such as diuretics that affect the handling of one electrolyte (eg, sodium) almost invariably alter the handling of other electrolytes as well (such as chloride, potassium, hydrogen, bicarbonate). Depending on the mechanism of action of the individual diuretic drugs, therefore, electrolyte or acid–base balance disturbances, or both, can develop during diuretic therapy. These electrolyte imbalances are responsible for many of the disturbing and occasionally serious side effects resulting from diuretic administration, and an understanding of the sites and mechanisms of action of the diuretics can aid in predicting the types of electrolyte changes expected with any one drug. The overall drug regimen can then be tailored to produce an optimal diuretic action with a minimal degree of electrolyte-induced side effects (eg, combining a drug that produces potassium loss with a potassium-sparing drug).

The effectiveness and safety of diuretics are greatly compromised in the presence of kidney disease. Most diuretics are of little value in patients with significantly impaired renal function, and in many instances they can be quite hazardous. These drugs should be prescribed to patients with known or suspected kidney impairment only after consideration of the potential risks.

A number of chemically dissimilar compounds have a diuretic action, and the diuretic drugs are usually classified on the basis of their predominant sites and mechanisms of action. The major categories of diuretics reviewed in this chapter are listed in Table 39-1, along with their principal sites of action in the kidney and the major electrolyte disturbances associated with each group. Refer to Chapter 38 for a discussion of the renal handling of water and ions; reference to Chapter 38 also will aid in understanding the sites and mechanisms outlined for each class of diuretics in the subsequent discussion.

Carbonic Anhydrase Inhibitors

Acetazolamide
Methazolamide
Dichlorphenamide

Compounds in the group of carbonic anhydrase inhibitors are sulfonamide derivatives that interfere with the activity of the enzyme carbonic anhydrase (CA), thus blocking the hydration of carbon dioxide (CO_2) to carbonic acid (H_2CO_3) and subsequent ionization to yield hydrogen (H^+) and bicarbonate (HCO_3^-) ions. In addition to their mild diuretic action, these agents reduce aqueous humor production and are often used adjunctively in the treatment of glaucoma. They are also used in treating some forms of epilepsy (see Chapter 27). The CA inhibitors are reviewed as a group, and individual drugs are listed in Table 39-2.

Mechanism

Decrease production of H^+ and HCO_3^- in renal tubules, thereby reducing HCO_3^- absorption in proximal tubule; increased distal delivery of HCO_3^- exceeds absorptive capacity of distal nephron, resulting in excretion of HCO_3^-, K^+, and water; sodium loss is minimal; diuretic effect of carbonic anhydrase inhibitors is transient, because tolerance develops as serum bicarbonate levels decline.

In the eye, carbonic anhydrase inhibitors reduce the rate of aqueous humor formation, thereby lowering intraocular pressure. These drugs also may reduce the frequency of seizures (especially petit mal), possible by lowering the pH of brain tissue.

Uses

Adjunctive treatment of drug-induced edema or edema due to congestive heart failure refractory to single-drug therapy (not indicated alone in edema)

Adjunctive treatment of glaucoma (open-angle, secondary glaucoma, preoperative in narrow-angle) to lower intraocular pressure

Adjunctive treatment of certain forms of epilepsy, especially petit mal

Prophylaxis of acute mountain sickness (eg, weakness, dizziness, nausea) at high altitudes (acetazolamide)

Dosage

See Table 39-2.

Fate

Readily absorbed from GI tract; onset of action after oral administration is 1 to 2 hours (longer with methazolamide); peak plasma levels occur in 2 to 4 hours (except sustained-release

Table 39-1. **Diuretic Drugs: Sites of Action and Electrolyte Disturbances**

Classes of Diuretics	*Major Sites of Action*	*Electrolyte Disturbances*
Carbonic anhydrase inhibitors (eg, **acetazolamide**)	Proximal tubule and (?) distal tubule	Hyponatremic acidosis Hyperchloremic acidosis Hypokalemia
Loop (high-ceiling) diuretics (eg, **furosemide**)	Thick ascending loop of Henle and (?) proximal tubule	Hypokalemia Hypochloremic alkalosis Hyponatremia (excessive diuresis) Hypocalcemia
Osmotics (eg, **mannitol**)	Proximal tubule, descending loop of Henle, and collecting tubule	Minimal
Potassium-sparing diuretics (eg, **triamterene**)	Collecting tubules	Hyperkalemia
Thiazides/sulfonamides (eg, **hydrochlorothiazide, chlorthalidone, indapamide**)	Distal convoluted tubule	Hypokalemia Hypochloremic alkalosis Hyponatremia Hypercalcemia

forms, which peak in 8–12 h); largely excreted within 24 hours, either as unchanged drug or *N*-dealkylated metabolites, some of which are active.

Common Side Effects

Paresthesias, drowsiness.

Significant Adverse Reactions

CNS: confusion, myopia, tinnitus, malaise, vertigo, headache, xerostomia, depression, nervousness, weakness, flaccid paralysis, convulsions, tremor, ataxia

Dermatologic/hypersensitivity: skin eruptions, urticaria, pruritus, melena, photosensitivity

Hepatic–renal: hepatic insufficiency, pancreatitis, polyuria, dysuria, glycosuria, hematuria, urinary frequency, ureteral colic

Electrolyte: hypokalemia, hyponatremia

Other: aplastic anemia, diarrhea, vomiting, anorexia, loss of taste and smell

NOTE: Drugs are sulfonamide derivatives. See Chapter 59 for other potential adverse reactions.

Table 39-2. **Carbonic Anhydrase Inhibitors**

Drug	*Usual Dosage Range*	*Nursing Considerations*
Acetazolamide *Dazamide, Diamox (CAN) Acetazolam, Apo-Acetazolamide*	*Glaucoma*: 250 mg orally, 1–4 times/d depending on response; children—10–15 mg/kg/d in divided doses every 6–8 h *Edema*: 250–375 mg orally, once daily in the morning for 1–2 d; then skip a day; children—5 mg/kg once daily in the morning; IV, 500 mg initially; then 125–250 mg every 4 h as needed in acute situation (500 mg/5 mL sterile water for injection) *Epilepsy*: Adults and children—8–30 mg/kg/d in divided doses *Acute mountain sickness*: 500–1000 mg daily in divided doses; initiate 24–48 h before ascent and continue as long as needed to control symptoms	Used for edema of congestive heart failure, certain forms of epilepsy, chronic open-angle glaucoma, and preoperatively in narrow-angle glaucoma; doses in excess of 1000 mg do not usually produce an increased effect; sustained-release form may be used on a twice-daily basis; reconstituted injection solution should be used within 24 h; *avoid* IM administration if possible because alkaline solution is painful when injected
Dichlorphenamide *Daranide*	100–200 mg initially, followed by 100 mg/12 h until desired response is achieved; maintenance 25–50 mg 1–3 times/d	Indicated as adjunctive treatment for open-angle glaucoma and preoperatively in narrow-angle glaucoma, together with miotics and osmotic diuretics
Methazolamide *Glauc-Tabs, Neptazane*	50–100 mg 2–3 times/d	Adjunctive therapy for both open-angle and narrow-angle glaucoma, with miotics and osmotic diuretics; contraindicated in severe or absolute glaucoma, hemorrhagic glaucoma, or that due to peripheral anterior synechiae; higher incidence of drowsiness than with other CA inhibitors

CA, carbonic anhydrase.

Contraindications

Severe liver or kidney disease, chronic pulmonary disease, adrenocortical insufficiency, hyperchloremic acidosis, electrolyte imbalances, sensitivity to sulfonamides, pregnancy, and chronic noncongestive angle-closure glaucoma. *Cautious use* in patients with impaired hepatic function, respiratory disease, diabetes, and gout.

Interactions

CA inhibitors make the urine alkaline and thus may enhance the action of amphetamines, catecholamines, procainamide, quinidine, tricyclic antidepressants, and any other basic drug by increasing their reabsorption.
CA inhibitors can decrease the effects of lithium, barbiturates, nitrofurantoin, salicylates, and other acidic substances by reducing their renal tubular reabsorption.
A reduced response to insulin and oral hypoglycemics has been reported with CA inhibitors.
Increased hypokalemia can result with combinations of CA inhibitors and other diuretics, corticosteroids, and amphotericin B.
CA-induced hypokalemia may augment digitalis toxicity.
Metabolic acidosis can occur if CA inhibitors are given together with salicylates.

Nursing Management

Pretherapy Assessment

Assess and record baseline data necessary for detection of adverse effects of carbonic anhydrase inhibitors: General: vital signs (VS), body weight, skin color and temperature, edema, weight; CNS: orientation, reflexes; Cardiovascular system (CVS): baseline electrocardiogram (ECG), muscle strength, intraocular pressure; GI: liver evaluation, bowel sounds; Genitourinary (GU): output patterns; Laboratory: complete blood count (CBC), serum electrolytes, liver and renal function tests, urinalysis.
Review medical history and documents for existing or previous conditions that:
a. require cautious use of carbonic anhydrase inhibitors: impaired hepatic function; respiratory disease; diabetes; gout.
b. contraindicate use of carbonic anhydrase inhibitors: allergy to sulfonamides; severe liver or kidney disease; chronic pulmonary disease; adrenocortical insufficiency; hyperchloremic acidosis; electrolyte imbalances; chronic, noncongestive, narrow-angle glaucoma; **pregnancy (Category C)**; lactation (safety not established).

Nursing Interventions

Medication Administration

Administer with food or milk if GI upset occurs.
Use caution if giving with other drugs whose excretion is pH dependent.
Administer by direct IV injection because intramuscular injection is painful.
Ensure ready access to bathroom facilities when diuretic effect occurs.
Provide small, frequent meals if GI upset occurs.

Surveillance During Therapy

Carefully monitor laboratory studies and patient for indications of adverse reactions: serum electrolytes and acid–base balance.
Provide skin care if rash or lesions occur.
Protect patient from sun or bright lights if photophobia occurs.
Interpret results of diagnostic tests and contact practitioner as appropriate.
Monitor for possible drug–drug and drug–nutrient interactions; see Interactions.
Provide for patient safety needs if CNS side effects occur.

Patient Teaching

Explain, as appropriate, that an alternate-day regimen (see Usual Dosage Range, Table 39-2) is used to minimize development of tolerance and loss of diuretic potency. If diuretic effect decreases, *reducing* dose or frequency of administration often restores effectiveness.
Teach patient to recognize and report symptoms of metabolic acidosis (nausea, vomiting, malaise, abdominal pain, hyperpnea, tinnitus, disorientation, dysuria, numbness in extremities). If signs occur, drug should be temporarily discontinued, and dosage should be reduced on resumption.
Instruct patient to inform practitioner immediately if signs of hypersensitivity (rash, fever) or possible blood dyscrasias (sore throat, bruising, mucosal ulceration) occur because CA inhibitors are sulfonamide derivatives. Periodic (4–6 mo) blood cell counts are recommended during prolonged therapy.
Warn patient that prolonged exposure to sunlight may cause photosensitivity.
Inform patient with diabetes that dosage of hypoglycemic drugs may need to be increased because CA inhibitors may raise blood glucose.

Loop (High-Ceiling) Diuretics

Bumetanide
Furosemide
Ethacrynic acid
Torsemide

Several diuretic drugs are classified as "high-ceiling" agents, inasmuch as their peak diuretic effect is much greater than that observed with other clinically available oral diuretic drugs. Moreover, they exhibit a prompt onset of action when given orally, their action is independent of acid–base disturbances, and they are effective in patients with impaired renal function, whereas most other diuretics are not. The term *loop* derives from their site of action, the thick ascending loop of Henle, where a significant fraction of the filtered sodium load is reabsorbed. They are potent diuretics, and can lead to significant electrolyte disturbances. Careful medical supervision is therefore essential whenever these drugs are used, and the dosage must be critically adjusted for each patient. The drugs in this category are reviewed together; information pertaining to each individual drug is presented in Table 39-3.

Table 39-3. **Loop (High-Ceiling) Diuretics**

Drug	Usual Dosage Range	Nursing Considerations
Bumetanide Bumex	Oral: 0.5–2 mg/day, as a single dose; maximum oral dose is 10 mg/d IV, IM: 0.5–1 mg; repeat at 2–3 h intervals to a maximum of 10 mg as needed	Drug is more chloruretic than natriuretic; hypokalemia may be less severe than with furosemide; cross-sensitivity with furosemide is rare; use *cautiously* in patients allergic to sulfonamides; use an intermittent dosage schedule for prolonged therapy; use parenteral solutions within 24 h; safety and efficacy in children younger than 18 y has not been established
Ethacrynic acid Edecrin	*Oral* Adults: initially 50–100 mg daily; maintenance dose 50–200 mg/d on an intermittent schedule Children: initially 25 mg/d; adjust dosage in 25-mg increments to achieve optimal response *IV* 0.5–1 mg/kg (usual adult dose 50 mg); a second dose of 50 mg at a different site may be required (maximum 100 mg/dose)	Reconstitute IV solution by adding 50 mL 5% dextrose injection or sodium chloride injection to vial; do *not* inject SC or IM, because pain and irritation may occur; direct IV injection should be made over several minutes; do not use solution if cloudy; discard within 24 h after preparation; when used IV, be alert for presence of pain in calf, chest, or pelvic area, possible signs of thromboembolic complications; safety and efficacy of ethacrynic acid in treating hypertension have not been established; hypoproteinemia may reduce response to ethacrynic acid; discontinue drug if diarrhea occurs
Furosemide Lasix (CAN) Apo-Furosemide, Furoside, Novasemide, Uritol	ORAL *Adults* Diuresis: 20–80 mg as a single dose; may increase by 20–40-mg increments to a maximum of 600 mg/d Hypertension: 40 mg twice a day; adjust according to response; usual maintenance dose 40–80 mg/d in 1 or 2 divided doses *Children* Initially 2 mg/kg as a single dose; may increase by 1–2-mg/kg increments to a maximum of 6 mg/kg/d PARENTERAL *Adults* 20–40 mg IV or IM as a single dose; may increase by 20-mg increments every 2–3 h until desired response is obtained Acute pulmonary edema: 40 mg IV over 1–2 min; may increase to 80 mg IV after 1 h *Children* 1 mg/kg IV or IM; may increase by 1 mg/kg no sooner than 2 h after previous dose; maximum 6 mg/kg	Oral doses should be given on an intermittent schedule where possible (eg, 2–4 d/wk); parenteral therapy is indicated for emergency situations only and should be replaced by oral therapy as soon as possible; do *not* mix parenteral solutions with highly acidic preparations; use mixture within 24 h of preparation and do *not* use if solution is yellow; use *cautiously* in patients allergic to sulfonamides, because cross-reactions can occur; when adding drug to an existing antihypertensive regimen, reduce dose of other drugs by half to avoid excessive drop in blood pressure and titrate furosemide dosage to obtain optimal hypotensive effect; in patients with impaired renal function, use controlled IV infusion (4 mg/min) to minimize danger of azotemia or oliguria; drug can stimulate renal synthesis of prostaglandin E_2, which can complicate the neonatal respiratory distress syndrome
Torsemide Demadex	*Hypertension*: 5–10 mg once daily *Congestive heart failure*: 10–20 mg once daily, oral or IV; titrate dose upward until desired effect *Hepatic cirrhosis*: 5–10 mg once daily, oral or IV; titrate dose upward to a maximum of 40 mg/day	Long-acting diuretic that may be given without regard to meals; oral and IV doses are equivalent, and patients may be switched without a dosage adjustment; use with caution in patients with sulfonamide allergy; not recommended in children

Mechanism

Inhibit active tubular reabsorption of sodium and chloride by blocking the sodium–potassium–chloride cotransport system in the thick ascending loop of Henle, resulting in excretion of large quantities of urine high in sodium chloride; also may block sodium and chloride reabsorption in the proximal tubule; magnesium and calcium excretion is increased secondarily, and prolonged use of loop diuretics can lead to hypomagnesemia and hypocalcemia; renal blood flow is increased (perhaps owing to increased production of vasodilatory prostaglandins), and left ventricular filling pressure is lowered; no effect on carbonic anhydrase or aldosterone.

Uses

- Treatment of severe edema associated with congestive heart failure, hepatic cirrhosis, and renal disease
- Relief of acute pulmonary edema (IV administration)
- Adjunctive treatment of hypertension (furosemide, torsemide)
- Management of ascites due to malignancy, idiopathic edema, and lymphedema (ethacrynic acid)
- Short-term management of pediatric patients with congenital heart disease or the nephrotic syndrome (ethacrynic acid)

Treatment of acute hypercalcemia (IV furosemide with normal saline infusion)

Dosage

See Table 39-3.

Fate

Onset of diuresis after oral administration is 30 to 60 minutes; peak effect occurs in 1 to 2 hours, and duration is 6 to 8 hours, except for bumetanide (3–6 h). IV injection produces a diuretic response within 5 to 10 minutes, which then peaks within 15 to 30 minutes and persists for 2 hours (up to 8 hours with torsemide). Drugs are highly bound to plasma proteins (94%–98%) and are rapidly excreted in the urine, both as metabolites and unchanged drug. Approximately one third of the dose is eliminated by way of the bile in the feces.

Common Side Effects

Bumetanide: abdominal discomfort, orthostatic hypotension
Ethacrynic acid: anorexia, abdominal discomfort
Furosemide: orthostatic hypotension (initial period of therapy)
Torsemide: headache, dizziness, rhinitis

Significant Adverse Reactions

All drugs

CAUTION

A dose-related *reversible* ototoxic effect, manifested as tinnitus, hearing impairment, and rarely deafness, can occur. This effect is usually associated with overzealous therapy (eg, rapid IV injection of large doses) in patients with reduced renal function.

GI: vomiting, diarrhea, dysphagia, acute pancreatitis, jaundice
CNS: headache, blurred vision, tinnitus, hearing loss, weakness, vertigo
Electrolyte: hypokalemia, hyponatremia, hypochloremic alkalosis, hypomagnesemia, hypocalcemia
Other: rash, pruritus, hyperglycemia, hyperuricemia, azotemia, increased serum creatinine, agranulocytosis, thrombocytopenia

Individual drugs

Bumetanide: Dry mouth, arthritic pain, muscle cramping, hives, premature ejaculation, ECG changes, chest pain, hyperventilation, breast tenderness
Ethacrynic acid: GI bleeding associated with corticosteroid treatment, *profuse* watery diarrhea, fever, chills, hematuria, neutropenia, confusion, fatigue, hypovolemia, hypocalcemia, orthostatic hypotension, muscle cramping, and nystagmus
Furosemide: GI irritation, constipation, paresthesias, leukopenia, anemia, urticaria, photosensitivity, erythema multiforme, exfoliative dermatitis, necrotizing angiitis, weakness, urinary frequency, urinary bladder spasm, and thrombophlebitis

Contraindications

Anuria, hepatic coma, dehydration, severe electrolyte depletion, early pregnancy, and in infants (ethacrynic acid). *Cautious use* in patients with hepatic cirrhosis, hearing impairment, orthostatic hypotension, diabetes, gout, or cardiogenic shock; in patients receiving digitalis drugs or potassium-depleting steroids, in elderly patients, and pregnant or nursing women.

Interactions

Loop diuretics may potentiate the action of other antihypertensive medications.
Loop diuretics may increase the toxicity of aminoglycoside antibiotics (ototoxicity), cisplatin (ototoxicity), cephalosporins (nephrotoxicity), salicylates, lithium, and cardiac glycosides.
Increased orthostatic hypotension can occur with combinations of loop diuretics and alcohol, narcotics, or barbiturates.
Increased potassium loss may occur when corticosteroids are given with loop diuretics.
Loop diuretics may reduce the effectiveness of uricosuric drugs by elevating serum uric acid levels.
Probenecid may reduce the diuretic effectiveness of bumetanide and furosemide.
Indomethacin, and possibly other nonsteroidal antiinflammatory drugs may impair the action of loop diuretics by decreasing prostaglandin synthesis.
Loop diuretics can potentiate the muscle-relaxing effects of the nondepolarizing neuromuscular-blocking drugs but may enhance the muscle-relaxing action of succinylcholine.
Increased requirements for oral hypoglycemic drugs or insulin may occur in patients taking loop diuretics, which can elevate blood glucose levels.
Furosemide (and possibly bumetanide) can potentiate the pharmacologic effects of theophylline.
Ethacrynic acid may displace oral anticoagulants from their protein-binding sites.

Nursing Management

Pretherapy Assessment

Assess and record baseline data necessary for detection of adverse effects of loop diuretics: General: VS, body weight, skin color and temperature, edema, weight; CNS: orientation, reflexes, hearing; CVS: baseline ECG, orthostatic blood pressure; GI: liver evaluation, bowel sounds; GU: output patterns; Laboratory: CBC, serum electrolytes (including calcium), liver and renal function tests, urinalysis, blood glucose, uric acid.

Review medical history and documents for existing or previous conditions that:

a. require cautious use of loop diuretics: hepatic cirrhosis; hearing impairment; orthostatic hypotension; diabetes; gout; cardiogenic shock; in patients receiving digitalis drugs or potassium-depleting steroids; use in elderly patients.
b. contraindicate use of loop diuretics: allergy to loop diuretics, sulfonamides; anuria; hepatic coma; dehydration; severe electrolyte depletion; use in infants (especially ethacrynic acid); **pregnancy**

(Category C); lactation (secreted in breast milk, use alternative approach to neonatal nutrition, safety not established).

Nursing Interventions

Medication Administration

Administer with food or milk if GI upset occurs.
Expect therapy to be initiated with small doses. Dosage should be adjusted carefully on the basis of serum electrolyte levels and clinical response.
Check blood pressure frequently, and monitor infusion rate, which should not exceed 4 mg/min, when giving IV. Check for signs of extravasation, which commonly causes pain and irritation.
Ensure ready access to bathroom facilities when diuretic effect occurs.
Provide small, frequent meals if GI upset occurs.
Seek clarification if diuretic is prescribed for patient in hepatic coma or a state of electrolyte deficiency. These underlying conditions should be corrected before diuretic therapy is initiated.

Surveillance During Therapy

Carefully monitor laboratory studies and patient for indications of adverse reactions: CO_2, blood urea nitrogen (BUN), white blood cell count, and liver function studies, which should be performed periodically.
Provide skin care if rash or lesions occur.
Protect patient from sun or bright lights if photophobia occurs.
Assess for signs of joint swelling, tenderness, or pain, which may signify onset of gout. If these occur, advise practitioner.
Interpret results of diagnostic tests and contact practitioner as appropriate.
Assess adequacy of glucose control in known and suspected diabetics. Advise practitioner of increased blood glucose or altered glucose tolerance.
Monitor for possible drug–drug and drug–nutrient interactions; see Interactions.
Provide for patient safety needs if CNS side effects occur.

Patient Teaching

Instruct patient to take drug with meals or food if GI irritation occurs.
Explain that an intermittent dosage schedule (eg, 3–4 days/wk interspersed with a rest period) is used when possible to allow electrolyte and acid–base balance to stabilize.
Instruct patient to report immediately any indication of impaired hearing (often preceded by vertigo and tinnitus). Dosage should be reevaluated because danger of permanent hearing loss exists with prolonged high-dose therapy.
Instruct patient to report any *weight gain*.
Inform patient that GI side effects occur most frequently after 1 to 2 months of therapy. Diarrhea or abdominal pain should be reported because dosage adjustment may be warranted.

Osmotic Diuretics

The term *osmotic diuretic* refers to any solute that is readily filtered by the kidney but poorly reabsorbed in the renal tubules. When these agents are taken, the large amount of nonreabsorbed material increases the osmotic pressure of the tubular fluid, causing an osmotically equivalent amount of water to be carried through the tubule with it, eventually to be excreted. Sodium excretion is not significantly increased, however, by normal therapeutic doses of the osmotic diuretics. For this reason, and because most of these diuretics must be administered IV in large doses, they are infrequently used for routine treatment of edema and are primarily indicated for the prevention of acute renal failure associated with a sharply reduced glomerular filtration rate.

Their osmotic effects are not confined to the kidney but extend to the bloodstream as well, where the presence of the drug in the circulation draws fluid from tissue spaces *into* the blood. This effect underlies their application in reducing elevated intraocular and intracranial pressures, actions important in treating cranial injuries and acute congestive glaucoma, and as an aid to neurosurgery.

• Glycerin

Osmoglyn

Mechanism

Elevates plasma osmotic pressure, thus drawing fluid from extravascular spaces; decreases intraocular and intracranial pressure.

Uses

Interruption of an acute attack of glaucoma
Reduction in intraocular pressure, either before or after surgery for glaucoma
Reduction of intracranial or intraocular pressure (investigational use for IV administration)

Dosage

Orally, 1 to 2 g/kg of a 50% solution 1 to 1.5 hours before surgery.

Fate

Rapidly absorbed when taken orally; intraocular pressure is reduced within 15 minutes, maximal effect occurring in 1 hour; action persists 4 to 6 hours; metabolized in the liver.

Significant Adverse Reactions

Nausea, vomiting, diarrhea, headache, disorientation, confusion. Rarely, arrhythmias, dehydration, hyperglycemia.

Contraindications

Anuria, severe dehydration, acute pulmonary edema, severe cardiac decompensation. *Cautious use* in people with hypervolemia, confusion, diabetes, or congestive heart disease, and in elderly or senile patients.

Isosorbide

Ismotic

Mechanism

Increases plasma osmotic pressure, thereby reducing elevated intraocular pressure by promoting redistribution of fluid toward the circulatory vessels.

Uses

Short-term reduction of elevated intraocular pressure before and after surgery for glaucoma or cataract to interrupt an acute attack of glaucoma.

Dosage

Initially, 1.5 g/kg orally 2 to 4 times a day; usual range is 1 to 3 g/kg 2 to 4 times a day.

Fate

Rapidly absorbed orally; onset of action is within 30 minutes; peak effect occurs in 1 to 1.5 hours and duration is 5 to 6 hours.

Significant Adverse Reactions

Nausea, vomiting, diarrhea, thirst, headache, dizziness, lightheadedness, lethargy, irritability, rash, hiccups, hypernatremia.

Contraindications

Anuria due to severe renal disease, severe dehydration, acute pulmonary edema, and hemorrhagic glaucoma. *Cautious use* in patients with hypertension, congestive heart failure.

Mannitol

Osmitrol

Mechanism

Not appreciably metabolized after IV injection, rapidly excreted by the kidneys; not reabsorbed in the renal tubules, hence raises the osmotic pressure of tubular fluid, thereby reducing reabsorption of water and increasing urine flow; may increase electrolyte excretion when used in large doses; decreases elevated intracranial and intraocular pressure by raising plasma osmotic pressure.

Uses

Prevention and treatment of the oliguric phase of acute renal failure before irreversible renal failure occurs
Treatment of cerebral edema and elevated intracranial pressure (eg, resulting from head injury or surgery)
Reduction of elevated intraocular pressure in acute congestive glaucoma
Treatment of acute chemical poisoning, by enhancing renal excretion of toxic substances
Measurement of glomerular filtration rate

Dosage

CAUTION

Use by IV infusion only: Carefully evaluate patient's cardiovascular status before administering mannitol solution IV, because sudden expansion of extracellular fluid volume may aggravate or precipitate congestive heart failure.

Acute renal failure: 50 to 100 g as a 5% to 25% solution
Reduction of intracranial pressure: 1.5 to 2 g/kg as a 15% to 25% solution over 30 to 60 minutes
Reduction of intraocular pressure: 1.5 to 2 g/kg as a 15% to 25% solution over 30 to 60 minutes.
Acute chemical poisoning: 100 to 200 g depending on fluid requirement and urinary output
Measurement of glomerular filtration rate: 100 mL of 20% solution diluted with 180 mL of sodium chloride injection infused at a rate of 20 mL/min
Test dose (patients with marked oliguria to determine drug's effectiveness): 0.2 g/kg infused over 3 to 5 minutes to produce a urine flow of at least 30 to 50 mL/h

Fate

Confined to extracellular space; only slightly metabolized and rapidly excreted by the kidneys (80% of a dose appears in the urine within 3 h); less than 10% is reabsorbed by the kidneys; diuresis occurs in 1 to 2 hours, and elevated cranial and ocular pressures are reduced within 30 minutes.

Significant Adverse Reactions

Infrequent—dry mouth, thirst, headache, blurred vision, nausea, vomiting, rhinitis, diarrhea, marked diuresis, electrolyte imbalance, acidosis, fever, chills, dizziness, hypotension, dehydration, tachycardia, angina-like pain.

Contraindications

Anuria, severe pulmonary edema or congestive heart failure, intracranial bleeding, severe dehydration, progressive renal disease after initiating mannitol therapy, and in children younger than 12 years of age. *Cautious use* in patients with marked cardiopulmonary or renal dysfunction and in pregnant women.

Urea

Ureaphil

Mechanism

Filtered but not reabsorbed by the kidney; increased osmotic pressure in tubular fluid prevents water reabsorption and increases rate and volume of urine flow; elevates osmotic pressure of blood, thus increasing movement of fluid from body tissues to bloodstream.

Uses

Reduction of intracranial and intraocular pressure (alternative drug *only*)
Induction of abortion (intraamniotic injection)—*investigational use*

Dosage

IV infusion *only* as a 30% solution; maximum infusion rate 4 mL/min; maximum dose 120 g/day.

Adults: 1 to 1.5 g/kg
Children: 0.5 to 1.5 g/kg
Infants: 0.1 to 0.5 g/kg

Fate

Onset of diuretic effect is 4 to 8 hours; intracranial–intraocular pressure is reduced within 1 to 2 hours; widely distributed by the bloodstream and excreted by the kidney essentially unchanged.

Common Side Effects

Headache, nausea.

Significant Adverse Reactions

Syncope, disorientation, confusion, agitation, pain, irritation, phlebitis and thrombosis at site of infusion, electrolyte imbalances, tachycardia, and hypotension.

Contraindications

Severely impaired renal function, marked dehydration, intracranial bleeding, and frank liver failure. *Cautious use* in patients with liver impairment or kidney disease, and in pregnant or lactating women.

Interactions

Urea may potentiate the action of anticoagulants.
Urea can reduce the effectiveness of lithium by increasing its excretion.

Nursing Management

Pretherapy Assessment

Assess and record baseline data necessary for detection of adverse effects of osmotic diuretics: General: VS, body weight, skin color and temperature, edema, hydration; CNS: orientation, reflexes, hearing; CVS: baseline ECG, orthostatic blood pressure; GI: liver evaluation, bowel sounds; GU: output patterns; Laboratory: CBC, serum electrolytes, liver and renal function tests, urinalysis.

Review medical history and documents for existing or previous conditions that:

a. require cautious use of osmotic diuretics: hypervolemia; confusion; diabetes; congestive heart disease; marked renal or cardiopulmonary function.
b. contraindicate use of osmotic diuretics: anuria; severe dehydration; acute pulmonary edema; severe cardiac decompensation; **pregnancy (Category B)**; lactation (safety not established).

Nursing Interventions

Medication Administration

Glycerin: Do not inject glycerin. It is for oral administration *only*. The 50% solution is lime flavored. The palatability of unflavored solutions may be improved by addition of lemon juice or other flavoring agents.

Isosorbide

Maintain proper fluid and electrolyte balance during prolonged administration.

Monitor urinary output. Drug should be discontinued if output continues to decrease because extracellular fluid overload can occur.

Pour medication over cracked ice and instruct patient to sip it to improve palatability.

Mannitol

Carefully assess patient's cardiovascular status before and during administration because congestive heart failure may occur.

Monitor urine output continually during infusion. Infusion should be terminated if output declines because accumulation of mannitol can result in expanded extracellular fluid volume, which may aggravate or precipitate congestive heart failure.

Monitor results of plasma electrolyte measurements, which should be performed if administration is prolonged. Infusion should be adjusted to prevent electrolyte imbalance.

Administer concurrently with whole blood only if at least 20 mEq/L of sodium chloride is added to mannitol solution to prevent pseudoagglutination.

Be prepared to administer test dose (see Dosage) in patient with severe renal impairment. A second test dose may be given if response to first is inadequate (urine flow less than 30 mL/h).

Adjust infusion rate to maintain urine flow of at least 30 to 50 mL/h.

Consult practitioner regarding allowable fluid intake.

If solution is crystallized (exposed to low temperatures), warm in hot water bath, then cool to body temperature before injecting. Do not administer if crystals are present.

Urea

Closely monitor intake and output during infusion. Comatose patient should have an indwelling bladder catheter. If diuresis does not occur within 6 to 12 hours after injection, or if BUN exceeds 75 mg/dL, drug should be discontinued, and renal function should be reevaluated.

Use extreme care to avoid extravasation of solution because irritation, thrombosis, and tissue necrosis can occur.

Do not infuse into veins of lower extremities in elderly patients because thrombosis and phlebitis of deep veins may result.

Do not infuse through the administration set used for blood infusion.

Keep infusion rate below 4 mL/min to avoid hemolysis.

Prepare solution by reconstituting it with 5% or 10% dextrose injection or 10% invert sugar in water. Use within a few hours if stored at room temperature (within 48 h if stored at 2°–8°C).

Discard unused portion.

Surveillance During Therapy

Carefully monitor laboratory studies and patient for indications of adverse reactions: urinary output; blood pressure regularly and frequently; serum electrolytes with prolonged therapy.

Interpret results of diagnostic tests and contact practitioner as appropriate.

Monitor for possible drug–drug and drug–nutrient interactions; see Interactions.

Patient Teaching

Instruct the patient that the following may occur as a result of drug therapy: increased urination; GI upset; dry mouth; headache; blurred vision.

Instruct patient to inform practitioner if any of the following occur: difficulty breathing; pain at the IV site; chest pain.

Potassium-Sparing Diuretics

Unlike most other major classes of diuretic drugs, the potassium-sparing diuretics do *not* cause a loss of potassium by way of the kidney but rather act to conserve potassium by reducing its distal tubular secretion in conjunction with sodium reabsorption. These agents are not potent diuretic drugs when used alone, and their use as single agents can result in significant hyperkalemia. Their principal application, therefore, is in combination with other oral diuretics (eg, thiazides, high-ceiling drugs) both to increase the excretion of sodium and water and, more important, to minimize the potassium loss normally induced by the more potent drugs. Because several important differences exist among the available potassium-sparing diuretics, they are reviewed individually.

CAUTION

When used alone, hyperkalemia occurs in about 10% of patients receiving potassium-sparing diuretics and if uncorrected, may be fatal! Symptoms include paresthesias, fatigue, muscle weakness, bradycardia, and flaccid paralysis in the extremities. The incidence of hyperkalemia is greater in the elderly or diabetic patient or in the patient with renal impairment. Serum potassium levels must be closely monitored and the drug discontinued if the levels exceed 5.5 to 6 mEq/L. Treatment of hyperkalemia includes IV sodium bicarbonate, oral or parenteral glucose, and sodium polystyrene sulfonate orally or by enema.

• Amiloride

Midamor

Mechanism

Acts principally on the distal tubule to inhibit active sodium reabsorption and potassium secretion across tubular membranes; inhibition of Na^+-K^+-adenosine triphosphatase enzyme may play a role in blocking transtubular transport of these ions; also decreases magnesium excretion, which occurs with thiazide and loop diuretics; possesses weak diuretic and blood pressure-lowering activity and does not significantly alter renal blood flow or glomerular filtration rate.

Uses

Adjunctive treatment with potassium-depleting diuretics (eg, thiazides, loop diuretics) to minimize potassium loss or restore normal serum potassium levels (rarely used alone)

Reduction of lithium-induced polyuria (does *not* increase lithium levels, as thiazide diuretics do)—*investigational use*

Dosage

Initially 5 mg/day orally as a single dose added to the diuretic regimen; increase if necessary in 5-mg increments. Maximum recommended dose is 20 mg/day for severe, persistent hypokalemia.

Fate

Onset of action with oral administration is 2 hours; peak effects occur between 6 and 10 hours; duration is 24 hours; plasma half-life is 6 to 9 hours; not metabolized, but excreted largely unchanged in both urine and feces in approximately equivalent amounts.

Common Side Effects

Nausea, anorexia, diarrhea, headache, vomiting, hyperkalemia (paresthesias, muscle weakness, fatigue, bradycardia).

Significant Adverse Reactions

GI: abdominal pain, dyspepsia, constipation, flatulence, GI bleeding

CNS: dizziness, encephalopathy, confusion, insomnia, tremors, depression

Respiratory: dyspnea, coughing

Musculoskeletal: muscle cramping; weakness; pain in joints, back, neck, shoulders

Other: impotence, polyuria, dysuria, arrhythmias, photosensitivity, skin rash, pruritus, alopecia, visual disturbances, nasal congestion, tinnitus, increased intraocular pressure

Contraindications

Hyperkalemia, impaired renal function, and concomitant use with other potassium-sparing diuretics or potassium supplements. *Cautious use* in patients with diabetes, renal impairment, cardiopulmonary disease; in pregnant women or nursing mothers; in children; and in elderly, debilitated, or severely ill patients.

Interactions

Hyperkalemia may be augmented by concomitant use of other potassium-sparing drugs (eg, spironolactone, triamterene), angiotensin-converting enzyme inhibitors or potassium supplements.

Amiloride can reduce the clinical effectiveness of digitalis drugs, but also reduces the risk of toxicity resulting from hypokalemia.

Nonsteroidal antiinflammatory agents may reduce the therapeutic effectiveness of amiloride.

Nursing Management

Pretherapy Assessment

Assess and record baseline data necessary for detection of adverse effects of amiloride: General: VS, body weight, skin color and temperature, edema, hydration; CNS: orientation, reflexes, muscle strength; CVS: baseline ECG, orthostatic blood pressure; GI: liver evaluation, bowel sounds; GU: output patterns; Laboratory: CBC, serum electrolytes, liver and renal function tests, urinalysis.

Review medical history and documents for existing or previous conditions that:

a. require cautious use of amiloride: diabetes; renal impairment; cardiopulmonary disease; use in children; use in elderly; severe illness of debilitated state.

b. contraindicate use of amiloride: hyperkalemia; impaired renal function; concomitant use with other potassium-sparing diuretics or potassium supplements; **pregnancy (Category B)**; lactation (safety not established).

Nursing Interventions

Medication Administration

Administer with food or milk to prevent GI upset.
Administer early in the day so increased urination does not disturb sleep.
Ensure ready access to bathroom facilities when diuretic effect occurs.
Avoid giving foods rich in potassium.

Surveillance During Therapy

Carefully monitor laboratory studies and patient for indications of adverse reactions: urinary output; blood pressure regularly and frequently; serum electrolytes with prolonged therapy.
Monitor results of BUN determinations, which should be performed frequently during extended therapy, and inform practitioner of change in renal function.
Interpret results of diagnostic tests and contact practitioner as appropriate.
Monitor for possible drug–drug and drug–nutrient interactions; see Interactions.

Patient Teaching

Suggest drug be taken with food to minimize GI upset.
Alert patient to avoid foods rich in potassium.
Instruct the patient that the following may occur as a result of drug therapy: increased urination; GI upset; dry mouth; headache; dizziness; blurred vision; decreased sexual function; increased thirst.
Instruct patient to inform practitioner if any of the following occur: weight loss or gain of more than 1.3 kg (3 lb) in 1 day; swelling in the ankles or fingers; dizziness; trembling; numbness; fatigue; muscle cramps or weakness.

• **Spironolactone** (*Pregnancy Category D*)

Aldactone

(CAN) Novospiroton, Sincomen

Mechanism

Competitive antagonist of the naturally occurring hormone aldosterone at distal tubular sites involved in sodium reabsorption and potassium excretion; aldosterone normally stimulates enzymes that supply energy for active sodium and potassium transport in the distal tubule; inhibition of aldosterone results in excretion of sodium and retention of potassium; does not appear to elevate serum uric acid or alter carbohydrate metabolism, but can interfere with testosterone synthesis, leading to increased estrogenic : androgenic activity ratio.

Uses

Management of edema associated with congestive heart failure, primary hyperaldosteronism, cirrhosis of the liver, and nephrotic syndrome
Treatment of essential hypertension, usually combined with other diuretics or antihypertensive drugs
Adjunctive therapy with other potent diuretics to minimize potassium loss
Diagnosis and treatment of primary hyperaldosteronism
Investigational uses include treatment of hirsutism, acne vulgaris, and relief of symptoms of premenstrual syndrome

Dosage

Oral administration *only*.

Edema: Adults, 25 to 200 mg/day in a single dose or divided doses; children, 3.3 mg/kg in a single dose or divided doses
Hypertension: 50 to 100 mg daily in a single dose or divided doses; maximum 200 mg/day
Diagnosis of hyperaldosteronism: 400 mg/day for 4 days; if serum potassium increases during this time, then falls when drug is stopped, a presumptive diagnosis of primary hyperaldosteronism may be considered
Treatment of hyperaldosteronism: 100 to 400 mg/day
Hypokalemia: 25 to 100 mg/day to prevent diuretic-induced potassium loss

Fate

Peak plasma levels occur in 3 to 4 hours after a single dose; maximal diuretic action is seen in 2 to 3 days and may persist for several days after therapy is discontinued; highly bound to plasma proteins; rapidly and extensively metabolized and excreted primarily in the urine, with small amounts in the bile.

Common Side Effects

Gynecomastia and breast tenderness (in men and women), GI upset, lethargy.

Significant Adverse Reactions

CAUTION

Spironolactone has been shown to be a tumorigen in chronic toxicity studies in rats at significantly higher-than-recommended doses. Its use should be restricted to those indications outlined previously for which other diuretic drugs are ineffective or inappropriate.

Cramping, diarrhea, vomiting, cutaneous eruptions, urticaria, fever, ataxia, drowsiness, confusion, impotence, hirsutism, irregular menses, voice deepening, postmenopausal bleeding, fluid and electrolyte disturbances (especially hyperkalemia and hyponatremia), mild acidosis, and elevated BUN.

Contraindications

Anuria, acute renal insufficiency or significantly impaired renal function, and hyperkalemia. *Cautious use* in decreased renal function and in pregnant or nursing women.

Interactions

Spironolactone may potentiate the effects of other diuretics and antihypertensive drugs.

Salicylates may reverse the effects of spironolactone.

Spironolactone may reduce the clinical effectiveness of digitalis drugs but also reduces the likelihood of digitalis-induced arrhythmias occurring as a result of hypokalemia.

The renal clearance of lithium may be reduced by spironolactone.

The effects of oral anticoagulants may be reduced owing to hemoconcentration of clotting factors resulting from diuretic action.

Ammonium chloride and other acidifying agents can induce systemic acidosis when given in combination with spironolactone.

Hyperkalemia may result if potassium supplements are used together with spironolactone, if patient is also on an angiotensin-converting enzyme inhibitor, or if patients consume a potassium-rich diet.

Nursing Management

Pretherapy Assessment

Assess and record baseline data necessary for detection of adverse effects of spironolactone: General: VS, body weight, skin color and temperature, edema, hydration; CNS: orientation, reflexes, muscle strength; CVS: baseline ECG, orthostatic blood pressure; GI: liver evaluation, bowel sounds; GU: output patterns, menstrual cycle; Laboratory: CBC, serum electrolytes, liver and renal function tests, urinalysis.

Review medical history and documents for existing or previous conditions that:

a. require cautious use of spironolactone: decreased renal function.
b. contraindicate use of spironolactone: allergy to spironolactone; hyperkalemia; impaired renal function; concomitant use with other potassium-sparing diuretics or potassium supplements; **pregnancy (Category D)**; lactation (secreted in breast milk, safety not established).

Nursing Interventions

Medication Administration

Administer with food or milk to prevent GI upset.

Administer early in the day so increased urination does not disturb sleep.

Ensure ready access to bathroom facilities when diuretic effect occurs.

Avoid giving foods rich in potassium.

Surveillance During Therapy

Carefully monitor laboratory studies and patient for indications of adverse reactions: urinary output; blood pressure regularly and frequently; serum electrolytes with prolonged therapy.

Interpret results of diagnostic tests and contact practitioner as appropriate.

Monitor for possible drug–drug and drug–nutrient interactions; see Interactions.

Patient Teaching

Instruct the patient that the following may occur as a result of drug therapy: increased urination; GI upset; dry mouth; headache; blurred vision; changes in the menstrual cycle; deepening of the voice; impotence; enlargement of the breasts.

Instruct patient to inform practitioner if any of the following occur: weight loss or gain of more than 1.3 kg (3 lb) in 1 day; swelling in the ankles or fingers; dizziness; trembling; numbness; fatigue; muscle cramps or weakness; enlargement of breasts; impotence.

• Triamterene

Dyrenium

Mechanism

Inhibits active reabsorption of sodium and secretion of potassium by distal tubular cells; does not appear to interfere with aldosterone but acts directly on the renal tubule.

Uses

Treatment of edema associated with congestive heart failure, cirrhosis of the liver, or the nephrotic syndrome, and in steroid-induced or idiopathic edema

Adjunctive therapy of hypertension, in combination with other diuretics, for its added diuretic effect as well as its potassium-conserving effect

Dosage

When used alone, 100 mg twice a day (maximum 300 mg/day); dosage should be reduced when given in combination with other diuretics.

Fate

Well absorbed from the GI tract; onset of action is 2 to 4 hours; maximal diuretic effect occurs within 6 to 8 hours; duration of action is approximately 16 hours after a single dose; 50% to 70% bound to plasma proteins; metabolized primarily in the liver and excreted by the kidneys.

Common Side Effects

GI upset, nausea, leg cramps.

Significant Adverse Reactions

Headache, weakness, metallic taste, dryness of the mouth, skin rash, photosensitivity, elevated BUN, hyperuricemia, hyperkalemia, hypotension, and blood dyscrasias (rare).

Contraindications

Anuria, severe hepatic disease, hyperkalemia, and severe or progressive kidney dysfunction (except nephrosis). *Cautious use* in patients with gout or gouty arthritis, reduced renal function, or hepatic cirrhosis, and in pregnant or nursing women.

Interactions

See Spironolactone. In addition:

Serum levels of digitalis glycosides may be increased by triamterene.

Acute renal failure has been reported when indomethacin was given with triamterene.

Nursing Management

Pretherapy Assessment

Assess and record baseline data necessary for detection of adverse effects of triamterene: General: VS, body weight, skin color and temperature, edema, hydration; CNS: orientation, reflexes, muscle strength; CVS: baseline ECG, orthostatic blood pressure; GI: liver evaluation, bowel sounds; GU: output patterns, menstrual cycle; Laboratory: CBC, serum electrolytes, liver and renal function tests, urinalysis, blood glucose, serum uric acid.

Review medical history and documents for existing or previous conditions that:

a. require cautious use of triamterene: gout or gouty arthritis; reduced renal function; hepatic cirrhosis.
b. contraindicate use of triamterene: allergy to triamterene; hyperkalemia; impaired renal function; anuria; severe hepatic disease; concomitant use with other potassium-sparing diuretics or potassium supplements; **pregnancy (Category B)**; lactation (secreted in breast milk, safety not established).

Nursing Interventions

Medication Administration

Administer with food or milk to prevent GI upset.

Administer early in the day so increased urination does not disturb sleep.

Ensure ready access to bathroom facilities when diuretic effect occurs.

Avoid giving foods rich in potassium.

Surveillance During Therapy

Carefully monitor laboratory studies and patient for indications of adverse reactions: urinary output; blood pressure regularly and frequently; serum electrolytes with prolonged therapy.

Monitor results of BUN and serum creatinine determinations, which should be performed periodically during extended therapy, especially in patients with kidney dysfunction as well as in elderly or diabetic patients. Note possible early signs of renal insufficiency (eg, fatigue, vomiting, stomatitis, confusion, bad taste in mouth).

Monitor diabetic patient for hyperglycemia because drug can elevate blood glucose.

Expect drug to be withdrawn *gradually* over several days to prevent excessive rebound potassium excretion.

Interpret results of diagnostic tests and contact practitioner as appropriate.

Monitor for possible drug–drug and drug–nutrient interactions; see Interactions.

Patient Teaching

Instruct the patient that the following may occur as a result of drug therapy; increased urination; GI upset; dry mouth; headache; blurred vision; sensitivity to sunlight.

Instruct patient to inform practitioner if any of the following occur; weight loss or gain of more than 1.3 kg (3 lb) in 1 day; swelling in the ankles or fingers; dizziness; trembling; numbness; fatigue; muscle cramps or weakness.

Instruct patient to report immediately the development of fever, sore throat, mucosal ulceration, extreme fatigue, or weakness, possible symptoms of a blood dyscrasia. If symptoms occur, blood counts should be performed.

Thiazides and Related Diuretics

Bendroflumethiazide
Benzthiazide
Chlorothiazide
Chlorthalidone
Hydrochlorothiazide
Hydroflumethiazide
Indapamide
Methyclothiazide
Metolazone
Polythiazide
Quinethazone
Trichlormethiazide

The largest group of orally effective diuretic drugs, thiazides and related compounds are structurally related to the sulfonamide antibacterial drugs; however, they possess no antiinfective properties. Most of these sulfonamide diuretics are derived from a benzothiadiazine nucleus and hence are commonly referred to as *thiazide diuretics*. A few other diuretics differ slightly in their chemical structure from the thiazides, although their pharmacologic and toxicologic properties are essentially similar, and these compounds are referred to as *thiazide-like* diuretics. Structural differences notwithstanding, all of these drugs possess parallel dose–response curves; that is, there is essentially no difference among them in their clinical efficacy, and all drugs in this category possess similar sites and mechanisms of diuretic action.

The thiazide and thiazide-like diuretics are the most widely used drugs for the treatment of edematous states and for the control of mild to moderate hypertension. Because of the similarity of action among the drugs in this class, they are reviewed as a group; individual drugs are listed in Table 39-4.

Mechanism

Diuretic: Impair active sodium and chloride reabsorption in the early portion of the distal segment of the renal tubule and also in the cortical thick ascending loop of Henle, resulting in excretion of these ions with an osmotically equivalent volume of water; possess weak carbonic anhydrase inhibitory activity, although the importance of this action to their diuretic effect is probably minimal; bicarbonate excretion is slightly increased, whereas calcium excretion is reduced; potassium is lost in conjunction with sodium reabsorption in the distal tubule.

Antihypertensive: May be the result of 1) reduction of plasma volume and sodium levels, 2) direct relaxation of arteriolar smooth muscle, and 3) decreased reactivity of vascular smooth muscle to endogenous pressor substances, possibly because of alterations in sodium content within the muscle fibers.

Table 39-4. Thiazide and Related Diuretics

Drug	*Usual Dosage Range*	*Nursing Considerations*
Bendroflumethiazide *Naturetin*	*Edema*: initially 5–20 mg/d; maintenance 2.5–5 mg/d *Hypertension*: initially 5–20 mg/d; maintenance 2.5–15 mg/d	Short-acting preparation (6–12 h); low doses do not appreciably alter serum electrolyte levels; available in fixed combinations with rauwolfia (Rauzide) and nadolol (Corzide)
Benzthiazide *Exna*	*Edema*: initially 50–200 mg/d; maintenance 50–150 mg/d *Hypertension*: initially 50–100 mg/d; maintenance 50 mg 2–4 times/d	Maximal effect in 4–6 h, with a duration of 12–18 h
Chlorothiazide *Diuril and various other manufacturers*	*Edema* Adults: 0.5–1 g 1–2 times a day, 3–5 d/wk Children: 22 mg/kg/d in 2 doses *Hypertension*: 0.5–1 g/d, adjusted to optimal response	After oral administration, onset within 2 h and duration of 6–12 h; IV solution prepared by adding 18 mL sterile water to vial; do *not* administer with plasma or whole blood nor give SC or IM; use IV *only* in emergency situations and avoid extravasation—IV injections are not recommended in children; solutions may be stored up to 24 h at room temperature; available with reserpine (Diupres) and methyldopa (Aldoclor) in oral form
Chlorthalidone *Hygroton, Thalitone, (CAN) Apo-Chlorthalidone, Novothalidone*	*Edema*: 50–100 mg/d *or* 100 mg/d 3 times/wk on alternate days *Hypertension*: initially 25–50 mg; adjust to optimal response; maximum 100 mg/d; children—3 mg/kg/d, 3 times/wk	Sulfonamide diuretic; onset 2–3 h and duration 24–48 h; given by single daily dosage in the morning; effective hypotensive agent, often used as initial therapy in mild hypertension; doses above 25 mg/d offer little additional antihypertensive action but increase potassium loss; may elevate plasma levels of cholesterol, triglycerides, and LDL; available with clonidine (Combipres), reserpine (Regroton, Demi-Regroton) and atenolol (Tenoretic)
Hydrochlorothiazide *Esidrix, Hydrodiuril, and several other manufacturers (CAN) Apo-Hydro, Novohydrazide, and other manufacturers*	*Edema*: initially 25–200 mg/d; maintenance 25–100 mg/d, usually on an intermittent schedule *Hypertension*: initially 25–100 mg/d; adjust to desired response; usual range 25–100 mg/d; children—2.2 mg/kg/d	Most widely used thiazide diuretic; onset 1–2 h and duration 6–12 h; available in fixed combination with many other antihypertensive drugs; oral absorption may be improved if taken with food
Hydroflumethiazide *Diucardin, Saluron*	*Edema*: initially 50–100 mg/d; usual maintenance dose 25–200 mg/d on an intermittent schedule *Hypertension*: 50 mg twice a day; adjust to desired response	Rapid onset (1–2 h) and short duration (6–12 h); do not exceed 200 mg/d; available with reserpine (Salutensin)
Indapamide *Lozol (CAN) Lozide*	*Edema*: 2.5 mg/d as a single daily dose; may increase to 5 mg/d after 1–4 wk if necessary *Hypertension*: 1.25 mg daily as a single dose; may increase to 2–5 mg daily after 1 wk	Indoline derivative used for hypertension and edema of congestive heart failure; increases serum uric acid an average of 1 mg/dL; doses greater than 5 mg/d do not provide additional therapeutic benefit but are associated with a greater degree of hypokalemia than smaller doses
Methyclothiazide *Aquatensen, Enduron (CAN) Duretic*	*Edema*: 2.5–10 mg daily *Hypertension*: 2.5–5 mg daily	Onset in 2 h and duration lasts about 24 h; do not exceed 10 mg/d; available with reserpine (Diutensen-R), deserpidine (Enduronyl)
Metolazone *Mykrox, Zaroxolyn*	*Zaroxolyn* *Edema*: 5–20 mg once daily *Hypertension*: 2.5–5 mg once daily *Mykrox* *Hypertension*: 0.5–1 mg daily	Rapid onset (1 h) and moderate duration (12–24 h) of action; dosage should be in upper end of range in patients with congestive heart failure to ensure diuretic effect for full 24 h; *not* recommended in children; profound volume and electrolyte depletion can occur in combination with furosemide; Mykrox is more quickly bioavailable; *not* interchangeable with Zaroxolyn at similar doses
Polythiazide *Renese*	*Edema*: 1–4 mg/d *Hypertension*: 2–4 mg/d	Onset 1–2 h and duration 24–36 h; available with reserpine (Renese-R) and prazosin (Minizide)
Quinethazone *Hydromox (CAN) Aquamox*	50–100 mg in a single daily morning dose; maximum 200 mg/d	Onset of 2 h and a duration of 18–24 h
Trichlormethiazide *Diurese, Metahydrin, Naqua*	*Edema*: 2–4 mg/d *Hypertension*: 2–4 mg/d	Onset 2 h and duration 24 h or longer; available with reserpine (Metatensin)

Other: Interfere with insulin release, possibly a result of hypokalemia, and compete with uric acid for renal tubular secretory sites, thus elevating serum uric acid levels; exert a paradoxic *anti*diuretic effect in diabetes insipidus, possibly by enhancing the action of antidiuretic hormone as a consequence of sodium depletion.

Uses

Treatment of edema associated with congestive heart failure, hepatic cirrhosis, renal dysfunction, and steroid or estrogen therapy

Management of all forms of hypertension, either alone (mild cases) or in combination with other antihypertensive drugs (moderate to severe cases)

Symptomatic treatment of diabetes insipidus to reduce polyuria

Investigational uses include prevention of formation and recurrence of calcium stones in hypercalciuria, either alone or with amiloride or allopurinol, and prevention of osteoporotic changes in postmenopausal women.

Dosage

See Table 39-4.

Fate

Well absorbed orally; onset of diuresis is usually 1 to 2 hours after oral administration (except cyclothiazide, 4–6 h); peak diuretic effect usually occurs in 4 to 6 hours, and duration ranges from 6 to 72 hours (average duration, 12–18 h); several days are necessary for development of the antihypertensive action, and peak antihypertensive effects usually occur after 2 to 4 weeks; many drugs are highly bound to plasma proteins; excreted in the urine, both as unchanged drug and metabolites.

Common Side Effects

Lightheadedness, hypokalemia (muscle weakness, dizziness, paresthesias, cramping), especially if potassium supplements are not used.

Significant Adverse Reactions

GI: nausea, GI irritation, vomiting, anorexia, dry mouth, diarrhea, cramping, bloating, jaundice, pancreatitis, sialoadenitis, hepatitis

CV: orthostatic hypotension, palpitation, irregular heartbeat, premature ventricular contractions, angina-like pain, hemoconcentration

CNS: headache, vertigo, blurred vision, syncope, fatigue, drowsiness, restlessness, depression

Hypersensitivity: rash, photosensitivity, fever, purpura, urticaria, vasculitis, Stevens-Johnson syndrome, dyspnea, pneumonitis, anaphylactic reactions

Hematologic: blood dyscrasias (rare)

Other: muscle spasm, chills, impotence, hyperglycemia, hyperuricemia, elevated BUN, hypercalcemia

Contraindications

Sulfonamide hypersensitivity, anuria, renal decompensation, IV administration in infants and children; metolazone is also contraindicated in patients with hepatic coma or precoma. *Cautious use* in patients with renal or hepatic disease, bronchial asthma, diabetes mellitus, gout, history of allergies or cardiac arrhythmias, lupus erythematosus, advanced arteriosclerosis, or advanced heart disease, and in elderly or debilitated people, patients receiving digitalis drugs, and pregnant women or nursing mothers.

Interactions

Thiazides potentiate the hypotensive action of other antihypertensive drugs and may increase the incidence of orthostatic hypotension associated with use of alcohol, narcotics, barbiturates and other CNS depressants, phenothiazines, and tricyclic antidepressants.

The effects of oral anticoagulants, vasopressors, hypouricemic drugs, and oral hypoglycemics may be antagonized by thiazide diuretics.

Hypokalemia may be intensified if thiazides are combined with corticosteroids.

Thiazide-induced hypokalemia may increase digitalis toxicity.

Indomethacin and the pyrazolones may reduce the diuretic efficacy of the thiazides owing to excessive fluid retention.

Hypercalcemia can occur if thiazides are given with calcium carbonate or other calcium-containing products.

Thiazides can potentiate amphetamines, quinidine, and lithium by decreasing their excretion.

Prolonged relaxation of skeletal muscle (including respiratory) may occur if thiazides are given together with nondepolarizing muscle relaxants.

Oral absorption of thiazides may be impaired by cholestyramine and colestipol.

Concurrent use of thiazides and diazoxide can increase the likelihood of hyperglycemia, hyperuricemia, and hypotension.

Nursing Management

Pretherapy Assessment

Assess and record baseline data necessary for detection of adverse effects of thiazide diuretics: General: VS, body weight, skin color and temperature, edema, hydration; CNS: orientation, reflexes, muscle strength; CVS: baseline ECG, orthostatic blood pressure; GI: liver evaluation, bowel sounds; GU: output patterns, menstrual cycle; Laboratory: CBC, serum electrolytes, liver and renal function tests, urinalysis, blood glucose, serum uric acid.

Review medical history and documents for existing or previous conditions that:

a. require cautious use of thiazide diuretics: renal or hepatic disease; bronchial asthma; diabetes mellitus; gout; history of allergies; cardiac arrhythmias; lupus erythematosus; advanced arteriosclerosis; advanced heart disease; use in elderly or debilitated people; patients receiving digitalis drugs.

b. contraindicate use of thiazide diuretics: allergy to thiazides, sulfonamides; anuria; renal decompensation; IV administration in infants and children; metolazone is also contraindicated in patients with hepatic coma or precoma; **pregnancy (Category B)**; lactation (secreted in breast milk, safety not established).

Nursing Interventions

Medication Administration

Administer with food or milk to prevent GI upset.

Administer early in the day so increased urination does not disturb sleep.

Ensure ready access to bathroom facilities when diuretic effect occurs.

Avoid giving foods rich in potassium.

Expect dose of each drug to be reduced by half to avoid excessive hypotension when a thiazide is added to an existing antihypertensive regimen. Dosage may then be slowly titrated to obtain maximal benefit.

Ensure that drug is discontinued for several days before parathyroid function tests because it may decrease calcium excretion.

Surveillance During Therapy

Monitor results of baseline and periodic determinations of BUN, CO_2, uric acid, blood glucose, and blood counts.

Carefully monitor for loss of drug effectiveness or development of toxic reactions if patient is taking a digitalis, hypouricemic, or oral hypoglycemic preparation. Dosage adjustments may be necessary.

Carefully monitor laboratory studies and patient for indications of adverse reactions: urinary output; blood pressure regularly and frequently; serum electrolytes with prolonged therapy.

Monitor diabetic patient for hyperglycemia because drug can elevate blood glucose.

Interpret results of diagnostic tests and contact practitioner as appropriate.

Monitor for possible drug–drug and drug–nutrient interactions; see Interactions.

Patient Teaching

Encourage patient to avoid high-sodium foods and to refrain from adding table salt to other foods.

Instruct the patient that the following may occur as a result of drug therapy; increased urination; GI upset; dry mouth; headache; dizziness; blurred vision; sensitivity to sunlight; decrease in sexual function.

Instruct patient to inform practitioner if any of the following occur: weight loss or gain of more than 1.3 kg (3 lb) in 1 day; swelling in the ankles or fingers; dizziness; trembling; numbness; fatigue; muscle cramps or weakness; unusual bleeding or bruising.

Selected Bibliography

Cody RJ: Clinical trials of diuretic therapy in heart failure: Research directions and clinical considerations. J Am Coll Cardiol 22(Suppl 4):165A, 1993

Dupont AG: The place of diuretics in the treatment of hypertension: A historical review of classical experience over 30 years. Cardiovasc Drugs Ther 7(Suppl 1):55, 1993

Rose BD: Diuretics. Kidney Int 39:336, 1991

Russo D, Memoli B, Andreucci VE: The place of loop diuretics in the treatment of acute and chronic renal failure. Clin Nephrol 38(Suppl 1):S69, 1992

Stanton BA: Cellular actions of thiazide diuretics in the distal tubule. J Am Soc Nephrol 1:832, 1990

Straand J, Fugelli P, Laake K: Withdrawing long-term diuretic treatment among elderly patients in general practice. Fam Pract 10(1):38, 1993

Vlay SC: Innovations in the management of ischemic cardiomyopathy. Am Heart J 127:235, 1994

Nursing Bibliography

Collins J: The treatment of mild to moderate hypertension in patients with diabetes. Nurse Practitioner 16(6):28, 1991

Dolleris P: Diuretic and vasopressor usage in acute renal failure: A synopsis. Critical Care Nursing Quarterly 14(4):28, 1992

Jessup M, et al: Managing CHF in the older patient. Patient Care 26(14): 65, 1992

Leffert C, Leucke L: Assessing and treating pulmonary edema. Nursing '93 23(7):54, 1993

Peppers M: Head trauma and osmotic diuretics. Emergency 25(5): 55, 1993

Sonnenblick M, et al: Diuretic induced severe hyponatremia. Chest 103:601, 1993

Winer N: Hypertensive crisis. Critical Care Nursing Quarterly 13(3): 23, 1990

V

Drugs Acting on the Endocrine Glands

40

The Endocrine Glands: A Review

The endocrine system functions in close harmony with the nervous system in regulating, coordinating, and integrating the wide range of metabolic and physiologic activities essential to the maintenance of homeostasis in an ever-changing environment.

The anatomically distinct and functionally diverse organs of the endocrine system participate in the regulation of the following basic activities: 1) energy metabolism, 2) electrolyte and water metabolism, 3) reproduction, 4) growth and development, and 5) response to stress.

The products of endocrine glands, the *hormones*, are characteristically produced in small amounts by specialized glandular cells and are secreted directly into the bloodstream, whereby they are transported to specific target tissues on which they exert regulatory control. In some cases, chemical messengers (*paracrine secretions*) may act locally, diffusing to nearby sites and exerting effects on neighboring cells.

Chemically, hormones may be

- Peptides (polypeptides, protein and glycoproteins, eg, insulin, growth hormone)
- Steroids (eg, aldosterone and cortisol)
- Amino acid derivatives (eg, epinephrine and thyroxine)

Transport and Metabolism of Hormones

Water-insoluble hormones, such as steroids and thyroid hormones, are transported through the blood bound to plasma proteins. Because only free (unbound) hormone is physiologically active and subject to biodegradation (metabolic transformation), protein binding affords a mechanism by which reserve hormones are readily available. Hormones may be inactivated by the liver or kidneys, or, more rarely, by the target tissues. Because of the great importance of the liver and kidneys in the metabolism and excretion of hormones, the state of hepatic and renal function should be established during the course of diagnosing specific endocrine dysfunctions.

Mechanisms of Hormone Action

The ability of a target cell to respond to a particular hormone is inherent in its hormone receptors. The cellular mechanisms whereby hormones exert their specific effects on target tissues vary.

Lipophilic hormones (steroids and thyroid hormones) easily penetrate the plasma membranes of their target cells and bind to intracellular receptors on the nuclear membrane or within the cell nucleus. The hormone:receptor interaction induces gene activation and transcription of messenger RNA, thereby modifying protein synthesis. Changes in the levels of specific proteins, in turn, lead to characteristic cellular responses associated with the hormone, eg, enhanced transport of a particular substrate.

Hydrophilic hormones (eg, peptides, catecholamines) bind to plasma membrane receptors on the surface of target cells. The hormone:receptor interaction leads to the formation or increased availability of a *second messenger*, which ultimately induces a specific cellular response, such as altered cellular permeability or enzyme activity.

Second Messenger Mechanisms

To date, three intracellular second messenger mechanisms have been identified:

1. *Cyclic AMP (cAMP)*, formed from adenosine triphosphate (ATP) through activation of *adenylate cyclase*
2. *Inositol triphosphate (IP_3)* and *diacylglycerol (DAG)*, formed from phosphatidylinositol biphosphate in cell membranes by activated *phospholipase C*.
3. *Calcium ions*, which gain entry into target cells *through* receptor-linked ion channels and activate calcium-dependent proteins such as calmodulin

The activities of adenylate cyclase and phospholipase C are coupled to membrane hormone receptors by guanosine triphosphate (GTP)-binding proteins called *G-proteins*. (For a more detailed discussion of G-proteins, refer to Chapter 11.)

Regulation of Hormone Secretion

Secretion of certain hormones is under the direct control of the nervous system. Other hormones are controlled by the blood level of an electrolyte (eg, calcium), a metabolite (eg, glucose) or another hormone (eg, tropic hormone). Typically, negative-feedback loops are involved in the regulation of hormone secretion. Figure 40-1 illustrates a complex negative feedback mechanism involving the brain (hypothalamus), anterior pituitary gland (adenohypophysis), and a target endocrine gland.

Pituitary Gland

The pituitary gland, formerly called the "master gland," secretes several polypeptide hormones that directly or indirectly regulate a wide variety of metabolic and physiologic processes essential to normal growth and development as well as to the maintenance of homeostasis. Many of the hormones secreted by the pituitary gland are critical to the activity of target glands, including the thyroid, adrenals, and gonads.

Anatomy

The pituitary gland (*hypophysis cerebri*) is located at the base of the brain, resting within the sella turcica of the sphenoid

Malseed, RT; Goldstein, FJ; and Balkon, N: PHARMACOLOGY: DRUG THERAPY AND NURSING CONSIDERATIONS, Fourth Edition. © 1995 J. B. Lippincott Company.

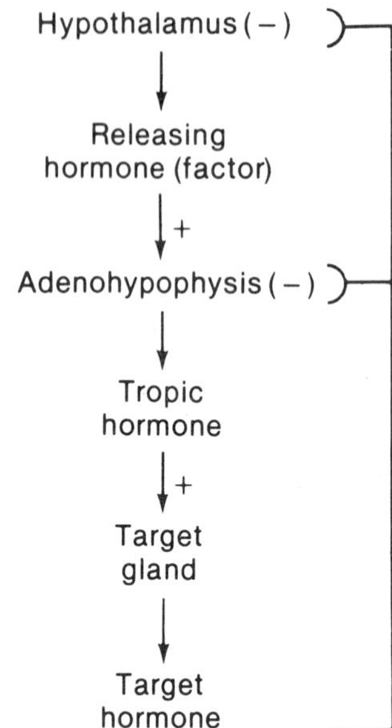

Figure 40-1. Negative-feedback mechanism regulating endocrine hormone secretion.

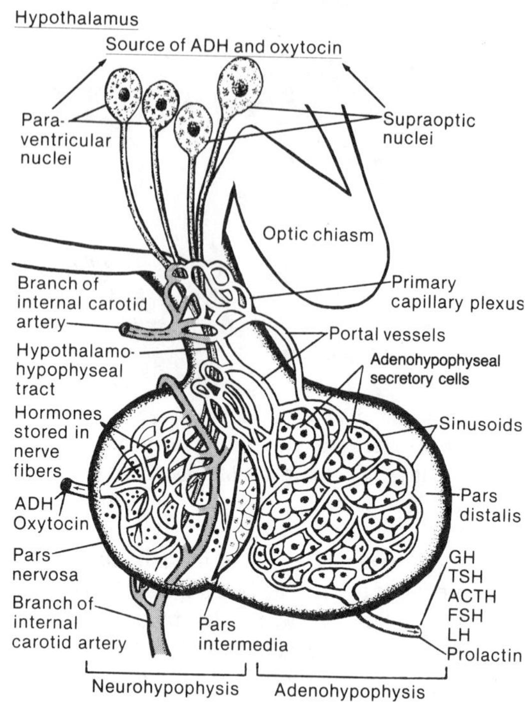

Figure 40-2. The pituitary gland (hypophysis) and its relationship with the hypothalamus.

bone. The pituitary gland maintains elaborate neural and vascular connections with the hypothalamus of the brain, which plays a central role in the integration of neuroendocrine activity (Fig. 40-2).

The pituitary gland has two major divisions: the neurohypophysis and the adenohypophysis.

Neurohypophysis

The *neurohypophysis*, which is connected directly to the hypothalamus by the *infundibular* (pituitary) *stalk*, is rich in nerve fibers of hypothalamic origin (the *hypothalamohypophyseal tract*).

Neurosecretory cells in the *supraoptic* and *paraventricular nuclei* of the hypothalamus produce two hormones: *antidiuretic hormone* (ADH or vasopressin) and *oxytocin*. These hormones are then transported along the axons of the hypothalamohypophyseal tract to the *pars nervosa* (posterior lobe) of the pituitary gland for storage and ultimate release under hypothalamic control.

Adenohypophysis

The *adenohypophysis* is served by an elaborate vascular system, including the *hypothalamohypophyseal portal system*, which transports hypothalamic regulating hormones (hypophyseotropic hormones) to the glandular cells of the adenohypophysis. The classification of cells in the adenohypophysis is based on specific immunohistochemical techniques. Accordingly, there are at least five recognized cell types:

1. *Somatotrophs*, which secrete growth hormone (hGH) or somatotropin.
2. *Lactotrophs*, which secrete prolactin (PRL).
3. *Corticotrophs*, which produce corticotropin (ACTH) and beta-lipotropin (beta-LPH) by splitting a large peptide prohormone, pro-opiomelanocortin (POMC).
4. *Thyrotrophs*, which secrete thyrotropin (TSH).
5. *Gonadotrophs*, which produce follicle stimulating hormone (FSH) and luteinizing hormone (LH)

There is also evidence that some adenohypophyseal cells may secrete more than one hormone, promoting the use of such terms as corticothyrotrophs, corticogonadotrophs, and mammosomatotrophs.

Hormones of the Neurohypophysis

Antidiuretic Hormone (ADH; Vasopressin)

Control of Secretion

Antidiuretic hormone (ADH) is a polypeptide hormone of hypothalamic origin (supraoptic and paraventricular nuclei) that is stored in and released from the neurohypophysis in response to a variety of stimuli. Included among these are increased plasma osmolality, reduced extracellular fluid (ECF) volume, pain, emotional stress, and such pharmacologic agents as morphine, nicotine, barbiturates, and certain general anesthetics.

Decreased plasma osmolality, increased ECF volume, and alcohol inhibit ADH secretion.

Osmoreceptors found in the anterior hypothalamus monitor changes in plasma osmolality, whereas ECF volume changes are detected by volume ("stretch") receptors located in the wall of the left atrium. The osmoreceptors and volume receptors work in concert to exert precise control over ADH secretion, thus forming a delicate homeostatic feedback mechanism for the regulation of ECF volume and concentration.

Actions

The principal physiologic role of ADH is to regulate extracellular fluid volume and osmolality by controlling the final volume and concentration of urine.

ADH, acting through the second messenger cyclic AMP, increases the permeability of the distal nephron (late distal convoluted tubules and collecting ducts) to water. The enhanced reabsorption of water from the renal tubules results in the production of a concentrated urine that is reduced in volume.

Pharmacologic amounts of ADH produce a *pressor* (hypertensive) effect that results from a direct constrictor action of the hormone on vascular smooth muscle.

The early observations that posterior pituitary extracts produce a marked elevation of arterial blood pressure led to the initial naming of this hormone as *vasopressin*.

Clinical States

Diabetes Insipidus

Inadequate ADH secretion leads to the excretion of large volumes of dilute urine (polyuria). Intense thirst and consumption of large amounts of liquid (polydipsia) are also characteristic of diabetes insipidus.

This disorder may be idiopathic, or it may follow trauma or cranial injury, central nervous system disease, infection, or emotional shock. The deficit may be related to the supraoptic or paraventricular nuclei, the hypothalamohypophyseal tract, or the neurohypophysis.

A rare ADH-resistant or *nephrogenic* diabetes also exists. In this inherited disorder, ADH secretion is normal, but the renal tubules are unresponsive to the hormone. Treatment of diabetes insipidus is discussed in Chapter 41.

Inappropriate ADH Syndrome

The inappropriate ADH syndrome (SIADH), a clinical state characterized by hypersecretion of ADH, may result from generalized infection, mediastinal tumors, metastatic tumors to the brain, pathologic CNS changes, or intracranial surgery.

Abnormal fluid retention leads to dilution of plasma sodium (dilutional hyponatremia), and urine becomes inappropriately concentrated. Fluid intake must be stringently restricted to minimize water intoxication.

Oxytocin

Control of Secretion and Actions

The two major physiologic actions of oxytocin are exerted on the female breast and uterus. Oxytocin binds to a G-protein coupled receptor that ultimately brings about elevated intracellular calcium levels.

Galactokinetic Action (Milk Ejection Reflex). The ejection of milk from a primed, lactating mammary gland follows a neuroendocrine reflex in which oxytocin serves as the efferent limb. The reflex is normally initiated by suckling, which stimulates cutaneous receptors in the areola of the breast. Afferent nerve impulses travel to the supraoptic and paraventricular nuclei of the hypothalamus to effect the release of oxytocin from the neurohypophysis. Oxytocin is carried by the blood to the mammary gland, where it causes contraction of *myoepithelial cells* surrounding the alveoli and lactiferous ducts to bring about the ejection of milk (milk letdown).

In lactating women, tactile stimulation of the breast areola, emotional stimuli, and genital stimulation may also lead to oxytocin release and activate the ejection of milk.

Oxytocic Action. Oxytocin acts directly on uterine smooth muscle to elicit strong, rhythmic contractions of the myometrium. Uterine sensitivity to oxytocin varies with its physiologic state and with hormonal balance. The gravid (pregnant) uterus is highly sensitive to oxytocin, particularly in the late stages of gestation. Uterine sensitivity to oxytocin is greatly enhanced by estrogen and inhibited by progesterone.

Oxytocin release appears to follow a neuroendocrine reflex initiated by genital stimulation. It has been suggested that oxytocin may facilitate sperm transport through the female genital tract.

Hormones of the Adenohypophysis

The secretion of hormones by the adenohypophysis is controlled by hypothalamic regulatory (hypophyseotropic) hormones that are transported to the pituitary gland by the hypothalamohypophyseal portal system illustrated in Figure 40-2.

There are six recognized hypophyseotropic hormones secreted from the median eminence of the hypothalamus:

- Growth hormone-releasing hormone (GHRH; somatocrinin)
- Growth hormone-inhibiting hormone (GHIH; somatostatin)
- Corticotropin-releasing hormone (CRH)
- Thyrotropin-releasing hormone (TRH)
- Gonadotropin-releasing hormone (GnRH)
- Prolactin-inhibiting hormone (PIH)

It is probable that a prolactin-releasing hormone (PRH) also exists; however, the exact substance has yet to be clearly identified.

Some hypophyseotropic hormones influence the secretion of more than one adenohypophyseal hormone. Gn-RH stimulates secretion of FSH and LH. TRH stimulates the secretion of TSH and prolactin. Somatostatin inhibits the secretion of growth hormone and TSH.

Growth Hormone (GH); Somatotropin (STH)

Human growth hormone (hGH) is a peptide hormone composed of 191 amino acids, and is secreted by the somatotrophs of the adenohypophysis primarily under hypothalamic control. The wide variety of factors that may affect GH secretion is summarized below.

Control of Secretion

Factors Promoting GH Secretion

GHRH (Somatocrinin)
Hypoglycemia and fasting
Elevated plasma levels of amino acids (eg, arginine)

Stress (physical or psychological)
Exercise
Deep sleep
Levodopa
Glucagon

Factors Inhibiting GH Secretion

GHIH (Somatostatin)
Hyperglycemia
Elevated plasma levels of free fatty acids
REM sleep
Cortisol
Alpha-adrenergic blocking agents
GH (negative feedback mechanism): GH secretion in response to hypoglycemia, fasting, and exercise appears to be reduced by obesity.

Actions

Effects on Growth. Growth is a complex phenomenon influenced by genetic, nutritional, and hormonal factors. In addition to growth hormone, the thyroid hormones, insulin, androgens, and estrogens play important roles in normal human growth and development at various times of the life cycle. GH accelerates overall body growth by increasing the mass of both skeletal and soft body tissues through hyperplasia (increased cell number) and hypertrophy (increased cell size).

The effects of GH are particularly evident in skeletal tissues where chondrogenesis (cartilage formation) and osteogenesis (bone formation) are enhanced, leading to an increase in linear growth and stature before epiphyseal closure and increased bone thickness following closure of the epiphyses.

Growth hormone stimulates certain tissues, notably the liver, to produce *somatomedins* or insulinlike growth factors (IGF-I and IGF-II). These low–molecular-weight peptides mediate the growth-promoting effects of GH, including the stimulation of collagen synthesis and chondrogenesis.

Metabolic Effects

- *Protein metabolism*: GH increases protein synthesis and nitrogen retention by enhancing the incorporation of amino acids into protein. The protein anabolic action results from 1) accelerated entry of amino acids into cells and 2) increased ribonucleic acid (RNA) synthesis. In muscle and liver, the protein anabolic effects are attributed directly to GH. However, in cartilage, bone, and other body tissues, the protein anabolic and growth-promoting actions are mediated by insulinlike growth factors (*somatomedins*).
- *Lipid metabolism*: GH stimulates the mobilization and utilization of fats by promoting lipolysis in adipose tissue, thus enabling the body to use stored fats as an energy source. The elevation of plasma levels of free fatty acids resulting from the hydrolysis of triglycerides (stored neutral fats) is potentially ketogenic.
- *Carbohydrate metabolism*: GH elevates blood glucose levels by increasing the hepatic output of glucose (gluconeogenesis) and impairing glucose transport into muscle and adipose tissue ("anti-insulin" action). Excessive secretion of GH may precipitate or increase the severity of clinical diabetes mellitus ("diabetogenic" effect).

Prolactin (PRL)

Control of Secretion

Prolactin (PRL) is a peptide hormone composed of 199 amino acids. Its secretion by the lactotrophs of the adenohypophysis is tonically suppressed by dopamine (also known as PIH) of hypothalamic origin. Dopamine antagonists (eg, antipsychotic drugs) promote PRL secretion by blocking dopamine receptors, whereas dopamine agonists (eg, bromocriptine) inhibit PRL secretion by activating dopamine receptors.

Secretion of PRL increases during pregnancy, peaking near the time of parturition. Suckling and tactile stimulation of the nipple increase PRL secretion.

Prolactin facilitates the secretion of dopamine in the hypothalamus, thereby regulating its own secretion by a negative feedback mechanism.

Actions

Prolactin initiates and maintains milk secretion from breasts primed for lactation by other hormones such as estrogens, progesterone, and insulin. It also appears to inhibit the effects of the gonadotropins and may prevent ovulation in lactating women. Excessive production of PRL (hyperprolactinemia), which may accompany some pituitary tumors, may cause anovulation and amenorrhea in women, and may lead to impotence and infertility in men.

Follicle-Stimulating Hormone (FSH)

Control of Secretion

Follicle-stimulating hormone (FSH) is a glycoprotein gonadotropic hormone whose secretion is stimulated by hypothalamic GnRH. *Inhibin*, a polypeptide produced by testicular Sertoli cells in the male and follicular granulosa cells in the female, acts directly on the adenohypophysis to inhibit FSH secretion.

Actions

Follicle-stimulating hormone directly stimulates the Sertoli cells in testicular seminiferous tubules, thereby promoting spermatogenesis in the male. In the female, FSH stimulates follicular growth and development within the ovaries. The actions of FSH are mediated by cyclic AMP.

Luteinizing Hormone (LH; Interstitial Cell Stimulating Hormone; ICSH)

Control of Secretion

Like FSH, LH is a glycoprotein hormone whose secretion is stimulated by GnRH. Testosterone inhibits LH secretion through a direct action on the adenohypophysis, as well as indirectly by inhibiting hypothalamic GnRH production.

The effects of female hormones on LH secretion are more complex. Constant, moderate levels of estrogen (without progesterone) have a negative feedback effect on LH, whereas high estrogen levels exert a positive feedback that leads to a surge in LH production. High levels of progesterone and estrogen (luteal phase of the ovulatory cycle) inhibit LH secretion.

Actions

In the male, this hormone stimulates testosterone production by testicular interstitial cells (of Leydig); hence the alternate name, interstitial cell stimulating hormone (ICSH).

In the female, LH promotes maturation of ovarian follicles and sustains their secretion of estrogens. LH is also responsible for ovulation and the formation of the corpus luteum. The actions of LH are mediated by cyclic AMP.

Thyroid-Stimulating Hormone (Thyrotropin; TSH)

Control of Secretion

Thyrotropin-releasing hormone (TRH) and cold (especially in infants) promote secretion of TSH by the thyrotrophs of the adenohypophysis. Elevated plasma levels of free thyroid hormones (T_3 and T_4) inhibit thyrotropin secretion as outlined in Figure 40-3. TSH secretion is inhibited by stress.

Actions

Thyroid-stimulating hormone maintains the structural integrity of the thyroid gland and promotes the synthesis and release of thyroid hormones thyroxine (T_4) and triiodothyronine (T_3). The actions of TSH on the thyroid gland are mediated by cyclic AMP, and they are detailed in the section on the thyroid gland.

Adrenocorticotropic Hormone (Corticotropin; ACTH)

Control of Secretion

Adrenocorticotropic hormone is a 39–amino-acid polypeptide derived from the prohormone pro-opiomelanocortin (POMC) produced by the corticotrophs of the adenohypophysis. Hydrolysis of POMC also produces beta-lipotropin, beta-endorphin, and melanocyte-stimulating hormone (MSH).

Adrenocorticotropic hormone (ACTH) is secreted in irregular bursts that follow a diurnal circadian rhythm, with peak production in the early morning. ACTH secretion is regulated by the hypophyseotropic hormone corticotropin-releasing hormone (CRH). The increased production of ACTH in response to many stressors appears to be mediated through the hypothalamus and CRH.

Elevated plasma free glucocorticoid (cortisol) levels inhibit both CRH and ACTH secretion.

Actions

Adrenocorticoptropic hormone exerts its tropic effects on the adrenal glands, promoting structural integrity and steroidogenesis in the adrenal cortex. The stimulation of corticosteroid production (steroidogenesis) in response to ACTH is mediated by the second messenger, cyclic AMP.

Disorders of the Adenohypophysis

Hypofunctional States

Hypopituitarism (Pituitary Insufficiency). In the adult, hypopituitarism may be manifested in a variety of forms, such as panhypopituitarism, Simmond's disease (pituitary cachexia), or Sheehan syndrome.

Pituitary insufficiency may be related to hypothalamic lesions, cysts or tumors affecting the pituitary, surgical hypophysectomy, infiltrative granulomatous disease, vascular collapse, or thrombosis.

The deficiency in the production of tropic hormones leads to functional deficiency and atrophy of target glands such as the adrenal cortex, thyroid, and gonads. Symptoms of pituitary insufficiency may include weakness; decreased resistance to stress, cold, and infection; sexual dysfunction (eg, infertility, amenorrhea, decreased secondary sex characteristics); sallow, dry, wrinkled skin; and hypotension.

Pituitary Dwarfism. The hallmark of hypopituitarism in children is growth retardation or dwarfism. Despite the small stature, the pituitary dwarf has normal body proportions. Hypoglycemia, hypogonadism, and hypothyroidism may also occur.

Hyperfunctional States

Gigantism and Acromegaly. Excessive secretion of growth hormone (GH) is usually caused by acidophilic adenomas. Hypersecretion of GH occurring before closure of the epiphyses leads to proportional but immense growth. An individual may grow to 7 or 8 feet in height; hence the term *gigantism*.

Excessive secretion of GH after epiphyseal closure results in *acromegaly*. Because the bones can no longer increase in length, overall height (stature) is not affected. However, the bones thicken considerably, an effect particularly noticeable in the face, hands, and feet. Overgrowth of the mandible results in prognathism (jaw protrusion) and separation of the lower teeth. The skeletal changes predispose to joint disorders such as osteoarthritis.

Increased sweating, thickening of the skin, and increased body hair (in women) are common. Hyperglycemia and glucose intolerance may be noted. Headaches and visual disturbances may result from pressure by the tumor.

Thyroid Gland

The hormones of the thyroid gland exert a wide spectrum of metabolic and physiologic actions that affect virtually every tissue in the body.

Anatomy

The thyroid gland is a bilobed organ overlying the trachea anteriorly. The thyroid gland is composed of numerous closely packed spheres or follicles.

Each follicle consists of a simple cuboidal epithelium (*follicular cells*) enclosing a lumen or cavity containing a viscous hyaline substance termed *colloid*. The chief constituent of the colloid is the iodinated glycoprotein *thyroglobulin*.

Interspersed among the follicles are small clusters of *parafollicular* (C) cells, which secrete *calcitonin*, a hormone affecting calcium metabolism.

Thyroid Hormones

The follicular cells of the thyroid gland secrete two hormones, thyroxine (3,3′, 5,5′-tetraiodothyronine or T_4) and 3,3′, 5-triiodothyronine (T_3). The plasma levels of these hormones are

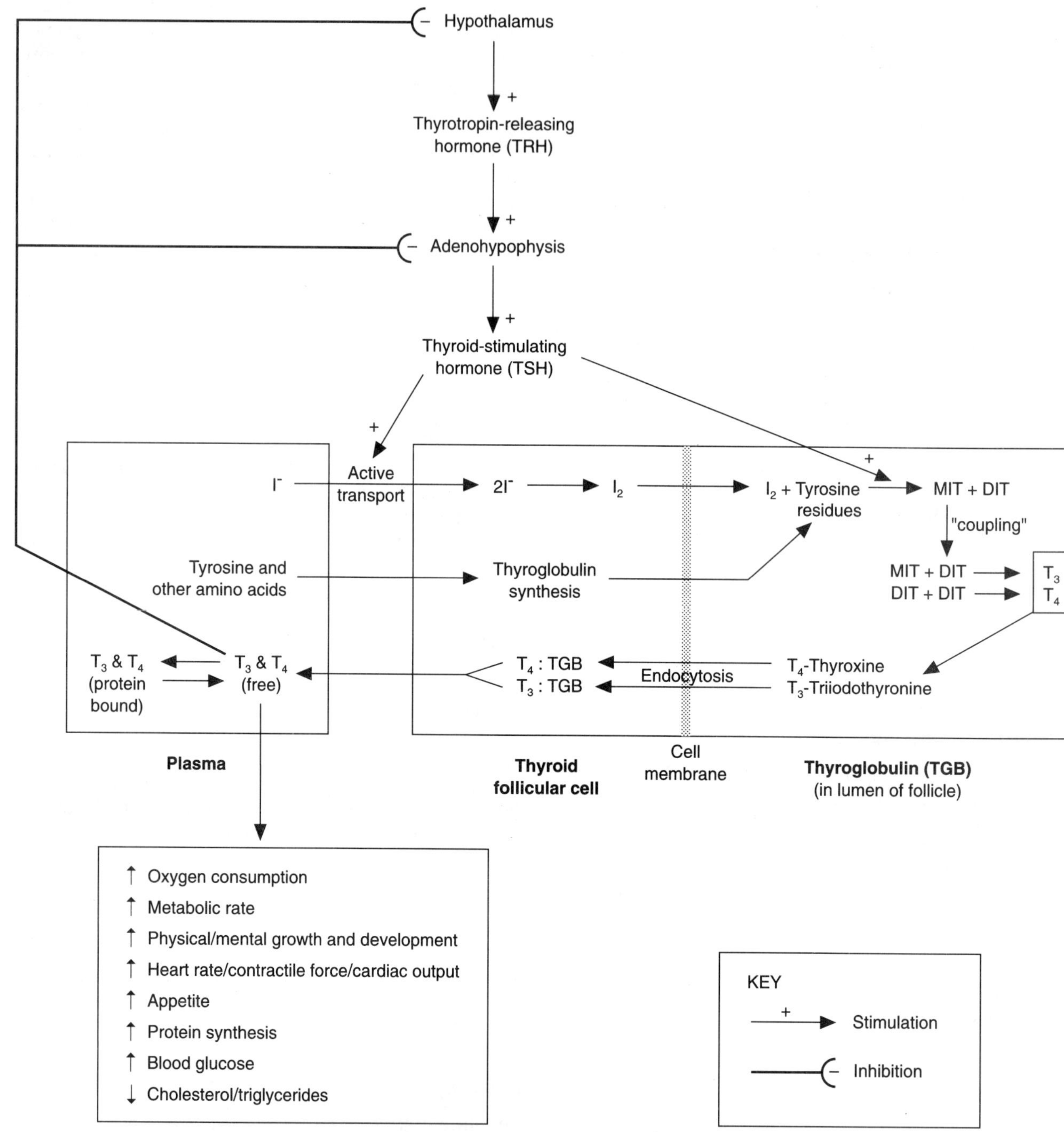

Figure 40-3. Synthesis, storage, release, and actions of thyroid hormones (see text for further information).

regulated by the hypothalamopituitary axis as outlined in Figure 40-3. Intrinsic (intrathyroidal) mechanisms, as well as bioavailability of iodine, influence thyroid hormone production.

Biosynthesis of Thyroid Hormones

1. *Iodide uptake*: Ingested iodine is readily absorbed from the GI tract in the reduced iodide state. Iodide ions are actively transported from the blood into the thyroid follicles by an energy-requiring "trapping" mechanism often called the *iodide pump*. The normal thyroid:serum ratio of iodide is 25:1. The uptake of iodide is enhanced by TSH and may be blocked by anions such as perchlorate and thiocyanate.
2. *Oxidation to iodine*: On entering the colloid, iodide is rapidly oxidized to iodine in the presence of peroxidase enzymes. Thiouracil appears to inhibit peroxidase activity.
3. *Iodination of tyrosine*: Free molecular iodine spontaneously combines with tyrosine residues on the thyroglobulin (TGB) to form 3-monoiodotyrosine (MIT) and 3,5-diiodotyrosine (DIT). This organic iodination is enhanced by TSH and blocked by agents such as

propylthiouracil and methimazole. Goitrogens found in cabbage, kale, and turnips, as well as cobalt and phenylbutazone, also block organification of iodine.
4. *Coupling reaction*: Two iodinated tyrosines combine to form either T_3 or T_4. The coupling occurs within the thyroglobulin molecule, and the reaction appears to be promoted by TSH.
5. *Storage and release of thyroid hormones*: T_3 and T_4 remain stored within the colloid bound to thyroglobulin until a stimulus for secretion arrives. On stimulation by TSH, portions of the TGB (colloid) are engulfed by microvilli that extend from the apical surface of the follicular cells. Droplets of the engulfed colloid fuse with lysosomes, and proteolytic enzymes release T_3 and T_4 from the TGB. The lipophilic hormones (T_3 and T_4) readily diffuse to nearby capillaries and enter the bloodstream.

Thyroid-stimulating hormone, acting through cyclic AMP, increases the production of thyroid hormones by promoting virtually every step in the biosynthetic process, including the synthesis of TGB and the eventual release of T_3 and T_4 from storage.

Transport

Circulating thyroid hormones bind specifically with *thyroxine-binding globulin* and *thyroxine-binding prealbumin*, and non-specifically with serum albumin. The extent of plasma protein binding can be measured as protein-bound iodine (PBI).

Only the small fraction of circulating thyroid hormones that is in the free (unbound) form is physiologically active and inhibitory to TSH secretion.

Several drugs, including phenytoin and the salicylates, compete for plasma protein-binding sites, thus lowering the PBI and increasing the percentage of free, active hormones. High levels of estrogen, such as those occurring in pregnancy or during oral contraceptive therapy, elevate plasma protein levels, thereby increasing PBI levels.

Fate

Thyroid hormones are inactivated by deiodination, deamination, decarboxylation, or conjugation with glucuronic acid or sulfate. Much of the iodine released during biodegradation is recycled and reused for synthesis of new hormones. The remainder is excreted in the urine. Metabolism occurs chiefly in the liver, and excretion is mainly through the kidneys. The conjugated hormones are excreted through the bile and eliminated in the feces.

Actions

The thyroid hormones increase the rate of metabolism, total heat production, and oxygen consumption in most body tissues. Exceptions include the adult brain, spleen, lymph nodes, uterus, and testes. The thyroid hormones promote normal physical growth and development, and they are essential for normal myelination and development of the nervous system in early life. Hypothyroid infants exhibit severe mental retardation and defective myelination of nerve fibers.

The thyroid hormones increase the number and affinity of beta-adrenergic cardiac receptors for catecholamines, thereby increasing heart rate, myocardial contractile force, and cardiac output.

The metabolic actions of the thyroid hormones are somewhat complex, being dependent on the level of the thyroid hormones, as well as on the presence of other hormones, for example, catecholamines and insulin. In normal physiologic amounts, the thyroid hormones stimulate protein synthesis, increase lipid turnover, lower plasma cholesterol, and promote GI absorption of glucose.

T_3 is more potent and more rapidly active than T_4; in fact, the latter may be considered a prohormone, since most target cells convert T_4 into T_3.

The pharmacologic uses of the thyroid hormones are discussed in Chapter 42.

Disorders of the Thyroid

Simple Goiter

Goiter, an enlargement of the thyroid gland, most commonly results from an insufficient dietary intake of iodine. The gland becomes hyperplastic and filled with colloid lacking in iodine. TSH levels are usually high because plasma levels of free thyroid hormones are insufficient to suppress TSH production by the adenohypophysis. More rarely, goiter may result from excessive intake of goitrogens (such as cabbage) or may be due to congenital lack of biosynthetic enzymes.

Transient simple goiter may occur during pregnancy or at the onset of puberty, when the demand for thyroid hormones increases.

Hypothyroidism

Hypothyroidism may result from primary disease of the thyroid gland itself, or it may be secondary to a deficiency of pituitary TSH or hypothalamic TRH.

Because thyroid hormones affect a wide range of physiologic and metabolic processes, including growth and development, the time of onset of a deficiency state is most important.

Cretinism (Congenital or Neonatal Hypothyroidism). Cretinism results from fetal or neonatal thyroid hormone deficiency, which may be caused by anatomic dysgenesis of the thyroid, iodine deficiency, or inborn errors of iodine metabolism.

Cretinism is characterized by mental retardation and dwarfism caused by delayed skeletal maturation. Other signs of this disorder include the presence of thick, dry skin; large, protruding tongue; and umbilical hernia. The child appears apathetic or lethargic and has a low body temperature. TSH and serum cholesterol levels are elevated.

Myxedema (Adult Hypothyroidism). Primary myxedema may follow thyroidectomy, eradication of the thyroid by radioactive iodine, ingestion of goitrogens, or chronic thyroiditis. Idiopathic atrophy, possibly involving autoimmune mechanisms, also may lead to hypothyroidism.

Early symptoms of myxedema include cold intolerance, weakness, fatigue, dryness of the skin, thinning hair, and thin brittle nails. Among later signs are weight gain, pallor, dyspnea, peripheral edema, anginal pain, bradycardia, and slow speech. Cardiac enlargement may result from pericardial effusion, and macrocytic anemia may occur.

The low turnover of protein leads to the accumulation of a protein-rich fluid under the skin, lending a puffiness and thickness to the skin.

Manifestations of personality changes and organic psychoses ("myxedema madness") may occur.

It is noteworthy that myxedematous patients are unusually sensitive to opiates and may die of average doses of these agents.

Hyperthyroidism (Thyrotoxicosis)

Hyperthyroid states are characterized by some degree of glandular hyperplasia and excessive thyroid hormone production. Nervousness, excessive sweating, heat intolerance, warm moist skin, weight loss despite increased appetite, restlessness, and tremor are common signs of hyperthyroidism. Tachycardia, high pulse pressure, and systolic hypertension frequently occur.

When associated with toxic diffuse goiter, elevated metabolic rate and exophthalmos, hyperthyroidism is termed *Graves' disease*. Graves' disease is an autoimmune disorder associated with the presence of autoantibodies exerting thyroid-stimulating activity.

The treatment of thyroid disorders is detailed in Chapter 42.

Calcitonin

Calcitonin (thyrocalcitonin) is a 32–amino-acid peptide hormone secreted by the parafollicular (C) cells of the thyroid gland in response to *hypercalcemia* (elevated blood calcium). Several gastrointestinal hormones (eg, gastrin, cholecystokinin [CCK], secretin) also stimulate calcitonin secretion.

Calcitonin lowers plasma calcium and phosphate levels by inhibiting osteoclastic activity, thereby decreasing the resorption of bone. Calcitonin also inhibits renal tubular reabsorption of calcium and phosphate, thus increasing urinary excretion of these ions. The actions of calcitonin are mediated by the second messenger, cyclic AMP. Because calcitonin is not the principal calcium-regulating hormone, no clinical syndromes are associated with abnormal rates of calcitonin secretion. Clinically, calcitonin may be useful for reducing the accelerated osteoclastic activity associated with Paget's disease and has also been employed to slow osteoporotic changes occurring after onset of menopause.

Parathyroid Glands

The parathyroid glands, usually four in number, are embedded in the dorsal surface of the thyroid gland.

In response to *hypocalcemia* (low plasma calcium), the chief cells of the parathyroid glands secrete a single 84–amino-acid polypeptide hormone known as *parathyroid hormone* (PTH).

Parathyroid hormone regulates serum calcium levels by exerting its effects on the following target tissues:

- *Bone*: PTH stimulates bone resorption by activating the bone-destroying osteoclasts. The demineralization of bone elevates plasma calcium and phosphate levels; however, the renal actions of PTH lead to a net *decrease* in plasma phosphate levels.
- *Kidneys*: PTH promotes renal tubular reabsorption of calcium and increases urinary excretion of phosphate by blocking its reabsorption. PTH also stimulates the activity of a renal enzyme that catalyzes the formation of *calcitriol*, an active metabolite of vitamin D (see Chapter 75). Calcitriol elevates plasma calcium and phosphate levels primarily by promoting the intestinal absorption of both ions, but also by increasing renal tubular reabsorption of calcium and phosphate.

The major actions of PTH are mediated by cyclic AMP. Calcium metabolism and the clinical uses of PTH and calcitonin are discussed in Chapter 43.

Disorders of the Parathyroid Glands

Hypoparathyroidism

Hypoparathyroidism, which may result from congenital absence, disease, injury, or removal of the parathyroid glands, causes *hypocalcemia* and *hyperphosphatemia*. Varying degrees of neuromuscular irritability, related to the extent of hypocalcemia, may be manifested, ranging from tingling sensations (paresthesias), muscular twitching and cramping, to tetany. Mental disturbances and respiratory difficulties that mimic asthma also may occur.

Hyperparathyroidism

Primary hyperparathyroidism may result from adenoma, carcinoma, or primary hyperplasia of the parathyroid glands. It also may be associated with ectopic production of PTH by carcinomas elsewhere in the body.

Signs and symptoms characteristic of hyperparathyroidism include *hyper*calcemia, anorexia, vomiting, thirst, polyuria, and renal calculi (kidney stones). Skeletal manifestations may range from simple joint or back pain to pathologic fractures and cystic bone lesions throughout the skeleton (osteitis fibrosa cystica). The skeletal abnormalities result from the excessive demineralization of bone, whereas the occurrence of kidney stones is related to excessive renal excretion of minerals (calcium and phosphate).

Pancreas

The endocrine functions of the pancreas are performed by the *islets of Langerhans* (also called pancreatic islets)—small, highly vascularized masses of cells scattered throughout the pancreas and representing only 1% to 3% of the entire organ.

The islets of Langerhans contain four types of secretory cells, as follows:

Alpha (A) cells, which secrete *glucagon*
Beta (B) cells, which secrete *insulin*
Delta (D) cells, which secrete *somatostatin*
PP (F) cells, which secrete *pancreatic polypeptide*

Insulin-secreting beta cells are the most numerous, making up to 75% of the islet cell population. The A cells containing glucagon comprise approximately 20% of islet cell mass, whereas the somatostatin-containing D cells account for 3% to 5% of pancreatic islet cells. The F cells make up less than 2% of islet cells and secrete a polypeptide that slows food absorption in humans, but whose exact physiologic significance is unclear.

A paracrine relationship exists within the pancreatic islets, with one hormone affecting the secretion of other pancreatic hormones. Somatostatin inhibits the secretion of insulin, glucagon, and pancreatic polypeptide. Insulin inhibits the secretion of glucagon, whereas glucagon stimulates the secretion of insulin and somatostatin.

Glucagon

Glucagon is a 29–amino-acid polypeptide hormone secreted by the alpha cells of the pancreatic islets primarily in response to *hypoglycemia* (low blood sugar). Glucagon is essentially a catabolic hormone that decreases carbohydrate and lipid energy stores and increases the amount of glucose and fatty acids available for oxidation.

Control of Secretion

The plasma glucose concentration is the major physiologic regulator of glucagon secretion. In addition to hypoglycemia and fasting, the following factors promote glucagon secretion: amino acids, exercise, stress, gastrin, cortisol, CCK, acetylcholine, and beta-adrenergic stimulation. The rate of glucagon secretion is inhibited by elevated blood levels of glucose and free fatty acids, and by somatostatin, insulin, secretin, phenytoin, and alpha-adrenergic stimulation.

Major Actions

- *Carbohydrate metabolism*: Glucagon stimulates hepatic glycogenolysis, thereby promoting the release of glucose from liver glycogen stores. This action is mediated by cyclic AMP, which stimulates protein kinase activity, leading to the activation of phosphorylase, the glycogenolytic enzyme. Glucagon also interacts with hormone receptors coupled to the activation of phospholipase C, which eventually leads to calcium influx and stimulation of glycogenolysis. In addition to stimulating hepatic glycogenolysis, glucagon inhibits glycogenesis and raises the rate of hepatic gluconeogenesis. The net effect is an elevation of blood glucose (*hyperglycemia*).
- *Lipid metabolism*: Glucagon stimulates lipolysis, thereby increasing the release of free fatty acids and glycerol from adipose tissue. Glucagon also enhances hepatic ketogenesis by facilitating conversion of fatty acids to ketone bodies.
- *Protein metabolism*: Glucagon exerts a catabolic action on hepatic proteins and inhibits the incorporation of amino acids into hepatic protein.
- *Cardiac effects*: Large amounts of exogenous glucagon produce a positive inotropic effect on the heart by increasing myocardial levels of cyclic AMP.

Insulin

Structure, Biosynthesis, and Secretion

Insulin is a polypeptide hormone composed of 51 amino acids arranged in two chains (A and B), linked by disulfide bridges.

Insulin is derived from a large polypeptide precursor—*proinsulin*—which is synthesized in the endoplasmic reticulum of beta cells and packaged into membrane-bounded granules within the Golgi complex.

A connecting (C) peptide is removed from the proinsulin molecule by proteolytic cleavage before the secretion of insulin in its biologically active form.

Insulin secretion occurs through exocytosis (emiocytosis), a calcium-dependent process that is enhanced by cyclic AMP and potassium. On entering the circulation, insulin is transported largely in free molecular form, not bound to plasma proteins.

Control of Secretion

The secretion of insulin is regulated primarily by the blood glucose level, with an elevation of blood glucose (hyperglycemia), increasing both production and release of insulin. Ingested glucose effects a far greater secretion of insulin than an equivalent amount of intravenously administered glucose because several gastrointestinal hormones, including gastrin, secretin, CCK, gastric inhibitory polypeptide (GIP), and glucagon, stimulate insulin secretion.

Insulin secretion is also increased by mannose, certain amino acids, vagal stimulation (acetylcholine), cyclic AMP, beta-adrenergic stimulation, potassium, and oral hypoglycemic drugs such as tolbutamide. Hyperglycemia, somatostatin, alpha-adrenergic stimulation, thiazide diuretics, phenytoin, and diazoxide inhibit insulin secretion.

Major Actions

- *Cellular membrane permeability*: Insulin facilitates the transport of glucose across selected cell membranes, thereby accelerating the entry of glucose into muscle, adipose tissue, fibroblasts, leukocytes, mammary glands, and the anterior pituitary. The transport of glucose into the liver, brain, renal tubules, intestinal mucosa, and erythrocytes is *independent* of insulin. Exercise and hypoxia mimic the effect of insulin on cellular permeability to glucose in skeletal muscle. The insulin requirements of diabetics engaging in strenuous exercise may be reduced substantially and therefore must be monitored carefully to avoid hypoglycemia. Insulin also increases cellular permeability to amino acids, fatty acids, and potassium, particularly in muscle and adipose tissue.
- *Carbohydrate metabolism*: Insulin effectively lowers the level of blood glucose by enhancing the transport and peripheral utilization of glucose. Insulin increases muscle and liver glycogen stores by activating enzymes involved in glycogenesis while inhibiting those that produce glycogenolysis. Glycolytic enzymes are also activated by insulin, whereas several enzymes involved in gluconeogenesis are inhibited.
- *Protein metabolism*: Insulin is strongly anabolic, increasing protein synthesis and inhibiting protein catabolism. Insulin increases the incorporation of amino acids into protein by accelerating the entry of amino acids into the cell and possibly by increasing RNA synthesis.
- *Lipid metabolism*: Insulin stimulates formation of triglycerides (*lipogenesis*) and inhibits their breakdown (*lipolysis*). Insulin accelerates synthesis of fatty acid and glycerol phosphate and enhances cellular permeability to fatty acids, leading to increased deposition of triglycerides in adipose tissue.

Pancreatic Somatostatin

Unlike glucagon and insulin, pancreatic somatostatin does not directly regulate intermediary metabolism. Rather, it slows digestion and absorption of nutrients by exerting several inhibitory effects on digestive processes (eg, reduced gastric acid secretion, decreased gastric emptying, and inhibition of CCK secretion and gallbladder contraction).

Pancreatic somatostatin secretion is stimulated by elevations in blood glucose and amino acid levels, as well as by glucagon and gastrointestinal hormones (eg, CCK). The paracrine actions of somatostatin in the pancreatic islets have been discussed previously.

Disorders of Glucose Metabolism

Hypoglycemia

Hypoglycemic states are characterized by the presence of an abnormally low blood glucose level. This represents a threat to the brain, which depends on glucose as its source of energy.

Normally, when the blood glucose falls below a critical level, insulin secretion is inhibited and release of glucagon, epinephrine, GH, and glucocorticoids is increased. Only the release of the catecholamine epinephrine leads to observable symptoms, such as sweating, palpitation, anxiety, and weakness.

Impairment of brain function, confusion, amnesia, bizarre behavior, or blurred vision may occur if the blood glucose decreases to below a level of 40 mg/dL. Severe hypoglycemia may ultimately lead to hypothermia, convulsions, and coma. Hypoglycemic disorders may be divided into two types: *fasting* (food-deprived) and *postprandial* (food-stimulated or reactive).

Possible causes of fasting hypoglycemia are:

- *Hyperinsulinism*: insulinomas (insulin-secreting tumors of the pancreas), overdosage with exogenous insulin or sulfonylurea drugs (oral hypoglycemic agents)
- *Endocrine disorders*: Addison's disease (adrenocortical insufficiency), hypopituitarism (eg, Simmond's disease), myxedema
- *Liver disease*: hepatic necrosis, malignancy, or advanced cirrhosis, which may lead to impairment of glycogenesis and gluconeogenesis, thereby reducing liver glycogen stores and hepatic output of glucose
- *Acute alcoholism*
- *Extrapancreatic tumors*

The possible causes of *postprandial (reactive) hypoglycemia* include early or alimentary hypoglycemia, which may follow gastric intestinal surgery or result from increased vagal tone, and late hypoglycemia (early or occult diabetes mellitus).

Diabetes Mellitus

Diabetes mellitus is a chronic disorder of metabolism characterized by carbohydrate intolerance and inappropriate hyperglycemia resulting from a deficiency of insulin secretion or a reduction in its biologic efficacy ("relative" insulin deficiency).

The insulin deficiency, be it absolute or relative, triggers a series of biochemical changes in the metabolism of carbohydrates, lipids, and proteins, as outlined in Figure 40-4. These metabolic abnormalities lead to the classic symptoms of diabetes mellitus—*polyuria* (frequent urination), *polydipsia* (excessive thirst), *polyphagia* (hunger), and fatigue.

Long-term, serious complications of diabetes mellitus include gangrene, visual impairment resulting from proliferative retinopathy, myocardial infarction, polyneuropathy, and uremia. Pathologic changes in the blood vessels, particularly in the microcirculation (microangiopathy), appear to underlie most of these complications.

Diabetes mellitus is a disorder of heterogenous origin. Predisposition to diabetes is inherited, although the genetic factors are complex. There are two generally recognized types of dia-

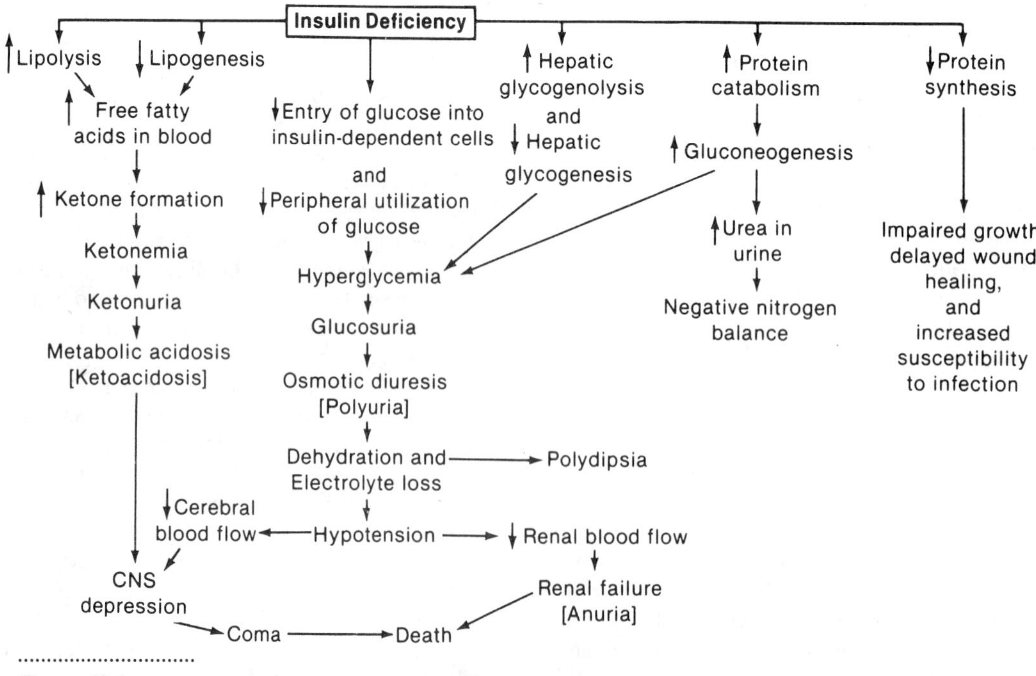

Figure 40-4. Metabolic consequences of severe insulin deficiency.

betes mellitus: type I (or *insulin dependent*), IDDM, and type II (or *non–insulin-dependent*), NIDDM.

Insulin-Dependent Diabetes Mellitus—Type I; IDDM. IDDM generally occurs in nonobese persons before the age of 30, most commonly in adolescence. Circulating insulin is virtually absent, and the beta pancreatic cells fail to respond to all normal stimuli for insulin secretion. The islet beta cell reserve is markedly reduced or totally absent, and ketosis usually develops in the course of the disease. Patients respond to exogenous insulin, which is required to reverse the hyperglycemia and the general catabolic state and to prevent ketosis.

Immunopathologic (autoimmune) mechanisms have been strongly implicated in this type of diabetes. Specific histocompatibility (HLA) antigens have been linked to this disorder, and circulating autoantibodies to islet cells have been detected in some patients early in the course of the disease.

Several viruses have been associated epidemiologically with the onset of type I diabetes. It is likely that genetic factors and environmental influences interact to trigger the autoimmune response that leads to beta cell destruction.

Non–Insulin-Dependent Diabetes Mellitus—Type II; NIDDM. This type of diabetes mellitus usually has its onset after the age of 40, although it may occur at any age. Obesity is a major risk factor to the development of NIDDM. Beta cell mass may be only moderately reduced, and autoimmunity is not demonstrable. There is no correlation with HLA antigens; however, there is a strong genetic component. Ketosis rarely occurs.

In at least some cases of NIDDM, a defect in insulin binding to cellular receptors is likely. Insulin apparently exerts a negative feedback control over its own receptors. In the presence of obesity, certain tissues (such as muscle and adipose tissue) display insensitivity to insulin. The hyperinsulinism that results from chronic excessive caloric intake and sustained beta cell stimulation apparently reduces (ie, "downregulates") the number of available insulin receptors and leads to glucose intolerance.

In addition to obesity and excessive carbohydrate intake, diabetes mellitus may be precipitated by pancreatitis, pregnancy, and endocrine disorders associated with overproduction of GH, glucocorticoids, or catecholamines.

Almost all forms of clinical and experimental diabetes mellitus are associated with increased secretion of glucagon, a potent hyperglycemic hormone whose glycogenolytic, gluconeogenic, lipolytic, and ketogenic actions are intensified by insulin deficiency.

Adrenal Glands

The *adrenal* (suprarenal) glands are paired yellowish masses of tissue situated at the superior pole of each kidney. Each gland consists of two distinct entities—an outer *adrenal cortex* and an inner *adrenal medulla*—that differ in embryologic origin, character, and function.

Adrenal Medulla

The *adrenal medulla* develops from the embryonic ectoderm. It remains functionally associated with the sympathetic nervous system, being essentially a modified sympathetic ganglion whose postganglionic neurons have lost their axons and become secretory.

Histologically, the adrenal medulla contains large, ovoid cells arranged in clumps or irregular cords around numerous blood vessels. The medullary cells, often termed *chromaffin cells* because their granules possess affinity for chromium salts, secrete the catecholamine hormones epinephrine (adrenaline) and norepinephrine (noradrenaline). The principal secretory product is epinephrine, with norepinephrine normally accounting for only 20% of the total secretion.

Adrenal medullary secretion of the catecholamines is physiologically controlled by the posterior hypothalamus. The hormones are stored in cellular granules, bound to adenosine triphosphate (ATP) and protein, and are released in response to the following stimuli: sympathetic nervous system activation, hypoglycemia, pain, hypoxia, hypotension, cold, emotional stress, acetylcholine, histamine, and nicotine.

Epinephrine and norepinephrine are rapidly metabolized to inactive products, principally by the liver and kidneys. Major products of biodegradation include metanephrine, normetanephrine, and vanillylmandelic acid (VMA). These appear in the urine and may be assayed during clinical diagnosis.

Actions of Adrenal Medullary Hormones

Epinephrine and norepinephrine mimic the effects of sympathetic nerve discharge, producing the following effects:

- Direct increase in cardiac rate and myocardial force of contraction
- Dilation of coronary and skeletal muscle blood vessels
- Constriction of the cutaneous and visceral vasculature
- Relaxation of respiratory smooth muscle
- Inhibition of GI motility
- Pupillary dilation (mydriasis)
- Glycogenolysis in liver and muscle
- Lipolysis

The cardiac excitatory effects and the metabolic actions of lipolysis and glycogenolysis are mediated by cyclic AMP, the latter involving the activation of phosphorylase enzyme by protein kinase.

The catecholamines also elevate the metabolic rate (calorigenic action), stimulate the central nervous system, increase alertness, and stimulate respiration.

Clinical Disorders

Adrenal medullary function is not essential to life; therefore, hyposecretion of adrenal medullary hormones does not constitute a recognized clinical entity.

Pheochromocytoma. Pheochromocytoma is a chromaffin-cell tumor of the sympathoadrenal system, most commonly involving one of the adrenal glands. It is characterized by hypersecretion of the catecholamines epinephrine and norepinephrine, the latter usually dominating. Clinical manifestations of pheochromocytoma include paroxysmal or persistent hypertension, severe headaches, tachycardia, profuse sweating, epigastric pain, nausea, irritability, and dyspnea. Metabolic signs of this disorder include hyperglycemia, increased basal metabolic rate, weight loss, and elevated levels of urinary catecholamines or their metabolites.

Adrenal Cortex

The adrenal cortex develops from the mesoderm during embryonic life. The cells of the adrenal cortex, which are arranged in continuous cords separated by capillaries, are characterized by an abundance of mitochondria, endoplasmic reticulum, and accumulation of lipid.

Adrenal cortical tissue is structurally arranged into three concentric regions or zones: a thin outer zona glomerulosa, a thick middle zona fasciculata, and an inner zona reticularis bordering on the adrenal medulla.

Chemically, the steroid hormones of the adrenal cortex, the *adrenocorticoids*, are all derivatives of cholesterol. The adrenocorticoid hormones are usually divided into three functional groups: the *mineralocorticoids*, such as aldosterone, which regulate electrolyte and water balance; the *glucocorticoids*, such as cortisol, which affect carbohydrate, protein, and fat metabolism; and the *adrenogenital steroids* or *sex hormones*.

The adrenogenital steroids are of three types: *androgens* (such as dehydroepiandrosterone), *estrogens* (such as estradiol), and *progestins* (such as progesterone).

Under normal physiologic conditions the adrenogenital steroids are secreted (under ACTH control) in minute amounts, and therefore they exert minimal effects on reproductive functions. Excessive secretion of adrenal androgens results in precocious pseudopuberty in boys, and causes masculinization of females (*adrenogenital syndrome*).

Mineralocorticoids

Control of Secretion and Actions. Aldosterone is the principal physiologic mineralocorticoid secreted by the zona glomerulosa. Its secretion is regulated primarily by the renin–angiotensin mechanism described in Chapter 30. The plasma concentrations of sodium and potassium are involved in the control of aldosterone secretion. Hyperkalemia (elevated plasma potassium) exerts a direct stimulating effect on the zona glomerulosa, whereas hyponatremia (low plasma sodium) activates the renin-angiotensin mechanism. Atrial natriuretic hormone (ANH) inhibits renin secretion, and it also reduces the responsiveness of the cells in the zona glomerulosa to angiotensin II.

Other factors contributing to the control of aldosterone secretion include blood volume and ACTH, the latter exerting a limited, nonselective stimulatory effect.

Aldosterone plays a major physiologic role in the maintenance of electrolyte and fluid balance by promoting the renal tubular reabsorption of sodium and the secretion of potassium and hydrogen. Aldosterone binds to nuclear receptors and stimulates DNA-directed RNA synthesis leading to increased formation of specific proteins involved in sodium and potassium transport.

A similar sodium-retaining, potassium-excreting action is exerted on other target tissues, including salivary glands and sweat glands.

Glucocorticoids

Control of Secretion and Actions. Glucocorticoid secretion, which occurs primarily in the zona fasciculata, is controlled by ACTH. A variety of stressful stimuli, including anxiety, fear, hypoglycemia, hypotension, and hemorrhage, increase secretion of adrenocorticotropic hormone–releasing hormone (CRH) from the hypothalamus. CRH promotes ACTH secretion by the adenohypophysis, and ACTH stimulates adrenal cortical secretory activity, thereby elevating blood levels of cortisol (the principal physiologic glucocorticoid). Elevated blood levels of free cortisol normally exert a negative feedback control over further secretion of CRH and ACTH. Prolonged ACTH secretion results in hypertrophy and hyperplasia of the adrenal cortex and excessive secretion of all adrenocorticoid hormones. The metabolic and physiologic actions of the glucocorticoids are summarized below. The pharmacologic actions and clinical uses of these hormones are discussed in Chapter 45.

- *Carbohydrate metabolism*: Glucocorticoids stimulate hepatic gluconeogenesis and inhibit peripheral uptake and utilization of glucose by skeletal muscle and adipose tissue, thereby promoting hyperglycemia. Hepatic glycogenesis is also enhanced.
- *Protein metabolism*: Glucocorticoids exert protein catabolic and antianabolic actions, promoting the breakdown of existing proteins while inhibiting the incorporation of amino acids into new proteins.
- *Lipid metabolism*: Glucocorticoids inhibit lipogenesis and favor mobilization of fats from adipose tissues. When present in large amounts, these hormones favor redistribution of adipose stores by promoting loss of fat from the extremities, and accumulation of fat depots in central body regions (eg, "moon face" and "buffalo hump" formation).
- *Permissive Actions*: Glucocorticoids are essential for normal vascular reactivity to the catecholamines. Other permissive effects include support for the metabolic actions (particularly lipolysis) of the catecholamines and glucagon.
- *Blood and immunologic effects*: Glucocorticoids inhibit the immune response, cause involution of lymphoid tissue, and reduce blood levels of lymphocytes, eosinophils, and basophils. These hormones also stimulate erythropoiesis and elevate circulating levels of platelets and neutrophils.
- *GI tract effects*: Glucocorticoid hormones stimulate gastric acid and pepsin secretion and inhibit the production of protective mucus, thereby favoring development of gastric ulcers.

Disorders of the Adrenal Cortex

Addison's Disease. *Addison's disease* (chronic adrenocortical insufficiency) may result from idiopathic adrenocortical atrophy, adrenocortical destruction by disease (eg, tuberculosis or cancer), or deficiency of ACTH or CRH secretion.

Weakness and fatigability are early signs of the disease, and weight loss, dehydration, and hypotension are characteristic. Emotional changes and GI disturbances (such as anorexia, nausea, vomiting, diarrhea) frequently occur. Hyperpigmentation is a major characteristic of primary adrenocortical insufficiency, with increased pigmentation being prominent on skin folds, pressure points (bony prominences), extensor surfaces, nipples, perineum, tongue, and buccal mucosa.

In Addison's disease, aldosterone (mineralocorticoid) deficiency results in increased excretion of sodium and retention of potassium. The salt and water depletion causes severe dehydration, reduced circulatory volume, hypotension, and eventual circulatory collapse.

Glucocorticoid (cortisol) deficiency leads to reduced gluconeogenesis, hypoglycemia, diminished hepatic glycogen, and extreme insulin sensitivity. The inability to withstand stress (such as infection, trauma, surgery) may result in acute adrenal insufficiency (adrenal crisis).

Cushing's Syndrome. This is a clinical state characterized by glucocorticoid excess resulting from adrenocortical tumors, hypersecretion of ACTH, or from the administration of large amounts of exogenous corticosteroids or ACTH.

Clinical manifestations of this syndrome include truncal obesity, moon face, and buffalo hump, resulting from the characteristic redistribution of fat from the extremities to central body regions (abdomen, face, and upper back). The increased central subcutaneous fat depots stretch the skin, rupturing the subdermal tissue and causing formation of purple striae.

Excessive protein catabolism results in protein depletion and causes thin skin, muscular wasting, easy bruising, and poor wound healing. Osteoporosis develops, predisposing the patient to fractures and skeletal deformities.

Increased gluconeogenesis and decreased peripheral utilization of glucose result in hyperglycemia and glucose intolerance, and frank diabetes mellitus may develop in genetically predisposed individuals.

Hypertension and renal calculi frequently occur, and psychiatric disturbances are common.

Primary Hyperaldosteronism (Conn's Syndrome). A clinical state resulting from excessive production of the mineralocorticoid aldosterone, this syndrome is generally characterized by potassium depletion, sodium retention, hypertension, polyuria, fatigue, and muscular weakness. Hypokalemic alkalosis and tetany also may be observed.

Gonadal Hormones

The physiologic and metabolic actions of the gonadal hormones, together with their clinical uses, are reviewed in Chapter 46 (Estrogens and Progestins) and Chapter 48 (Androgens and Anabolic Steroids). The menstrual (endometrial) cycle is presented schematically in Chapter 47, Figure 47-1.

41
Hypophysial Hormones

Hormones of the Adenohypophysis

- Adrenocorticotropic hormone
- Growth Hormone
- Thyroid-stimulating hormone

Gonadotropin-Releasing Hormones

- Nafarelin
- Histrelin

Hormones of the Neurohypophysis

- Vasopressin
- Desmopressin
- Lypressin
- Oxytocin

Nonhypophysial Oxytocics

- Ergonovine
- Methylergonovine

The *hypophysis*, or pituitary gland, is composed of two major divisions, the *adenohypophysis* (anterior lobe), which contains at least six hormones, and the *neurohypophysis* (posterior lobe), which contains two hormones. Virtually no bodily function is exempt from the influence of at least one of these eight hypophysial hormones, which collectively serve to regulate and integrate the physiologic processes necessary for the maintenance of homeostasis. The synthesis, storage, release, and function of these hormones are reviewed in Chapter 40.

Hormones of the Adenohypophysis

Of the six principal hormones of the adenohypophysis, growth hormone (GH), adrenocorticotropic hormone (ACTH), and thyroid-stimulating hormone (TSH) are available clinically as purified preparations. GH is a purified polypeptide of recombinant DNA origin containing the identical sequence of the 191 amino acids constituting endogenous growth hormone. ACTH is a 39–amino-acid polypeptide extracted from pituitary glands of animals. TSH is a purified extract of the hormone from bovine pituitary glands. Because these three hormones are peptides, they must be given parenterally, because they would be quickly destroyed in gastric juice if taken by mouth. Further, because ACTH and TSH are naturally derived products, their use is associated with the possibility of allergic reactions. GH is now prepared synthetically and is virtually devoid of hypersensitivity problems.

The two adenohypophysial gonadotropins, *follicle-stimulating hormone (FSH)* and *luteinizing hormone (LH)*, are extracted from the urine of pregnant and postmenopausal women. The commercial preparation, human menopausal gonadotropin (HMG), is used in the treatment of infertility and cryptorchidism (undescended testes), and is discussed in Chapter 47. Two synthetic gonadotropin-releasing hormone analogues, nafarelin and histrelin, are also available clinically and are used in treating precocious puberty in adolescents. The remaining adenohypophysial hormone, *prolactin* (luteotropic hormone [LTH]), is unavailable for therapeutic use.

All adenohypophysial hormones except GH exert their effects on *selective* target organs, such as the adrenal cortex, thyroid gland, or gonads. For many of the reasons mentioned previously, replacement therapy in cases of hormonal deficiency states usually is best accomplished by supplying the individual target gland hormones (thyroxine, hydrocortisone, estrogen, progesterone) instead of the pituitary hormones. In the case of the gonadal hormones, moreover, the individual purified hypophysial hormones are not clinically available.

Adrenocorticotropic Hormone (ACTH)

- ***Corticotropin Injection***

ACTH, Acthar

- ***Repository Corticotropin Injection***

ACTH 40, ACTH 80, H.P. Acthar Gel

- ***Corticotropin Zinc Injection***

Cortrophin-Zinc

A polypeptide containing 39 amino acids, ACTH is extracted from the pituitary glands of several animals. The preparation is commercially available either as a stable aqueous solution for injection, an aqueous solution containing gelatin to delay absorption and prolong the action, or a zinc hydroxide complex to prevent tissue destruction, which also prolongs the effect. A synthetic subunit (ie, 24 amino acids) of ACTH, available as cosyntropin, is used to test for adrenocortical insufficiency. Cosyntropin is reviewed in Chapter 80. A second diagnostic agent, metyrapone, can also be used to ascertain whether pituitary secretion of ACTH is adequate, and is likewise considered in Chapter 80.

Mechanism

Stimulates the adrenal cortex to produce and secrete all of its hormones; activates adenyl cyclase in adrenal cortical tissue, thus increasing cyclic AMP levels, which enhances the synthesis of adrenal steroids, principally cortisone and hydrocortisone.

Uses

- Management of acute exacerbations of multiple sclerosis
- Treatment of nonsuppurative thyroiditis, tuberculous meningitis (with appropriate antibacterial therapy), trichinosis with neurologic or myocardial involvement, and hypercalcemia associated with cancer
- Diagnostic testing of adrenocortical function (cosyntropin is the preferred agent; see Chapter 80)
- Treatment of rheumatic, collagen, dermatologic, allergic,

hematologic, respiratory, edematous, and neoplastic disorders, *only as an alternative* to more specific glucocorticoid therapy (see Chapter 45)

Dosage

Adrenal responsiveness must first be verified: a normal response after an injection of ACTH is an increase in plasma cortisol greater than 20 μg/dL. A lesser response indicates adrenal insufficiency.

Diagnosis: 10 to 25 U/500 mL 5% dextrose by IV infusion over 8 hours
Treatment of deficiency states:
Regular injection: 20 U four times a day IM or SC
Repository injection: 40 to 80 U every 1 to 3 days IM or SC

CAUTION

Do not administer zinc preparations SC.

Multiple sclerosis (acute exacerbations): 80 to 120 U/day for 2 to 3 weeks IM

Fate

Readily absorbed from injection sites; effects are rapid after IM or IV injection and persist for 2 to 4 hours. Duration with repository injection is 24 to 48 hours. Half-life after IV injection is 20 to 30 minutes; excreted largely by the kidney.

Significant Adverse Reactions

Usually observed with prolonged use:

GI: ulceration and hemorrhage (cause-and-effect relationship not established), pancreatitis, abdominal distention
Musculoskeletal: weakness, osteoporosis, steroid myopathy, loss of muscle mass, vertebral compression fractures
Dermatologic: erythema, petechiae, ecchymoses, delayed wound healing, sweating, hyperpigmentation, acneiform reactions, thinning skin
CNS: convulsions, vertigo, headache, insomnia, depression, mood swings, euphoria, personality alterations
Endocrine: menstrual irregularities, hirsutism, diabetes, decreased carbohydrate tolerance, growth suppression
Electrolyte: hypernatremia, hypokalemia, hypocalcemia, fluid retention
CV: hypertension, necrotizing angiitis
Other: subcapsular cataracts, increased intraocular pressure, exophthalmos, negative nitrogen balance, allergic reactions

Contraindications

Osteoporosis, scleroderma, systemic fungal infections, ocular herpes simplex, recent surgery, congestive heart failure, hypertension, IV use (except diagnostic testing), alone in active tuberculosis, and sensitivity to proteins of porcine origin. *Cautious use* in patients with diabetes, hypothyroidism, cirrhosis, peptic ulcer, infections, diverticulitis, renal insufficiency, myasthenia gravis, in pregnant and lactating women, and in emotionally unstable patients.

CAUTION

Undertake immunization procedures with extreme caution during ACTH therapy because lack of antibody response and neurologic complications have been reported. Do not vaccinate against smallpox during treatment with ACTH.

Interactions

Increased requirements for hypoglycemic agents may occur with use of ACTH, owing to the hyperglycemic action of corticosteroids.
ACTH may enhance the hypoprothrombinemic action of aspirin.
Potassium loss with diuretics or amphotericin B may be enhanced with concurrent use of ACTH.
The ulcerogenic effects of aspirin and antiinflammatory drugs may be increased by ACTH.
Side effects from administration of viral vaccines may be enhanced by ACTH (see previous CAUTION).

Nursing Management

Pretherapy Assessment

Assess and record baseline data necessary for detection of adverse effects of ACTH: General: vital signs (VS), body weight, skin color and temperature, edema, hydration; CNS: orientation, reflexes, muscle strength; Cardiovascular system (CVS): peripheral perfusion, vein status; GI: liver evaluation, bowel sounds; Genitourinary (GU): output patterns, menstrual cycle; Laboratory: complete blood count (CBC), serum electrolytes, thyroid function tests, urinalysis, 2-hour postprandial blood glucose.

Review medical history and documents for existing or previous conditions that:

a. require cautious use of ACTH: diabetes; hypothyroidism; cirrhosis; peptic ulcer; infections; diverticulitis; renal insufficiency; myasthenia gravis; emotional instability.
b. contraindicate use of ACTH: allergy to pork, pork products; osteoporosis; scleroderma; systemic fungal infections; ocular herpes simplex; recent surgery; congestive heart failure; hypertension; IV use (except diagnostic testing); alone in active tuberculosis; **pregnancy (Category C)**; lactation (safety not established).

Nursing Interventions

Medication Administration

Question administration of full therapeutic doses if adrenal responsiveness has not been verified by a rise in plasma or urinary corticosteroid values after an IM or SC test injection.

Be prepared to assist with skin sensitivity test, which should be performed in any patient with suspected sensitivity to proteins of porcine origin. Observe patient closely for sensitivity reaction during IV infusion or immediately after IM or SC injection.

Ensure that ACTH therapy is not abruptly discontinued. The dosage should be reduced gradually to minimize the relative adrenal cortical insufficiency that can result from prolonged ACTH therapy. Full dosage should be reinstituted if periods of stress occur during withdrawal.

Inject repository forms deeply IM. They should not be administered IV. The zinc repository form should not be given SC.

Reconstitute prepared powder with sterile water for injection or sterile saline solution. Refrigerate. Discard unused portion after 24 hours.

Do not administer live virus vaccines while patient is on this drug.

Provide for small, frequent meals or arrange for antacids to minimize GI distress.

Surveillance During Therapy

Assess patient frequently for signs of electrolyte imbalances (eg, thirst, weakness, muscle cramping), sodium or water retention, or psychic changes (eg, mood swings, insomnia, depression, euphoria).

Monitor blood pressure regularly during therapy.

Keep in mind that it may take several days for maximal therapeutic effects to develop in evaluating patient's response. If an immediate effect is desired, more rapidly acting steroids should be used.

Carefully monitor laboratory studies and patient for indications of adverse reactions.

Interpret results of diagnostic tests and contact practitioner as appropriate.

Monitor for possible drug–drug and drug–nutrient interactions; see Interactions.

Provide for patient safety needs if CNS or musculoskeletal effects occur.

Patient Teaching

Instruct the patient that the following may occur as a result of drug therapy: GI distress; menstrual dysfunction; headache; mood swings; high blood pressure; increased sweating.

Instruct patient to inform practitioner if any of the following occur: unusual weight gain; swelling of the lower extremities; muscle weakness; abdominal pain; worsening of symptoms for which the drug is being taken.

Emphasize the importance of notifying practitioner if illness or infection develops because ACTH can induce immunosuppression. Proper antiinfective therapy should be administered in the presence of an infection.

Instruct patient to report any weight gain or signs of edema.

Synthetic Growth Hormone

- ***Somatrem***

Protropin

- ***Somatropin***

Humatrope, Nutropin

Somatrem and somatropin are synthetic, purified polypeptide hormones obtained by a recombinant DNA technique. Somatrem contains the identical sequence of 191 amino acids comprising endogenous GH *plus* an additional amino acid, methionine. Somatropin contains the *exact* amino acid sequence of human GH. These products are useful in treating growth retardation in young children lacking endogenous GH.

In addition, GH is being used in older patients to facilitate healing, for example after surgery or trauma and also experimentally to slow the aging process. These uses presently are somewhat controversial.

Mechanism

Increases linear bone growth in a manner therapeutically equivalent to that of endogenous human GH; skeletal growth is enhanced and the length of long bones is increased at the epiphyses; increases number and size of skeletal muscle cells and red cell mass; enhances cellular protein synthesis and nitrogen retention and decreases blood urea nitrogen; increases synthesis of chondroitin sulfate and collagen, and elevates serum levels of phosphate; facilitates urinary calcium excretion and enhances GI absorption of calcium, and thus serum calcium levels are relatively unchanged. Potassium and sodium retention can also occur; large doses may raise blood glucose levels, lower glucose tolerance, and decrease sensitivity to exogenous insulin, leading to a diabetogenic state; anabolic effects of GH are apparently mediated by a group of substances termed *somatomedins*, peptides whose hepatic synthesis is stimulated by GH; somatomedins promote uptake of sulfate into cartilage and appear to be the mediators of cellular processes involved with bone growth.

Uses

Treatment of growth failure due to a deficiency of pituitary GH (hypopituitary dwarfism)

Treatment of growth failure in children associated with chronic renal insufficiency, up to the time of renal transplantation (Nutropin only)

Investigational uses include aid in healing after surgery, burns and other catabolic states and slowing of physiologic deterioration in advancing age

Dosage

Somatrem: Up to 0.1 mg/kg (0.26 U/kg) IM three times a week for 6 to 36 months

Somatropin:

Humatrope: Up to 0.06 mg/kg (0.16 U/kg) SC or IM 3 times a week for 6 to 36 months

Nutropin: 0.04–0.05 mg/kg (0.11–0.13 U/kg) by daily SC injection

CAUTION

Before initiating treatment, document GH deficiency by failure of serum GH concentration to rise above 5 to 7 mg/mL in response to at least two standard stimuli (eg, insulin-induced hypoglycemia, IV arginine [see Chapter 80]).

Significant Adverse Reactions

Myalgia, pain and swelling at injection site, hyperglycemia, ketosis, hypothyroidism.

Contraindications

Patients with closed epiphyses, progressive intracranial lesions or tumors. *Cautious use* in patients with diabetes.

Interactions

Accelerated epiphyseal closure (fusion of ends of long bones) can occur if GH is combined with androgens or thyroid hormones.

Hydrocortisone and other antiinflammatory steroids may reduce the response to GH.

Growth hormone may decrease responsiveness to insulin or to oral hypoglycemic agents by increasing blood glucose levels.

Nursing Management

Pretherapy Assessment

Assess and record baseline data necessary for detection of adverse effects of growth hormone: General: VS, body weight, skin color and temperature; CNS: orientation, reflexes, muscle strength; CVS: peripheral perfusion, vein status; GI: liver evaluation, bowel sounds; GU: output patterns; Laboratory: thyroid function tests, urinalysis, blood glucose.

Review medical history and documents for existing or previous conditions that:

a. require cautious use of growth hormone: diabetes.

b. contraindicate use of growth hormone: closed epiphyses; progressive intracranial lesions or tumors; **pregnancy (Category C)**; lactation (safety not established).

Nursing Interventions

Medication Administration

Reconstitute each vial with 5 mL of bacteriostatic water for injection. Do *not* shake vial vigorously. Store in refrigerator. Discard after 1 month.

Surveillance During Therapy

Monitor for toxicity.

Check results of bone age assessments, which should be performed annually, especially in patients receiving concurrent thyroid or androgen therapy, because premature epiphyseal closure can occur.

Monitor patient for possible development of hypotension, tachycardia, or atrial arrhythmias.

Be alert for indications of hypercalciuria (eg, flank pain, renal colic, chills, fever, urinary frequency, hematuria), especially during first 2 to 3 months of therapy.

Monitor results of thyroid function tests, which should be performed periodically.

Carefully monitor laboratory studies and patient for indications of adverse reactions.

Interpret results of diagnostic tests and contact practitioner as appropriate.

Monitor for possible drug–drug and drug–nutrient interactions; see Interactions.

Patient Teaching

Instruct the patient regarding the goal of therapy with growth hormone.

Thyroid-Stimulating Hormone

- ***Thyrotropin***

Thytropar

A purified extract of TSH isolated from bovine pituitary glands, thyrotropin is used for the differential diagnosis of primary from secondary hypothyroidism and for the diagnosis of decreased thyroid reserve. The drug is considered in Chapter 80.

Gonadotropin-Releasing Hormones

- **Nafarelin Acetate** *(Pregnancy Category X)*

Synarel

- **Histrelin Acetate** *(Pregnancy Category X)*

Supprelin

Nafarelin and histrelin are synthetic gonadotropin-releasing hormone agonists that, when administered daily, gradually decrease secretion of gonadal steroids. In time, ovarian and testicular function is diminished and secondary sexual characteristics regress. Skeletal maturation and linear growth are also impaired. The principal indication for these agents is the control of the manifestations of central precocious puberty in children of both sexes. In addition, nafarelin may also be useful in treating endometriosis in women 18 years of age and older.

Nafarelin is available as a nasal spray, whereas histrelin is given by subcutaneous injection. In treating precocious puberty, 2 sprays of nafarelin are administered into each nostril morning and night, whereas a single injection of histrelin is given daily at alternating sites. For treatment of endometriosis, 1 or 2 sprays of nafarelin are given morning and night.

The drugs are contraindicated in pregnant or nursing mothers. Carcinogenicity studies in animals have shown an increase in tumors of hormonally responsive tissues, such as the pituitary, mammary glands, pancreas, stomach, and gonads. In addition, a wide range of adverse effects has been reported with these drugs, most common of which are vasodilation, "hot flashes," headache, vaginal bleeding, and local reactions at the injection site. Patients receiving these drugs must be closely monitored and a thorough physiologic and endocrinologic evaluation is required before initiating therapy.

Hormones of the Neurohypophysis

The *neurohypophysis*, or posterior lobe of the pituitary, secretes two hormones, oxytocin and vasopressin, both of which are available for clinical use. Vasopressin is also referred to as the antidiuretic hormone (ADH) because it promotes reabsorption of water from the distal tubules and collecting ducts of the kidney. Its other pharmacologic effects include contraction of vascular smooth muscle, especially of the portal and splanchnic (visceral) vessels, and a direct spasmogenic effect on gastrointestinal smooth muscle. Available preparations of vasopressin include a synthetic derivative of the naturally occurring hormone possessing marked pressor and antidiuretic activity and two structural analogues, desmopressin and lypressin, which exhibit relatively selective antidiuretic activity with minimal pressor effects. These drugs are reviewed individually in this chapter.

Oxytocin exerts two principal actions in the body: contraction of uterine smooth muscle (oxytocic effect) and contraction of the myoepithelial cells surrounding the ducts of the mammary gland, resulting in ejection of milk (galactokinetic effect). The sensitivity of the uterus to the effects of oxytocin depends on both the stage of gestation (maximal at term and immediately postpartum) and the existing balance of female sex hormones (increased in the presence of estrogen and reduced in the presence of progesterone). Clinically available oxytocin is a synthetic derivative used to stimulate uterine contractions during labor. Two other non–oxytocin-related drugs, ergonovine and methylergonovine, also exert a uterine spasmogenic action and are considered in this chapter as well.

• Vasopressin

Pitressin Synthetic

(CAN) Pressyn

A synthetic compound structurally identical to naturally occurring vasopressin, possessing vasopressor and antidiuretic activity, vasopressin injection is available as an aqueous solution containing 20 pressor units (U) per milliliter. The principal indication for vasopressin is the treatment of diabetes insipidus, a condition characterized by excretion of excessive quantities of dilute urine (polyuria) and extreme thirst (polydipsia). Insufficient antidiuretic hormone secretion from the neurohypophysis is often the cause of this condition, and vasopressin provides replacement therapy to correct the symptoms. Occasionally, however, the problem is unresponsiveness of the renal tubules to the action of vasopressin, and, in these cases, vasopressin is ineffective in treating the condition. Successful therapy of this latter type of diabetes insipidus is difficult, but clinical benefit has been reported with use of thiazide diuretics and chlorpropamide. Other uses for vasopressin are listed below.

Mechanism

Increases distal tubular reabsorption of water by increasing the permeability of the tubular epithelium by activation of cyclic AMP in cells of the renal collecting ducts; enhances contraction of vascular and nonvascular smooth muscle, thereby decreasing peripheral blood flow and increasing GI, urinary, and uterine smooth muscle spasm; constriction of coronary arteries may precipitate or worsen existing angina.

Uses

Treatment of diabetes insipidus of central (hypophysial) origin

Prevention and treatment of postoperative abdominal distention

Dispersion of gas shadows to aid abdominal roentgenography

Control of bleeding esophageal varices and hemorrhage due to abdominal surgery

Dosage

Diabetes insipidus: 5 to 10 U 2 to 3 times a day IM, SC, or intranasally on cotton pledgets

Abdominal distention: 5 U IM initially; increase to 10 U every 3 to 4 hours as necessary

Abdominal roentgenography: 10 U IM 2 hours and 0.5 hour before films are exposed

Esophageal bleeding episodes: 20 U by IV infusion (or occasionally intraarterially) over 5 to 10 minutes

Fate

Duration of action with aqueous injection is 2 to 8 hours; rapidly removed from the plasma (half-life 15 min); inactivated by the liver and kidneys and excreted in the urine as metabolites and unchanged drug.

Common Side Effects

Facial pallor, nausea, GI disturbances, and abdominal or uterine cramping.

Significant Adverse Reactions

Vertigo, sweating, headache, vomiting, urticaria, bronchoconstriction, hypersensitivity reactions, anaphylactic reaction, and anginal pain.

After nasal insufflation: congestion, irritation, rhinorrhea, headache, conjunctivitis, and mucosal ulceration.

Contraindications

Chronic nephritis, advanced arteriosclerosis, and severe coronary artery disease. *Cautious use* in patients with epilepsy, asthma, migraine, heart failure, angina, renal disease, goiter, and in elderly, very young, or pregnant patients.

Interactions

Action of vasopressin may be potentiated by hypoglycemics, acetaminophen, fludrocortisone, ganglionic blocking agents, neostigmine, and general anesthetics.

Antidiuretic activity can be increased by chlorpropamide, clofibrate, or carbamazepine.

Antidiuretic action of vasopressin may be reduced by alcohol, epinephrine, cyclophosphamide, heparin, and lithium.

Nursing Management

Pretherapy Assessment

Assess and record baseline data necessary for detection of adverse effects of vasopressin: General: VS, body weight, skin color and temperature; CNS: orientation, reflexes, affect; CVS: rhythm, edema, baseline electrocardiogram; GI: liver evaluation, bowel sounds; GU: output patterns; Laboratory: renal function tests, urinalysis, serum electrolytes.

Review medical history and documents for existing or previous conditions that:

a. require cautious use of vasopressin: epilepsy; asthma; migraine; heart failure; angina; renal disease; goiter; use in elderly, very young.

b. contraindicate use of vasopressin: chronic nephritis; advanced arteriosclerosis; severe coronary artery disease; **pregnancy (Category C)**; lactation (safety not established).

Nursing Interventions

Medication Administration

Have appropriate treatment available (eg, nitroglycerin, oxygen, antiarrhythmics) if used for patient with coronary artery disease because anginal attacks and myocardial infarction can occur.

Obtain baseline values for blood pressure, weight, and intake–output ratio before therapy is initiated. Monitor values regularly (daily, if possible) during therapy, and report any sudden changes.

Warm injection to body temperature before administering. Observe for development of allergic reactions to both vasopressin and the vehicle.

Administer 1 or 2 glasses of water with a large dose of vasopressin to reduce side effects such as cramping, skin blanching, and nausea.

Assess patient for appearance of peristaltic sounds, passage of flatus, and return of normal pattern of bowel movements when drug is used to relieve abdominal distention. Abdominal measurements should be obtained before and during treatment.

Surveillance During Therapy

Be alert for early symptoms of water intoxication (nausea, vomiting, drowsiness, listlessness, headache, confusion) because convulsions and coma can occur. If symptoms appear, drug should be withdrawn, and fluid intake should be restricted until specific gravity of urine is at least 1.015 and polyuria occurs. Diuretics may be used with caution.

Carefully monitor laboratory studies and patient for indications of adverse reactions.

Interpret results of diagnostic tests and contact practitioner as appropriate.

Monitor for possible drug–drug and drug–nutrient interactions; see Interactions.

Patient Teaching

Inform the patient that the following may occur as a result of vasopressin therapy: GI cramping, flatulence; anxiety, tinnitus, vision changes; nasal irritation.

Instruct patient to report any of the following to the practitioner: swelling; difficulty breathing; chest tightness; palpitations; runny nose; painful nasal passages.

• Desmopressin Acetate

Concentraid, DDAVP

A synthetic analogue of vasopressin, desmopressin acetate is used as an intranasal spray or solution or by SC or direct IV injection; it possesses prolonged, potent antidiuretic activity with little vasopressor or oxytocic action at normal doses.

Mechanism

Provides replacement therapy for antidiuretic hormone in treating polyuria and polydipsia; reduces urine volume and increases urine osmolality; elicits a dose-related increase in blood clotting factor VIII levels.

Uses

Treatment of diabetes insipidus of central (hypophysial) origin

Treatment of polyuria and polydipsia associated with trauma or surgery of the pituitary gland

Treatment of hemophilia A and certain forms of von Willebrand disease in which factor VIII levels are at least 5% or greater (parenteral administration)

Treatment of nocturnal enuresis (bedwetting)—intranasal use *only*

Test for renal concentration capacity (Concentraid nasal solution)

Dosage

NOTE: Desmopressin injection has a 10-fold greater antidiuretic effect than that of an equivalent intranasal dose.

Inhalation

Solution: Drug is supplied with a flexible calibrated plastic tube (rhinyle); desired quantity of solution is drawn into tube, one end is inserted into nostril, and patient blows on other end to deposit drug deep into nasal cavity; infants and young children may require assistance (eg, air-filled syringe attached to tube).

Adults: 0.1 to 0.4 mL/day, either as a single dose or in 2 or 3 divided doses

Children (younger than 12 y): 0.05 o 0.3 mL/day in a single or 2 divided doses

Nasal Spray: each spray = 10 µg

Adults: 1 to 4 sprays daily

Children: 1 to 2 sprays daily

IV, SC

Diabetes insipidus: 0.5 to 1.0 mL daily in 2 divided doses

Hemophilia A–von Willebrand disease: 0.3 µg/kg by slow IV infusion over 15 to 30 minutes. In adults, use 50 mL of sterile saline diluent; in children less than 10 kg, use 10 mL diluent

Fate

Antidiuretic effect persists for 8 to 20 hours; increases in factor VIII levels are evident within 30 minutes, and levels are maximal within 90 to 120 minutes; drug is metabolized by the liver and kidney and excreted in the urine.

Common Side Effects

Nasal irritation and congestion with inhalation.

Significant Adverse Reactions

Usually with high doses only—headache, nausea, flushing, rhinitis, abdominal cramping, vulval pain, and hypertension; erythema, swelling, and burning have occurred at the site of injection.

Contraindications

Hemophilia B, type IIB von Willebrand disease (platelet aggregation may be increased). *Cautious use* in patients with coronary artery disease or hypertension, and in pregnant or nursing women and the elderly.

Nursing Management

See **Vasopressin**. In addition:

Nursing Interventions

Medication Administration

Assist patient in planning a schedule for fluid intake if oral fluids must be reduced to decrease the possibility of water intoxication and hyponatremia. A diuretic may be administered if excessive fluid retention occurs.

Patient Teaching

Provide complete instructions for administering medication (see Dosage), and ensure that patient understands how to use the calibrated plastic tube (rhinyle).

• Lypressin

Diapid

A synthetic vasopressin, lypressin possesses little or no vasopressor or oxytocic activity. It is stable in aqueous solution and administered in the form of a nasal spray containing 50 USP posterior pituitary pressor units per milliliter. It provides replacement therapy for antidiuretic hormone, and is used to treat symptoms of diabetes insipidus in patients who are unresponsive to or intolerant of other forms of replacement therapy, or who experience allergic reactions or other adverse reactions with systemically administered vasopressin.

One or two sprays are administered in each nostril 4 times a day, with an additional dose at bedtime to eliminate nocturia if needed (one spray provides approximately 2 USP posterior pituitary pressor U). Administering more than 2 or 3 sprays in each nostril usually results in waste, with the unabsorbed excess draining into the digestive tract to be inactivated. If a higher dosage is indicated, increase frequency of use rather than number of sprays with each use. Instruct patient to clear nasal passages before administering, hold bottle upright when spraying, and keep head in an upright position.

The maximal antidiuretic effect occurs within 30 to 60 minutes and effects usually persist for 4 to 6 hours. Side effects are mild and infrequent; nasal irritation, congestion, pruritus, and rhinorrhea have been reported. Systemic adverse effects are minimal; however, large or frequent doses may eventually cause headache, heartburn, abdominal cramping, drowsiness, and dyspnea. Cautious use is necessary in patients with coronary artery disease. The effectiveness of intranasal lypressin may be impaired in the presence of nasal congestion, allergic rhinitis, or upper respiratory infections, because absorption may be reduced; larger doses may be required.

• Oxytocin, parenteral

Pitocin, Syntocinon

• Oxytocin, nasal

Syntocinon

Oxytocin is a synthetic peptide possessing the pharmacologic effects of the endogenous hormone. It is available as an injection for IM or IV use containing 10 U/mL, and as a nasal spray containing 40 U/mL.

Mechanism

Exerts a spasmogenic effect on uterine smooth muscle; increases permeability of the cell membranes of myofibrils to sodium ions, thereby augmenting contractile activity; also contracts myoepithelial cells surrounding the ducts and alveoli of the mammary gland, facilitating ejection of milk from the properly primed gland; large doses may exhibit antidiuretic activity.

Uses

Initiation or augmentation of uterine contractions to assist in delivery of the fetus for *valid fetal or maternal reasons only*, such as the following:
- Maternal diabetes
- Rh problems
- Uterine inertia
- Premature rupture of membranes
- Preeclampsia or eclampsia

Facilitation of uterine contractions during third stage of labor

Control of postpartum hemorrhage

Management of inevitable, incomplete, or missed abortion

Aid in milk let-down during breast-feeding or relief of postpartum breast engorgement (*only* indication for the nasal spray)

Dosage

Injection

Induction or enhancement of labor: 0.001 to 0.002 U/min (0.1–0.2 mL/min of a 1:1000 dilution; see below) by IV infusion; increase gradually in 0.001- to 0.002-U/min increments at 15- to 30-minute intervals until a desirable contraction pattern has been established; adjust rate according to uterine response; *dilution*—1-mL ampule (10 U) added to 1000 mL of 0.9% aqueous sodium chloride or other suitable IV fluid; use constant-infusion pump to accurately control dose

Postpartum uterine bleeding: IV—10 to 40 U/1000 mL diluent infused at a rate to control bleeding; IM—10 U after delivery of the placenta

Incomplete abortion: 10 U/500 mL diluent infused IV at a rate of 0.020 to 0.040 U/min

Nasal Spray

One spray into one nostril or both nostrils 2 to 3 minutes before nursing or pumping of breasts

Fate

Onset of effect is within 1 minute with IV infusion, 3 to 7 minutes with IM injection, and 5 to 10 minutes with nasal spray; nasal absorption is erratic; short plasma half-life (several minutes); rapidly cleared from the plasma by the liver, kidney, and mammary gland; primarily excreted as metabolites by the kidney, with small amounts as active drug.

Significant Adverse Reactions

Fetus: Bradycardia, arrhythmias, neonatal jaundice, hypoxia, and trauma from too-rapid expulsion

Mother: Arrhythmias, nausea, vomiting, pelvic hematoma, afibrinogenemia, uterine hypertonicity or spasm, uterine rupture, anaphylactic reaction, subarachnoid hemorrhage, hypertension, water intoxication, convulsions, and postpartum hemorrhage

Contraindications

Unfavorable fetal position, significant cephalopelvic disproportion, fetal distress where delivery is not imminent, hypertonic uterine patterns, undilated cervix, prolonged use in uterine inertia or severe toxemia, conditions in which vaginal delivery is contraindicated (eg, prolapsed cord, total placenta previa, vasa previa), previous cervical or uterine surgery, invasive cervical carcinoma, dead fetus, and abruptio placentae. *Cautious use*: except in unusual circumstances, do not use in prematurity, partial placenta previa, previous surgery on the cervix or uterus, overdistention of the uterus, grand multiparity, or history of uterine sepsis.

Interactions

Severe persistent hypertension can occur if oxytocin is given in the presence of other vasopressor drugs (eg, epinephrine, ephedrine, methoxamine, or metaraminol)

Estrogens may augment and progestins may decrease the uterine spasmogenic action of oxytocin

Nursing Management

Pretherapy Assessment

Assess and record baseline data necessary for detection of adverse effects of oxytocin: General: VS, body weight, skin color and temperature, fetal heart rate, fetal positions, fetus–pelvis proportions, uterine tone, timing and rate of contractions; CNS: orientation, reflexes, affect; CVS: rhythm, edema; Laboratory: CBC, urinalysis, serum electrolytes.

Review medical history and documents for existing or previous conditions that:

a. require cautious use of oxytocin: prematurity; partial placenta previa; previous surgery on the cervix or uterus; overdistention of the uterus; grand multiparity; history of uterine sepsis.

b. contraindicate use of oxytocin: unfavorable fetal position; significant cephalopelvic disproportion; fetal distress where delivery is not imminent; hypertonic uterine patterns; undilated cervix; prolonged use in uterine inertia or severe toxemia; conditions in which vaginal delivery is contraindicated (eg, prolapsed cord, total placenta previa, vasa previa); previous cervical or uterine surgery; invasive cervical carcinoma; dead fetus; abruptio placentae.

Nursing Interventions

Medication Administration

Ensure that oxytocin used for induction of labor is given only by IV infusion and administered by trained personnel. A practitioner should be readily available at all times to manage complications.

Carefully regulate infusion flow rate to obtain optimal contractions. If contractions are frequent (less than 2-min intervals), prolonged, or excessive (greater than 50 mm Hg), the infusion should be stopped to prevent fetal anoxia, the patient should be placed on her side, and oxygen should be ready for administration. Effects diminish rapidly because oxytocin is short acting.

Do not administer *undiluted* solution IV, nor give oxytocin by more than one route of administration at any one time.

Begin IV infusion with non–oxytocin-containing solution (eg, physiologic electrolytc solution). Oxytocin solution is then added to the system. A constant-infusion pump is used to regulate infusion rate accurately. Flow rate should not exceed 2 mL/min.

Have magnesium sulfate available to relax myometrium if necessary when drug is given IM (deep deltoid injection).

Surveillance During Therapy

Monitor uterine contractions, fetal heart rate, and maternal blood pressure and pulse regularly during infusion.

Assess patient for early signs of water intoxication (confusion, headache, and drowsiness) due to antidiuretic hormone effect of oxytocin during prolonged infusion. Intake–output ratio should be checked during labor, and edema and anuria should be promptly noted.

Be alert for development of severe hypertension if local anesthetics containing epinephrine are used during labor in patient receiving oxytocin. Symptoms may include throbbing headache, palpitations, sweating, fever, vomiting, stiff neck, photophobia, and chest pain.

Monitor neonate for occurrence of jaundice.

Monitor postpartum women for blood pressure changes and evidence of excessive bleeding.

Carefully monitor laboratory studies and patient for indications of adverse reactions.

Interpret results of diagnostic tests and contact practitioner as appropriate.

Monitor for possible drug–drug and drug–nutrient interactions; see Interactions.

Patient Teaching

The patient receiving parenteral oxytocin usually is receiving the drug as part of an immediate medical intervention or facilitation; teaching is focused on providing information about the procedures to be used and their outcomes.

In the circumstance of nasal application:

Instruct patient using nasal spray to clear nasal passages before spraying, to hold bottle upright, and to maintain a sitting or standing position.

Instruct the patient to inform the practitioner if any of the following occur: sores in the nostrils; palpitations; unusual bleeding or bruising.

Nonhypophysial Oxytocics

In addition to oxytocin, other compounds also possess a uterine spasmogenic action and are used for some of the same indications as oxytocin, particularly to control postpartum atony and hemorrhage. Ergonovine, an alkaloid obtained from ergot, a fungus that grows on the rye plant, and methylergonovine, a semisynthetic derivative of ergonovine, exert a somewhat more prolonged oxytocic action than oxytocin itself, and appear to be more selective spasmogens for uterine smooth muscle.

• Ergonovine

Ergotrate

Mechanism

Direct stimulating effect on smooth muscle of the uterus; small doses increase force and frequency of uterine contractions, but normal relaxant phase follows; larger doses produce sustained, forceful contractions, with markedly elevated resting tone; cerebral vasoconstriction is moderate, although less than that observed with ergotamine, a related alkaloid used in migraine (see Chapter 16).

Uses

Management of postpartum or postabortion hemorrhage or uterine atony

Investigational uses include facilitation of incomplete abortion, and diagnosis of Prinzmetal's variant (vasospastic) angina during coronary arteriography (provokes reversible coronary artery spasms)

Dosage

Oral: 0.2 to 0.4 mg 2 to 4 times a day until danger of atony has passed (usually 48 h)

IM: 0.2 mg after placental delivery; may repeat in 2 to 4 hours as needed

IV: 0.2 mg for excessive uterine bleeding

Diagnosis of Prinzmetal's angina: 0.05 mg IV; repeat every 5 minutes until chest pain occurs (maximum dose = 0.4 mg)

Fate

Well absorbed orally, sublingually, and parenterally; onset of action is 30 to 60 seconds IV, 3 to 7 minutes IM, and 8 to 10 minutes orally; uterine contractions may continue for up to 3 to 4 hours.

Significant Adverse Reactions

Most frequent with IV administration—nausea, vomiting, weak and rapid pulse, paresthesias, allergic reactions (including shock), hypertension, tinnitus, headache, dyspnea, cramping, dizziness, confusion, decreased lactation, and muscle weakness.

Contraindications

Threatened spontaneous abortion, severe hypertension, toxemia of pregnancy; *not* to be used for induction of labor. *Cautious use* in patients with heart disease, mild to moderate hypertension, mitral valve stenosis, renal or hepatic impairment, obliterative vascular disease, or sepsis.

Interactions

Blood pressure may be further elevated if ergonovine is combined with vasopressors, other oxytocics, nicotine, bromocriptine and general anesthetics.

Oxytocic action may be reduced by a decrease in calcium levels.

Nursing Management

Pretherapy Assessment

Assess and record baseline data necessary for detection of adverse effects of ergot alkaloids: General: VS, body weight, skin color and temperature, uterine tone; CNS: orientation, reflexes, affect; CVS: rhythm, edema; Laboratory: CBC, urinalysis, serum electrolytes.

Review medical history and documents for existing or previous conditions that:

a. require cautious use of ergot alkaloids: heart disease; mild to moderate hypertension; mitral valve stenosis; renal or hepatic impairment; obliterative vascular disease; sepsis.
b. contraindicate use of ergot alkaloids: allergy to ergot derivatives; threatened spontaneous abortion; severe hypertension; toxemia of pregnancy; *not* to be used for induction of labor; **pregnancy (Category C)**; lactation (may be given for up to 1 wk postpartum).

Nursing Interventions

Medication Administration

Expect to administer IV only in extreme emergencies because danger of hypertension and severe nausea and vomiting is increased with IV use.

Store injection in cool place, and do not use solution over 60 days old.

Surveillance During Therapy

Monitor blood pressure, pulse, vaginal blood flow, and uterine response after injection until condition has stabilized. Report marked changes in pulse or blood pressure.

Monitor patient for early symptoms of ergot poisoning (ergotism) such as vomiting, cramping, headache, or confusion. To avoid development of ergotism, the drug should not be used for prolonged periods.

Evaluate degree of cramping experienced. Although cramping is usually an indication of drug effectiveness, persistent or severe cramping may indicate a need for dosage reduction.

Use with extreme caution before delivery of the placenta, and only in the presence of a staff member well versed in the use of ergonovine, because very high uterine tone may be produced.

Carefully monitor laboratory studies and patient for indications of adverse reactions.

Interpret results of diagnostic tests and contact practitioner as appropriate.

Monitor for possible drug–drug and drug–nutrient interactions; see Interactions.

Patient Teaching

Inform the patient that the following may occur as a result of ergot therapy: nausea, vomiting, dizziness, headache, ringing in the ears.

Instruct the patient to inform the practitioner if any of the following occur: difficulty breathing; headache; numb or cold extremities; severe abdominal cramping.

• Methylergonovine

Methergine

Mechanism

Direct spasmogenic action on uterine smooth muscle; weak cerebral vasoconstrictive action.

Uses

Management of postpartum atony, hemorrhage, or subinvolution of the uterus after delivery of the placenta
Facilitation of labor (given in the second stage after delivery of the anterior shoulder)

Dosage

Oral: 0.2 mg 3 or 4 times a day for a maximum of 1 week
IM, IV: 0.2 mg after delivery of the anterior shoulder, after delivery of placenta, or during the puerperium; may repeat as required at 2- to 4-hour intervals

Fate

Well absorbed orally or parenterally; onset of action is 5 to 10 minutes orally and IM, and almost immediate with IV injection.

Significant Adverse Reactions

Nausea, vomiting, hypertension, dizziness, tinnitus, sweating, palpitation, chest pain, and dyspnea.

Contraindications

See Ergonovine.

Interactions

See Ergonovine.

Nursing Management

See **Ergonovine**. In addition:

Medication Administration

Administer slowly and monitor blood pressure closely when drug is used IV. Drug should not be administered IV routinely because risk of hypertension and cerebral vascular accident is increased.
Discard solution if discolored. Store in cool place, and protect from light.

Selected Bibliography

Casper RF: Clinical uses of gonadotropin-releasing hormone analogues. Can Med Assoc J 144:153, 1991
Conn PM, Crowley WF: Gonadotropin-releasing hormone and its analogs. Ann Rev Med 45:391, 1994
Jorgensen JO: Human growth hormone replacement therapy: Pharmacological and clinical aspects. Endocrinol Rev 12:189, 1991
Malseed RT: Growth Hormone: Not just for the young anymore. Med Surg Nurs 1(1):66, 1992
Neely EK, Rosenfeld RG: Use and abuse of human growth hormone. Ann Rev Med 45:407, 1994
North WG, Moses AM, and Share L (eds): The Neurohypophysis: A Window on Brain Function (Symposium). Ann NY Acad Sci 689, 1993
Plotsky PM: Pathways to the secretion of adrenocorticotrophin: A view from the portal. J Neuroendocrinol 3:1, 1991
Renaud LP and Bourque CW: Neurophysiology and neuropharmacology of hypothalamic neurons secreting vasopressin and oxytocin. Prog Neurobiol 36:131, 1991
Rudman D, Feller AG, et al: Effects of human growth hormone in men over 60 years old. N Engl J Med 323:1, 1990

Nursing Bibliography

Gaedeke M: Evaluating TSH. Nursing '93 23(10):72, 1993
Kelsey S: Recombinant growth factors and the neutropenic patient. Care of the Critically Ill 9(1):5, 1993
Loos F: Understanding diabetes insipidus: Recognition and management in critical care. Journal of the Canadian Association of Critical Care Nurses 3(3):18, 1992
Roberts G: Growth hormone therapy for short stature. Journal of Pediatric Health Care 5:327, 1991
Seoud M, et al: Electrical breast stimulation: Oxytocin, prolactin and uterine response. J Reprod Med 38:438, 1993

42

Thyroid Hormones and Antithyroid Drugs

Thyroid Hormones
Antithyroid Drugs
Radioactive Iodide
Iodine/Iodide Products

The endogenous thyroid hormones thyroxine (T_4) and triiodothyronine (T_3) are important in normal physical and mental growth and development and in regulating the metabolic activity of essentially every cell of the body. They affect a wide range of physiologic activities, including central nervous system (CNS), cardiovascular (CV), and gastrointestinal (GI) function; carbohydrate, lipid, and protein metabolism; temperature regulation; muscle activity; water and electrolyte balance; and reproduction. Unlike many other hormones, however, they do not act on discrete target organs but exert a diffuse effect throughout the body. Their onset of action is slow and their activity prolonged; thus, they generally provide long-term regulation of bodily functions rather than moment-to-moment control.

The synthesis, storage, and release of the thyroid hormones by the thyroid gland are regulated in large part by the thyroid-stimulating hormone (TSH) of the adenohypophysis; this schema is discussed in the review of endocrine function in Chapter 40. The principal clinical application of the thyroid hormones is in the treatment of *hypo*thyroidism. This disease, characterized by reduced or absent secretion of endogenous thyroid hormones, can be clinically subdivided into cretinism (fetal or neonatal hypothyroidism) and myxedema (adult hypothyroidism), and each of these conditions is reviewed in Chapter 40. It should be noted that use of thyroid hormones in hypothyroidism merely constitutes replacement therapy and does not effect a cure. Because normal thyroid function is usually not reestablished, clinical benefit is attained only so long as thyroid hormones are supplied.

Several types of thyroid hormone preparations are available, both natural extracts of animal thyroid glands and synthetic derivatives. The natural animal extracts exhibit more variation in potency than the synthetic derivatives and are much less frequently used today.

The available thyroid preparations are:

- *Desiccated thyroid*: powdered, dried thyroid glands of domesticated animals, standardized on the basis of iodine content
- *Levothyroxine sodium*: sodium salt of the synthetic L-isomer of thyroxine (T_4)
- *Liothyronine sodium*: sodium salt of the synthetic L-isomer of triiodothyronine (T_3)
- *Liotrix*: combination of levothyroxine sodium and liothyronine sodium in a 4:1 ratio, on a weight basis

Secretion of excessive amounts of thyroid hormones reflects a *hyper*thyroid state, the most common cause of which is overstimulation of the gland by circulating immunoglobulins synthesized by B lymphocytes. One such antibody is thyroid-stimulating immunoglobulin (TSI), also known as long-acting thyroid stimulator (LATS), which interacts with receptor sites in the thyroid cell to stimulate hormonal output.

Therapy of hyperthyroidism includes surgical removal of a part of the gland (subtotal thyroidectomy), use of radioactive iodide (^{131}I) to destroy thyroid tissue, or administration of antithyroid drugs that interfere with synthesis and release of thyroid hormones. Principal advantages and disadvantages of each of these three procedures are outlined in Table 42-1.

Effective treatment of thyroid disorders depends on accurate assessment of the thyroid state. Several laboratory parameters used to ascertain thyroid functioning are listed below, with average (normal) values given beside each test.

Commonly Used. NOTE: All values are decreased in hypothyroidism except TSH, which is increased in primary hypothyroidism.

Free thyroxine index: (FT_4I): 1.3 ng/dL to 4.2 ng/dL
Resin uptake of radioactive T_3 in vitro (RT_3U): 25% to 35% uptake of T_3
Radioimmunoassays for T_3 and *T_4*:
Serum T_3—80 to 180 ng/dL (adults)
Total T_4—5 to 12 μg/dL (adults)
TSH levels: 0.4 to 4.8 μU/mL
Other infrequently used thyroid function tests include measurement of the *Basal metabolic rate (BMR)*: (±10%), *Protein-bound iodine (PBI)*:(4 μg/dL to 8 μg/dL), *Radioactive iodine uptake*: (5% to 10% at 2 hours; 10% to 20% at 6 hours; 20% to 40% at 24 hours), *Thyroxine-binding globulin levels*: 10 μg/dL to 26 μg/dL and *Free T_3 index* (FT_3I): 20 ng/dL to 60 ng/dL

Because of the possibility of false increases or decreases in the readings of any one of these tests related to other medications taken by the patient (Table 42-2) or the presence of certain disease states (eg, hepatitis, nephrosis), *several* tests should be performed before a diagnosis is made, and the results should be used only in combination with a thorough clinical assessment of the patient.

The pharmacologic actions of the thyroid hormones are reviewed as a group; individual drugs are then listed in Table 42-3. Likewise, the antithyroid drugs are considered together, then presented individually in Table 42-4. Certain types of thyroid disorders can also be effectively treated with elemental iodine preparations, and these products are considered at the end of the chapter.

Two other thyroid-related drugs are protirelin, a synthetic thyrotropin-releasing hormone, and thyrotropin itself, a highly purified form of thyroid stimulating hormone of bovine origin. These two agents are used for diagnosis of thyroid dysfunction and are reviewed in Chapter 80 along with other diagnostic drugs.

Table 42-1. **Approaches to the Treatment of Hyperthyroidism**

Treatment	*Advantages*	*Disadvantages*
Antithyroid drugs (propylthiouracil, methimazole)	No thyroid tissue damage Effects are reversible Rapid control of symptoms Dose is adjustable Can be given to pregnant women and to children	Relapse is common. Prolonged therapy is required. Blood dyscrasias can occur. Many side effects are possible.
Radioactive iodide (^{131}I)	Limited tissue damage Relapse is rare Multiple dosing usually not required	Dosage determination is not precise. Myxedema is common, requiring thyroid supplementation. Contraindicated in pregnancy.
Thyroidectomy (subtotal)	Provides rapid benefit Suspicious lesions can be removed Very effective if gland is greatly enlarged	Requires surgical skill Loss of thyroid function is irreversible. Discomfort and pain Complications can involve parathyroid glands and vocal cords.

Thyroid Hormones

- ***Levothyroxine***
- ***Liothyronine***
- ***Liotrix***
- ***Thyroid, dessicated***

Mechanism

Incompletely understood, but multiple sites and mechanisms are probably involved; probably bind to receptors on cellular surfaces, increasing uptake of glucose and amino acids; may also diffuse into cells and interact with receptors on mitochondria and chromatin material; increased mRNA synthesis can occur, leading to accelerated protein synthesis; appear to stimulate sodium-potassium-ATPase (adenosine triphosphatase) enzyme, thus facilitating membrane transport of sodium and potassium and increasing cellular utilization of oxygen; effects of these hormones include increases in body temperature, respiratory rate, heart rate, cardiac output, blood volume, carbohydrate, fat and protein metabolism, and enzymatic activity; conversely, serum cholesterol levels may be reduced

Table 42-2. **Effects of Drugs on Thyroid Function Tests**

Test	*Drugs That Increase Values*	*Drugs That Decrease Values*
Serum T_4	clofibrate estrogens insulin methadone phenothiazines topical betadine	androgens antidiabetics barbiturates carbamazepine diazepam heparin nitroprusside phenytoin salicylates sulfonylureas
Serum T_3	estrogens methadone thiazide diuretics	androgens corticosteroids phenytoin propranolol salicylates
T_3 uptake	anabolic steroids corticosteroids danazol phenylbutazone salicylates	estrogens fluorouracil methadone
Free thyroxine index	heparin propranolol	aminosalicylic acid barbiturates carbamazepine lithium phenylbutazone phenothiazines

Uses

- Replacement therapy of *primary* hypothyroidism (eg, cretinism; myxedema; nontoxic goiter; hypothyroid state of childhood, pregnancy, or old age) or of *secondary* hypothyroidism (eg, surgery, radiation, drug-induced)
- Adjuncts to thyroid-inhibiting agents when they are used to reduce release of thyrotropic hormones in treatment of thyrotoxicosis (Thyroid drugs prevent development of goiter and hypothyroidism.)
- Differentiation of hyperthyroidism from euthyroidism, that is, normal thyroid function (T_3 only—T_3 suppression test)
- Prevention or treatment of euthyroid goiters such as thyroid nodules, multinodular goiter, or chronic, lymphocytic thyroiditis
- Adjunctive therapy of follicular and papillary carcinoma of the thyroid, in conjunction with radioactive iodine

Dosage

See Table 42-3.

Fate

Oral absorption is variable, T_3 being absorbed to a greater extent (95% within 4 hours) than T_4 (50%–75%). Onset of action is within 6 to 8 hours for T_3 but much slower with T_4 (2 to 3 days). Peak effects may require up to 8 to 10 days to develop, however. Plasma half-lives are 1 to 2 days for T_3 and 6 to 7 days for T_4. Both hormones are highly bound (99%–100%) to plasma proteins (thyroxine-binding globulin, thyroxine-binding prealbumin, and albumin). Approximately 35% of T_4 is deiodinated in the periphery to T_3. Drugs are metabolized by the liver and in other

Table 42-3. **Thyroid Hormones**

Drug	***Usual Dosage Range***	***Nursing Considerations***
Thyroid, desiccated *Armour Thyroid, S-P-T, Thyrar*	*Adults* Myxedema: 16 mg/day for 2 wk; 32 mg/day for 2 wk; then 65 mg/day; increase daily dosage at monthly or greater intervals on basis of laboratory tests; usual range 65–195 mg/day Hypothyroidism without myxedema; 65 mg/day increased by 65 mg every 30 days until desired response *Children* Dosage regimen same as adults, with increments made at 2-wk intervals; maintenance doses may be higher in growing child than in adult	Dessicated animal thyroid glands containing active thyroid hormones (T_3 and T_4) in their natural state and ratio; potency can vary significantly from lot to lot; clinical effects develop slowly and are very prolonged; caution in transferring patient from thyroid to T_3 alone—discontinue thyroid, begin T_3 at very low doses, and gradually increase dosage levels; drug should be stored in dark, moisture-free bottles
Levothyroxine sodium—T_4 *Levo-T, Levothroid, Levoxine, Synthroid, (CAN) Eltroxin*	*Oral* Adults: 0.1 mg/day initially; increased by 0.05–0.1-mg increments every 1–3 wk until desired response is obtained; in elderly, myxedematous, or cardiovascular patients, initial dose 0.025 mg with 0.025–0.05-mg increments as needed; usual range, 0.1–0.2 mg/day Children: 0.025–0.05 mg initially, with increments of 0.05–0.1 mg/day at 1–3 wk intervals until desired response is obtained; usual range, 0.2–0.4 mg/day *Parenteral* Myxedematous coma: 0.2–0.5 mg IV first day; 0.1–0.3 mg second day if necessary; daily injections maintained until patient can accept a daily oral dose	Synthetic monosodium salt of the naturally occurring L-isomer of thyroxine; 0.1 mg is equivalent to 65 mg desiccated thyroid; used orally for hypothyroid replacement therapy and IV for treatment of myxedema coma or stupor demanding immediate replacement; may be given IM when oral route is not feasible; slower onset and longer duration than synthetic T_3; discontinue T_4 before switching to T_3; conversely, begin T_4 several days before stopping T_3; parenteral solution is prepared with sodium chloride injection and shaken until clear, use immediately; administer IV cautiously to patients with heart disease; inject slowly in small doses and carefully observe patient
Liothyronine sodium—T_3 *Cytomel, Triostat*	*Adults and children older than 3 yr* Mild hypothyroidism: 25 μg/day initially; increase by 12.5–25 μg/day every 1–2 wks; usual maintenance is 25–75 μg/day in divided doses Myxedema: 5 μg/day initially; increased by 5–10 μg/day every 1–2 wk; usual maintenance is 50–100 μg/day Simple nontoxic goiter: refer to **Myxedema** T_3 suppression test: 75–100 μg/day for 7 days; then repeat ^{131}I uptake test; in hyperthyroid patient, uptake is not affected; in normal patient, uptake will decrease to less than 20% *Children younger than 3 yr* Cretinism: initially 5 μg/day; increase by 5 μg every 3–4 days until desired response is achieved; infants a few months old require about 20 μg/day; at 1 yr, 50 μg/day is required	Synthetic form of the naturally occurring L-triiodothyronine (T_3); 25 μg is equivalent to 65 mg desiccated thyroid; possesses similar actions and uses of other thyroid hormones but has a more rapid onset of maximal effect and shorter duration (half-life, 1–2 days), allowing quicker dosage adjustments; serum TSH levels are most reliable laboratory index for monitoring T_3 replacement; also used in T_3 suppression test to differentiate borderline hyperthyroid from euthyroid (normal); useful in patients allergic to naturally extracted derivatives; be alert for possible additive effects caused by residual action of longer-acting thyroid drugs when T_3 is substituted for them; drug may be cardiotoxic—use with caution in patients with cardiac disease
Liotrix *Thyrolar*	Dosage given in thyroid equivalents Initially, 15–30 mg/day; increased gradually every 1–2 wks until desired response is obtained Replacement therapy for other thyroid products is based on the equivalency: 60 mg liotrix = 65 mg desiccated thyroid or thyroglobulin = 0.1 mg T_4 = 25 μg T_3	A constant mixture of synthetic T_4 and T_3 in a fixed 4:1 ratio by weight; although the product is claimed to more closely approximate the endogenous ratio of T_4:T_3, when differences in potency, absorption, binding, peripheral conversion of T_4 to T_3, and metabolism are considered, the fixed ratio offers *no* apparent advantage over other thyroid hormones used at optimal doses (except in those few intolerant persons); tablets have a shelf life of 2 yr

tissues and excreted in the urine (70%–80%) or bile (20%–30%) both as free drug and conjugated metabolites

Common Side Effects

(If dosage is excessive) Palpitations, nervousness, sweating, tachycardia

Significant Adverse Reactions

(Usually result of overdosage or too-rapid increase in dosage) Headache, diarrhea, fever, arrhythmias, anginal pain, tremors, insomnia, menstrual irregularities, heat intolerance, allergic skin reactions, congestive heart failure, shock

Contraindications

Thyrotoxicosis, nephrosis, hypogonadism, hyperthyroidism, hypoadrenalism, cardiovascular diseases uncomplicated by hypothyroidism; also not indicated for treating obesity, infertility, or depression, because there is no conclusive evidence of benefit in these conditions. *Cautious use* in the presence of

Table 42-4. **Antithyroid Drugs**

Drug	*Usual Dosage Range*	*Nursing Considerations*
Methimazole *Tapazole*	Adults: 15–60 mg initially, depending on degree of hyperthyroidism, in 3 daily doses at 8-h intervals; maintenance is 5–15 mg/day Children: 0.4 mg/kg initially in 3 divided doses at 8-h intervals; maintenance is ½ initial dose	More potent than propylthiouracil, longer duration of action, and somewhat more toxic; skin rash is an indication for discontinuing drug
Propylthiouracil *(CAN) Propyl-Thyracil*	Adults: 100 mg initially 3 times/day every 8 h; maintenance is 100–150 mg/day Children (older than 10 yr): 50–100 mg 3 times/day every 8 h Children (6–10 yr): 50–150 mg/day in divided doses	Least toxic antithyroid drug; administer with meals to reduce GI distress; monitor prothrombin time regularly during therapy, because drug can cause hypoprothrombinemia

angina, arrhythmias, diabetes mellitus, or adrenocortical insufficiency.

Interactions

Thyroid hormones can enhance the cardiovascular effects of catecholamines, possibly resulting in angina or arrhythmias.

Highly protein-bound drugs may compete with thyroid hormones for plasma protein binding sites, resulting in increased plasma levels of thyroid hormones.

Thyroid hormones can potentiate the effects of oral anticoagulants by increasing catabolism of vitamin K–dependent clotting factors.

Thyroid hormones may increase blood sugar levels, thus increasing requirements for insulin and oral hypoglycemic drugs.

Estrogens may decrease plasma levels of free T_4 by increasing levels of thyroid-binding globulin.

Thyroid hormone therapy may decrease the effectiveness and increase the likelihood of toxicity of the digitalis glycosides.

The activity of tricyclic antidepressants can be enhanced by thyroid hormones, possibly resulting in cardiac arrhythmias.

Tachycardia and hypertension may occur with ketamine in patients receiving thyroid hormones.

Nursing Management

Pretherapy Assessment

Assess and record baseline data necessary for detection of adverse effects of thyroid hormones: General: vital signs (VS), body weight, skin color and temperature, uterine tone; CNS: orientation, reflexes, muscle tone; CVS: baseline electrocardiogram (ECG); Lab: thyroid function tests.

Review medical history and documents for existing or previous conditions that:

a. require cautious use of thyroid hormones: angina; arrhythmias; diabetes mellitus; adrenocortical insufficiency

b. contraindicate use of thyroid hormones: allergy to active or extraneous components of the drug; thyrotoxicosis; nephrosis; hypogonadism; hyperthyroidism; hypoadrenalism; cardiovascular diseases uncomplicated by hypothyroidism; **pregnancy (Category A)**, lactation (secreted in breast milk; use caution)

Nursing Interventions

Medication Administration

Expect therapy to be initiated with small doses because hypothyroid patient is extremely sensitive to thyroid hormone. Dosage changes should be made gradually. Earliest clinical responses in adult are usually diuresis, increased appetite, and increased pulse.

Administer oral drug as a single daily dose before breakfast.

Provide comfort measures if headache, GI effects, or sweating occur.

Surveillance During Therapy

Assess cardiovascular status frequently for indications of possible complications (eg, chest pain, dyspnea) in patient with cardiovascular disease, including hypertension. Therapy should be initiated with small doses.

Monitor patient for development of signs of overdosage, such as irritability, nervousness, sweating, tachycardia, increased bowel motility, or menstrual irregularities. If these occur, the drug should be stopped for several days, then reinstituted at a lower dosage.

Monitor sleeping pulse and basal morning temperature, as indicated, because they are important guides to treatment, and the maintenance dosage may be higher in an actively growing child than in an adult.

Monitor pulse rate and rhythm during periods of dosage adjustment. Notify practitioner if rate exceeds 100 or if there is a marked change in rate or rhythm because drug may need to be withheld.

Test urine of diabetic patient regularly during therapy because dosage of antidiabetic drugs may need to be increased.

Evaluate effects when drug is used with oral anticoagulants. Their action may be enhanced by thyroid hormone, necessitating a dosage reduction.

Carefully monitor laboratory studies and patient for indications of adverse reactions.

Interpret results of diagnostic tests and contact practitioner as appropriate.

Monitor for possible drug–drug and drug–nutrient interactions: Refer to **Interactions**.

Patient Teaching

Suggest taking drug, which is used once a day, in the morning, if possible, to minimize the possibility of sleep disturbances.

Stress the importance of taking drug regularly even when feeling well. Replacement therapy is usually a lifelong requirement.

Warn juvenile hypothyroid patient and parents that initial response to therapy may be dramatic (excessive hair loss, rapid growth, assertiveness). These reactions tend to abate with continued therapy.

Instruct parents of juvenile taking thyroid hormone to monitor growth regularly. Too-rapid increases in height can result in premature closure of epiphyses and resultant skeletal deformities.

Explain, as appropriate, that both pharmacologic and toxicologic effects may persist for 10 to 14 days after withdrawal of T_3 and for 4 to 6 weeks after withdrawal of T_4.

Instruct the patient to inform the practitioner if any of the following occur: difficulty breathing; headache; numb or cold extremities; severe abdominal cramping.

Antithyroid Drugs (Thioamides)

- **Methimazole** *(Pregnancy Category D)*
- **Propylthiouracil** *(Pregnancy Category D)*

The antithyroid drugs impair the synthesis of the thyroid hormones T_3 and T_4 in the thyroid gland and are used in the treatment of hyperthyroid states. Unlike other means of hyperthyroid therapy, such as subtotal thyroidectomy or treatment with ^{131}I, antithyroid drugs do not tend to damage thyroid tissue beyond repair and thus are usually the initial treatment of choice. Long-term therapy may produce remission of the disease in some cases, but relapse is not uncommon. Patients who fail to respond fully to drug therapy or who show evidence of relapse should be considered as candidates for either surgery or radioisotope therapy.

Because the antithyroid drugs do not interfere with the release or activity of previously formed thyroid hormones, their clinical effects are often delayed for several weeks, until body stores of preformed T_4 and T_3 are exhausted. Likewise, the action of exogenously administered thyroid hormones is unimpaired by antithyroid drugs.

Several kinds of compounds are capable of exerting an antithyroid effect. Large amounts of the iodide ion (6–10 mg/day) can suppress release of thyroid hormones from the gland and are thus occasionally used for treating acute hyperthyroidism and for reducing the size and vascularity of the gland before surgical removal. Certain monovalent inorganic anions (eg, perchlorate, thiocyanate, periodate) block uptake of iodide by the gland and can exert an antithyroid action. They are rarely used clinically, however, because more effective and less toxic drugs are available. The principal antithyroid agents are the thioamide derivatives methimazole and propylthiouracil and they are discussed below, then summarized in Table 42-4.

Mechanism

Inhibit the biosynthesis of thyroid hormones by inhibiting the peroxidase enzyme system that catalyzes the conversion of iodide to iodine thus reducing the concentration of free iodine available for reaction with tyrosine. The drugs may also block oxidative coupling of mono- and diiodotyrosine to form T_3 and T_4 (see Chapter 40) and partially inhibit conversion of T_4 to T_3 in the periphery. They do *not* inactivate existing T_3 and T_4 nor interfere with the action of exogenously administered thyroid hormones.

Drug-induced depression of circulating hormone levels results in compensatory increase in TSH release from the adenohypophysis. Excess TSH activity can increase the size and vascularity of the thyroid gland, resulting in the development of *goiter* (refer to **Adverse Reactions**).

Uses

Treatment of hyperthyroidism (most effective in milder cases in which thyroid gland is not excessively enlarged)

Preparation for subtotal thyroidectomy or radioactive iodide therapy (to reduce hyperthyroidism and to lessen surgical risks)

Dosage

See Table 42-4.

Fate

Well absorbed orally and oral bioavailability is high; concentrated in the thyroid gland; peak serum levels occur within 1 hour; plasma half-lives are relatively short (2–3 hours) but do *not* reflect duration of antithyroid effect, which is due to action within the thyroid gland; dosing frequency is every 6 to 8 hours; propylthiouracil is excreted by the kidneys more quickly than methimazole

Common Side Effects

Skin rash, itching, nausea, epigastric distress

Significant Adverse Reactions

Paresthesias, arthralgia, myalgia, loss of taste, loss of hair, dizziness, drowsiness, neuritis, edema, skin pigmentation, lymphadenopathy, sialadenopathy, jaundice

Less commonly:

Agranulocytosis (0.5%), granulocytopenia, thrombocytopenia, drug fever, lupuslike reaction, hepatitis, periarteritis, hypoprothrombinemia, bleeding

Goitrogenic action is indicated by enlarged thyroid, periorbital edema, fatigue, paresthesias, muscle cramps, cool skin, sensitivity to cold, and bradycardia.

Contraindications

Nursing mothers. *Cautious use* in patients with liver dysfunction or bleeding tendencies and in pregnant women.

Interactions

Antithyroid drugs can magnify the effects of oral anticoagulants by causing hypoprothrombinemia.

Use cautiously in the presence of other drugs known to cause agranulocytosis (eg, antidepressants, carbamazepine, clofibrate, indomethacin, methyldopa, meprobamate, phenothiazines, phenylbutazone, procainamide, quinidine, and tolbutamide).

Nursing Management

Pretherapy Assessment

Assess and record baseline data necessary for detection of adverse effects of antithyroid drugs: General: VS, body weight, skin color and temperature, uterine tone; CNS: orientation, reflexes, muscle tone; CVS: baseline ECG; Lab: complete blood count (CBC), differential prothrombin time (PT), liver and renal function tests.

Review medical history and documents for existing or previous conditions that:

a. require cautious use of antithyroid drugs: liver dysfunction; bleeding tendencies
b. contraindicate use of antithyroid drugs: allergy to antithyroid products; **pregnancy (Category D)**, lactation (secreted in breast milk; avoid use)

Nursing Interventions

Medication Administration

Expect to use smallest effective dose during pregnancy because drugs readily cross placental barrier and may produce goiter and cretinism in developing fetus. The drug should be discontinued, if possible, 2 to 3 weeks before delivery. Thyroid hormones and antithyroid drugs are often given concurrently during pregnancy to prevent hypothyroidism in mother and fetus.

Expect to administer iodine (eg, Lugol's solution, potassium iodide solution) for 7 to 10 days before thyroidectomy, in patient receiving antithyroid drug, to reduce size and vascularity of the thyroid gland.

Administer in three equally divided doses at 8-hour intervals.

Provide small frequent meals if GI upset occurs.

Surveillance During Therapy

Monitor results of prothrombin times, which should be performed regularly during therapy, for hypoprothrombinemia.

Carefully monitor laboratory studies and patient for indications of adverse reactions.

Interpret results of diagnostic tests and contact practitioner as appropriate.

Monitor for possible drug–drug and drug–nutrient interactions: See **Interactions**.

Patient Teaching

Stress the importance of adhering to prescribed dosage regimen.

Warn patient that use of over-the-counter (OTC) preparations containing iodide (eg, cough syrups, asthma preparations) may interfere with effectiveness of antithyroid drug.

Teach patient how to monitor pulse and weight. Increased pulse, weight loss, anxiety, or tremor, possible indications of inadequate response, should be reported to drug prescriber.

Instruct patient to report development of sore throat, rash, fever, headache, or malaise immediately because these may be early indications of developing blood dyscrasia. If they occur, drug should be discontinued and hematologic studies should be performed.

Instruct patient to report appearance of petechiae, ecchymoses, or any other unexplained bleeding because drugs can cause hypoprothrombinemia.

Instruct patient and family to be alert for indications of overdosage (eg, depression, nonpitting edema, cold intolerance) and to notify practitioner if any occur.

Instruct mother taking antithyroid drug not to nurse infant.

Inform patient that thyroid hormone may be added to the regimen to prevent goiter when euthyroid state is attained.

Explain that therapy usually lasts 1 to 2 years, whereupon about 50% of patients have attained remission.

Instruct patient in remission to continue monitoring pulse and weight and to report any significant changes.

Radioactive Iodide

• Radioactive Sodium Iodide–^{131}I *(Pregnancy Category X)*

Iodotope

Of the several radioactive isotopes of iodine, ^{131}I is the most widely used clinically. Although its major indication is the treatment of certain types of hyperthyroidism, it has also been successfully employed for therapy of thyroid carcinoma.

Mechanism

Rapidly and efficiently taken up by the thyroid gland, incorporated into T_3 and T_4 and stored in the follicle of the gland; emits both beta-radiation, which penetrates only a few millimeters of tissue and thus remains localized in the thyroid gland, and small amounts of longer-wavelength gamma-radiation, which can be detected and measured externally; beta-radiation destroys thyroid tissue, leading to a gradual reduction in thyroid hormone secretion; some degree of *hypo*thyroidism almost always occurs

Uses

Treatment of hyperthyroidism, especially in patients older than 30 years of age whose condition does not respond to other antithyroid medications

Treatment of thyroid carcinoma and metastases (effectiveness is questionable in all cases because some thyroid neoplasms, eg, giant cell, spindle cell, and amyloid solid carcinomas, do *not* concentrate sufficient iodide ion)

Dosage

Dose is measured in millicuries (mCi) and varies depending on indication, size of the thyroid, uptake of a small initial tracer dose, and rate of release of radioactive iodine from the gland. Average doses are:

Hyperthyroidism: 4 to 10 mCi as a single dose; a second dose may be given 6 to 12 months later, depending on thyroid status

Thyroid carcinoma: 50 to 150 mCi

Usually administered orally as a solution (colorless and tasteless) or as capsules

Fate

Rapidly absorbed when taken orally, and quickly and efficiently concentrated by the thyroid gland as well as by the stomach and salivary glands; radioactivity can be detected in the thyroid within minutes. Half-life of ^{131}I isotope is 8 days. Thyroid function begins to decrease within 2 weeks; maximum effects are observed in 8 to 12 weeks; excreted mainly by the kidneys

Common Side Effects

Hypothyroidism (see Nursing Management), tenderness and soreness over the thyroid area, nausea, dysphagia, cough

Significant Adverse Reactions

Vomiting, sialoadenitis, thinning of the hair, acute thyroid crisis, chromosomal abnormalities, bone marrow depression, leukemia, anemia, leukopenia, thrombocytopenia

Destruction of excessive thyroid tissue can lead to symptoms of hypothyroidism such as:

- Weakness, fatigue, cold intolerance, peripheral edema, bradycardia, dyspnea, puffiness of the skin, anginalike pain

Contraindications

Pregnant and nursing mothers, very young children, preexisting vomiting and diarrhea, and persons with recent myocardial infarction. *Cautious use* in women of childbearing age.

Interactions

Uptake of ^{131}I by thyroid gland can be impaired by recent intake of iodine in any form (eg, x-ray contrast media; see Chapter 80) or by use of thyroid or antithyroid drugs

Nursing Management

Pretherapy Assessment

Assess and record baseline data necessary for detection of adverse effects of radioactive iodine: General: VS, body weight, skin color and temperature, uterine tone; CNS: orientation, reflexes, muscle tone; CVS: baseline ECG; Lab: CBC, differential PT, liver and renal function tests.

Review medical history and documents for evidence of existing or previous medical history related to conditions that:

a. require cautious use of radioactive iodine: women of childbearing age

b. contraindicate use of radioactive iodine: allergy to iodine; preexisting vomiting and diarrhea; recent myocardial infarction; **pregnancy (Category X)**, lactation (secreted in breast milk; avoid use)

Nursing Interventions

Medication Administration

Observe proper procedures for handling and administering radioactive materials.

Provide small frequent meals if GI upset occurs.

Surveillance During Therapy

Monitor results of thyroid function studies, which should be performed periodically to detect possible development of hypothyroidism.

Expect antithyroid drug therapy to be discontinued for 3 to 4 days before administration of radioiodide.

Note that solution may darken on standing, but this does not affect potency.

Carefully monitor laboratory studies and patient for indications of adverse reactions.

Interpret results of diagnostic tests and contact practitioner as appropriate.

Monitor for possible drug–drug and drug–nutrient interactions: Refer to **Interactions**.

Patient Teaching

Explain that several treatments with ^{131}I may be required to adequately control hyperthyroidism. If therapy is inadequate, it is usually apparent within 2 to 3 months (patient remains hyperthyroid).

Reassure patient that, with usual doses, no special radiation precautions are necessary because radioactivity is minimal.

Explain that thyroid hormone replacement therapy may be needed after treatment with ^{131}I to minimize the incidence and severity of hypothyroidism. Hypothyroidism often develops insidiously, but it probably occurs in *almost everyone* receiving ^{131}I. It may not, however, become manifest for years. Stress the importance of continuing thyroid replacement therapy for as long as necessary if hypothyroidism develops.

Iodine/Iodide Compounds

- **Potassium Iodide** *(Pregnancy Category D)*
- **Strong Iodine Solution** *(Pregnancy Category D)*

At one time, iodine and iodide were commonly used for treatment for hyperthyroidism. Despite their rapid beneficial action, effects were short-lived, and within a few weeks symptoms usually returned and in many instances were intensified. Largely for this reason, these drugs have only a limited therapeutic application today; they are primarily used adjunctively to reduce the size and vascularity of the thyroid gland *before thyroidectomy*. In addition, potassium iodide is used in radiation emergencies to block uptake of radioactive iodide by the thyroid gland. Available compounds include strong iodine solution (5% iodine and 10% potassium iodide), saturated solution of potassium iodide (SSKI), and tablets or solution containing potassium iodide in varying amounts. The pharmacology of these agents is discussed in general terms and individual drugs are then listed in Table 42-5. In addition, certain iodide-containing products useful as expectorants are detailed in Chapter 56.

Mechanism

Not completely established; may suppress release of thyroid hormones from thyroglobulin and interfere with synthesis of thyroid hormones; improvement in symptoms is rapid, hence these drugs are of value in treating thyroid storm; reduce size and vascularity of the thyroid gland and increase quantity of bound iodine within the gland

Uses

Preparation for thyroidectomy in hyperthyroid patients, in conjunction with an antithyroid drug (reduce size and vascularity of gland)

Table 42-5. **Iodine/Iodide Compounds**

Drug	*Usual Dosage Range*	*Nursing Considerations*
Potassium iodide *PIMA, Thyro-Block**	Expectorant: 300–1000 mg 2–3 times/day Radiation emergency: Adults: 130 mg daily Children (younger than age 1): 65 mg daily	Useful for hyperthyroidism, thyrotoxic crisis (with antithyroid drugs), preoperatively for thyroidectomy, and to facilitate bronchial drainage and cough in chronic pulmonary diseases; also used in radiation emergencies to block uptake of radioactive iodine by the thyroid gland; discontinue if skin rash appears; *see also* Chap. 56
Saturated solution potassium iodide *SSKI*	0.3–0.6 mL 4–12 times/day diluted in water, juice, or milk	Used presurgically for reducing size and fragility of thyroid gland; do not allow to stand uncovered for prolonged periods because solution may evaporate; slight discoloration of solution does not affect potency
Strong iodine solution *Lugol's solution*	0.1–0.3 mL (approximately 2–6 drops) 3 times/day (usually for 10–14 days before thyroidectomy)	Principally used to prepare thyroid gland for surgery; also used with an antithyroid drug for treating thyrotoxic crisis; discontinue if signs of iodism appear (metallic taste, stomatitis, swollen salivary glands, vomiting); administer solution diluted in juice, milk, or water, preferably after meals

* Available only to state and federal agencies for radiation emergencies

Acute treatment of thyrotoxic crisis (thyroid storm) or neonatal thyrotoxicosis

Provide a thyroid-blocking action in a radiation emergency

Symptomatic treatment of pulmonary diseases characterized by accumulation of excessive mucus (see Chapter 56)

Dosage

See Table 42-5.

Fate

Well absorbed when taken orally; effects usually noted within 24 to 48 hours and maximal effect occurs within 10 to 14 days; cleared from plasma primarily by thyroid uptake; eliminated in either urine or feces by way of the bile

Common Side Effects

Unpleasant metallic taste, GI distress

Significant Adverse Reactions

Gum soreness, mucosal ulceration, salivary gland enlargement, excessive salivation, rhinitis, fever, joint pain, dyspnea, edema, skin rash, vomiting, headache, goiter

IV administration can result in acute iodide poisoning, characterized by

Edema (bronchial, laryngeal), mucosal hemorrhaging, serum sickness, acneiform, maculopapular, vesicular or bullous eruptions, generalized inflammation

Contraindications

Potassium iodide is contraindicated in hyperkalemia. *Cautious use* in pregnant women.

Interactions

Lithium may enhance the hypothyroid action of potassium iodide

Estrogens and progestins can increase protein-bound iodine

Nursing Management

Nursing Interventions

Medication Administration

Question administration of ^{131}I to patient recently treated with iodine/iodides because the thyroid gland will be saturated and unable to take up the radioiodide.

Surveillance During Therapy

Be alert for development or exacerbation of hyperthyroidism if ^{131}I is given after iodine solution because large amounts of stored hormone may be released if gland is destroyed by radiation.

Observe patient for development of goiter. Withdrawal of iodide or administration of thyroid hormone will correct the condition, although the mechanism is incompletely understood.

Patient Teaching

Warn patient not to indiscriminately use OTC drugs containing iodides (eg, cough or asthma preparations, salt substitutes) because they may increase response to iodide therapy.

Stress the importance of adhering to prescribed dosage regimen when drug is used before thyroidectomy to avoid possible loss of iodide effectiveness and gland enlargement.

Advise patient to consult practitioner concerning need for restriction of iodine-rich foods (eg, seafoods, vegetables) or iodized salt.

Selected Bibliography

Dauncey MJ: Thyroid hormones and thermogenesis. Proceedings of the Nutrition Society 49(2):203, 1990

DeGroot LJ: Mechanism of thyroid hormone action. Adv Exp Med Biol 299:1, 1991

Feldt-Rasmussen U, Glinoer D, Orgiazzi I: Reassessment of antithyroid therapy of Graves' disease. Ann Rev Med 44:323, 1993

Franklyn JA: Syndromes of thyroid hormone resistance. Clin Endocrinol 34(3):237, 1991
Loosen PT: Effects of thyroid hormones on central nervous system in aging. Psychoneuroendocrinology 17(4):355, 1992
McDougall R: Graves' disease: Current concepts. Med Clin North Am 75:97, 1991
Schimke RN: Hyperthyroidism: The clinical spectrum. Postgrad Med 91:229, 1992
Stein SA, Adams PM, et al: Thyroid hormone control of brain and motor development: Molecular, neuroanatomical and behavioral studies. Adv Exp Med Biol 299:47, 1991
Weiss RE, Refetoff S: Thyroid hormone resistance. Annu Rev Med 43:363, 1992
Wolf PG, Meek JC: Practical approach to the treatment of hypothyroidism. Am Fam Physician 45:722, 1992

Nursing Bibliography

Isley W: Thyroid disorders. Critical Care Nursing Quarterly 13(3):39, 1990
Lammon C, et al: Action STAT! Recognizing thyrotoxic storm. Nursing '93 23(4):33, 1993
Mallet L: Hypothyroid treatment requires accurate diagnosis and follow up. Provider 19(1):49, 1993
Pines A, et al: Thyrotropin, menopause and hormone replacement. Journal of Women's Health 2(2):197, 1993

43
Parathyroid Drugs, Calcitonin, and Calcium

Calcitonin
Etidronate
Pamidronate
Plicamycin
Oral Calcium Salts

Calcium, the most abundant cation in the body, plays an important role in many vital physiologic processes, including bone formation, blood coagulation, muscle contraction, nerve conduction, hormone secretion, and enzyme activity. The level of free calcium and phosphate in the blood is dependent on a complex series of interactions among several substances, most important of which are parathyroid hormone (PTH) and vitamin D. PTH is a polypeptide synthesized by the parathyroid glands and is secreted in response to reductions in serum calcium. PTH elevates plasma calcium levels by increasing resorption of calcium ions from bone, by promoting renal tubular reabsorption of calcium, and by enhancing calcium absorption from the GI tract (see Chapter 40). *Vitamin D* is the term commonly applied to two biologically similar substances, ergocalciferol (D_2) and cholecalciferol (D_3). Its major actions on calcium metabolism are essentially identical to those of PTH, namely, increased resorption from bone and enhanced GI absorption. A third endogenous substance, *calcitonin*, can also influence calcium and phosphate metabolism. Calcitonin is a polypeptide secreted by the parafollicular (C) cells of the thyroid gland in response to an increase in serum calcium levels. It lowers serum calcium by inhibiting bone resorption and promotes renal excretion of calcium, probably by interfering with renal tubular reabsorption of the ion.

Serum levels of calcium are normally maintained within a narrow range (10 ± 1 mg/dL), and deviation from this level results in the appearance of symptoms of either hypercalcemia or hypocalcemia. *Hyper*calcemia may be related to hyperparathyroidism, excessive vitamin D intake, malignant tumors, or hyperthyroidism. It is characterized by vomiting, constipation, muscle weakness, electrocardiographic abnormalities, and deposition of calcium in soft tissues such as the kidney. Significant elevations in serum calcium can lead to progressive loss of sensation and eventually coma. Principal causes of *hypo*calcemia are hypoparathyroidism, inadequate vitamin D levels, and dietary calcium deficiency. Symptoms include muscle twitching, tetanic spasms, and convulsions.

Drugs discussed in this chapter are used to regulate body calcium stores, provide replacement for inadequate calcium, and to treat Paget's disease, a decalcification of bone leading to skeletal deformities, joint impairment, and development of vascular fibrous tissue in marrow spaces. Two forms of synthetic calcitonin and two nonhormonal biphosphonate compounds, etidronate and pamidronate, are used in moderate to severe forms of Paget's disease and are reviewed below. Mention is also made of plicamycin, an antibiotic used to treat hypercalcemia and hypercalciuria in patients whose condition is not responsive to conventional treatment. Plicamycin is also used to treat testicular tumors, and that aspect of its pharmacology is reviewed in Chapter 74. Several oral calcium salts, employed as dietary supplements for calcium deficiency states, are also considered in this chapter. Preparations with vitamin D–like activity (calcifediol, calcitriol, dihydrotachysterol) can be used to control hypocalcemic states related to a number of conditions, and these agents are discussed with the other fat-soluble vitamins in Chapter 75.

Synthetic Calcitonin

- ***Calcitonin, salmon***

Calcimar, Miacalcin, Osteocalcin

- ***Calcitonin, human***

Cibacalcin

The calcitonin products available for clinical use are synthetic compounds that resemble the polypeptide hormones of salmon calcitonin and human calcitonin. Salmon calcitonin is considerably more potent in humans than is human calcitonin, and it is also longer acting, perhaps because it is cleared from the circulatory system more slowly. However, circulating antibodies to calcitonin can form, and its efficacy may decline with continued use. The risk of reduced effectiveness caused by antibody formation appears to be less with synthetic *human* calcitonin, and this product may be effective in patients who have developed resistance to *salmon* calcitonin.

Mechanism

Decreases serum calcium levels by directly inhibiting osteoclastic bone resorption (effects become less intense with prolonged administration—possibly because of development of neutralizing antibodies); bone turnover rate is slowed and serum alkaline phosphatase levels decrease; increases excretion of calcium and phosphorus by blocking their renal tubular reabsorption; transiently but markedly reduces output of gastric and pancreatic secretions such as hydrochloric acid, gastrin, trypsin, and amylase

Uses

Treatment of moderate to severe Paget's disease (osteitis deformans)
Treatment of hypercalcemia, especially hypercalcemic emergencies
Adjunctive treatment of postmenopausal osteoporosis, in conjunction with adequate calcium and vitamin D intake

Dosage

Salmon Calcitonin

Prior skin testing for allergy: 0.1 mL of a 10-U/mL-dilution intracutaneously of the forearm; appearance of more than mild erythema or wheal indicates a positive allergic response

Paget's disease: initially 100 U/day SC (preferred) or IM; maintenance 50 U to 100 U daily or on alternate days

Hypercalcemia: initially 4 U/kg/12 hours SC or IM; may increase to 8 U/kg/12 hours after 1 day to 2 days, then to a maximum of 8 U/kg/6 hours if response is still unsatisfactory

Postmenopausal osteoporosis: 100 U/day SC or IM in conjunction with supplemental calcium and an adequate vitamin D intake

Human Calcitonin

Paget's disease: initially 0.5 mg/day SC; usual dosage range is 0.25 mg/day to 0.5 mg 2 to 3 times a week: more severe cases may require 0.5 mg twice a day; treatment may be continued for 6 months

Fate

Calcium-lowering effect occurs within 2 hours after injection and persists for 6 to 8 hours; when given every 12 hours, the calcium-lowering effect lasts for up to 8 days. Calcitonin is rapidly converted to smaller fragments in the kidneys, blood, and other organs, and these fragments are excreted in the urine.

Common Side Effects

Nausea, vomiting, local inflammatory reaction at injection site, facial flushing, paresthesias, urinary frequency

Significant Adverse Reactions

Diuresis, urticaria, skin rash, diarrhea, abdominal pain, salty taste, chills, dyspnea, dizziness, hypocalcemic tetany

Because calcitonin is a protein, systemic allergic reactions can occur and are more common with salmon calcitonin. In addition, antibodies to calcitonin may form with repeated use, reducing its efficacy. This latter effect is also seen more frequently with salmon calcitonin than with human calcitonin.

Contraindications

In young children, pregnancy, and nursing mothers. *Cautious use* in osteoporosis *without adequate calcium and vitamin D supplementation*, and in persons with renal dysfunction or pernicious anemia.

Interactions

Calcitonin may antagonize the hypercalcemic action of PTH, dihydrotachysterol, and vitamin D.

The effects of calcitonin can be augmented by androgens.

Nursing Management

Pretherapy Assessment

Assess and record baseline data necessary for detection of adverse effects of calcitonin products: General: vital signs (VS), body weight, skin color and temperature; central nervous system (CNS): muscle tone; Lab: urinalysis, serum calcium, serum alkaline phosphatase, urinary hydroxyproline.

Review medical history and documents for existing or previous conditions that:

a. require cautious use of calcitonin products: osteoporosis *without adequate calcium and vitamin D supplementation*, and in persons with renal dysfunction or pernicious anemia
b. contraindicate use of calcitonin products: allergy to salmon calcitonin; **pregnancy (Category C [human], Category B [salmon])**, lactation (secreted in breast milk; may inhibit lactation, avoid use)

Nursing Interventions

Medication Administration

Ensure that proper materials (eg, epinephrine, antihistamines, oxygen) are available to treat allergic reactions. Have parenteral calcium available to treat hypocalcemic tetany that may develop, especially during initial stages of therapy.

Surveillance During Therapy

Help evaluate drug effect by monitoring results of serum alkaline phosphatase and 24-hour urinary hydroxyproline levels, which should be measured periodically, and assessing patient for symptoms. Biochemical abnormalities and bone pain should decrease during the first few months of therapy. Dosages beyond 100 U/day of salmon calcitonin or 1 mg/day of human calcitonin usually do not result in improved clinical response.

Carefully monitor laboratory studies and patient for indications of adverse reactions.

Interpret results of diagnostic tests and contact practitioner as appropriate.

Monitor for possible drug–drug and drug–nutrient interactions: Refer to **Interactions**.

Patient Teaching

Teach patient proper technique for handling and injecting drug at home.

Reassure patient that the nausea and vomiting that may occur during initial stages of therapy disappear as treatment continues.

Stress the importance of continuing therapy even when clinical symptoms have abated.

Biphosphonates

- **Etidronate**

  Didronel

- **Pamidronate**

  Aredia

Biphosphonates are nonhormonal substances that inhibit both normal and abnormal bone resorption, and are used primarily in treating Paget's disease and controlling other hypercalcemic states.

Mechanism

Exact mechanism is not understood; may inhibit osteoclastic activity as well as dissolution of hydroxyapatite crystals; etidronate can decrease subsequent bone formation, thus slowing bone turnover rate in disease states.

Uses

Treatment of moderate to severe Paget's disease (osteitis deformans); symptomatic improvement occurs in approximately three of five patients (etidronate)
Reduction of heterotopic bone ossification caused by spinal cord injury or that complicating total hip replacement (etidronate)
Treatment of hypercalcemia of malignancy (etidronate or pamidronate given IV with adequate hydration and use of loop diuretics, if needed, to restore urine output)
Unlabeled uses include treatment of postmenopausal or glucocorticoid-induced osteoporosis, hyperparathyroidism, and reduction of bone pain in patients with prostatic carcinoma or multiple myeloma

Dosage

Etidronate

Oral:
Paget's disease: Initially 5 mg to 10 mg/kg/day for up to 6 months or 11 mg to 20 mg/kg/day for up to 3 months (maximum dose, 20 mg/kg/day); retreatment at the same doses may be initiated after at least a 3-month drug-free period if reactivation of the disease has occurred
Heterotopic ossification due to spinal cord injury: 20 mg/day for 2 weeks, followed by 10 mg/kg/day for 10 weeks, instituted as soon as possible after the injury
Heterotopic ossification complicating total hip replacement: 20 mg/kg/day for 1 month preoperatively; then 20 mg/kg/day for 3 months postoperatively
IV infusion:
Hypercalcemia of malignancy: 7.5 mg/kg/day for 3 successive days, given over at least 2 hours. Daily dosage is diluted in at least 250 mL sterile saline; may repeat after 7 days. Oral tablets may be started the day after the last infusion at a dose of 20 mg/kg/day for up to 30 days

Pamidronate

IV infusion:
Hypercalcemia of malignancy: 60 to 90 mg given over 24 hours; may repeat in 7 days if hypercalcemia recurs.

Fate

Etidronate is very poorly absorbed if taken orally (1% at 5 mg/kg); cleared from the blood within 6 hours; one half absorbed dose is excreted in the urine within 24 hours, the remainder being adsorbed onto bone and very slowly eliminated; half-life on bone is 3 to 6 months; unabsorbed drug is eliminated in the feces; approximately half of an infused dose is adsorbed onto bone and slowly eliminated; the remainder is excreted unchanged in the urine within 72 hours.

Common Side Effects

Loose stools, nausea, altered taste, fever (with pamidronate)

Significant Adverse Reactions

Increased bone pain at previously asymptomatic sites, demineralization of bone leading to fractures, hypersensitivity reactions (rash, pruritus, urticaria), electrolyte abnormalities (hypophosphatemia, hypokalemia, hypomagnesemia)

Contraindications

Etidronate is contraindicated if serum creatinine is less than 5 mg/dL. *Cautious use* in patients with renal impairment, enterocolitis, long-bone fractures (may retard fracture healing), in children, and in pregnant or nursing women.

Nursing Management

Pretherapy Assessment

Assess and record baseline data necessary for detection of adverse effects of biphosphonates: General: VS, body weight, skin color and temperature; CNS: muscle tone, bone pain; Lab: urinalysis, serum calcium.
Review medical history and documents for existing or previous conditions that:
a. require cautious use of biphosphonates: renal impairment; enterocolitis; long-bone fractures (may retard fracture healing); in children
b. contraindicate use of biphosphonates: allergy to biphosphonates; serum creatinine less than 5 mg/dl; **pregnancy (Category B)**, lactation (secreted in breast milk; may inhibit lactation, avoid use)

Nursing Interventions

Medication Administration

Administer etidronate 2 hours before meals, with fruit juice or water; if GI upset occurs, divide into two equal doses.
Do not administer foods high in calcium, vitamins with mineral supplements, or antacids high in metals within 2 hours of dosing.
Provide ready access to bathroom facilities, small frequent meals if GI upset occurs.
Seek verification if recommended dosage regimen is exceeded because the incidence of untoward reactions (eg, GI distress, bone pain, fractures) increases dramatically at elevated doses.
Question prophylactic use in asymptomatic patient because there is no evidence to support this. Most patients with mild symptoms can be effectively treated with analgesics.
Expect drug to be discontinued if a fracture occurs, and resumed only after fracture heals completely.

Surveillance During Therapy

Monitor results of urinary hydroxyproline and serum alkaline phosphatase tests, which should be performed periodically during therapy. Usually, the first evidence of clinical benefit is reduced urinary hydroxyproline excretion. Serum alkaline phosphatase is also lowered by 30% in most patients.

Carefully monitor laboratory studies and patient for indications of adverse reactions.
Interpret results of diagnostic tests and contact practitioner as appropriate.
Monitor for possible drug–drug and drug–nutrient interactions: Refer to **Interactions**.

Patient Teaching

Instruct patient to take etidronate on an empty stomach, 2 hours before meals, unless GI distress is extreme, because food impairs absorption.
Inform patient that response to therapy is gradual and continues for months after drug is stopped. Consequently, dosage is usually increased cautiously, treatment is usually not resumed until evidence of disease recurrence is clear, and therapy should not be reinstituted before at least 3 drug-free months have passed.
Stress the need to maintain an adequate intake of calcium and vitamin D through dietary sources, calcium supplementation, or both.

- ***Plicamycin***

Mithracin

Plicamycin (also known as mithramycin) is an antibiotic produced by *Streptomyces plicatus*. It is employed by IV infusion to treat hypercalcemia and hypercalciuria in patients whose condition is not responsive to conventional therapy, such as those with advanced neoplasms. Because of its potential to elicit serious toxicity (thrombocytopenia, hemorrhage, liver or kidney dysfunction), however, the drug's potential benefit must be carefully weighed against the risk. Plicamycin is contraindicated in patients with thrombocytopenia, coagulation disorders, increased susceptibility to bleeding, and bone marrow depression. Platelet counts, prothrombin time, and bleeding time must be determined frequently during therapy and for several days after the last dose. Epistaxis or hematemesis may be early indications of a developing hemorrhagic syndrome and should be reported immediately. GI symptoms (nausea, diarrhea, anorexia, stomatitis) represent the most frequent side effects. The recommended dose is 25 μg/kg/day by IV infusion over 4 to 6 hours for 3 or 4 days. If the desired degree of reversal of hypercalcemia is not attained, the dosage may be repeated at intervals of 1 week or more. Normal calcium balance can often be maintained with single weekly doses or 2 to 3 doses/week. Rapid IV injections should be avoided, because the incidence of GI disturbances is much greater with this method. Extravasation of the solution should be avoided, because local irritation, cellulitis, and possibly thrombophlebitis can occur. Moderate heat applied to the site of extravasation may help disperse the compound and minimize discomfort.

Plicamycin is also employed in the treatment of testicular neoplasms, and that application is considered in detail in Chapter 74. NOTE: for Nursing Management refer to Chapter 74.

Oral Calcium Salts

- ***Calcium acetate***
- ***Calcium carbonate***
- ***Calcium citrate***
- ***Calcium glubionate***
- ***Calcium gluconate***
- ***Calcium lactate***
- ***Tricalcium phosphate***

Adequate intake of calcium is essential for normal homeostasis and is particularly critical during periods of active bone growth—for example, during childhood, adolescence, pregnancy, or lactation. In addition, sufficient calcium intake is necessary for the prevention and treatment of disease-induced calcium deficiency states such as hypoparathyroidism, postmenopausal osteoporosis, and tetany of the newborn. The use of oral calcium supplements, particularly as they apply to the adjunctive treatment of calcium deficiency states resulting from hypoparathyroidism, is discussed here. In contrast, parenteral therapy with calcium is indicated for treatment of hypocalcemic states requiring a *prompt* elevation in plasma calcium, for example, neonatal tetany, severe vitamin D deficiency, and systemic alkalosis. Parenteral calcium therapy is reviewed along with other parenteral electrolytes in Chapter 76. The pharmacology of the oral calcium preparations is described for the group, then individual drugs are listed in Table 43-1.

Mechanism

Replace deficient calcium stores in the body; presence of sufficient calcium is essential for bone development, blood coagulation, muscle contraction, cardiac functioning, and many other physiological processes

Uses

Prevention or treatment of calcium deficiency states, such as those associated with hypoparathyroidism, osteoporosis, rickets, and osteomalacia
Supplementation of dietary calcium insufficiency such as may occur during childhood, pregnancy, lactation, and in the postmenopausal woman

Dosage

See Table 43-1.

Fate

Absorption is good when taken orally, provided adequate levels of vitamin D and PTH are present; solubility (and thus absorption rate) is increased in acidic pH; excretion occurs largely in urine

Common Side Effects

Occasional GI distress

Significant Adverse Reactions

Hypercalcemia (nausea, vomiting, abdominal pain, constipation, polyuria, fatigue, muscle weakness, bradycardia, arrhythmias, confusion), hypercalciuria

Contraindications

Renal calculi, hypercalcemia. *Cautious use* in persons with a history of renal stones, cardiac arrhythmias, or renal insuffi-

Table 43-1. **Oral Calcium Salts**

Drug	*Usual Dosage Range*	*Nursing Considerations*
Calcium acetate *Phos-Ex, PhosLo*	2–4 tablets with each meal (each tablet contains 167 mg or 250 mg elemental calcium)	Contains 25% calcium; used for control of hyperphosphatemia in end-stage renal failure; do not give other calcium supplements concurrently; serum calcium × phosphate product should not exceed 66
Calcium carbonate *Several manufacturers*	1–1.5 g 3 times/day (maximum, 8 g/day)	Contains 40% calcium; very potent antacid (*see* Chap. 50); high incidence of constipation; tablet may be chewed before swallowing or dissolved in mouth and followed by water
Calcium citrate *Citracal*	1–2 tablets 2–4 times/day	Contains 21% calcium; effervescent tablets contain phenylalanine
Calcium glubionate *Neo-Calglucon*	Adults: 15 mL, 3 times/day Pregnant women: 15 mL 4 times/day Children: 10 mL 3 times/day Infants: 5 mL 5 times/day	Contains 6.5% calcium; GI disturbances are rare; administer before meals to enhance absorption
Calcium gluconate	Adults:1–2 g orally 3–4 times/day	Contains 9% calcium; GI irritation is minimal, but drug may be constipating
Calcium lactate	325 mg–1.3 mg 3 times/day	Contains 13% calcium; tablets may be dissolved in hot water, then cool water added to taste; absorption may be enhanced by lactose; administer with meals
Tricalcium phosphate *Posture*	1–2 tablets 2–4 times/day	Contains 39% calcium

ciency and to persons receiving digitalis glycosides (refer to **Interactions**).

Interactions

Gastrointestinal absorption of calcium can be enhanced by vitamin D and impaired by corticosteroids, phosphorus (eg, milk, dairy products), oxalic acid (eg, spinach, rhubarb), and phytic acid (eg, bran cereals).

Calcium may reduce the muscle-relaxing effects of neuromuscular blocking agents.

Elevated serum calcium levels may increase digitalis toxicity.

Oral calcium products can retard the oral absorption of atenolol, tetracyclines, phenytoin, and iron salts.

Calcium may antagonize the action of calcium channel blocking drugs (see Chapter 34).

Nursing Management

Nursing Interventions

Patient Teaching

Advise patient to take oral calcium half hour before meals or 1 to 1.5 hours after meals to increase utilization.

Explain that frequent blood and urine tests may be required during prolonged therapy to avoid hypercalcemia and hypercalciuria.

Selected Bibliography

Bilczikain JP: Management of acute hypercalcemia. N Engl J Med 326: 1196, 1992

Canfield RE, Siris ES: Use of etidronate in Paget's disease of bone. In Summit L (ed): Diphosphonates: The First Decade. Williamsburg, Va, Virginia Commonwealth University, 1988

Deftos LJ, Parthemore JG, Stabile BE: Management of primary hyperparathyroidism. Ann Rev Med 44:19, 1993

Hodsman AB, Fraher LJ: Biochemical responses to sequential human parathyroid hormone and calcitonin in osteoporotic patients. Bone Mineral 9(2):137, 1990

Horowitz E, Miller JL, Rose LI: Etidronate for hypercalcemia of malignancy and osteoporosis. Am Fam Physician 43(6):2155, 1991

Overmyer RH: New studies show that etidronate has much potential as a treatment for osteoporosis. Modern Med 59:118, 1991

Recker RR: Current therapy for osteoporosis. J Clin Endocrinol Metab 76:14, 1993

Riggs BL: Treatment of osteoporosis with sodium fluoride or parathyroid hormone. Am J Med 91:37S, 1991

Watts NB, Harris ST, et al: Intermittent cyclical etidronate treatment of postmenopausal osteoporosis. N Engl J Med 323:73, 1990

Nursing Bibliography

Hawthorne J, et al: Common electrolyte imbalances associated with malignancy. Clinical Issues in Critical Care Nursing 3(3):714, 1992

Long K, et al: Current treatment concepts for osteoporosis. Nursing Practice Forum 2(4):214, 1991

Meythaler K, et al: Successful treatment of immobilization hypercalcemia using calcitonin with didronate. Arch Phys Med Rehabil 64(3):316, 1993

Norris M: Evaluating serum calcium levels. Nursing '93 23(2): 69, 1993

Urrows S, et al: Profiles in osteoporosis. Am Nurs 91(12): 32, 1991

44

Antidiabetic and Hyperglycemic Agents

Insulins
Oral antidiabetics

Glucose

Glucagon
Diazoxide, oral

Alterations in blood glucose levels can occur in a variety of disease states as well as with the use of many drugs; in most cases these changes represent undesired side effects of the compounds. A few drugs, however, are employed specifically for their ability to lower or raise blood glucose levels and thus are termed *hypoglycemic* and *hyperglycemic agents*, respectively.

Hypoglycemic drugs produce a decline in blood and urinary levels of glucose and are used principally in the treatment of diabetes mellitus, a chronic metabolic disorder characterized by a deficiency of *functional* insulin and elevated levels of glucose in the blood (hyperglycemia) and urine (glycosuria). The causes and types of diabetes mellitus and the associated metabolic disturbances are reviewed in Chapter 40. Drug therapy of diabetes mellitus may be undertaken by either providing replacement insulin or by oral administration of synthetic sulfonamide-related hypoglycemic drugs (sulfonylureas), which increase release of endogenous insulin and enhance the binding of insulin to receptors on body cells.

The antidiabetic drugs considered in this chapter include the various insulin preparations, which are indicated in insulin-deficient forms of diabetes (type I, insulin-dependent diabetes; see Chapter 40) and the oral hypoglycemic drugs, which are used mainly in milder diabetes, frequently associated with obesity, in which insulin levels are near normal but the hormone is relatively ineffective (type II, non–insulin-dependent diabetes; see Chapter 40).

Successful treatment of diabetes mellitus, however, requires more than mere drug therapy. Among the many adjunctive measures that should be considered when necessary in properly managing the diabetic state are:

- Weight reduction
- Regulation of the diet
- Proper amounts of exercise
- Maintenance of good hygiene
- Education of the patient about proper monitoring procedures to avoid untoward effects.

In fact, milder forms of type II diabetes can be adequately controlled in many instances without resorting to drugs, simply through weight loss and careful regulation of the diet. Drug treatment of diabetes mellitus, when necessary, is a highly individual matter and requires accurate diagnosis, continual monitoring of the patient, and proper drug dosage modifications as necessitated by changes in patient status.

Conversely, drugs that elevate blood glucose levels can be employed to reverse hypoglycemia resulting from diseases (such as pancreatic carcinoma, hormonal imbalances, liver and kidney dysfunction) or antidiabetic drug overdosage. Parenteral glucose is the most effective agent for elevating blood glucose levels and should be employed in acute situations whenever feasible. Glucagon, a purified peptide extracted from pancreatic alpha (A) cells; diazoxide, a thiazide derivative that blocks insulin release; and oral administration of glucose as a gel or chewable tablet also may be employed. These compounds are also reviewed in this chapter.

Insulins

- ***Insulin injection***
- ***Insulin zinc suspension***
- ***Insulin zinc suspension, extended***
- ***Isophane insulin suspension***

Endogenous insulin is a 51–amino-acid polypeptide hormone secreted by the beta (β) cells of the islets of Langerhans of the pancreas. It is composed of two amino acid chains joined together by disulfide linkages. Insulin is the principal hormone that regulates glucose utilization by human cells. The clinically available insulin preparations include purified extracts from beef or pork pancreas that possess biologic effects qualitatively identical to those of human insulin, differing structurally from human insulin by only three (beef) or one (pork) amino acid in the sequence. In addition, *"human"* insulin (ie, a preparation having the *exact* amino acid sequence of endogenous insulin) is now available; it is derived by either a recombinant DNA technique using strains of *Escherichia coli* or chemical modification of animal-extracted pork insulin to replace the lone amino acid that is different from that of human insulin.

All commercially available insulins extracted from animal sources contain certain quantities of the prohormone proinsulin and possibly other proteins or substances resulting from incomplete conversion of the prohormone. These "contaminants" may contribute to the immunogenic reactions that some insulin users experience, such as lipodystrophy and local and systemic allergic reactions. All commercially available insulins in the United States contain no more than 25 parts per million (ppm) of proinsulin. Newer purification techniques used to remove the allergenic contaminants have been refined to the point that a number of "purified insulins" are now available that contain less than 10 ppm proinsulin. These "purified" insulins elicit even fewer allergic reactions than the older insulins. Finally, the "human" insulins, as indicated above, are prepared synthetically and are virtually free of contaminants. They appear to be as effective as the conventional insulins and may be slightly less antigenic than the beef or pork insulins in certain patients because of their lack of contaminants.

Most diabetic patients do equally well on conventional or human insulin. Generally, candidates for the human insulins are those patients who exhibit local or systemic allergic reactions or severe lipodystrophy with conventional insulin preparations. A few patients may require dosage adjustments when switched from conventional to purified or human insulins, because the latter preparations are less bound by insulin antibodies. All stabilized diabetic patients being switched to a different insulin preparation should be monitored closely to determine if a dosage modification is required. Human insulin is probably viewed as the insulin of choice in patients displaying insulin resistance or insulin allergy, as well as in pregnant diabetics. Should the methods for synthesizing human insulins become more cost-effective than animal-extraction procedures over time, the use of human insulin products will probably increase.

Several types of chemically modified insulin preparations are available in addition to regular insulin. These modified forms of insulin have been formulated to display differences in onset, peak, and duration of action, thereby allowing the physician to carefully control the response in each patient. The time course of action of the various insulins is largely dependent on the composition of the different preparations, such as the presence of conjugating metals or proteins (eg, zinc, protamine), the types of buffers used, and the pH of the medium. Thus, insulin preparations can conveniently be divided into three groups according to their onset and duration of action. This classification is outlined in Table 44-1, where several characteristics of the different insulins are listed. All available insulin preparations are presented in Table 44-2, where specific indications and other pertinent information are given for each individual drug.

Insulin preparations are standardized on the basis of their hypoglycemic action in fasted rabbits, and doses are measured in units (U). One insulin unit (U) possesses the activity of 1/24 mg Zinc Insulin Crystals Reference Standard. Insulin is marketed in 10-mL vials containing 100 U/mL as well as a 20-mL concentrated solution containing 500 U/mL. Most insulin preparations are stable at room temperature, provided they are not subject to temperature fluctuations or direct sunlight. However, it is advisable to store any extra bottles in the refrigerator until needed.

The mixing of certain types of insulins in the same syringe can be accomplished without incompatibility problems (see Table 44-1 and Dosage). In addition, several fixed combinations of insulins are now available and are listed in Table 44-2.

Mechanism

Facilitates uptake of glucose by cells of striated muscle and adipose tissue, probably by activating a carrier system for transport of glucose across the cell membrane; stimulates glycogen synthesis in muscle and liver by increasing enzyme activity, and suppresses gluconeogenesis; enhances formation of triglycerides and retards release of free fatty acids from adipose tissue; facilitates incorporation of amino acids into muscle protein and may thus promote protein synthesis. Restoration of efficient glucose utilization decreases hyperglycemia, reduces glucosuria, and prevents diabetic acidosis and coma

Uses

Treatment of diabetes mellitus, especially the insulin-dependent (type I) type and complicated forms of non–insulin-dependent (ie,type II) diabetes not adequately controlled by diet, exercise, and weight loss

Emergency treatment of severe ketoacidosis or diabetic coma (regular insulin given IM or IV)

Dosage

Must be individually titrated on the basis of blood glucose, urinary glucose, and ketone determinations. The various insulin preparations are listed in Table 44-2 along with their source and nursing considerations. The drug is given SC, and sites of administration are rotated to minimize the occurrence of lipodystrophy (localized hollowing of the skin at injection sites, presumably because of alterations in lipid metabolism).

Preparations available as suspensions should be rolled gently between the hands before administration to facilitate uniform dispersion; vigorous shaking should be avoided, because frothing may lead to withdrawal of improper amounts of drug for injection.

Compatibility of Admixtures

Certain types of insulin may be mixed in the same syringe. If regular insulin is used, it should always be drawn into the syringe first. Mixtures of regular insulin with NPH or lente insulins should be injected immediately after mixing, because some regular insulin is bound to either protamine or zinc within the first 15

Table 44-1. **Characteristics of Insulin Preparations**

Drug	*Synonym*	*Onset*	*Peak Action*	*Duration*	*Compatibility*
Rapid Acting					
Insulin Injection	Regular insulin	1/2–1 hour	2–4 hours	6–8 hours	All others
Intermediate Acting					
Insulin zinc suspension	Lente insulin	1–2 hours	8–15 hours	18–24 hours	Regular, Ultralente
Isophane insulin suspension	NPH insulin	1–1 1/2 hours	4–12 hours	18–24 hours	Regular
Long Acting					
Insulin zinc suspension, extended	Ultralente insulin	4–8 hours	12–24 hours	>36 hours	Regular, Lente

Note: A 70/30 mixture of isophane insulin suspension and regular insulin injection is also available; onset is 1/2 hour, peak effect is within 4 to 8 hours, and duration is 18 to 24 hours. In addition, a 50/50 mixture of regular insulin injection and isophane insulin suspension is available providing faster peak blood levels and a shorter duration of action than the 70/30 mixture.

Table 44-2. **Insulin Preparations**

Drug	Preparations and Sources	Nursing Considerations
RAPID ACTING		
Insulin injection *Regular Insulin, Regular Iletin I*	Injection: 100 U/mL (pork, beef and pork)	Short acting; solution is clear; may be administered SC 15–30 min before meals for control of diabetes or IV (only insulin suitable for IV use) for severe ketoacidosis or diabetic coma; give 1 g dextrose/U insulin when administered IV, and monitor blood sugar, blood pressure, and intake/output ratio every hour until stable; be alert for development of rapid hypoglycemia and insulin shock
Purified *Regular Purified Pork, Regular Iletin II*	Purified injection: 100 U/mL (pork)	
Human *Novolin R, Humulin R, Velosulin Human*	Human: 100 U/mL	
Insulin injection, concentrated *Regular Concentrated Iletin II*	Purified injection: 500 U/mL (pork)	Indicated for control of diabetes in patients with marked insulin resistance; may be administered SC or IM: concentrated from pork pancreas, solution is clear and colorless; accuracy in dosage is essential because of potency; marked hypoglycemia can occur
INTERMEDIATE ACTING		
Insulin zinc suspension *Lente Iletin I, Lente Insulin*	Injection: 100 U/mL (beef, beef and pork)	Cloudy suspension containing a mixture of 30% prompt zinc suspension and 70% extended zinc suspension; contains no proteins, thus allergic reactions are rare; administered SC 30–60 min before breakfast; action closely approximates that of NPH insulin, although duration of action may be slightly longer; see Table 44-1 for compatibilities
Purified *Lente Iletin II, Lente L*	Purified injection: 100 U/mL (pork)	
Human *Humulin L, Novolin L*	Human: 100 U/mL	
Isophane insulin suspension *NPH insulin, NPH Iletin I*	Injection: 100 U/mL (beef, beef and pork)	Suspension of protamine zinc insulin crystals; administered SC 30 min before breakfast; a second injection in the evening may be required; may be mixed with regular insulin injection, but not lente forms; available in fixed combination with regular insulin injection as a 70%/30% mixture as Novolin 70/30 and Humulin 70/30; also available in a 50%/50% mixture as Humulin 50/50
Purified *NPH Iletin II, NPH-N*	Purified injection: 100 U/mL (pork)	
Human *Humulin N, Novolin N*	Human: 100 U/mL	
LONG ACTING		
Insulin zinc suspension, extended *Ultralente U*	Injection: 100 U/mL (beef)	Cloudy suspension of large particles of zinc insulin, which delay absorption and prolong effects; no protein and low incidence of allergic reactions; administered SC 30–90 min before breakfast; may be mixed with other lente preparations
Human *Humulin U, Ultralente U*	Human: 100 U/mL	

minutes, possibly altering the onset and duration of action. Lente and ultralente insulins may be combined in any proportion, because they are chemically identical.

Insulin can adsorb onto plastic IV infusion sets; the extent of adsorption is approximately 20% to 30% and is inversely proportional to the concentration of insulin. If insulin is administered in this manner, the patient's response should be closely monitored.

Fate

Inactivated when taken orally; absorbed at varying rates from SC injection sites (see Table 44-1 for onset, peak action, and duration of effect); bioavailability of insulins is identical when administered SC; plasma half-life ($T_{1/2}$) is less than 10 minutes; metabolized by both the liver and the kidneys and excreted in the feces and to a small extent in the urine

Common Side Effects

Mild hypoglycemia (fatigue, headache, drowsiness, nausea, mild tremor), local allergic reactions at injection site (itching, swelling, erythema)

Significant Adverse Reactions

Marked hypoglycemia (sweating, tremor, hypothermia, weakness, hunger, palpitations, nervousness, paresthesias, irritability, blurred vision, numbness in mouth, confusion, delirium, convulsions, and loss of consciousness), systemic allergic reactions (urticaria, angioedema, anaphylactic episodes), lipodystrophy at injection sites, insulin resistance, visual disturbances

Contraindications

Hypersensitivity to specific animal proteins (eg, bovine, porcine)

Interactions

Hypoglycemia may be augmented by alcohol, anabolic steroids, anticoagulants, beta-blockers (can also mask early symptoms of hypoglycemia), clofibrate, oral hypoglycemics, antineoplastics, monoamine oxidase (MAO) inhibitors, guanethidine, phenylbutazone, tetracyclines, and salicylates.

The hypoglycemic effects of insulin can be antagonized by corticosteroids, thiazide diuretics, dextrothyroxine, diltiazem, dobutamine, diazoxide, epinephrine, estrogens, glucagon, oral contraceptives, phenytoin, and thyroid preparations.

Insulin may lower serum potassium levels and can increase the toxicity of digitalis glycosides.

Nursing Management

Pretherapy Assessment

Assess and record baseline data necessary for detection of adverse effects of insulin: General: vital signs (VS), body weight, skin color and temperature; central nervous system (CNS): orientation, reflexes, peripheral sensation; Lab: urinalysis, blood glucose.

Review medical history and documents for existing or previous conditions that:

a. require cautious use of insulin: none
b. contraindicate use of insulin: allergy to beef, pork products; **pregnancy (Category B)**, lactation (not secreted in breast milk; requirements may drop during lactation).

Nursing Interventions

Medication Administration

Closely monitor patient receiving insulin through a plastic IV infusion set to ensure adequate response because the plastic surface can adsorb 25% to 50% of the dose.

Store insulin vials in a cool place. Avoid freezing or high temperatures and protect from strong light.

Avoid injecting cold insulin because lipodystrophy and reduced absorption can result.

Rotate vial and invert end to end several times just before withdrawing each dose to ensure proper dispersion of particles in suspension preparations. Do *not* shake vigorously because frothing may occur, which could result in withdrawal of an inadequate dose. Regular insulin, which is a solution, does not contain particles.

Withdraw appropriate volume of regular insulin first to avoid contaminating vial of regular insulin, which does not contain protein (ie, protamine), with insulin that does contain protein (see Table 44-1 for mixture compatibility of different insulins), when mixing regular insulin with another insulin in one syringe.

Use immediately, if regular insulin is mixed with NPH or lente insulin, because mixture may not be stable beyond 10 to 15 minutes.

Administer insulin 15 to 90 minutes before a meal, depending on type (see Table 44-1). If a dose is withheld for any reason, decrease food intake and increase fluid intake.

Inject SC into areas with substantial fatty layers.

Systematically rotate injection sites to minimize trauma and lipodystrophy at particular sites.

Observe injection site for local allergic reaction. Although symptoms usually disappear with continued use, an antihistamine may be used to alleviate local discomfort. Allergic reactions can also be minimized by using pork insulin instead of either beef or mixtures of beef and pork (or vice versa). Switching to the corresponding purified or human insulin are additional alternatives.

Discard discolored or clumped solutions or partially used vials that have been open for several weeks.

Surveillance During Therapy

Monitor urine and blood glucose levels frequently to determine effectiveness and dosage.

Carefully monitor laboratory studies and patient for indications of adverse reactions.

Interpret results of diagnostic tests and contact practitioner as appropriate.

Monitor for possible drug–drug and drug–nutrient interactions: Refer to **Interactions**.

Patient Teaching

Teach patient techniques involved in insulin administration.

Advise patient to carry a sufficient supply of syringes and needles when traveling and to store insulin vial in a cool place.

Inform patient that visual disturbances may occur during initial therapy. Eyeglass prescriptions should not be changed for at least several weeks after therapy has been initiated.

Warn patient not to use any other medications without consulting the primary healthcare provider.

Instruct patient in the procedures for monitoring blood/urine glucose or ketones.

Instruct the patient to report to the practitioner any of the following if they occur: fever; sore throat; vomiting; hypoglycemic or hyperglycemic reactions; skin rash.

Oral Antidiabetic Drugs

- ***Acetohexamide***
- ***Chlorpropamide***
- ***Glipizide***
- ***Glyburide***
- ***Tolazamide***
- ***Tolbutamide***

The orally effective antidiabetic agents are sulfonamide derivatives, termed sulfonylureas, that are devoid of antibacterial activity. The clinically useful oral antidiabetics have similar mechanisms of action, that is, release of endogenous insulin from functional beta cells in the pancreas and enhanced sensitivity of insulin receptor sites on cellular membranes. However, they display significant differences in the duration of their hypoglycemic action. These differences are detailed in Table 44-3, which lists the available drugs and other pertinent characteristics.

The principal indication for the oral antidiabetic agents is management of mild, stable, non–insulin-dependent (type II) diabetes that cannot be adequately controlled by diet alone. They are of no value in type I, insulin-dependent diabetes, nor in those forms of diabetes complicated by ketoacidosis.

This cautious approach to oral antidiabetic drug therapy has evolved from earlier reports of increased cardiovascular mortality in patients receiving oral antidiabetic drugs compared with patients being controlled with diet or diet plus insulin. Although the conclusions of this study conducted in a number of American clinics some years ago have been challenged, largely on the basis of faulty experimental design, the status of oral antidiabet-

Table 44-3. Oral Antidiabetic Drugs

Drug	Usual Dosage Range	Nursing Considerations
FIRST GENERATION		
Acetohexamide *Dymelor* *(CAN) Dimelor*	250–1500 mg/day in a single dose or 2 divided doses if over 1000 mg/day	Intermediate-acting drug (duration 12–24 h); possesses significant uricosuric activity at therapeutic doses; metabolized to active intermediate by the liver (2.5 times as potent as parent compound); use with caution in renal insufficiency
Chlorpropamide *Diabinese* *(CAN) Apo-Chlorpropamide, Novopropamide*	Initially 250 mg/day (100–125 mg/day in older patients); maintenance 100–500 mg/day (usual, 250 mg/day); depending on condition	Longest-acting oral antidiabetic drug (duration up to 60 h); more potent and generally more toxic than other oral drugs; also indicated for treatment of polyuria of diabetes insipidus; may enhance effects of ADH; give as a single morning dose, with food, to minimize GI upset; if hypoglycemia occurs, give frequent feedings or glucose for at least 3–5 days, as drug is very long acting, and observe patient closely during this time may cause disulfiramlike reaction with alcohol (see text)
Tolazamide *Tolinase*	Initially 100–250 mg/day in a single dose depending on fasting blood sugar; maintenance, 100–500 mg/day	Intermediate-acting drug (duration, 10–14 h); may be effective in patients who do not respond to other sulfonylureas or in some patients with a history of ketoacidosis or coma; close observation of these patients is required; converted to several weakly active metabolites by the liver
Tolbutamide *Orinase* *(CAN) Apo-Tolbutamide, Mobenol, Novobutamide*	Initially 1–2 g/day orally; maintenance 0.25–2 g/day, usually in divided doses IV: 1 g given over 2–3 min	Short-acting drug (duration, 6–12 h); mildly goitrogenic at high doses and may reduce radioactive iodide uptake after prolonged administration without producing clinical hypothyroidism; rapidly metabolized to inactive metabolites; useful in patients with kidney disease; Orinase IV is used to diagnose islet cell adenoma (see Chap. 80); in presence of tumor, there is a rapid, marked drop in blood glucose that persists for up to 3 h; IV injection may produce local irritation or thrombophlebitis
SECOND GENERATION		
Glipizide *Glucotrol*	Initially 5 mg before breakfast; increase in 2.5–5 mg increments every 7 days until optimal response; maximum daily dose is 40 mg	Peak plasma concentrations occur in 1–3 h. Elimination half-life is 2–4 h, but blood sugar control persists for up to 24 h. Liver metabolism is rapid and extensive. Daily doses greater than 15 mg should be divided and given before meals. Reduce dosage in elderly, debilitated, or malnourished persons, and in the presence of impaired renal or hepatic function
Glyburide *Diabeta, Glynase, Micronase* *(CAN) Euglucon*	Initially 2.5–5 mg before breakfast; usual maintenance dose is 5–20 mg daily in a single dose or two divided doses; maximum daily dose is 20 mg Micronized tablets (Glynase): Initially, 1.5–3 mg once daily; maintenance dose is 0.75–12 mg daily	Peak plasma levels with regular tablets are attained within 4 h, and effects persist for at least 24 h. Elimination half-life is approximately 10 h; micronized tablets (Glynase) have a faster onset of action (1 h) and shorter half-life (4 h) but a similar duration of action. Excreted in the bile and urine, 50% by each route, thus, can be used in patients with renal impairment with greater safety than other oral antidiabetics

ic drugs still remains somewhat uncertain. General guidelines for use of oral antidiabetic drugs in type II diabetes are onset of diabetes at age 40 or older, duration of diabetes of less than 5 years, absence of ketoacidosis and renal or hepatic dysfunction, fasting serum glucose of less than 200 mg/dL, and insulin requirements of less than 40 U/day.

Although the pharmacology of all the oral sulfonylurea drugs is rather similar, certain distinctions can be made among some of the drugs. Therefore, they have been categorized as first-generation (acetohexamide, chlorpropamide, tolazamide, tolbutamide) and second-generation (glipizide, glyburide) drugs. Second-generation drugs are more lipophilic and possess a higher intrinsic potency (ie, are used in lower doses), and they appear to be less easily displaced from protein binding sites than the first-generation drugs. Thus, the second-generation drugs may provide a more stable plasma insulin level. The following discussion pertains to all of the sulfonylurea agents; individual drugs are then listed in Table 44-3.

Mechanism

Stimulate release of preformed endogenous insulin from functional beta cells in the pancreas; also appear to increase the number of insulin receptors and enhance the binding of insulin to the receptors; may inhibit hepatic glucose production and reduce serum glucagon concentrations

Uses

Treatment of stable, nonketotic, or nonacidotic type II (non–insulin-dependent) diabetes mellitus not adequately controlled by diet and weight reduction

Adjunct to insulin in certain types of *non–insulin-dependent* diabetes to improve symptom control

Diagnosis of pancreatic islet cell adenoma (see Chapter 80)

Adjunctive treatment of nephrogenic diabetes insipidus (chlorpropamide *only*)

Refer to Chapter 40.

Dosage

See Table 44-3.

Fate

Drugs are well absorbed orally, *tolazamide* being the most slowly absorbed and having the slowest onset of action (4–6 hours) compared with the other drugs (1–2 hours); all are highly bound to plasma proteins, the first-generation agents being less strongly bound than the second-generation drugs; metabolized in the liver to both active and inactive metabolites, which are excreted primarily in the urine, except for *glyburide*, whose metabolites are eliminated equally in both the bile and urine. *Tolbutamide* is the shortest-acting oral hypoglycemic drug (6–12 hours) and is given 2 to 3 times a day. The duration of action of *chlorpropamide* is up to 60 hours, whereas the remaining drugs exhibit durations of action ranging from 12 to 24 hours.

Common Side Effects

Mild hypoglycemia (fatigue, drowsiness, headache, weakness, hunger, nervousness), GI distress (anorexia, nausea, abdominal cramps, heartburn)

Significant Adverse Reactions

Severe hypoglycemia (tachycardia, vomiting, diarrhea, sweating, blurred vision, irritability, delirium, convulsions)
Dermatologic: urticaria, pruritus, photosensitivity, morbilliform or maculopapular rash, erythema multiforme, exfoliative dermatitis
Hepatic: cholestatic jaundice, altered liver function tests, hepatic porphyria
Hematologic (rare): thrombocytopenia, leukopenia, mild anemia, eosinophilia, agranulocytosis
Other: dizziness, edema, hyponatremia

Contraindications

Insulin-dependent diabetes; severe hepatic or renal dysfunction; uremia; diabetes complicated by ketoacidosis or pregnancy; *severe* cases of stress, fever, infection, or trauma; *Cautious use* in patients with cardiac impairment or adrenal or thyroid dysfunction, in women of childbearing age, in elderly or debilitated patients, and in alcoholics.

Interactions

Effects of oral antidiabetic drugs may be prolonged or enhanced by many other drugs, including androgens, oral anticoagulants, alcohol, allopurinol, anti-inflammatory drugs, chloramphenicol, clofibrate, histamine-2 antagonists, insulin, MAO inhibitors, probenecid, salicylates, sulfonamides, tricyclic antidepressants, and other highly protein-bound drugs.

Effects of oral antidiabetic drugs may be reduced by beta-blockers, calcium channel blockers, diazoxide, estrogens, glucocorticoids, phenobarbital, phenothiazines, phenytoin, sympathomimetics, thiazide diuretics, and thyroxine.

Alcohol may elicit a mild disulfiram-like reaction (facial flushing, dyspnea; see Chapter 81) in patients taking oral antidiabetics, especially chlorpropamide.

Chlorpropamide and possibly other sulfonylureas may prolong the effects of barbiturates.

Oral antidiabetic drugs may increase the serum levels of digoxin.

Nursing Management

Pretherapy Assessment

Assess and record baseline data necessary for detection of adverse effects of oral antidiabetic drugs: General: VS, body weight, skin color and temperature; CNS: orientation, reflexes, peripheral sensation; Lab: urinalysis, blood urea nitrogen (BUN), serum creatinine, liver function tests, blood glucose.

Review medical history and documents for existing or previous conditions that:

a. require cautious use of oral antidiabetic drugs: cardiac impairment, adrenal or thyroid dysfunction, in women of childbearing age, in elderly or debilitated patients, and in alcoholics
b. contraindicate use of antidiabetic drugs: allergy to sulfonylureas; insulin-dependent diabetes; severe hepatic or renal dysfunction; uremia; thyroid or endocrine impairment; diabetes complicated by ketoacidosis or pregnancy; *severe* cases of stress, fever, infection, or trauma; **pregnancy (Category C)**, lactation (secreted in breast milk; avoid use in mothers because of risk of hypoglycemia in the infant)

Nursing Interventions

Medication Administration

Administer drug in the morning before breakfast; if severe GI upset occurs, dose may be divided.

Transfer patients from one oral antidiabetic drug to another with no transitional period or priming dose.

Assure ready access to bathroom facilities if diarrhea occurs.

Surveillance During Therapy

Monitor urine and blood glucose levels frequently to determine effectiveness and dosage.

Collaborate with patient and healthcare team to carefully weigh benefit versus risk before oral antidiabetic drugs are prescribed. Although its controversial results have not been replicated, results of one study showed a higher mortality from cardiovascular disease in patients receiving oral antidiabetic agents than in those treated with diet alone or diet plus insulin.

Carefully monitor results of blood and urine glucose tests, which should be obtained daily, when therapy is begun in an elderly patient. Dosage should be adjusted accordingly. Low dosages should be used initially because hyperresponsiveness has been reported.

Observe patient closely if patient is being transferred from insulin to oral antidiabetic drug. Dosages should be adjusted gradually to avoid precipitating ketosis, acidosis, or coma unless insulin dosage has been 20 U/day or less, in which case it may be discontinued abruptly. Urine should be tested frequently during transition. No transitional period is required when switching between different oral antidiabetic agents. Oral antidiabetic agents are *not*, however, insulin substitutes and should never be employed alone in insulin-dependent diabetes.

Carefully monitor laboratory studies and patient for indications of adverse reactions.

Interpret results of diagnostic tests and contact practitioner as appropriate.

Monitor for possible drug–drug and drug–nutrient interactions: Refer to **Interactions**.

Patient Teaching

Instruct patient in the procedures for monitoring blood/urine glucose or ketones.

Instruct patient to report immediately any indications of hypersensitivity or hepatic dysfunction (eg, itching, rash, fever, sore throat, dark urine, light-colored stools, diarrhea, vomiting).

Advise patient beginning therapy to avoid excessive sunlight because photosensitivity reactions can occur. Exposure to sun should be gradual until effects of drug are known.

Instruct the patient to report to the practitioner any of the following if they occur: fever; sore throat; vomiting; hypoglycemic or hyperglycemic reactions; skin rash.

Hyperglycemic Agents

Although the most effective means of elevating the blood sugar level in cases of severe hypoglycemia is direct IV injection of glucose, this method is not always available or feasible. Alternatives include the oral administration of *glucose*, as a gel or chewable tablet, or *diazoxide*, a thiazidelike drug that inhibits release of insulin from the pancreas and is used in the management of hypoglycemia due to hyperinsulinism. Also, the parenteral use of *glucagon*, a polypeptide produced by pancreatic alpha cells, can increase conversion of glycogen to glucose and stimulate hepatic gluconeogenesis, thereby elevating blood glucose levels.

Most drug-induced hypoglycemic episodes are mild and generally can be reversed by oral ingestion of some form of glucose (such as candy, soda, sweetened orange juice). Only in those instances in which the hypoglycemic response is severe (insulin shock) or prolonged (when symptoms persist longer than 30 minutes after oral consumption of glucose) is the use of IV glucose or glucagon indicated.

• Glucose, oral

B-D Glucose, Glutose, Insta-Glucose

(CAN) Glucosal

Although glucose may be administered by IV infusion (see Chapter 76) to provide an immediate source in acute hypoglycemic episodes, symptoms of mild hypoglycemic reactions can often be controlled by the oral use of glucose as either chewable tablets or a 40% liquid gel-like solution. Glucose is rapidly absorbed from the GI tract, and a rapid increase (ie, 5–10 minutes) in blood glucose concentration occurs after oral administration. The recommended dose is 10 to 20 g, which may be repeated in 10 minutes if required. Glucose is *not* absorbed from the buccal cavity and therefore must be swallowed to be effective. Thus, whenever possible, other drugs should be employed to treat hypoglycemia in the *unconscious* patient, because the swallowing reflex does not always occur, and the absence of the normal gag reflex can lead to aspiration. Occasional reports of nausea have appeared, but the drug is virtually nontoxic when taken as directed. It is not recommended in children younger than 2 years of age.

• Glucagon

Mechanism

Accelerates breakdown of liver glycogen by increasing synthesis of cyclic AMP, promotes uptake of amino acids into liver, and stimulates hepatic gluconeogenesis, all of which result in elevation of blood glucose; also inhibits conversion of glucose to glycogen; exerts effects on heart similar to catecholamines, that is, increased rate and force of contraction

Uses

Treatment of severe drug-induced hypoglycemic reactions in diabetic patients or persons undergoing insulin shock therapy (only effective if liver glycogen is available—minimal effectiveness in states of starvation, adrenal insufficiency, or chronic hypoglycemia)

Production of GI hypotonia as a diagnostic aid for radiologic examination of stomach, duodenum, small intestine, and colon

Investigational uses include treatment of beta-blocker overdose and relief of GI disturbances associated with spasm

Dosage

Hypoglycemia: 0.5 to 1 mg SC, IM, or IV; repeat once or twice at 10- to 20-minute intervals if no response has occurred; IV glucose may also be needed to prevent cerebral hypoglycemia

Children: 0.025 mg/kg (maximum, 1 mg) SC, IM or IV

Insulin shock therapy: 0.5 to 1 mg SC, IM, or IV after 1 hour of coma; if no response within 15 to 25 minutes, repeat the dose

Diagnostic aid: 0.25 to 2 mg IV or IM, depending on speed of onset and duration of action desired

Fate

Blood glucose begins to increase and consciousness is restored within 5 to 20 minutes; duration of action is approximately 1 to 2 hours; metabolized in the liver, kidneys, and plasma

Significant Adverse Reactions

(Rare) Nausea, vomiting, and hypersensitivity reactions. Hypokalemia in large doses

Contraindications

No absolute contraindications. *Cautious use* in patients with a history of insulinoma (increased *hypo*glycemia can occur) and pheochromocytoma (increased blood pressure can occur).

Interaction

Glucagon may potentiate the action of oral anticoagulants.

Nursing Management

Pretherapy Assessment

Assess and record baseline data necessary for detection of adverse effects of glucagon: General: VS, body weight, skin color and temperature; CNS: orientation, reflexes, peripheral sensation; Lab: blood and urine glucose, serum potassium.

Review medical history and documents for existing or previous conditions that:

a. require cautious use of glucagon: insulinoma; pheochromocytoma

b. contraindicate use of glucagon: **pregnancy (Category B)**, lactation (safety not established, use with caution in nursing mothers).

Nursing Interventions

Medication Administration

Be prepared to administer supplemental carbohydrates, as needed, to an insulin-dependent (type I) diabetic, who usually does not respond to glucagon with as large an increase in blood glucose as a non–insulin-dependent (type II) diabetic. Also, glucagon is of little benefit in states of starvation, adrenal insufficiency, chronic hypoglycemia, or other conditions in which liver glycogen is unavailable. IV glucose should be available and must be used if patient is in a deep coma or fails to respond to glucagon.

Expect to begin oral carbohydrates as soon as possible after consciousness is regained to restore liver glycogen and prevent secondary hypoglycemia.

Be alert for indications of possible hypersensitivity reactions because drug is a protein.

Do not mix glucagon solution with solutions containing sodium, potassium, or calcium chlorides because precipitation will occur. Glucagon does not precipitate in dextrose solution.

Surveillance During Therapy

Carefully monitor laboratory studies and patient for indications of adverse reactions.

Interpret results of diagnostic tests and contact practitioner as appropriate.

Monitor for possible drug–drug and drug–nutrient interactions: Refer to **Interactions**.

Patient Teaching

Because this agent is used in the emergency management of acute hypoglycemia, patient information is likely to be limited to drug information and effects.

• Diazoxide, oral

Proglycem

Diazoxide is used orally for the management of persistent hypoglycemia caused by hyperinsulinism, for example, resulting from pancreatic cell hyperplasia or carcinoma. It is also available for IV injection as Hyperstat for treating hypertensive emergencies (see Chapter 33). The drug inhibits secretion of insulin from the pancreas and may increase glycogen synthesis. Its effect on insulin release is antagonized by alpha-adrenergic blocking agents. As an antihypertensive agent, diazoxide directly relaxes vascular smooth muscle; however, its effects on blood pressure are minimal when it is used orally in therapeutic doses. The initial dosage is 3 mg/kg/day in three divided doses every 8 hours. Maintenance dosage is 3 mg/kg to 8 mg/kg/day in divided doses. The drug should be discontinued if a response is not observed within 2 to 3 weeks. Side effects can include sodium and fluid retention (sometimes severe), hirsutism, GI distress (nausea, diarrhea, abdominal pain), loss of taste, palpitations, tachycardia, hyperuricemia, skin rash, headache, and weakness. Many other adverse reactions have been reported and patients should be closely monitored during therapy. Diazoxide oral should be used cautiously in patients with diabetes, renal dysfunction, impaired cerebral or cardiac circulation, or history of gout, in children and pregnant women, and in persons taking corticosteroids. The effects of diazoxide, oral can be potentiated by antihypertensives, chlorpromazine, diuretics and protein-bound drugs (eg, anti-inflammatory agents, anticoagulants, barbiturates, phenytoin, sulfonamides)

Nursing Management

Pretherapy Assessment

Refer to **Diazoxide**, Chapter 33. In addition:

Nursing Interventions

Surveillance During Therapy

Closely monitor intake/output ratio and check frequently for appearance of edema. Drug can cause significant fluid retention, which may be hazardous in cardiac patient. Conventional diuretic therapy usually controls fluid retention.

Be alert for development of ketoacidosis, which may lead to coma, in cases of overdosage. Overdosage responds promptly to insulin and restoration of fluid and electrolyte balance. Observe patient closely for at least 7 days after suspected overdosage because diazoxide is long-acting.

Monitor results of serum electrolyte determinations, which should be performed often, in patient with impaired renal function and in whom dosage should be reduced.

Collaborate in evaluation of drug effects. Clinical response and blood glucose levels should be monitored frequently until condition is stable. The drug formulation should be changed cautiously because blood levels may be higher with the liquid than with the capsule formulation. Diazoxide should be discontinued if response is not satisfactory within 2 to 3 weeks.

Patient Teaching

Teach patient to monitor urine for sugar and ketones. Abnormalities should immediately be reported to practitioner.

Instruct patient to report any changes in vision because transient cataracts have occurred.

Reassure patient that the hirsutism that may occur (mainly on forehead, back, and limbs, especially in children and women) is reversible on withdrawal of the drug.

Selected Bibliography

Bressler R, Johnson D: New pharmacological approaches to therapy of NIDDM. Diabetes Care 15(6):792, 1992

Carlisle BA: Treatment of diabetes in the elderly. J Pract Nurs 43(1): 23, 1993

Groop LC: Sulfonylureas in NIDDM. Diabetes Care 15(6):737, 1992

Haas LB: Drug therapy for diabetes. Nurse Pract Forum 2(3):166, 1991

Melkus GD: Type II non-insulin-dependent diabetes mellitus. Nurs Clin North Am 28(1):25, 1993

Morley JE, Perry HM: The management of diabetes mellitus in older individuals. Drugs 41(4):548, 1991

Peters AL, Davidson MB: Insulin plus a sulfonylurea agent for treating type-2 diabetes. Ann Intern Med 115(1):45, 1991

Reed RL, Mooradian AD: Treatment of diabetes in the elderly. Am Fam Physician 44(3):915, 1991

Shamoon H: Pathophysiology of diabetes: A review of selected recent developments and their impact on treatment. Drugs 44(suppl 3): 1, 1992

Shlossberg AH: Treating non-insulin dependent diabetes: Oral agents or insulin? Can Family Physician 39:119, 1993

Steil CF, Deakins DA: Oral hypoglycemics: What you and your patient need to know. Nursing 22(11):34, 1992

Nursing Bibliography

Collo M, Johnson J, Kabadi L: Combination sulfonyluria and insulin therapy in non-insulin dependent diabetes mellitus. Nurse Practitioner, 18(7):40, 1993

Graves L: Diabetic ketoacidosis and hyperosmolar hyperglycemic nonketotic coma. Critical Care Nursing Quarterly 13(3):50, 1990

Hardway D, Weatherly K, Bonheur B: Diabetes education on wheels. Journal of Nursing Staff Development 9(3): 1993

Spollett G: Intensive insulin therapy in insulin dependent diabetes and combination therapy. Nurse Practitioner 18(7):27, 1993

Steil C, Deakins D: Oral hypoglycemics: What you and your patient need to know. Nursing '92 22(11):34, 1992

45 Adrenal Cortical Steroids

Fludrocortisone

Glucocorticoids

Aminoglutethimide
Trilostane

The adrenal cortex secretes a large number of steroidal compounds possessing a variety of physiologic actions. These substances are termed *adrenocorticoids*, or simply *corticoids*. According to their predominant action in the body, they may be divided into one of the three following categories:

- Mineralocorticoids (eg, aldosterone)
- Glucocorticoids (eg, hydrocortisone)
- Adrenogenital corticoids (eg, dehydroepiandrosterone)

The *mineralocorticoids*, of which aldosterone is the major endogenous representative, exert their principal action on electrolyte and water metabolism, especially in the kidney; there they facilitate the reabsorption of sodium and water from the urine by the ionic exchange mechanisms in the distal segments of the renal tubules. Aldosterone itself is not available for therapeutic use, and the clinically available mineralocorticoid is fludrocortisone.

The *glucocorticoids* are those compounds that primarily influence carbohydrate, fat, and protein metabolism and thus can elicit varied effects in the body and alter the body's immune response to diverse stimuli. Hydrocortisone and cortisone are the major endogenous glucocorticoids. Metabolic actions of the glucocorticoids include gluconeogenesis, increased protein catabolism in connective tissue, muscle, and fat (which increases hepatic concentrations of amino acids required for glucose synthesis), and increased lipolysis, all of which contribute to increased glucose levels. In addition, they suppress the inflammatory process through a combination of actions that include inhibition of leukocyte and macrophage activity, reduction in circulating lymphocytes, eosinophils and basophils, increased neutrophil levels, and inhibition of prostaglandin and leukotriene synthesis. These actions are responsible for one of their major clinical applications, the control of symptoms of inflammation. Naturally occurring glucocorticoids (such as cortisone, hydrocortisone) as well as synthetic glucocorticoids (eg, dexamethasone, prednisone) are available for therapeutic use, and they differ primarily in potency and degree of side effects.

The *adrenogenital corticoids* are male and female sex hormones (such as estrogen, progesterone, testosterone) found in very small amounts in the adrenal cortex. Other than dehydroepiandrosterone, a precursor of both testosterone and the estrogens, the adrenogenital corticoids are present in the adrenal cortex in amounts too small to be of clinical significance. The sex hormones are discussed in Chapters 46 to 48.

Although the classification of the major adrenal corticoids into mineralocorticoids and glucocorticoids is convenient for discussion purposes, it represents an oversimplification from a functional standpoint. With the exception of a few potent synthetic glucocorticoids, *complete* separation of mineralocorticoid from glucocorticoid activity has not been achieved, and considerable overlapping of activity exists with most compounds, especially when employed in large doses. This overlapping is responsible for many of the side effects associated with adrenal corticosteroid therapy, although in some cases it may represent a desirable extension of the clinical activity of a particular drug. For example, in the treatment of primary adrenal cortical hypofunction (Addison's disease), the mineralocorticoid action (salt and water retention) of glucocorticoid compounds such as hydrocortisone is desirable from a therapeutic point of view. In fact, mineralocorticoid supplementation is often provided with glucocorticoid therapy in the treatment of Addison's disease. Conversely, a mineralocorticoid action might prove undesirable in the cardiac patient, because salt and water retention may aggravate the already compromised cardiac function.

Regulation of adrenal corticosteroid secretion is reviewed in Chapter 40. Synthesis of adrenal corticoids is controlled primarily by adrenocorticotropic hormone (ACTH) (corticotropin) released from the adenohypophysis. ACTH itself is used in certain clinical situations and is discussed in Chapter 41; the remaining adrenal cortical drugs are reviewed in this chapter. In addition, aminoglutethimide and trilostane, drugs used in the treatment of adrenal cortical *hyper*function (Cushing's syndrome) are considered at the end of the chapter.

Mineralocorticoids

Mineralocorticoids possess actions qualitatively similar to those of the major endogenous agent aldosterone; that is, they facilitate the reabsorption of sodium and water from the distal segment of the nephron. The only clinically available drug is fludrocortisone, an orally effective, potent synthetic mineralocorticoid indicated as partial replacement therapy for adrenocortical insufficiency and for treatment of salt-losing adrenogenital syndrome.

• *Fludrocortisone Acetate*

Florinef

Mechanism

Promotes sodium and water reabsorption in the distal tubule of the nephron, which occurs in conjunction with hydrogen and potassium excretion; may also enhance sodium retention in sweat and salivary glands; small doses can cause marked sodium retention and elevated blood pressure; large doses inhibit adrenal cortical secretion and promote hepatic deposition of glycogen and may induce a negative nitrogen balance unless protein intake is adequate; also exhibits effects on carbohydrate, fat, and protein metabolism (refer to Mechanism under **Glucocorticoids**).

Uses

Partial replacement therapy for primary and secondary adrenocortical insufficiency in Addison's disease
Treatment of salt-losing adrenogenital syndrome
Management of severe orthostatic hypotension (eg, Shy-Drager syndrome); *investigational use only*

Dosage

Addison's disease: 0.1 mg 3 times/week orally to 0.2 mg/day (usually 0.1 mg/day); dose should be reduced to 0.05 mg/day if transient hypertension develops
Salt-losing adrenogenital syndrome: 0.1 mg/day to 0.2 mg/day
Orthostatic hypotension: 0.1 mg to 0.4 mg/day; dosage is titrated to clinical response or development of ankle edema

Fate

Readily absorbed orally; metabolized in the liver and excreted mainly in the urine; effects persist 24 to 48 hours

Common Side Effects

Hypokalemia (muscle weakness, paresthesias, fatigue), fluid retention

Significant Adverse Reactions

(See also under **glucocorticoids**)

Hypertension, pulmonary congestion, cardiac arrhythmias, headaches, arthralgia, muscle paralysis, hypersensitivity reactions

Contraindications

Treatment of conditions other than those specifically indicated (see Uses), systemic fungal infections. *Cautious use* in the presence of hypertension, cardiac disease, stress, trauma or severe infection or other illness and in pregnant or nursing women.

Interactions

Refer to **Glucocorticoids**. In addition:

Potassium loss resulting from fludrocortisone may be enhanced by diuretics.
Toxicity of digoxin may be increased secondary to fludrocortisone-induced potassium loss
The risk of edema with androgens or anabolic steroids may be augmented by fludrocortisone.

Nursing Management

Refer to **Glucocorticoids** (oral use). In addition:

Nursing Interventions

Medication Administration

Ensure that weight, blood pressure, and electrolyte levels are obtained before initiation of therapy and periodically during extended therapy. The practitioner should be advised of any significant changes.

Surveillance During Therapy

Assess patient for indications of excessive hypokalemia (eg, muscle cramping or weakness, paresthesias, palpitations, fatigue, nausea, polyuria) or drug overdosage (weight gain, edema, hypertension, pulmonary congestion, insomnia). Supplemental potassium therapy may be indicated.

Patient Teaching

Stress the importance of controlling salt intake for optimal drug effects. Excess salt intake increases sodium retention and potassium excretion, reducing drug efficacy and necessitating potassium supplementation.
Stress the need to maintain a diet adequate in protein.

Glucocorticoids

Alclometasone
Amcinonide
Beclomethasone
Betamethasone
Budesonide
Clobetasol
Clocortolone
Cortisone
Desonide
Desoximetasone
Dexamethasone
Diflorasone
Flunisolide
Fluocinolone
Fluocinonide
Fluorometholone
Flurandrenolide
Fluticasone
Halcinonide
Halobetasol
Hydrocortisone
Medrysone
Methylprednisolone
Mometasone
Prednisolone
Prednisone
Triamcinolone

The glucocorticoids encompass a large number of naturally occurring and synthetic steroids possessing similar pharmacologic actions but differing widely in potency and the type and severity of side effects. The principal naturally occurring adrenal cortical steroids are cortisone and hydrocortisone, and they exhibit both mineralocorticoid (salt-retaining) as well as glucocorticoid (anti-inflammatory) effects. As such, they are primarily used as replacement therapy for adrenocortical deficiency states.

Synthetic glucocorticoids are characterized by their greater glucocorticoid potency compared with natural adrenal cortical steroids and by their reduced (and in some cases complete absence of) mineralocorticoid action. The synthetic drugs are used principally for their potent anti-inflammatory action and are available in many different dosage forms. The relative potencies of the various systemically employed glucocorticoids are listed in Table 45-1, which compares their oral effectiveness, anti-inflammatory activity, and mineralocorticoid potency.

It is important to recognize that most adverse reactions associated with glucocorticoid use occur after the systemic use of these compounds. When a local effect is desired, the drug may be applied topically in several dosage forms (eg, ointment, cream, lotion, aerosol, nasal spray, ophthalmic drops) or administered by an intralesional or intra-articular injection. A number of different corticosteroids are used topically, and the relative potency of topical steroids is dependent on several factors, including the concentration of drug applied, the basic characteristics of the drug molecule, and the type of vehicle used. For example, fluorinated derivatives (eg, betamethasone, fluocinonide, halcinonide) are more potent than nonfluorinated agents (eg, hydrocortisone, desonide), but may have a higher incidence of local adverse effects. A relative potency ranking of the various topical steroid preparations is presented in Table 45-2.

The discussion of glucocorticoids below focuses mainly on their systemic pharmacology. Following this general review of glucocorticoids, individual drugs, both systemic and local, are listed in Table 45-3; the available dosage forms are given along with recommended dose levels for each dosage form, and nursing considerations pertaining to each drug are presented.

Mechanism

Mechanism of anti-inflammatory action is complex and not completely established, but may include several of the following actions:

- Stabilization of lysosomal membranes, reducing release of tissue-destructive enzymes and other mediators of inflammation
- Reduction of dilation and permeability of inflamed capillaries and decreased leukocyte migration into inflammatory site
- Inhibition of accumulation of inflammatory cells (leukocytes, macrophages) at sites of inflammation and impaired phagocytosis
- Inhibition of fibroblast formation and collagen deposition
- Decreased synthesis of membrane phospholipid-derived mediators of inflammation, such as prostaglandins and leukotrienes
- Suppression of cell-mediated immune reactions (eg, binding of immunoglobulins to cell surface receptors)
- Reduction in the number of T-lymphocytes, monocytes, and eosinophils

Drugs may also enhance the responsiveness of the cardiovascular system to circulating catecholamines, thereby increasing cardiac output as well as local perfusion pressure. Derivatives possessing mineralocorticoid activity exert effects on fluid and electrolyte balance as well (refer to **Mechanism** for fludrocortisone earlier in the chapter)

Uses

NOTE: The following is a representative listing of the indications for glucocorticoid drugs in general; the literature accompanying the individual drug products should be consulted for specific indications for each drug.

Replacement therapy in primary or secondary adrenal cortical insufficiency (hydrocortisone is drug of choice)

Treatment of congenital adrenal hyperplasia

Symptomatic treatment of various inflammatory, allergic, or immunoreactive disorders including the following:

Rheumatic: rheumatoid arthritis, bursitis, osteoarthritis, acute gouty arthritis, tenosynovitis, synovitis, ankylosing spondylitis

Collagen: acute rheumatic carditis, systemic lupus erythematosus

Allergic: allergic rhinitis, bronchial asthma, status asthmaticus, dermatitis, serum sickness, drug hypersensitivity

Dermatologic: erythema multiforme (Stevens-Johnson syndrome) exfoliative dermatitis, severe psoriasis, angioedema, urticaria, chronic eczema

Ophthalmic: conjunctivitis, keratitis, iritis, uveitis, acute optic neuritis, chorioretinitis, allergic corneal marginal ulcers

Gastrointestinal: ulcerative colitis, regional enteritis

(*text continues on page 476*)

Table 45-1. **Comparative Activities of Systemic Glucocorticoids**

Drug	Equivalent Oral Doses (mg)	Relative Anti-inflammatory Activity	Relative Mineralocorticoid Potency
Short Acting			
Cortisone	25	0.8	+ +
Hydrocortisone	20	1	+ +
Intermediate Acting			
Prednisone	5	3–4	+
Prednisolone	5	4	+
Methylprednisolone	4	5	0
Triamcinolone	4	5	0
Long Acting			
Dexamethasone	0.75	20–30	0
Betamethasone	0.6	20–30	0

Table 45-2. **Relative Potencies of Topically Applied Corticosteroids**

Generic Name	*Trade Names*	*Dosage Form*	*Strength (%)*
I. Very high potency			
Augmented betamethasone dipropionate	Diprolene	Ointment	0.05
Clobetasol propionate	Temovate	Cream, ointment	0.05
Diflorasone diacetate	Florone, Maxiflor, Psorcon	Ointment	0.05
Halobetasol propionate	Ultravate	Cream, ointment	0.05
II. High potency			
Amcinonide	Cyclocort	Cream, lotion, ointment	0.1
Augmented betamethasone dipropionate	Diprolene	Cream	0.05
Betamethasone dipropionate	Diprosone, Maxivate	Cream, ointment	0.05
Betamethasone valerate	Betatrex, Valisone	Ointment	0.1
Desoximetasone	Topicort	Cream, ointment, Gel	0.25 0.05
Diflorasone diacetate	Florone, Maxiflor, Psorcon	Cream, ointment (emollient base)	0.05
Fluocinolone acetonide	Synalar-HP	Cream	0.2
Fluocinonide	Lidex	Cream, ointment, gel	0.05
Halcinonide	Halog	Cream, ointment	0.1
Triamcinolone acetonide	Aristocort, Kenalog	Ointment	0.1
III. Medium potency			
Betamethasone benzoate	Uticort	Cream, gel, lotion	0.025
Betamethasone dipropionate	Diprosone, Maxivate	Lotion	0.05
Betamethasone valerate	Betatrex, Valisone	Cream	0.1
Clocortolone pivalate	Cloderm	Cream	0.1
Desoximetasone	Topicort	Cream	0.05
Fluocinolone acetonide	Fluorosyn, Synalar	Cream, ointment	0.025
Flurandrenolide	Cordran	Cream, ointment Cream, ointment, lotion Tape	0.025 0.05 4 mcg/cm^2
Fluticasone propionate	Cutivate	Cream Ointment	0.05 0.005
Hydrocortisone butyrate	—	Ointment, solution	0.1
Hydrocortisone valerate	Westcort	Cream, ointment	0.2
Mometasone furoate	Elocon	Cream, ointment, lotion	0.1
Triamcinolone acetonide	Aristocort, Kenalog	Cream, ointment, lotion Cream, ointment, lotion Cream, ointment	0.025 0.1 0.5
IV. Low potency			
Aclometasone dipropionate	Aclovate	Cream, ointment	0.05
Desonide	Des Owen, Tridesilon	Cream	0.05
Dexamethasone	Decaspray	Aerosol Aerosol	0.01 0.04
Dexamethasone sodium phosphate	Decadron	Cream	0.1
Fluocinolone acetonide	Fluonid, Synalar	Cream, solution	0.01
Hydrocortisone	various manufacturers	Lotion Cream, ointment, lotion, aerosol Cream, ointment, lotion, solution Cream, ointment, lotion	0.25 0.5 1 2.5
Hydrocortisone acetate	various manufacturers	Cream, ointment Cream, ointment	0.5 1

Adapted from Facts and Comparisons, JB Lippincott Co., 1993

Table 45-3. **Glucocorticoids**

Drug	*Preparations*	*Usual Dosage Range*	*Nursing Considerations*
Alclometasone *Aclovate*	Ointment: 0.05% Cream: 0.05%	Apply to affected area 2–3 times/day	Synthetic corticosteroid used for treatment of inflammatory and pruritic manifestations of steroid-responsive dermatoses; side effects include localized itching, burning, erythema, dryness, irritation, and rash
Amcinonide *Cyclocort*	Cream: 0.1% Ointment: 0.1% Lotion: 0.1%	Apply 2–3 times/day	Effective against steroid-responsive dermatoses; cream and lotion are formulated in nonsensitizing hydrophilic base
Beclomethasone *Beclovent, Beconase, Vancenase, Vanceril* *(CAN) Propaderm*	Aerosol for oral inhalation: 42 μg/dose Aerosol for intranasal inhalation: 42 μg/dose	*Oral inhalation* Adults: 2 inhalations 3–4 times/day (maximum, 20/day) Children: 1–2 inhalations 3–4 times a day (maximum, 10/day) Nasal inhalation: 1 inhalation 2–4 times a day	Synthetic corticosteroid related to prednisolone; used by oral inhalation for long-term management of bronchial asthma (see Chap. 57); dry mouth, hoarseness, and localized fungal infections of mouth and pharynx can occur; danger of adrenal insufficiency if patients are transferred from oral to inhaled steroids too quickly or during periods of stress; oral steroids should be available at all times; *not* indicated for relief of acute asthmatic attack; intranasal solution is used for relief of symptoms of seasonal or perennial rhinitis, minimal systemic effects; do not use in children younger than 12; nasal irritation and dryness are most common side effects; effects are evident only with several days use; patients with blocked nasal passages should use a decongestant (see Chap. 14) before administration
Betamethasone *Celestone* *(CAN) Betnelan*	Tablets: 0.6 mg Syrup: 0.6 mg/5 mL	Oral: 0.6–7.2 mg/day IM, (phosphate only): up to 9 mg/day IM, IV (respository): 0.5–9.0 mg/day Intraarticular: 2–8 mg (0.25–2 mL), depending on joint size and disease Topical: 1–3 times/day	Long-acting agent with no mineralocorticoid activity; phosphate salt has a prompt onset of action and is given IV or IM; may be combined with acetate salt (prolonged action) for repository IM injections, given every 3–10 days into joints, lesions, or bursae; up to 2 mL may be injected into very large joints; *not used* in Addison's disease where salt- and water-retaining action is desirable; used topically for dermatoses, pruritis, and psoriatic lesions; use aerosol *cautiously* because systemic absorption may be substantial, resulting in increased adverse effects. Dipropionate (augmented) is available in a specially formulated vehicle that enhances drug absorption (Diprolene) very high potency product, thus do not use occlusive dressings.
Betamethasone Phosphate *Betameth, Celestone Phosphate, Cel-U-Jec, Selestoject* *(CAN) Betnesol*	Injection: 4 mg/mL Repository injection: 3 mg acetate and 3 mg phosphate/mL Cream: 0.01%, 0.025%, 0.05%, 0.1%		
Betamethasone Benzoate *Uticort* *(CAN) Beben*	Cream: 0.025% Lotion: 0.025% Gel: 0.025%		
Betamethasone Dipropionate *Alphatrex, Diprosone, Maxivate, Telador*	Ointment: 0.05% Cream: 0.05% Lotion: 0.05% Aerosol: 0.1%		
Betamethasone Dipropionate, Augmented *Diprolene*	Ointment: 0.05% Cream: 0.05% Gel: 0.05% Lotion: 0.05%		
Betamethasone Valerate *Betatrex, Beta-Val, Valisone,* *(CAN) Betacort, Betaderm, Betnovate, Celestoderm, Ectosone, Metaderm, Novobetamet*	Ointment: 0.1% Cream: 0.1% Lotion: 0.1% Powder		
Clobetasol *Temovate* *(CAN) Dermovate*	Cream: 0.05% Ointment: 0.05% Lotion: 0.05%	Apply twice a day	Very potent topical corticosteroid; limit treatment to 14 days; adrenal suppression has occurred with doses as low as 2 g/day; use very sparingly and *do not* cover with occlusive dressings
Clocortolone *Cloderm*	Cream: 0.1%	Apply 1–3 times/day	Indicated for relief of inflammatory manifestations of corticosteroid-responsive dermatoses

(continued)

Table 45-3. **Glucocorticoids (Continued)**

Drug	*Preparations*	*Usual Dosage Range*	*Nursing Considerations*
Cortisone *Cortone*	Tablets: 5 mg, 10 mg, 25 mg	Oral: 25–300 mg/day; reduce to lowest effective dosage	Short-acting glucocorticoid with prominent mineralocorticoid activity; it is largely converted to hydrocortisone, which is responsible for most of its pharmacologic action
Desonide *Des Owen, Tridesilon*	Cream: 0.05% Ointment: 0.05% Lotion: 0.05%	Apply 2–3 times/day	Possesses anti-inflammatory, antipruritic, and vasoconstrictive activity; discontinue if irritation develops; less potent than most other topical steroids
Desoximetasone *Topicort*	Cream: 0.05%, 0.25% Gel: 0.05% Ointment: 0.25%	Apply 1–2 times/day	Higher strength (0.25%) cream and ointment are very potent; weaker-strength cream (Topicort LP) is of moderate potency
Dexamethasone *Decadron, Hexadrol and other manufacturers* *(CAN) Deronil, Dexasone, Oradexon, Spersadex*	Tablets: 0.25 mg, 0.5 mg, 0.75 mg, 1.0 mg, 1.5 mg, 2 mg, 4 mg, 6 mg Oral solution: 0.5 mg/5 mL Elixir: 0.5 mg/5 mL Drops: 0.5 mg/0.5 mL Injection: 4 mg/mL, 10 mg/mL, 20 mg/mL, 24 mg/mL Repository injection: (acetate salt): 8 mg/mL, 16 mg/mL Ophthalmic solution: 0.1% Ophthalmic suspension: 0.1% Ophthalmic ointment: 0.05%, 0.1% Cream: 0.1% Aerosol: 0.01%, 0.04% Aerosol (Respihaler): 12.6 g (84 μg/dose) Aerosol (Turbinaire): 12.6 g (84 μg/dose)	Oral: 0.75–9 mg/day Children: 0.2 mg/kg/day Parenteral: 1/3–1/2 oral dose/12 h (usual range, 0.5–5 mg/day) Repository injection: 8–16 mg IM every 1–3 wk Intraarticular, intralesion, or soft-tissue injection: 0.4–6 mg, depending on area Ophthalmic: 1–2 drops *or* thin film of ointment 3–4 times/day Topical: 2–4 times/day as needed Respihaler: 2–3 inhalations 3–4 times/day Turbinaire: 2 sprays in nostril 2–3 times/day	Widely used, potent corticosteroid; long-acting, and *not* recommended for alternate-day dosing; phosphate salt is freely soluble and is given IM or IV; prompt onset of action; acetate salt is highly insoluble and has a prolonged effect when given IM; aerosol therapy may result in nasal or bronchial irritation, drying of mucosa, rebound congestion, asthmatic-like reaction, and other systemic effects; Turbinaire aerosol is used for nasal inflammation, whereas Respihaler aerosol is indicated for bronchial asthma; available with lidocaine for soft-tissue injection (eg, bursitis, tenosynovitis); systemic adverse effects may follow long-term or high-dose topical intralesional, or inhalation therapy; *protect eyes* from topical spray in the face area; discontinue ophthalmic use if eye irritation develops
Diflorasone *Florone, Maxiflor, Psorcon* *(CAN) Flutone*	Ointment: 0.05% Cream: 0.05%	Apply 2–3 times/day	Used in steroid-responsive dermatoses; cream is in an emulsified hydrophilic base; ointment in an emollient occlusive base
Flunisolide *AeroBid, Nasalide* *(CAN) Bronalide, Rhinalar*	Aerosol: 7 g (250 μg/dose) Nasal spray: 25 μg/dose	*Oral inhalation* Adults: 2 inhalations twice/day (maximum, 2 mg/day) Children (age 6–15): 1–2 inhalations twice/day (maximum, 1 mg/day) *Nasal inhalation* Adults: 2 sprays each nostril 2–3 times/day Children (age 6–14): 1 spray 3 times/day or 2 sprays twice/day	Oral inhalation used to control bronchial asthma—see Chap. 57 (*not* for relief of acute attacks); transfer from oral steroids should be done *gradually*; during periods of stress or severe asthma attacks, oral steroids should be reinstituted; side effects include cough, dry mouth, hoarseness, and local fungal infections; nasal spray is used to relieve symptoms of rhinitis; *not* recommended in children younger than age 6; discontinue after 3 wk if no improvement is noted; after clinical effect is observed, reduce to lowest effective maintenance dosage
Fluocinolone *Derma-Smooth/FS, Fluonid, Flurosyn, FS Shampoo, Synalar, Synemol* *(CAN) Dermalar, Fluoderm, Fluolar*	Ointment: 0.025% Cream: 0.01%, 0.025%, 0.2% Solution: 0.01% Shampoo: 0.01% Oil: 0.01%	Apply 2–4 times/day in a thin layer	Possesses moderate anti-inflammatory and antipruritic activity; high-potency cream (0.2%) should be used for short periods only; shampoo is a 12-mg capsule which is mixed with a shampoo base; cream is also available with neomycin (Neo-Synalar)
Fluocinonide *Fluonex, Lidex, Lidex-E* *(CAN) Lidemol, Lyderm, Topsyn*	Ointment: 0.05% Cream: 0.05% Gel: 0.05% Solution: 0.05%	Apply 3–4 times/day	Used for anti-inflammatory action in steroid responsive dermatoses; one of the more potent topical corticosteroids; available in several different vehicles

(*continued*)

Table 45-3. **Glucocorticoids (Continued)**

Drug	*Preparations*	*Usual Dosage Range*	*Nursing Considerations*
Fluorometholone *Flarex, Fluor-Op, FML Liquifilm*	Ophthalmic suspension: 0.1% Ophthalmic ointment: 0.1%	Ophthalmic: 1–2 drops or small ribbon of ointment 3–4 times/day	Be alert for ocular irritation and discontinue drug; transient burning may occur when first applied
Flurandrenolide *Cordran* *(CAN) Drenison*	Ointment: 0.025%, 0.05% Cream: 0.025%, 0.05% Lotion: 0.05% Tape: 4 μg/cm²	Apply 2–3 times/day Tape: Cut tape to size of area; apply to clean dry skin and replace every 12 h	Good anti-inflammatory, antipruritic, and vasoconstrictive activity; tape is usually removed every 12 h but may be left in place for 24 h if well tolerated; if irritation or infection develops, remove tape and inform physician
Fluticasone *Cutivate*	Ointment: 0.05% Cream: 0.05%	Apply 2–3 times/day	Moderately effective topical steroid; ointment is 1/10 as potent as cream
Halcinonide *Halog, Halog E*	Ointment: 0.1% Cream: 0.025%, 0.1% Solution: 0.1%	Apply 2–3 times/day in a thin film	Similar to most other topical corticosteroids; ointment is formulated in a polyethylene and mineral oil gel base; cream (0.1%) is available in a vanishing base (Halog E)
Halobetasol *Ultravate*	Ointment: 0.05% Cream: 0.05%	Apply 2–3 times/day	Highly potent steroid; not intended for prolonged use
Hydrocortisone *Cort-Dome, Cortef, and several other manufacturers* *(CAN) Cortamed, Cortiment, Emocort, Unicort*	Tablets: 5 mg, 10 mg, 20 mg Oral suspension: 10 mg/5 mL Injection: 50 mg/mL; 100 mg/vial, 250 mg/vial, 500 mg/vial, 1000 mg/vial Respository injection (acetate): 25 mg/mL, 50 mg/mL Enema: 100 mg/60 mL Rectal foam aerosol: 90 mg/application Ointment: 0.2%, 0.5%, 1%, 2.5% Cream: 0.2%, 0.5%, 1%, 2.5% Lotion: 0.25%, 0.5%, 1%, 2%, 2.5% Gel: 0.5%, 1% Aerosol spray: 0.5%, 1%	Oral: 20–240 mg/day in divided doses Parenteral: 1/3–1/2 oral dose every 12 h *Acute adrenal insufficiency* Adults: 100 mg IV followed by 100 mg/8 h in IV fluids Children: 1–2 mg/kg IV bolus, then 150–250 mg/day IV in divided doses Enema: 100 mg/night for 21 days Intralesional, intraarticular, or soft-tissue injection: 5–50 mg depending on area Ophthalmic: A thin film of ointment 3–4 times/day Topical: Apply 2–4 times/day	Short-acting corticosteroid possessing mineralocorticoid activity; similar in action but less potent than many other synthetic derivatives; local injection as acetate provides long-lasting effect owing to low solubility; phosphate and succinate salts are water soluble and may be given IV; topical hydrocortisone preparations of 1.0% or weaker are available over-the-counter; available with neomycin in cream and ointment (Neo-Cort-Dome, Neo-Cortef)
Medrysone *HMS Liquifilm*	Ophthalmic suspension: 1%	1–2 drops 2–4 times/day as needed	Used for steroid-responsive inflammatory conditions of the eye; discontinue drug if irritation develops; prolonged use has resulted in cataract formation; shake suspension well before using
Methylprednisolone *Medrol and other manufacturers*	Tablets: 2 mg, 4 mg, 8 mg, 16 mg, 24 mg, 32 mg Injection: 40 mg/mL, 125 mg/2 mL, 500 mg/8 mL, 1000 mg/16 mL Repository injection (acetate): 20 mg/mL, 40 mg/mL, 80 mg/mL Powder for injection: 2000 mg/vial Enema: 40 mg	*Adults* Oral: 4–48 mg/day in divided doses Repository injection: 40–120 mg IM every 1–4 wk, depending on condition Intra-articular: 4–80 mg, depending on joint size Injection: 10–40 mg IV over several minutes; subsequent doses may be given IM or IV *Children* No less than 0.5 mg/kg/day	Available as base (tablets), sodium succinate (rapid-acting injection) or acetate (repository injection, topical ointment); use alternate-day regimen when administered over extended periods; do *not* inject acetate salt IV

(*continued*)

Table 45-3. **Glucocorticoids (Continued)**

Drug	Preparations	Usual Dosage Range	Nursing Considerations
Mometasone *Elocon*	Cream: 0.1% Ointment: 0.1% Lotion: 0.1%	Apply once daily	Topical steroid used for steroid-responsive dermatoses; do *not* use occlusive dressings
Prednisolone *Several manufacturers*	*Oral* Tablets: 5 mg Oral liquid: 5 mg/5 mL *Injection* Sodium phosphate: 20 mg/mL Acetate: 25 mg/mL, 50 mg/mL, Tebutate: 20 mg/mL *Ophthalmic drops*: 0.12%, 0.125%, 0.5%, 1%	Oral: 5–60 mg/day up to 200 mg/day for acute exacerbation of multiple sclerosis Systemic injection: IM (acetate, sodium phosphate) or IV (sodium phosphate *only*)—4–60 mg/day Intralesional, intraarticular, or soft-tissue injection: 4–30 mg (tebutate) *or* 5–100 mg (acetate) Ophthalmic: 1–2 drops into conjunctival sac every 4 h	Synthetic derivative of hydrocortisone, approximately 5 times more potent; administer orally with meals to minimize GI irritation; sodium and water retention is minimal with normal doses; alternate-day therapy is advisable with prolonged use to reduce incidence of adverse effects; ophthalmic use may increase intraocular pressure; *frequent ocular examinations* are advisable during extended therapy; injections are available as phosphate (rapid onset; short duration), acetate (prolonged action), tebutate (prolonged action), and a combination of acetate and phosphate (prompt onset and prolonged effect)
Prednisone *Several manufacturers*	Tablets: 1 mg, 2.5 mg, 5 mg, 10 mg, 20 mg, 50 mg Syrup: 5 mg/5 mL Oral concentrate: 5 mg/mL	Adults: 5–60 mg/day in divided doses Children: 0.1–0.15 mg/kg/day divided every 12 h	Synthetic derivative of hydrocortisone; therapeutic action is due to metabolism to prednisolone; use with *caution* in patients with liver disease; may induce sodium and water retention and potassium loss, especially at high doses; administer on alternate days during prolonged therapy; frequently combined with antineoplastic drugs in certain forms of carcinoma (see Chap. 74)
Triamcinolone *Aristocort, Azmacort, Kenalog, and other manufacturers* *(CAN) Triaderm, Trianide*	Tablets: 1 mg, 2 mg, 4 mg, 8 mg Syrup: 2 mg/5 mL, 4 mg/5 mL Suspension: 3 mg/mL Injection: 25 mg/mL, 40 mg/mL Repository injection: 3 mg/mL, 5 mg/mL, 10 mg/mL, 20 mg/mL, 40 mg/mL Ointment: 0.025%, 0.1%, 0.5% Cream: 0.025%, 0.1%, 0.5% Dental paste: 0.1% Lotion: 0.025%, 0.1% Topical spray: approximately 0.2 mg per spray Oral inhaler: approximately 100 μg are delivered with each activation	Oral: 4–60 mg/day depending on condition Repository injection (IM): 40 mg once a week Intralesional, intraarticular injection: Diacetate: 5–40 mg Acetonide: 2.5–15 mg Hexacetonide: 2–20 mg Topical: 2–4 times/day as needed Inhalation: 2 inhalations 3–4 times/day	Synthetic corticosteroid approximately 5 times more potent than hydrocortisone; no significant mineralocorticoid activity at normal doses; diacetate has an intermediate onset and moderate duration of action; acetonide and hexacetonide derivatives possess a slow onset and prolonged duration of action; do *not* use in children; injections should be made IM—do *not* administer IV; oral inhalation (Azmacort) is used in steroid-responsive bronchial asthma (see Chap. 57)

Hematologic/neoplastic: thrombocytopenic purpura, hemolytic anemia (autoimmune), erythroblastopenia, leukemias, Hodgkin's disease, multiple myeloma

Other: nephrotic syndrome, gout, hypercalcemia, multiple sclerosis, acute myasthenic episodes, anaphylactic shock, tuberculous meningitis, nonsuppurative thyroiditis

Testing of adrenal cortical hyperfunction and treatment of cerebral edema associated with brain tumors, craniotomy, or trauma (dexamethasone only)

Treatment of pulmonary emphysema with bronchospasm and edema, treatment of diffuse interstitial pulmonary fibrosis, control of postoperative dental inflammatory reactions, and in conjunction with diuretics in refractory congestive heart failure (triamcinolone *only*)

Investigational uses include prevention of cisplatin-induced vomiting (dexamethasone), prevention of respiratory distress syndrome in premature neonates (betamethasone), treatment of septic shock (methylprednisolone IV), prevention or treatment of acute mountain sickness (dexamethasone), acute spinal cord injury (methylprednisolone), severe alcoholic hepatitis (methylprednisolone), prevention of hearing loss in bacterial meningitis (dexamethasone), Duchenne's muscular dystrophy (prednisone) and diagnosis of depression (dexamethasone)

Dosage

See Table 45-3.

Fate

Most drugs are well absorbed from the GI tract and circulate in the blood partially bound to plasma proteins; duration of action varies among derivatives; metabolized in the liver and excreted largely by the kidneys in conjugated form; induction of hepatic enzymes will increase the metabolic clearance of glucocorticoids; renal clearance is accelerated when plasma levels are increased. (See Table 45-3 for specific data for individual drugs.)

Common Side Effects

Mild GI distress, salt and water retention, restlessness, increased appetite

Significant Adverse Reactions

CAUTION

The incidence of adverse reactions with glucocorticoids generally increases with frequency of administration and duration of therapy.

GI: vomiting, peptic ulcer, pancreatitis, abdominal distention, ulcerative esophagitis
CV: hypertension, arrhythmias, congestive heart failure, shock, thrombophlebitis, fat embolism
Dermatologic: petechiae, ecchymoses, purpura, hirsutism, acne, thinning of skin, striae, fatty redistribution in subcutaneous layers, impaired wound healing, abnormal pigmentation
Musculoskeletal: osteoporosis, muscle weakness, tendon rupture, vertebral compression fractures, spontaneous fractures, steroid myopathy
Neurologic: vertigo, headache, syncope, personality changes, irritability, insomnia, convulsions, catatonia
Fluid/electrolyte: hypokalemia, hypocalcemia, alkalosis
Endocrine: menstrual irregularities, growth retardation, decreased carbohydrate tolerance, steroid diabetes
Ophthalmic: posterior subcapsular cataracts, glaucoma, exophthalmos
Other: increased susceptibility to or masking of infections, fatty embolism, negative nitrogen balance, hypersensitivity and anaphylactic reactions, renal stones, leukocytosis

Contraindications

Systemic glucocorticoids are contraindicated in the presence of active peptic ulcer, systemic fungal infection, active tuberculosis, and in combination with any live virus vaccine; *IM* administration is contraindicated in thrombocytopenic purpura; *ocular and topical* administration are contraindicated in the presence of herpes simplex, tubercular, or other viral infections of the eye or skin. *Cautious use* in patients with hypothyroidism, ulcerative colitis, fresh intestinal anastomoses, diverticulitis, cirrhosis, active or latent peptic ulcer, diabetes mellitus, chronic nephritis, hypertension, congestive heart failure, osteoporosis, renal insufficiency, thrombophlebitis, glaucoma, myasthenia gravis, convulsive disorders, metastatic carcinoma, pyogenic infections, Cushing's syndrome, vaccinia or varicella infections, and in pregnant or nursing women

CAUTION

Steroids should not be injected into a joint suspected of being infected or unstable, because frequent intra-articular injections can damage joint.

Interactions

The pharmacologic effects of corticosteroids may be reduced by barbiturates, phenytoin, ephedrine, and rifampin, drugs that enhance the metabolic clearance of steroids.
Corticosteroids may increase the dosage requirements for insulin and oral antidiabetic agents, isoniazid, salicylates, and oral anticoagulants.
Increased intraocular pressure can result from combinations of corticosteroids and anticholinergics, tricyclic antidepressants, or adrenergics.
Excessive hypokalemia has resulted from concomitant use of corticosteroids and potassium-depleting diuretics or amphotericin.
Corticosteroids can increase digitalis toxicity as a result of potassium loss.
The anti-inflammatory action of corticosteroids may be enhanced by estrogens because of reduced hepatic clearance.
Gastrointestinal absorption of corticosteroids can be impaired by cholestyramine and colestipol.
Corticosteroids may increase the pharmacologic effects of theophylline.
Concurrent use of corticosteroids and salicylates may result in reduced salicylate levels and increased likelihood of gastric ulceration.

Nursing Management

Pretherapy Assessment

Assess and record baseline data necessary for detection of adverse effects of glucocorticoids: General: vital signs (VS), body weight, skin color and temperature; central nervous system (CNS): orientation, reflexes, bilateral grip strength; cardiovascular system (CVS): peripheral perfusion, discoloration; genitourinary (GU): upper GI x-ray, liver palpation; Lab: complete blood count (CBC), serum electyrolytes, 2-hour postprandial blood glucose, urinalysis, thyroid function tests, serum cholesterol.

Review medical history and documents for existing or previous conditions that:

a. require cautious use of glucocorticoids: hypothyroidism; ulcerative colitis; fresh intestinal anastomoses; diverticulitis; cirrhosis; active or latent peptic ulcer; diabetes mellitus; chronic nephritis; hypertension; congestive heart failure; osteoporosis; renal insufficiency; thrombophlebitis; glaucoma; myasthenia gravis; convulsive disorders; metastatic carcinoma; pyogenic infections; Cushing's syndrome; vaccinia or varicella infections

b. contraindicate use of glucocorticoids: *systemic* glucocorticoids: active peptic ulcer; systemic fungal infection; active tuberculosis; any live virus vaccine; *IM* administration; thrombocytopenic purpura; *ocular and topical* administration: herpes simplex; tubercular; other viral infections of the eye or skin; **pregnancy (Category C)**, lactation (secreted in breast milk, do not nurse).

Nursing Interventions

Medication Administration

Systemic:

Administer once a day before 9:00 AM to mimic normal peak diurnal corticosteroid levels and minimize hypothalamic-pituitary-adrenal (HPA) suppression.

Do not give IM injections if patient has thrombocytopenic purpura.

Use minimum doses for a minimum duration of time to reduce adverse effects.

Arrange to taper doses when discontinuing high-dose or long-term therapy.

Use alternate day maintenance therapy with short-acting agents when possible.

Provide antacids between meals to help avoid peptic ulcer.

Topical:

Use caution with occlusive dressings as these can enhance systemic availability.

Avoid prolonged use, especially near eyes, in genital and rectal areas, on the face, and in skin creases.

Surveillance During Therapy

Be alert for possibility of hypersensitivity reactions with parenteral use. Severe anaphylactic reactions have been reported.

Assess patient's mental status carefully for signs of change (eg, euphoria, insomnia, depression, mood swings) because emotional aberrations may occur. Glucocorticoids should be used cautiously in persons with a history of emotional instability.

Ensure that baseline values for blood pressure, weight, intake/output ratio, blood glucose, and serum potassium are obtained before therapy is initiated. These values should also be determined at regular intervals thereafter.

Collaborate with healthcare team in evaluating drug effects. Dosage should be individually adjusted for each patient on the basis of the disease state being treated and the clinical response. Initial dosage should be adjusted and then maintained until a satisfactory response is evident. Dosage may then be gradually reduced to lowest effective level. Alternate-day therapy is generally preferred, where feasible, to minimize adrenal suppression.

Monitor diabetic patients closely because hyperglycemia can occur.

Monitor weight and height of pediatric patient because drugs can suppress normal growth pattern.

Determine if patient has a history of excessive use of over-the-counter (OTC) topical corticosteroid preparations if signs and symptoms of toxicity occur without obvious cause.

Carefully monitor laboratory studies and patient for indications of adverse reactions.

Interpret results of diagnostic tests and contact practitioner as appropriate.

Monitor for possible drug–drug and drug–nutrient interactions: Refer to **Interactions**.

Patient Teaching

Instruct patient to take drug with food or milk in a single daily morning dose, preferably before 9:00 AM. Corticosteroids suppress adrenal function least when given at the time of maximal adrenocortical activity, which is early morning.

Provide patient with schedule of doses to be taken each day to effect a changeover from daily to alternate-day dosing. Alternate-day therapy is usually accomplished by administering twice the daily maintenance dose every other morning. Long-acting drugs should *not* be employed in alternate-day therapy.

Reassure patient that sudden worsening of condition during periods of dosage adjustment is temporary.

Inform patient that drug requirements may be increased during periods of stress. Supplementary doses of a rapid-acting agent should be administered during these periods.

Emphasize the importance of trying to avoid infections and of notifying practitioner immediately if one is suspected (eg, slow wound healing, prolonged inflammation, persistent fever, sore throat). Glucocorticoids may mask some signs of infection, encourage their spread, and decrease patient's resistance. Appropriate antibiotic therapy is essential.

Instruct patient receiving long-term therapy to obtain periodic ophthalmic examinations and to report any visual disturbances immediately because cataracts, glaucoma, or optic nerve damage may occur.

Urge patient to advise practitioner if gastric distress is severe or persistent because gastric ulceration may occur. Supplemental antacids may alleviate GI distress.

Encourage patient to use a firm mattress and bedboard and to report persistent backache or chest pain, which may indicate the presence of spontaneous vertebral or rib fractures.

Instruct patient to notify practitioner if excessive weight gain, edema, hypertension, muscle weakness, or bone pain occurs.

Ensure that patient undergoing high-dose therapy understands that immunizations are contraindicated (antibody response is impaired, and neurologic complications could occur).

Inform female patients that menstrual irregularities may develop.

Stress the importance of adhering to prescribed dosage regimen and the danger of sudden termination of usage. After extended therapy, corticosteroids should be withdrawn gradually to minimize the risk of adrenal suppression.

Teach patient symptoms of adrenal insufficiency (eg, nausea, dyspnea, fever, hypotension, myalgia, hypoglycemia) and instruct patient to notify practitioner if they occur. Supplementary steroids may be needed to reverse the symptoms.

Suggest that patient carry information describing condition treated and drug and dosage taken.

Warn patient not to overuse an injected joint after cessation of pain because the inflammatory focus may still be present, and further deterioration may occur with overactivity.

Instruct patient to moderate salt intake.

Encourage patient to regularly include potassium-rich foods in diet, especially if taking a glucocorticoid with significant mineralocorticoid activity (see Table 45-1).

Warn patient to avoid licorice because it may intensify hypokalemia.

Adrenal Steroid Inhibitors

Two drugs, aminoglutethimide and trilostane, that inhibit the synthesis of adrenal steroids, are available for treating selected cases of Cushing's syndrome (adrenocortical hyperfunction). They are reviewed below.

• Aminoglutethimide *(Pregnancy Category D)*

Cytadren

Mechanism

Inhibits the conversion of cholesterol to delta-5-pregnenolone, thus impairing normal synthesis of adrenal steroids; probably acts by binding to the drug-metabolizing enzyme cytochrome P-450; also inhibits conversion of androgens to estrogens in peripheral tissues

Uses

Suppression of adrenal function in selected patients with adrenocortical hyperfunction (Cushing's syndrome). Usually given only until more definitive therapy (ie, surgery) can be undertaken

Investigational uses include treatment of postmenopausal metastatic breast cancer and prostatic carcinoma unresponsive to hormonal or surgical therapy

Dosage

Initially 250 mg 4 times a day; may increase in increments of 250 mg/day at intervals of 1 to 2 weeks to a total daily dose of 2 g; may be necessary to provide mineralocorticoid replacement therapy (eg, fludrocortisone) because of reduced aldosterone production

Fate

Well absorbed orally; plasma half-life is initially 12 to 16 hours but decreases to 6 to 8 hours with continued therapy; eliminated as both unchanged drug and metabolites in the urine

Common Side Effects

Drowsiness, skin rash, nausea, anorexia, headache, dizziness

Significant Adverse Reactions

Hematologic: neutropenia, transient leukopenia, pancytopenia, thrombocytopenia

CV: orthostatic hypotension, tachycardia

GI: vomiting

Dermatologic: pruritus, urticaria

Other: adrenal insufficiency, hypothyroidism, hirsutism, fever, myalgia, altered liver function tests, cholestatic jaundice

Contraindications

Sensitivity to glutethimide (Doriden). *Cautious use* in patients with hypothyroidism, liver disease, or acute illness and in pregnant or nursing women.

Interactions

Aminoglutethimide can decrease the effects of dexamethasone, digitoxin, medroxyprogesterone, oral contraceptives and theophylline.

Aminoglutethimide can reduce the anticoagulant effectiveness of warfarin.

Concurrent use of alcohol may potentiate the effects of aminoglutethimide.

Nursing Management

Nursing Interventions

Surveillance During Therapy

Monitor results of serum cortisol levels. Either drug overdosage or increased levels of stress may induce adrenal insufficiency.

Assess patient carefully for indications of adrenocortical hypofunction (eg, fatigue, nausea, vomiting, anorexia, diarrhea), especially under conditions of stress, trauma, surgery, or acute illness. It may be necessary to administer a mineralocorticoid (refer to **Dosage**).

Monitor results of thyroid function tests, which should be performed at regular intervals, and observe for clinical signs of hypothyroidism (fatigue, hypotension, weakness). Supplementary thyroid drugs may be required.

Monitor blood pressure because orthostatic hypotension may occur.

Ensure that baseline hematologic studies are performed. They should also be repeated at regular intervals during therapy.

Monitor results of liver function tests and serum electrolyte determinations, which should be obtained periodically during therapy.

Patient Teaching

Instruct patient to perform hazardous tasks cautiously because dizziness, faintness, ataxia, or weakness may occur.

Teach patient appropriate interventions to minimize symptoms of orthostatic hypotension.

Inform patient that nausea and loss of appetite can occur during early therapy. If these effects are pronounced or prolonged, the practitioner should be consulted.

Instruct patient to notify practitioner if side effects (eg, skin rash, drowsiness) become severe because a dosage reduction or temporary discontinuation of drug may be warranted.

- ***Trilostane** (Pregnancy Category D)*

Modrastane

Mechanism

Lowers circulating glucocorticoid levels by inhibiting enzyme systems essential for their production; exhibits *no* intrinsic hormonal activity.

Use

Temporary treatment of adrenocortical hyperfunction (Cushing's syndrome) until more definitive measures (eg, surgery) can be undertaken.

Dosage

Initially, 30 mg 4 times/day; increase gradually at 3-day to 4-day intervals; doses generally do not exceed 360 mg/day; discontinue therapy if no response occurs within 2 weeks.

Common Side Effects

Abdominal discomfort, cramping, diarrhea, headache, flushing, burning sensation of the oral or nasal mucosa

Significant Adverse Reactions

Nasal stuffiness, bloating, belching, lacrimation, muscle and joint pain, skin rash, erythema, fever, paresthesias, fatigue

Contraindications

Adrenal insufficiency, severe renal or hepatic disease, pregnancy. *Cautious use* in patients with acute illness, in nursing mothers and in persons receiving other drugs that may suppress adrenal function.

Interactions

Concurrent use of trilostane and aminoglutethimide or mitotane can cause severe adrenocortical hypofunction.

Nursing Management

Refer to **Aminoglutethimide**.

Selected Bibliography

Bailey JM: New mechanisms for effects of anti-inflammatory glucocorticoids. Biofactors 3(2):97, 1991

Boumpas DT, Paliogianni F, et al: Glucocorticosteroid action on the immune system: Molecular and cellular aspects. Clin Exp Rheumatol 9(4):413, 1991

Cook DM: Safe use of glucocorticoids. How to monitor patients taking these potent agents. Postgrad Med 91(3):145, 1992

Holland EG, Taylor AT: Glucocorticoids in clinical practice. J Fam Pract 32(5):512, 1991

Jadoul M, Ferrant A, et al: Mineralocorticoids in the management of primary adrenocortical insufficiency. J Endocrinol Invest 14(2): 87, 1991

Kimberly RP: Mechanisms of action, dosage schedules and side effects of steroid therapy. Curr Opin Rheumatol 3(3):373, 1991

Kimberly RP: Glucocorticoid therapy for rheumatic diseases. Curr Opin Rheumatol 4(3):325, 1992

Krane SM: Some molecular mechanisms of glucocorticoid action. Br J Rheumatol 32(suppl 2):3, 1993

Lacomis D, Samuels MA: Adverse neurologic effects of glucocorticosteroids. J Gen Intern Med 6(4):367, 1991

Lozewicz S, Wang J, et al: Topical glucocorticoids inhibit activation by allergen in the upper respiratory tract. J Allerg Clin Immunol 89(5): 951, 1992

Reasner CA: Adrenal disorders. Crit Care Nurs Q 13(3):67, 1990

Scudeletti M, Castagnetta L, et al: New glucocorticoids. Mechanisms of immunological activity at the cellular level and in the clinical setting. Ann NY Acad Sci 595:368, 1990

Nursing Bibliography

Hardy E: Steroid management in orthopaedic patients. Orthopedic Nursing 11(6):27, 1992

McPherson M: The use of topical corticosteroids. Journal of Home Health Care Practice 5(3):50, 1993

Plutkin M, et al: Fatigue and edema in steroid therapy. Hosp Prac 28(4):322, 1993

Reasner C: Adrenal disorders. Critical Care Nursing Quarterly 13(3): 67, 1990

Stumpf J, Mitrzyk B: Management of orthostatic hypotension. Am J Hosp Pharm 51:59, 1994

Wilson B: Understanding corticosteroids: Pharmacologic and adverse effects. Med Surg Nurse 2(4):322, 1993

Wrona S, Tankanow R: Corticosteroids in the management of alcoholic hepatitis J Hosp Pharm 51:74, 1994

46

Estrogens and Progestins

The female hormones may be categorized into two types—estrogens and progestins. Both groups consist of steroidal compounds secreted by the ovaries, beginning around the time of puberty, as well as by the placenta during pregnancy, and in much lesser amounts by the adrenal cortex. The female sex hormones play a major role in the development and maintenance of the reproductive system and also affect the functioning of many other physiologic systems.

Estrogens *(Pregnancy Category X)*

Chlorotrianisene
Conjugated estrogens
Dienestrol
Diethylstilbestrol
Esterified estrogens
Estradiol
Estrone
Estropipate
Ethinyl estradiol
Mestranol
Polyestradiol phosphate
Quinestrol

The *estrogens* are a group of both naturally occurring and synthetic derivatives that exhibit similar pharmacologic and toxicologic effects, differing primarily in suitability for a particular route of administration, potency, and therapeutic indications. One useful classification for the estrogens divides them into the following categories:

- *Natural (endogenous) estrogens* (eg, estradiol, estriol, estrone)
- *Esters and conjugates of natural estrogens* (eg, estradiol valerate, estropipate, polyestradiol phosphate, conjugated estrogens)
- *Semisynthetic and synthetic estrogens* (eg, ethinyl estradiol, chlorotrianisene, dienestrol, diethylstilbestrol)

The *naturally occurring estrogens* are synthesized principally in the ovary and are secreted during the early phase of the menstrual cycle through the synergistic action of follicle-stimulating hormone (FSH) and luteinizing hormone (LH) on the maturing ovarian follicle. The *endogenous* estrogens are composed of several related substances, the principal one being estradiol, which is the most potent. Estradiol is rapidly converted to estrone, which is approximately one half as potent. Estrone in turn is metabolized to estriol, the weakest in action of the three. These endogenous estrogens promote the growth and development of the endometrium and exert a wide range of effects on other body structures (refer to **Mechanism**).

Naturally occurring estrogens are adequately absorbed when administered orally, but are rapidly metabolized and quickly eliminated, and thus are largely unsuited for oral therapy. Estradiol is available for injection as either the cypionate or valerate salt in an oily vehicle (long-acting), whereas estrone is available as an aqueous suspension. Crystalline estrone sulfate stabilized with piperazine (estropipate) can be used as a vaginal cream, as can dienestrol, a synthetic estrogen. Orally effective estrogens include micronized estradiol, estropipate, conjugated estrogens, esterified estrogens, and a number of semisynthetic and synthetic derivatives. In addition, two very potent orally effective semisynthetic estrogens, ethinyl estradiol and mestranol, are the only estrogens found in the combination oral contraceptive formulations, and these products are reviewed in Chapter 47. Estradiol is also available in the form of a transdermal patch, which yields higher blood levels than oral administration, thus requiring smaller doses.

Principal indications for use of estrogens include relief of the symptoms of menopause, symptomatic management of atrophic vaginitis, treatment of primary female hypogonadism and ovarian failure, palliation of certain types of carcinoma, suppression of lactation, relief of postpartum breast engorgement, and control of abnormal uterine bleeding caused by hormonal imbalance. In addition, certain estrogens are used in combination with progestins for contraception. Of these uses, the control of menopausal symptoms has been a somewhat controversial application for estrogens, and a division of opinion still exists on the safety and efficacy of oral estrogen replacement therapy for menopausal symptoms.

There is fairly general agreement that *low-dose* oral estrogen therapy can reduce the incidence and severity of vasomotor symptoms associated with the menopause (such as sweating, flushing, "hot flashes") and alleviate sleep disorders that often accompany them. Topical application is likewise effective in retarding the atrophic changes in the vaginal epithelium (as in senile vaginitis). Conversely, the use of estrogens to retard the progression of osteoporosis in postmenopausal women has been the subject of some debate; however, the current consensus seems to favor use of *low doses* of estrogen together with supplemental calcium as a safe and effective means of retarding bone loss and reducing the incidence of spontaneous fractures. The estrogen, usually conjugated estrogens, is given for 25 days each month and a progestin is added for the last 12 days of the cycle to decrease the risk of endometrial carcinoma (refer to **Significant Adverse Reactions**, below). Most clinicians prescribe supplemental calcium as well, and it appears that the dosage necessary to maintain a positive calcium balance in postmenopausal women is 1.0 to 1.5 g elemental calcium per day. Concurrent use of vitamin D, which facilitates calcium absorption from the gastrointestinal tract, is also recognized as safe and effective, but dosage should be restricted to 400 U/day or less. Large doses of vitamin D have actually been demonstrated to *increase* bone resorption. Use of other therapeutic agents, such as calcitonin, etidronate, pamidronate, or sodium fluoride, currently represent alternative approaches to pre-

Malseed, RT; Goldstein, FJ; and Balkon, N: PHARMACOLOGY: DRUG THERAPY AND NURSING CONSIDERATIONS, Fourth Edition. © 1995 J. B. Lippincott Company.

venting osteoporotic changes and are discussed elsewhere in the text.

Evidence indicates that estrogen therapy is probably most effective if begun as soon as possible after the onset of menopause, because early menopause is characterized by fairly rapid bone loss. Further, estrogen supplementation, once begun, may have to be continued indefinitely, because menopausal symptoms usually recur shortly after the estrogen is stopped. Some reports even indicate that bone loss may be *accelerated* after withdrawal of estrogen after prolonged use. Still other reports have suggested that estrogen replacement therapy is associated with a *decreased* risk of ischemic heart disease and myocardial infarction and may also have a favorable effect on the lipid profile.

The principal hazards associated with estrogen replacement therapy are thromboembolic complications, gallbladder disease, hypertension, and, most critically, endometrial and possibly breast carcinoma. In general, the risk of these adverse reactions is largely proportional to the dose of estrogen and the duration of therapy. Current recommendations call for use of small doses of estrogens (ie, 0.3–0.625 mg conjugated estrogens) in conjunction with calcium and addition of a progestin from days 13 to 25 of the dosage cycle. Progestin treatment has been shown to reduce (and perhaps even eliminate) the risk of endometrial carcinoma, but can increase the frequency of cyclic withdrawal bleeding.

The use of estrogens in postmenopausal women must be undertaken cautiously, minimal effective doses must be used, and cyclic administration in conjunction with progestins should be employed in women who still have an intact uterus. Appropriate laboratory tests and a physical examination should be performed before initiating therapy and at regular intervals thereafter. Therapy should be reevaluated periodically and dosage adjustments made if necessary.

The discussion of the estrogens considers the agents as a group. Individual drugs and dosages are listed in Table 46-1, along with nursing implications pertaining to each individual drug.

Mechanism

Produce thickening and increase development of blood vessels and glands of the endometrium; increase volume and acidity of cervical and vaginal secretions; promote growth and cornification of vaginal epithelium and enhance glycogen deposition; accelerate uterine motility; assist growth and development of the duct system of the mammary glands; increase sensitivity of uterus to oxytocin; metabolic actions include a protein anabolic action, accelerated closure of the epiphyses, decreased bone resorption rate, increased serum triglycerides, decreased serum cholesterol and low-density lipoproteins, and enhanced sodium and water retention; reduce platelet adhesiveness and increase levels of vitamin K–dependent clotting factors; *large doses* reduce release of FSH and prolactin from the anterior pituitary by negative feedback, thus inhibiting follicular maturation and lactation; appear to increase release of LH, assisting ovulation; biochemical actions of estrogens are apparently attributable to their binding to tissue-specific receptor proteins on estrogen-responsive tissues (eg, pituitary, breasts, genitalia); as a result, there is increased synthesis of DNA, RNA, and several proteins that alter the function of these tissues; receptor effects are blocked by inhibitors of RNA or protein synthesis.

Uses

See Table 46-1 for specific indications for each drug.

- Relief of vasomotor and atrophic symptoms of the menopause and prevention of osteoporotic changes
- Treatment of atrophic vaginitis and kraurosis vulvae (dryness and pruritus of female genitalia)
- Replacement therapy in female hypogonadism, female castration, and primary ovarian failure
- Palliative treatment of advanced prostatic carcinoma, and mammary carcinoma in women who are at least 5 years postmenopausal (see Chapter 74)
- Relief of postpartum breast engorgement (benefit versus risk must be critically weighed)
- Control of abnormal uterine bleeding caused by lack of estrogen secretion
- Relief of severe acne resistant to more conventional therapy (investigational use in female patients only)
- Postcoital contraception (*emergency* use only; refer to **Diethylstilbestrol**, Table 46-1)

Dosage

See Table 46-1.

Fate

Estradiol is metabolized to estrone and further to estriol in vivo, then is conjugated and excreted in the urine. Natural estrogens are rapidly inactivated in the GI tract. Esterification of natural estrogens delays metabolism and prolongs action. Aqueous solution of estrogens provides rapid onset and relatively short duration of action. Suspensions or solutions in oil allow slower absorption from IM injection sites, delayed onset, and prolonged duration of action. Oral absorption of synthetic estrogens is good, and they are less rapidly inactivated than natural derivatives. They circulate in both free and conjugated forms, which are 50% to 75% protein bound. Metabolism of estrogens occurs primarily in the liver; less active conjugated products are produced. Estrogens are excreted largely in the urine, although some excretion occurs by way of the bile.

Common Side Effects

Nausea, fluid retention, "breakthrough" (midcycle) menstrual bleeding, change in menstrual flow, breast fullness or tenderness, erythema and irritation at transdermal application sites

Significant Adverse Reactions

CAUTION

Use of estrogens is associated with an increased risk of endometrial carcinoma. The risk is dose and duration dependent, and is estimated to be between 5 and 14 times that of nonusers. There appears to be no difference in risk between "natural" and synthetic estrogens. Cyclical progestin therapy (ie, days 13 to 25) appears to largely eliminate this risk. There may be a *slightly* higher risk of breast cancer in women older than 50 years of age who have taken estrogen for at least 7 to 10 years; cyclical progestin use does *not* appear to protect against the development of breast cancer. Use of estrogens during early pregnancy may damage the fetus. Female offspring exposed in utero to diethylstilbestrol display an increased incidence of cervical or vaginal adenocarcinoma. Congenital deformities have also

Table 46-1. **Estrogens**

Drug	*Usual Dosage Range*	*Nursing Considerations*
Chlorotrianisene *Tace*	*Menopause*: 12–25 mg/day cyclically for 30 days *Hypogonadism*: 12–25 mg/day cyclically for 21 days, followed by oral progestin last 5 days of cycle *Prostatic carcinoma*: 12–25 mg/day *Breast engorgement*: 12 mg 4 times/day for 7 days *or* 50 mg every 6 h for 6 doses	Synthetic estrogen with delayed onset and prolonged duration of action; stored in adipose tissue; drug is *not* recommended for mammary carcinoma, because it induces uterine bleeding and endometrial hyperplasia (see Chap. 74)
Conjugated Estrogens *Premarin* *(CAN) C.E.S., Conjugated Estrogens C.S.D.*	*Menopause*: 0.3–0.625 mg/day cyclically with progestins on days 13–25 *Hypogonadism, ovarian failure*: 2.5–7.5 mg/day in divided doses for 20 days; oral progestin during last 5 days *Prostatic carcinoma*: 1.25–2.5 mg 3 times/day for several weeks (maintenance, 1/2 initial dose) *Breast cancer*: 10 mg 3 times/day for 2–5 mo as needed to obtain desired response *Vaginitis, kraurosis vulvae*: Insert vaginal cream 1–2 times/day *Abnormal uterine bleeding*: 25 mg IV or IM; repeat in 6 h if necessary	Water-soluble mixture of conjugated estrogens (sodium estrone sulfate, 50%–65%, and sodium equilin sulfate, 20%–35%) obtained from the urine of pregnant mares; most commonly used orally for menopausal symptoms; also for palliation of breast and prostatic carcinoma (see Chap. 74); vaginal cream is employed for atrophic vaginitis and pruritus vulvae; injection can be used to control abnormal uterine bleeding due to hormonal imbalance; perform IV injection slowly to minimize flushing; do *not* use if solution is darkened or a precipitate is noted; solution is incompatible with other solutions having an acid pH; also available in combination with meprobamate as PMB.
Dienestrol *DV, Ortho Dienestrol*	*Atrophic vaginitis, kraurosis vulvae*: 1–2 applicators of cream daily for 1–2 wk, then 1 applicator every other day	Synthetic estrogen employed vaginally; systemic absorption may be significant during prolonged use
Diethylstilbestrol (DES)	*Prostatic carcinoma*: 1–3 mg/day *Breast cancer*: 15 mg/day *Postcoital contraception*: 25 mg twice a day for 5 days (*emergency use only*)	Potent synthetic estrogen given orally; frequently produces nausea, vomiting, and headache; contraindicated during pregnancy, because drug has been implicated in causing vaginal and cervical cancer in offspring of women receiving the drug during first trimester; as a postcoital contraceptive, must be given within 24–72 h of intercourse
Diethylstilbestrol Diphosphate *Stilphostrol* *(CAN) Honvol*	*Advanced prostatic carcinoma*: 50–200 mg orally 3 times/day *or* 0.5 g by IV infusion first day, then 1 g/day on subsequent 5 days; maintenance 0.25–0.5 g 1–2 times/wk	High-dose diethylstilbestrol used for treatment of prostatic carcinoma unresponsive to other estrogens; be alert for early signs of thrombotic complications; for IV administration, dissolve 0.5–1 g drug in 300 mL saline or dextrose and infuse *slowly* (20–30 drops a min) during first 10–15 min; adjust rate thereafter so that entire amount is given over 1 h (see Chap. 74)
Esterified Estrogens *Estratab, Menest* *(CAN) Neo-Estrone*	*Menopause*: 0.3–0.625 mg/day *Hypogonadism, ovarian failure*: 2.5–7.5 mg/day in divided doses for 20 days, then stop for 10 days *Prostatic carcinoma*: 1.25–2.5 mg 3 times/day; maintenance—reduce by half after several weeks *Breast cancer*: 10 mg 3 times/day for 3 mo	Mixture of sodium estrone sulfate (75%–85%) and sodium equilin sulfate (6%–15%); action is similar to conjugated estrogens; also available with chlordiazepoxide as Menrium
Estradiol, Oral *Estrace*	*Hypogonadism, ovarian failure, menopause*: 1–2 mg/day orally for 3 wk; then 1 wk off *Breast cancer*: 10 mg 3 times/day for 3 mo *Prostatic carcinoma*: 1–20 mg 3 times/day *Osteoporosis*: 0.5 mg/day for 3 wk, then 1 wk off; repeat monthly	Estrogenic hormone derived from estrone but more potent; readily absorbed orally; available in salt form for injection (see below), providing slow onset and more prolonged duration of action
Estradiol Cypionate *Depo-Estradiol, and other manufacturers*	*Menopause*: 1–5 mg IM every 3–4 wk *Hypogonadism*: 1.5–2 mg once a month	Salt of estradiol in cottonseed oil providing a depot effect; duration of action 3–6 wk; administered IM only

(*continued*)

Table 46-1. **Estrogens (Continued)**

Drug	Usual Dosage Range	Nursing Considerations
Estradiol Valerate *Delestrogen, and other manufacturers* *(CAN) Femogex*	*Hypogonadism, ovarian failure, menopause*: 10–20 mg IM every 4 wk *Prostatic carcinoma*: 30 mg every 1–2 wk	Salt of estradiol in sesame or castor oil provides 2–3 wk estrogenic activity after a single IM dose (see also Chap. 74)
Estradiol Transdermal System *Estraderm*	Apply patch to skin twice weekly; usually given on a cyclic schedule (ie, 3 wk on, 1 wk off)	Transdermal patch available in 2 strengths; used to control vasomotor symptoms of the menopause, atrophic vaginitis, kraurosis vulvae, and symptoms of primary ovarian failure and female hypogonadism; also used to prevent osteoporosis; system is placed on a clean, dry area of skin, preferably the abdomen; do not apply to breasts; rotate application sites; apply patch immediately after opening pouch; ensure good contact between patch and skin
Estrone *Theelin Aqueous, and other manufacturers* *(CAN) Femogen Forte*	*Senile vaginitis*: 0.1–0.5 mg IM 2–3 times/wk *Hypogonadism, ovarian failure*: 0.1–2 mg/wk IM in single or divided doses *Inoperable prostatic carcinoma*: 2–4 mg IM 2–3 times/wk	Estrogenic hormone derived from both natural and synthetic sources; response to therapy for prostatic carcinoma should become apparent within 3 mo; if response occurs, continue drug until disease again becomes progressive (see Chap. 74)
Estropipate *Ogen, Ortho-Est*	*Menopause*: 0.625–5 mg/day cyclically each month *Hypogonadism, ovarian failure*: 1.25–7.5 mg/day for 3 wk, followed by 8–10-day rest period; repeated as needed *Atrophic vaginitis*: 2–4 g vaginal cream daily for 3 wk, then 1 wk off	Crystalline form of estrone solubilized as sulfate and stabilized with piperazine, making preparation orally effective; tablets contain 83% sodium estrone sulfate equivalent; formerly known as piperazine estrone sulfate
Ethinyl Estradiol *Estinyl*	*Menopause*: 0.02–0.05 mg/day for 21 days cyclically each month *Hypogonadism*: 0.05 mg 1–3 times/day for 2 wk, followed by an oral progestin for 2 wk *Breast cancer*: 1 mg 3 times/day *Prostatic carcinoma*: 0.15–2 mg/day	Potent, orally effective synthetic estrogen; found in many oral contraceptives (see Chap. 47); also used for menopausal symptoms, female hypogonadism, and certain carcinomas (see Chap. 74)
Polyestradiol Phosphate *Estradurin*	*Advanced prostatic carcinoma*: 40–80 mg IM every 2–4 wk	Provides a stable level of active estrogen over a prolonged period; quickly cleared from blood (24 h) and passively stored in reticuloendothelial system; estradiol levels are maintained constant by continuous replacement from storage sites; increasing the dose prolongs the duration of action but does not significantly enhance the response; may produce temporary burning at IM injection site; clinical response should be evident within 3 mo; continue drug until disease becomes progressive (see Chap. 74)
Quinestrol *Estrovis*	*Menopause, hypogonadism, ovarian failure, kraurosis vulvae, atrophic vaginitis*: 100 μg once daily for 7 days, then 100 μg to 200 μg once a week thereafter	A derivative of ethinyl estradiol that is stored in body fat and slowly released, thus providing a prolonged duration of action; once-weekly administration is as effective as cyclic therapy with shorter-acting estrogens, and may improve patient compliance

been reported in male offspring whose mothers ingested the drug. Patients using estrogens must be apprised of the risks of becoming pregnant while taking these drugs.

GI: vomiting, abdominal cramps, bloating, diarrhea, anorexia, cholestatic jaundice, colitis

Dermatologic: skin rash, pruritus, hirsutism, chloasma, melasma, erythema multiforme, erythema nodosum, alopecia, acne

CNS: irritability, depression, headache, migraine attacks, dizziness, insomnia, paresthesias

Genitourinary: in women, dysmenorrhea, amenorrhea, vaginal candidiasis, increased cervical secretions, cystitis-like reaction, endometrial hyperplasia, increase in size of uterine fibromyomata; in men, feminization of genitalia, testicular atrophy, impotence

Other: gallbladder disease, thromboembolic complications, hepatic adenoma, hypertension, hypercalcemia, decreased carbohydrate tolerance, aggravation of porphyria, changes in libido, pain at injection site, sterile abscess

Refer also to **Oral Contraceptives**, Chapter 47.

Contraindications

Pregnancy **(Category X)**, known or suspected breast cancer in premenopausal women, estrogen-dependent neoplasia, undiagnosed genital bleeding, a history of or active thromboembolic disease, incomplete bone growth, or epiphyseal closure. *Cautious use* in persons with cerebrovascular or coronary artery disease, severe hypertension, epilepsy, migraine, renal or hepatic dysfunction, diabetes mellitus, depression or other emotional disturbances, gallbladder disease, metabolic bone disease associated with hypercalcemia, thyroid dysfunction, endometriosis, and in patients with a history of jaundice or a family history of breast or genital cancer.

Interactions

Refer to **Oral Contraceptives**, Chapter 47. In addition:

Estrogens may reduce the effectiveness of oral anticoagulants and insulin, thereby increasing dosage requirements.

The incidence of adverse effects with tricyclic antidepressants may be increased by estrogens.

The effects of estrogens may be attenuated by phenobarbital, phenytoin, carbamazepine, primidone, rifampin, and other drugs that can induce hepatic microsomal enzymes, thus accelerating the metabolism of estrogens.

Estrogens increase the effects of oxytocin on the uterus.

Estrogens can alter many laboratory values; for example, they may increase prothrombin, thyroid-binding globulin, serum triglycerides, phospholipids, sulfobromophthalein retention, and norepinephrine-induced platelet aggregability, and they may decrease serum folate levels, glucose tolerance, pregnanediol excretion, antithrombin III levels, and triiodothyronine (T_3) uptake; in addition, estrogens may cause an impaired response to the metyrapone test.

Nursing Management

Pretherapy Assessment

Assess and record baseline data necessary for detection of adverse effects of estrogenics: General: vital signs (VS), body weight, skin color and temperature; central nervous system (CNS): orientation, reflexes; cardiovascular system (CVS): peripheral perfusion; genitourinary (GU): liver palpation, bowel sounds; Lab: serum calcium, phosphorus, liver and renal function tests, Pap smear, glucose tolerance test.

Review medical history and documents for existing or previous conditions that:

a. require cautious use of estrogenics: cerebrovascular or coronary artery disease; severe hypertension; epilepsy; migraine; renal or hepatic dysfunction; diabetes mellitus; depression or other emotional disturbances; gallbladder disease; metabolic bone disease associated with hypercalcemia; thyroid dysfunction; endometriosis; history of jaundice; family history of breast or genital cancer

b. contraindicate use of estrogenics: known or suspected breast cancer in premenopausal women; estrogen-dependent neoplasia; undiagnosed genital bleeding; a history of or active thromboembolic disease; incomplete bone growth; epiphyseal closure; **pregnancy (Category X)**, lactation (secreted in breast milk, do not nurse).

Nursing Interventions

Medication Administration

Ensure that a comprehensive patient history and physical examination are completed before therapy is initiated. If therapy is prolonged, physical examination should be repeated at regular intervals. Estrogen should be administered very cautiously to patients with a family history of breast cancer or thromboembolic or other cardiovascular disorders.

Arrange for concomitant use of progestin therapy during chronic estrogen therapy in women to mimic normal physiologic cycling and allow for cyclical uterine bleeding.

Provide appropriate comfort measures for headache, abdominal discomfort, injection site pain, breast tenderness if these occur.

Surveillance During Therapy

Carefully monitor laboratory studies and patient for indications of adverse reactions.

Interpret results of diagnostic tests and contact practitioner as appropriate.

Monitor for possible drug–drug and drug–nutrient interactions: refer to **Interactions**.

Patient Teaching

Strongly encourage patient to curtail smoking during therapy because the risk of cardiovascular complications increases with amount of smoking (and age).

Explain to menopausal patient that the lowest effective dose is used to control symptoms and that estrogen is administered on a cyclic schedule whenever possible to minimize untoward reactions. If therapy is extended, patient should obtain Pap smear periodically and report abnormal vaginal bleeding immediately.

Explain to postmenopausal woman taking estrogen *cyclically* that withdrawal bleeding is normal and does not indicate return of fertility.

Reassure patient that the nausea that often occurs early in therapy will disappear within 1 to 2 weeks.

Teach patient signs of embolic disorders (eg, severe headache, chest pains, dyspnea, calf pain, leg swelling, visual disturbances). If these occur, drug should be discontinued and practitioner should be notified immediately.

Stress the importance of healthcare supervision during treatment because the potential for adverse reactions is considerable, and early detection is important.

Instruct female patients to inform practitioner immediately if pregnancy is suspected. Estrogen use should be avoided during pregnancy because fetal abnormalities have occurred.

Alert patient and significant others to note behavioral

changes or signs of depression. If any occur, unless the drug is absolutely necessary, it should be discontinued to avoid further psychological deterioration.

Instruct patient to be alert for signs of developing jaundice (yellow skin or sclera, itching, darkened urine, light-colored stools) and to discontinue drug if they occur.

Advise patient to report symptoms of abdominal distress because gallbladder disease and benign hepatic adenomas can occur.

Instruct patient to inform practitioner if fluid retention or weight gain occur because dose may have to be adjusted.

Warn diabetic patient that estrogen may increase hypoglycemic drug requirements by decreasing glucose tolerance.

Inform female patients that vaginal candidiasis may occur and should be treated with an appropriate antifungal agent. Symptoms include thick, whitish vaginal secretion and local inflammation.

Reassure male patients that signs of feminization and impotence that may occur during therapy are reversible on cessation of drug.

Progestins *(Pregnancy Category X)*

Hydroxyprogesterone
Levonorgestrel
Medroxyprogesterone
Megestrol
Norethindrone
Norgestrel
Progesterone

The term *progestins* refers to a group of naturally occurring and synthetic steroids having the physiologic effects of progesterone, the principal endogenous progestational hormone. Progesterone is normally secreted by the corpus luteum and also by the placenta during pregnancy, and it elicits a variety of actions in the body, which are reviewed under **Mechanism**. Because it is rapidly inactivated after oral ingestion, progesterone is administered IM only, in either an aqueous or an oily vehicle. A number of synthetic progestational steroids are also available. These drugs exhibit effects qualitatively similar to progesterone itself but differ from the endogenous progestin in that they possess greater potency, longer duration of action, and in some cases, oral or sublingual effectiveness.

Primary indications for the various progestins are amenorrhea, abnormal uterine bleeding, endometriosis, and endometrial carcinoma. In addition, several orally effective synthetic derivatives (desogestrel, ethynodiol, levonorgestrel, norethindrone, norgestimate) are used either alone or in fixed combinations with estrogen for the prevention of conception. A discussion of the oral contraceptive agents is presented in Chapter 47.

Progestins were formerly employed during the first trimester of pregnancy in an attempt to prevent habitual abortion or to treat threatened abortion. There is no conclusive evidence that such treatment is effective, however, and several reports have suggested that fetal damage (ie, congenital heart or limb-reduction defects) and delayed spontaneous abortion of defective ova can result from use of progestational agents during early pregnancy. If inadvertently exposed to progestins during the initial stages of pregnancy, patients should be apprised of the potential risks to the fetus.

The discussion of the progestational drugs treats them as a group, inasmuch as their pharmacology is similar. Individual drugs are listed in Table 46-2.

Mechanism

Induce biochemical changes in the endometrium in preparation for implantation of the fertilized egg; inhibit secretion of pituitary gonadotropins (primarily LH), preventing maturation of the follicle and ovulation; stimulate cervical mucus secretion; decrease sensitivity of uterus to oxytocin and facilitate development of secretory apparatus in mammary gland; metabolic actions include increased body temperature, decreased plasma level of amino acids, and elevated basal insulin levels

Uses

Refer to Table 46-2 for specific indications for each drug.

Treatment of primary and secondary amenorrhea and dysmenorrhea

Control of abnormal uterine bleeding due to hormonal imbalance, in the absence of organic pathology

Treatment of endometriosis

Palliative and adjunctive treatment of advanced, inoperable, or metastatic breast or endometrial carcinoma (see Chapter 74)

Prevention of conception (alone or combined with estrogens; see Chapter 47)

Investigational uses include use of medroxyprogesterone acetate for relief of menopausal symptoms and to stimulate respiration in obstructive sleep apnea, use of progesterone suppositories or oral progestins for treatment of premenstrual syndrome (PMS), and use of norethindrone in treating hyperparathyroidism with hypercalcemia in postmenopausal women.

Dosage

See Table 46-2.

Fate

Progesterone is quickly inactivated when given orally. Other derivatives are rapidly absorbed after oral administration or aqueous IM injection; metabolized by the liver and excreted both in the urine and feces

Common Side Effects

Fluid retention, breakthrough bleeding

Significant Adverse Reactions

(Usually seen with prolonged use or high doses) Menstrual flow irregularities, amenorrhea, cervical erosion, changes in cervical secretion, altered libido, masculinization of the female fetus, edema, weight gain, breast tenderness, hirsutism, alopecia, rash, melasma, decreased glucose tolerance, photosensitivity, cholestatic jaundice, pruritus, diarrhea, depression, nervousness, migraine, coughing, dyspnea, allergic reactions, retinal vascular lesions, thromboembolic episodes with medroxyprogesterone

Refer also to **Oral Contraceptives**, Chapter 47.

Table 46-2. **Progestins**

Drug	*Usual Dosage Range*	*Nursing Considerations*
Hydroxyprogesterone Caproate *Duralutin and other manufacturers*	*Amenorrhea, uterine bleeding*: 375 mg IM; if no bleeding after 21 days, begin cyclic therapy with estradiol and repeat every 4 wk for 4 cycles *Uterine adenocarcinoma*: 1 g or more IM initially; repeat 1 or more times each week (maximum 7/g/wk; stop when relapse occurs or after 12 wk with no response) *Test for endogenous estrogen production*: 125–250 mg IM on 10th day of cycle; repeat every 7 days; bleeding 7–14 days after injection indicates presence of endogenous estrogen	Long-acting synthetic progestin, available in either sesame oil or castor oil; duration of action is approximately 10–17 days; devoid of estrogenic activity and does not prevent conception; may produce dyspnea, coughing, constriction of the chest, and allergic-like reactions, especially at high doses; solution should be protected from light and stored at room temperature (see also Chap. 74)
Levonorgestrel Implants *Norplant*	Implant 6 capsules subdermally in upper arm during first 7 days of onset of menses	Used for long-term (5 yr) prevention of pregnancy; may alter menstrual bleeding patterns (see Chap. 47)
Medroxyprogesterone Acetate *Amen, Curretab, Cycrin, Depo-Provera, Provera*	*Amenorrhea*: 5–10 mg/day orally for 5–10 days *Uterine bleeding*: 5–10 mg/day for 5–10 days beginning on 16th or 21st day of cycle *Endometrial or renal carcinoma*: 400–1000 mg/wk IM; maintenance therapy after improvement is 400 mg a month *Prevention of pregnancy*: 150 mg (Depo-Provera) IM every 3 mo	Synthetic progestin used orally for inducing secretory changes in the estrogen-primed endometrium and IM in a depot-injectable form for prevention of pregnancy and as adjunctive therapy of inoperable, recurrent, or metastatic endometrial or renal carcinoma; also has been used orally to stimulate respiration in obstructive sleep apnea; has produced malignant mammary nodules in dogs; the human significance of this finding is not established (see Chaps. 47 and 74)
Megestrol Acetate *Megace, Palace*	*Breast or endometrial carcinoma*: 40–80 mg 4 times/day for at least 2 mo *Stimulate appetite in AIDS patients*: up to 800 mg/day (oral suspension)	Orally effective synthetic progestin indicated for palliative treatment of advanced breast or endometrial carcinoma; malignant breast tumors have occurred in megestrol-treated dogs; no serious side effects have been reported in humans in doses as high as 800 mg/day (see Chap. 74)
Norethindrone *Micronor, Norlutin, Nor-Q.D.*	*Amenorrhea, uterine bleeding*: 5–20 mg/day from day 5–25 of cycle *Endometriosis*: 10 mg/day for 2 wk, then increase by 5 mg/day every 2 wk to 30 mg/day *Contraception*: 0.35 mg daily	Synthetic progestin possessing androgenic, anabolic, and *anti*estrogenic properties, especially in high doses; component of several oral contraceptive products and used alone (0.35 mg) as well as a progestin-only contraceptive (see Chap. 47)
Norethindrone Acetate *Aygestin, Norlutate*	*Amenorrhea, uterine bleeding*: 2.5–10 mg/day from day 5–25 of cycle *Endometriosis*: 5 mg/day for 2 wk; then increase by 2.5 mg/day every 2 wk to 15 mg/day	Potent synthetic progestin possessing androgenic, anabolic, and *anti*estrogenic activity; component of several oral contraceptive drugs (see Chap. 47)
Norgestrel *Ovrette*	*Contraception*: 0.075 mg/day	Potent progestational hormone used as a progestin-only oral contraceptive ("mini-pill") (see Chap. 47)
Progesterone	*Amenorrhea*: 5–10 mg IM for 6–8 consecutive days *Uterine bleeding*: 5–10 mg/day IM for 6 days	Endogenous progestin possessing *anti*estrogenic activity; large doses may have a catabolic action and produce loss of sodium and chloride; warm solution before injecting to ensure dissolution of all particles; should not be used for diagnosis of pregnancy; suppositories have been used for treatment of premenstrual syndrome (PMS) and to decrease spontaneous abortions in previous aborters but are *not* approved for these indications

Contraindications

CAUTION

Progestins should not be administered during the first 4 months of pregnancy, because there is evidence that they may be harmful to the fetus.

Thromboembolic disorders, markedly impaired liver function, known or suspected genital or breast malignancy, undiagnosed vaginal bleeding, missed abortion, cerebral bleeding

Not to be used as a diagnostic test for pregnancy. *Cautious use* in patients with diabetes, migraine, epilepsy, cardiac or renal disease, asthma, psychoses and in nursing mothers.

Interactions

Progestins can reduce the effectiveness of hypoglycemic agents by decreasing glucose tolerance

The effects of progestins may be reduced by barbiturates, phenylbutazone, phenytoin, and rifampin.

Nursing Management

Pretherapy Assessment

Assess and record baseline data necessary for detection of adverse effects of progestins: General: VS, body weight, skin color and temperature; CNS: orientation, reflexes; CVS: peripheral perfusion, edema; GI: liver palpation, bowel sounds; Lab: liver and renal function tests, Pap smear, glucose tolerance test.

Review medical history and documents for existing or previous conditions that:

a. require cautious use of progestins: diabetes; migraine; epilepsy; cardiac or renal disease; asthma; psychoses

b. contraindicate use of progestins: allergy to progestins; thromboembolic disorders; markedly impaired liver function; known or suspected genital or breast malignancy; undiagnosed vaginal bleeding; missed abortion; cerebral bleeding; **pregnancy (Category X)**, lactation (secreted in breast milk, do not nurse)

Nursing Interventions

Medication Administration

Ensure that a comprehensive patient history and physical examination are completed before therapy is initiated. If therapy is prolonged, physical examination should be repeated at regular intervals. Progestins should be administered very cautiously to patients with a family history of breast cancer or thromboembolic or other cardiovascular disorders.

Arrange to discontinue medication if: sudden partial or complete loss of vision occurs; papilledema or retinal vascular lesions are present; at the first sign of thromboembolic disease (leg pain; swelling; peripheral perfusion changes; shortness of breath).

Protect patient from exposure to sun or ultraviolet light if photosensitivity occurs.

Surveillance During Therapy

Carefully monitor laboratory studies and patient for indications of adverse reactions.

Interpret results of diagnostic tests and contact practitioner as appropriate.

Monitor for possible drug–drug and drug–nutrient interactions: Refer to **Interactions**.

Provide for patient safety needs if CNS effects occur.

Patient Teaching

Discuss the need for pretreatment and periodic follow-up examinations of the breast and pelvic region, including a Pap smear. Teach breast self-examination.

Suggest that oral progestin be taken with food to minimize GI distress.

Alert patient receiving IM injection that pain or local allergic reaction can occur, but that these side effects are generally transient.

Explain the difference between normal withdrawal bleeding (3–4 days after discontinuation of drug) and breakthrough bleeding or spotting (during course of drug therapy). The latter type of bleeding should be reported because dosage may need to be adjusted.

Teach patient how to recognize and stress the importance of immediately reporting early manifestations of thromboembolic complications (eg, chest or calf pain, dyspnea, numbness in arm or leg, edema, dizziness, visual disturbances). Drug should be discontinued if these occur.

Apprise patient of danger to fetus if a progestin is taken during initial months of pregnancy. Healthcare provider should be informed immediately if pregnancy is suspected in a woman taking progestin.

Instruct patient to note, and report to practitioner, occurrence of any visual changes, diplopia, ptosis, or headache. If ophthalmic examination shows retinal vascular lesions or papilledema, drug should be discontinued.

Instruct patient to observe for symptoms of jaundice (dark urine, pruritus, yellowish skin or sclera) and to report them immediately.

Teach patient to monitor weight regularly and to observe for signs of edema. Significant weight variations should be reported.

Explain that vaginal itching or burning may indicate local candidal infection, which should be treated with appropriate antifungal medication (see Chapter 72).

Instruct diabetic patient to monitor urine or blood sugar carefully and to report any changes because progestins may reduce glucose tolerance.

Advise significant others to closely observe patient with a history of depression for mood changes or signs of recurring depression.

Selected Bibliography

Duursma SA, Raymakers JA: Estrogen and bone metabolism. Obstet Gynecol Surg 47:38, 1992

Levin R: The prevention of osteoporosis. Hosp Pract 5:77, 1991

L'Hermite M: Sex hormones and cardiovascular risk. Acta Cardiol 46(3): 357, 1991

Mitlak BH, Nussbaum SR: Diagnosis and treatment of osteoporosis. Ann Rev Med 44:265, 1993

Refn H, Kjaer A, et al: Metabolic changes during treatment with two different progestogens. Am J Obstet Gynecol 163:374, 1990

Riggs BL: Overview of osteoporosis. West J Med 1(154):63, 1991

Schiff I: Keys to balancing thc risks and benefits of estrogen therapy for postmenopausal women. Mod Med 61:72, 1993

Stampfer MJ et al: Postmenopausal estrogen therapy and cardiovascular disease: Ten-year follow-up from the Nurses' Health Study. N Engl J Med 325:756, 1991

Whitcroft SI, Stevenson JC: Hormone replacement therapy: Risks and benefits. Clin Endocrinol 36:15, 1992

Nursing Bibliography

Maddox M: Women at midlife: Hormone replacement. Nurs Clin North Am 27(4):959, 1992

Malseed R: Estrogen's potential role in auto immune diseases. Med Surg Nurse 2(4):324, 1993

Marten S: Complications of menopause and the risks and benefits of estrogen replacement therapy. J Am Acad Nurse Practitioners 5(2): 55, 1993

Miller C: Estraderm for osteoporosis. Geriatr Nurs 13(6): 337, 1992

Youngkin E: Progestogens: A look at the other hormone. The Nurse Practitioner 18(11):28, 1993

47
Drugs Used in Fertility Control

Estrogen–progestin contraceptives
Progestin-only contraceptives
Clomiphene
Gonadorelin acetate
Menotropins
Urofollitropin
Human chorionic gonadotropin
Prostaglandin abortifacients
Sodium chloride, hypertonic

Several different kinds of pharmacologic agents are employed to regulate female fertility. They may be grouped according to their action as the following:

- *Steroid contraceptives* (eg, estrogen–progestin combinations, progestin-only contraceptives)
- *Ovulation stimulants* (eg, clomiphene, gonadorelin acetate, menotropins)
- *Abortifacients* (eg, prostaglandins, sodium chloride 20%)

Steroid contraceptives are the most effective drug-based means of preventing conception and are widely used. They are discussed in detail below. Ovulation stimulants are drugs capable of inducing ovulation in infertile women, provided ovarian responsiveness is adequate. These agents are likewise considered in detail in this chapter. Drugs used to abort a fetus include two prostaglandin derivatives as well as hypertonic sodium chloride solution. These agents are also reviewed in this chapter.

Steroid Contraceptives

Estrogen-progestin combination products are widely used in the prevention of pregnancy. These combinations are commonly referred to as oral contraceptives or "the pill," and are the most effective means for preventing pregnancy in fertile women. The many fixed-combination products differ both in the amount and potency of the two components and in the relative estrogen–progestin activity ratio.

Three basic types of combination oral contraceptives are currently available:

- *Monophasic*: a fixed dose of estrogen and progestin in every tablet; most oral contraceptives are of this type
- *Biphasic* (eg, Ortho-Novum 10/11, Nelova 10/11): a fixed amount of estrogen in every tablet; the amount of progestin in the first 10 tablets is half the amount in the remaining 11 tablets
- *Triphasic* (eg, Ortho-Novum 7/7/7, Tri-Norinyl, Triphasil): ratio of estrogen *and* progestin vary throughout the tablets

The latter two types, biphasic and triphasic, are formulated to deliver the hormones in a manner that more closely resembles their physiologic secretion than is possible with the monophasic preparations. However, contraceptive efficacy is *equivalent* for all three types of products, and the potential advantages of phasic delivery of the hormones remains to be definitively established.

One of two estrogens is found in all of the oral contraceptives, either ethinyl estradiol or mestranol, and they are essentially equivalent in their activity. They are present in varying amounts in the different products, as indicated in Table 47-1. The most popular products are those that contain relatively low amounts of estrogens (ie, 35 μg ethinyl estradiol or 50 μg mestranol), because they are associated with a lower incidence of estrogen-related side effects than combinations containing 50 to 100 μg estrogen and are equally effective.

The progestin component of these preparations, however, may comprise one of several different compounds, which vary not only in potency but also in degree of estrogenic, antiestrogenic, and androgenic activity. Although contraceptive efficacy varies little among the currently available oral contraceptive combinations, frequency and severity of side effects are often related to the relative ratio of the estrogen versus progestin component. Achieving the proper hormonal balance of estrogen to progestin activity in each individual can often significantly reduce the degree of untoward effects and thus maximize patient compliance. Table 47-2 presents the important side effects resulting from either estrogen or progestin excess and provides a listing of currently available oral contraceptives grouped according to their relative estrogen to progestin ratio.

Although the estrogen–progestin combination products are generally recognized as being the most effective nonsurgical means of contraception, other types of steroidal and nonsteroidal products are used to prevent conception. Progestin-only contraceptives are available in several dosage forms. Oral progestins, such as norethindrone or norgestrel, are also known as the "mini-pill," and are claimed to elicit fewer adverse effects than the combination products, but are also somewhat less effective, having approximately a threefold higher incidence of pregnancy than the estrogen–progestin combinations.

Another progestin-only preparation is the intrauterine progesterone contraceptive system, a T-shaped device containing a reservoir of progesterone that is continuously released in small amounts into the uterine cavity after implantation. The unit is effective for up to 1 year. Contraceptive efficacy is equivalent to that of progestin-only drugs. A second type of progestin-implantable product is levonorgestrel implants, six small elongated capsules that are surgically implanted beneath the skin of the upper arm and provide a contraceptive effect for up to 5 years. Finally, IM injection of medroxyprogesterone acetate can inhibit ovulation and follicular maturation for up to 3 months and is also useful as a contraceptive agent.

Diethylstilbestrol (DES), a synthetic estrogen (see Chapter 46), has been effective as a postcoital contraceptive in large doses (25 mg twice a day for 5 days), provided the drug is given

Table 47-1. **Oral Contraceptives**

Drug	*Estrogen*	*Progestin*
INTERMEDIATE ESTROGEN–LOW PROGESTIN		
Norlestrin 1/50	ethinyl estradiol 50 μg	norethindrone 1 mg
Ovcon-50	ethinyl estradiol 50 μg	norethindrone 1 mg
INTERMEDIATE ESTROGEN–INTERMEDIATE PROGESTIN		
Demulen 1/50	ethinyl estradiol 50 μg	ethynodiol diacetate 1 mg
Nelulen 1/50E	ethinyl estradiol 50 μg	ethynodiol diacetate 1 mg
Norlestrin 2.5/50	ethinyl estradiol 50 μg	norethindrone 2.5 mg
Ovral	ethinyl estradiol 50 μg	norgestrel 0.5 mg
LOW ESTROGEN–LOW PROGESTIN		
Monophasic		
Brevicon	ethinyl estradiol 35 μg	norethindrone 0.5 mg
Desogen	ethinyl estradiol 30 μg	desogestrel 0.15 mg
GenCept 0.5/35	ethinyl estradiol 35 μg	norethindrone 0.5 mg
GenCept 1/35	ethinyl estradiol 35 μg	norethindrone 1.0 mg
Genora 0.5/35	ethinyl estradiol 35 μg	norethindrone 0.5 mg
Genora 1/35	ethinyl estradiol 35 μg	norethindrone 1 mg
Genora 1/50	mestranol 50 μg	norethindrone 1 mg
Loestrin 1/20	ethinyl estradiol 20 μg	norethindrone 1 mg
Modicon	ethinyl estradiol 35 μg	norethindrone 0.5 mg
N.E.E.	ethinyl estradiol 35 μg	norethindrone 1 mg
Nelova 0.5/35E	ethinyl estradiol 35 μg	norethindrone 0.5 mg
Nelova 1/35E	ethinyl estradiol 35 μg	norethindrone 1 mg
Nelova 1/50E	mestranol 50 μg	norethindrone 1 mg
Nelulen 1/35E	ethinyl estradiol 35 μg	ethynodiol diacetate 1 mg
Norcept-E 1/35	ethinyl estradiol 35 μg	norethindrone 1 mg
Norethin 1/35E	ethinyl estradiol 35 μg	norethindrone 1 mg
Norethin 1/50M	mestranol 50 μg	norethindrone 1 mg
Norinyl 1 + 50	mestranol 50 μg	norethindrone 1 mg
Norinyl 1 + 35	ethinyl estradiol 35 μg	norethindrone 1 mg
Ortho-Cept	ethinyl estradiol 30 μg	desogestrel 0.15 mg
Ortho-Novum 1/50	mestranol 50 μg	norethindrone 1 mg
Ortho-Novum 1/35	ethinyl estradiol 35 μg	norethindrone 1 mg
Ovcon-35	ethinyl estradiol 35 μg	norethindrone 0.4 mg
Biphasic		
GenCept 10/11	ethinyl estradiol 35 μg	norethindrone (10 tablets 0.5 mg; 11 tablets 1.0 mg)
Jenest-28	ethinyl estradiol 35 μg	norethindrone (7 tablets 0.5 mg; 14 tablets 1.0 mg; 7 inert tablets)
Nelova 10/11	ethinyl estradiol 35 μg	norethindrone (10 tablets 0.5 mg; 11 tablets 1 mg)
Ortho-Novum 10/11	ethinyl estradiol 35 μg	norethindrone (10 tablets 0.5 mg; 11 tablets 1 mg)
Triphasic		
Ortho Tri-Cyclen	ethinyl estradiol 35 μg	norgestimate (7 tablets 0.18 mg; 7 tablets 0.215 mg; 7 tablets 0.25 mg)
Ortho-Novum 7/7/7	ethinyl estradiol 35 μg	norethindrone (7 tablets 0.5 mg; 7 tablets 0.75 mg; 7 tablets 1.0 mg)
Tri-Levlen, Triphasil	ethinyl estradiol (6 tablets 30 μg; 5 tablets 40 μg; 10 tablets 30 μg)	levonorgestrel (6 tablets 0.05 mg; 5 tablets 0.075 mg; 10 tablets 0.125 mg)
Tri-Norinyl	ethinyl estradiol 35 μg	norethindrone (7 tablets 0.5 mg; 9 tablets 1 mg; 5 tablets 0.5 mg)
LOW ESTROGEN–INTERMEDIATE PROGESTIN		
Demulen 1/35	ethinyl estradiol 35 μg	ethynodiol diacetate 1 mg
Levlen	ethinyl estradiol 30 μg	levonoregestrel 0.15 mg
Loestrin 1.5/30	ethinyl estradiol 30 μg	norethindrone 1.5 mg
Lo/Ovral	ethinyl estradiol 30 μg	norgestrel 0.3 mg
Nordette	ethinyl estradiol 30 μg	levonorgestrel 0.15 mg
PROGESTIN ONLY		
Micronor		norethindrone 0.35 mg
Nor-Q.D.		norethindrone 0.35 mg
Ovrette		norgestrel 0.075 mg

Table 47-2. **Hormonal Balance of Oral Contraceptive Products and Relation to Adverse Effects**

Hormone Balance

Intermediate estrogen–low progestin: Norlestrin 1/50, Ovcon-50

Intermediate estrogen–intermediate progestin: Demulen 1/50, Nelulen 1/50E, Norlestrin 2.5/50, Ovral

Low estrogen–low progestin: Brevicon, Desogen, GenCept 0.5/35, 1/35, 10/11, Genora 0.5/35, Genora 1/35, 1/50, Jenest-28, Loestrin 1/20, Modicon, N.E.E., Nelova 0.5/35E, 1/35E, Nelova 1/50E, Nelulen 1/35E, Norcept-E 1/35, 10/11, Norethin 1/35E, 1/50M, Norinyl 1 + 35 and 1 + 50, Ortho-Cept, Ortho-Novum 1/35, 1/50, 10/11 and 7/7/7, Ortho Tri-Cyclen, Ovcon-35, Tri-levlen, Triphasil, Tri-Norinyl

Low estrogen–intermediate progestin: Demulen 1/35, Levlen, Loestrin 1.5/30, Lo/Ovral, Nordette

Adverse Effects

Estrogen excess: Cervical mucorrhea, edema, nausea, bloating, breast tenderness, migraine, hypertension, chloasma

Estrogen deficiency: Early or midcycle breakthrough bleeding, spotting, nervousness, hypomenorrhea

Progestin excess: Acne, depression, hirsutism, fatigue, increased appetite, weight gain, monilial vaginitis, oily skin, pruritis, hypomenorrhea

Progestin deficiency: Late-cycle bleeding, dysmenorrhea, delayed withdrawal bleeding

within 72 hours after intercourse. At these dosages, DES apparently blocks implantation of the fertilized ovum. Because of the hazards of such large doses of DES, this method of contraception is no longer approved for routine use but may be employed in emergency situations, such as rape or incest. Other estrogens have also been evaluated for postcoital contraception.

Many other chemical (spermicidal foams, gels, and creams) and mechanical (diaphragm, intrauterine device, condom) methods of contraception are available. Although usually somewhat less reliable than steroidal drugs, these methods do not present as great a risk of serious untoward reactions as does the use of steroid drugs. Choice of a contraceptive method is a highly personal one, and the advantages and disadvantages of the available methods should be clearly understood by both prescriber and user before a decision is reached.

Fertility control is commonly practiced and is highly successful in most instances. However, serious and occasionally fatal adverse effects have occurred in some women taking these drugs. Proper dosing of fertility control drugs is essential for their safe and effective use, and these drugs should always be prescribed and monitored by persons aware of their pharmacologic actions and toxicologic potential as well as the pituitary hormone–ovarian relationship. A graphic representation of the menstrual (endometrial) cycle and the hormonal influences on ovarian function and endometrial growth and development is presented in Figure 47-1. In addition, patient education is a vital component of a safe and successful contraceptive regimen (refer to **Nursing Management**), and all persons receiving contraceptives for the first time should be given the literature included in the package, and encouraged to read it.

The oral contraceptives are discussed as a group, inasmuch as they are similar in their pharmacologic action. A complete list of available products is given in Table 47-1, along with their respective estrogen and progestin content. A review of the progestin-only products is also presented.

• *Estrogen–progestin contraceptives*

Mechanism

Interfere with follicular maturation (estrogen decreases release of follicle-stimulating hormone [FSH]) and inhibit ovulation (progestin suppresses release of luteinizing hormone [LH]) (see Fig. 47-1); induce structural and biochemical changes in the endometrium, making it unfavorable for implantation of the fertilized ovum; progestins reduce the amount and increase the viscosity of cervical mucus, thus interfering with motility of sperm cells; many also impair the ciliary and peristaltic activity of the fallopian tubes, impeding movement of the ova.

Uses

Prevention of pregnancy
Treatment of menstrual irregularities (refer to **Progestins**, Chap. 46)

Dosage

CAUTION

Because of the association between the dose of estrogen and the risk of thromboembolism and possibly hypertension, the dose of estrogen should be the equivalent of 50 μg mestranol or 35 μg ethinyl estradiol or less.

Estrogen–progestin combinations: 1 tablet daily for 21 days, beginning on cycle day 5 (day 1 is first day of bleeding); stop for 7 days, then begin a new course of therapy whether or not withdrawal bleeding has stopped; some products are supplied as 28-tablet packs, the last 7 tablets being inert or containing only iron, allowing continuous daily dosage for the entire 28-day cycle;
Progestin-only products: 1 tablet daily without interruption

Although the likelihood of ovulation is minimal if one tablet is missed, it increases with each succeeding day that a dose is missed. If *one* tablet is missed, it may be taken later that day or two tablets may be taken the following day. If tablets are missed for 2 consecutive days, two tablets should be taken daily for the next 2 days before resuming the regular schedule. If 3 consecutive days of therapy are missed, a new package of tablets should be started 7 days after the last tablet was taken and alternative means of birth control should be used until resumption of therapy.

Fate

Ethinyl estradiol is rapidly absorbed and undergoes significant first-pass hepatic metabolism; *mestranol* is converted to ethinyl estradiol, which is highly bound to plasma proteins (97%–98%); plasma half-life ranges from 6 to 18 hours; the drugs are excreted in both the bile and the urine.

Progestins are well absorbed orally. Norethynodrel and ethynodiol diacetate are converted to norethindrone. Peak plasma levels occur in 0.5 to 3 hours. Progestins are bound to plasma proteins and are primarily metabolized in the liver

Common Side Effects

(Depends to a large extent on the estrogen–progestin ratio—see Table 47-2) Nausea, vomiting, headache, fluid retention, weight

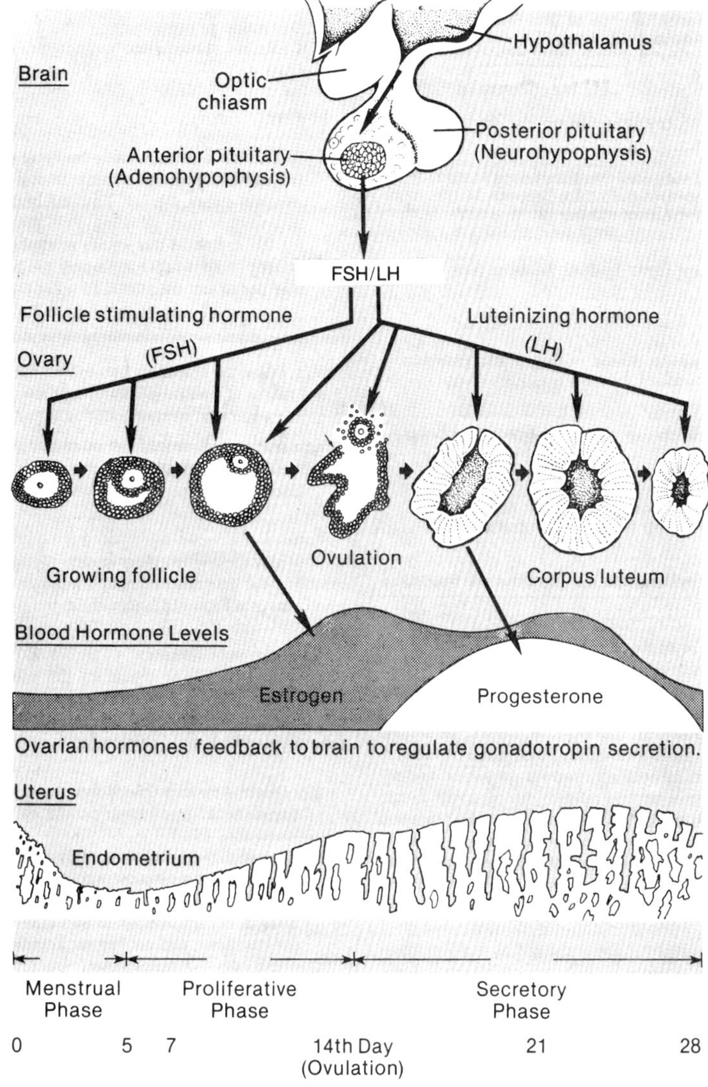

Figure 47-1 The menstrual (endometrial) cycle.

gain, dizziness, breast tenderness, breakthrough bleeding, leg cramps

Significant Adverse Reactions

CAUTION

Use of oral contraceptives has been associated with increased risk of thromboembolic episodes, hemorrhagic stroke, hypertension, myocardial infarction, hepatic tumors, visual disturbances, gallbladder disease, and fetal abnormalities. In addition, cigarette smoking *significantly* increases the risk of cardiovascular side effects, especially in women older than 35 years of age.

GI/hepatic: abdominal cramping, diarrhea, benign adenomas and other hepatic lesions, cholelithiasis, and cholestatic jaundice

Genitourinary: dysmenorrhea, amenorrhea, infertility after discontinuation, change in cervical secretions, increased urinary tract and vaginal infections

Ophthalmic: neuroocular lesions (eg, retinal thrombosis, optic neuritis), papilledema, change in corneal curvature, intolerance to contact lenses

CNS: migraine, depression, menstrual tension, fatigue

Other: rash, chloasma, reduced lactation, impaired carbohydrate tolerance, altered laboratory values (eg, liver function, thyroid function, serum triglycerides, blood glucose)

Contraindications

Thromboembolic disorders, coronary artery or cerebrovascular disease, myocardial infarction or history of these disorders, known or suggested breast or other estrogen-dependent carcinoma, undiagnosed vaginal bleeding, known or possible pregnancy, severe liver disease, or liver tumors. *Cautious use* in women with diabetes, hypertension, obesity, migraine, depression, anemia, amenorrhea, and porphyria.

CAUTION

(Pregnancy Category X) Pregnancy must be ruled out before beginning an oral contraceptive regimen, because fetal damage can occur if these agents are used during early pregnancy.

Interactions

Refer to **Estrogens and Progestins**, Chapter 46. In addition:

Increased incidence of breakthrough bleeding and possibly reduced contraceptive efficacy may occur with barbiturates, penicillin, ampicillin, chloramphenicol, sulfonamides, tetracyclines, primidone, phenytoin, carbamazepine, rifampin, isoniazid, meprobamate, griseofulvin, phenylbutazone, or nitrofurantoin.

Oral contraceptives may impair the effectiveness of anticonvulsants, anticoagulants, antihypertensives, tricyclic antidepressants, hypoglycemics, and certain vitamins (folic acid, B_6).

Oral contraceptives may impair the metabolism of benzodiazepines, caffeine, corticosteroids, metoprolol, imipramine, phenytoin, phenylbutazone, and theophylline

The clearance of lorazepam, oxazepam, and salicylates may be accelerated by oral contraceptives.

Use of aminocaproic acid with oral contraceptives may increase clotting factors, leading to a hypercoagulable state.

Concurrent use of troleandomycin and oral contraceptives may result in jaundice.

Nursing Management

Refer to **Estrogens and Progestins**, Chapter 46. In addition:

Nursing Interventions

Surveillance During Therapy

Assess patient for indications of hormonal imbalance. If a certain pattern of side effects persists (see Table 47-2), the oral contraceptive formulation may need to be changed.

Patient Teaching

Discuss the need to rule out pregnancy before therapy is initiated or before therapy is continued if pregnancy is suspected.

Inform patient that the combination with the lowest effective and tolerable estrogen content is usually prescribed because a positive correlation exists between dosage of estrogen and risk of both thromboembolism and endometrial carcinoma.

Explain that pregnancy should always be suspected if withdrawal bleeding does not occur after each course of therapy.

Provide user with patient information contained in each package. Carefully review material with patient to ensure that she understands it.

Suggest that patient use an additional method of contraception during first week of administration in initial cycle of therapy.

Suggest that medication be taken at the same time every day to minimize possibility of missing a dose.

Explain actions to be taken if doses of medication are missed (refer to information at end of **Dosage** section, above).

ɛplain to patient taking progestin-only product that breakthrough bleeding and altered menstrual pattern are more likely to occur than with a combination product.

Instruct patient to report any abnormal vaginal bleeding immediately. If bleeding is sparse (eg, spotting), medication may be continued uninterrupted, but practitioner should be notified if spotting continues past the second month. If flow is heavy (eg, menstrual-like), patient should discontinue medication and begin a new package of tablets on the fifth day after the start of new bleeding.

Alert patient that menstrual flow may be greatly reduced after several months of therapy.

Instruct patient to terminate oral contraceptives and use alternative means of birth control for an additional 3 months to minimize risk of congenital abnormalities from residual effects of steroidal hormones when pregnancy is desired.

Progestin-only Contraceptives

- ***Intrauterine Progesterone Contraceptive System*** *(Pregnancy Category X)*

Progestasert

The intrauterine progesterone contraceptive system is a T-shaped intrauterine device (IUD) containing 38 mg progesterone dispersed in silicone oil. After insertion of the unit into the uterine cavity, progesterone is continuously released at an average rate of 65 μg/day. The contraceptive effectiveness approximates that of progestin-only tablets and is retained for a period of 1 year, after which the system must be replaced. The system acts to suppress proliferation of endometrial tissue, creating an environment unfavorable for implantation; it also may decrease sperm survival time, possibly by altering cervical mucus; it does *not* appear to prevent ovulation.

The intrauterine progesterone system is contraindicated in the presence of pregnancy or suspicion of pregnancy, previous ectopic pregnancy, pelvic inflammatory disease, sexually transmitted disease, previous pelvic surgery, uterine abnormalities, uterine or cervical malignancy, vaginal bleeding of undetermined origin, and acute cervicitis.

Adverse reactions associated with the system include dysmenorrhea, amenorrhea, cervical erosion, pelvic infection, vaginitis, endometritis, spotting, prolonged menstrual flow, delayed menses, dyspareunia, septicemia, septic abortion, cervical or uterine perforation, ectopic pregnancy, and pain, bleeding, bradycardia, or syncope on insertion.

The device should be inserted during or immediately after menstruation to ensure that pregnancy has not occurred. An increased risk of pelvic inflammatory disease (PID) is associated with the use of intrauterine devices. Users should be apprised of the usual symptoms of PID (fever, nausea, vomiting, abdominal pain, malaise, purulent vaginal discharge) and if these are present, should report to their physician.

Nursing Management

See **Progestins**. In addition:

Nursing Interventions

Surveillance During Therapy

Provide emotional support as needed if pregnancy occurs with the system in place, and explain that the device will be removed by its threads if possible. Termination of the pregnancy should be considered if the system cannot be removed because risk of spontaneous abortion and sepsis is considerable.

Be alert for delayed menses, unilateral pelvic pain, and falling hematocrit, possible indications of an ectopic fetus, because incidence of ectopic pregnancy is higher in patient with an IUD in place.

Patient Teaching

Instruct patient not to pull on threads or to attempt to remove unit once it is inserted.

Explain that reexamination is required within 3 months after insertion to ensure that unit is in place.

• **Levonorgestrel Implant Contraceptive System** *(Pregnancy Category X)*

Norplant System

The levonorgestrel implant system consists of a set of six flexible capsules, 34 mm in length and 2 mm in diameter, each containing 36 mg levonorgestrel. The capsules are implanted under sterile conditions beneath the dermis in the midportion of the upper arm in a fanlike pattern; implantation is done during the first 7 days of the cycle or immediately after an abortion. The rate of levonorgestrel absorption is initially approximately 85 μg/day, but declines slowly to approximately 30 μg/day within 2 to 3 years. The system may be replaced every 5 years if continuing contraception is desired. Blood levels are substantially below those resulting from use of oral contraceptive products containing either norgestrel or levonorgestrel.

The implant system is contraindicated in patients with active thromboembolic disorders, acute liver disease or liver tumors, undiagnosed genital bleeding, and known or suspected breast carcinoma. Most women experience some alteration in menstrual bleeding patterns during the early stages of use, but these irregularities diminish over time. Other side effects commonly noted during the first year of use include amenorrhea, spotting, breast discharge, abdominal discomfort, vaginitis, and musculoskeletal pain. Infection at the implantation site is uncommon, provided that aseptic techniques have been followed. Capsules should be removed if jaundice develops or if clinically significant depression occurs.

Refer to the discussion of oral contraceptives earlier in the chapter and to Chapter 46 for a complete review of potential adverse effects, cautions and interactions of progestins.

• **Medroxyprogesterone Contraceptive Injection** *(Pregnancy Category X)*

Depo-Provera

Medroxyprogesterone is a synthetic progestin (see Chapter 46) that is available as a depot injection for IM administration containing 150 mg/mL. Given at 3-month intervals, medroxyprogesterone is an effective contraceptive that prevents follicular maturation, inhibits ovulation, and produces endometrial thinning. The injection is administered during the first 5 days after the onset of a menstrual period or within 5 days postpartum if not breastfeeding. Contraindications, precautions, and adverse reactions are similar to those outlined for Norplant above.

Ovulation Stimulants

Although an infrequent cause of infertility, anovulation, when it occurs, has responded to the use of ovulation-stimulating drugs, and conception has been made possible in previously anovulatory women. Because therapy with these agents is expensive, often tedious, and potentially hazardous, selection of patients with a reasonable expectation for success is important. Thus, women with primary ovarian failure, uterine abnormalities, fallopian tube obstruction, or endometrial carcinoma should be excluded as potential candidates. Likewise, impaired or absent sperm production in the partner should be ruled out. When careful patient selection is observed, 25% to 50% of women completing a course of therapy can be expected to conceive. However, treatment with ovulation-inducing drugs is not without its hazards, such as ovarian enlargement, often accompanied by pain and ascites. The incidence of early abortion is increased with use of these drugs, and the occurrence of multiple pregnancies with recommended dosage schedules has been estimated to be as high as 20%.

Ovulation-inducing agents include clomiphene, an antiestrogen drug capable of increasing release of FSH and LH from the adenohypophysis, gonadorelin acetate, a synthetic gonadotropin-releasing hormone, and human menopausal gonadotropins (hMG) and urofollitropin, two preparations that are purified extracts of FSH and LH. Clomiphene and gonadorelin acetate are used alone, whereas hMG and urofollitropin therapy are followed by an injection of human chorionic gonadotropin (hCG) to induce ovulation. These drugs are reviewed individually below.

• **Clomiphene** *(Pregnancy Category X)*

Clomid, Milophene, Serophene

A nonsteroidal synthetic estrogen possessing weak estrogenic as well as antiestrogenic activity, clomiphene stimulates release of FSH and LH from the adenohypophysis and thus requires both a functioning pituitary and a responsive ovary for its therapeutic effect. A single ovulation is induced by each 5-day course of treatment, and most patients who are going to respond do so with the first course of therapy. A second and third course may be tried if conception has not occurred, but treatment beyond three courses in patients exhibiting no evidence of ovulation or who do not conceive is not recommended. Approximately 30% to 40% of women with ovulatory dysfunction conceive with a course of clomiphene therapy.

Mechanism

Binds to estrogenic receptors in the cytoplasm, thus decreasing the number of available estrogenic receptor sites (antiestrogenic action); action is interpreted by the hypothalamus and pituitary as a sign that estrogen levels are low, and the secretion of FSH and LH is increased in response to the removal of the negative feedback; increased release of FSH and LH stimulates maturation of the follicle, ovulation, and development of the corpus luteum

Uses

Treatment of ovulatory failure in properly selected patients (refer to **Contraindications**) desiring pregnancy, whose partners are fertile

Treatment of male infertility (investigational use)

Dosage

Female infertility: beginning on the fifth day of the cycle, 50 mg/day for 5 days (therapy may be started anytime in amenorrheic women); if ovulation does not occur, a second and third course of therapy (at 100 mg/day for 5 days) may be tried, with a minimum 30-day interval between treatment courses. Treatment beyond three courses of therapy is *not* recommended

Male infertility: 25 mg/day for 25 days or 100 mg 3 times a week (eg, Monday, Wednesday, and Friday)

Fate

Well absorbed when taken orally; metabolized in the liver and excreted largely in the feces, both as metabolites and unchanged drug

Common Side Effects

Ovarian enlargement, abdominal discomfort, bloating, vasomotor symptoms (eg, hot flashes, flushing), breast tenderness

Significant Adverse Reactions

Nausea, vomiting, diarrhea, visual disturbances (eg, blurring, photophobia, diplopia, scotomata), headache, nervousness, lightheadedness, vertigo, insomnia, depression, abnormal uterine bleeding, ovarian hemorrhage, urinary frequency, rash, dermatitis, fluid retention, weight gain; increased incidence of early abortion and multiple births (approximately 7%)

Contraindications

NOTE: Therapy is ineffective in patients with primary pituitary or ovarian failure.

Pregnancy, liver dysfunction or history of liver disease, ovarian cysts, thrombophlebitis, and abnormal uterine or vaginal bleeding. *Cautious use* in thyroid disorders (refer to **Interactions**)

Interactions

Clomiphene can elevate levels of serum thyroxine and thyroxine-binding globulin

Nursing Management

Nursing Interventions

Medication Administration

Ensure that recommended procedures (eg, complete pelvic examination, endometrial biopsy, liver function tests) have been completed and the cause of any abnormal bleeding has been determined before initiating administration.

Question dosage that exceeds 100 mg/day for 5 days because effectiveness is not enhanced with higher doses, but the incidence of untoward reactions and the danger of multiple births is increased.

Patient Teaching

Teach patient how to use a basal thermometer to ascertain time of ovulation.

Explain the importance of properly timed sexual intercourse for conception.

Instruct patient to report development of any visual disturbances. If they occur, treatment should be discontinued, and a complete ophthalmologic examination should be performed.

Caution patient against engaging in hazardous activities because blurred vision, dizziness, and lightheadedness may occur.

Instruct patent to report development of pelvic or abdominal pain. Patient should be examined for ovarian enlargement if this occurs.

• Gonadorelin acetate

Lutrepulse

Gonadorelin acetate is a synthetic peptide with the identical amino-acid sequence of endogenous gonadotropin-releasing hormone. It stimulates the synthesis and release of FSH and LH from the anterior pituitary, resulting in maturation of the follicle and ovulation. Gonadorelin hydrochloride (Factrel) is a similar preparation used for evaluating pituitary responsiveness and residual gonadotropic function (see Chapter 80).

Uses

Induction of ovulation in women with primary hypothalamic amenorrhea

Dosage

5 μg every 90 minutes, given over a 1-minute period by a battery-driven pump (Lutrepulse pump). The 8 mL reconstituted gonadorelin acetate solution supplies pulsatile doses every 90 minutes for approximately 7 days. Recommended treatment interval is 21 days. Dosage may be raised cautiously in stages up to 20 μg. if there is no response after three treatment intervals.

Fate

After IV administration, gonadorelin is rapidly metabolized to inactive peptide fragments which are excreted in the urine.

Significant Adverse Reactions

Ovarian hyperstimulation (abdominal pain, ascites, pleural effusion), multiple pregnancies, anaphylaxis, inflammation and infection at infusion site

Contraindications

Any condition that could be worsened by increased levels of reproductive hormones; anovulation from causes other than those of hypothalamic origin, such as ovarian cysts; nursing mothers. Gonadorelin acetate should not be used together with other ovulation stimulants.

Nursing Management

Pretherapy Assessment

Assess and record baseline data necessary for detection of adverse effects of gonadorelin: General: vital signs (VS), body weight, skin color and temperature; central nervous system (CNS): orientation, reflexes; genitourinary (GU): Pap smear, pelvic examination; Lab: pregnancy test.

Review medical history and documents for existing or previous conditions that:

a. require cautious use of gonadorelin: use of estrogens, progestins, or glucocorticoids; phenothiazines

b. contraindicate use of gonadorelin: allergy to gonadorelin; **pregnancy (Category B)**, lactation (safety not established)

Nursing Interventions

Medication Administration

Confirm cause of amenorrhea before treatment is undertaken.
Provide comfort measures for local effect, headache, or GI discomfort.

Surveillance During Therapy

Carefully monitor laboratory studies and patient for indications of adverse reactions.
Interpret results of diagnostic tests and contact practitioner as appropriate.

Patient Teaching

Advise patient of risk of multiple pregnancies.
Teach the patient that ovulation may occur within 2 to 3 weeks; if pregnancy does occur, therapy will be continued for 2 weeks to help maintain the pregnancy.
Teach the patient that the following side effects may occur: headache; abdominal discomfort; multiple pregnancies; pain or discomfort at the injection site.
Instruct the patient to report any of the following to the practitioner if they occur: difficulty breathing; rash; fever; severe abdominal pain; redness, swelling or pain at the injection site.

• Menotropins (human menopausal gonadotropins–hMG)
(Pregnancy Category X)

Pergonal

A purified preparation of gonadotropins extracted from the urine of postmenopausal women, menotropins is biologically standardized for FSH and LH activity. It is frequently referred to as human menopausal gonadotropins or hMG and provides an exogenous source of pituitary gonadotropins and thus, unlike clomiphene, does not require the presence of functional hypophyseal gonadotropins for its activity. Treatment with menotropins usually results only in follicular growth and maturation; subsequent ovulation is effected by sequential administration of hCG (refer to **Chorionic Gonadotropin**, below) when sufficient follicular maturation has occurred.

Mechanism

Provides a source of FSH and LH, thus promoting growth of ovarian follicles in women who do not have primary ovarian failure (see Fig. 47-1); does not usually elicit ovulation, which must be induced by injection of hCG, a polypeptide possessing significant LH activity (see below)

Uses

In combination with hCG for the induction of ovulation in anovulatory women (*not* effective in primary ovarian failure)
Stimulation of spermatogenesis in men who have primary or secondary hypogonadotropic hypogonadism

Dosage

Women (must be individually adjusted): usually 75 U each of FSH and LH activity (1 ampule menotropins) given IM for 9 to 12 days, followed by hCG, 10,000 U IM 1 day after the last dose of hMG; if ovulation occurs without pregnancy, may repeat course of therapy twice with same dosage levels at monthly intervals. If ovulation does not occur, dosage may be increased to 150 U each of FSH and LH for 9 to 12 days, followed by 10,000 U hCG IM. Do *not* exceed 150 U/day.
Men (to increase spermatogenesis): hCG alone (5,000 IU 3 times/week for 4–6 mo); then, 1 ampule of menotropins IM 3 times/wk and hCG, 2,000 IU, twice a week for 4 months

Common Side Effects

Mild uncomplicated ovarian enlargement, with or without abdominal pain (20% incidence)

Significant Adverse Reactions

(Usually with larger doses) Ovarian hyperstimulation syndrome (eg, abdominal pain, ascites, pleural effusion, sudden ovarian enlargement), fever, nausea, vomiting, diarrhea, hemoperitoneum, arterial thromboembolism (rare), ovarian cysts, multiple births have occurred with hMG–hCG treatment, occasional gynecomastia in men

Contraindications

Primary ovarian failure, pregnancy, ovarian cysts, or enlargement *not* due to polycystic ovary syndrome, thyroid or adrenal dysfunction, intracranial lesion, abnormal bleeding of unknown origin, and infertility due to factors other than anovulation.
In men, primary testicular failure and infertility *not* due to hypogonadotropic hypogonadism.
Cautious use in persons with thromboembolic disorders.

Nursing Management

Pretherapy Assessment

Assess and record baseline data necessary for detection of adverse effects of menotropins: General: VS, body weight, skin color and temperature, masculinization (men); GU: testicular examination, pelvic examination; Lab: serum gonadotropins, 24-hour urinary estrogen, estriol, serum testosterone.
Review medical history and documents for existing or previous conditions that:

a. require cautious use of menotropins: thromboembolic disorders
b. contraindicate use of menotropins: allergy to menotropins; primary ovarian failure; pregnancy; ovarian cysts or enlargement *not* due to polycystic ovary syndrome; thyroid or adrenal dysfunction; intracranial lesion; abnormal bleeding of unknown origin; infertility due to factors other than anovulation; in men, primary testicular failure and infertility *not* due to hypogonadotropic hypogonadism;

pregnancy (Category X), lactation (safety not established)

Nursing Interventions

Medication Administration

Provide comfort measures for local effect, headache, or GI discomfort.

Surveillance During Therapy

Carefully monitor laboratory studies and patient for indications of adverse reactions.

Interpret results of diagnostic tests and contact practitioner as appropriate.

Patient Teaching

Advise patient of risk of multiple pregnancies.

Advise patient that administration of hMG–hCG or urofollitropin–hCG (see below) should be undertaken only by persons trained in their use, knowledgeable about the necessary estrogen and progesterone assays required to monitor hormonal status, and thoroughly familiar with treatment of female infertility.

Explain that a thorough gynecologic examination and endocrinologic evaluation are performed before therapy is initiated. Pregnancy and primary ovarian failure must be ruled out and the cause of any abnormal vaginal bleeding determined. Evaluation of the male partner is likewise essential.

Teach patient signs of ovarian hyperstimulation (refer to **Significant Adverse Reactions**). Advise patient to notify practitioner if signs occur and to refrain from sexual intercourse. Mild ovarian enlargement generally regresses within 2 to 3 weeks.

Inform patient that she will probably be examined every other day during treatment and for at least 2 weeks after treatment for signs of excessive ovarian stimulation. Most ovarian hyperstimulation is noted 7 to 10 days after ovulation.

Explain that hCG should not be administered if ovaries are abnormally enlarged or if estrogen excretion is greater than 100 μg/24 h on the last day of hMG (or urofollitropin) therapy because risk of excessive ovarian stimulation is greatly increased.

Encourage patient to have sexual intercourse daily beginning the day hCG is administered until ovulation has occurred, as indicated by indices of increased progesterone production.

• Urofollitropin *(Pregnancy Category X)*

Metrodin

Urofollitropin is a purified preparation of gonadotropin extracted from the urine of postmenopausal women.

Mechanism

Stimulates ovarian follicular growth in women who do not have primary ovarian failure; treatment results in follicular growth and maturation only; ovulation is effected by subsequent administration of hCG (see below) where laboratory assessment indicates that sufficient follicular maturation has occurred.

Uses

Induction of ovulation in patients with polycystic ovarian disease who display elevated LH:FSH ratio and whose condition has not responded to clomiphene therapy; treatment with urofollitropin must be followed by administration of hCG to induce ovulation from the mature follicle.

Dosage

75 U/day IM for 7 to 12 days followed by 5,000 to 10,000 U hCG 1 day after the last urofollitropin dose

If there is evidence of ovulation but no pregnancy, the above course of therapy may be repeated at least twice at monthly intervals before increasing the dose of urofollitropin to 150 U/day for three additional monthly treatments. Do *not* increase the dose further.

Common Side Effects

Abdominal pain and distention, ovarian enlargement, rash, pain, swelling, irritation at injection site

Significant Adverse Reactions

Nausea, vomiting, diarrhea, abdominal cramping, bloating, headache, breast tenderness, fever, muscle aching, chills, malaise, fatigue, dry skin, hair loss, ectopic pregnancy. Thromboembolic episodes have occurred with the similar-acting drug menotropins and must be considered a possibility with urofollitropin as well. Multiple births have occurred, with a frequency estimated to be in the range of 15% to 20%. *Sudden* ovarian enlargement, occasionally accompanied by ascites and pleural effusion, has been reported in approximately 5% of treated patients.

Contraindications

Presence of high levels of FSH or LH, indicating primary ovarian failure; thyroid or adrenal dysfunction; intracranial lesions; abnormal bleeding of undetermined origin; ovarian cysts; pregnancy. *Cautious use* in persons with thromboembolic disorders and in nursing mothers.

Nursing Management

Refer to **Menotropins**.

• Human Chorionic Gonadotropin (hCG)

A.P.L., Chorex, Chorigon, Choron 10, Follutein, Glukor, Gonic, Pregnyl, Profasi HP

(CAN) Autuitrin

A purified polypeptide hormone, hCG is produced by the human placenta and extracted from the urine of women during the first trimester of pregnancy. The effect of hCG is due primarily to its LH-like activity, although it exhibits a slight degree of FSH-like activity as well.

Mechanism

Stimulates the corpus luteum of the ovaries to produce progesterone, and triggers ovulation from FSH-primed follicles. In men, stimulates the interstitial cells of the testes to produce androgens, thus promoting development of secondary sex characteristics and descent of the testicles.

Uses

Induction of ovulation in the anovulatory female who has been properly pretreated with hMG or urofollitropin
Treatment of cryptorchidism (undescended testes) in instances *not* due to anatomic obstruction; therapy is usually instituted between the ages of 4 and 9 years
Treatment of male hypogonadism secondary to a pituitary deficiency

Dosage

(Highly individualized; IM only; dosage measured in USP units)

Induction of Ovulation

5,000 to 10,000 U 1 day after last dose of hMG or urofollitropin

Cryptorchidism

4,000 U 3 times a week for 3 weeks *or*
5,000 U every other day for four injections *or*
15 injections of 500 to 1,000 U over 6 weeks *or*
500 U 3 times a week for 4 to 6 weeks; if unsuccessful, repeat after 1 month with 100 U per injection

Hypogonadism

500 to 1,000 U 3 times a week for 3 weeks, then twice a week for 3 weeks *or*
1,000 to 2,000 U 3 times a week *or*
4,000 U 3 times a week for 6 months to 9 months, then 2,000 U 3 times a week for 3 months

Common Side Effects

Headache, restlessness

Significant Adverse Reactions

Depression, fatigue, ovarian hyperstimulation, thromboembolism, fluid retention, gynecomastia, pain at injection site, sexual precocity in prepubertal patients

Contraindications

Androgen-dependent neoplasms (eg, prostatic cancer), precocious puberty. *Cautious use* in patients with cardiac or renal disease, asthma, migraine, or epilepsy.

Nursing Management

Nursing Interventions

Medication Administration

Question prescription of hCG for treatment of obesity. Although drug is sometimes used to treat obesity, there is no substantial evidence that hCG alters fat mobilization or distribution, retards appetite, or reduces hunger associated with low-calorie diets.

Surveillance During Therapy

Assess patient being treated for cryptorchidism for signs of precocious puberty. Drug should be discontinued if signs appear.

Patient Teaching

Explain to child and parents that cryptorchidism that does not respond to hCG within a reasonable period (6–12 weeks) usually requires surgical intervention because excessive treatment with hCG may damage a mechanically obstructed undescended testis.
Instruct patient to notify practitioner if edema becomes problematic. Dosage reduction usually eliminates fluid retention.

Abortifacients

Termination of pregnancy can be accomplished by both mechanical and pharmacologic methods. During the early weeks of pregnancy, there is no safe and reliable method for pharmacologically inducing fetal expulsion, and suction curettage is the commonly performed procedure. Beginning at approximately the start of the second trimester, however, pharmacologic methods are usually employed; these consist of injections of hypertonic saline solution into the amniotic sac, IM administration of a prostaglandin salt, or use of a prostaglandin (E_2) vaginal suppository. Certain prostaglandins (PGE_2, $PGF_{2\alpha}$) have been detected in amniotic fluid during labor or spontaneous abortion and appear to play a role in fetal expulsion by facilitating myometrial contractions. These observations have led to the development of prostaglandin preparations for the induction of second trimester elective abortion. These agents are preferable to intra-amniotic injection of hypertonic sodium chloride (see below) because they have a more rapid onset of action and a lower incidence of side effects. The prostaglandins used as abortifacients are reviewed as a group, followed by a listing of individual drugs and dosages, in Table 47-3.

Dinoprostone (Prepidil) is also available as a gel (0.5 mg/2.5 mL), which is indicated for ripening the cervix at or near term in women with a need for labor induction. It is introduced through a catheter into the cervical canal. A second dose may be given after 6 hours if necessary. A 6- to 12-hour interval should be allowed before administration of oxytocin.

Prostaglandin Abortifacients

- **Carboprost Tromethamine**

  Hemabate

- **Dinoprostone**

  Prostin E_2

Mechanism

Elicit contractions of the gravid uterus, probably by a direct stimulation of the myometrium; may produce a regression of corpus luteum function; also increase contractile activity of the GI tract and other smooth muscle, especially after systemic injection

Uses

Termination of pregnancy from the 12th through the 20th gestational week
Production of uterine evacuation in cases of missed abortion or fetal death up to 28 weeks' gestational age (dinoprostone only)
Management of nonmetastatic gestational trophoblastic disease (benign hydatidiform mole)—dinoprostone only

Table 47-3. **Prostaglandin Abortifacients**

Drug	Usual Dosage Range	Nursing Considerations
Carboprost Tromethamine *Hemabate*	Initially 250 μg IM; repeat at 1.5–3.5-h intervals; may increase to 500 μg per dose if necessary; maximum dose, 12 mg *Refractory postpartum bleeding*: Initially, 250 μg IM; if necessary, additional doses, may be given at 15–90-min intervals to a maximum of 2 mg	Administer deeply IM; abortion is incomplete in about 20% of cases; may produce transient elevation in body temperature (1°–3°F), which persists only as long as drug is being given; forced fluids are recommended during hyperpyrexia; an optional test dose of 100 μg (0.4 mL) may be given initially to ascertain hypersensitivity to drug
Dinoprostone *Prostin E2*	Insert 1 suppository high into vagina; repeat at 3–5-h intervals until abortion occurs	Keep patient supine for at least 10 min after insertion; vomiting occurs in about two thirds of all patients, and diarrhea in approximately half, provide assistance as needed; nausea, headache, chills, and hypotension (20 mm Hg–30 mm Hg) have also been noted frequently

Induction of labor and initiation of cervical ripening before induction of labor (low-dose dinoprostone vaginal suppositories or gel)

Dosage

Refer to Table 47-3.

Fate

After IM injection, drug is widely distributed in both fetal and maternal bodies; half-life in amniotic fluid is several hours, but much shorter in plasma; metabolized by maternal liver and excreted largely in the urine, 80% of the dose within 5 to 10 hours

Common Side Effects

Vomiting, diarrhea, nausea, headache, shivering, chills, hyperthermia, flushing, abdominal cramps

Significant Adverse Reactions

(Not all are clearly drug related)

GI: hiccups, dry throat, choking sensation, pharyngitis, laryngitis, taste alterations
CNS: paresthesia, weakness, drowsiness, tremor, dizziness, lethargy, anxiety, blurred vision, tinnitus, vertigo, sleep disorders
CV: hypertension (*hypo*tension with dinoprostone), chest pain, arrhythmias, bradycardia, palpitations, congestive heart failure, cardiac arrest
Respiratory: coughing, wheezing, dyspnea, hyperventilation, asthmalike reactions, pulmonary embolism
Genitourinary: endometritis, urinary tract infection, perforated cervix or uterus, uterine or vaginal pain, urinary incontinence, hematuria
Other: sweating, hot flashes, muscle pain, leg cramps, joint pain, stiff neck, diplopia, polydipsia, rash, aggravation of diabetes, uterine infections

Contraindications

Acute pelvic inflammatory disease; active cardiac, pulmonary, hepatic, or renal disease. *Cautious use* in patients with asthma, hypertension, heart disease, diabetes, glaucoma, epilepsy, renal or hepatic impairment, anemia, jaundice, vaginitis, and cervicitis.

CAUTION

Prostaglandin-induced abortion is not always complete. If incomplete, other measures should be taken to ensure complete expulsion (eg, hypertonic sodium chloride; see below)

Interactions

Aspirin and other anti-inflammatory drugs may prolong the time required for fetal expulsion with prostaglandins
The activity of oxytocin may be enhanced by prostaglandin abortifacients

Nursing Management

Nursing Interventions

Medication Administration

Administer drugs only in a hospital or other healthcare facility where trained personnel, intensive care, and acute surgical facilities are available.
Anticipate the possibility of a liveborn fetus, especially if drugs are given near the end of the second trimester, because prostaglandins, unlike hypertonic saline, are not usually lethal to the fetus.
Expect pregnancy to be terminated by other means, such as hypertonic sodium chloride (see below), if these drugs fail because prostaglandins can damage the fetus.
Be prepared for the possibility of transient pyrexia with IM injection of carboprost. Temperature elevations greater than 2°F have been noted in approximately one eighth of patients receiving the drug. Supplemental fluids are recommended, but other modes of treatment are usually unnecessary because temperature reverts to normal shortly after therapy is discontinued.
Advocate pretreatment of patient with antiemetic and antidiarrheal medication to minimize incidence of nausea, vomiting, and diarrhea, as appropriate.

After drug administration, monitor uterine activity, and monitor cardiovascular status for signs of vasomotor disturbance (eg, bradycardia, pallor, rapid decrease in blood pressure).

Patient Teaching

Teach the patient that the following side effects may occur: nausea; vomiting; diarrhea; uterine/vaginal pain; fever; headache; weakness; dizziness.

Instruct the patient to report any of the following to the practitioner: severe pain; difficulty breathing; palpitations; eye pain; rash.

• Sodium Chloride

20% sodium chloride solution

Intra-amniotic injection of hypertonic sodium chloride can be used for second trimester abortion but has been largely replaced by the prostaglandins, which are both safer and more effective. The principal indication for sodium chloride injection is in the patient desiring abortion who has not responded successfully or completely to one of the prostaglandins. When prostaglandin-induced abortion is incomplete, however, injection of hypertonic saline should be delayed until the uterus is no longer contracting. The volume of solution instilled should not exceed the volume of amniotic fluid removed. Injection should be performed at a relatively slow rate and fluid samples taken at regular intervals to ensure that the injection catheter remains in the amniotic cavity. The maximum dose is considered to be 250 mL. Inadvertent intravascular injection should be avoided, because sudden, severe hypernatremia may result, possibly leading to cardiovascular shock, extensive hemolysis, and renal necrosis. The drug should be administered only in a medical unit with intensive care facilities readily available. If labor has not begun within 48 hours after instillation, a reevaluation of the patient's status is indicated.

Selected Bibliography

Chi I: The safety and efficacy issues of progestin-only oral contraceptives: An epidemiologic perspective. Contraception 47:1, 1993

Coe FL, Parks JH: The risks of oral contraceptives and estrogen replacement therapy. Perspect Biol Med 33:86, 1989

Derman RJ: An overview of the noncontraceptive benefits and risks of oral contraception. Int J Fertil 37:19, 1992

Hoppe G: Clinical relevance of oral contraceptive pill-induced plasma lipid changes: Facts and fiction. Am J Obstet Gynecol 163:388, 1990

L'Hermite M: Sex hormones and cardiovascular risk. Acta Cardiol 46: 357, 1991

Paul C, Skegg DC, Spears GF: Oral contraceptives and risk of breast cancer. Int J Cancer 46(3):366, 1990

Rosenberg MJ, Long SC: Oral contraceptives and cycle control: A critical review of the literature. Adv Contracept 8:35, 1992

Sondheimer SJ: Update on the metabolic effects of steroidal contraceptives. Endocrinol Metab Clin North Am 20:911, 1991

Thorogood M, Vessey MP: An epidemiologic survey of cardiovascular disease in women taking oral contraceptives. Am J Obstet Gynecol 163:274, 1990

Wynn V: Oral contraceptives and coronary heart disease. J Reprod Med 36:219, 1991

Nursing Bibliography

Klitsch M: The new pill: Awaiting the next generation of oral contraceptives. Family Planning Perspectives 24(5):226, 1992

Mastrioianni L, Courtland R: Contraception in the 1990's. Patient Care 107:84, 1994

Milhan D: DES exposure: Implications for childbearing. International Journal of Childbirth Education 7(4):21, 1992

"Morning after" pills compared. Nurses Drug Alert 17(1):4, 1993

Williams R: Benefits and risks of oral contraceptive use. Postgrad Med 92(7):155, 1992

48

Androgens and Anabolic Steroids

Androgens
Anabolic steroids

Finasteride

Danocrine

The term *androgen* refers to a number of naturally occurring or synthetic steroidal compounds exhibiting the masculinizing and tissue-building (anabolic) actions of testosterone, the principal endogenous physiologic androgenic hormone. Testosterone is produced in and secreted by the interstitial (Leydig) cells of the testes under the stimulus of interstitial cell–stimulating hormone (ICSH), which is identical to the luteinizing hormone (LH) of the female.

Testosterone is responsible for the development and support of the male sex organs and the appearance of the male secondary sex characteristics (eg, deep voice, body hair), at the time of puberty. In addition, testosterone exerts a protein anabolic action, thus stimulating growth of skeletal muscle tissue; it also reduces excretion of sodium, potassium, chloride, nitrogen, and phosphorus and enhances growth of long bones in prepubertal males. However, testosterone also accelerates the ossification (hardening) process at the ends of long bones, eventually resulting in a conversion of cartilage into bone in the active growth areas (epiphyses) and cessation of further bone growth. For this reason, use of large amounts of androgens in young boys may actually cause a *reduction* of full potential growth by inducing a premature closing of the epiphyses after an initial growth spurt. Likewise, androgenic therapy in young males can result in precocious puberty, that is, premature development of the male sex organs and secondary sex characteristics, with possible attendant psychological trauma.

Other physiologic actions of testosterone include increased sebaceous gland activity, thickening of the vocal cords, darkening of the skin, loss of subcutaneous fat, and increased skin vascularization. In addition, psychologic and behavioral changes occur as production of testosterone is increased.

Testosterone itself, although adequately absorbed from the GI tract, is not administered orally because it is rapidly inactivated in the gut and liver, approximately one-half of a dose being metabolized on first pass through the liver. Thus, very large oral doses (eg, 400 mg/day) are needed to provide clinically effective blood levels. Testosterone may be given by IM injection (aqueous suspension, propionate in oil suspension); however, these preparations are relatively short acting when administered by this route, again because of rapid metabolism. However, two esters of testosterone (cypionate, enanthate) exhibit greater stability and slower metabolism and, when injected IM in an oily vehicle, display a prolonged duration of action (2–4 weeks). Other structural modifications of testosterone (eg, methyltestosterone, fluoxymesterone) not only increase potency but also confer resistance to hepatic metabolism, thus permitting use by the oral or buccal route. In addition, a testosterone transdermal patch is available for replacement therapy in congenital or acquired hypogonadal states. The transdermal system is applied daily to the scrotal sac for 6 to 8 weeks, after which another form of testosterone replacement therapy should be provided if the response is inadequate.

A group of synthetic steroids structurally related to testosterone have been developed that display some separation of anabolic from androgenic activity, although the degree of separation is incomplete and variable. These compounds are termed *anabolic steroids* and have been used for a variety of conditions in which an anabolic activity is desired, such as corticosteroid-induced osteoporosis, debilitation resulting from trauma, surgery, or chronic infections, and certain types of anemias (eg, aplastic).

Much attention has been focused in recent years on the use of anabolic steroids by athletes for the purpose of enhancing their performance. In conjunction with sufficient caloric and protein intake, anabolic steroids can increase muscle mass and decrease healing time after muscle injury. They also appear to increase aggressiveness, and may provide a competitive edge in those athletic activities that depend on strength. However, the serious health hazards associated with steroid use, such as hepatotoxicity, fluid retention, endocrine disorders, and blood lipid changes, argue strongly against the use of these agents strictly for athletic purposes. Any gain in performance with use of anabolic steroids is achieved at the expense of incurring serious and potentially life-threatening physiologic damage and there can be no justification for the use of steroids in otherwise healthy athletes.

Chronic use of anabolic steroids frequently leads to an addiction syndrome, resulting in incessant craving and difficulty in stopping despite the appearance of side effects. At his point, decreased levels of these substances in the body are often associated with withdrawal symptoms, resembling those seen during alcohol or narcotic withdrawal. Steroid abuse commonly results in behavioral instability and extreme aggressiveness, and the effects of these drugs often persist for months after the last dose. As of early 1991, anabolic steroids were reclassified as Schedule III controlled substances because of their abuse potential.

Although these compounds exhibit a higher anabolic: androgenic ratio than testosterone or methyltestosterone, excessive dosage or prolonged administration is associated with most of the same untoward effects as seen with testosterone itself. Thus, the clinical use of anabolic steroids, especially in women and children, should be closely supervised and restricted to those valid medications listed below.

Other steroids that bear structural resemblance to testosterone but exhibit reduced androgenic activity are used in the treatment of advanced or metastatic breast cancer in postmenopausal women. These drugs, dromostanolone and testolactone, are reviewed in Chapter 74. The rest of the androgenic and anabolic steroids are discussed here as a group and then are listed in Table 48-1 with their specific indications and recommended dosages. An androgen hormone inhibitor, finasteride, used to reduce the size of the prostate gland, is also reviewed in this chapter, as is danazol, a synthetic androgen possessing antigonadotropic and androgenic activity and used in the treatment of endometriosis.

Androgens and Anabolic Steroids

(Pregnancy Category X)

- ***Fluoxymesterone***
- ***Methyltestosterone***
- ***Nandrolone***
- ***Oxandrolone***
- ***Oxymetholone***
- ***Stanozolol***
- ***Testosterone***

Mechanism

Increase synthesis of RNA and cellular protein; testosterone is converted to its active metabolite dihydrotestosterone in many tissues, whereas at other sites it is active itself; other derivatives also enhance RNA and protein synthesis directly; stimulate growth of muscle, bone, skin, and hair and accelerate closure of epiphyses at ends of long bones; increase production of red blood cells; cause retention of nitrogen, phosphorus, sodium, and probably also calcium and potassium; temporarily arrest progression of estrogen-dependent carcinomas; *large doses* can suppress pituitary gonadotropin secretion, and decrease spermatogenesis through feedback inhibition of follicle-stimulating hormone (FSH)

Uses

Refer to Table 48-1 for specific indications.

Replacement therapy in androgen deficiency states, such as testicular hypofunction, pituitary dysfunction, eunuchism (complete testicular failure), eunuchoidism (partial testicular failure), cryptorchidism, castration, or male climacteric

Treatment of low sperm count or impotence caused by androgen deficiency (low doses only)

Palliative therapy of androgen-responsive inoperable breast cancer in 1- to 5-year postmenopausal women

Induction of a positive nitrogen balance in those conditions in which an anabolic action is desired, for example, osteoporosis, anemia, corticosteroid-induced catabolism, and debilitation resulting from injury, trauma, infection, and other causes

Table 48-1. **Androgens and Anabolic Steroids**

Drug	*Usual Dosage Range*	*Nursing Considerations*
ANDROGENS		
Fluoxymesterone (C-III) *Halotestin*	*Hypogonadism, impotence*: 5–20 mg/day *Breast cancer*: 10–40 mg/day in divided doses *Postpartum breast engorgement*: 2.5 mg shortly after delivery; thereafter, 5–10 mg/day in divided doses for 4–5 days	Potent, orally effective, short-acting derivative of testosterone, approximately 5 times more active than testosterone itself; minimal sodium and water retention but frequent GI distress (administer drug with food); be alert for symptoms suggestive of peptic ulcer; confirmatory tests should be performed
Methyltestosterone (C-III) *Android, Oreton, Testred, Virilon*	*Male hypogonadism, impotence, male climacteric*: 10–40 mg/day (oral) *or* 5–20 mg/day (buccal) *Cryptorchidism*: 30 mg/day (oral) *Postpartum breast pain and engorgement*: 80 mg/day (oral) for 3–5 days *Breast cancer*: 200 mg/day (oral) *or* 100 mg/day (buccal)	Orally effective, short-acting androgen somewhat less effective than testosterone esters; does not produce full sexual maturation in prepubertal testicular failure unless patient has been pretreated with testosterone; creatinuria is a common finding, although its significance is not known; buccal tablets should be placed between cheek and gum and allowed to dissolve, *not* chewed or swallowed, patient should avoid eating, drinking, or smoking for at least 1 h after ingestion; instruct patient to report any inflammation or pain in oral cavity after drug usage; good oral hygiene should be stressed to reduce infection or irritation
Testosterone, Aqueous (C-III) *Andro 100, Histerone, Tesamone* *(CAN) Malogen*	*Male hypogonadism, impotence, male climacteric*: 25–50 mg IM 2–3 times/wk *Postpartum breast engorgement*: 25–50 mg/day for 3–4 days *Breast cancer*: 50–100 mg 3 times/wk *Delayed puberty*: 40–50 mg/m^2/dose once a month for 6 months	Male sex hormone used as replacement therapy in deficiency states, for relief of breast engorgement and treatment of mammary carcinoma in women; inject IM only deep into gluteal muscle; if crystals are present in the vial, warming and shaking will disperse them; absorption is slow and effects persist for several days; do *not* administer more frequently than recommended; regression of mammary tumors should be apparent within 3 mo; occasionally, acceleration of tumor growth is encountered, in which case discontinue immediately; in some of these cases, estrogens will then cause regression

(continued)

Table 48-1. **Androgens and Anabolic Steroids (Continued)**

Drug	Usual Dosage Range	Nursing Considerations
Testosterone Transdermal System (C-III) *Testoderm*	Apply one system to scrotal sac daily	Used for replacement therapy in testosterone-deficient states; must be applied to shaved scrotal skin; determine serum testosterone after 3 to 4 weeks of daily use; do not use longer than 8 wk if desired results have not occurred
Testosterone Propionate (C-III) *Testex* *(CAN) Malogen in Oil*	IM: see Testosterone, aqueous	Ester of testosterone formulated in an oily vehicle; absorption may be somewhat slower than testosterone aqueous, but duration of action is comparable
Testosterone Cypionate (C-III) *Andro-Cyp, Andronate, depAndro, Depo-Testosterone, Depotest, Duratest, Testred Cypionate* **Testosterone Enanthate** *Andro-L.A., Andropository, Delatest, Delatestryl, Durathate, Everone, Testone L.A., Testrin-P.A.* *(CAN) Malogex*	*Hypogonadism, male climacteric*: 50–400 mg IM every 2–4 wk *Delayed puberty*: 50–200 mg every 2–4 wk *Inoperable mammary cancer*: 200–400 mg every 2–4 wk	Long-acting esters of testosterone providing a therapeutic effect for approximately 4 wk with single injection; *not* recommended for use in treating *metastatic* breast carcinoma; inject *deep* into gluteal muscle; shaking and warming of vial will redissolve any crystals that have formed; use of a wet needle or syringe may cloud solution but potency is unaffected
ANABOLIC STEROIDS		
Nandrolone Decanoate (C-III) *Androlone-D, Deca-Durabolin, Hybolin, Neo-Durabolic*	Adults: 50–200 mg IM every 3–4 wk Children: 25–50 mg every 3–4 wk	Long-acting ester of nandrolone (duration 3–4 wk); indicated for management of anemia of renal insufficiency; increases red cell mass; inject deeply IM
Nandrolone Phenpropionate (C-III) *Durabolin, Hybolin Improved*	*Metastatic breast cancer*: 50–100 mg/wk IM	Synthetic androgen with high anabolic–androgenic ratio; effects persist 1–3 wk; injection should be made deeply into gluteal muscle in adults; intermittent therapy is recommended, with 4–8 wk rest periods every 4 mo
Oxandrolone (C-III) *Oxandrin*	*Osteoporosis, tissue building* Adults: 2.5 mg orally 2–4 times/day (up to 20 mg a day) for 2–4 wk; repeat after a rest period if desired Children: 0.1 mg/kg/day	Synthetic anabolic steroid with low androgenic activity; used frequently to help promote weight gain after trauma, severe illness, major surgery, or prolonged corticosteroid administration; do not administer longer than 3 mo
Oxymetholone (C-III) *Anadrol-50* *(CAN) Anapolin*	*Anemias*: (adults and children): 1–2 mg/kg/day orally to a maximum of 5 mg/kg/day (highly individual)	Synthetic anabolic steroid used primarily for anemias due to deficient red cell production, congenital or acquired aplastic anemia, and anemias resulting from administration of myelotoxic drugs; a minimum of 3–6 mo should be allowed, because response is often slow; after remission, some patients may be able to stop drug, and others may require a minimum daily dosage
Stanozolol (C-III) *Winstrol*	*Hereditary angioedema* (adults): Initially 2 mg 3 times/day; decrease gradually to maintenance dosage of 2 mg/day	Primarily used to decrease frequency and severity of attacks of hereditary angioedema; exhibits minimal androgenic effects at normal doses; administer with meals to decrease GI distress

CAUTION

Anabolic steroids are dangerous drugs that can cause serious adverse effects, and their use has resulted in death. Although muscle mass and muscle strength may increase, the increased body weight and muscle size noted with use of these drugs is partially the result of increased sodium and fluid retention. In addition, increases in muscle mass are *not* accompanied by increases in tendon strength, and ruptured tendons are common if the muscle mass becomes too great for the tendon to support under higher physical demand.

Nitrogen retention and increased body mass can occur with *females* taking anabolic steroids, but the inevitable virilizing side effects must be recognized and seem a high price to pay for possible improvement in athletic performance. Moreover, use of other drugs with anabolic steroids, such as diuretics to reduce fluid retention, can further increase the likelihood of toxicity, and resultant electrolyte imbalances may have serious adverse consequences. Use of anabolic steroids for improving athletic prowess should be *strongly* discouraged.

Dosage

See Table 48-1.

Fate

Testosterone is adequately absorbed when given orally, but as much as 50% of a dose undergoes first-pass hepatic metabolism, and very high doses are necessary to achieve effective plasma levels. Synthetic androgens are less extensively metabolized and exhibit longer half-lives. Esterification of testosterone increases its stability, and when administered in an oily vehicle it possesses a long duration of action (2–4 weeks). Testosterone is highly (98%) bound to plasma proteins, especially testosterone-estradiol–binding globulin. Androgens are metabolized in the liver, and conjugated metabolites are excreted largely in the urine

Common Side Effects

Female virilization (eg, hirsutism, voice changes, clitoral enlargement), amenorrhea, changes in libido, flushing, nausea with oral preparations, gynecomastia in males

Significant Adverse Reactions

CAUTION

Use of androgens or anabolic steroids can result in development of peliosis hepatis, a condition in which the liver and spleen may become engorged with blood-filled cysts. Liver failure has resulted, and intra-abdominal hemorrhage has also occurred. Liver cell tumors have been reported, and although these are usually benign, fatal malignant tumors can occur. Adverse serum lipid changes, such as decreased high-density lipoproteins and elevated low-density lipoproteins, have also been noted with androgen therapy. Cholestatic hepatitis and jaundice can occur with fluoxymesterone and methyltestosterone at relatively low doses; the drug-induced jaundice is reversible when the medication is discontinued

Males

Prepubertal: phallic enlargement, increased erections, premature closing of epiphyses

Postpubertal: impotence, testicular atrophy, bladder irritability, decreased sperm count, epididymitis, chronic priapism

Females

Male pattern baldness, menstrual irregularities, suppression of ovulation or lactation

Both sexes

Acne, oily skin, excitation, insomnia, anxiety, depression, headache, paresthesia, chills, leukopenia, polycythemia, hypercalcemia, pain, swelling, urticaria, irritation at injection sites, jaundice, hepatic necrosis, sodium and water retention, increased serum cholesterol

In addition, *oral* preparations may cause vomiting and ulcer symptoms.

Alterations can occur in many clinical laboratory tests.

Contraindications

Pregnancy, lactation, known or suspected prostatic or breast cancer in males; in addition, *anabolic hormones* are also contraindicated in prostatic hypertrophy, pituitary insufficiency, history of myocardial infarction, hepatic dysfunction, nephrosis, hypercalcemia, and in elderly asthenic men, who may react adversely to overstimulation. *Cautious use* in persons with hypertension, coronary artery disease, gynecomastia, renal dysfunction, hypercholesterolemia, and in prepubertal males.

Interactions

Androgens may enhance the effects of oral anticoagulants

Barbiturates and other hypnotics, phenytoin, and phenylbutazone may decrease the action of androgens by accelerating their metabolic breakdown

Androgens can antagonize the action of calcitonin and parathyroid hormone

Corticosteroids may increase the severity of androgen-induced edema

Anabolic steroids may decrease blood glucose in diabetics, reducing insulin or oral hypoglycemic drug requirements

Nursing Management

Pretherapy Assessment

Assess and record baseline data necessary for detection of adverse effects of androgens: General: vital signs (VS), body weight, skin color and temperature; central nervous system (CNS): affect, orientation, peripheral sensation; GI: abdominal exam, liver evaluation; Lab: serum electrolytes, cholesterol, liver function tests, glucose tolerance test, thyroid function tests.

Review medical history and documents for existing or previous conditions that:

a. require cautious use of androgens: hypertension; coronary artery disease; gynecomastia; renal dysfunction; hypercholesterolemia; use in prepubertal males
b. contraindicate use of androgens: pregnancy; lactation; known or suspected prostatic or breast cancer in males; prostatic hypertrophy; pituitary insufficiency; history of myocardial infarction; hepatic dysfunction; nephrosis; hypercalcemia; use in elderly asthenic males who may react adversely to overstimulation; **pregnancy (Category X)**, lactation (safety not established, do not use in nursing mothers)

Nursing Interventions

Medication Administration

Inject deeply into gluteal muscle.

Do not administer frequently, because these drugs are typically slow-onset, long-acting agents.

Surveillance During Therapy

Provide copious fluids to prevent formation of renal calculi if symptomatic hypercalcemia occurs (eg, vomiting, constipation, loss of muscle tone, polyuria, lethargy). The drug should be discontinued, and symptoms should be treated with appropriate medications. All patients should be tested regularly for development of hypercalcemia, which occurs mainly in patients who are bedridden or immobilized or those who have metastatic breast cancer. In the latter, elevated calcium levels usually indicate bone metastases.

Notify practitioner if liver tests are abnormal, signs of excessive sexual stimulation occur (eg, priapism), or vaginal bleeding develops because the drug should be discontinued. Observe for signs of jaundice (yellow skin or sclerae, itching) or excessive stimulation in the elderly patient.

Monitor results of liver function tests, serum cholesterol determinations, and tests for serum calcium levels, which should be performed periodically during therapy.

Assist with evaluation of drug effects. Anabolic steroids should not be administered for longer than 90 days without careful patient reassessment.

Cautiously interpret results of the following laboratory tests because androgens may alter their values: liver function, thyroid function, glucose tolerance, blood coagulation, creatinine excretion, serum cholesterol, and the metyrapone test.

Carefully monitor laboratory studies and patient for indications of adverse reactions.

Interpret results of diagnostic tests and contact practitioner as appropriate.

Monitor for possible drug–drug and drug–nutrient interactions: Refer to **Interactions**.

Patient Teaching

Suggest that oral tablets be taken with food to minimize GI distress. Buccal tablets should be allowed to dissolve between gum and cheek or under the tongue, but should not be swallowed. Instruct patient not to eat, drink, or smoke while tablet is in place.

Instruct female patient to report signs of virilization (refer to **Common Side Effects**) to practitioner because they may necessitate termination of therapy. Some changes (eg, voice deepening, hirsutism) may be irreversible when drug is discontinued.

Advise male patient to notify practitioner if priapism, reduced ejaculatory volume, impotence, or gynecomastia occurs. These symptoms may be controlled by dosage reduction or temporary cessation of therapy.

Instruct parents to carefully observe for signs of premature sexual development when an anabolic steroid is given to a prepubertal male. Rate of bone growth and maturation should be periodically checked radiologically to minimize danger of premature fusion of epiphyses.

Instruct patient on prolonged therapy to note signs of development of excessive fluid retention (eg, edema, weight gain). If these occur, the drug should be temporarily withdrawn or a diuretic administered.

Instruct diabetic patient to be alert for signs of hypoglycemia (sweating, tremor, anxiety, vertigo) and to adjust antidiabetic drug dosage accordingly.

Instruct patient taking anticoagulants to report signs of bleeding (eg, petechiae, ecchymoses) because dosage of anticoagulant drug may have to be reduced.

Encourage bedridden patient to perform exercises regularly to minimize development of hypercalcemia.

When appropriate, explain that anabolic steroids do not significantly enhance athletic ability and should not be used to improve performance or stamina because the risk far outweighs the potential benefit.

Androgen Hormone Inhibitor

- ***Finasteride*** *(Pregnancy Category X)*

Proscar

Mechanism

Competitively inhibits the enzyme steroid 5-alpha-reductase, thereby blocking conversion of testosterone to 5-alpha-dihydrotestosterone (DHT). The reduction in DHT serum levels results in a gradual decrease in the size of an enlarged prostate gland. Improved urinary flow is observed in approximately one-half of patients receiving the drug for 12 months. The plasma lipid profile is unchanged.

Uses

Treatment of benign prostatic hyperplasia (BPH)

Investigational uses include treatment of male pattern baldness, acne, and hirsutism

Dosage

5 mg once a day. At least 6 to 12 months of therapy may be needed to determine whether a beneficial effect has occurred.

Fate

Maximum plasma levels occur within 1 to 2 hours after dosing. Mean plasma half-life is 6 to 8 hours. Approximately 90% bound to plasma proteins. Drug accumulates slowly with repeated dosing. Excreted approximately one third in the urine and the remainder in the feces.

Significant Adverse Reactions

Decreased libido, impotence

Contraindications

Pregnancy, nursing mothers, children. *Cautious use* in patients with liver function abnormalities, obstructive uropathy.

Interactions

Finasteride can increase theophylline clearance

Finasteride decreases serum levels of prostate-specific antigen (PSA), which is used as a screening test for prostate cancer.

Nursing Management

Pretherapy Assessment

Assess and record baseline data necessary for detection of adverse effects of finasteride: General: VS, body weight, skin color and temperature; CNS: affect, orientation; GU: normal output, voiding pattern, prostate examination, reproductive function profile; Lab: serum prostatic specific antigen test.

Review medical history and documents for existing or previous conditions that:

a. require cautious use of finasteride: liver function abnormalities, obstructive uropathy

b. contraindicate use of finasteride: allergy to any

component of the medication; pregnancy; children; **pregnancy (Category X)**, lactation (safety not established, do not use in nursing mothers)

Nursing Interventions

Medication Administration

May be administered with or without meals

Crushed tablets should not be handled by a woman who is pregnant or may become pregnant because of reproductive risk

Surveillance During Therapy

Carefully monitor laboratory studies and patient for indications of adverse reactions.

Interpret results of diagnostic tests and contact practitioner as appropriate.

Monitor for possible drug–drug and drug–nutrient interactions: Refer to **Interactions**.

Patient Teaching

Patient should be advised to wear a condom during sexual activity to prevent exposure of his sexual partner to his semen.

Inform the patient that ejaculatory volume may be decreased as a result of this medication.

• Danazol

Danocrine

(CAN) Cyclomen

A synthetic derivative of 17-alpha-ethinyl testosterone, danazol inhibits the release of gonadotropins from the pituitary gland and exhibits a weak androgenic effect. No estrogenic or progestational activity has been demonstrated. Danazol provides alternative therapy for endometriosis in those women who cannot tolerate or who fail to respond to other forms of treatment, and it may also be employed in severe fibrocystic breast disease and hereditary angioedema.

Mechanism

Suppresses release of FSH and LH from the adenohypophysis; inhibits enzymes necessary for biosynthesis of gonadal hormones; may also compete with sex steroids for binding sites on body tissues; lack of ovulation and associated amenorrhea results in atrophy of endometrium and resolution of endometrial lesions.

Uses

Treatment of endometriosis in those patients who cannot tolerate or who fail to respond to other means of therapy (*not* indicated in cases in which surgery is the treatment of choice)

Symptomatic treatment of severe fibrocystic breast disease

Prevention of attacks of all types (eg, cutaneous, laryngeal, abdominal) of hereditary angioedema

Treatment of gynecomastia, infertility, and menorrhagia (investigational use only)

Dosage

CAUTION

Begin therapy during menstruation, if possible, to ensure that patient is not pregnant. Otherwise, perform pregnancy test before initiating therapy if possibility of pregnancy exists. Also, rule out carcinoma of the breast before initiating therapy for fibrocystic breast disease. If any nodule persists or enlarges during therapy, discontinue drug and perform appropriate tests

Endometriosis

200 to 400 mg twice a day for 3 to 9 months; may reinstitute therapy if symptoms recur

Fibrocystic Breast Disease

100 to 400 mg/day in two divided doses for 3 to 6 months

Hereditary Angioedema

Initially, 200 mg 2 to 3 times/day; reduce dosage at 1- to 3-month intervals if clinical response is favorable.

Common Side Effects

Flushing, sweating, vaginitis

Significant Adverse Reactions

Virilization (acne, oily skin, hirsutism, deepening of the voice, decrease in breast size, clitoral hypertrophy), vaginal bleeding, edema, weight gain, nervousness

Other effects for which a direct causal relationship has not been established are loss of hair, changes in libido, pelvic pain, muscle cramps, back, neck, or leg pain, skin rash, nasal congestion, nausea, vomiting, gastroenteritis, dizziness, headache, tremor, paresthesias, visual disturbances

Contraindications

Pregnancy, lactation, undiagnosed vaginal bleeding, and markedly impaired cardiac, hepatic, or renal function. *Cautious use* in patients with migraine, epilepsy, hypertension, cardiac disease, and mild to moderate renal dysfunction.

Interactions

Danazol may prolong prothrombin time in patients stabilized on warfarin.

Therapy with danazol may increase insulin requirements and result in abnormal glucose tolerance tests.

Nursing Management

Refer to **Androgens**. In addition:

Nursing Interventions

Patient Teaching

Reassure patient that drug-induced anovulation and amenorrhea are reversible within 60 to 90 days after therapy is terminated.

Instruct patient to inform practitioner if signs of virilization develop. Some of these may be irreversible.

Selected Bibliography

Bahrke MS, Yesalis CE, Wright JE: Psychological and behavioural effects of endogenous testosterone levels and anabolic-androgenic steroids among males: A review. Sports Med 10:303, 1990

Bardin CW, Swerdloff RS, Santen RJ: Androgens: Risks and benefits. J Clin Endocrinol Metab 73:4, 1991

Friedl KE: Reappraisal of the health risks associated with the use of high doses of oral and injectable androgenic steroids. NIDA Res Monogr 102:142, 1990

Gillmer MD: Mechanism of action/effects of androgens on lipid metabolism. Int J Fertil 37(suppl 2):83, 1992

Katz DL, Pope HG: Anabolic-androgenic steroid-induced mental status changes. NIDA Res Monogr 102:215, 1990

Lombardo JA: Anabolic-androgenic steroids. NIDA Res Monogr 102:60, 1990

Lukas SE: Current perspectives on anabolic-androgenic steroid abuse. Trends Pharmacol Sci 14:61, 1993

Rockhold RW: Cardiovascular toxicity of anabolic steroids. Annu Rev Pharmacol 33:497, 1993

Nursing Bibliography

Anabolic steroids and domestic violence. Nurse's Drug Alert 17(3):24, 1993

Cheever K, et al: Cardiovascular implications of anabolic steroid abuse. J Cardiovasc Nurs 6(2):19, 1992

Medical or nonmedical uses of anabolic androgenic steroids. JAMA 264(22):2923, 1990

Porterfield L: Steroid abuse advances in clinical care 6(2):44, 1991

Spindler J: Female androgenic alopecia: A review. Dermato Nurs 4(2):93, 1992

VI

Drugs Acting on Gastrointestinal Function

49 Gastrointestinal Physiology: A Review

The digestive system functions to provide body cells with water, electrolytes, vitamins, and nutritive substances. During passage through the gastrointestinal (GI) tract, ingested carbohydrates, fats, and proteins are converted into smaller, absorbable units by the action of digestive enzymes aided by specialized secretions such as bile and hydrochloric acid.

The luminal contents of the digestive tract are transported and effectively mixed with digestive secretions and mucus by specialized muscular movements. GI motility and secretion are affected by a complex interaction of intrinsic and extrinsic neural influences and by several peptide hormones. This chapter briefly reviews the important anatomic features of the GI tract, and provides an overview of the principal physiologic functions of the digestive system.

Organization of the Digestive System

Gastrointestinal Tract

The GI tract (digestive tract or alimentary canal) is a continuous muscular tube lined with mucous membrane, extending from the mouth to the anus, with regional anatomic and functional modifications as outlined in Tables 49-1 and 49-2. The digestive tract includes the mouth, pharynx, esophagus, stomach, and the small and large intestines.

Accessory Organs of Digestion

The salivary glands, pancreas, liver, and gallbladder contribute exocrine secretions essential to the chemical breakdown of food. Digestion is also aided mechanically by the teeth, tongue, and cheeks.

General Histology of the Gastrointestinal Tract

The walls of the organs making up the digestive tract contain four basic layers (tunics) of tissue. From the lumen outward they are as depicted in the following sections.

Tunica Mucosa

The tunica mucosa or mucous membrane consists of a lining *epithelium*, which is in direct contact with the luminal contents. The epithelium may be protective, secretory, or absorptive. Histologically, the epithelium is stratified squamous in the mouth, pharynx (except for the nasopharynx), esophagus, and anal canal. It is simple columnar in the stomach and intestines.

A connective tissue, the *lamina propria*, supports the epithelium and binds it to the underlying smooth muscle, the *muscularis mucosae*.

Tunica Submucosa

This connective tissue layer contains blood vessels, lymphatics, and the nerve *plexus of Meissner* (submucosal plexus).

Tunica Muscularis (Muscularis Externa)

Characteristically, the tunica muscularis is composed of two layers of smooth muscle, an inner, somewhat thicker circular layer and an outer longitudinal layer. Between these lies the *plexus of Auerbach* (myenteric plexus), which contains autonomic nerve fibers and ganglia.

Tunica Serosa or Adventitia

Generally, the outermost tunic is a serous membrane or *serosa* (visceral peritoneum) composed of loose connective tissue covered by a layer of squamous mesothelial cells. In certain parts of the digestive tract (such as the esophagus and rectum) where the connective tissue is not covered by mesothelial cells, the outer tunic is termed the *adventitia*.

Functional Overview

The principal activities of the digestive system include 1) motility, 2) secretion, 3) digestion, and 4) absorption.

Motility

Muscular movements propel materials through the digestive tract, aid in the mechanical breakdown of food, promote mixing of luminal contents with mucus and digestive secretions, and facilitate absorption by renewing the absorptive surface.

The motor functions of the alimentary canal are of two basic types: *mixing* and *propulsive*. These movements are subject to intrinsic and extrinsic neural influences as well as to hormonal regulation.

The alimentary canal is extensively innervated by autonomic nerve fibers belonging to both the sympathetic and parasympathetic divisions. Autonomic elements are represented in the intrinsic nerve supply, the submucosal plexus (of Meissner) and more extensively in the myenteric plexus (of Auerbach). The nerves maintain muscle tone and regulate the force and velocity of muscular contractions.

Gastrointestinal motility is generally increased by parasympathetic (vagal and sacral nerve) stimulation and inhibited by sympathetic activation. Only the sphincters respond in an opposite manner, being relaxed by parasympathetic stimulation and contracted by sympathetic stimulation.

The motor functions of individual digestive organs are summarized in Table 49-2.

Table 49-1. **Anatomic and Histologic Features of the Major Organs of the Digestive Tract**

Organ	Gross Anatomic Features	Histologic Features
Esophagus	Muscular tube continuous with the pharynx	Mucosal epithelium is nonkeratinizing *stratified squamous*. Composition of the tunica muscularis: upper one-third—striated muscle; middle one-third—striated and smooth muscle; and lower one-third—smooth muscle. Outer layer—adventitia
Stomach	*Cardia*—portion surrounding the lower esophageal sphincter *Fundus*—rounded upper portion lying above the entrance of the esophagus *Body*—dilated (major) central region *Pylorus*—tapering distal portion terminating at the pyloric sphincter *Greater curvature*—Large convex curvature on the lateral border *Lesser curvature*—smaller, concave curvature on the medial border The empty (contracted) stomach exhibits longitudinal folds of mucosa termed *rugae*	Mucosal epithelium is *simple columnar*. Tunica muscularis contains three layers of smooth muscle; an inner *oblique*, a middle *circular*, and an outer *longitudinal* Outer layer is a *serosa* formed by the visceral peritoneum, which reflects from the greater and lesser curvatures as the greater and lesser omenta.
Small Intestine	*Duodenum*—first 25 cm, which receives the common bile duct and the pancreatic ducts *Jejunum*—middle segment representing about two fifths of the small intestine *Ileum*—remaining three fifths, rich in lymphatic aggregates (Peyer's patches)	Mucosal epithelium is *simple columnar*. Submucosa of duodenum contains Brunner's glands. Outer layer is a *serosa* (except in duodenum) Absorptive surface area is increased by the following structural features: • *Plicae circulares* (valves of Kerckring)—circular folds of the mucosa and submucosa projecting into the lumen • *Villi*—fingerlike projections of mucous membrane containing a blood capillary and a lacteal (lymphatic) • *Microvilli*—microscopic projections of the free surfaces of lining epithelial cells
Large Intestine	*Cecum*—blind pouch from which the vermiform appendix is suspended *Colon* (ascending, transverse, descending and sigmoid) Rectum Anal canal	Mucosal epithelium is *simple columnar* Outer layer is a *serosa* except for the rectum and anal canal, which are covered by adventitia. Prominent morphologic features include: • *Taeniae coli*—three straplike bands of longitudinal smooth muscle • *Haustra*—sacculations or pouches giving the colon a scalloped appearance • *Epiploic appendages*—fat-filled tabs suspended from the taeniae coli

Secretion

The major secretions of the digestive system are saliva, gastric juice, intestinal juice, pancreatic juice, and bile. These are produced by specialized exocrine glands associated with specific components of the digestive tract. Basically, each secretion consists of water, electrolytes, and one or more active organic constituents. *Mucin*, the active constituent of mucus, is produced by all segments of the digestive tract. Mucus lubricates and protects each region of the alimentary canal from chemical and mechanical irritation.

Digestive secretions are produced in response to both mechanical and chemical stimulation. Nervous and humoral (hormonal) mechanisms control the rate and, in some instances, the relative composition of secretions. Generally, parasympathetic activity promotes GI secretion.

The major digestive secretions are characterized in Table 49-2.

Control of Gastric Secretion

Gastric secretion, which occurs in three phases, cephalic, gastric, and intestinal, is controlled by neural and humoral mechanisms.

The *cephalic phase*, which occurs before food enters the stomach, may be initiated by the thought, sight, smell, or taste of food. This phase is mediated by the vagus (10th cranial) nerve, which stimulates HCl and pepsinogen production by directly activating gastric parietal and chief cells, as well as indirectly by first stimulating the secretion of gastrin.

The *gastric phase* of secretion, which is mediated mainly by the hormone gastrin, takes place while food is present in the stomach. Gastrin is released from the pyloric antrum in response to mechanical distention or chemical stimulation (eg, protein digestion products, alcohol, caffeine). Gastrin release is a major stimulus to HCl secretion and pepsinogen production by the parietal and chief cells, respectively. In the absence of a

Table 49-2. **Major Activities of the Digestive Tract**

Organ	*Motor Activity*	*Secretion*	*Digestion*	*Absorption*
Mouth	Chewing (mastication)—ingested food is subdivided into small particles by the teeth and mixed with saliva to form a bolus. Swallowing (deglutition)—oral phase of swallowing is initiated voluntarily as the tongue forces the bolus toward the oropharynx.	Saliva is secreted by buccal and salivary glands (parotid, submaxillary, and sublingual) in response to the sight, smell, or taste of food. Saliva moistens the mucous membranes, cleanses the mouth and teeth, lubricates the food to facilitate chewing and swallowing, and enhances the taste of food.	Digestion of complex carbohydrates (starches) is initiated by salivary amylase (ptyalin).	Certain drugs (eg, nitroglycerin) are absorbed sublingually.
Pharynx	Swallowing (pharyngeal phase)—swallowing proceeds reflexly as the bolus enters the oropharynx and continues through the laryngopharynx into the esophagus.			
Esophagus	Swallowing (esophageal phase)—swallowing continues reflexly, coordinated by a swallowing center in the medulla. Bolus passes along the esophagus into the stomach through peristalsis.	Esophageal glands secrete mucus to facilitate passage of bolus and protect the mucosa.		
Stomach	Receptive relaxation—stomach adapts to increased volume without an increase in intragastric pressure Reservoir function—stomach stores contents ingested in a meal and allows partial digestion and gradual emptying into the intestine. Mixing function—mixing waves, aided by peristaltic waves, macerate the bolus, mix it with gastric juice, and reduce it into chyme. Propulsive function—peristaltic waves force the chyme through the pyloric sphincter into the duodenum. Gastric emptying—chyme leaves the stomach at a rate consistent with the most effective rates of digestion and absorption by the small intestine. The rate of gastric emptying is influenced by the physical and chemical composition of chyme (eg, volume, viscosity, acidity, osmotic pressure). Hormonal and neural factors, including emotional state, can affect the gastric emptying rate.	Gastric juice contains: *Mucus* (secreted by mucous cells)—protects the stomach wall from autodigestion *Hydrochloric acid* (secreted by parietal or oxyntic cells) denatures proteins, converts pepsinogen into active pepsin; provides optimal pH for pepsin activity; inactivates ptyalin; bacteriostatic action *Pepsinogen*: (secreted by chief or zymogenic cells)—inactive form of the proteolytic enzyme pepsin *Intrinsic factor* (secreted by oxyntic or parietal cells)—forms a complex with vitamin B_{12} to allow intestinal absorption	Protein digestion—pepsin begins the digestion of proteins by attacking certain amino-acid linkages and reducing proteins into peptides Fat digestion—gastric lipase acts principally on tributyrin and is not considered to contribute significantly to the digestion of fats. Lingual lipase acts in the stomach, converting triglycerides into fatty acids and monoglycerides	Certain organic molecules and drugs (eg, alcohol, aspirin), some water, and a few electrolytes are absorbed from the stomach.
Small intestine	Segmentation—these fairly regular localized contractions of the circular smooth muscle mix the chyme with pancreatic, intestinal, and hepatobiliary secretions.	*Succus entericus* (intestinal juice)—intestinal glands secrete a slightly alkaline fluid containing water, mucus, and enzymes that complete the digestion of carbohydrates, fats, and proteins.	*Fats* are emulsified by bile and are digested principally by pancreatic lipase. *Carbohydrates* are digested by pancreatic amylase and by intestinal disaccharidases. Proteolytic enzymes produced by the pancreas and the small intestine digest *proteins* (see Table 49-4)	Water, electrolytes, vitamins, and nutrients (products of carbohydrates, fat, and protein digestion) are absorbed readily from the small intestine (particularly the duodenum and jejunum), as are most orally administered drugs.

(continued)

Table 49-2. **Major Activities of the Digestive Tract (Continued)**

Organ	Motor Activity	Secretion	Digestion	Absorption
	Peristalsis—peristaltic waves propel the intestinal contents onward at a rate suitable for optimal absorption.	*Bile* (produced by the liver and concentrated by the gallbladder) and *pancreatic juice* are delivered to the duodenum by the common bile duct and pancreatic ducts, respectively.	Enterokinase converts pancreatic trypsinogen into active trypsin. Nucleic acids are broken down by pancreatic and intestinal nucleases.	Bile salts and vitamin B_{12} are absorbed from the ileum.
Large intestine	Haustral churning—haustral (segmenting) contractions promote water and electrolyte absorption. Peristalsis—peristaltic waves move the contents along the length of the large intestine. Mass peristalsis—strong propulsive contractions drive the luminal contents into the sigmoid colon and rectum; occur 3–4 times a day Defecation—reflex evacuation of the bowel initiated by distention of the rectum; reflex is integrated by the sacral segments of the spinal cord.	*Mucus* is secreted to protect the mucosa from chemical and mechanical trauma, and to lubricate the colonic contents, thereby facilitating passage of feces.		Water is absorbed, thereby reducing the contents from a semifluid to a semisolid mass. Some electrolytes and certain vitamins (B and K) synthesized in the colon are absorbed. Organic products of bacterial action (eg, indole and skatole) are absorbed and transported to the liver for biotransformation to less toxic substances. Rectally administered drugs are absorbed from the rectum.

basal level of histamine, gastrin alone has little effect on HCl secretion. The parietal (oxyntic) cells contain separate receptors for gastrin, acetylcholine, and histamine, suggesting a synergistic effect. The histamine receptors on the parietal cells are blocked by the histamine-2 (H_2) antagonists (see Chapter 16). Other actions of gastrin are listed in Table 49-3.

Excessive gastric acidity (pH less than 2) inhibits gastrin (and therefore HCl) secretion. The buffering actions of proteins and polypeptides in the stomach help prevent a rapid decline in gastric pH, thereby promoting the secretion of gastrin.

The *intestinal phase* of gastric secretion regulation is largely inhibitory. Both neural and hormonal mechanisms are involved in this control of gastric secretion and gastric emptying. Distention of the duodenum and the arrival of acidic chyme, hyper-

Table 49-3. **Major Hormones and Regulatory Peptides of the Digestive Tract**

Hormone	Source	Stimulus for Secretion	Action
Gastrin	Gastric mucosa of pyloric antrum	Peptides; amino acids Vagal stimulation Pyloric distention	Stimulates acid (HCl) secretion Stimulates pepsinogen production Promotes antral motility Increases gastric emptying Promotes growth of gastric and intestinal mucosa (trophic effect)
Secretin	Mucosa of upper small intestine	Acid chyme	Stimulates secretion of a watery, $NaHCO_3$-rich pancreatic juice Stimulates secretion of $NaHCO_3$-rich bile by liver Inhibits gastric secretion and motility
Cholecystokinin (CCK)	Mucosa of upper small intestine	Peptides; amino acids Long-chain fatty acids	Stimulates gallbladder contraction and relaxes sphincter of Oddi to promote bile flow into duodenum Stimulates secretion of pancreatic enzymes Exerts trophic effect on exocrine pancreatic acini Inhibits gastric secretion and gastric emptying
Gastric inhibitory peptide (GIP)	Mucosa of upper small intestine	Fatty acids; Glucose	Stimulates insulin secretion Inhibits gastric emptying and gastric acid secretion

Note: Other gut regulatory peptides/hormones include: gastrin-releasing peptide (GRP), vasoactive intestinal peptide (VIP), motilin, pancreatic polypeptide (PP), somatostatin, substance P, and neurotensin.

tonic or hypotonic fluid, and protein digestion products trigger the enterogastric reflex, which inhibits gastric secretion and gastric motility. The above-mentioned stimuli, as well as the presence of fats, also promote the release of intestinal hormones (secretin, cholecystokinin, gastric inhibitory peptide) that reduce gastric secretory activity.

Digestion

Most substances ingested in the diet are structurally complex carbohydrates, fats, or proteins, which cannot be absorbed and used by the body in their natural states. During the process of digestion these complex organic constituents are chemically broken down into molecules that can be absorbed readily into body fluids. Specific digestive enzymes from the salivary glands, stomach, small intestine, and pancreas hydrolyze 1) complex carbohydrates into simple sugars; 2) fats into monoglycerides, fatty acids, and glycerol; and 3) proteins into amino acids.

The digestion of carbohydrates is initiated in the mouth by salivary amylase and is completed in the small intestine by pancreatic amylase and intestinal disaccharidases. Proteins are broken down by the combined actions of gastric, pancreatic, and intestinal proteolytic enzymes. Fats are emulsified by bile and are hydrolyzed mainly by pancreatic lipase.

The major digestive enzymes are presented in Table 49-4.

Absorption

Absorption involves the transport of substances (water, electrolytes, vitamins, and products of digestion) across the wall of the digestive tract into the blood or lymph. Mechanisms of transport include diffusion, osmosis, active transport, pinocytosis, and endocytosis.

The proximal small intestine is the major site of absorption of vitamins, water, electrolytes, and nutrients. With the exception of vitamin B_{12} (cyanocobalamin) and the bile salts, which are absorbed mainly from the terminal ileum, most substrates are absorbed from the duodenum and upper jejunum. Intestinal villi, richly endowed with blood capillaries and lymphatic vessels (lacteals), provide an extensive surface area that greatly facilitates absorption. Epithelial cells lining the small intestine exhibit microvilli that further increase the absorptive surface. Finally, the epithelium of the small intestine contains a variety of specialized transport systems for certain substrates (such as amino acids and glucose).

Absorption through the gastric mucosa is limited. Aspirin and alcohol are, however, rapidly absorbed from the stomach.

Absorption of Carbohydrates

Carbohydrates are absorbed mainly in the form of monosaccharides (pentoses or hexoses), principally from the duodenum

Table 49-4. **Major Digestive Enzymes**

Source	*Enzyme*	*Activator*	*Substrate*	*Products*
Lingual (Ebner's) glands	Lingual lipase		Triglycerides	Fatty acids and monoglycerides
Salivary glands	Salivary amylase (ptyalin)	Chloride ion	Polysaccharides Starch	Oligosaccharides, maltotriose, and maltose
Gastric glands (chief cells)	Pepsin (Pepsinogen*)	HCl	Proteins	Peptides
	Gastric lipase		Triglycerides	Fatty acids and glycerol
Exocrine pancreas (acinar cells)	Trypsin (Trypsinogen*)	Enterokinase	Proteins	Peptides
	Chymotrypsin (Chymotrypsinogen*)	Trypsin	Proteins	Peptides
	Carboxypeptidase (Procarboxypeptidase*)	Trypsin	Polypeptides	Smaller peptides and amino acids
	Pancreatic amylase	Chloride ion	Polysaccharides Starch	Oligosaccharides, maltotriose and maltose
	Pancreatic lipase		Triglycerides	Fatty acids and monoglycerides
	Ribonuclease		RNA	Nucleotides
	Deoxyribonuclease		DNA	Nucleotides
	Phospholipase	Trypsin	Phospholipids (Lecithin)	Fatty acids; Lysolecithin
	Cholesterol esterase		Cholesterol esters	Cholesterol
Intestinal mucosa (brush border)	Enterokinase		Trypsinogen	Trypsin
	Aminopeptidase		Polypeptides	Peptides and amino acids
	Dipeptidase		Dipeptides	Amino acids
	Sucrase		Sucrose	Glucose and fructose
	Lactase		Lactose	Glucose and galactose
	Maltase		Maltose	Glucose
	Nuclease		Nucleotides	Pentoses; phosphates, purine and pyrimidine bases

* Zymogen (Inactive form of enzyme).

and upper jejunum. Glucose and galactose are absorbed by a sodium-dependent cotransport mechanism. Fructose is transported by facilitated diffusion, whereas pentoses are transported by simple passive diffusion.

Absorption of Fats (Lipids)

The products of fat digestion—fatty acids and monoglycerides—are absorbed mainly in the proximal segments of the small intestine. Fatty acids containing fewer than 12 carbons are transported directly into the portal blood. Those containing more than 12 carbons are esterified into triglycerides and then transported into the lymphatics (lacteals) in the form of chylomicrons.

Glycerol may pass into the liver to be used for glycogen synthesis, it may be oxidized by the intestinal mucosal cells, or it may be used for intracellular resynthesis of triglycerides.

Certain essential fat-soluble substances and vitamins A, D, E, and K require bile for their absorption. Water-soluble aggregates containing fatty acids, monoglycerides, and bile salts are called *micelles*.

Absorption of Proteins

Ingested proteins are absorbed mainly as amino acids from the duodenum and jejunum. There are several carriers that cotransport specific amino acids with sodium. At least two sodium-independent carrier mechanisms also exist, one for basic and another for neutral amino acids. Dipepetides and tripeptides are transported by separate active carrier systems.

Occasionally, whole proteins may be absorbed from the intestine through endocytosis. For example, gamma-globulins (antibodies) ingested by a suckling infant are absorbed intact in this manner.

Absorption of Water

The net absorption of water from the intestines is variable, being greatly affected by the osmotic pressure and electrolyte composition of the intestinal contents. The transport of water occurs through osmosis, with the driving force for water absorption being generated by the absorption of various solutes (such as glucose, amino acids, and electrolytes). Water is absorbed principally in the upper small intestine and to a limited extent in the ileum and colon. Saline cathartics are poorly absorbed salts (eg, magnesium sulfate) that remain in the intestinal lumen and pull in an osmotic equivalent of water, thereby creating a laxative effect.

Absorption of Electrolytes

The electrolytes absorbed from the intestine include minerals ingested in the diet and electrolyte constituents of various digestive juices.

Sodium is actively absorbed throughout the small and large intestines. As noted above, the absorption of such nutrients as glucose and amino acids is associated with sodium transport.

Glucose facilitates the absorption of sodium (this is the rationale for treating severe diarrhea with oral administration of glucose and sodium chloride). Potassium, magnesium, zinc, chloride, bicarbonate, iodide and phosphate ions are also absorbed, some actively and others passively.

Calcium and iron are absorbed by special mechanisms largely in accordance with the body's needs. The rate of calcium absorption from the upper small intestine is greatly enhanced by calcitriol. Iron is absorbed best in the reduced, ferrous (Fe^{+2}) state, and its absorption is increased when the body's iron stores are low and erythrocyte production is increased.

Dietary factors, such as the presence of anions (eg, phosphates, oxalates) in the intestine may inhibit absorption of both calcium and iron by forming insoluble salts with those ions.

Absorption of Vitamins

The water-soluble vitamins (B and C) are readily absorbed in the upper portions of the small intestine. Vitamin B_{12} (cyanocobalamin), however, is absorbed in the ileum and requires a special mechanism for absorption. Vitamin B_{12} forms a complex with *intrinsic factor*, a glycoprotein produced by the gastric parietal cells. The vitamin B_{12}–intrinsic factor complex is taken up by the mucosal cells through pinocytosis, and the vitamin B_{12} is then liberated for uptake into the blood. Failure to elaborate intrinsic factor impairs absorption of vitamin B_{12} and results in pernicious anemia.

The fat-soluble vitamins (A, D, E, and K) require bile for proper absorption. Lack of bile or pancreatic lipase may impair adequate absorption of these fat-soluble vitamins.

Vomiting (Emesis)

Vomiting is the reflex expulsion of the gastric contents through the mouth. Vomiting involves a complex sequence of visceral and somatic events coordinated by a *vomiting center* in the medulla.

The medullary vomiting center may be stimulated through several pathways:

- The chemoreceptor trigger zone (CTZ)
- Cortical stimulation
- Disturbances of the inner ear
- Visceral stimulation
- Nodose ganglion stimulation

Chemoreceptor Trigger Zone

Located in the floor of the fourth ventricle of the brain near the vomiting center, the CTZ may be stimulated by the following:

- Drugs, chemicals, and toxins (eg, cardiac glycosides and apomorphine)
- Pathologic states (eg, uremia and diabetic ketoacidosis)
- Variations in gonadotropin and progesterone levels (eg, pregnancy)
- Radiation

The CTZ exerts a tonic influence on the vomiting center, maintaining a state of excitability to other incoming vestibular impulses (see below).

Drug-, chemical-, or toxin-induced neuronal excitation of the CTZ is probably mediated by the release of dopamine from surrounding cells (eg, astrocytes) that form synaptic connections with the neurons of the CTZ.

Cortical Stimulation

Emesis may follow cortical stimulation induced by *psychic factors*, such as unpleasant scenes or disagreeable odors, or *increased intracranial pressure*, for example, hydrocephalus, brain tumors, or inflammation.

Disturbances of the Inner Ear (Labyrinth)

Motion (through mechanical stimulation of receptors in the labyrinths of the ear) and disorders affecting the vestibular apparatus may produce emesis. Impulses are carried by the vestibulocochlear (8th cranial) nerve and are transmitted through the cerebellum and CTZ to the vomiting center. Acetylcholine is thought to be the neurotransmitter involved with impulse transmission along the labyrinthine pathway to the vomiting center.

Visceral Stimulation

Afferent impulses from the abdominal viscera may be generated by *visceral distention* or *visceral irritation*, and these impulses can *directly* stimulate the vomiting center. Destruction of the CTZ abolishes vomiting of labyrinthine origin (suggesting a modulatory role for the CTZ in vestibular activation of the vomiting center) but does not alter the emetic effect of visceral stimulation.

Nodose Ganglion

Certain drugs may produce vomiting by stimulating the nodose ganglion of the vagus (10th cranial) nerve.

Mechanism of Vomiting

After stimulation of the vomiting center, the esophagus, the lower esophageal sphincter, and the body of the stomach relax, while the pyloric antrum and duodenum contract. Forced inspiration follows, and sudden, powerful contraction of the diaphragm and abdominal muscles generates increased intragastric pressure that propels the gastric contents through the esophagus and pharynx into the mouth. Reflex elevation of the soft palate prevents the vomitus from entering the nasopharynx, and closure of the glottis prevents pulmonary aspiration.

Emesis is often preceded by nausea and profuse salivary secretion. Severe nausea may be accompanied by sweating, pallor of the skin, and dizziness.

50
Antacids and Antiulcer Drugs

Antacids

Sucralfate
Omeprazole
Bismuth subsalicylate

Misoprostol

Antiflatulents

Simethicone
Charcoal

The drugs reviewed in this chapter—antacids, other antiulcer drugs, and antiflatulents—represent the most widely used group of medications for the treatment of upper gastrointestinal (GI) disorders, ranging from mild indigestion and heartburn to peptic ulcer.

The principal action of antacids is to neutralize acidity, thus raising gastric pH. Increasing the pH results in progressive inhibition of the proteolytic activity of pepsin, thereby reducing its digestive action on the gastric mucosa. Consequently, antacids can reduce pain that results when mucosal nerve endings are activated by excessive gastric acid. They can also promote healing of damaged or ulcerated mucosa by protecting it from the destructive effects of pepsin.

The efficacy of antacids depends on many factors, most importantly their acid-neutralizing capacity, formulation, and dosage schedule. Among the commercially available antacid preparations, there is nearly a 20-fold difference in acid-neutralizing capacity. Sodium bicarbonate and calcium carbonate possess the greatest neutralizing capacity, whereas aluminum phosphate and magnesium trisilicate are considerably weaker.

It is important to recognize, however, that the most potent preparation may not always be the most suitable in terms of potential toxicity (diarrhea, constipation, hypercalcemia, systemic alkalosis), patient acceptance (taste, consistency), sodium content (danger in cardiovascular conditions), or cost. For example, persons with conditions such as edema, hypertension, or congestive heart failure, in which low salt intake is required, should be given antacid preparations containing little or no sodium such as Riopan Plus or Rolaids Sodium Free. Magnesium-containing antacids may cause central nervous system (CNS) toxicity in patients with renal failure and may intensify chronic diarrhea; thus they should be avoided in these conditions. Antacids containing aluminum require cautious use in the presence of constipation or gastric outlet obstruction because they may further reduce gastric emptying. Preparations containing calcium carbonate or sodium bicarbonate are indicated only for short-term therapy, because their side effects (eg, systemic alkalosis, rebound hyperacidity, milk–alkali syndrome) are significantly enhanced during prolonged treatment.

Aluminum-containing antacids bind phosphate ions in the intestine, causing accelerated elimination with the danger of hypophosphatemia. Clinical advantage is taken of this property in the use of aluminum carbonate gel for prevention of phosphatic urinary stones or in the management of hyperphosphatemia associated with advanced renal failure.

Product formulation (suspension, tablet, powder) may also be a determining factor in the effectiveness and acceptance of antacids—liquid suspensions generally providing the best neutralizing action. Dosage schedules should be based on the type and severity of the condition being treated; both the frequency and duration of therapy should be sufficient to provide maximum therapeutic benefit with minimal untoward reactions.

Failure of antacid therapy is frequently related to poor selection, inadequate dosage, or improper administration and can be avoided in most cases by judicious choice of an agent appropriate for both the patient and the condition. Selection of an appropriate antacid regimen requires consideration of many factors, and persons should be cautioned against indiscriminate use of these widely available and easily obtainable products.

Antacids are usually administered as one of the many available combination products, inasmuch as these products generally provide good acid-neutralizing activity with a reduced incidence of side effects as compared with the individual components themselves. A popular pairing of antacids is aluminum hydroxide and magnesium hydroxide, a mixture that reduces the occurrence of the constipation and diarrhea frequently observed with aluminum (constipation) and magnesium (diarrhea) alone.

Antacid drugs are discussed as a group, then listed individually in Table 50-1, in which the major uses and characteristics (including acid-neutralizing capacity [ANC], where established) of each drug are presented. Because most antacid preparations are combination products, the composition of the most commonly used combination products, including sodium content and ANC, is given in Table 50-2. Other antiulcer drugs discussed in this chapter include *sucralfate*, a sulfated sucrose–aluminum hydroxide complex that appears to form a protective barrier over the ulcerated area, *omeprazole*, an inhibitor of the proton-pump in gastric cellular membranes, and *bismuth subsalicylate*. In addition, *misoprostol*, a synthetic prostaglandin E derivative, is useful in preventing gastric ulceration resulting from use of nonsteroidal anti-inflammatory drugs and is also reviewed here. Finally, a discussion of simethicone, an antiflatulent drug used to relieve symptoms associated with excessive production of gas in the digestive tract, and charcoal, an adsorbent, are presented at the end of the chapter.

Several other classes of drugs have been employed in treating peptic ulcer disease and are discussed in previous chapters. Thus, anticholinergics may be found in Chapter 13, the histamine$_2$ receptor blockers, perhaps the most frequently employed antiulcer drugs, are reviewed in Chapter 16, and the tricyclic antidepressants are considered in Chapter 26.

Although the belief that most ulcers either result from or are exacerbated by excess secretion of gastric acid has been prevalent for many years, more recent evidence has implicated a bacterium as a major cause of peptic ulcer disease. *Helicobacter pylori*, a spiral-shaped organism found only in gastric epithelium, can be isolated in approximately 90% of patients with

(*text continues on page 523*)

Table 50-1. **Antacids**

Drug	Preparations	Sodium Content	Acid Neutralizing Capacity (mEq)	Usual Dosage Range	Nursing Considerations
Aluminum Carbonate Gel, Basic *Basaljel*	Suspension (equivalent to 400 mg of aluminum hydroxide per 5 mL)	0.58 mg/mL	14	*Antacid*: 2 capsules or tablets, or 2 tsp of regular suspension 4–8 times a day *Prevention of phosphate stones*: 2 capsules or tablets 1 h after meals and at bedtime *or* 1–2 tbsp suspension in water or juice 1 h after meals and at bedtime	Used as an antacid and for preventing development of urinary phosphate stones; exhibits strong phosphate-binding capacity, increasing fecal and decreasing urinary phosphate excretion; periodic determinations of serum electrolytes, especially calcium and phosphate, should be performed; low-phosphate diet is recommended; excessive doses can lead to phosphate depletion (weakness, tremors, bone pain, demineralization); be alert for signs of urinary infection (fever, chills, dysuria); high fluid intake should be maintained
	Capsules and swallow tablets (equivalent to 500 mg of aluminum hydroxide)	2.8 mg/capsule 2.8 mg/tablet	12 13		
Aluminum Hydroxide Gel *ALternaGEL, Alu-Cap, Alu-Tab, Amphojel, Dialume*	Suspension: 320 mg/5 mL	0.5 mg/mL	10	500–1800 mg 3–6 times/day between meals and at bedtime *Hypophosphatemia in children*: 50–150 mg/kg/24 h in divided doses every 4–6 h	Antacid with moderate acid-neutralizing capacity; does not produce acid rebound or alkalosis; possesses phosphate-binding capacity although to a lesser degree than aluminum carbonate; constipation is a frequent side effect; do *not* use for prolonged periods in patients with low-serum phosphate or those on a low-sodium diet
	Concentrated suspension: 600 mg/5 mL	0.5 mg/mL	16		
	Capsules: 475 mg, 500 mg	1 mg/capsule	10		
	Tablets: 300 mg, 600 mg	300 mg–1.8 g 600 mg–2.9 g	8 16		
Aluminum Phosphate Gel *Phosphaljel*	Suspension: 233 mg/5 mL	1.4 mg/mL		15–30 mL every 2 h between meals and at bedtime	No longer labeled for use as an antacid; only used to reduce fecal excretion of phosphates
Calcium Carbonate *Alka-Mints, Chooz, Dicarbosil, Tums, and various other manufacturers (CAN) Apo-Cal, Calcite*	Tablets: 650 mg, 1250 mg Chewable tablets—350 mg, 420 mg, 500 mg, 750 mg, 850 mg	Less than 2 mg/tablet	350 mg—7 500 mg—10 750 mg—15	0.5–1.5 g 3–6 times a day as needed	Very effective antacid, possessing high neutralizing capacity, rapid onset, and relatively prolonged duration of action; does not cause systemic alkalosis but is constipating and may elicit acid rebound and gastric hypersecretion; converted to calcium chloride by gastric acid, which may be absorbed in sufficient quantities to produce hypercalcemia with prolonged treatment; long-term use with foods high in vitamin D (eg, milk) may lead to milk–alkali syndrome (see Significant Adverse Reactions); contains 40% calcium; use with caution in persons receiving thiazide diuretics, which may reduce calcium excretion
	Liquid: 1 g/5 mL	Less than 1 mg/mL			

(continued)

Table 50-1. **Antacids (Continued)**

Drug	Preparations	Sodium Content	Acid Neutralizing Capacity (mEq)	Usual Dosage Range	Nursing Considerations
Dihydroxyaluminum Sodium Carbonate *Rolaids*	Chewable tablets: 334 mg	53 mg/tablet	7–8	1–2 tablets 3–6 times/day as needed	Converted to aluminum hydroxide in the presence of gastric acid, releasing carbon dioxide; gives rapid but transient neutralizing effect; because of high sodium content, use with caution in sodium-restricted patients
Magaldrate *Lowsium, Riopan*	Suspension: 540 mg/5 mL Tablets: 480 mg Chewable tablets: 480 mg Extra-strength liquid: 1,080 mg/5 mL	Less than 0.1 mg/5 mL Less than 0.1 mg/ tablet or chewable tablet Less than 0.3 mg/5 mL	13–14 13–14 30	480–1,080 mg between meals and at bedtime	A *chemical* combination of magnesium and aluminum hydroxides equivalent to 28%–39% magnesium oxide and 17%–25% aluminum oxide; has somewhat lower neutralizing capacity than a physical mixture of the two ingredients; does not elicit acid rebound or systemic acidosis; has a low incidence of diarrhea and constipation, and very low sodium content; available with simethicone as Riopan Plus
Magnesium Hydroxide *Milk of Magnesia*	Tablets: 325 mg Liquid: 390 mg/5 mL	0.1 mg/5 mL	10–14	*Antacid*: 5–15 mL *or* 2–4 tablets 4 times/day *Cathartic* Adults: 15–30 mL Children: 5–30 mL	Used as an antacid in small doses or as a cathartic in slightly higher doses; elicits prompt and sustained neutralization of gastric acid without marked acid rebound or systemic alkalosis; however, laxative action is commonly observed at higher doses, thus drug is often combined with aluminum or calcium antacids; also available as an emulsion containing mineral oil (Haley's MO); laxative dose should be given at bedtime, followed by a full glass of water (see Chap. 52)
Magnesium Oxide *Mag-Ox 400, Uro-Mag*	Tablets: 400 mg, 420 mg Capsules: 140 mg		21	400–840 mg daily	Slow-acting antacid with prolonged effects; high neutralizing capacity, but frequently elicits nausea and diarrhea; in large doses has been used as a cathartic
Sodium Bicarbonate *Bell/ans, Soda Mint*	Tablets: 325 mg, 520 mg, 650 mg	27% sodium		0.3–2 g as needed 1–4 times a day	Systemic, absorbable antacid, with a short duration of action; *its use should be discouraged* because it frequently elicits acid rebound, belching (owing to liberated carbon dioxide), and gastric distention and may cause systemic alkalosis; high sodium content precludes its use in patients with hypertension or cardiac or renal disease; large doses may cause phosphaturia

Table 50-2. **Antacid Combinations**

Trade Name	Dosage Form	Aluminum Hydroxide	Calcium Carbonate	Magnesium Oxide or Hydroxide	Simethicone	Other	Sodium Content	Acid Neutralizing Capacity (mEq)
Alka-Seltzer	Tablet					Sodium bicarbonate 958 mg; citric acid 832 mg; potassium bicarbonate 312 mg	311 mg/tablet	10–11
Alkets	Tablet		780 mg	65 mg		Magnesium carbonate 130 mg		
Almacone	Tablet	200 mg		200 mg	20 mg			
	Liquid	40 mg/mL		40 mg/mL	4 mg/mL		0.15 mg/mL	10
Almacone II	Liquid	80 mg/mL		80 mg/mL	6 mg/mL		0.3 mg/mL	20
Alma-Mag	Liquid	40 mg/mL		40 mg/mL	5 mg/mL			
Aludrox	Tablet	233 mg		83 mg			1.4 mg/tablet	10
	Liquid	61.4 mg/mL		20.6 mg/mL			0.46 mg/mL	12
Bromo Seltzer	Granules					Sodium bicarbonate 2.8 g/dose; citric acid 2.2 g/dose; acetaminophen 0.325 g/dose	0.75 g/dose	
Camalox	Liquid	45 mg/mL	50 mg/mL	40 mg/mL			0.24 mg/mL	18
Citrocarbonate	Effervescent powder					Sodium citrate 1.82 g and sodium bicarbonate 0.78 g per 3.9-g dose	700 mg/dose	
Di-Gel	Liquid	40 mg/mL		40 mg/mL	4 mg/mL		1 mg/mL	11
Di-Gel, Advanced	Tablet		280 mg	128 mg	20 mg			
ENO	Powder					Sodium tartrate 324 mg/g and sodium citrate 235 mg/g	104 mg/g	
Foamicon	Tablet	80 mg				Magnesium trisilicate 20 mg; plus alginic acid and calcium stearate		
Gaviscon	Tablet	80 mg				Magnesium trisilicate 20 mg plus alginic acid and sodium bicarbonate	19 mg/tablet	0.5
Gaviscon-2	Tablet	160 mg				Magnesium trisilicate 40 mg plus alginic acid and sodium bicarbonate	37 mg/tablet	
Gaviscon	Liquid	6.3 mg/mL				Magnesium carbonate 27.5 mg/mL plus alginic acid	2.6 mg/mL	1
Gaviscon Extra Strength	Tablet	160 mg				Magnesium carbonate 105 mg plus alginic acid and sodium bicarbonate	30 mg/tablet	5–7
	Liquid	51 mg/mL				Magnesium carbonate 48 mg/mL		
Gelusil	Tablet	200 mg		200 mg	25 mg		0.8 mg/tablet	11
	Liquid	40 mg/mL		40 mg/mL	5 mg/mL		0.14 mg/mL	12
Gelusil-II	Tablet	400 mg		400 mg	30 mg		2.1 mg/tablet	21
	Liquid	80 mg/mL		80 mg/mL	6 mg/mL		0.26 mg/mL	24
Gelusil-M	Tablet	300 mg		200 mg	25 mg		1.3 mg/tablet	12–13
	Liquid	60 mg/mL		40 mg/mL	5 mg/mL		0.24 mg/mL	15
Genaton	Tablet	80 mg				Magnesium trisilicate 20 mg; plus alginic acid and sodium bicarbonate		
Kudrox Double Strength	Liquid	100 mg/mL		90 mg/mL	8 mg/mL		0	20–25

(continued)

Table 50-2. **Antacid Combinations (Continued)**

Trade Name	Dosage Form	Aluminum Hydroxide	Calcium Carbonate	Magnesium Oxide or Hydroxide	Simethicone	Other	Sodium Content	Acid Neutralizing Capacity (mEq)
Kolantyl	Wafer	180 mg		170 mg			2 mg/tablet	10–11
	Liquid	30 mg/mL		30 mg/mL			< 1 mg/mL	10–11
Lowsium Plus	Tablet				20 mg	Magaldrate 480 mg		
	Liquid				4 mg/mL	Magaldrate 96 mg/mL		
Maalox	Liquid	45 mg/mL		40 mg/mL			0.27 mg/mL	13–14
Maalox HRF	Liquid	28 mg/mL				Magnesium carbonate 35 mg/mL		
Maalox	Tablet	200 mg		200 mg			0.7 mg/tablet	9–10
Maalox Extra Strength	Tablet	400 mg		400 mg			1.4 mg/tablet	18
Maalox TC	Liquid	120 mg/mL		60 mg/mL			0.16 mg/mL	28
	Tablet	600 mg		300 mg			0.5 mg/tablet	28
Maalox Plus	Tablet	200 mg		200 mg	25 mg		0.8 mg/tablet	11–12
	Liquid	45 mg/mL		40 mg/mL	5 mg/mL		0.26 mg/mL	13–14
Maalox Plus Extra Strength	Liquid	100 mg/mL		90 mg/mL	8 mg/mL		0	
Magnatril	Tablet	260 mg		130 mg		Magnesium trisilicate 455 mg		
	Liquid	52 mg/mL		26 mg/mL		Magnesium trisilicate 52 mg/mL		
Marblen	Tablet		520 mg			Magnesium carbonate 400 mg	3.2 mg/tablet	18
	Liquid		104 mg/mL			Magnesium carbonate 80 mg/mL	0.6 mg/mL	18
Mylanta	Tablet	200 mg		200 mg	20 mg		0.77 mg/tablet	11–12
	Liquid	40 mg/mL		40 mg/mL	4 mg/mL		0.14 mg/mL	12–13
Mylanta Double Strength	Tablet	400 mg		400 mg	40 mg		1.3 mg/tablet	23
	Liquid	80 mg/mL		80 mg/mL	8 mg/mL		0.23 mg/mL	25–26
Mylanta Gelcaps	Tablet		311 mg			Magnesium carbonate 232 mg		
Riopan Plus	Tablet				20 mg	Magaldrate 480 mg	0.1 mg/tablet	13–14
	Liquid				4 mg/mL	Magaldrate 180 mg/mL	< 0.02 mg/mL	15
Riopan Plus 2	Liquid				6 mg/mL	Magaldrate 216 mg/mL	< 0.06 mg/mL	30
	Tablet				20 mg	Magaldrate 1080 mg	0.1 mg/tablet	30
Rulox No. 1	Tablet	200 mg		200 mg				
Rulox No. 2	Tablet	400 mg		400 mg				
Rulox	Liquid	45 mg/mL		40 mg/mL			0.16 mg/mL	12
Tempo	Tablet	133 mg	414 mg	81 mg	20 mg		2.5 mg/tablet	14
Titralac	Tablet		420 mg			Glycine 150 mg	< 0.3 mg/tablet	7–8
Titralac Plus	Liquid		100 mg/mL		4 mg/mL		0	11
Tums Plus	Tablet		500 mg		20 mg		< 2 mg	
Win-Gel	Tablet	180 mg		160 mg			2.5 mg/tablet	12
	Liquid	36 mg/mL		32 mg/mL			0.5 mg/mL	11–12

duodenal or gastric ulcers and has been strongly implicated not only in the development of ulcers but also in their frequent recurrence. Eradication of the organism from the gastrointestinal tract by use of antibiotic therapy has been shown not only to improve healing rates of ulcers but, perhaps more importantly, to significantly decrease ulcer recurrence rates. Current treatment recommendations for *Helicobacter pylori* infections consist of a 2-week course of therapy with tetracycline (500 mg 4 times a day), metronidazole (250–500 mg 3 times a day) and bismuth subsalicylate (2 tablets or tablespoonfuls 4 times a day). Amoxicillin may be substituted for tetracycline in similar doses and some clinicians prefer to add the acid-secreting blockers ranitidine or prilosec to the above regimen. Eradication of the organism from the gastric epithelium is difficult, and combination therapy, as outlined above, seems to provide the most effective results.

Antacids

- **Aluminum carbonate**
- **Aluminum hydroxide**
- **Aluminum phosphate**
- **Calcium carbonate**
- **Dihydroxyaluminum sodium carbonate**
- **Magaldrate**
- **Magnesium hydroxide**
- **Magnesium oxide**
- **Sodium bicarbonate**

Mechanism

Neutralize gastric acidity and usually elevate gastric pH above 3 to 4; proteolytic activity of pepsin on gastric mucosa is suppressed above pH 4 and totally abolished above pH 7 to 8; elevated pH also induces the pyloric antrum to release gastrin; acid neutralization may increase lower esophageal sphincter tone; antacids do not appear to "coat" the mucosal barrier but can bind bile acids (especially the aluminum products), although the contribution of this latter action to the therapeutic effects of the drugs is unclear.

Uses

Symptomatic treatment of GI symptoms associated with hyperacidity (eg, heartburn, acid indigestion)
Treatment of hyperacidity associated with gastritis, peptic ulcer, hiatal hernia, esophagitis
Prophylaxis of GI bleeding or stress ulcers
Reduction of phosphate absorption in hyperphosphatemia and chronic renal failure (investigational use for aluminum hydroxide and aluminum carbonate)

Dosage

See Table 50-1.

Fate

Most preparations (except sodium bicarbonate) are not appreciably absorbed from the GI tract and are excreted largely in the feces. Calcium and magnesium products can form chloride salts by reaction with hydrochloric acid, which may be partly absorbed and require elimination by the kidneys. The presence of food can prolong the action of antacids. Thus, antacids taken on an empty stomach have a duration of action of 30 minutes, whereas if they are taken 1 hour after meals, their duration is approximately 3 hours.

Common Side Effects

Diarrhea (magnesium products), constipation (aluminum and calcium products)

Significant Adverse Reactions

Aluminum: intestinal impaction, phosphate depletion (anorexia, weakness, impaired reflexes, depression, tremors, bone pain, osteomalacia)
Magnesium: profound diarrhea, dehydration, hypermagnesemia (nausea, vomiting, impaired reflexes, hypotension, respiratory depression—high risk in patients with impaired renal function), bradyarrhythmias, renal stones (magnesium trisilicate)
Calcium carbonate: rebound hyperacidity, milk–alkali syndrome (metabolic alkalosis, hypercalcemia, vomiting, confusion, headache, renal insufficiency), renal calculi, neurologic impairment, GI hemorrhage, fecal impaction
Sodium bicarbonate: systemic alkalosis, sodium overload, milk–alkali syndrome, rebound hypersecretion

Contraindications

Depend on individual product (see Table 50-1). *Cautious use* of magnesium-containing products in renal insufficiency and of aluminum-containing products in gastric outlet obstruction. Products high in sodium (see Tables 50-1 and 50-2) must be used cautiously in hypertension, congestive heart failure, and in persons on sodium-restricted diets.

Interactions

CAUTION

Because of the adsorptive capacity of most antacids and their ability to alter gastric pH, other drugs should not be administered within 1 to 2 hours of antacid ingestion, if possible.

Antacids (especially magnesium–aluminum combinations) can impair the absorption of tetracyclines, digoxin, phenothiazines, indomethacin, phenylbutazone, isoniazid, benzodiazepines, captopril, chloroquine, cimetidine, valproic acid, corticosteroids, phenytoin, oral iron products, salicylates, and many other drugs.
Antacids can increase the effects of pseudoephedrine, levodopa, and meperidine by *facilitating* their intestinal absorption, and can enhance the effects of amphetamines and quinidine by decreasing their urinary excretion.

Nursing Management

Refer to Table 50-1 for specific information on each drug.

Pretherapy Assessment

Assess and record baseline data necessary for detection of adverse effects of antacids: General: vital signs (VS), body weight, skin color and temperature; CNS: affect, orientation; cardiovascular system (CVS): peripheral perfusion; GI: abdominal examination, bowel sounds; Lab: serum electrolytes, phosphorus, fluoride.
Review medical history and documents for existing or previous conditions that:
a. require cautious use of antacids: magnesium-con-

taining products in renal insufficiency; aluminum-containing products in gastric outlet obstruction; products high in sodium (see Tables 50-1 and 50-2) must be used cautiously in hypertension, congestive heart failure, and in persons on sodium-restricted diets

b. contraindicate use of antacids: depends on constituents of each product; **pregnancy (Category C)**, lactation (safety not established, do not use in nursing mothers)

Nursing Interventions

Medication Administration

Administer drug hourly for the first 2 weeks when used in the treatment of acute peptic ulcer; during the healing stage, administer 1 to 3 hours after meals and at bedtime.

Do not administer oral drugs within 1 to 2 hours of antacid administration.

Have patient chew drug thoroughly before swallowing; follow with a glass of water.

Surveillance During Therapy

Carefully monitor laboratory studies and patient for indications of adverse reactions.

Interpret results of diagnostic tests and contact practitioner as appropriate.

Monitor for possible drug–drug and drug–nutrient interactions: Refer to **Interactions**.

Patient Teaching

Inform patient that the efficacy of liquid antacid is significantly greater than that of tablets or capsules. If drug is taken in tablet form, instruct patient to chew *thoroughly* before swallowing and to drink a small amount of water afterward.

Explain that antacid is optimally effective during long-term therapy if administered 1 to 3 hours after meals and at bedtime. Food acts as a buffer to gastric acid for approximately 60 minutes, and the presence of food can enhance the action of antacids. Thus, the duration of action of antacids taken on an empty stomach is 30 minutes, whereas it is approximately 3 hours if they are taken 1 hour after meals.

Urge patient to report GI pain that persists longer than 72 hours or the presence of tarry stools because these symptoms may indicate ulcer perforation, gastric hemorrhage, or other serious complications.

Inform patient that diarrhea or constipation may occur, depending on particular antacid used, and should be treated early.

Advise patient on restricted or low-sodium diet (eg, for hypertension, congestive heart failure, edema, pregnancy) that a low-sodium preparation should be used.

Warn patient with significant renal impairment that magnesium- or calcium-containing products are contraindicated because hypermagnesemia and hypercalcemia can occur. Refer to **Significant Adverse Reactions** for symptoms.

Explain that milk has no antacid properties and may increase acid production.

Instruct patient to avoid coffee, other caffeine-containing beverages, and alcohol. The value of bland diets, other than during the acute symptomatic period, is unproven. A *reasonable* diet is far more acceptable than a bland diet, and compliance is accordingly better.

Suggest small, frequent meals or snacks. They may be tolerated better than larger meals consumed twice a day, and they result in less gastric acid secretion.

• Sucralfate

Carafate

(CAN) Sulcrate

Sucralfate is a complex of sulfated sucrose and aluminum hydroxide used orally for the short-term treatment of duodenal ulcers. Because it is not absorbed from the GI tract, it is virtually free of systemic side effects. It requires an acidic environment for optimal activity, so it should not be administered simultaneously with antacids or H_2 antagonists, because its effectiveness may be somewhat reduced.

Mechanism

Not completely established; possible actions include formation of an ulcer-adherent complex with exudative material at the ulcer site, thus protecting the ulcerated area from further attack by acid, pepsin, and bile salts; may also inhibit activity of pepsin; does not appear to neutralize gastric acid

Uses

Short-term (ie, up to 8 weeks) treatment of duodenal ulcers

Maintenance therapy of duodenal ulcer

Other uses can include treatment and prophylaxis of gastric ulcers, treatment of reflux esophagitis, treatment of nonsteroidal anti-inflammatory drug-induced mucosal damage, and prevention of stress ulcers.

Dosage

1 g (1 tablet) 4 times a day on an empty stomach for 4 to 8 weeks

Maintenance therapy: 1 g twice a day

Fate

Minimally absorbed from GI tract and eliminated primarily in the feces; absorbed fraction is excreted principally in the urine

Common Side Effect

Constipation

Significant Adverse Reactions

(Rare) Diarrhea, nausea, GI distress, indigestion, dry mouth, rash, pruritus, dizziness, vertigo, sleepiness

Interactions

Sucralfate may reduce GI absorption of tetracyclines, theophylline, cimetidine, digoxin, phenytoin, ranitidine, and probably many other drugs if given concurrently.

Nursing Management

Pretherapy Assessment

Assess and record baseline data necessary for detection of adverse effects of sucralfate: General: VS, body weight, skin color and temperature; CNS: affect, orientation; GI: abdominal examination, bowel sounds

Review medical history and documents for existing or previous conditions that:

a. require cautious use of sucralfate: chronic renal failure, dialysis

b. contraindicate use of sucralfate: allergy to sucralfate; **pregnancy (Category B)**, lactation (safety not established, do not use in nursing mothers)

Nursing Interventions

Medication Administration

Administer drug on an empty stomach, 1 hour before or 2 hours after meals and at bedtime.

Administer antacids between sulcralfate doses, not within a ½-hour of the sucralfate dose.

Provide small, frequent meals if GI upset occurs.

Surveillance During Therapy

Monitor bowel function, provide corrective measures for constipation.

Interpret results of diagnostic tests and contact practitioner as appropriate.

Monitor for possible drug–drug and drug–nutrient interactions: Refer to **Interactions**.

Patient Teaching

Inform patient that sucralfate tablets should be taken at least 1 hour before meals and at bedtime to obtain maximal benefit.

Advise patient that antacids may be used to control pain, but they should not be used within ½-hour of sucralfate.

• Omeprazole

Prilosec

(CAN) Losec

Mechanism

Inhibits the H^+/K^+ adenosine triphosphatase (ATPase) enzyme system in the membranes of gastric parietal cells, thereby blocking the final step in gastric acid production; decreases both basal and stimulated gastric acid secretion. The drug does not exhibit anticholinergic or antihistaminic activity, nor affect pepsin output; however, when gastric pH is elevated above 4, pepsin activity is reduced.

Uses

Short-term (4–8 weeks) treatment of active duodenal ulcer, severe erosive esophagitis and gastroesophageal reflux disease (GERD)

Treatment of pathological hypersecretory conditions

Dosage

Duodenal ulcer, esophagitis, GERD: 20 mg daily for 4 to 8 weeks

Pathologic hypersecretory conditions: initially, 60 mg once daily; up to 120 mg 3 times a day have been used

Fate

Absorption is rapid, with peak plasma levels in 1 to 3 hours. Onset of action occurs within 1 hour. Plasma half-life ($T_{1/2}$) is less than 1 hour, but antisecretory effect persists for up to 72 hours because of prolonged binding to ATPase enzyme. Maximum inhibitory effect on acid secretion is attained within 4 days. Protein binding is approximately 95%. Most of a dose is excreted in the urine as several metabolites.

Common Side Effects

Headache, diarrhea, abdominal pain

Significant Adverse Reactions

Nausea, vomiting, dizziness, cough, rash, back pain, flatulence

CAUTION

Long-term studies in animals have demonstrated a dose-related increase in gastric carcinoid tumors; while human studies await final results, omeprazole should be prescribed only for the indications listed above and only in the dosages and for the durations listed.

Contraindications

No absolute contraindications. *Cautious use* in patients with liver impairment, and in the elderly, young children, and pregnant or nursing mothers.

Interactions

Omeprazole may prolong the $T_{1/2}$ of diazepam, phenytoin, and warfarin, increasing the effects.

Omeprazole can decrease the oral absorption of other drugs that depend on a low gastric pH for adequate absorption (eg, iron salts, ampicillin, ketoconazole).

Nursing Management

Pretherapy Assessment

Assess and record baseline data necessary for detection of adverse effects of omeprazole: General: VS, body weight, skin color and temperature; CNS: affect, reflexes; GI: abdominal examination, bowel sounds.

Review medical history and documents for existing or previous conditions that:

a. require cautious use of omeprazole: liver impairment; use in the elderly, young children

b. contraindicate use of omeprazole: allergy to omeprazole; **pregnancy (Category C)**, lactation (safety not established, do not use in nursing mothers)

Nursing Interventions

Medication Administration

Administer drug on an empty stomach before meals; caution patient not to open, chew, or crush capsules.

Administer antacids concomitant with omeprazole doses.

Provide small, frequent meals if GI upset occurs.

Surveillance During Therapy

Monitor bowel function, provide corrective measures for constipation.

Carefully monitor laboratory studies and patient for indications of adverse reactions.

Interpret results of diagnostic tests and contact practitioner as appropriate.

Monitor for possible drug–drug and drug–nutrient interactions: Refer to **Interactions**.

Patient Teaching

Inform patient that drug should be taken before meals.
Advise patient that antacids may be used to control pain.

• Bismuth subsalicylate

Bismatrol, Pepto-Bismol

Although usually classed as an antidiarrheal agent, bismuth subsalicylate does have both antisecretory and antimicrobial effects as well as GI adsorptive and coating properties. It is commonly used for indigestion, nausea, and control of diarrhea, including "traveler's diarrhea." Of recent interest has been the finding that many peptic ulcers may be caused by a bacterium, (*Helicobacter pylori*), found in the gastric mucosa of ulcer patients. Bismuth subsalicylate, administered together with antibiotics (eg, tetracycline, metronidazole, amoxicillin) in a dosage regimen as outlined in the introduction to this chapter is effective in eradicating *Helicobacter pylori* from the GI tract and in decreasing the likelihood of ulcer recurrence. Its use as an antidiarrheal drug is considered further in Chapter 53.

• Misoprostol *(Pregnancy Category X)*

Cytotec

Misoprostol is a synthetic prostaglandin E_1 analogue that possesses both an acid antisecretory as well as a mucosal cytoprotective effect in the stomach. It increases mucus and bicarbonate production while inhibiting basal and nocturnal acid secretion. Misoprostol is used orally for preventing gastric ulceration resulting from administration of nonsteroidal anti-inflammatory agents, including aspirin. The drug is taken 4 times a day for the duration of nonsteroidal drug therapy. In addition, the drug may also be useful in treating duodenal ulcers unresponsive to conventional antiulcer therapy, such as histamine-2 antagonists; however, it does not appear to *prevent* non–steroidal-induced duodenal ulcers. The drug is contraindicated in pregnant women and women of childbearing potential because of its strong uterine spasmogenic action, which can lead to increased uterine bleeding and miscarriage. The most frequent side effects are diarrhea, abdominal pain, headache, nausea, and flatulence.

Antiflatulents

Drugs used to reduce the symptoms resulting from excess production of gas in the GI tract are termed *antiflatulents*. Simethicone is a silicone derivative commonly found in combination with antacids (see Table 50-2), although it is also available alone in tablet and liquid form. Charcoal is an adsorbent used as tablets or capsules for a variety of indications, including the relief of indigestion and bloating resulting from accumulation of intestinal gas.

• Simethicone

Gas-X, Mylicon, Phazyme, and others

(CAN) Ovol

Mechanism

Alters the surface tension of gas bubbles, causing coalescence of the gas, thereby facilitating its elimination by belching or flatus

Uses

Adjunctive treatment of conditions associated with retention of excessive gas (eg, dyspepsia, peptic ulcer, spastic colon, diverticulitis, or postoperative gaseous retention)

Dosage

Capsules or tablets: 40 to 125 mg 4 times a day
Drops: 40 mg 4 times a day

Nursing Management

Nursing Interventions

Patient Teaching

Inform patient that drug should be taken after each meal and at bedtime. Tablets should be chewed thoroughly because complete particle dispersion facilitates the antiflatulent action.
Advise patient to consult healthcare provider if symptoms are not relieved within several days because continual passage of gas may indicate a more serious underlying condition.

• Charcoal

CharcoCaps

Mechanism

Absorbs toxins and gas onto surface of carbon particles, thereby relieving cramping, diarrhea, and flatulence

Uses

Temporary relief of indigestion, bloating, cramping, and flatulence
Prevention of nonspecific pruritus associated with kidney dialysis treatment

NOTE: Refer also to **Activated Charcoal**, Chapter 81, as an antidote; charcoal may be "activated" by exposing it to an oxidizing gas at high temperatures; this activated product is used as a powder or suspension for emergency treatment of poisoning with many drugs and other chemicals.

Dosage

520 mg (2 capsules) 3 or 4 times a day; repeat as needed up to 4.16 g daily.

Interactions

Charcoal can adsorb other drugs it comes into contact with in the GI tract, thereby interfering with their absorption; administer 2 hours before or 1 hour after other drugs.

Nursing Management

Nursing Interventions

Patient Teaching

Warn patient not to take for more than 3 days and to use only when condition is acute. Charcoal can absorb nutrients, digestive enzymes, and other essential substances.

Instruct parent(s) or guardian(s) to administer to children younger than 3 years of age only if directed by a healthcare provider.

Selected Bibliography

Axon AT: Helicobacter pylori therapy: Effect on peptic ulcer disease. J Gastroenterol Hepatol 6(2):131, 1991

Cave DR: Therapeutic approaches to recurrent peptic ulcer disease. Hosp Pract 27(9A):33, 43, 47, 1992

Hixson LJ, Kelley CL, Jones WN, Tuohy CD: Current trends in the pharmacotherapy for peptic ulcer disease. Arch Intern Med 152(4): 726, 1992

Hunt RH: Treatment of peptic ulcer disease with sucralfate: A review. Am J Med 91(2A):102S, 1991

Pajares JM, Carballo F, Blanco M: Treatment of peptic ulcer disease: Is *Helicobacter pylori* a consideration. Hepato-Gastroenterol 39(suppl 1)1:40, 1992

Peterson WL: *Helicobacter pylori* and peptic ulcer disease. N Engl J Med 324:1043, 1991

Walt RP, Langman MJ: Antacids and ulcer healing: A review of the evidence. Drugs 42(2):205, 1991

Ziller SA, Netchvolodoff CV: Uncomplicated peptic ulcer disease. An overview of formation and treatment principles. Postgrad Med 93(4):126, 131, 137, 1993

Nursing Bibliography

Bezzarro E: Changing perspectives of H_2 antagonists for stress ulcer prophylaxis. Critical Care Nursing Clinics of North America 5(2):325, 1993

Bozymski E: Pathophysiology and diagnosis of gastroesophageal reflux disease. Am J Hosp Pharm 50:107, 1993

Keithley J: Histamine H_2-receptor antagonists. Nurs Clin North Am 26(2):361, 1991

Mamel J: Clinical pharmacology of commonly used drugs in G.I. practice. Part 2. Gastroenterology Nurse 4:156, 1993

Prevost S, et al: Stress ulceration in the critically ill patient. Critical Care Nursing Clinics of North America 5(1):163, 1993

Quillen T: Myths and facts . . . about peptic ulcers. Nursing '93 23(5): 111, 1993

Schentag J, Goss T: Pharmacokinetics and pharmacodynamics of acid-suppressive agents in patients with gastroesophageal reflux disease. Am J Hosp Pharm 50:34, 1993

Soll A: Confronting and combating NSAID-induced ulceritis. Consultant 33(2):45, 1993

51

Digestants and Gallstone-Solubilizing Agents

Dehydrocholic acid
Glutamic acid
Pancreatin
Pancrelipase

Chenodiol
Monoctanoin
Ursodiol

Digestants are substances that assist the physiologic process of food digestion in the gastrointestinal (GI) tract. The major endogenous digestive enzymes, along with their source and action, are listed in Table 49-4, Chapter 49. The usefulness of most enzymes (eg, amylase, lipase, protease, cellulose) as *exogenous* digestive aids is probably greatly overstated, inasmuch as symptoms of GI distress can rarely be attributed to an actual deficiency of endogenous digestive chemicals. Nevertheless, certain digestive substances, especially the pancreatic enzymes pancreatin and pancrelipase, have proved valuable as replacement therapy in elderly or debilitated persons or in persons with conditions such as GI surgery, achlorhydria, chronic pancreatitis, or gastric carcinoma, in whom there exists a definite lack of one or more of these digestive substances. In such cases, however, the deficient chemicals must be replaced in sufficient amounts to restore digestive activity, and it should be recognized that many commercially available products contain amounts *too small* to provide the required quantity of digestant. Thus, empiric use of combination or "shotgun" digestive products has no place in rational pharmacotherapy. Moreover, the inclusion of anticholinergics, antihistamines, or barbiturates in these formulations merely increases the likelihood of untoward reactions.

The digestive aids most frequently employed clinically may be grouped as follows:

- Gastric acidifiers (eg, glutamic acid hydrochloride)
- Digestive enzymes (eg, pepsin, pancreatin, pancrelipase)
- Bile salts and bile acids (eg, dehydrocholic acid)

Gastric hydrochloric acid deficiency (*achlorhydria*) can occur in association with various pathologic conditions such as pernicious anemia or gastric carcinoma, as well as in the absence of observable disease. Dilute solutions (10%) of hydrochloric acid were previously used to aid digestion in patients with achlorhydria and to relieve complaints such as belching, nausea, and epigastric distress. Today, glutamic acid hydrochloride is used as a source of hydrochloric acid, because it it available in capsule form and offers a safer and more convenient mode of therapy. However, glutamic acid does not yield as much free acid as does hydrochloric acid.

Pepsin is a proteolytic enzyme activated by gastric acid, and thus it is sometimes administered with glutamic acid to stimulate digestion. It is of doubtful benefit in most instances, because absolute lack of pepsin is relatively rare, except perhaps in gastric carcinoma and occasionally in pernicious anemia, and the acid deficiency is usually of far greater consequence. Conversely, deficiency of pancreatic enzymes is a frequent occurrence, especially in cases of pancreatitis and duct obstruction, and of course following pancreatectomy. In these instances, replacement therapy with either pancreatin, a powdered concentrate of bovine, porcine, or vegetable origin containing amylase, lipase, and protease activity, or pancrelipase, a more concentrated mixture of pancreatic enzymes of porcine origin, is indicated.

Natural bile contains a series of organic acids, secreted as sodium salts, that lower the surface tension of fat globules, breaking them into small droplets. Bile further aids fat digestion by stimulation of pancreatic secretions and activation of pancreatic lipase. Exogenous bile salts (eg, ox bile extract) have previously been used as replacement therapy in patients with partial biliary obstruction or after removal of the gallbladder (cholecystectomy), but their effectiveness was minimal and they have been removed from the market. Bile salts also exhibit a choleretic action; that is, they stimulate the outflow of bile. Certain bile salts, especially the synthetic derivative dehydrocholic acid, markedly increase the output of a thin, watery bile and are termed *hydrocholeretics*. Dehydrocholic acid may be used to facilitate flushing and drainage of partially obstructed bile ducts, thereby minimizing infections and preventing biliary calculi from lodging in the duct.

Several drugs that have become available in recent years can solubilize recently formed gallstones. They are indicated for the dissolution of radiolucent, noncalcified gallstones in patients in whom elective surgery may prove hazardous. These gallstone-solubilizing drugs are reviewed in this chapter.

Hydrocholeretics

• *Dehydrocholic acid*

Cholan-HMB, Decholin

(CAN) Dycholium

Dehydrocholic acid, a semisynthetic derivative of cholic acid, is termed a hydrocholeretic agent because its principal pharmacologic action is to increase the volume of dilute bile output without markedly altering the amount of solid bile constituents. It can be used to facilitate biliary tract drainage in cases of biliary stasis and may also be employed for temporary relief of constipation (maximum duration of therapy is 1 week). Recommended dosage is 250 to 500 mg 3 times a day after meals. A bowel movement normally ensues within 6 to 12 hours.

Adverse reactions are rare at recommended oral doses, although diarrhea and hypersensitivity reactions have been reported. Contraindications include jaundice, severe hepatitis, advanced cirrhosis, cholelithiasis, and complete obstruction of the common or hepatic bile ducts or GI or urinary tract. The use of dehydrocholic acid as an adjunct to diuretics, or when abdominal pain, nausea, or vomiting is present should also be avoided.

Gastric Acidifiers

• *Glutamic Acid HCl*

Glutamic acid hydrochloride is a source of hydrochloric acid that may aid digestion in conditions associated with reduced (hypoacidity) or absent (achlorhydria) gastric acid. It is used as a hydrochloride salt of glutamic acid in capsule form that releases hydrochloric acid in the stomach, thus minimizing oral mucosal irritation and damage to dental enamel. Hydrochloric acid facilitates conversion of pepsinogen to pepsin and provides an optimal pH for the action of pepsin. It also stimulates pancreatic secretions and neutralizes bicarbonates in gastrointestinal fluid, helping to maintain electrolyte balance. Increased acidity may also inhibit growth of putrefactive organisms in ingested food. Recommended dosage is 1 to 3 capsules (340 mg each) 3 times a day before meals. Occasional GI irritation can occur and overdosage may lead to systemic acidosis. The drug is contraindicated in gastric hyperacidity states and peptic ulcer.

Patients should be instructed to prevent the capsules from becoming wet because hydrochloric acid is released on contact with water.

Pancreatic Enzymes

• *Pancreatin*

Dizymes, Donnazyme, Entozyme, Hi-Vegi-Lip, Pancrezyme 4X

• *Pancrelipase*

Cotazym, Ilozyme, Ku-Zyme HP, Pancrease, Ultrase, Viokase, Zymase

Mechanism

Pancreatic enzyme concentrates of bovine or porcine origin containing lipase, protease, and amylase activity; provide enzymatic activity necessary to assist in the digestion of carbohydrates, fats, and proteins; exert their primary effects in the duodenum and upper jejunum; pancrelipase has greater lipase activity than does pancreatin and can be used in lower doses to control steatorrhea (refer to **Uses** below).

Uses

Replacement therapy in pancreatic enzyme deficiency states, such as chronic pancreatitis or pancreatic insufficiency, steatorrhea of malabsorption syndrome, cystic fibrosis, postgastrectomy, or postpancreatectomy

Test for pancreatic function, especially in pancreatic insufficiency attributable to chronic pancreatitis

Dosage

NOTE: Tablets, capsules, and powder packets of different manufacturers contain different amounts of lipase, protease, and amylase.

Pancreatin: 1 to 2 tablets (600–45,000 U lipase activity) with meals or snacks;

Pancrelipase: 1 to 2 tablets or capsules (4,000–48,000 U lipase activity) before or with meals or snacks

Significant Adverse Reactions

(Usually with high doses) Nausea, diarrhea, cramping, vomiting, anorexia, hypersensitivity reactions (sneezing, rash, lacrimation), perianal irritation

Contraindications

Hypersensitivity to beef or pork products, acute pancreatitis. *Cautious use* in patients with asthma (attacks may be precipitated), hyperuricemia and in pregnant or nursing mothers.

Interactions

Pancreatic enzymes may retard the absorption of orally ingested iron.

Availability of pancreatin in the duodenum may be enhanced by histamine$_2$ antagonists (see Chapter 16).

Antacids containing magnesium hydroxide or calcium carbonate may reduce the effects of the enzymes.

Nursing Management

Nursing Interventions

Medication Administration

Rule out previous hypersensitivity to beef or pork products before administering pancreatic enzymes because they are derived from either bovine or porcine sources.

Evaluate patient's response to drug by noting appearance of stools, monitoring weight, and checking results of periodically determined fecal fat and nitrogen.

Patient Teaching

Instruct patient to take drug with meals. Enteric-coated tablets should be swallowed whole. Powder or granules may be added to milk or water or sprinkled on food.

Refer patient for dietary consultation as needed to ensure that intake of starch, protein, and fat is balanced during therapy to minimize indigestion.

Inform patient that supplemental antacid may be used to control refractory steatorrhea. Antacid should not, however, be taken within 1 hour of pancreatic medication (refer to **Interactions**).

Gallstone-Solubilizing Agents

When cholesterol is present in bile in concentrations that exceed the capacity of bile acids and lecithin to solubilize it, crystals can precipitate and eventually coalesce into gallstones. Dissolution of these gallstones can now be effected in several ways by a number of drugs. The clinically available gallstone-solubilizing agents are considered individually below.

• Chenodiol (Chenodeoxycholic acid)

(Pregnancy Category X)

Chenix

Mechanism

Blocks hepatic synthesis of cholesterol and cholic acid, thereby reducing biliary cholesterol levels and gradually dissolving radiolucent cholesterol gallstones; drug has no apparent effect on radiopaque, calcified gallstones or on bile pigment stones; likelihood of stone dissolution decreases as the size and number of stones increase. Stones have recurred in approximately 50% of patients within 5 years. Retreatment with chenodiol has proved effective in dissolving newly reformed stones, but the long-term toxic effects of repeated therapy remain to be established.

Uses

Treatment of patients with radiolucent gallstones in well-opacified gallbladders, in whom surgery is not feasible because of age or presence of systemic disease

Dosage

Initially 250 mg twice a day for 2 weeks; increase by 250 mg/day each week thereafter until the recommended dose (ie, 13–16 mg/kg/day) or the maximally tolerated dose is attained

CAUTION

Doses less than 10 mg/kg/day are usually ineffective and may be associated with an *increased* risk that cholecystectomy will be necessary.

Fate

Well absorbed orally but undergoes extensive first-pass hepatic clearance; converted in the colon to lithocholic acid, which is excreted largely (80%) in the feces; the remainder is absorbed and metabolized in the liver; in patients unable to form hepatic sulfate conjugates of lithocholic acid, liver toxicity can occur; fecal bile acids are increased threefold to fourfold.

Common Side Effects

Diarrhea, elevated serum aminotransferase, biliary pain

Significant Adverse Reactions

Abdominal cramping, nausea, vomiting, anorexia, elevated serum cholesterol and high-density lipoprotein (HDL), decreased white cell count

Contraindications

Intrahepatic cholestasis, primary biliary cirrhosis, sclerosing cholangitis, radiopaque bile pigment stones, acute cholecystitis, gallstone pancreatitis, biliary GI fistula, and pregnancy

Interactions

Bile acid sequestering agents (cholestyramine, colestipol) and aluminum-based antacids may reduce absorption of chenodeoxycholic acid.

Estrogens, oral contraceptives, clofibrate, and other lipid-lowering drugs may decrease the effectiveness of chenodeoxycholic acid by increasing biliary cholesterol secretion.

Nursing Management

Nursing Interventions

Surveillance During Therapy

Monitor results of serum aminotransferase determinations, which should be performed frequently during therapy. If serum alanine aminotransferase (ALT) levels increase to over 3 times the upper limit of normal, the drug should be discontinued. If levels increase to 1.5 to 3 times the limit, the drug should be stopped temporarily and resumed only after levels return to normal. Enzyme levels return to normal after drug discontinuation.

Patient Teaching

Supportively discuss the possibility of fetal damage if a female patient becomes pregnant while taking the drug. The drug is a potential teratogen and should not be used by a woman who is or is likely to become pregnant.

Inform patient that serum cholesterol levels are usually monitored at 4- to 6-month intervals because the drug should be discontinued if levels increase to above the age-adjusted limit.

Instruct patient to report persistent or severe diarrhea. A temporary dosage reduction may be needed to alleviate it.

Inform patient that a prophylactic dosage has not been established. Stones have recurred on dosages as high as 500 mg/day; therefore, the drug is usually discontinued after stones have dissolved. Serial cholecystograms should be performed to monitor for recurrence, which occurs in approximately 50% of patients within 5 years.

Encourage patient to maintain low cholesterol, low carbohydrate diet after stone dissolution and to reduce weight to minimize stone recurrence.

Explain that the likelihood of successful therapy is greatly reduced if partial stone dissolution is not evident within 9 to 12 months. Treatment will probably be discontinued if there is no response after 15 to 18 months.

• Monoctanoin

Moctanin

Monoctanoin is a semisynthetic esterified glycerol that acts as a solubilizing agent for cholesterol gallstones in the biliary tract. Treatment with monoctanoin results in complete stone dissolution in approximately one third of patients, especially those with single stones. Another one third of patients show reduction in stone size, and approximately one third of patients are not benefited.

Mechanism

Acts as a solubilizing agent for cholesterol stones when perfused through the common bile duct; complete dissolution is most often achieved when a single stone is present

Uses

Solubilization of radiolucent gallstones in the biliary tract following cholecystectomy, when other means of removal are inappropriate

Dosage

NOTE: Drug is administered as a continuous perfusion through a catheter inserted into the common bile duct or through a T-tube or nasobiliary tube.

3 to 5 mL per hour infused continuously for up to 10 days (average duration, 5 days). Infusion solution should be maintained at body temperature (37°C)

Fate

Drug is readily hydrolyzed by pancreatic or other digestive lipases, and the resultant fatty acids are either absorbed and metabolized or excreted intact.

Common Side Effects

Abdominal pain or discomfort, nausea, vomiting, diarrhea, anorexia, fever

Significant Adverse Reactions

Indigestion, elevated serum amylase, bile shock, leukopenia, pruritus, fatigue, chills, diaphoresis, headache, allergic reactions, hypokalemia, metabolic acidosis, depression, (*rarely*) acute pancreatitis, cholangitis, hematemesis

Contraindications

Jaundice, biliary tract infection, acute pancreatitis, impaired hepatic function, recent duodenal ulcer, or jejunitis. *Cautious use* in pregnant or nursing women and in children.

Nursing Management

Nursing Interventions

Medication Administration

Administer infusion with a positive pressure or peristaltic perfusion pump equipped with an overflow manometer to avoid complications associated with use of excessive pressure. Pressure should not exceed 15 cm H_2O.

Monitor flow rate carefully. GI side effects usually worsen when rate is too rapid.

Surveillance During Therapy

Assess patient for GI side effects, particularly nausea and diarrhea. These effects must be controlled to prevent nutritional inadequacy and fluid/electrolyte imbalance.

Consider interrupting the perfusion for 1 to 2 hours at mealtimes if GI side effects persist. Aspiration of the biliary tract may also relieve GI discomfort. Abdominal pain does not, however, appear to correlate with either dosage or perfusion rate.

Monitor patient for indications of ascending cholangitis (elevated temperature, chills, severe right upper quadrant abdominal pain, jaundice). Notify practitioner if these occur.

Monitor patient for indications of leukopenia (decreased white blood cell count [WBC], sore throat, fever, chills). Notify practitioner if these occur.

Patient Teaching

Explain to patient and family that therapy often continues for 10 or more days.

Teach patient and family how to operate the infusion pump they will use in the home if treatment is to be administered at home.

• Ursodiol (Ursodeoxycholic acid)

Actigall

Ursodiol is a naturally occurring bile acid found in small quantities in normal human bile. The drug is used orally to dissolve radiolucent gallstones.

Mechanism

Suppresses hepatic synthesis and secretion of cholesterol and inhibits intestinal absorption of cholesterol; ursodiol-rich bile solubilizes cholesterol by raising the concentration level at which saturation of cholesterol occurs; may also cause dispersion of cholesterol as liquid crystals in an aqueous medium; does not appear to significantly alter the secretion of bile acids or phospholipids into bile.

Uses

Facilitate dissolution of radiolucent, noncalcified gallbladder stones less than 20 mm in diameter in persons presenting an increased surgical risk or who decline surgery.

Treatment of primary biliary cirrhosis (*investigational use*)

Dosage

8 to 10 mg/kg/day orally in 2 or 3 divided doses. Treatment generally requires months of therapy, and complete dissolution does not occur in all patients. Recurrence of stones within 5 years has occurred in 50% of patients.

Fate

Well absorbed orally; extracted from the portal circulation by the liver, conjugated with glycine or taurine, and secreted into hepatic bile ducts; concentrated in the gallbladder and secreted into the duodenum through the cystic and common bile ducts; small amounts are found in the systemic circulation and excreted in the urine; after enterohepatic recirculation, most of a dose is eliminated in the feces.

Common Side Effects

Nausea, dyspepsia, metallic taste

Significant Adverse Reactions

Diarrhea, vomiting, abdominal pain, biliary pain, cholecystitis, stomatitis, flatulence, headache, fatigue, sleep disturbances, cough, anxiety, depression, arthralgia, myalgia, rash, pruritus, urticaria, dry skin, sweating

Contraindications

Chronic liver disease, biliary obstruction, pancreatitis, acute cholecystitis, cholangitis, bile acid allergy. *Cautious use* in persons with altered liver function values, in pregnant or nursing women, and in children.

Interactions

Oral absorption of ursodiol may be impaired by aluminum-containing antacids, cholestyramine resin, and colestipol.

Estrogens, oral contraceptives, and clofibrate may counteract the effectiveness of ursodiol by increasing the hepatic secretion of cholesterol.

Nursing Management

Nursing Interventions

Patient Teaching

Instruct patient to report persistent or severe diarrhea. A temporary dosage reduction may be needed to alleviate it.

Inform patient that the drug is usually discontinued if stones have dissolved, but serial cholecystograms should be performed to monitor for recurrence, which occurs within 5 years in approximately 50% of patients.

Encourage patient to maintain low-cholesterol, low-carbohydrate diet after stone dissolution and to reduce weight to minimize stone recurrence.

Selected Bibliography

Fisher RL et al: The lack of relationship between hepatotoxicity and lithocholic-acid sulfation in biliary bile acids during chenodiol therapy in the National Cooperative Gallstone Study. Hepatology 14(3): 454, 1991

Hofmann AF: Primary and secondary prevention of gallstone disease: Implications for patient management and research priorities. Am J Surg 165(4):541, 1993

Leuschner V: Oral bile acid treatment of biliary cholesterol stones. Recent Prog Med 83(7-8):392, 1992

Peine CJ: Gallstone-dissolving agents. Gastrointest Clin North Am 21(3): 715, 1992

Roupon RE, Roupon R: Ursodeoxycholic acid for the treatment of cholestatic diseases. Prog Liver Dis 10:219, 1992

Nursing Bibliography

Krumberger J: Acute pancreatitis. Critical Care Nursing Clinics of North America 5(1):188, 1993

Orally administered gallbladder therapeutic agents: Chenix. Part 1. Gastroenterology Nursing 15(5):208, 1993

Orally administered gallbladder therapeutic agents: Actigall. Part 2. Gastroenterology Nursing 15(6):254, 1993

52
Laxatives

Bisacodyl	Methylcellulose
Cascara sagrada	Mineral oil
Castor oil	Nondiastatic barley malt
Docusate calcium	Phenolphthalein
Docusate potassium	Polycarbophil
Docusate sodium	Polyethylene glycol electrolyte solution
Glycerin	Psyllium
Lactulose	Senna
Magnesium citrate	Sodium biphosphate
Magnesium hydroxide	Sodium phosphate
Magnesium sulfate	

A laxative is an agent that facilitates evacuation of the bowel. The valid indications for use of such drugs are few, and laxatives are frequently misused and abused by a large number of persons suffering from constipation, a condition characterized by a reduced frequency of fecal elimination. Diagnosis of constipation is difficult because there is a tremendous variation in the "normal" frequency of bowel movements, estimated to range from as low as three per week to as high as three per day. Given this inherent variability, constipation cannot be characterized strictly in terms of bowel frequency but must be viewed in relation to previous bowel habits, presence of disease states, or to other drug therapy, diet, and other conditions.

Chronic simple constipation can frequently be relieved by proper diet, adequate fluid intake, and sufficient exercise; it does not usually require drug therapy. When indicated, laxative therapy should be short-term (that is, 1–2 weeks) and should be discontinued once bowel regularity has returned. Prolonged use of laxative drugs should be strongly discouraged because regular use of most laxatives can lead to dependence on the drug rather than on the natural defecation reflex to achieve bowel movements. Persistent constipation is most often a result of improper diet, chronic disease states, prolonged laxative use, or a mental outlook or behavioral pattern adversely affecting bowel function. As such, drug therapy is usually ineffective and frequently harmful and should *not* be employed in lieu of determining and correcting the underlying cause of the dysfunction.

In contrast, *acute constipation* is often amenable to drug therapy, especially in those individuals who do not have a history of bowel irregularities. Certain laxative products (eg, stimulants, saline, or osmotics) are also indicated for rapid lower bowel evacuation in preparation for radiographic or endoscopic examination of the intestinal tract or in cases of poisoning.

There are a variety of laxative products available that function by a number of different mechanisms. The choice of a laxative product is dependent on many factors, including speed and intensity of evacuation desired (eg, chronic, mild constipation versus preradiologic intestinal flushing), presence of other disease states (eg, cardiac impairment, anorectal disorders), or need for sodium restriction.

A classification of laxatives based on their respective mechanisms of action is presented in Table 52-1. In general, bulk-producing agents (eg, methylcellulose) are considered the safest and most "physiologic" type of laxative and are the preferred agents for short-term treatment of most types of mild constipation. Emollients or fecal softeners are likewise relatively safe and are widely used in conditions in which hard or dry stools might prove painful or dangerous, such as after rectal or anal surgery, or in the presence of hemorrhoids and other conditions in which straining is undesirable (eg, heart disease, hernias).

The laxative products are discussed as a group, and are followed by a tabular listing of each product with nursing considerations. It should be noted that in addition to the products reviewed here, dehydrocholic acid, a hydrocholeretic (see Chapter 51) has also been employed for the symptomatic treatment of mild, uncomplicated constipation, although its efficacy has been questioned.

Mechanism

See Table 52-1.

Uses

- Short-term treatment of constipation
- Evacuation of the lower intestinal tract in preparation for surgery or endoscopic or radiologic examination
- Removal of toxic substances from the lower intestinal tract
- Prevention of straining where such action is painful or hazardous (eg, anorectal disorders, hernia, cardiac disease)
- Management of constipation associated with irritable bowel syndrome (especially psyllium)

NOTE: Irritable bowel syndrome may be accompanied by diarrhea as well, in which case laxatives are inappropriate.

Dosage

See Table 52-2.

Fate

(See Table 52-2 for specific information) Administered orally or rectally; systemic absorption is minimal in most cases; onset of action ranges from 5 to 10 minutes with many suppositories or rectal enemas, from 30 to 60 minutes with most oral products, and from 24 to 72 hours with some bulk-forming products; excreted largely unchanged in the feces, although a number of drugs may be partially metabolized upon systemic absorption and eliminated by the kidneys, often producing a colored urine.

Common Side Effects

(Incidence varies among different preparations) Excessive bowel activity, cramping, nausea, unpleasant taste

Malseed, RT; Goldstein, FJ; and Balkon, N: PHARMACOLOGY: DRUG THERAPY AND NURSING CONSIDERATIONS, Fourth Edition.

Table 52-1. Classification of Laxatives

Bulk-Forming (eg, Methylcellulose, Polycarbophil, Psyllium)

Cellulose derivatives that swell in intestinal fluid, stimulating peristalsis by retaining water in the stool; considered the safest and most physiologic type of laxative; each dose should be taken with sufficient water to minimize risk of intestinal or esophageal obstruction; onset of action is usually 12–24 h

Emollients/Fecal Softening (eg, Docusate Sodium)

Anionic surfactants that increase the wetting efficiency of intestinal water, thus softening the fecal mass by facilitating mixture of aqueous and fatty substances; most useful in conditions in which straining is hazardous (eg, heart disease, perianal disease, hypertension, hernia, rectal surgery); may require several days before an effect is seen

Lubricant (eg, Mineral Oil)

Softens fecal matter by lubricating the intestinal mucosa, facilitating passage of the stool; may prevent absorption of fat-soluble vitamins and nutrients and delay gastric emptying; do *not* administer with meals; effects usually occur within 6–8 h

Saline/Osmotic (eg, Magnesium Citrate, Sodium Phosphate, Polyethylene Glycol-Electrolyte Solution, Lactulose)

Nonabsorbable cations (magnesium), anions (phosphate), or sugars (lactulose) that retain water in the intestinal lumen, thus mechanically stimulating peristalsis and altering stool consistency; action is rapid (0.5–2 h); should be used only for acute bowel evacuation, except for lactulose, which may be administered in chronic constipation

Stimulant (eg, Bisacodyl, Castor Oil, Phenolphthalein)

Increase intestinal propulsion by either a direct irritant effect on the mucosa or an activation of sensory nerve endings in intestinal smooth muscle; may produce excessive catharsis, leading to fluid and electrolyte disturbances; prolonged use can result in habituation and laxative dependency; onset of action is generally 6–8 h orally

Hyperosmolar (eg, Glycerin)

Produce dehydration of exposed mucosal tissue, resulting in irritation and subsequent evacuation; laxative effect occurs within 30 min

Significant Adverse Reactions

(Not associated with all drugs and usually observed with excessive or prolonged use)

Vomiting, profound diarrhea, perianal irritation; electrolyte imbalance (especially with saline/osmotic laxatives) resulting in weakness, fainting, dizziness, palpitations, sweating; hypersensitivity reactions (especially with phenolphthalein); esophageal, intestinal, or rectal obstruction (particularly with bulk laxatives), discoloration of urine or rectal mucosa, laxative dependence

Contraindications

Presence of abdominal pain, nausea, vomiting, or other signs of acute appendicitis, diverticulitis, colitis, or regional enteritis; acute surgical abdomen, fecal impaction, intestinal obstruction or perforation, acute hepatitis, or late pregnancy.

In addition, use of magnesium or potassium salts is contraindicated in patients with renal dysfunction, use of sodium salts is contraindicated in patients requiring sodium restriction, and use of emollients and mineral oil together is contraindicated altogether. *Cautious use* in persons with rectal bleeding, and in pregnant women or young children.

CAUTION

Bulk-forming laxatives should *not* be swallowed as a dry powder but should be taken in a large glass of water followed by a second glass; refer to Patient Education. Esophageal impaction could result from dry ingestion.

Interactions

Systemic absorption of mineral oil or danthron can be enhanced by emollient (ie, fecal softening) laxatives.

Mineral oil may impair the gastrointestinal (GI) absorption of fat-soluble vitamins (A, D, E, K) or nutrients.

Laxatives (particularly bulk-forming) may reduce absorption of other drugs present in the GI tract, either by chemically combining with them or by hastening their passage through the intestinal tract.

Antacids, other alkaline substances, or histamine-2 antagonists may prematurely dissolve the enteric coating on bisacodyl tablets, reducing the laxative action, and leading to gastric or duodenal stimulation.

Nursing Management

Nursing Interventions

Patient Teaching

Stress the importance of adequate bulk and roughage (fiber) in the diet to minimize the occurrence and severity of constipation. Desirable foods include whole grain bread and cereal, raw and cooked vegetables, plums, and prunes. Adequate fluid intake is likewise important.

Suggest that patient include sufficient roughage in the diet, maintain adequate fluid intake, and undergo a normal exercise routine instead of relying on laxative drugs if constipation occurs only occasionally.

Help patient plan time of administration so that maximum effect occurs at the most convenient time (eg, drug with a 6–8-hour onset of action should be taken at bedtime for morning evacuation).

Instruct patient to take bulk laxatives in a large glass of water followed by a second glass of water to prevent esophageal impaction.

Instruct patient to notify primary healthcare provider immediately if rectal bleeding, severe abdominal pain, or a sudden change in bowel function occurs during therapy.

Explain that the cause of constipation should be ascertained and relieved; symptomatic treatment may mask an underlying disorder.

Inform patient that laxatives should not be used for more than 1 or 2 weeks without consulting primary healthcare provider. Dosage should be adjusted to provide sufficient but not excessive bowel activity, and the drug should be discontinued when bowel regularity is achieved. Dosage increases should be avoided if the product is ineffective because laxative dependence or electrolyte imbalance can develop.

Instruct patient to report signs of electrolyte imbalance, such as muscle cramping, weakness, or dizziness. Electrolytes should be monitored regularly during prolonged therapy.

(text continues on page 538)

Table 52-2. **Laxatives**

Drug	*Usual Dosage Range*	*Nursing Considerations*
BULK-FORMING		
Methylcellulose *Citrucel, Unifiber*	Adults: 5 mL to 20 mL *or* 1 tbsp of powder in 8 oz water 3 times/day with water Children: 1 tsp in 4 oz water 3 or 4 times a day	Used orally for constipation; also available in ophthalmic drops for relief of dry, irritated eyes and as an ocular lubricant for artificial eyes and contact lenses; oral doses should be taken with 1 or more glasses of water for each dose, and additional fluids are indicated throughout the day to prevent fecal impaction; sodium carboxymethylcellulose is available in capsule form with dioctyl sodium sulfosuccinate (Disoplex, Disolan Forte)
Nondiastatic Barley Malt Extract *Maltsupex*	*Tablets* Adults only: 4 tablets with meals and at bedtime; 4 times a day with liquid *Powder/liquid* Adults: 2 tbsp twice a day for 3 to 4 days; then 1 to 2 tbsp at bedtime Children: 1 tbsp to 2 tbsp in milk 1 to 2 times a day	Useful in treating functional constipation in infants and children, as well as in adults, including those with laxative dependence; also may provide relief from itching in pruritis ani; use with caution in diabetic patients because preparations contain 14 g carbohydrates/tbsp and 0.6 g/tablet; mixes more easily with cold liquids when first stirred with a little hot water; available in combination with powdered psyllium seed as Syllamalt
Polycarbophil Calcium *Fiberall, Fiber-Con, Fiber-Lax, Equalactin, Mitrolan*	Adults: 1 g 1–4 times a day Children (6–12 y): 500 mg 1–3 times a day Children (3–6 y): 500 mg 1–2 times a day	A hydrophilic agent that is used for treating both diarrhea and constipation; claimed to restore a more normal moisture level and to provide bulk in the GI tract; as a laxative, retains free water in the lumen of the intestine; a full glass of water or other liquid should be taken with each dose; discontinue use after 1 wk if desired effects are not noted; also used for controlling simple diarrhea (see Chap. 53)
Psyllium *Effersyllium, Konsyl, Metamucil, Serutan and other manufacturers* *(CAN) Karacil, Novomucilax, Siblin*	1 or 2 rounded teaspoons of powder, *or* 1 packet of powder in a glass of liquid 1 to 3 times a day (check package instructions for individual dosage recommendations)	Natural products derived from the blond psyllium seed (*Plantago ovata*); available in several dosage forms, many containing dextrose as a dispersing agent; contact with water in GI tract produces a bland, nonirritating bulk that aids peristalsis; sodium content is usually less than 10–30 mg/dose; some preparations (eg, Konsyl) are sodium free; drug should be taken with adequate water to prevent esophageal, gastric, intestinal, or rectal obstruction; each dose should be followed by a second full glass of water; do not attempt to swallow dry; available in combination with barley malt extract (Syllamalt) or senna (Perdiem Granules)
EMOLLIENT		
Docusate Calcium–Dioctyl Calcium Sulfosuccinate *DC, Sulfalax, Surfak, Pro-Cal-Sof* *(CAN) PMS-Docusate Calcium*	Adults: 240 mg/day Children: 50–150 mg/day	Similar in action to docusate sodium (see below) but does not contain sodium, which may be hazardous in patients with hypertension, congestive heart failure, edema, impaired renal function, or in persons on sodium-restricted diets; do not use in combination with mineral oil, because drug may enhance systemic absorption of the oil; available in combination with phenolphthalein (Doxidan)
Docusate Sodium–Dioctyl Sodium Sulfosuccinate *Colace, Doxinate, D-S-S, Modane Soft, and various other manufacturers* *(CAN) Laxagel, Regulex*	Adults: 50–500 mg Children (6–12 y): 40–120 mg Children (3–6 y): 20–60 mg Children (younger than 3 y): 10–40 mg Larger doses may be given initially, then adjusted to optimal response	A surface-wetting agent that increases the wetting efficiency of intestinal water, thus facilitating the mixing of aqueous and fatty substances to soften the fecal mass for easier passage; effect on stools is apparent 1–3 days after first dose; does not exert a laxative action itself, but is mainly used as adjunctive treatment in constipation associated with hard, dry stools or in patients who should avoid straining (eg, with cardiac disease, hernia, anorectal disorders); should not be used regularly by patients who must restrict sodium intake; may increase systemic absorption of mineral oil if given in combination; available in combination with casanthranol (eg, Peri-Colace), senna concentrate (eg, Senokot S), phenophthalein (eg, Correctol, Dialose Plus, Feen-a-Mint Pills, Unilax), sodium carboxymethylcellulose (eg, Disoplex), and various other laxatives
Docusate Potassium–Dioctyl Potassium Sulfosuccinate *Dialose, Diocto-K, Kasof*	Adults: 100–300 mg/day with a full glass of water Children (younger than 6 y): 100 mg/day	See docusate sodium; may be used where sodium restriction is necessary; available in capsules combined with casanthranol (Diocto-K Plus)

(*continued*)

Table 52-2. **Laxatives (Continued)**

Drug	*Usual Dosage Range*	*Nursing Considerations*
LUBRICANTS		
Mineral Oil *Agoral Plain, Fleet Mineral Oil Enema, Kondremul Plain, Liqui-Doss, Milkinol, Neo-Cultol*	*Oral* Adults: 5–45 mL at bedtime Children: 5–20 mL at bedtime *Rectal* Adults: 120 mL Children: 30–60 mL	Useful to maintain soft stools to avoid straining; coats fecal contents, preventing colonic absorption of water; probably not as effective or safe as emollients; may interfere with absorption of fat-soluble vitamins and nutrients, therefore administer on an empty stomach; do not use during pregnancy or with emollients; use of enema may avoid interference with nutrient absorption, but oil seepage from rectum can stain clothing; use *cautiously* in the very old, debilitated, or very young (younger than 2 yr), because danger of aspiration and possible development of lipid pneumonia is increased; emulsified preparations (eg, Agoral, Kondremul) mask the objectionable consistency of plain oil and may be slightly more effective but tend to increase systemic absorption of oil and are significantly more expensive; avoid prolonged or excessive use; available in combination with phenolphthalein (Agoral, Kondremul with Phenolphthalein) and magnesium hydroxide (Haley's M-O)
SALINE/OSMOTIC		
Lactulose *Cephulac, Cholac, Chronulac, Constilac, Constulose, Duphulac, Enulose, Evalose, Heptalac* *(CAN) Acilac, Lactulax*	*Laxative*: 15–30 mL/day to a maximum of 60 mL/day *Portal–systemic encephalopathy*: 30–45 mL 3–4 times a day May also be given to comatose patient by means of retention enema as 300 mL in 700 mL of water or saline for acute hepatic coma; dosage is adjusted to minimize diarrhea and may be repeated every 4–6 h	A complex sugar that is not hydrolyzed in the GI tract, but enters the colon unchanged; there it is broken down primarily to lactic acid by colonic bacteria; this elevates the osmotic pressure, increasing stool water content and softening the fecal matter; may require 24–48 h to produce a bowel movement; use cautiously in pregnant or nursing women, in elderly or debilitated patients, and in diabetic patients; initial doses may produce flatulence and cramping; may be mixed with fruit juice or milk to improve palatability; reduces blood ammonia levels by 25%–50% and is also used for prevention and treatment of portal–systemic encephalopathy, including the stages of hepatic precoma and coma; may be administered long-term for this indication, dosage is usually adjusted to produce 2 or 3 soft stools a day
Magnesium Citrate *Citrate of Magnesia, Citro-Nesia* *(CAN) Citro-Maq, National Laxative*	Adults: 200–250 mL (1 glass) at bedtime Children: 100–125 mL (½ glass) at bedtime	Chilling liquid improves the taste; do *not* use in patients with renal impairment; observe for signs of magnesium toxicity (thirst, drowsiness, dizziness); available in several bowel evacuation kits (Evac-Q-Kit, Evac-Q-Kwik, Tridrate Bowel Evacuation Kit)
Magnesium Hydroxide *Milk of Magnesia*	Adults: 15–30 mL regular liquid or 10–20 mL concentrated liquid at bedtime Children: 5–30 mL regular liquid, depending on age	Recommended for *short-term use only* because accumulation of magnesium ions can result in serious toxicity (CNS or neuromuscular depression, fluid and electrolyte imbalances); tablets are less effective than liquid as a laxative; concentrated liquid (233 mg/mL) is lemon flavored to improve palatability; do *not* use in patients with renal impairment; also used as an antacid (see Chap. 50); available in emulsion form containing mineral oil (Haley's M-O)
Magnesium Sulfate *Epsom salt*	Adults: 10–15 g in a glass of water or fruit juice Children: 5–10 g in a glass of water	Administer in a flavored vehicle if necessary to mask the salty taste; effects are noted within several hours; infrequently used as a laxative
Polyethylene Glycol-Electrolyte Solution *Co-Lav, Colovage, CoLyte, Go-Evac, GoLYTELY, Nulytely, OCL*	Adults: 4 L solution orally (240 mL every 10 min) before GI examination	Orally administered solution used to cleanse bowel before radiologic examination; contains PEG 3350, a nonabsorbable solution that acts as an osmotic agent in the intestines; electrolytes prevent any change in ion concentration following evacuation of bowel; transient bloating, nausea, and cramping may occur; patient should fast 3–4 h before ingestion of solution; first bowel movement occurs within 1 h after ingestion is complete; flavorings and other ingredients should not be added; tap water may be used to reconstitute solution
Sodium Phosphate and Sodium Biphosphate *Fleet Enema, Phospho-Soda*	*Oral* Adults: 20–30 mL in ½ glass of water Children: 5–15 mL *Rectal* Adults: 118 mL Children: 60 mL	Indicated only for acute evacuation of the bowel (eg, before rectal or bowel examinations); high sodium content (4.4 g/dose); available in packaged forms with bisacodyl tablets, suppositories, or enema (Fleet Barium Enema Prep Kits)

(continued)

Drug	Usual Dosage Range	Nursing Considerations
STIMULANTS		
Bisacodyl *Bisco-Lax, Dulcagen, Dulcolax, Fleet Bisacodyl,* *(CAN) Apo-Bisacodyl, Bisacolax, Laxit*	*Oral* Adults: 10–15 mg Children: 5–10 mg *Rectal (suppository)* Adults: 10 mg after each bowel movement Children: 5 mg *Rectal enema* 1 container (30 mL)	Increases peristalsis, probably by a direct effect on sensory nerve endings in colonic mucosa; used to relieve constipation and to evacuate the bowel before examination; onset of action is 6–10 h orally and 15–60 min after insertion of suppository; tablets should not be crushed or chewed, and milk or antacids should not be consumed within 1 h of the drug because they may prematurely dissolve the enteric coating on the tablet; rectal burning and itching may follow use of suppositories; no untoward systemic effects have been observed with either oral or rectal use; habituation can occur, with gradual loss of effectiveness
Bisacodyl Tannex *Clysodrast*	Cleansing enema: 2.5 g in 1 L warm water Barium enema: 2.5–5 g in 1 L barium suspension (maximum, 4 packets in 72 h)	A nonabsorbable complex of bisacodyl and tannic acid used as a colonic evacuant; tannic acid is claimed to reduce intestinal secretions and when used with barium suspension, to improve the adherence of barium to intestinal walls; *contraindicated* in pregnant women and in children younger than 10 y; tannic acid may be hepatotoxic if sufficient quantities are absorbed; use *cautiously* if multiple enemas are being administered and in elderly or debilitated patients
Cascara Sagrada	1 tablet *or* 5 mL aromatic fluid extract at bedtime	Direct chemical irritant that increases propulsive movements in the colon; onset of action is 6–10 h; urine may be colored reddish to yellow brown, and rectal mucosa may become discolored; prolonged use should be avoided because habituation can result; available with aloe (Nature's Remedy) and senna (Herbal Laxative)
Castor Oil *Emulsoil, Fleet Castor Oil, Purge* *(CAN) Unisoil*	*Adults:* 15–60 mL Children Older than 2 y: 5–15 ml Younger than 2 y: 1–5 mL (depending on strength of emulsion)	Natural product that is broken down in small intestine to glycerol and ricinoleic acid, a local irritant; stimulates intestinal activity, resulting in production of liquid stools; primarily used for prompt evacuation of bowel before radiologic examination or in cases of poisoning; onset is 2–6 h; do *not* use in pregnant women or in treating worm infestation, because systemic absorption may be increased
Phenolphthalein *Alophen, Espotabs, Ex-Lax, Feen-A-Mint, Modane, and other manufacturers* *(CAN) Alphen, Fructines-Vichy*	60–194 mg at bedtime	Stimulant laxative similar to bisacodyl in most respects; onset of action is 6–8 h; may color urine red to yellow brown; effects may be prolonged for several days because of enterohepatic circulation; allergic skin reactions can occur—drug should be discontinued at first sign of rash; some preparations are fruit or chocolate flavored—keep out of reach of children, because serious toxicity can result if large quantities are consumed; available in combination with docusate sodium (eg, Correctol, Disolan, Modane Plus), docusate calcium (Doxidan), and mineral oil (eg, Agoral, Kondremul w/Phenolphthalein)
Senna Concentrate *Gentlax, Senexon, Fletcher's Castoria, Senokot, Senna-Gen, Senolax*	*Constipation* Adults: 2 tablets, 1 tsp granules, or 1 suppository at bedtime Children: 1/2 adult dose	Natural product prepared from species of *Cassia*, having a similar but more potent laxative action than cascara; concentrate may provide a more uniform effect than other preparations, with less colic; onset of action is usually 6–12 h, but may require 24 h in some cases; may impart a yellow-brown to red color to the urine or feces
Senna Equivalent *Black-Draught*	Adults: 2 tablets or 1/4 tsp to 1/2 tsp granules with water	
Sennosides A & B—Calcium Salts *Ex-Lax Gentle Nature* *(CAN) Glysennid*	Adults: 1–2 tablets at bedtime Children: 1 tablet at bedtime	
HYPEROSMOLAR		
Glycerin *Fleet Babylax, Sani-Supp*	1 suppository or 4 mL liquid inserted high into the rectum	Produces dehydration of exposed mucosal tissue, leading to irritation and subsequent evacuation; laxative effect occurs within 15–30 min

- Inform patient that certain laxatives (eg, cascara, danthron, phenolphthalein, senna) may discolor urine (pink to red to yellow-brown) as well as rectal mucosa.
- Instruct patient taking laxative product before endoscopic or radiologic examination to carefully follow instructions concerning timing of doses to achieve maximal bowel evacuation.
- Inform parents that stimulant cathartics or laxative enemas should not be administered to children younger than 2 years of age.

Selected Bibliography

Castle SC, Cantrell M, Israel DS, Samuelson MJ: Constipation prevention: Empiric use of stool softeners questioned. Geriatrics 46(11):84, 1991

Heaton KW, Cripps HA: Straining at stool and laxative taking in an English population. Dig Dis Sci 38(6):1004, 1993

Korkis AM, Miskovitz PF, Yurt RW, Klein H: Rectal prolapse after oral cathartics. J Clin Gastroenterol 14(4):339, 1992

Kune GA: Laxative use not a risk for colorectal cancer: Data from the Melbourne Colorectal Cancer Study. Z Gastroenterol 31(2):140, 1993

Perkins SL, Livesey JF: A rapid HPLC urine screen for laxative abuse. Clin Biochem 26(3):179, 1993

Toskes PP, Connery KL, Ritchey TW: Calcium polycarbophil compared with placebo in irritable bowel syndrome. Aliment Pharmacol Ther 7(1):87, 1993

Yakabowich M: Prescribe with care: The role of laxatives in the treatment of constipation. J Gerontol Nurs 16(7):4, 1990

Zanolli MD, McAlvany J, Krowchuk DP: Phenolphthalein-induced fixed drug eruption: A cutaneous complication of laxative use in a child. Pediatrics 91(6):1199, 1993

Nursing Bibliography

Antacids and laxatives don't mix with other meds. Consumer Reports Health 4(5):38, 1992

Beverley L: Constipation: Proposed natural laxative mixtures. Journal of Gerontological Nursing 18(10):5, 1992

Gruber M, et al: Palatability of colonic lavage solution is improved by addition of artificially sweetened flavored drink mixes. Gastroenterology Nursing 14(3):135, 1991

Murray S, et al: How do you prep the bowel without enemas? Am J Nurs 92(8):66, 1992

53
Antidiarrheal Drugs

Difenoxin and atropine sulfate
Diphenoxylate and atropine sulfate
Loperamide

Opium tincture, camphorated

Locally acting antidiarrheal combinations

Diarrhea, the passage of excessive, watery stools, is generally viewed as a *symptom* of an underlying pathologic condition rather than as a disease entity in itself. Distinction must be made, however, between acute and chronic diarrhea, because significant differences exist between the two conditions with respect to cause, potential danger to the patient, and preferred treatment. *Acute diarrhea*, characterized by sudden onset of frequent, watery stools, often accompanied by fever, pain, vomiting, and weakness, may have several causes, including viral or bacterial infection, food or drug poisoning, or radiation exposure. The major danger of severe acute diarrhea is that it can quickly lead to dehydration and electrolyte imbalances, especially in infants and children. Fortunately, most episodes of acute diarrhea are self-limiting, that is, once the offending organisms, foods, or medications are removed, the symptoms soon subside.

Chronic diarrhea likewise may be related to any of a number of causative factors, such as secondary disease states (eg, ulcerative colitis, diverticulitis, irritable colon, hyperthyroidism, gastric carcinoma), surgery (such as subtotal gastrectomy, vagotomy, ileal resection), or presence of excessive amounts of hormones, bile acids, or other substances in the GI tract. Chronic diarrhea may also be of psychogenic origin, a most difficult type to treat.

Whatever the type of diarrhea, every effort should be made to determine and remove the underlying cause of the distress. For example, diarrhea resulting from the presence of an infectious organism may best be treated by use of an appropriate antibiotic. Likewise, drug-induced diarrhea can often be corrected by simply discontinuing the offending drug. Successful treatment of secondary disease states associated with diarrhea usually reduces or eliminates the accompanying episodes of diarrhea. In those instances in which the cause of the diarrhea is not readily apparent or cannot be successfully eliminated by other means, use of antidiarrheal drugs for symptomatic relief should be considered on a short-term basis. In no instance, however, should the use of antidiarrheal agents be substituted for attempts to eradicate the cause of the condition, nor should these drugs be administered over prolonged periods except in unusual circumstances, because many of the more effective antidiarrheals have the potential to elicit a wide range of side effects and may become habituating.

The most effective antidiarrheal medications are the opiates (such as paregoric), related opiate derivatives (eg, difenoxin, diphenoxylate) and loperamide, which is chemically related to the antipsychotic haloperidol. These are systemically acting agents that reduce intestinal hypermotility and slow peristalsis. Anticholinergics have also been used to reduce GI motility by impairing parasympathetic nerve stimulation to intestinal smooth muscle; although these drugs are possibly effective in some forms of diarrhea, the dosages required to slow peristalsis effectively are quite high, which often results in a wide range of unacceptable side effects. Anticholinergic drugs are reviewed in detail in Chapter 13 and are not discussed here.

Several locally acting drugs have been employed for the symptomatic relief of diarrhea, frequently in combination form. Among the pharmacologic products used in this way are adsorbents (kaolin, pectin, attapulgite), astringents (zinc phenolsulfonate), antacids (aluminum hydroxide, bismuth salts), and bacterial cultures (*Lactobacillus acidophilus*). These substances are relatively safe for normal use, but there is insufficient clinical evidence to establish their effectiveness for the intended purpose. Nevertheless, they are available without prescription and are widely used by the general public. Every product carries a warning against use for longer than 2 days, in the presence of high fever or in children younger than 3 years of age except on physicians' orders.

Treatment of most types of diarrhea, with the possible exception of severe acute diarrhea in infants and children, is usually best carried out conservatively. One of the locally acting drug combinations (such as kaolin and pectin) is usually satisfactory for the symptomatic management of mild, episodic diarrhea. More intense acute diarrhea may require addition of one of the opiate derivatives plus the ingestion of large amounts of fluids or electrolyte solutions (eg, Lytren, Pedialyte; see Chapter 76) to prevent dehydration and electrolyte depletion. Persistent or recurrent diarrhea generally signifies an underlying pathologic condition that should be identified and corrected. Routine use of antidiarrheal drugs for extended periods should be confined to certain conditions (such as chronic inflammatory bowel disease, GI carcinoma, intestinal surgery, radiation therapy), undertaken only after careful examination, and closely supervised by a physician. Continuous self-use of antidiarrheal drug formulations by persons with mild, intermittent, or episodic diarrhea should be strongly discouraged, because the drug may not only elicit untoward reactions but can mask the symptoms of a more severe underlying disease.

The potent systemically active antidiarrheal drugs are reviewed individually, followed by a brief, general discussion of the principal locally acting antidiarrheal agents and a listing of commonly used antidiarrheal combination products.

Systemic Antidiarrheals

The systemic antidiarrheals comprise the opiates, principally camphorated tincture of opium (paregoric), two opiate (meperidine) derivatives, difenoxin and diphenoxylate, and loperamide, which is claimed to have a lower incidence of CNS effects and less addiction liability than the opiates.

• Difenoxin HCl with Atropine Sulfate (C-IV)

Motofen

• Diphenoxylate HCl with Atropine Sulfate (C-V)

Lomotil and other manufacturers

Difenoxin and diphenoxylate are structural analogues of meperidine with a relatively low risk of dependence at normal doses, although typical opiate effects (such as euphoria) may occur with high doses. Prolonged ingestion can lead to habituation. These drugs are combined with a subtherapeutic amount of atropine to discourage deliberate abuse; excessive doses lead to a variety of atropine-induced adverse effects that are distinctly unpleasant (refer to **Significant Adverse Reactions**).

Mechanism

Slow intestinal motility, probably by a direct inhibitory action on circular and longitudinal GI smooth muscle; may exert an antisecretory action as well; prolong intestinal transit time, increase viscosity and density of intestinal contents, and reduce daily fecal volume; little or no analgesic effect

Uses

Adjunctive treatment of diarrhea

Dosage

Difenoxin

2 mg initially, then 1 mg after each loose stool or every 3 to 4 hours as needed; maximum dose is 8 mg/24 hours

Diphenoxylate

Adults: 5 mg 4 times a day; reduce when symptoms are controlled
Children: Initially 0.3 to 0.4 mg/kg/day in divided doses. Average daily dosages:
2–5 years: 4 mL (2 mg) 3 times a day
5–8 years: 4 mL (2 mg) 4 times a day
8–12 years: 4 mL (2 mg) 5 times a day

Fate

Drugs are well absorbed when taken orally; onset of action is 30 to 60 minutes. Diphenoxylate is quickly and extensively metabolized to diphenoxylic acid (difenoxin), the major active circulating metabolite. The plasma half-life of the parent drug is 2 to 3 hours, and the elimination half-life of difenoxin is 12 to 15 hours; difenoxin is metabolized to an inactive metabolite and both the parent drug and its metabolites are excreted in the feces (approximately 50%) and the urine.

Common Side Effects

Dry mouth, drowsiness, nausea, dizziness, headache

Significant Adverse Reactions

(Usually with large doses)

Abdominal discomfort, vomiting, anorexia, restlessness, depression, malaise, numbness of extremities, pruritus, urticaria, angioneurotic edema, paralytic ileus, toxic megacolon, respiratory depression, hypotonia, miosis, nystagmus, blurred vision

Atropine side effects are more common in children and include flushing, diminished secretions, hyperthermia, tachycardia, urinary retention

Contraindications

Diarrhea associated with organisms that can penetrate the intestinal mucosa (eg, toxigenic *Escherichia coli, Salmonella, Shigella*), pseudomembranous colitis, obstructive jaundice, and in children younger than 2 years old. *Cautious use* in patients with cirrhosis or other advanced liver disease, ulcerative colitis, or glaucoma, in addiction-prone persons, and in pregnant or nursing women.

Interactions

Refer to **Anticholinergics**, Chapter 13. In addition:

Diphenoxylate and difenoxin may potentiate the depressant effects of barbiturates, alcohol, narcotics, and other tranquilizers or sedatives.

Concurrent use with monoamine oxidase (MAO) inhibitors may precipitate a hypertensive crisis.

Nursing Management

Refer to **Anticholinergics** (Chapter 13). In addition:

Nursing Interventions

Surveillance During Therapy

Monitor patient, especially a young child, for signs of atropine overdosage (refer to **Atropine Side Effects** under **Significant Adverse Reactions**). Notify primary healthcare provider if they occur because dosage should be reduced or drug should be discontinued.

Observe patient for potential respiratory depression for at least 48 hours after last dose has been administered because respiratory depression may not occur for some time if overdosage occurs. Naloxone (Narcan) is the drug of choice for reversing respiratory depression.

Assess patient's abdomen frequently. Abdominal distention or pain is a possible indication of developing toxic megacolon, which is caused by delayed intestinal transit. The drug should be discontinued if these signs occur.

Assist in evaluating drug effects. Administration for acute diarrhea should be discontinued if clinical improvement is not noted within 48 hours.

Follow proper procedures for handling controlled substances (see Chapter 10).

Patient Teaching

Instruct patient taking liquid preparation to use only the calibrated dropper provided with the bottle.

Warn patient not to exceed recommended dosage because incidence of adverse effects greatly increase at high doses, and the danger of habituation is enhanced.

Instruct patient to avoid alcohol or other CNS depressants because an additive depressant effect can result.

• Loperamide

Imodium and other manufacturers

A structural analogue of haloperidol, loperamide is similar to diphenoxylate and difenoxin in action but possesses a reduced risk of dependence at recommend doses. Further, it is not combined with atropine, so anticholinergic side effects are eliminated. Opiate-like effects have not occurred with prolonged treatment, and tolerance to the antidiarrheal effect has not occurred. The liquid and tablet dosage forms are available over-the-counter, whereas the capsules are to be dispensed only on prescription.

Mechanism

Slows intestinal motility and inhibits peristalsis by a direct depressant effect on intestinal smooth muscle; minimal action on the CNS at recommended dosage levels.

Uses

Control of acute nonspecific diarrhea and chronic diarrhea associated with inflammatory bowel disease
Control of "traveler's diarrhea"
Reduction of volume of discharge from ileostomies

Dosage

Adults

Acute diarrhea: initially 4 mg, followed by 2 mg after each loose stool; maximum dose 16 mg/day
Chronic diarrhea: as above for acute diarrhea, then reduce to an effective maintenance dose; usual dosage range 4 to 8 mg/day

Children (2–12 years of age)

2 to 5 years: 1 mg 3 times a day
6 to 8 years: 2 mg twice a day
8 to 12 years: 2 mg 3 times a day

Fate

Approximately 40% absorbed when taken orally; onset is 30 to 60 minutes, and duration is 4 to 5 hours; elimination half-life is approximately 10 to 12 hours; metabolized by the liver and excreted mainly in the feces as both unchanged drug and metabolites with small amounts in the urine.

Significant Adverse Reactions

Abdominal distention and discomfort, constipation, drowsiness, dizziness, nausea, vomiting, skin rash, CNS depression

Contraindications

Patients in whom constipation should be avoided (eg, severe cardiac disease, intestinal obstruction). *Cautious use* in persons with ulcerative colitis or hepatic dysfunction, in pregnant or nursing women, and in young children.

Interactions

Loperamide may enhance the sedative effects of other CNS depressants (eg, barbiturates, alcohol, narcotics, hypnotics).

Nursing Management

Pretherapy Assessment

Refer to **Difenoxin/diphenoxylate**.

Nursing Interventions

Surveillance During Therapy

If clinical benefit is not obtained at a dosage of 16 mg/day for 10 days, question further administration because it is unlikely to be effective. However, drug may be continued as a supplement to diet or specific treatment (eg, antibiotics).

• Opium Tincture, Camphorated (C-III)

Paregoric

Camphorated opium tincture contains 2 mg morphine equivalent per 5 mL, together with other ingredients (eg, camphor, anise oil, benzoic acid) in 45% alcohol. Its antidiarrheal effectiveness is attributable to its morphine content. Opium tincture, camphorated, should not be confused with *opium tincture, deodorized*, which contains 25 times the morphine equivalency and should not be used for treating diarrhea (refer to the discussion of opiates in Chapter 20).

Mechanism

Decreases GI motility and peristalsis, reduces digestive secretions, and increases intestinal smooth muscle tone, thereby slowing passage of intestinal contents

Uses

Treatment of acute diarrhea
Relief of abdominal cramping
Treatment of neonatal withdrawal syndrome (tremulousness, irritability, excessive crying, decreased sleeping time)

Dosage

Diarrhea and/or Cramping

Adults: 5 to 10 mL (2–4 mg morphine equivalent) after loose bowel movements, up to 4 times a day
Children: 0.25 to 0.5 mL/kg up to 4 times a day

Neonatal Withdrawal Syndrome

Usually 4 to 6 drops every 3 to 6 hours; adjust dosage to control withdrawal symptoms; once stabilized, reduce dosage gradually over several weeks

Common Side Effects

Drowsiness, lightheadedness

Significant Adverse Reactions

Allergic reactions (eg, rash, urticaria, pruritus), vomiting, dizziness, sweating, constipation, habituation

In addition, because the drug is a narcotic, large doses or prolonged administration can result in symptoms of narcotic overdosage (scc Chapter 20 for other possible untoward reactions).

Contraindications

Diarrhea resulting from poisoning. *Cautious use* in the presence of hepatic disease, prostatic hypertrophy, bronchial asthma, and in persons with a history of drug dependence.

Interactions

Paregoric can enhance the depressive effects of alcohol, barbiturates, tranquilizers, and other CNS depressants

Nursing Management

Nursing Interventions

Surveillance During Therapy

Monitor vital signs and intake and output during treatment of neonatal withdrawal syndrome.

Increase infant's intake of fluids and calories in proportion to severity of withdrawal symptoms (vomiting, diarrhea, sweating, increased motor activity) during treatment of neonatal withdrawal syndrome.

Follow proper procedure for handling a schedule III drug (see Chapter 10). Note that small amounts of powdered opium equivalent are contained in several antidiarrheal combination preparations (Table 53-1) that are schedule V products, but that paregoric alone is a schedule III preparation.

Patient Teaching

Suggest that drug be taken with water to facilitate passage through the GI tract.

Stress the importance of adhering closely to recommended dosage. Prolonged use or excessive doses may lead to habituation and dependence.

Discuss the need for adequate fluid replacement during periods of diarrhea to prevent dehydration and electrolyte imbalance.

Instruct patient to discontinue drug as soon as symptoms of diarrhea are controlled. Primary healthcare provider should be notified if diarrhea persists longer than 48 hours or if fever or abdominal pain develops.

Locally Acting Antidiarrheals

A large number of compounds exhibiting diverse pharmacologic effects have been employed in the treatment of diarrhea. Except for those drugs previously discussed in this chapter,

Table 53-1. **Antidiarrheal Combination Products**

Trade Name	*Dosage Form*	*Opiate Derivative*	*Adsorbents/Astringents*	*Anticholinergics*	*Other Ingredients*
Bacid	Capsules				*Lactobacillus acidophilus*, sodium carboxymethylcellulose
Children's Kaopectate	Chewable tablets Liquid		Activated attapulgite		
Devrom	Chewable tablets		Bismuth subgallate		
Diar Aid	Tablets		Activated attapulgite, pectin		
Diasorb	Tablets Liquid		Activated attapulgite		
Donnagel	Suspension Chewable tablets		Activated attapulgite		
Kaodene Nonnarcotic	Suspension		Kaolin, pectin, bismuth subsalicylate, sodium carboxymethylcellulose		
Kaopectate advanced formula	Suspension		Activated attapulgite		
Kaopectate Caplets	Tablets		Activated attapulgite, pectin		
Kapectolin	Suspension		Kaolin, pectin		
Kapectolin PG (C-V)	Suspension	Powdered opium	Kaolin, pectin	Hyoscyamine, atropine, scopolamine	
Kao-Spen	Suspension		Kaolin, pectin		
K-C	Suspension		Kaolin, pectin, bismuth subcarbonate		
K-Pek	Suspension		Activated attapulgite		
Lactinex	Granules Tablets				*Lactobacillus bulgaricus* *Lactobacillus acidophilus*
Mitrolan	Chewable tablets				Calcium polycarbophil
Parepectolin	Suspension		Activated attapulgite		
Pepto-Bismol	Suspension Chewable tablets		Bismuth subsalicylate		
Rheaban	Tablets		Activated attapulgite		

most frequently used antidiarrheal agents are locally acting drugs; that is, they are primarily nonabsorbable chemicals that act within the lumen of the GI tract by a variety of mechanisms. The most commonly employed classes of locally acting antidiarrheal drugs are the adsorbents and bacterial cultures, although astringents, antacids, bulk laxatives, digestive enzymes, and electrolytes have all been tried in the treatment of diarrhea. These locally acting agents, although essentially safe in recommended doses, have not been conclusively demonstrated to be clinically effective. Nevertheless, they are widely available without prescription, usually as combination products containing several different locally acting ingredients. Because they are readily available and relatively safe, they are most often the initial agents tried in cases of occasional, uncomplicated diarrhea, and in many instances they provide sufficient relief. The warning that appears on every product should be heeded, however, and these agents should not be used for longer than 2 to 3 days, nor should they be used when high fever is present. Further, children younger than 3 years should be given these drugs only by prescription from a physician.

A general review of the pharmacology of the most frequently used locally acting antidiarrheals is presented here, followed by a listing of the ingredients of the commonly employed combination products in Table 53-1.

Adsorbents

The adsorbents are most frequently used for the treatment of mild diarrhea. Commercial products usually contain two or more adsorbents, occasionally combined with small amounts of opium derivatives or anticholinergics, or both. These compounds have the ability to bind toxins, bacteria, and other irritants that may be present in the GI tract to their particle surface; in addition, some adsorbents (eg, pectin) may also exert a soothing demulcent action on the mucosal surface of the irritated bowel. The adsorptive activity of these compounds is not selective for irritants or toxins, however, and they may also bind drugs or food products found in the intestinal tract at the same time. Thus, adsorbents can potentially interfere with the normal GI absorption of many drugs or foodstuffs, and this possibility should be noted whenever an adsorbent substance is given to a patient receiving medications for other conditions.

The most frequently encountered adsorbents in commercial preparations are kaolin, pectin, activated attapulgite, and certain bismuth salts (eg, subgallate, subsalicylate). Cholestyramine, an anion-exchange resin discussed in Chapter 35, has also been employed in some cases of severe diarrhea. It is thought to complex with bacterial toxins in the GI tract. Anion-exchange resins are not approved as antidiarrheal drugs, and their use in this manner is strictly experimental.

Bacterial Cultures

Cultures of viable strains of *Lactobacillus acidophilus* and *Lactobacillus bulgaricus* have been used in the treatment of diarrhea resulting from a disruption of normal intestinal microorganism balance. Seeding the bowel with bacterial cultures is believed to reestablish the normal intestinal flora and suppress the growth of undesired microorganisms, thus improving those GI disturbances, including diarrhea, resulting from an altered intestinal flora. Although possibly effective in those cases of diarrhea induced by treatment with antibiotics that can upset the normal bacterial population of the GI tract, lactobacillus preparations are not recommended for most episodes of diarrhea, inasmuch as they are somewhat more costly than other locally acting drugs, and there is no conclusive evidence that modification of intestinal flora has a beneficial effect in acute diarrhea.

Other

Among the other types of locally acting products that have been used in the treatment of diarrhea are the bulk-producing laxatives or hydrophilic colloids (eg, carboxymethylcellulose, polycarbophil, psyllium seed). The rationale behind this apparent paradoxical action is that these substances have the ability to absorb excess fecal fluid as they swell in the intestinal tract, thus aiding in the production of formed stools. Their suitability for most forms of diarrhea, however, remains speculative.

An important facet of the adjunctive treatment of persistent or severe, acute diarrhea is replenishment of fluid and electrolyte loss, especially in infants and young children. The parenteral fluids and electrolyte solutions available for this purpose are reviewed in Chapter 76.

Selected Bibliography

Brown KH: Dietary management of acute childhood diarrhea: Optimal timing of feeding and appropriate use of milks and mixed diets. J Pediatr 118:S592, 1991

Butler T et al: Treatment of acute bacterial diarrhea: A multicenter international trial comparing placebo with fleroxacin given as a single dose or once daily for 3 days. Am J Med 94(3A):187S, 1993

Dukes GE: Over-the-counter antidiarrheal medications used for the self-treatment of acute nonspecific diarrhea. Am J Med 88(6A):24S, 1990

Ellett ML, Fitzgerald JF, Winchester M: Dietary management of chronic diarrhea in children. Gastroenterol Nurs 15(4):170, 1993

Figueroa-Quintanilla D et al: A controlled trial of bismuth subsalicylate in infants with acute watery diarrheal disease. N Engl J Med 328(23): 1653, 1993

McCarron MM, Challoner KR, Thompson GA: Diphenoxylate-atropine (Lomotil) overdose in children: An update. Pediatrics 87(5):694, 1991

Petruccelli BP et al: Treatment of traveler's diarrhea with ciproflaxacin and loperamide. J Infect Dis 165(3):557, 1992

Toskes PP, Connery KL, Ritchey TW: Calcium polycarbophil compared with placebo in irritable bowel syndrome. Aliment Pharmacol Ther 7(1):87, 1993

Nursing Bibliography

Carpenter D, et al: How do you treat and control *C. difficile* infection? Am J Nurs 92(9):22, 1992

Losonsky G: Diarrhea and gastroenteritis. Curr Opin Infect Dis 5(4):576, 1992

Norfloxain for bacterial diarrhea. Emer Med 25(1)L150, 1993

Robinson B: Be alert to an avoidable problem: Management and prevention of antibiotic acquired diarrhea. Prof Nurse 8(8):510, 1993

54

Gastrointestinal Stimulants, Emetics, and Antiemetics

Metoclopramide
Cisapride
Dexpanthenol
Ipecac
Benzquinamide
Diphenidol
Dronabinol
Ondansetron
Granisetron
Phosphorated carbohydrate solution
Thiethylperazine
Trimethobenzamide

Several drugs that possess the ability to stimulate motility in the gastrointestinal (GI) tract are available for treating gastroesophageal reflux and delayed gastric emptying and for the relief of intestinal atony after surgery. Other drugs can enhance vomiting reflex mechanisms through both a peripheral (ie, local gastric mucosal irritation) and central (ie, stimulation of medullary chemoreceptor trigger zone) action and are termed *emetics*. They are used primarily to induce vomiting in cases of drug overdosage or poisoning with other types of chemicals or toxins.

Antiemetics are agents that reduce the hyperreactive vomiting reflex, largely by a central action, at the level of the vomiting center or chemoreceptor trigger zone (CTZ), or on the vestibular apparatus in the inner ear. The mechanisms that may be involved in eliciting the vomiting reflex are reviewed in Chapter 49.

GI Stimulants

• Metoclopramide

Maxolon, Octamide PFS, Reglan

(CAN) Emex, Maxeran

Metoclopramide is a smooth-muscle stimulant that acts largely on the upper GI tract. It increases gastric contractions and peristalsis of the duodenum and jejunum but relaxes the pyloric sphincter and duodenal bulb, thus accelerating gastric emptying and upper intestinal transit. Metoclopramide has little if any effect on colonic or gallbladder motility or on intestinal, biliary, or pancreatic secretions. It is used either orally or IV for a number of indications as listed below under Uses.

Mechanism

Stimulates upper GI motility and decreases normal inhibitory tone, by blocking dopamine receptors and sensitizing tissues to the action of acetylcholine; action is not dependent on intact vagal innervation and can be reversed by anticholinergic drugs; produces sedation and can elicit extrapyramidal reactions (refer to **Significant Adverse Reactions**); antiemetic action is attributable to blockade of central and peripheral dopamine receptors.

Uses

Symptomatic treatment of acute or chronic diabetic gastroparesis (gastric stasis). Symptoms of delayed gastric emptying, such as nausea, vomiting, anorexia, and abdominal fullness are progressively relieved over several weeks

Treatment of gastroesophageal reflux (short-term [ie, 4–12 wk], course of therapy in patients who do not respond to conventional therapy)

Prevention of postoperative nausea and vomiting or that associated with cancer chemotherapy

Facilitation of small bowel intubation in patients in whom the tube does not pass the pylorus by conventional measures

Stimulation of gastric emptying and intestinal transit of barium where delayed emptying interferes with radiologic examination

Investigational uses include facilitation of lactation and symptomatic treatment of gastric ulcers, anorexia nervosa, and nausea and vomiting due to pregnancy or a variety of other causes; also treatment of atonic bladder and esophageal variceal bleeding

Dosage

Diabetic Gastroparesis

10 mg orally 30 minutes before each meal and at bedtime for 2 to 8 weeks; severe symptoms may necessitate IM or IV administration

Gastroesophageal Reflux

10 mg to 15 mg orally up to four times/day 30 minutes before meals and at bedtime *or* 20 mg as a single dose before the provoking situation

Chemotherapy-Induced Emesis

Initially, 1 mg/kg to 2 mg/kg by slow infusion at least 30 minutes before beginning cancer chemotherapy; dose may be repeated every 2 hours for two doses, then every 3 hours for three doses; the higher dosage should be used when highly emetogenic antineoplastic drugs such as cisplatin or dacarbazine are used.

Small Bowel Intubation

Adults: 10 mg by slow IV injection (1–2 min)
Children 6 to 14 years: 2.5 to 5 mg as above
Children younger than 6 years: 0.1 mg/kg as above

Fate

Onset of action is 1 to 2 minutes IV, 10 to 15 minutes IM, and 30 to 60 minutes orally; effects persist for 1 to 2 hours; protein binding is minimal; drug is primarily excreted in the urine (80% in 24 h) as both unchanged drug or metabolites; elimination half-life ($T_{1/2}$) is 3 to 6 hours

Common Side Effects

Drowsiness, fatigue, restlessness, nausea, diarrhea

Significant Adverse Reactions

CNS: extrapyramidal reactions (acute dystonia, torticollis, facial grimacing, rhythmic tongue protrusion), parkinsonian-like symptoms, tardive dyskinesias, akathisia, dizziness, anxiety, insomnia, headache, depression

Endocrine: galactorrhea, gynecomastia, amenorrhea, impotence

Other: hypertension, tachycardia, urinary frequency, visual disturbances, neuroleptic malignant syndrome

Contraindications

Gastrointestinal obstruction, perforation or hemorrhage, pheochromocytoma, and epilepsy. *Cautious use* in the presence of depression, diabetes, galactorrhea, or gynecomastia and in pregnant women or nursing mothers.

Interactions

The action of metoclopramide can be antagonized by anticholinergics and narcotic analgesics.

Metoclopramide may impair absorption of drugs from the stomach (eg, digoxin, cimetidine) and increase absorption of drugs from the small intestine (eg, acetaminophen, ethanol, tetracyclines, levodopa).

Increased sedation may be observed when metoclopramide is given with alcohol, barbiturates, narcotics, or other sedatives and hypnotics.

Metoclopramide may alter insulin requirements by influencing the timing of food delivery to the intestines.

Nursing Management

Pretherapy Assessment

Assess and record baseline data necessary for detection of adverse effects of metoclopramide: General: vital signs (VS), body weight, skin color and temperature; central nervous system (CNS): orientation, reflexes, affect; GI: bowels sounds, normal output; Lab: electroencephalogram (EEG).

Review medical history and documents for existing or previous conditions that:

a. require cautious use of metoclopramide: depression; diabetes; galactorrhea; gynecomastia; previously detected breast cancer
b. contraindicate use of metoclopramide: allergy to metoclopramide; GI obstruction; perforation or hemorrhage; pheochromocytoma; epilepsy; **pregnancy (Category B)**, lactation (secreted in breast milk, avoid use).

Nursing Interventions

Medication Administration

Have diphenhydramine (50 mg, IM) available in case extrapyramidal symptoms occur, especially dystonias.

Inject slowly (1–2 min) to minimize restlessness and anxiety when giving IV push; these effects are often intense if injection is rapid. IV doses greater than 10 mg should be diluted and infused over 15 minutes.

Cover solution to protect it from light during IV infusion.

Note that the drug is usually given only when the small bowel tube has not passed the pylorus within 10 minutes with conventional maneuvers when used to facilitate small bowel intubation.

Assure ready access to bathroom facilities with high doses or when diarrhea occurs.

Surveillance During Therapy

Ensure that baseline data are obtained for weight, vital signs, state of hydration, and for a diabetic patient, serum glucose before long-term therapy is initiated.

Monitor diabetic patients and arrange for alteration in insulin dose or timing as diabetic control is compromised by changes in timing of food absorption.

Monitor patient for possible sodium retention and hypokalemia, particularly if congestive heart failure or cirrhosis is present.

Be alert for development of extrapyramidal reactions, especially in children, young adults, or the elderly or when high dosages are used. Symptoms (eg, restlessness, facial grimacing, involuntary movements), which occur both early and late in therapy, may take months to regress. If symptoms appear, notify the practitioner, discontinue the drug, and administer anticholinergic or antiparkinsonian drugs, as ordered, to control symptoms.

Carefully monitor laboratory studies and patient for indications of adverse reactions.

Interpret results of diagnostic tests and contact practitioner as appropriate.

Monitor for possible drug–drug and drug–nutrient interactions: Refer to **Interactions**.

Provide for patient safety needs if CNS effects occur because the drowsiness and dizziness that may occur after administration can last for several hours.

Patient Teaching

Inform the patient not to use alcohol, sleep remedies, and other over-the-counter (OTC) medications without the expressed consent of the practitioner.

Inform the patient that the following effects may occur as a result of therapy with this drug: dizziness; drowsiness; restlessness; anxiety; depression; headache; insomnia; nausea; diarrhea.

Instruct the patient to report the occurrence of any of the following to the practitioner: involuntary movement of the eyes, face, or limbs; severe depression; severe diarrhea.

• Cisapride

Propulsid

Cisapride is a GI stimulant that accelerates gastric emptying and increases lower esophageal peristalsis. It is indicated for the treatment of nocturnal heartburn due to gastroesophageal reflux. The mechanism of action appears to be enhancement of acetylcholine release in the GI tract. Cisapride, unlike metoclopramide, does not possess a significant dopamine receptor blocking action nor does it alter basal gastric acid secretion. Oral dosage is 10 mg four times a day before meals and at bedtime. Onset of action is within 30 to 60 minutes, and the drug is extensively metabolized before elimination. Plasma protein binding is approximately 98%. As with metoclopramide, the accelerated gastric emptying can alter the absorption of other drugs present at the same time. The most frequently encountered adverse effects are headache, diarrhea, abdominal pain, nausea, constipation, and rhinitis. The drug does not appear to affect psychomotor function nor cause sedation itself, but may potentiate the sedative effects of alcohol and other CNS depressants. Coagulation times with anticoagulants may be increased in the presence of cisapride and the absorption of cimetidine and ranitidine can be enhanced in patients receiving cisapride. **Pregnancy Category C**. Cisapride is excreted in breast milk and should not be used in nursing mothers.

• Dexpanthenol

Ilopan, Panthoderm

Dexpanthenol is an analog of pantothenic acid, a precursor of coenzyme A, which serves as a cofactor in the synthesis of acetylcholine. It is available as an IM injection solution (Ilopan) for prevention of postoperative paralytic ileus or intestinal atony, as an oral tablet (combined with choline bitartrate, Ilopan-Choline) for relief of gas retention, and as a cream (Panthoderm) for the relief of itching and minor skin irritation. IM doses are 250 to 500 mg, repeated in 2 hours and then every 6 hours until normal motility has returned. Orally, 2 to 3 tablets are taken 3 times a day, and the cream is applied once or twice daily. Side effects resulting from systemic use include itching, difficulty in breathing, generalized dermatitis, urticaria, diarrhea, and hypotension. Agitation has occurred in the elderly. If signs of hypersensitivity are noted, the drug should be discontinued.

Emetics

Vomiting is an efficient means of removing unabsorbed drugs or toxins from the stomach; thus, emetics are frequently used in instances of drug overdosage or accidental ingestion of toxic chemicals or other substances. Prompt administration is essential to remove as much of the toxin as possible before significant amounts are absorbed into the system. Emetics generally should not be used, however, in certain types of poisoning—for example, with corrosive or caustic agents or petroleum products—because the expulsion of these substances by vomiting can severely irritate or damage the epithelium of the upper digestive tract. Likewise, patients who are comatose or semiconscious or who demonstrate hyperactive or convulsive activity should not receive emetics. Whenever possible, adjunctive drugs and other measures (eg, materials for gastric lavage or suction, oxygen, specific antidotes to the common poisons) should be available and employed when necessary. Drug overdosage or chemical poisoning is a potentially serious problem, and everyone, especially parents, should have ready access to a poisoning chart giving explicit instructions for handling poisoning emergencies. The phone number of the closest poison prevention center should be posted, because speed of recognition and treatment is very often a critical factor for successful recovery.

• Ipecac syrup

An alkaloidal mixture containing principally emetine and cephaline, ipecac exerts its emetic effect by a direct irritant action on the GI tract as well as a central stimulatory action on the chemoreceptor trigger zone (CTZ) in the medulla. Ipecac syrup is available in quantities up to 30 mL without prescription; larger sizes require a prescription.

CAUTION

Ipecac *syrup* must not be confused with Ipecac *fluid extract*, which is 14 times more potent and can be fatal if given in the same dosage as the syrup.

Mechanism

Elicits emesis by a direct irritative action on the gastric mucosa and an activation of the CTZ; possesses an expectorant action, possibly by increasing bronchial secretions

Uses

Induction of vomiting, primarily to remove unabsorbed drugs and poisons

Dosage

Adults and children older than 1 year: 15 mL syrup followed by one or two glasses of water; may be repeated in 20 to 30 minutes if vomiting has not occurred

Children younger than 1 yr: 5 mL to 10 mL followed by one half to one glass of water

Fate

Vomiting occurs within 15 to 30 minutes, and effects may persist for another 20 to 30 minutes

Common Side Effects

Diarrhea, mild CNS depression

Significant Adverse Reactions

(Usually with large doses) Bloody diarrhea, myopathy, arrhythmias, cardiotoxicity, shock, convulsions

Contraindications

In semiconscious, unconscious, or convulsing patients; shock; poisoning with corrosive or caustic substances, strychnine, petroleum distillates, or volatile oils. *Cautious use* in pregnant or nursing women.

Interactions

Activated charcoal may absorb ipecac syrup, nullifying its emetic effect

Nursing Management

Pretherapy Assessment

Assess and record baseline data necessary for detection of adverse effects of ipecac syrup: General: VS, body weight, skin color and temperature; CNS: orientation, reflexes, affect; GI: bowel sounds.

Review medical history and documents for existing or previous conditions that:

a. require cautious use of ipecac: none
b. contraindicate use of ipecac: use in semiconscious, unconscious, or convulsing patients; shock; poisoning with corrosive or caustic substances, strychnine, petroleum distillates, or volatile oils; **pregnancy (Category C)**, lactation (secreted in breast milk, avoid use)

Nursing Interventions

Medication Administration

Administer drug to conscious patients only.
Administer with adequate amounts of water.
Arrange for use of activated charcoal if vomiting of ipecac does not occur or if overdose of ipecac occurs.
Assure ready access to bathroom facilities if diarrhea occurs.

Surveillance During Therapy

Monitor for possible drug–drug and drug–nutrient interactions: Refer to **Interactions**.

Patient Teaching

Instruct patient not to take drug with milk or carbonated beverages, because they may reduce its effectiveness.
Advise patient to drink 200 to 300 mL water after taking drug.
Instruct patient to contact a practitioner or emergency room immediately if vomiting does not occur within 20 minutes after the second dose, because cardiotoxicity may occur from the amount of the alkaloid emetine that is absorbed.

Table 54-1. **Antiemetic Drugs**

Phenothiazines (eg, Chlorpromazine, Perphenazine, Prochlorperazine, Promethazine, Thiethylperazine)

Potent antiemetic drugs acting by inhibition of CTZ through a dopaminergic blocking action; primarily effective for drug-induced emesis and nausea and vomiting associated with surgery, anesthesia, radiation, carcinoma, and severe infections; little usefulness in motion sickness, because drugs do not affect the vestibular apparatus; possibility of numerous side effects (some serious); thus recommended for short-term use only; most drugs also used as antipsychotic agents (except thiethylperazine; see Chap. 24)

Antihistamines (eg, Buclizine, Cyclizine, Dimenhydrinate, Meclizine)

Act by decreasing sensitivity of vestibular apparatus of inner ear, thus most effective in treating nausea and vomiting of motion sickness, Meniere's disease, or labyrinthitis; all elicit varying degrees of drowsiness and may have significant anticholinergic activity (see Chap. 16)

Anticholinergics (eg, Scopolamine)

Depress the vestibular apparatus and inhibit cholinergic activation of the vomiting center; very effective in preventing motion sickness; high incidence of side effects limits oral usefulness, but scopolamine is also available as Transderm-Scop in the form of a circular, flat disk that adheres to the skin behind the ear and provides for a continuous steady rate of drug release over 3 days (5 μg/h) with minimal side effects (see Chap. 13)

Miscellaneous (eg, Benzquinamide, Diphenidol, Dronabinol, Ondansetron, Granisetron, Trimethobenzamide)

Both centrally and peripherally acting antiemetics possessing several mechanisms of action; individual drugs are discussed in this chapter

Antiemetics

The mechanisms involved in the vomiting reflex can involve several pathways and are outlined in detail in Chapter 49. To briefly review, the vomiting center in the medulla may be stimulated by the chemoreceptor trigger zone (CTZ), also in the medulla, by the vestibular nuclei through the labyrinthine apparatus in the inner ear, and also directly by GI irritation. Dopamine appears to be the major neurotransmitter in the CTZ, whereas acetylcholine is believed to be the neurotransmitter involved with impulse transmission along the labyrinthine pathway to the vomiting center.

A variety of drugs have been successfully employed for the prophylaxis and treatment of nausea and vomiting of diverse etiology. Although vomiting may have many causes (for example, drug or chemical poisoning, motion sickness, radiation exposure, bacterial or viral infection, pregnancy, endocrine disorders, neurologic or psychic disturbances), most successful antiemetic drugs act mainly by inhibition of the CTZ or by depression of vestibular apparatus sensitivity in the inner ear. The major groups of drugs used to control nausea and vomiting are the phenothiazines, anticholinergics, antihistamines, and sedatives, along with a group of miscellaneous drugs, most of which also exhibit a central mechanism of action. These agents are listed in Table 54-1, with brief descriptions of their pharmacologic effects. In addition, a variety of other drugs, predominantly local acting, have been used in the treatment of nausea and vomiting; examples include antacids, adsorbents, antiflatulents, demulcents, and local anesthetics. The efficacy of most of these locally acting antiemetic drugs is subject to considerable debate; nevertheless, the placebo effect of such medications cannot always be discounted, and their occasional use to settle an "upset stomach" is probably not harmful in the otherwise healthy patient.

Many clinically useful antiemetic drugs are considered elsewhere in this text. Thus, the phenothiazines, which are potent dopamine-blocking agents and therefore very effective against drug-induced emesis at the level of the CTZ, are discussed in Chapter 24. Antihistamines, which are primarily useful in preventing the nausea and vomiting of motion sickness, because they apparently reduce vestibular activation of the vomiting center, are reviewed in Chapter 16. Scopolamine, a highly effective antinauseant for motion sickness, is frequently used as a transdermal patch, which provides a prolonged action (ie, 3 days) and produces fewer side effects than oral administration of the drug. Scopolamine is considered in Chapter 13.

A number of other drugs exhibiting an antiemetic action do not fit any of the above categories and therefore are reviewed individually in this chapter. One of these, metoclopramide, a drug with several GI indications, including antineoplastic drug–induced nausea and vomiting has been reviewed earlier in the chapter. Dronabinol, the psychoactive principle in marijuana, has been demonstrated to be effective in controlling refractive cases of nausea and vomiting accompanying cancer chemotherapy and is reviewed below. In addition, ondansetron, a selective serotonin-3 receptor antagonist useful in preventing postoperative and chemotherapy-induced nausea and vomiting is also considered here.

Another natural product recently studied for its antiemetic properties is ginger (*Zingiber officinale*). Long known as a spice and "medical food," it also has carminitive, stimulant, and diuretic properties. Clinical studies have shown that ginger can ameliorate the effects of motion sickness in the gastrointestinal tract itself and, although it is slower acting, it is comparable to dimenhydrinate (Dramamine) in activity.

• Benzquinamide

Emete-Con

Benzquinamide is believed to depress the CTZ and reduce activation of the vomiting center. It also possesses antihistaminic, anticholinergic, antiserotonin, and sedative action. The drug is used by IM or IV injection for the prevention and treatment of nausea and vomiting associated with anesthesia or surgery. Recommended dosage is 50 mg IM, which may be repeated in 1 hour and again every 3 to 4 hours as needed. The recommended IV dose is 25 mg given slowly over several minutes; subsequent doses should be given IM. Common side effects are drowsiness and dry mouth. Many other adverse reactions have been reported, including restlessness, headache, excitement, fatigue, insomnia, weakness, tremors hypotension, dizziness, atrial fibrillation, premature ventricular contractions, anorexia, nausea, and allergic reactions (rash, chills, fever, urticaria). Sudden increases in blood pressure and onset of arrhythmias have occurred after IV injection. The drug should be used cautiously in elderly or debilitated patients and in persons with arrhythmias. Benzquinamide may increase the pressor effects of other drugs and enhance the effects of other CNS depressants.

Nursing Management

Pretherapy Assessment

Assess and record baseline data necessary for detection of adverse effects of benzquinamide: General: VS, body weight, skin color and temperature; CNS: orientation, reflexes, affect; GI: bowel sounds.

Review medical history and documents for existing or previous conditions that:

a. require cautious use of benzquinamide: use in the elderly; arrhythmias

b. contraindicate use of benzquinamide: allergy to benzquinamide; use in young children; IV administration in cardiac patients; **pregnancy (Category C)**, lactation (secreted in breast milk, avoid use)

Nursing Interventions

Medication Administration

Administer drug 15 minutes before recovery from anesthesia when used to control postanesthesia nausea and vomiting.

Seek clarification if prescribed IV for patient with cardiovascular disease because the danger of sudden hypertension or arrhythmias is high.

Consider possible causes underlying nausea and vomiting because the drug may mask signs of overdosage with other drugs or prevent accurate diagnosis of conditions associated with nausea and vomiting (eg, intestinal obstruction, carcinoma, brain tumors).

Inject deeply into large muscle when giving IM.

Surveillance During Therapy

Carefully monitor laboratory studies and patient for indications of adverse reactions.

Interpret results of diagnostic tests and contact practitioner as appropriate.

Monitor for possible drug–drug and drug–nutrient interactions: Refer to **Interactions**.

Patient Teaching

Because this drug is employed as a postanesthetic agent to control nausea and vomiting, patient teaching is likely to focus on possible postanesthetic side effects.

• Diphenidol

Vontrol

Diphenidol depresses the excitability of the vestibular apparatus and the CTZ and exhibits relatively weak antihistaminic, anticholinergic, and CNS depressant activity. It is used orally for the control of nausea and vomiting due to surgery, vestibular disturbances, infectious diseases, neoplasms, and radiation therapy, and also for the treatment of vertigo due to Meniere's disease, labyrinthitis, or middle or inner ear surgery. Usual adult dosage is 25 to 50 mg every 4 hours; children may be given 0.4 mg/lb up to 25 mg every 4 hours. Adverse effects include drowsiness, indigestion, dry mouth, malaise, depression, insomnia, dizziness, headache, skin rash, slight hypotension, and mild jaundice.

CAUTION

Diphenidol may cause confusion, disorientation, and hallucinations and should be used only in professionally supervised persons. The drug is eliminated almost entirely in the urine, and cumulation can occur in patients with reduced renal function. Cautious use is warranted in patients with glaucoma, prostatic hypertrophy, obstructive lesions of the GI or urinary tracts, or hepatic disease, and in nursing mothers. Additive CNS-depressant effects can occur in combination with other sedative or hypnotic drugs.

Nursing Management

Nursing Interventions

Medication Administration

Administer only to hospitalized patients or those under close medical supervision because drug has caused auditory and visual hallucinations, disorientation, and confusion. The drug should be discontinued if such reactions occur (incidence approximately 0.5%; onset usually within 3 days after starting therapy; symptoms subside within several days after discontinuation of therapy).

Consider possible causes underlying nausea and vomiting because drug may mask signs of drug overdosage or underlying pathology.

Provide frequent mouth care if patient is unable to take fluids for relief of dry mouth.

Patient Teaching

Warn patient that drowsiness can occur and may interfere with performance of tasks.

• Dronabinol

Marinol

Dronabinol is delta-9-tetrahydrocannabinol (THC), the principal psychoactive substance found in *Cannabis sativa* or marijuana. It is effective in controlling nausea and vomiting due to cancer chemotherapy, but its use should be reserved for those patients not helped by conventional antiemetic therapy, because the drug is capable of causing profound CNS effects. The drug has also been used for stimulating appetite in patients with acquired immunodeficiency syndrome (AIDS). Cannabinoid administration has been associated with extreme mood changes (euphoria, anxiety, depression, panic, paranoia), altered states of reality, impaired memory, distorted perception, and hallucinations. In addition, tachycardia is noted frequently, and orthostatic hypotension and fainting have been reported. Dronabinol is strongly habituating and is classified as a Schedule II controlled substance (refer to Chapter 10).

Mechanism

Not completely established; may depress the vomiting mechanism in the brain stem; other nonrelated effects include increased heart rate, decreased blood pressure (mainly orthostatic), reduced body temperature, and profound CNS changes (see above)

Uses

Treatment of nausea and vomiting due to cancer chemotherapy in patients who have not responded to more conventional antiemetic therapy

Treatment of anorexia and weight loss in patients with AIDS

Dosage

Antiemetic:

Initially, 5 mg/m^2 of body surface, orally, 1 to 3 hours before chemotherapy, then every 2 to 4 hours thereafter to a maximum of 6 doses/day; increase in 2.5 mg/m^2 increments, as needed, to a maximum of 15 mg/m^2

Appetite Stimulant: 2.5 mg orally twice a day before lunch and supper; may increase up to 10 mg twice daily if tolerated

Fate

Oral absorption is good, although there is extensive first-pass hepatic metabolism; peak effect occurs within 2 to 4 hours; psychoactive effects last for 4 to 6 hours, but the appetite stimulant effect may persist for 24 hours or longer; plasma protein binding is high (97%); within 72 hours, approximately one half of an oral dose is recovered in the feces, biliary excretion being the major route of elimination; smaller amounts are excreted in the urine; prolonged use may result in drug accumulation to toxic amounts

Common Side Effects

Drowsiness, elation, giddiness, euphoria, dizziness, impaired thinking ability, decreased coordination, tachycardia, weakness, depression

Significant Adverse Reactions

Paresthesias, visual distortions, confusion, memory impairment, disorientation, depression, paranoia, tinnitus, nightmares, speech difficulty, flushing, sweating, hypotension, fainting, diarrhea, muscle pain

Contraindications

No absolute contraindications. *Cautious use* in patients with hypertension, heart disease, depression, schizophrenia, mania, and in patients receiving other psychoactive drugs.

Interactions

Enhanced CNS effects may occur with combined use of cannabinoids and alcohol, sedatives, hypnotics, or other psychotomimetic substances

Dronabinol may increase theophylline metabolism, decreasing its effectiveness.

Increased risk of tachycardia and drowsiness can occur with use of dronabinol and tricyclic antidepressants, antihistamines, anticholinergics, and adrenergic amines.

Nursing Management

Pretherapy Assessment

Assess and record baseline data necessary for detection of adverse effects of dronabinol: General: VS, body weight, skin color and temperature; CNS: orientation, reflexes, bilateral grip strength, affect; cardiovascular system (CVS): orthostatic blood pressure (BP); GI: bowel sounds.

Review medical history and documents for existing or previous conditions that:

a. require cautious use of dronabinol: hypertension; heart disease; depression; schizophrenia; mania; use of other psychoactive drugs
b. contraindicate use of dronabinol allergy to dronabinol or sesame oil vehicle; nausea and vomiting arising from any other cause other than cancer chemotherapy; **pregnancy (Category B)**, lactation (concentrated in breast milk, avoid use)

Nursing Interventions

Medication Administration

Ensure that patient will remain under close supervision of a responsible adult while using drug (inpatient therapy is recommended).

Implement interventions to prevent injury resulting from CNS and systemic effects (refer to introductory section, **Common Side Effects**, and **Significant Adverse Reactions**) until reactions to drug are evident and thereafter as indicated.

Follow procedures for administration of schedule II substances (see Chapter 10).

Be aware of the drugs' potential effects on mood and behavior and be prepared to deal with these if they occur.

Surveillance During Therapy

Monitor patient's mental and emotional status frequently. Cannabinoids induce some change in virtually all patients.

Place patient in quiet environment and provide supportive measures, including reassurance, if disturbing psychiatric symptoms occur. Such reactions, which occur more commonly with higher dosages, disappear spontaneously (within 24 hours with dronabinol) without specific therapy.

Monitor blood pressure and cardiac status of patient with hypertension or heart disease because hypotension, usually orthostatic, and tachycardia frequently occur.
Monitor for toxicity.
Carefully monitor laboratory studies and patient for indications of adverse reactions.
Interpret results of diagnostic tests and contact practitioner as appropriate.
Monitor for possible drug–drug and drug–nutrient interactions: Refer to **Interactions**.
Provide for patient safety needs if CNS, visual, or hypotensive effects occur.

Patient Teaching

Carefully prepare patient for the kinds of CNS reactions that may occur.
Caution patient not to drive or perform other potentially hazardous tasks because CNS functions are typically altered, and orthostatic hypotension may occur.
Warn patient that additive CNS depression occurs when cannabinoids are used in conjunction with other drugs that depress the CNS (refer to **Interactions**).
Inform patient that use with other substances that induce psychotomimesis (eg, mixed opiate agonist–antagonists) may increase the likelihood of psychotic reactions.
Teach patient control measures if orthostatic hypotension occurs.

• Ondansetron

Zofran

Ondansetron is a selective 5-HT_3 receptor antagonist used for prevention of nausea and vomiting associated with cancer chemotherapy or that occurring postoperatively. The serotonin receptors of the 5-HT_3 type occur both peripherally on vagal nerve terminals and centrally in the chemoreceptor trigger zone of the brain stem. Chemotherapy-induced nausea and vomiting may be due to release of serotonin (5-HT) from enterochromaffin cells in the small intestine. The resultant stimulation of vagal afferents (via the 5-HT_3 receptors) may instigate the vomiting reflex.

Mechanism

Not completely understood; selectively blocks 5HT_3 receptors, which blunts the vomiting reflex elicited by cancer chemotherapeutic agents; appears to decrease stimulation of vagal afferents resulting from released serotonin.

Uses

Prevention of nausea and vomiting associated with initial and repeat courses of emetogenic cancer chemotherapy, including high-dose cisplatin.
Prevention of postoperative nausea and vomiting

Dosage

Cancer Chemotherapy
IV:
Adults: Three 0.15 mg/kg doses; usually the first dose is infused over 15 minutes, beginning 30 minutes before the start of emetogenic chemotherapy. Following doses are given 4 and 8 hours after the first dose. Alternately, 32 mg as a single dose infused over 15 minutes, beginning 30 minutes before the start of emetogenic chemotherapy
Children (older than 3 y): as above for adults in three doses; few data are available on dosage in children younger than 3 years of age.
Orally:
Adults: 8 mg 3 times a day
Children (4–12 y): 4 mg 3 times a day

Postoperative

4 mg undiluted IV over 2 to 5 minutes

Fate

After IV injection, elimination $T_{1/2}$ is 3 to 5 hours. Orally, drug is well absorbed, and absorption is increased in the presence of food; peak effects occur in 1.5 to 2 hours; elimination $T_{1/2}$ is approximately 3 hours. Plasma protein binding is 70% to 75%.

Common Side Effects

Headache, diarrhea, dizziness, muscular pain, drowsiness

Significant Adverse Reactions

Constipation, rash, fever, abdominal pain, weakness, shivering, malaise, urinary retention
Rarely, bronchospasm, tachycardia, angina, hypokalemia, electrocardiographic alterations, grand mal seizures

Contraindications

No absolute contraindications. *Cautious use* in patients with impaired liver function, and in pregnant and nursing mothers.

Nursing Management

Pretherapy Assessment

Assess and record baseline data necessary for detection of adverse effects of ondansetron: General: VS, body weight, skin color and temperature; CNS: orientation, reflexes, bilatral grip strength, affect, ophthalmic examination; CVS: orthostatic BP; GI: bowel sounds.
Review medical history and documents for existing or previous conditions that:
a. require cautious use of ondansetron: impaired liver function
b. contraindicate use of ondansetron: allergy to ondansetron; **pregnancy (Category B)**, lactation (concentrated in breast milk, avoid use)

Nursing Interventions

Medication Administration

Administration of the drug with food increases the extent of absorption of the drug.

Surveillance During Therapy

Monitor for toxicity; headache; constipation; abdominal pain; weakness; dry mouth.
Carefully monitor laboratory studies and patient for indications of adverse reactions.
Interpret results of diagnostic tests and contact practitioner as appropriate.
Monitor for possible drug–drug and drug–nutrient interactions: refer to **Interactions**.

Provide for patient safety needs if CNS, visual, or hypotensive effects occur.

Patient Teaching

Teach patient that the following effects may occur as a result of drug therapy: headache; weakness; dizziness; drowsiness; diarrhea; muscular pain.

Instruct the patient to report any of the following to the practitioner if they occur: rash; fever; weakness; shivering; malaise; urinary retention; bronchospasm; tachycardia; angina; seizures.

• Granisetron

Kytril

Granisetron, like ondansetron, is a selective serotonin (5-HT_3) receptor antagonist with little or no activity at other serotonin receptors. It is indicated for the prevention of nausea and vomiting associated with initial or repeat courses of emetogenic cancer chemotherapy. The recommended dosage is 10 μg/kg, infused IV over 5 minutes beginning 30 minutes prior to initiation of chemotherapy. The most frequently reported adverse effects are headache, diarrhea, somnolence, and asthenia. Elevations in liver enzymes have occurred in 2%–4% of patients. Refer to the discussion of ondansetron for additional information and nursing considerations.

• Phosphorated Carbohydrate Solution

Emetrol, Naus-A-Way, Nausetrol

These products are hyperosmolar solutions of different carbohydrates (eg, sucrose, dextrose, levulose) with phosphoric acid. The phosphorated carbohydrate solutions are locally acting antiemetics that probably exert a direct action on the wall of the GI tract to reduce smooth muscle contraction and delay gastric emptying. They are used for the symptomatic relief of nausea and vomiting. Adults receive 15 to 30 mL undiluted solution, whereas infants and young children are given 5 to 10 mL. A dose may be taken every 15 minutes until vomiting ceases. For prevention of morning sickness, a dose may be taken every 3 hours or as needed. To prevent regurgitation in infants, 5 to 10 mL are given 10 to 15 minutes before feeding. Side effects are infrequent, although large doses can produce diarrhea and abdominal pain. Because they contain a high content of carbohydrates, these preparations should not be taken by diabetic patients.

Nursing Management

Nursing Interventions

Patient Teaching

Inform patient that drug is quite safe when taken as directed, is virtually free of side effects, and will not mask symptoms of underlying pathology.

Instruct patient *not* to dilute drug or ingest fluids immediately before or for at least 15 minutes after administration.

Advise patient to consult primary healthcare provider if symptoms are not relieved or recur after drug treatment.

• Thiethylperazine

Torecan

A phenothiazine derivative used exclusively as an antiemetic–antivertigo agent, thiethylperazine is claimed to have less tranquilizing action than other phenothiazines. It may be used either orally, rectally, or by IM injection at a dose of 10 to 30 mg a day in divided doses for the relief of nausea and vomiting. The onset of action is 30 to 60 minutes with oral or rectal administration and 15 to 30 minutes after IM injection. Drowsiness is a frequent side effect. Because the drug is a phenothiazine derivative, many other adverse effects are possible; refer to the discussion of phenothiazine antipsychotics in Chapter 24 for a listing of these other possible adverse reactions. Contraindications to use of thiethylperazine include severe CNS depression, comatose states, pregnancy, and children younger than 12 years of age. *Cautious use* is necessary in patients with renal or hepatic disease, in nursing mothers, and after intracardiac or intracranial surgery.

Nursing Management

Refer to **Phenothiazines**, in Chapter 24. In addition:

Nursing Interventions

Medication Administration

Administer deeply into large muscle mass of recumbent patient when giving IM. Keep patient in bed for at least 1 hour after injection to minimize orthostatic hypotension.

Assess patient for allergy to tartrazine and sulfite because the oral form contains tartrazine and the parenteral form contains metabisulfite.

Patient Teaching

Urge caution in driving or performing hazardous tasks because drug can cause drowsiness, dizziness, and blurred vision.

Teach patient how to recognize and report extrapyramidal reactions (eye movements, difficulty speaking, unusual body movements, gait disturbances). If they should occur, dosage should be reduced or drug discontinued.

• Trimethobenzamide

Tigan and other manufacturers

Mechanism

Not established; may directly depress the CTZ and interfere with vestibular activation of the CTZ or the vomiting center; does not appear to block *direct* activation of the vomiting center; possesses weak antihistamine activity

Uses

Symptomatic control of nausea and vomiting (combined with other antiemetics if vomiting is severe)

Dosage

Oral

Adults: 250 mg 3 or 4 times a day
Children: 100 mg to 200 mg 3 or 4 times a day

Rectal

Adults: 200 mg 3 or 4 times a day

Children: 100 mg to 200 mg 3 or 4 times a day

IM

Adults *only*: 200 mg 3 or 4 times a day

Fate

Onset of action after oral or rectal administration is 15 to 45 minutes, with duration of 3 to 4 hours; after IM injection, onset is 15 minutes and duration is 2 to 3 hours; metabolized in liver and excreted principally in the urine

Significant Adverse Reactions

Hypersensitivity reactions, hypotension (especially with IM use), blurred vision, depression, diarrhea, dizziness, drowsiness, jaundice, muscle cramping, blood dyscrasias

In addition, during acute fever, gastroenteritis, dehydration, or electrolyte imbalance. Drug has also produced CNS reactions such as opisthotonos (tetanic spasm of back muscles), convulsions, extrapyramidal symptoms (rigidity, akathisia, tremor), and coma.

After IM injection, redness, irritation, stinging, swelling, or burning at injection site have occurred.

Contraindications

Parenteral use in children; rectal administration in newborns, premature infants, or persons hypersensitive to benzocaine or other local anesthetics. *Cautious use* during acute febrile illnesses, in pregnant or nursing women, elderly or debilitated patients, and in persons receiving other centrally acting drugs.

Interactions

Additive depressant effects can occur with other CNS-depressant drugs (eg, narcotics, alcohol, barbiturates).

Extrapyramidal reactions, convulsions, and other CNS disturbances may be enhanced if trimethobenzamide is given together with phenothiazines or barbiturates.

Nursing Management

Pretherapy Assessment

Assess and record baseline data necessary for detection of adverse effects of trimethobenzamide: General: VS, body weight, skin color and temperature; CNS: orientation, reflexes, affect, ophthalmic examination; CVS: orthostatic BP; GI: bowel sounds; GU: prostate examination; Lab: CBC, electrolytes.

Review medical history and documents for existing or previous conditions that:

a. require cautious use of trimethobenzamide: acute febrile illnesses, use in the elderly or debilitated; with other CNS drugs; conditions aggravated by anticholinergic therapy.

b. contraindicate use of trimethobenzamide: allergy to trimethobenzamide, benzocaine, other amide local anethetics; parenteral use in children; rectal administration in newborns, premature infants; **pregnancy (Category C)**, lactation (secreted in breast milk, avoid use)

Nursing Interventions

Medication Administration

Consider possible causes of nausea and vomiting because antiemetic drugs can mask symptoms of a more serious underlying disorder or impair diagnosis of a pathologic condition (eg, appendicitis).

Assure ready access to bathroom facilities in case diarrhea occurs.

Assure adequate hydration.

Provide adequate skin care and protection from sunlight if dermatologic effects occur.

Inject deeply into upper outer quadrant of gluteal region and avoid escape of the solution along the injection route to minimize irritation and pain with IM injection.

Do *not* administer IM in children of any age and do not use rectal suppositories in premature or full-term newborns.

Surveillance During Therapy

Observe patient for signs of CNS toxicity (eg, disorientation, lethargy, tremors), particularly if patient is receiving other centrally acting drugs (eg, phenothiazines, barbiturates, anticholinergics). Drug should be discontinued if signs occur.

Ensure that if signs of extrapyramidal reactions appear they are carefully evaluated. They can be confused with symptoms of certain CNS disorders that may be responsible for the vomiting, such as encephalopathy or Reye's syndrome.

Observe patient for abrupt onset of vomiting, confusion, lethargy, or irrational behavior, possible signs of Reye's syndrome (refer to **Significant Adverse Reactions** for salicylates, Chapter 21). Immediate medical attention is imperative if such symptoms occur. Although Reye's syndrome has not been *definitely* linked to trimethobenzamide and other antiemetic drugs, it has been associated with their use during febrile periods.

Monitor blood pressure after parenteral administration because hypotension can occur.

Carefully monitor laboratory studies and patient for indications of adverse reactions.

Interpret results of diagnostic tests and contact practitioner as appropriate.

Monitor for possible drug–drug and drug–nutrient interactions: refer to **Interactions**.

Provide for patient safety needs if CNS, visual, or hypotensive effects occur.

Patient Teaching

Inform patient to use caution in performing hazardous tasks (driving, operating machinery) because drug may induce drowsiness, dizziness, and loss of orientation.

Instruct patient to report development of rash, itching, or other signs of hypersensitivity. Drug should be discontinued if they occur.

Teach patient that the following effects may occur as a result of drug therapy: weakness; dizziness; drowsiness; diarrhea; blurred vision.

Instruct the patient to report any of the following to the practitioner if they occur: difficulty breathing; muscle spasms; unusual bleeding or bruising; sore throat; visual disturbances; irregular heartbeat; yellowing of the skin or eyes.

Selected Bibliography

Barisano A, Mehl B, Bradbury K: Serotonin antagonists: Treatment of chemotherapy-induced emesis. Mount Sinai J Med 59(5):433, 1992

Bone ME et al: Ginger root-a new antiemetic: The effect of ginger root on postoperative nausea and vomiting after major gynaecological surgery. Anaesthesia 45(8):669, 1990

Brunberg SM, Hesketh PJ: Control of chemotherapy-induced emesis. N Engl J Med 329:1790, 1993

Marty M: Future trends in cancer treatment and emesis control. Oncology 50(3):159, 1993

Mitchelson F: Pharmacological agents affecting emesis: A review (Parts I and II). Drugs 43:295, 443, 1992

Ojind N, Katz N: Update on the pharmacology of anti-emetic drugs used in cancer chemotherapy. Pharmindex 35(1):6, 1993

Ondansetron: A new concept in the management of emesis. Semin Oncol 19(4 Suppl 10):1, 1992

Pisters KM, Kris MG: Management of nausea and vomiting caused by anticancer drugs: State of the art. Oncology 6(2 Suppl):99, 1992

Nursing Bibliography

Distasio S: Zofran makes chemo bearable. RN 56(5):56, 1993

Knapman J: Controlling emesis after chemotherapy. Nursing Standard 7(15-16):38, 1993

Lewis M, Fishman D: Ondansetron for post operative nausea and vomiting: Decision in the absence of comparative trials. Am J Hosp Phar 51:98, 1994

Lichter I: Which antiemetic . . . ? Journal of Palliative Care 9(1):42, 1993

VII

Drugs Acting on Respiratory Function

55
Respiratory Physiology: A Review

Normal metabolism requires the continual supply of oxygen (O_2) and removal of carbon dioxide (CO_2). The respiratory system functions in concert with the cardiovascular system to supply all body tissues with O_2 for cellular oxidative metabolism and to remove CO_2, a major metabolic waste product.

The respiratory system also plays a critical role in the regulation of acid–base balance, adjusting its activities rapidly to maintain a constant pH of the internal environment.

Respiration, which may be broadly defined as the exchange of gases (O_2 and CO_2) between a living organism and its external environment, consists of five interrelated phases that operate continuously:

- *Pulmonary ventilation:* the periodic flow of air into and out of the lungs
- *Pulmonary exchange of gases:* the diffusion of O_2 from the alveoli into the pulmonary capillaries and the diffusion of CO_2 out of the blood into the alveoli
- *Transport of gases:* the transport of O_2 by the blood from the lungs for distribution to all body tissues and the return of CO_2 from the tissues to the lungs for expiration
- *Blood–tissue exchange of gases:* the exchange of gases at the tissue level, with O_2 diffusing from the blood into the tissue cells and CO_2 diffusing from the cells into the blood
- *Cellular respiration:* the cellular utilization of O_2 for oxidative metabolism with the production of CO_2

Anatomy/Histology Overview

The respiratory system can be divided into two major functional divisions: the conducting division and the respiratory division.

Conducting Division

The components of the *conducting division* serve primarily as air conduits to the gas-exchanging areas of the lungs. During its passage through the upper segments of the conducting division, the air is filtered, warmed, and humidified. Components of the conducting division are the nose, pharynx, larynx, trachea, bronchi, bronchioles, and terminal bronchioles.

Respiratory Division

The respiratory bronchioles, alveolar ducts, alveolar sacs, and alveoli form the respiratory division of the lungs wherein the oxygen-rich, water-saturated air is exposed to the blood for gaseous exchange.

The Respiratory Tree

During *inspiration* the air passes through the nose (or mouth), pharynx, and larynx before entering the trachea. The trachea is structurally characterized by the presence of 16 to 20 C-shaped rings of hyaline cartilage (completed posteriorly by smooth muscle and connective tissue), which support the trachea and keep it patent. The tissue lining the trachea is pseudostratified cilated columnar epithelium with goblet cells. The trachea terminates in the thorax by dividing into two primary bronchi that pass to the roots of the lungs. The right bronchus is shorter, wider, and more vertical than the left and is therefore more likely to retain inhaled foreign particles.

Within the lungs, the primary bronchi undergo successive branching to form a treelike arrangement of smaller bronchi and bronchioles, often called the *bronchial tree*. The branching within the bronchial tree results in the formation of successively narrower tubes that collectively offer a greater total cross-sectional area of the lumina than the parent tubes.

The following histologic modifications occur with progressive branching:

1. The rings of cartilage are replaced by irregular plates of cartilage that gradually become smaller and finally disappear in the bronchioles.
2. As the amount of cartilage decreases the amount of smooth muscle progressively increases. The smooth muscle layer is crucial in determining the airway resistance because it governs the caliber of the bronchioles (which no longer have cartilage rings to maintain tubular patency).
3. The pseudostratified ciliated columnar epithelium loses its goblet cells and then its cilia, eventually thinning to simple cuboidal epithelium in the terminal bronchioles.

Arising from the terminal bronchioles are the first components of the respiratory division—the *respiratory bronchioles*—whose free terminations open into *alveolar ducts*. The alveolar ducts communicate with spaces called *alveolar sacs*, which in turn open into a number of pocketlike expansions, the *alveoli*.

Histologically, the smooth muscle prominent in the latter segments of the conducting division is replaced by elastic connective tissue within the respiratory division.

The respiratory epithelium gradually loses its cilia and eventually thins to a simple squamous configuration, thus allowing gaseous exchange to occur. Increasing vascularity and a greater cross-sectional surface area further promote efficient exchange of gases. It has been estimated that human lungs contain approximately 300 million alveoli and provide a total surface area of 70 m^2 for gaseous exchange. Alveolar walls are lined with type I pneumocytes, which are the principal lining cells, and type II (granular) pneumocytes, which secrete surfactant.

The Lungs

All of the components of the respiratory tract beyond the primary bronchi are contained within the lungs. The lungs are cone-shaped, paired structures located in the thoracic cavity, surrounded by a cagelike framework composed of the sternum, costal cartilage, ribs, and vertebrae. The muscular, dome-shaped diaphragm serves as the floor of the thoracic cage.

Blood vessels, lymphatics, nerves, and the bronchi enter the lungs at the *hilus* and form the root of the lung. The *parietal pleura*, which lines the thoracic cavity, and the *visceral pleura*, which covers the lung surface, are continuous serous membranes that reflect upon each other at the root of each lung. The potential space between these two membranes (the *pleural cavity*) contains a thin film of lubricating fluid that minimizes friction during respiratory movements.

The right lung contains three lobes and the left lung has two lobes, each of which is supplied by a *secondary* (or lobar) *bronchus*. Each lung is further subdivided into *bronchopulmonary segments* supplied by *tertiary* (or segmental) *bronchi*.

Each bronchopulmonary segment contains smaller anatomical units called *lobules*, supplied by a terminal bronchiole, arteriole, venule, and lymphatic vessel.

Blood Supply

The pulmonary artery and its branches carry blood from the right ventricle of the heart to the respiratory tissue of the lung for oxygenation and removal of CO_2. *Venules*, arising from the vast network of pulmonary capillaries that surround the alveoli, collect oxygenated blood, which is then returned to the left atrium of the heart by the *pulmonary veins*.

Oxygenated blood reaches the visceral pleura and other portions of the lung through the *bronchial arteries* and their branches. Some *bronchial veins* empty into the superior vena cava through the azygos system, whereas others drain into the pulmonary veins.

In contrast to the systemic circulation, the pulmonary circulation is a low-pressure, low-resistance circuit.

Nerve Supply

The bronchial tree is innervated by fibers from both divisions of the autonomic nervous system. Activation of parasympathetic (vagal) nerve fibers causes contraction of respiratory smooth muscle, whereas sympathetic stimulation brings about relaxation.

Autonomic nerves also supply pulmonary and bronchial blood vessels.

Respiratory Defense Mechanisms

Large particulate matter inhaled through the *nares* (nostrils) is filtered by the coarse hairs lining the nasal vestibule. A blanket of mucus (secreted by goblet cells and mucous glands in the upper respiratory tract) traps dust and fine particulate matter. The mucus and entrapped materials are swept toward the mouth by ciliary movements. The cough reflex provides a more forceful mechanism for the expulsion of secretions and particulate matter from the respiratory tract.

Alveolar macrophages ("dust cells") provide a major defense against bacterial invasion of the lungs. These unique phagocytic cells migrate freely over the alveolar surface, engulfing and lysing bacteria and other particulate matter.

Pulmonary Ventilation

Pulmonary ventilation operates on the principle (Boyle's Law) that the pressure and volume of a closed cavity are inversely related. Therefore, if the volume of a closed cavity increases, the pressure within it will fall.

The lungs lie in separate airtight cavities within the thorax, surrounded by the pleura. The elastic recoil of the lungs tends to pull them away from the thoracic wall, creating a partial vacuum within the pleural cavity. The flow of air through the respiratory tract follows pressure gradients between the atmosphere and the lungs. Just before inspiration, the pressure inside the lungs (the *intrapulmonary pressure*) is equal to atmospheric pressure, whereas the pressure within the pleural cavity (the *intrapleural pressure*) is always subatmospheric.

Inspiration is an active process resulting from the expansion of the thorax. It is initiated by neural activity leading to the contraction of respiratory muscles. During normal quiet inspiration, the contraction and descent of the *diaphragm* increases the vertical dimensions of the thoracic cavity, whereas contraction of the *external intercostal muscles* widens the thorax by elevating the ribs and sternum. The lungs expand as they follow the movements of the thoracic wall because the serous fluid in the pleural cavity causes the visceral and parietal pleura to adhere closely, much as two moist plates of glass resist separation.

As the lungs expand and the pulmonary volume increases, the intrapulmonary (intra-alveolar) pressure falls below atmospheric, creating a pressure gradient that causes air to flow from the atmosphere through the conducting passageways into the lungs. As the lungs expand, elastic components of the lung stretch and develop tension.

Quiet expiration occurs passively through relaxation of the inspiratory muscles. As the diaphragm ascends and the ribs and sternum return to their resting positions, the size of the thoracic cavity decreases. As the thorax assumes its original size, the potential energy stored in the elastic elements of the lung is converted into kinetic energy. These events cause the intrapulmonary pressure to temporarily exceed the atmospheric pressure, thus reversing the flow of air.

Accessory muscles of respiration include the scalene, sternomastoid, and the pectoralis minor, which contract during forceful inspiration to further expand the thorax. During active, forceful expiration, coughing, and vomiting, the internal intercostal muscles contract to pull the ribs downward and inward, while the abdominal muscles contract to push the diaphragm upward.

Respiratory Compliance

Respiratory compliance, which may be defined as the lung volume change per unit change in pressure, is a term often used to describe the ease with which the lungs may be inflated. The high content of elastic tissue in the lungs resists distension. However, the elasticity of the lungs and other thoracic structures facilitates expiration.

A major factor affecting pulmonary compliance is the surface tension of the alveolar lining fluid.

Surface Tension

Surface tension results from the forces of attraction between molecules on a fluid surface at a liquid–gas interface. The inner surface of the alveoli is coated with a thin film of fluid that exerts a surface tension tending to impair expansion of alveoli on inspiration (and to favor collapse on expiration).

According to the law of LaPlace, the pressure created by surface tension is greater in smaller alveoli. In the absence of surfactant, the smaller alveoli would therefore collapse and empty their air into larger alveoli.

Normally, the type II alveolar cells (pneumocytes) secrete a lipoprotein *surfactant* that reduces the surface tension and lowers the resistance of the alveoli to expansion on inspiration. Pulmonary surfactant therefore increases respiratory compliance and reduces the work required for breathing.

A deficiency of pulmonary surfactant characterizes *respiratory distress syndrome* (also known as *hyaline membrane disease*), a condition often afflicting premature infants. Thyroid hormones and glucocorticoids enhance surfactant production, with surfactant activity, while two newer drugs, beractant and colfosceril, are available for treating infants with surfactant deficiency.

Resistance to Airflow

Any obstruction or resistance to the flow of air would increase the force required to bring air into the alveoli. Airway resistance is encountered chiefly in the bronchi and bronchioles. It can be increased by the contraction of respiratory smooth muscle (*bronchoconstriction*) or by swelling of the respiratory mucosa (*mucosal edema*).

Reflex bronchoconstriction may follow mechanical or chemical stimulation of airway receptors. Parasympathetic stimulation, acetylcholine, and histamine cause bronchoconstriction. Sympathetic stimulation, epinephrine, and isoproterenol relax bronchiolar smooth muscle.

Bronchial asthma is an inflammatory bronchospastic disease (frequently allergic in origin) characterized by great airway resistance. Major factors contributing to the heightened airway resistance are respiratory muscle spasm and mucosal edema leading to excessive accumulation of mucus.

The important mechanisms involved in bronchial constriction and relaxation are summarized in Figure 55-1.

Volumes of Air Exchanged

The amount of air exchanged during normal, quiet respiration (*eupnea*) varies with the age, sex, and size of the person. In the average adult the *tidal volume* (volume of air inspired or expired) is approximately 500 mL. The product of *tidal volume* and *respiratory rate* equals the *minute respiratory volume*, which represents the volume of air entering the lungs in 1 minute.

A critical factor in the total process of pulmonary ventilation is *alveolar ventilation*. Alveolar ventilation (the volume of air that enters the alveoli per minute) is a fraction of the total ventilation because with each breath some air remains in the conducting passages and is therefore unavailable to the alveoli for gaseous exchange. The total internal volume of these conducting passages is termed *anatomic dead space*, estimated to be 150 mL. The *physiologic dead space*, which in normally functioning lungs is essentially equal to the anatomical dead space, is more variable (and larger) if nonfunctioning alveoli are present.

Exchange and Transport of Respiratory Gases

In a mixture of gases (such as the atmosphere), the portion of the total pressure contributed by a particular gas in the mixture is termed the *partial pressure* or *tension*. The partial pressure exerted by each individual gas varies directly with its concentration in the mixture and with the total pressure of the mixture. For example, O_2, which makes up approximately 21% of atmospheric air, exerts a partial pressure (PO_2) of 160 mm Hg under standard total atmospheric pressure of 760 mm Hg, that is, $0.21 \times 760 = 160$.

Atmospheric (inspired) air is composed predominantly of nitrogen and O_2 with very small amounts of CO_2, water vapor, and inert gases. Alveolar air differs from atmospheric air in composition because the inspired air becomes saturated with water vapor and mixed with old anatomic dead space air during its passage through the conducting components of the respiratory tract. *Alveolar* PO_2 is 100 mm Hg in contrast with the *atmospheric* PO_2 of 160 mm Hg.

The exchange of gases within the body occurs through diffusion, with each gas diffusing according to its partial pressure gradient. As shown in Figure 55-2, pressure gradients cause O_2 to diffuse from the alveoli into the blood, and from the blood into the tissues. The pressure gradients are reversed for CO_2, causing it to diffuse from the tissues into the blood and subsequently into the alveoli.

Within the alveoli, large volumes of water-saturated air are exposed to a vast volume of blood to effect efficient exchange of gases. Pulmonary venous blood is not maximally oxygenated because alveolar ventilation and perfusion are not uniform throughout the lung. During normal ventilation (in an upright person at rest) the lower (basal) segments of the lungs receive a relatively greater blood flow than the upper (apical) portions because of gravitational forces. Many respiratory disorders are characterized by even greater ventilation–perfusion inequalities. Possible pathologic causes of uneven ventilation include obstruction of airways (as in asthma), altered elasticity of airways (as in advanced emphysema), and reduced pulmonary expansion (as in atelectasis). Uneven capillary perfusion may result from shunts, embolization, and compression of pulmonary blood vessels. Pulmonary arterioles constrict when alveolar PO_2 is low and dilate when PO_2 is high to better match perfusion to ventilation. This autoregulatory mechanism serves to reduce overperfusing poorly ventilated alveoli and minimizes diluting the PO_2 in blood leaving the lungs.

During pulmonary exchange of gases, O_2 and CO_2 must diffuse across a functional respiratory membrane composed of 1) alveolar membrane, 2) interstitial fluid, 3) capillary endothelium and basement membrane, 4) plasma, and 5) erythrocyte (red blood cell) membrane.

The rate of gaseous exchange across the respiratory membrane is affected by the following factors: 1) the partial pressure gradient of each gas, 2) the total functional surface area of the alveolar and capillary membranes, 3) the thickness of the respiratory membrane, and 4) the diffusion coefficient (a constant related to the molecular weight of the gas and its solubility in plasma). The diffusion coefficient of CO_2 is about 20 times greater than that of O_2 because of the greater solubility of CO_2.

Erythrocytes play an essential role in the transport of both O_2 and CO_2 because mere physical solution of these gases in blood plasma would not be adequate to meet even minimal body needs. The gas-carrying capacity of blood is greatly increased by rapidly reversible chemical reactions that remove O_2 and CO_2 from solution, thus steepening their gradients for diffusion.

Oxygen Transport

The amount of O_2 in the blood is essentially determined by three factors: 1) the amount of O_2 dissolved in the plasma, 2) the

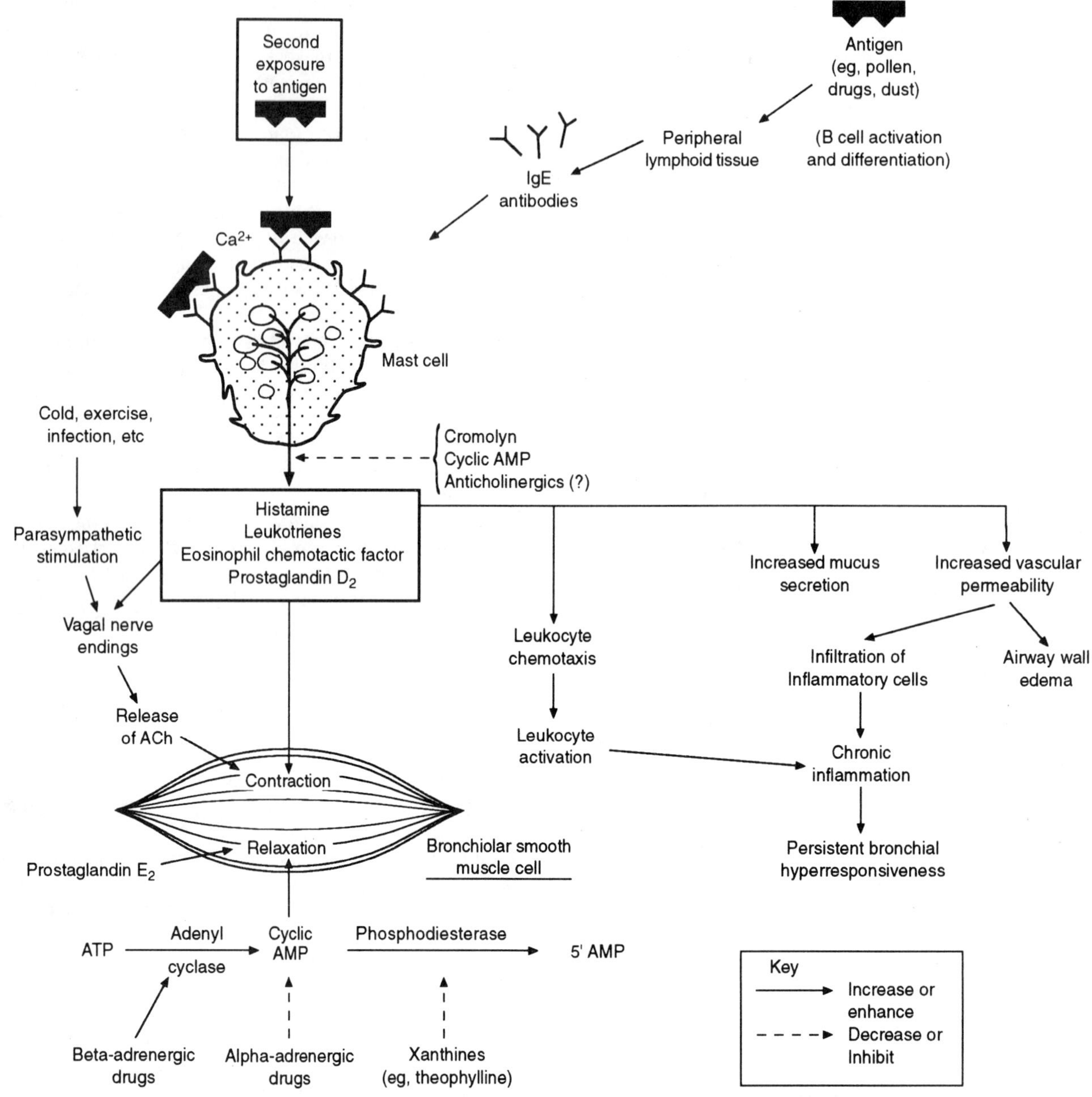

Figure 55-1. Factors regulating bronchial smooth muscle tone and responsiveness. On exposure to an antigen, lymphoid tissue forms IgE antibodies, which then attach to the surface of mast cells. Reexposure to antigen triggers an antigen–antibody reaction on the mast cell surface (termed IgE bridging), resulting in release of endogenous mediators from the mast cell, probably by way of increased calcium influx. The mediators elicit contraction of bronchiolar smooth muscle cells either by a direct action on the cells or by activating parasympathetic pathways. In addition, an inflammatory reaction is provoked in the bronchioles, resulting in infiltration of inflammatory cells and development of persistent bronchial hyperresponsiveness.

amount of *hemoglobin* (Hb) in the blood, and 3) the affinity of Hb for O_2.

Normally, the amount of O_2 physically dissolved in plasma is very small because of its low solubility in this fluid. Approximately 98.5% of the O_2 in the blood is transported in combination with Hb, a conjugated protein present in erythrocytes. Hemoglobin has four ferrous iron–containing heme groups, each of which can reversibly bind one molecule of oxygen. Although the oxygenation of Hb occurs in a stepwise fashion, the overall process is generally represented by the simple equation:

$$\underset{\text{hemoglobin}}{\text{Hb}} + \underset{\text{oxygen}}{O_2} \rightleftharpoons \underset{\text{oxyhemoglobin}}{\text{HbO}_2}$$

When fully saturated with the gas, each gram of Hb can hold 1.34 mL O_2. At an average Hb concentration of 15 g per dL of

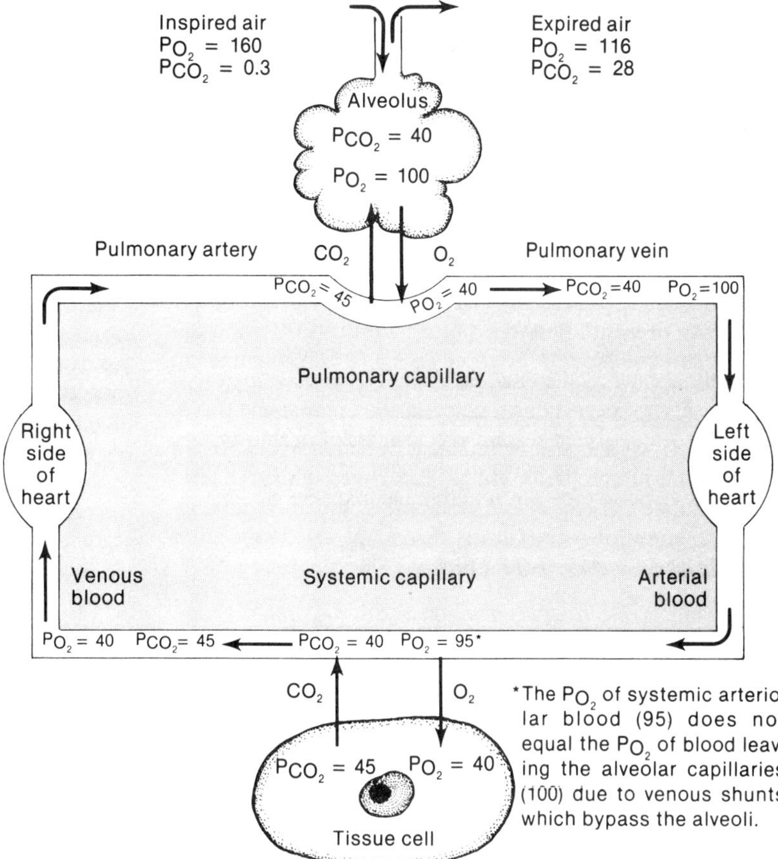

Figure 55-2. Gaseous exchange according to partial pressure gradients.

blood, the O_2-carrying capacity of Hb is 20.1 volumes percent (15 × 1.34).

In arterial blood Hb is 97% saturated with O_2, whereas in venous blood the degree of saturation decreases to 75%. The color of Hb reflects the degree of its saturation with O_2. HbO_2 is bright crimson, which explains the bright red color of arterial blood; reduced Hb is dark purple, imparting a port wine color to venous blood.

The affinity of Hb for O_2 is greatly affected by the Po_2. When the Po_2 is high, as it is in the lungs, Hb binds large amounts of O_2 and becomes nearly saturated with it. In the tissue capillaries, where Po_2 is substantially lower, the affinity of Hb for O_2 is reduced, and O_2 is released for diffusion into the tissues.

The amount of O_2 in combination with Hb also depends on the Pco_2, pH, and temperature of the blood. Under conditions of increased Pco_2, low pH, or elevated temperature of the blood, the amount of O_2 that binds to hemoglobin at any given Po_2 is diminished.

The reduced affinity of Hb for O_2 that occurs when blood pH decreases is termed the *Bohr effect*. The pH of the blood decreases as its CO_2 content increases because CO_2 combines with water to form carbonic acid (H_2CO_3), which rapidly dissociates into hydrogen (H^+) and bicarbonate ions (HCO_3^-), as shown below:

$$CO_2 + H_2O \rightleftharpoons H_2CO_3 \rightleftharpoons H^+ + HCO_3^-$$

Another metabolic factor that favors the dissociation of O_2 from Hb is 2,3 diphosphoglycerate (2,3 DPG), an organic phosphate present in erythrocytes that binds to Hb and decreases its affinity for O_2. Erythrocyte 2,3 DPG concentration increases during prolonged exercise, anemia, and in diseases marked by chronic hypoxia.

As the O_2 dissociates from Hb, it becomes available for diffusion into tissue cells. Metabolically active tissues tend to accumulate CO_2 and acidic metabolites and to undergo temperature elevation—conditions that favor O_2 dissociation from Hb and increase availability of O_2 to the tissue cells.

Carbon Dioxide Transport

Carbon dioxide (CO_2), a principal end-product of cellular metabolism, diffuses from the tissues into the blood for transport to the lungs (for elimination). It is transported by the blood in three forms as follows:

- *Dissolved* in the plasma
- As *carbamino compounds*
- As *bicarbonate ions*

Carbon dioxide is highly soluble in plasma, and nearly 10% of the total CO_2 in the blood is carried in physical solution within the plasma.

Approximately 20% of blood CO_2 combines with *amino* groups of several blood proteins (principally Hb) to form *carbamino compounds*. Some of the CO_2 that diffuses from the plasma into the erythrocytes combines with Hb to form the compound *carbaminohemoglobin*. However, most of the CO_2 in the erythrocytes is readily hydrated in the presence of carbonic anhydrase enzyme, forming H_2CO_3. H_2CO_3 rapidly dissociates into H^+ and HCO_3^- ions. The H^+ ions are buffered, principally by Hb, whereas the HCO_3^- ions diffuse into the plasma. Electrochemical neutrality is maintained by the rapid diffusion of chloride (Cl^-) ions into the erythrocytes (the so-called *chloride shift*). Approximately 70% of the CO_2 in the blood is transported in the form of HCO_3^- ions.

Regulation of Respiration

Neural Control of Respiration

The rhythmic pattern of normal respiration is maintained by the cyclic discharge of neurons located in the brain stem. Three bilateral interconnected respiratory "centers" (located in the medulla and pons) are generally recognized: the medullary center, the apneustic center, and the pneumotaxic center.

Medullary Respiratory Center

The *medullary respiratory center* consists of two anatomic aggregates of neurons: the *dorsal respiratory group* (DRG), containing mostly inspiratory neurons and the *ventral respiratory group* (VRG), composed of both inspiratory and expiratory neurons. During normal quiet respiration, the neurons of the VRG remain inactive. The inspiratory neurons of the DRG exhibit spontaneous bursts of activity during which the expiratory neurons are inhibited by the operation of oscillating negative feedback circuits.

Simultaneously, impulses originating in the inspiratory neurons travel along the phrenic and intercostal nerves to the diaphragm and external intercostal muscles, respectively, causing their contraction and the subsequent enlargement of the thorax, leading to inspiration. The medullary respiratory center receives afferent (sensory) input from central chemoreceptors, from several kinds of peripherally located receptors, and from higher brain centers (including the apneustic and pneumotaxic centers of the pons). The afferent input can modify the basic rhythmic discharge of the medullary respiratory neurons. For example, impulses originating in the cerebral cortex allow voluntary interruption of the normal breathing cycle for activities such as speaking, laughing, and breath-holding.

Pontine Respiratory Centers

The *pneumotaxic center*, located in the superior pons, limits inspiration and facilitates expiration by inhibiting both the apneustic center and the medullary inspiratory neurons of the DRG.

The *apneustic center*, located in the reticular formation of the lower pons, provides tonic stimulation to the medullary inspiratory neurons of the DRG, thereby facilitating and prolonging inspiration. The apneustic center is not necessary for the maintenance of a basic respiratory rhythm, and its level of activity can be modified (inhibited) by afferent input from the more dominant pneumotaxic center.

Chemical Control of Respiration

The CO_2, O_2, and H^+ ion levels of the blood (and other body fluids) are of major importance in the control of respiration. CO_2 is the most potent physiologic stimulant of respiration, exerting its effects chiefly through central chemoreceptors. It must be noted, however, that very high concentrations of CO_2 (in excess of 30% in inspired air) produce central nervous system (and respiratory) depression and may be lethal.

Central Chemoreceptors

The ventral surface of the medulla contains chemosensitive cells that respond to elevations of CO_2 and H^+ ions in arterial blood and cerebrospinal fluid by stimulating the medullary respiratory center.

Carbon dioxide readily diffuses from the blood plasma into the cerebrospinal fluid, where it combines with water to form H_2CO_3, which then dissociates into H^+ and HCO_3^- ions.

Because cerebrospinal fluid is not as well buffered as the blood, the H^+ ion concentration rises quickly, effectively stimulating the central chemoreceptors and thereby increasing pulmonary ventilation.

Peripheral Chemoreceptors

Located peripherally in the *carotid* and *aortic bodies* are chemoreceptors neurally connected to the medullary respiratory center by afferent glossopharyngeal and vagal nerve fibers.

These peripheral chemoreceptors are sensitive only to low arterial O_2 levels (below 60 mm Hg), and they serve as an important emergency mechanism of respiratory stimulation in states of severe oxygen deprivation.

Carotid and aortic chemoreceptors respond weakly to elevations in arterial P_{CO_2} and H^+ ion concentrations, mechanisms of some importance in acidosis.

Reflex Regulation of Respiration

In addition to chemoreceptors, there are a number of peripheral receptors whose stimulation initiates reflex changes in respiration.

Sensory modalities such as pain, temperature, and touch affect respiration, with pain exerting a strong excitatory effect on the medullary respiratory center.

Movements of joints, whether active or passive, stimulate respiration by way of afferent pathways originating in the proprioceptors of muscles, tendons, and joints. These pathways, which converge on the medullary respiratory center, augment pulmonary ventilation during exercise.

Sneezing and coughing are reflex, modified respiratory responses to irritants of the respiratory mucosa.

Inflation of the lungs stimulates pulmonary stretch receptors that lead to vagally mediated inhibition of inspiration. This "inflation reflex" (also termed the *vagal* or *Hering–Breuer reflex*) does not appear to be of great importance during normal respiration in humans.

56

Antitussives, Expectorants, and Mucolytics

Antitussives

Codeine
Hydrocodone
Hydromorphone
Dextromethorphan
Benzonatate
Diphenhydramine

Expectorants

Guaifenesin
Iodine products
Ammonium chloride
Terpin hydrate

Mucolytics

Acetylcysteine

Lung surfactants

Beractant
Colfosceril

Coughing is a protective mechanism initiated by chemical or mechanical stimulation of the tracheobronchial tree by which the body attempts to remove foreign particles or accumulated secretions from the respiratory tract. The cough reflex may be initiated by a number of factors, such as local inflammation of the bronchioles (eg, smoking), mechanical or physical obstruction (eg, foreign bodies, emboli), local or systemic disease states (eg, pulmonary edema, bronchogenic carcinoma, or congestive heart failure), and emotional stress. To the extent that the cough is annoying or debilitating, proper drug therapy should be undertaken to eliminate the condition. Not all coughing is undesirable, however, and the productive type of cough that aids in removing excessive bronchiolar mucus in the form of sputum generally should not be suppressed. Of course, if the cough is secondary to some other disease, every effort should be made to identify and eliminate the underlying pathologic condition, such as pneumonia, bronchitis, or tuberculosis.

The most frequently employed drugs for the control of coughing may be divided into the antitussives and the expectorants. *Antitussives* are cough suppressants that may act centrally at the level of the "cough center" in the brain stem or peripherally at several sites along the tracheobronchial tree. Antitussives are primarily indicated in the treatment of annoying, dry, unproductive coughing, especially where it interferes with other functions (eg, talking, sleeping) or leads to excessive weakness or progressive irritation.

Expectorants, in contrast, increase and liquefy bronchial secretions so that they can be more easily expelled. These drugs act either on the secretory glands of the respiratory tract or by irritation of the gastric mucosa, which reflexively increases respiratory secretions. They find their major clinical application in the treatment of obstructive pulmonary diseases associated with accumulation of excessive, tenacious mucus; they may reduce the viscosity of bronchial secretions, thus facilitating elimination. There is doubt, however, as to the efficacy of the usual amounts of expectorants found in over-the-counter cough formulations in reducing bronchial irritation or lessening the severity of nonproductive coughing. Exposure to humidified air and especially adequate fluid intake have proved as effective as most expectorants in relieving nonproductive coughing, liquefying thick, tenacious mucus, and facilitating removal of respiratory secretions.

In addition to antitussives and expectorants, a number of cough syrup formulations contain flavor ingredients (citrus flavors, fruit flavors), mild cooling or antiseptic agents (camphor, menthol), sweeteners (sucrose, sorbitol), and preservatives (methylparaben, propylparaben). Although these are intended to generally enhance the effectiveness of cough syrup formulations overall, they may occasionally be a problem in terms of specific ingredient hypersensitivity reactions or palatability problems with certain patients. For this reason, alternative or generic products containing the same main ingredients but different ancillary agents may be employed.

Mucolytic agents also have the ability to liquefy mucus and thus facilitate its removal from the respiratory passages by normal physiologic processes such as ciliary action, bronchiolar peristalsis, and coughing, or through suction. Although numerous proteolytic enzymes and detergents have been tried as mucolytic agents, most exhibited undesirable side effects and were unsuitable for clinical use. The only currently available mucolytic drug is acetylcysteine, an amino acid derivative that disrupts the molecular structure of mucus. It is relatively nontoxic when used by inhalation for adjunctive therapy of a number of bronchoobstructive conditions resulting from excessive or highly viscous mucus.

Antitussives

The antitussive drugs are used to reduce the frequency of dry, unproductive coughing, and most act to depress the cough reflex by a direct inhibition of the cough center in the medulla. Drugs possessing antitussive activity can be divided into two groups, the narcotic and the nonnarcotic cough suppressants. Although many opiate drugs possess a cough-suppressive action, most are deemed unsuitable for controlling simple coughing because they exhibit a significant danger of habituation and their use is associated with many undesirable side effects. Of the many opiates available, only codeine and hydrocodone are routinely used for the relief of coughing, and usually as a component of a combination product (Table 56-1). Hydromorphone, a potent opiate analgesic, is also available with guiafenesin, an expectorant for the relief of severe coughing.

The nonnarcotic antitussives are a structurally diverse group of pharmacologic agents that possess both central and peripheral mechanisms of action. In most cases, they are nearly as effective as codeine, with perhaps a somewhat lower incidence of disturbing side effects. They are considered individually below.

Table 56-1. **Representative Codeine-Containing Cough Preparations**

Trade Name	Other Ingredients
Actifed with Codeine	pseudoephedrine, triprolidine
Ambenyl	bromodiphenhydramine
Cheracol	guaifenesin
Dimetane-DC	brompheniramine, phenylpropanolamine
Isoclor Expectorant	guaifenesin, pseudoephedrine
Naldecon-Cx	guaifenesin, phenylpropanolamine
Novahistine Expectorant	guaifenesin, pseudoephedrine
Nucofed	pseudoephedrine
Phenergan with Codeine	promethazine
Phenergan VC with Codeine	promethazine, phenylephrine
Robitussin A-C	guaifenesin
Tussar-2	guaifenesin, pseudoephedrine
Tussi-Organidin	iodinated glycerol

Narcotic Antitussives

Codeine is the most commonly used narcotic antitussive because it is very effective in reducing the frequency of coughing but is less likely to depress respiration or lead to habituation than most other narcotic agents. Although it is available in tablet form, it is most frequently administered as a component of liquid cough preparations, in which it may be combined with antihistamines, decongestants, expectorants, or analgesics (see Table 56-1).

Hydrocodone (dihydrocodeinone) is comparable to codeine in efficacy but may be somewhat more habituating. It is not available for use alone but like codeine, is found in a number of cough preparations in combination with expectorants, antihistamines, and/or decongestants. It is considered briefly in this chapter; however, the general information presented for codeine below applies to hydrocodone as well.

• Codeine (C-II)

(CAN) Paveral

Mechanism

Suppresses cough reflex by a direct depressant effect on the cough center in the medulla

Uses

Suppression of nonproductive coughing

Relief of mild to moderate pain, usually in combination with aspirin or acetaminophen (see Chapter 20)

Dosage

Adults: 10 to 20 mg every 4 to 6 hours; maximum, 120 mg/day

Children 6 to 12 years: 5 to 10 mg every 4 to 6 hours; maximum, 60 mg/day

Children 2 to 6 years: 2.5 to 5 mg every 4 to 6 hours; maximum 30 mg/day

Fate

Well absorbed when taken orally; onset of action is 15 to 30 minutes; duration of action is 3 to 4 hours; metabolized in the liver and excreted largely in the urine

Common Side Effects

(Frequent at *excessive* doses) Lightheadedness, dizziness, sedation, sweating, nausea

Significant Adverse Reactions

GI: dry mouth, anorexia, vomiting, constipation, biliary spasm

CNS: euphoria, weakness, insomnia, headache, anxiety, fear, mood changes, disorientation, agitation, tremors, impaired physical performance, psychological dependence, delirium, hallucinations, coma, visual disturbances, respiratory and cardiovascular depression (especially with large doses)

CV: flushing, tachycardia, palpitations, hypotension

Other: allergic reactions (rash, urticaria, pruritus, edema), urinary retention, decreased libido, impotence, faintness, syncope, ureteral spasm

Contraindications

Patients with known or suspected narcotic addiction. *Cautious use* in patients with asthma or other pulmonary diseases, cardiac disease (including arrhythmias), convulsive disorders, renal or hepatic impairment, prostatic hypertrophy, severe CNS depression, toxic psychoses, head injuries, intracranial lesions, hypothyroidism, or Addison's disease, and in alcoholics and pregnancy.

Interactions

Profound sedation, hypotension, and respiratory depression may occur with combinations of codeine and other narcotics, sedatives, hypnotics, alcohol, phenothiazines, tricyclic antidepressants, general anesthetics, and other CNS depressants (refer to **Narcotic Analgesics**, Chapter 20)

Nursing Management

Refer to **Nursing Considerations Related to Opiate Usage** (Chapter 20) for those applicable to use of codeine as an antitussive. In addition:

Nursing Interventions

Medication Administration

Note that codeine alone in tablet form is a schedule II drug, but codeine is most commonly used in combination with other agents in cough syrups. Depending on the amount of codeine contained in the mixture, these combination antitussives may be schedule III or schedule V products. Follow proper procedures for handling controlled substances (see Chapter 10).

Patient Teaching

Instruct patient to take medication undiluted and *not* to drink water immediately afterwards when syrup is used.

Warn patient not to exceed recommended dosage because antitussive effect is not significantly enhanced, but untoward reactions and danger of habituation are increased.
Inform patient that drug may cause drowsiness, but that restlessness, anxiety, or nervousness sometimes occur instead, especially with large doses.
Suggest that patient drink large amounts of fluids (eg, 2 L/day), which may help decrease the tenacity of bronchial secretions, and use a humidifier or vaporizer during the night.
Advise patient to use hard candy, gum, or throat lozenges to soothe pharyngeal mucosa irritated by constant coughing.

• Hydrocodone (C-III)

(CAN) Robidone

Hydrocodone (dihydrocodeinone) is a relatively weak analgesic and a strong antitussive found in combination with other agents such as expectorants and antihistamines in many cough formulations. Most of these products are schedule III controlled substances. It exhibits a relatively low degree of respiratory depression and physical dependence, although the likelihood of habituation appears to be greater than that of codeine. Commercial preparations containing hydrocodone include:

Hycodan (with homatropine)
Hycomine (with phenylpropanolamine)
Tussionex (with chlorpheniramine)
Entuss-D (with pseudoephedrine)

The recommended dosage for hydrocodone in these preparations is 5 mg 3 to 4 times a day or 10 mg twice a day. Refer to the preceding discussion of codeine for additional information regarding side effects, precautions, interactions, and nursing management.

• Hydromorphone (C-II)

Dilaudid Cough Syrup

Hydromorphone is a centrally acting opiate antitussive that acts directly on the cough reflex center. It is available in combination with guaifenesin (glyceryl guaiacolate), which reduces the viscosity of secretions, hence increasing the efficiency of the cough reflex and of ciliary action in expelling accumulated mucous from the bronchi and trachea. Dilaudid cough syrup is indicated for the control of *persistent exhausting* cough, because it is very potent and has a higher addiction potential than other opiate cough preparations. It is contraindicated where patients have hypersensitivity to narcotics; in any increased intracranial pressure situation; and whenever bronchial or ventilatory function is depressed. Each 5 mL contains 1 mg hydromorphone and 100 mg quaifenesin in a flavored syrup containing 5% alcohol. The usual adult dosage is one teaspoonful every 3 to 4 hours.

Nonnarcotic Antitussives

The principal nonnarcotic antitussive is dextromethorphan, which is reviewed in detail below. Other less frequently used nonnarcotic drugs are considered briefly.

• Dextromethorphan

Benylin DM, Delsym, Hold, Pertussin, and other manufacturers

(CAN) Balminil D.M., DM Syrup, Koffex, Ornex DM, Robidex, Sedatuss

Dextromethorphan is the *d*-isomer of the codeine analogue of levorphanol. It exhibits minimal CNS depressant action and has no analgesic effect, and its administration is unlikely to produce constipation or lead to significant tolerance. It is commonly found in over-the-counter cough formulations, frequently combined with antihistamines, decongestants, and expectorants. A 30-mg dose is approximately equivalent to 15 mg codeine.

Mechanism

Not conclusively established; appears to depress the cough center in the medulla.

Uses

Temporary relief of nonproductive coughing

Dosage

Lozenges/Syrup/Liquid

Adults: 10 to 30 mg every 4 to 8 hours; maximum, 120 mg/24 h
Children 6 to 12 years: 5 to 10 mg every 4 hours *or* 7.5 to 15 mg every 6 to 8 hours; maximum, 60 mg/24 h
Children 2 to 6 years: 2.5 to 5 mg every 4 hours *or* 3.75 to 7.5 mg every 6 to 8 hours; maximum, 30 mg/24 h

Controlled-Release Liquid (Delsym)

Adults: 60 mg twice a day
Children 6 to 12 years: 30 mg twice a day
Children 2 to 6 years: 15 mg twice a day

Fate

Onset of action is 15 to 30 minutes and antitussive effects persist 3 to 6 hours, depending on the dose (up to 12 hours with controlled release liquid).

Significant Adverse Reactions

Dizziness, GI distress, drowsiness

Contraindications

Patients taking monoamine oxidase (MAO) inhibitors (refer to **Interactions**, below). *Cautious use* in persons with chronic cough or cough associated with excessive secretions, chronic obstructive pulmonary disease, high fever, persistent headache, vomiting.

Interactions

Combinations of dextromethorphan and MAO inhibitors can result in hyperpyrexia, muscular rigidity, and laryngospasm

Nursing Management

Refer to **Codeine**. In addition:

Nursing Interventions

Medication Administration

Note that the drug's antitussive activity is comparable to that of codeine, and, in therapeutic doses, the drug does not induce tolerance, hypnosis, respiratory depression, or analgesia. Also, constipation is much less frequent than with codeine.

Note that drug is available in throat lozenge form alone and combined with benzocaine (eg, Formula 44 Cough Control Discs, Spec-T Sore Throat Cough Suppressant, Vick's Cough Silencers) for control of spasmodic coughing. Lozenges are not as effective as the syrup.

Patient Teaching

Instruct parents not to administer to children younger than 2 years of age except under medical supervision.

Instruct patient to take syrup undiluted to enhance its local effect.

Inform patient that increasing the dose increases the duration of action.

Advise patient to consult practitioner if coughing persists longer than 7 days with dextromethorphan or any other antitussive therapy.

• Benzonatate

Tessalon Perles

Benzonatate is structurally related to tetracaine and exerts a local anesthetic action on stretch receptors in the respiratory passages, lungs, and pleural cavity. As a result, the activity of these receptors is suppressed and the cough reflex is dampened. The drug does not appear to alter the function of the respiratory center at recommended doses. It is used as capsules for relief of nonproductive coughing, at a dosage of 100 mg three times a day; effects persist for 3 to 6 hours.

Adverse reactions may include sedation, dizziness, nasal congestion, constipation, nausea, GI upset, pruritus, skin eruptions, burning in the eyes, a "chilly" sensation, and numbness in the chest. Large doses can lead to CNS stimulation (restlessness, tremor, convulsions).

Benzonatate is contraindicated in persons who are allergic to tetracaine or related local anesthetics. The drug should be used *cautiously* in pregnant women or nursing mothers. Capsules should be swallowed whole and not chewed because release of the drug in the mouth can anesthetize the oral mucosa.

Nursing Management

Refer to **Codeine**. In addition:

Nursing Interventions

Medication Administration

Observe carefully for possible development of pneumonitis from aspiration if drug is used in patient who is vomiting.

Note that benzonatate is reportedly as effective as codeine in controlling nonproductive coughing and does not lead to habituation.

Patient Teaching

Instruct patient to swallow the capsule (perle) whole because release of drug in the mouth can produce temporary anesthesia in the oral mucosa.

Encourage patient to use interventions (eg, adequate hydration, hard candy or gum, cessation of smoking, air humidification) that help control nonproductive coughing.

• Diphenhydramine

Benylin and other manufacturers

Diphenhydramine is an antihistamine (see Chapter 16) that is used as a syrup to control coughing from colds or allergies. Oral dosage is 25 mg every 4 hours for adults, and 6.25 to 12.5 mg every 4 hours for children. The major side effect with diphenhydramine is drowsiness. The drug is also found in 25-mg and 50-mg strengths as the principal ingredient in over-the-counter sleep aids such as Nytol, Sleep-Eze 3, Sominex 2, Compoz, and Twilite.

Expectorants

Expectorants are claimed to facilitate removal of viscous mucus from the respiratory tree and to provide a soothing, demulcent action on the respiratory mucosa by stimulating secretion of a lubricating fluid. Although large doses of certain prescription-only expectorants (such as potassium iodide) may decrease the tenacity of mucus associated with chronic obstructive pulmonary disease, the efficacy of most nonprescription expectorants is subject to considerable debate. They are probably no more effective in providing relief of bronchial irritation or facilitating mucus liquefaction than high fluid intake, that is, 6 to 10 glasses/day, and humidification of the environment. There is little support for the claim that expectorants relieve dry, irritative coughing by increasing production of a soothing fluid any more than would be produced by use of a cough drop or throat lozenge. Therefore, their inclusion in cough/cold formulations containing antitussives, antihistamines, and decongestants among other medications apparently adds little to the overall therapeutic efficacy of such preparations.

Conversely, adverse reactions are rare at usual therapeutic doses, the most frequent problem being GI distress. Thus the drugs are quite safe when taken as directed, and if patients believe the compounds are effective, it may be difficult to convince them otherwise.

Guaifenesin and several iodine-containing products are the most commonly employed expectorants and are discussed in detail. Other infrequently used expectorants are briefly considered.

• Guaifenesin

Breonesin, Humibid, Robitussin, and other manufacturers

(CAN) Balminil Expectorant, Resyl

Guaifenesin is available as a syrup as well as both regular and long-acting (sustained-release) tablets and capsules. There is no conclusive evidence that one type of preparation is any more effective than any other type of preparation.

Mechanism

May increase output of respiratory tract fluid by reducing its adhesiveness and surface tension, thus facilitating removal of mucus; increased fluid flow is also claimed to soothe dry, irritated membranes, thereby relieving dry, hacking cough

Use

Symptomatic relief of dry, unproductive coughing associated with common respiratory disorders, such as colds, bronchitis, bronchial asthma (efficacy not conclusively established)

Dosage

Adults: 100 to 400 mg every 3 to 6 hours; maximum 2.4 g/day
Children 6 to 12 years: 100 to 200 mg every 4 hours; maximum, 1.2 g/day
Children 2 to 6 years: 50 to 100 mg every 4 hours; maximum, 600 mg/day

Significant Adverse Reactions

(Usually with large doses) Nausea, vomiting, GI distress, drowsiness

Contraindications

No absolute contraindications. *Cautious use* in persons with persistent cough, high fever, persistent headache, or rash.

Interactions

Guaifenesin may decrease platelet aggregation, thus increasing the risk of bleeding with anticoagulants
Guaifenesin may cause a color interference with laboratory determinations of vanillylmandelic acid (VMA) and 5-hydroxyindoleacetic acid (5-HIAA)

Nursing Management

Nursing Interventions

Medication Administration

Note that although drug is widely used alone or in combination with other cough suppressants, antihistamines, analgesics, and other drugs, convincing evidence that it is a clinically effective expectorant is lacking.

Patient Teaching

Encourage patient to employ adjunctive interventions (eg, high fluid intake, humidification of room air) that facilitate liquefaction of mucus and relieve dry, nonproductive cough.

Iodine Products

- **Iodinated glycerol**

Organidin and other manufacturers

- **Potassium iodide**

Pima and other manufacturers

Several iodine-containing preparations are used as expectorants, although their clinical efficacy is subject to doubt. In addition, they have the potential to cause a number of adverse reactions, and many persons display allergic reactions to iodine-containing drugs. Iodinated glycerol is claimed to be less irritating to the GI tract than other iodides but is probably less effective as well.

Mechanism

Enhance secretion of respiratory fluid and decrease viscosity and tenacity of mucus; may also facilitate breakdown of fibrous material at inflammatory sites

Uses

Adjunctive treatment of respiratory conditions associated with increased mucus, such as bronchitis, asthma, emphysema, and cystic fibrosis, and after surgery to help prevent atelectasis (efficacy not conclusively established)

Dosage

Potassium Iodide
Adults: 300 to 600 mg every 4 to 6 hours
Children: 150 to 300 mg every 4 to 6 hours

Iodinated Glycerol
Adults: 60 mg 4 times a day
Children: Up to one-half adult dosage based on weight

Fate

Oral absorption is adequate; iodides are absorbed in conjunction with amino acids; attain high levels in gastric and salivary secretions; excretion is primarily by way of the kidney

Common Side Effects

GI distress

Significant Adverse Reactions

Epigastric pain, sore throat, metallic taste, mucosal ulceration, sneezing, coryza, increased salivation, diarrhea, hypersensitivity reactions (arthralgia, fever, angioedema, lymph node enlargement, cutaneous bleeding, eosinophilia), large doses may cause goiter, thyroid adenoma, or myxedema

Contraindications

Hyperthyroidism, hyperkalemia, Addison's disease, kidney disease, sensitivity to iodides, tuberculosis, and acute bronchitis. *Cautious use* in persons with goiter, high fever, persistent cough, inflammatory bowel lesions, cystic fibrosis, acne, or dermatoses, and in pregnant women or nursing mothers.

Interactions

The hypothyroid and goitrogenic effects of potassium iodide may be potentiated by lithium or other antithyroid drugs.
Hyperkalemia can be intensified by potassium supplements or potassium-sparing diuretics.

Nursing Management

Refer to **Chapter 42** for additional information on iodide products.

Nursing Interventions

Medication Administration

Assess patient's abdomen often because small-bowel lesions resulting in obstruction, hemorrhage, and perforation have occurred if enteric-coated tablets are administered. Dosage form should be discontinued immediately if abdominal pain or distention, vomiting, or GI bleeding occurs.

Seek clarification if prescription exceeds recommended dosage or iodide is administered for extensive period because prolonged use can lead to hypothyroidism and iodide-induced goiter.

Surveillance During Therapy

Interpret results cautiously if laboratory determinations of protein-bound iodine and 17-hydroxycorticosteroids are performed. Iodide preparations may elevate values of the former and interfere with results of the latter.

Patient Teaching

Instruct patient to dilute the preparation liberally with water or another vehicle before swallowing if a liquid drug form is used. Tablets should be taken with food or milk to minimize GI distress.
Encourage increased fluid intake, cessation of smoking, and use of humidifier to increase expectorant action of iodides.
Instruct patient to stop taking iodide if signs of iodism appear (eg, skin rash, fever, sore throat, metallic taste, vomiting, epigastric pain, parotid gland swelling).

• *Ammonium Chloride*

Ammonium chloride is used predominantly as a systemic and urinary acidifier to treat metabolic alkalosis, to correct chloride depletion, and to assist in the urinary excretion of certain basic drugs. These indications are considered in Chapter 76. The drug has also been used as an expectorant and is found in a number of over-the-counter cough preparations, although its efficacy is subject to considerable doubt and its use in this manner should be discouraged.

The drug appears to exert an irritative action on the GI mucosa, leading to reflex stimulation of respiratory secretions. The average adult expectorant dose is 100 to 400 mg several times a day.

Gastrointestinal upset is common with oral administration of ammonium chloride. Large doses can cause metabolic acidosis, which is characterized by vomiting, thirst, weakness, lethargy, confusion, and hyperventilation. The drug must be used cautiously in persons with chronic heart disease.

The excretion of basic drugs (eg, amphetamines, antidepressants, antihistamines, antianxiety agents, catecholamines, narcotic analgesics, quinidine, theophylline) may be enhanced by ammonium chloride, whereas the systemic actions of acidic drugs (eg, barbiturates, clofibrate, mercurial diuretics, pyrazolones, salicylates, oral antidiabetics, thyroid hormones) may be potentiated by ammonium chloride, because their renal excretion may be retarded.

• *Terpin Hydrate*

Terpin hydrate is used in liquid form to stimulate respiratory secretions, presumably by a direct action on respiratory tract secretory glands. Recommended dosage is 85 mg every 3–4 h for minor bronchial irritations. This preparation contains approximately 40% alcohol and may cause drowsiness. Gastric upset can occur, especially if it is given on an empty stomach. A glass of water should be taken after each dose to facilitate loosening of mucus.

Mucolytics

• *Acetylcysteine (N-Acetylcysteine)*

Mucomyst, Mucosil

(CAN) Airbron, Parvolex

Acetylcysteine decreases the viscosity of pulmonary mucus and may be administered by nebulization, using a face mask or mouthpiece, or if large volumes are required, by use of a tent or croupette. The drug may also be instilled directly into the bronchial tree through a tracheostomy tube or intratracheal cannula. However, when it is administered by an ordinary aerosol nebulizer, its effectiveness is often compromised by its inability to penetrate deeply enough into the obstructed bronchiolar passages. Acetylcysteine is *not* indicated for routine use in bronchial asthma patients with mucus accumulation, because it is frequently irritating and may elicit reflex bronchospasm, further impairing the patient's respiratory function.

Prompt removal of the liquefied secretions is necessary after use of a mucolytic agent. When coughing is unsuccessful in eliminating the liquefied mucus, or in the case of elderly or debilitated patients who are unable to encourage productive coughing, the airway must be kept clear by mechanical suction.

Acetylcysteine is also employed to prevent or to minimize hepatotoxicity associated with acetaminophen overdosage by blocking the formation of toxic metabolites (see Chapter 21). The drug is given orally for this indication, and the dosage is outlined below.

Mechanism

Breaks disulfide linkages in the mucoprotein structure of mucus, thus lowering its viscosity; mucolytic activity increases with increasing pH and is optimal between pH 7 and 9. In acetaminophen overdosage, retards formation of a hepatotoxic metabolite by serving as an alternative substrate for conjugation of the metabolite

Uses

Adjunctive therapy for the relief of abnormal, viscous mucus accumulation associated with a variety of chronic respiratory conditions, such as emphysema, asthmatic bronchitis, bronchiectasis, tuberculosis, or amyloidosis of the lung
Minimization of bronchiolar obstructive complications associated with tracheostomy, cystic fibrosis, atelectasis, surgery, anesthesia, or trauma
Facilitation of diagnostic bronchial studies
Prevention of hepatotoxicity due to acetaminophen overdosage
Investigational uses include ophthalmic administration for treatment of keratoconjunctivitis sicca (dry eye) and as an enema for treating bowel obstruction due to meconium ileus

Dosage

Nebulization (face mask, mouthpiece, tracheostomy): 1 to 10 mL (20% solution) *or* 2 to 20 mL (10% solution)

every 2 to 6 hours; usual dose is 6 to 10 mL 10% solution 3 to 4 times a day

Nebulization (tent, croupette): volume of 10% to 20% solution sufficient to maintain a *heavy* mist in the area for the desired period

Direct instillation: 1 to 2 mL of 10% to 20% solution every 1 to 4 hours through a tracheostomy tube or tracheal cannula

Diagnostic bronchography: 1 to 2 mL (20% solution) *or* 2 to 4 mL (10% solution) by nebulization or direct instillation before diagnostic procedure

Antidote to acetaminophen overdosage (oral use: 20% is diluted with soft drinks to a final concentration of 5%; dilutions should be used within 1 hour; undiluted solutions may be kept refrigerated up to 96 hours) Initially, 140 mg/kg is given as a loading dose followed by 70 mg/kg every 4 hours thereafter for a total of 17 doses, *unless* an acetaminophen assay shows a nontoxic plasma level

CAUTION

If the patient vomits within 1 hour of any dose, the dose should be repeated. Refer to the package instructions for further diluting and dosing instructions.

Significant Adverse Reactions

Nausea, vomiting, rhinorrhea, stomatitis, fever, tracheal and bronchial irritation, chest tightness, bronchospasm, dermal eruptions

Contraindications

No absolute contraindications. *Cautious use* in patients with bronchial asthma, and in elderly or debilitated patients with respiratory insufficiency.

Interactions

Acetylcysteine is incompatible in solution with many antibiotics (eg, tetracyclines, amphotericin B, sodium ampicillin, erythromycin) and should not be mixed in the same solution

Nursing Management

Pretherapy Assessment

Assess and record baseline data necessary for detection of adverse effects of *N*-acetylcysteine: General: vital signs (VS), body weight, skin color and temperature; CNS: orientation, reflexes, affect, ophthalmic exam; cardiovascular system (CVS): orthostatic blood pressure (BP); GI: bowel sounds, liver palpation; Lab: in use for acetaminophen OD; acetaminophen levels.

Review medical history and documents for existing or previous conditions that:

a. require cautious use of *N*-acetylcysteine: bronchial asthma, use in elderly with respiratory insufficiency, esophageal varices, peptic ulcer
b. contraindicate use of *N*-acetylcysteine: allergy to *N*-acetylcysteine; **pregnancy (Category B)**, lactation (safety unknown, use caution)

Nursing Interventions

Medication Administration

Use only nebulizers that have a compressed air source. Ordinary hand-held bulb nebulizers should not be used because output is too small and particle size of drug is too large.

Dilute nebulizing solution if indicated. The 20% solution may be diluted with sterile normal saline or sterile water for injection, whereas the 10% solution is usually used undiluted.

Ensure that patient clears airway by productive coughing before inhaling drug.

Prepare patient for the disagreeable, rotten egg–like odor that may be noticeable initially but will soon become less apparent.

Be prepared to assist patient if odor causes nausea or vomiting.

Dilute the nebulizing solution to prevent extreme concentration, which might impair proper drug delivery, during prolonged nebulization.

Wash patient's face, the mask, and the container with water, after use, because drug leaves a sticky coating.

Avoid contact of drug solution with rubber, iron, or copper because they can discolor solution and possibly reduce its potency.

Store unused portion of solution in refrigerator and use within 96 hours to minimize contamination. A light purple color may appear, but it does not impair drug's effectiveness.

Administer the following separately because they are incompatible with acetylcysteine solutions: tetracyclines; erythromycin; amphotericin; trypsin; hydrogen peroxide.

Do not administer diuretics when acetylcysteine is used antidotally.

Surveillance During Therapy

Closely observe asthmatic patient. Drug should be discontinued at first sign of bronchospasm. If necessary, a bronchodilator may be given by inhalation.

Ensure that patient expectorates liquefied secretions. If coughing is inadequate, mucus may be aspirated mechanically.

Administer as soon as possible after ingestion of acetaminophen when used to prevent acetaminophen-induced hepatotoxicity. Effectiveness is greatly reduced if given later than 18 hours after acetaminophen poisoning.

Carefully monitor laboratory studies and patient for indications of adverse reactions.

Interpret results of diagnostic tests and contact practitioner as appropriate.

Monitor for possible drug–drug and drug–nutrient interactions: Refer to **Interactions**.

Patient Teaching

Inform the patient that the following may occur as a result of treatment: increased productive cough; nausea; GI upset.

Instruct the patient to report any of the following to the practitioner: difficulty breathing, nausea.

Combination Cough Mixtures

Although this chapter has dealt largely with individual antitussive and expectorant drugs, the most frequent use of these products is in combination cough mixtures. Such formulations may contain several other types of drugs in addition to an antitussive and an expectorant. The most commonly used of these additional agents are listed below, along with the rationale for their inclusion.

- *Analgesics*. For example, aspirin, acetaminophen, sodium salicylate; used to provide relief of headache, fever, and muscle aches often accompanying an upper respiratory condition (see Chapter 21)
- *Anticholinergics*. For example, atropine, belladonna alkaloids, methscopolamine; employed for their drying action on mucous membranes, thus are only beneficial in conditions characterized by excessive secretions (eg, rhinorrhea); should be avoided in chronic obstructive pulmonary diseases (see Chapter 13)
- *Antihistamines*. For example, chlorpheniramine, pyrilamine; provide symptomatic relief of running nose, sneezing, itching, watery eyes; may be effective in relieving chronic cough resulting from postnasal drip (eg, allergic rhinitis, chronic sinusitis); exhibit an anticholinergic (drying) action, therefore should not be used in respiratory conditions characterized by excessive congestion; most have a sedative effect (see Chapter 16)
- *Bronchodilators*. For example, ephedrine, theophylline; relax bronchiolar smooth muscle, thus are of greatest benefit in conditions characterized by excessive bronchiolar muscle tone (eg, asthma) rather than mucus accumulation (see Chapter 57)
- *Decongestants*. For example, phenylephrine, phenylpropanolamine, pseudoephedrine; used to reduce mucosal congestion by activating alpha-adrenergic receptor sites, thus eliciting vasoconstriction; probably not significantly effective and can lead to systemic side effects (eg, hypertension; see Chapter 14)

The principal disadvantage of combination products is that the fixed dosage ratio of the ingredients precludes adjusting the dosage of each drug according to the needs of the patient. Moreover, the "shotgun" approach to drug therapy—inclusion of several different kinds of drugs in one preparation—is usually unnecessary from a therapeutic standpoint and most often simply increases the likelihood of untoward reactions without significantly improving the *desired* therapeutic effect. Finally, the cost of combination formulas is frequently in excess of the cost of the necessary individual ingredients used separately. Nevertheless, antitussive and expectorant combinations remain the most widely used over-the-counter preparations for the relief of cough, and it is essential that users of such medications be advised of the potential hazards inherent in the indiscriminate consumption of these readily available cough mixtures.

Lung Surfactants

- ***Beractant***

  Survanta

- ***Colfosceril (DPPC)***

  Exosurf Neonatal

Two pulmonary surfactants (ie, surface tension reducing agents), beractant and colfosceril, are used via intratracheal administration for the prevention and/or treatment of infant respiratory distress syndrome (RDS), also known as hyaline membrane disease. A deficiency of natural surfactant in the lungs of newborns is an important factor in the development of RDS. These two agents replenish the surfactant, thus lowering the surface tension on alveolar surfaces during respiration, preventing collapse.

For prophylactic treatment in premature or low–birth-weight infants or neonates with evidence of surfactant deficiency, the drugs should be given through a trachea tube as soon as possible after birth, preferably within 15 minutes. Audiovisual instructional materials are available that describe the proper dosing and administration procedures and should be viewed by healthcare providers who will be using these drugs. Only clinicians experienced in neonatal intubation and ventilatory management should administer these surfactants.

Selected Bibliography

Bernard GR: *N*-acetylcysteine in experimental and clinical acute lung injury. Am J Med 91(3c):545, 1991

Eccles R, Morris S, Jawad M: Lack of effect of codeine in the treatment of cough associated with acute upper respiratory tract infection. J Clin Pharmacol Ther 17(3):175, 1992

Hatch RT, Carpenter GB, Smith LJ: Treatment options in the child with a chronic cough. Drugs 45(3):367, 1993

Hendeles L: Efficacy and safety of antihistamines and expectorants in nonprescription cough and cold preparations. Pharmacotherapy 13(2):154, 1993

Lurie A et al: Methods of clinical assessment of expectorants: A critical review. Int J Clin Pharmacol Res 12(1):47, 1992

Petty TL: The National Mucolytic Study: Results of a randomized, double-blind placebo-controlled study of iodinated glycerol in chronic obstructive bronchitis. Chest 97(1):75, 1990

Nursing Bibliography

Hagen N: An approach to cough in cancer patients. Journal of Pain and Symptom Management 6(4):257, 1991

Irwin R, et al: The treatment of cough: A comprehensive review. Chest 99(6):1477, 1991

Louie K, et al: Management of intractable cough. Journal of Palliative Care 8(4):46, 1992

57

Bronchodilators and Other Antiasthmatics

Xanthine bronchodilators
Inhaled corticosteroids
Anticholinergics
Cromolyn sodium
Nedocromil

Drugs capable of relaxing bronchiolar smooth muscle have their principal clinical application in the common respiratory disorder bronchial asthma. Asthma is a disease that is characterized by airway hyperresponsiveness, airway inflammation, and reversible airway obstruction. Major factors contributing to the heightened airway resistance are respiratory muscle spasm, thickening of the respiratory mucosa related to edema, and excessive secretion of viscous mucus. Symptoms of asthma, such as coughing, wheezing, and dyspnea, often occur as a result of exposure to provoking factors such as dust and pollen, which trigger, by way of an antigen–antibody reaction, release of endogenous allergenic mediators (eg, histamine, leukotrienes, eosinophil chemotactic factor) from mast cells (see Fig. 55-1). These substances then interact with bronchiolar smooth muscle cells to cause contraction.

Asthmatic symptoms can appear without any exposure to a provoking agent, however. Asthma of this type is sometimes termed *atopic asthma*, because it is often associated with other allergic disorders. It is commonly noted in younger persons and usually becomes progressively more severe. A second important mechanism contributing to bronchospasm is activation of parasympathetic reflex pathways, which appear to become hypersensitive in many persons with asthma. This reflex parasympathetic response triggers release of acetylcholine (ACh) from vagal nerve endings and may be elicited by the allergens extruded from the mast cells, although many other nonimmunologic factors, such as cold, stress, infection, or exercise, can also trigger an attack. ACh constricts bronchiolar smooth muscle cells, thereby narrowing the airways.

In recent years, increasing attention has been directed toward the role of airway inflammation as a principal cause of asthmatic symptoms. Inflammatory changes in airway walls, resulting from mast cell degranulation and lymphocyte infiltration and typified by migration of inflammatory cells and edema, are noted in almost all types of asthma and are believed to be a prime trigger for the airway hyperresponsiveness and subsequent bronchoconstriction. In fact, many researchers believe that inflammation is the critical causative factor in asthma, ultimately responsible for all other facets of the disease. This view is reflected in the increased use of locally acting anti-inflammatory drugs in treating asthma, which act to reduce the degree of airway hyperresponsiveness. Thus, because asthma does not appear to be simply a bronchospastic disease, effective control of asthmatic symptoms requires judicious use of both bronchodilating as well as anti-inflammatory drugs.

Distinction must be made between the therapeutic aims in treating acute versus chronic bronchospastic conditions. Patients with mild attacks are usually effectively managed with one of the inhaled adrenergic bronchodilators (see Chapter 14). More severe attacks frequently require the concurrent use of an adrenergic bronchodilator, intravenous infusion of aminophylline and perhaps a corticosteroid. Maintenance therapy of the asthmatic patient, however, is directed toward decreasing the overall tone and responsiveness of bronchiolar smooth muscle, which is usually considerably higher in the asthmatic person as compared with the nonasthmatic. Further, treatment is also intended to help keep the respiratory passages free of obstructions, thus reducing the incidence and severity of acute bronchospastic attacks. To accomplish these aims, a variety of pharmacologic agents are often employed, including oral or inhaled bronchodilators (eg, theophylline, beta-adrenergic agonists, anticholinergics), anti-inflammatory agents (corticosteroids, cromolyn, nedocromil), expectorants, and mucolytics. In addition, persons with bronchospastic disorders should employ adjunctive measures such as adequate hydration, cessation of smoking, and avoidance of precipitating factors such as irritants, cold, and allergens to minimize the disturbing symptoms associated with these diseases and to avoid potentially dangerous complications.

Most drugs useful in bronchial asthma, such as xanthines, inhaled corticosteroids, ipratropium, cromolyn, and nedocromil are considered in this chapter. The adrenergic bronchodilators are reviewed in detail in Chapter 14, and expectorants and mucolytics, sometimes employed adjunctively, are discussed in Chapter 56.

Xanthine Derivatives

Aminophylline
Dyphylline
Oxtriphylline
Theophylline

The methylated xanthine derivatives (methylxanthines) include theophylline, its soluble salts (eg, aminophylline, oxtriphylline), and a chemically related derivative, dyphylline. These products are available in a number of different dosage forms. Theophylline, as the base, has been used as an bronchodilator for more than a quarter of a century, although, owing to its rather narrow safety margin, frequent side effects and lowered effectiveness compared with other antiasthmatic drugs, its use has decreased in recent years. Clinical efficacy, as well as frequency of side effects, are a direct function of theophylline plasma levels, and the desired therapeutic range has traditionally been given as 10 to 20 μg/mL. Adverse effects begin to occur at levels of approximately 15 μg/mL and become common above 20 μg/mL. Because recent studies indicate there is little additional bronchodilation above 10 to 12 μg/mL, many clinicians are maintaining theophylline plasma levels at these lower values to reduce the incidence of adverse effects.

Principal reasons for the variation in theophylline plasma levels are:

- Variations in anhydrous theophylline content among different preparations
- Varying rates of absorption, metabolism, and elimination
- Altered availability of theophylline from different dosage forms
- Age and health status of the patient.

A closer look at some of these factors is presented below.

Because of differences in anhydrous theophylline base content, the available salt preparations are not therapeutically equal on a weight basis, and equivalent doses of the theophylline products can differ by as much as 100%. Table 57-1 lists the percentage of theophylline base and approximate equivalent doses for each clinically available preparation. These differences become important if patients are transferred from one theophylline product to another, because the plasma concentration, and thus clinical efficacy, varies directly with the intake of *theophylline base*.

Oral absorption of theophylline appears to be related primarily to the dosage form. Most data indicate that theophylline is inherently well absorbed, tablet disintegration being the major rate-limiting step. Thus, oral liquids are the most rapidly absorbed form of theophylline, followed very closely by uncoated tablets. Sustained-release forms of the drug are somewhat more slowly absorbed but provide more consistent serum drug levels for up to 12 hours, resulting in better symptom control, especially with nocturnal asthma, in which the duration of action of most *inhaled* bronchodilators is often too short to provide adequate nighttime control.

The presence of food generally has little effect on theophylline availability, although oral absorption may be somewhat slower when food is present than from an empty stomach. Rectal absorption in adults is generally considered to be slow and unreliable, and this route of administration should be avoided if possible. IM administration yields effective serum levels about equal to those of oral dosing, although not quite so rapidly as with use of oral liquids.

Rates of metabolism and excretion of theophylline also vary widely. Hepatic metabolism is extensive (80%–90%), and the major metabolite is 3-methylxanthine, which exhibits approximately one-third to one-half the bronchodilator activity of theophylline itself. The plasma elimination half-life ($T_{1/2}$) can range from 3 to 12 hours in adults and 1½ to 9 hours in children (refer to **Fate**). Decreased clearance is noted in patients with heart failure, liver dysfunction, respiratory infections, prolonged fever, obesity, and pulmonary edema, whereas smoking enhances plasma clearance. Children older than 9 years of age generally respond to theophylline in a manner similar to adults, and should be given comparable doses. Younger children require higher infusion rates and larger oral doses of theophylline than adults to maintain effective plasma concentrations. However, some children are unusually sensitive to the CNS-stimulating effects of theophylline, and caution is recommended when administering this drug to pediatric patients.

Dosage must, of course, be individually adjusted and carefully titrated, and serum levels maintained in the range of 10 to 20 μg/mL for optimal therapeutic effect. To achieve a rapid effect, an initial loading dose can be given, although many clinicians prefer to start at lower doses and gradually increase the dosage based on the response. Dosage adjustments are usually made on the basis of clinical signs and careful monitoring of toxicity. Once the plasma levels have stabilized, they tend to remain constant so long as the dose and dosage form are kept consistent. Dosage intervals with immediate-release products are usually maintained at 6 hours in children and nonsmoking adults to provide stable blood levels, whereas sustained-release formulations may be given to nonsmokers every 12 hours. Smokers, however, may require sustained-release dosage forms every 8 hours because of the increased rate of theophylline clearance. IV administration of aminophylline is usually accomplished by giving an initial loading dose over a 20- to 30-minute period, followed by a continuous maintenance infusion (refer to **Dosage**, below).

Because of the difficulties in individualizing theophylline dosage, the use of fixed-combination bronchodilator products (eg, theophylline, ephedrine, sedatives, or expectorants) should be strongly discouraged. Such combination formulations do not allow the dosage flexibility necessary in bronchodilator therapy, and they may increase the overall incidence of untoward reactions. Moreover, inclusion of barbiturates in these preparations may enhance the hepatic metabolism of theophylline, necessitating use of larger doses to maintain steady-state blood levels.

Table 57-1. **Theophylline Content of Xanthine Derivatives**

Preparation	*Percent Theophylline Base*	*Equivalent Dosage (mg)*
Theophylline, anhydrous	100	100
Aminophylline anhydrous†	86	115
Aminophylline dihydrate	79	127
Dyphylline*	N/A	N/A
Oxtriphylline	64	156
Theophylline sodium glycinate†	49	204

* A derivative of theophylline that is approximately 70% theophylline by molecular weight ratio but is *not* a theophylline salt; the amount of dyphylline equivalent to a given amount of theophylline is not known.
† Components of various combination products; not used alone.

Ephedrine, another inclusion in such formulations, may potentiate the CNS-excitatory action of the methylxanthines and increase the risk of cardiovascular toxicity.

Mechanism

Not completely established; appear to competitively antagonize the action of adenosine at its receptors, diminishing its bronchoconstrictive action; other postulated mechanisms include prostaglandin antagonism, stimulation of endogenous catecholamine release, and an agonistic action at beta$_2$ receptors in the bronchioles; also believed to inhibit the enzyme phosphodiesterase, thus increasing levels of cyclic AMP, a bronchodilator; this latter action, however, is probably negligible at therapeutic plasma levels; other actions include myocardial stimulation, mild diuresis, CNS excitation, increased respiration and gastric acid secretion, glycogenolysis, lipolysis, and release of epinephrine from the adrenal medulla

Uses

Symptomatic relief or prevention of bronchial asthma and bronchospasm associated with chronic bronchitis, emphysema, and other obstructive pulmonary diseases

Treatment of bradycardia and apnea in premature infants (investigational use only)

Dosage

Highly individual and adjusted on the basis of theophylline serum levels (optimal range, 10–20 μg/mL).

NOTE: The following doses are for *anhydrous theophylline*—refer to Table 57-1 for conversion factors.

Acute Therapy (patients not receiving theophylline)

Adults: 5 mg/kg as a loading dose, then 3 mg/kg every 6 hours for 2 doses, then 3 mg/kg every 8 hours

Older adults: 5 mg/kg as a loading dose, then 2 mg/kg every 6 for 2 doses, then 2 mg/kg every 8 hours

Adults with congestive heart failure: 5 mg/kg as a loading dose, then 2 mg/kg every 8 hours for 2 doses, then 1 to 2 mg/kg every 12 hours

Children 9 to 16 years of age and adult smokers: 5 mg/kg as a loading dose, then 3 mg/kg every 4 hours for three doses, then 3 mg/kg every 6 hours

Children younger than 9 years: 5 mg/kg as a loading dose, then 4 mg/kg every 4 hours for three doses, then 4 mg/kg every 6 hours

Acute Therapy (patients currently receiving theophylline)

Initially 2.5 mg/kg; subsequent doses based on serum theophylline levels; each 0.5 mg/kg will raise the serum theophylline concentration approximately 1.0 μg/mL

Prolonged Therapy

Initially 16 mg/kg/day or 400 mg/day (whichever is less) in divided doses every 6 to 8 hours; increase in approximately 25% increments at 2- to 3-day intervals, if tolerated, until optimal response or maximum dose is attained; maximum doses are the following:

Adults: 13 mg/kg/day, or 900 mg
Children 12 to 16 years: 18 mg/kg/day
Children 9 to 12 years: 20 mg/kg/day
Children younger than 9 years: 24 mg/kg/day

See Table 57-2 for recommended dosage schedules for individual preparations.

Fate

Well absorbed orally, except for enteric-coated and some sustained-release dosage forms; rectal absorption from suppositories is slow and unreliable, but concentrated rectal solutions yield good absorption; peak effects differ among preparations and dosage forms, ranging from 1 hour with most liquids to 10 hours with sustained-release tablets and capsules; plasma elimination $T_{1/2}$ of theophylline averages 7 to 9 hours in adult nonsmokers, 4 to 5 hours in adult smokers, and 3 to 5 hours in children; decreased plasma clearance occurs in patients with congestive heart failure, liver dysfunction, pulmonary edema, cor pulmonale, respiratory infections, and in alcoholism; metabolized in the liver to several metabolites, which are excreted largely in the urine; less than 15% of the drug is eliminated unchanged

Common Side Effects

GI upset, nausea, nervousness, urinary frequency

Significant Adverse Reactions

GI: vomiting, hematemesis, diarrhea, intestinal bleeding, activation of ulcer pain

CNS: restlessness, dizziness, insomnia, muscle twitching, headache, reflex hyperexcitability, depression, speech difficulties, tonic or clonic convulsions

CV: palpitations, tachycardia, flushing, hypotension, extrasystoles, circulatory failure

Renal: diuresis, dehydration, proteinuria

Other: tachypnea, respiratory arrest, fever, hyperglycemia, rectal irritation and strictures with use of suppositories

Rapid IV injection can result in flushing, palpitations, dizziness, hyperventilation, hypotension, and anginalike pain.

Contraindications

Severe peptic ulcer, active gastritis, and in patients in whom myocardial stimulation might prove dangerous. *Cautious use* in patients with acute cardiac disease, renal or hepatic disease, severe hypoxemia, hypertension, myocardial damage, congestive heart failure, glaucoma, hyperthyroidism, diabetes, prostatic hypertrophy; in pregnant or nursing mothers, and in children and alcoholics.

Interactions

Xanthines may increase the CNS stimulation seen with amphetamines, ephedrine, and other sympathomimetic drugs

Increased theophylline plasma levels (decreased clearance) may occur with use of allopurinol, beta-blockers, calcium-channel blockers, cimetidine, corticosteroids, ephedrine, influenza virus vaccine, interferon, macrolide antibiotics, mexilitene, oral contraceptives, quinolone antibiotics, thiabendazole.

The plasma levels of theophylline may be decreased by aminoglutethimide, barbiturates, hydantoins (eg, phenytoin), ketoconazole, rifampin, smoking, sulfinpyrazone, and sympathomimetics.

Xanthines can increase the excretion of lithium and phenytoin, and decrease their effectiveness.

Table 57-2. **Xanthine Bronchodilators**

Drug	Usual Dosage Range	Nursing Considerations
Aminophylline *Phyllocontin, Truphylline* *(CAN) Corophyllin, Palaron*	*Oral* Adults: 500 mg initially, then 200–300 mg every 6–8 h Children: 7.5 mg/kg initially, then 5–6 mg/kg every 6–8 h *Timed-release tablets* Adults and children 12 and over: 1–2 tablets every 8–12 h before meals and at bedtime *Rectal* Adults: 500 mg 1–2 times a day Children: 7 mg/kg *IV* (In patients *not* currently receiving theophylline) Initially: 6-mg/kg loading dose at a rate not exceeding 25 mg/min For continuous infusion: rates (mg/kg/h) are as follows: (see rates table below)	Ethylenediamine salt of theophylline with similar pharmacologic properties; may be used IV for acute attacks of bronchial asthmas; sensitivity reactions and dermatitis have occurred, especially with parenteral use; suppositories may produce rectal irritation; use only diluted solutions (25 mg/mL) for IV injection and warm to room temperature; inject very slowly (maximum 25 mg/min) to avoid cardiovascular disturbances, and closely monitor vital signs during infusion. Timed-release tablets are *not* recommended in children younger than 12; drug is incompatible in IV fluids with ascorbic acid, chlorpromazine, corticotropin, dimenhydrinate, hydralazine, hydroxyzine, insulin, meperidine, methadone, morphine, oxytetracycline, penicillin G potassium, phenobarbital, phenytoin, prochlorperazine, promethazine, tetracycline, and vancomycin
Dyphylline *Dilor, Dyflex, Lufylin, Neothylline* *(CAN) Protophylline*	*Oral* Adults: up to 15 mg/kg every 6 h depending on response *IM* Adults: 250–500 mg every 6 h	A chemically related derivative of theophylline that is *not* metabolized to theophylline in vivo; equivalent to approximately 70% theophylline by molecular weight ratio; claimed to produce less GI upset and fewer overall side effects, but blood levels and activity are somewhat lower than theophylline; safety and efficacy have not been established in children; inject drug *slowly* IM and aspirate to avoid inadvertent IV injection; excreted essentially unchanged in the urine; specific dyphylline blood levels must be used to monitor therapy; serum *theophylline* levels are *not* indicative of dyphylline levels
Oxtriphylline *Choledyl* *(CAN) Apo-Oxtriphylline, Novotriphyl*	Adults: 4.7 mg/kg orally every 8 h Children (9–16 y): 4.7 mg/kg every 6 h Children (1–9 y): 6.2 mg/kg every 6 h	Choline salt of theophylline containing 64% theophylline; claimed to be more uniformly absorbed and more stable than theophylline and to produce less GI distress and tolerance; regular tablets are partially enteric coated, which delays onset but not completeness of absorption
Theophylline *Aerolate, Bronkodyl, Elixophyllin, Slo-Phyllin, Theo-Dur and other manufacturers* *(CAN) Pulmophylline, Theochron, PMS Theophylline*	*Oral* Adults: 100–250 mg every 6 h *or* 1–2 timed-release preparations every 8–12 h Children: 4 mg/kg to 6 mg/kg every 6 h (See Dosage under general discussion of xanthines)	Standard xanthine derivative widely used as a bronchodilator; available in several dosage forms, allowing flexibility in dosing; sustained-release preparations provide for gradual release of active drug so that they may be given every 8–12 h, depending on formulation; a 24-h timed-release preparation is available (Theo-24), but plasma levels may not remain constant for the entire time; liquid formulations may be hydro-alcoholic elixirs or alcohol-free syrups or suspensions; aqueous solutions provide similar serum levels as alcoholic elixirs but lack CNS-depressant effects and are better tasting; some timed-release products may exhibit unpredictable absorption; drug is found in many combination products with ephedrine, phenobarbital, and/or expectorants; fixed-combination preparations do *not* allow individual dosage adjustments that are often necessary to obtain optimal action; inclusion of ephedrine or phenobarbital is probably unnecessary and potentially harmful; also available as an injection solution in 5% dextrose for rapid dosing.

Aminophylline continuous IV infusion rates (mg/kg/h):

	0–12 h	>12 h
Nonsmoking adults	0.7	0.5
Smoking adults and children 9–16 y	1.0	0.8
Children 6 mo–9 y	1.2	1.0
Older patients	0.6	0.3
Patients with congestive heart failure	0.5	0.1–0.2

Xanthines and beta-adrenergic blocking agents may be mutually antagonistic.

Xanthines can enhance the diuretic action of other types of diuretics.

The sedative effects of benzodiazepines may be antagonized by theophylline.

Concurrent use of theophylline and tetracyclines may result in an increased incidence of GI side effects.

Dosage requirements for nondepolarizing muscle relaxants (eg, pancuronium) may be increased by concurrent use of theophylline.

Antacids can retard the *rate* of absorption of orally administered theophylline, but *not* the overall extent.

An increased likelihood of cardiac arrhythmias is associated with concurrent use of theophylline and halothane.

Nursing Management

Pretherapy Assessment

Assess and record baseline data necessary for detection of adverse effects of methylxanthines: General: vital signs (VS), body weight, skin color and temperature; CNS: orientation, reflexes, affect, bilateral grip strength; cardiovascular system (CVS): perfusion; GI: bowel sounds, liver palpation; genitourinary (GU): frequency, pattern, output; Lab: electroencephalogram (EEG), electrocardiogram (ECG), thyroid, liver, kidney function tests.

Review medical history and documents for existing or previous conditions that:

a. require cautious use of methylxanthines: acute cardiac disease; renal, hepatic disease; severe hypoxemia; hypertension; myocardial damage; congestive heart failure; glaucoma; hyperthyroidism; diabetes; prostatic hypertrophy

b. contraindicate use of methylxanthines: allergy to methylxanthines; **pregnancy (Category C)**, lactation (excreted in breast milk, use caution)

Nursing Interventions

Medication Administration

Monitor vital signs and observe closely for development of untoward reactions such as hypotension, arrhythmias, or convulsions, with IV infusion, which may be the *initial* signs of toxicity.

Question use of liquid formulation containing alcohol because alcohol is *not* necessary for absorption and may be potentially harmful, especially in younger patient.

Advocate use of another route of administration when appropriate because IM injection is usually quite painful.

Insert suppositories, if used, before meals and keep patient recumbent for 15 to 20 minutes or until defecation reflex subsides. Because rectal absorption is much faster in children than in adults, suppositories should be used very cautiously in children.

Carefully check compatibilities before mixing with any other drugs in solution because many incompatibilities exist (refer to **Nursing Considerations for Aminophylline** in Table 57-2).

Caution patient not to chew or crush sustained-release preparations.

Do not administer sustained-release preparations with food; these should be administered on an empty stomach.

Have diazepam available in event of seizures.

Assure ready access to bathroom facilities in case GI effects occur.

Surveillance During Therapy

Observe patient for early signs of possible overdose (refer to **Significant Adverse Reactions**). Notify practitioner if they occur.

Assist with evaluation of drug efficacy. Dosage adjustments should be made carefully on the basis of clinical response (eg, respiratory function, pulse rate, urine output) and plasma levels, if possible. When blood is difficult to obtain, saliva levels (approximately 60% of simultaneous plasma levels) may be used.

Expect appropriate dosage adjustments to be based on content of theophylline base (see Table 57-1) when one xanthine preparation is used instead of another.

Carefully monitor laboratory studies and patient for indications of adverse reactions.

Interpret results of diagnostic tests and contact practitioner as appropriate.

Monitor for possible drug–drug and drug–nutrient interactions: refer to **Interactions**.

Patient Teaching

Instruct patient to take oral preparation with a full glass of water and with food, if necessary, to minimize GI upset.

Warn patient not to chew or crush enteric-coated or sustained-release formulation because premature release of drug or release of excessive amounts of drug may result.

Instruct patient to avoid indiscriminate use of over-the-counter (OTC) preparations containing medications that can alter respiratory function (eg, adrenergics, expectorants, antitussives).

Inform patient that cigarette smoking may shorten the drug's duration of action, necessitating dosage adjustment (refer to **Dosage**).

Recommend use of adjunctive measures such as adequate fluid intake, humidification of room air, breathing exercises, postural drainage to remove secretions, and avoidance of smoking, irritants, and cold weather to improve respiratory function.

Explain that charcoal-broiled foods may increase theophylline elimination.

Recommend moderation in consumption of caffeine-containing beverages (eg, coffee, tea, cocoa, soft drinks) because large amounts may increase the side effects of theophylline.

Inform the patient that the following may occur as a result of treatment: nausea; loss of appetite; difficulty sleeping; depression; emotional lability.

Instruct the patient to report any of the following to the practitioner: nausea; vomiting; severe GI pain; restlessness; convulsions; irregular heartbeat.

Inhaled Corticosteroids

Beclomethasone
Flunisolide
Dexamethasone
Triamcinolone

Several corticosteroids are available for inhalation in the treatment of bronchial asthma. These agents are synthetic steroids with glucocorticoid activity, and the basic pharmacology of glucocorticoids is reviewed in detail in Chapter 45. This discussion is limited to their application in treating bronchial asthma, and a listing of the drugs, with recommended doses and pertinent remarks, is given in Table 57-3.

Inhaled corticosteroids can improve pulmonary function in asthmatics and reduce the need for adrenergic bronchodilators or other antiasthmatic medications. They are not bronchodilators per se, but decrease bronchial reactivity to substances, such as allergens, which can induce contraction of bronchial smooth muscle. Inhaled corticosteroids are being increasingly prescribed, as chronic therapy, in patients with mild asthma, with the inhaled adrenergic bronchodilators being reserved for ameliorating acute bronchospastic episodes. The reasons for this are twofold. First, *chronic* use of adrenergic bronchodilators has been reported, in some cases, to result in an actual *worsening* of asthmatic symptoms and an increase in morbidity and mortality. Although these reports are still somewhat controversial, they nevertheless caution against the routine use of inhaled sympathomimetic bronchodilators in all asthmatics. Second, inflammation of the respiratory tree has been well established to play a significant role in the increased susceptibility of bronchiolar smooth muscle to various spasmogens. Thus, drugs that decrease the local inflammatory process in the bronchioles enhance the effectiveness of other drugs that reduce bronchiolar smooth muscle tone. The advantage of inhaled corticosteroid therapy over oral corticosteroid therapy, which is indicated for control of severe asthmatic conditions not responsive to inhalation therapy, is a reduced incidence of adverse effects. Most common side effects with the inhaled steroids are throat irritation, coughing, dry mouth, and hoarseness. Oral and pharyngeal fungal infections have occurred but can be minimized by thorough gargling and washing of the mouth after each inhalation. These fungal infections respond promptly to appropriate antifungal medication. An inhaled bronchodilator can be administered several minutes before inhalation of the steroid to enhance its penetration into the lungs. The beneficial effect of orally inhaled corticosteroids usually becomes evident within 2 to 4 weeks after beginning therapy.

Asthmatic patients transferred from systemic to inhaled corticosteroids are at risk for adrenal insufficiency, particularly if the oral steroid has been used for any length of time. Chronic systemic steroid therapy suppresses hypothalamic–pituitary–adrenal (HPA) function through a negative-feedback mechanism. However, systemic steroid levels remain high because of the presence of the exogenously administered steroid. After withdrawal of systemic steroids, many months are often required for HPA function to return to normal, and the inhaled steroid can no longer supply the high plasma concentrations of exogenous steroid. During this period (ie, while patients are being transferred from systemic steroid to inhaled steroid and for several months thereafter), symptoms of adrenal insufficiency can occur if a sudden demand is made on adrenal function, such as with trauma, stress, severe infection, or surgery. Thus, during periods of stress or in the event of an acute asthmatic attack, patients receiving only inhaled corticosteroids should *immediately* resume systemic steroid treatment and contact their physician for further instructions. Although the inhaled steroid is usually sufficient to control asthmatic symptoms during transfer periods, it can *not* provide the systemic steroid necessary in these emergencies.

Transfer from systemic to inhaled steroid must be accomplished gradually. The aerosol should be initiated while the patient is still receiving normal maintenance doses of systemic steroids. After 1 week, the systemic steroid dosage should be reduced gradually at 1- to 2-week intervals while the patient is

Table 57-3. **Inhaled Corticosteroids Used in Bronchial Asthma**

Drug	Usual Dosage Range	Nursing Considerations
Beclomethasone *Beclovent, Vanceril*	Adults: 2 inhalations 3 or 4 times a day or 4 inhalations twice a day, up to 20 inhalations/day in severe asthma Children: 1–2 inhalations 3 or 4 times a day or 2–4 inhalations twice a day up to 10 inhalations a day	Systemic absorption is rapid, and drug and metabolites are eliminated primarily in the feces; improvement in symptoms is noted in 1–4 wk; not recommended in children younger than 6 y
Dexamethasone *Decadron*	Adults: 3 inhalations 3 or 4 times a day (maximum, 3/dose and 12/day) Children: 2 inhalations 3–4 times a day (maximum, 2/dose and 8/day)	Dosage is gradually reduced when a favorable response is noted; aerosolized particles dissolve rapidly in bronchial secretions; systemic absorption is about 50% (higher with larger dosages or more frequent inhalation)
Flunisolide *AeroBid* *(CAN) Bronalide, Rhinalar*	Adults: 2 inhalations twice a day (maximum, 4 inhalations twice a day) Children (6–15 y): 2 inhalations twice a day	Systemic absorption is approximately 40%; rapidly and extensively metabolized during first-pass through the liver; half-life is about 2 h; *not* recommended in children younger than 6 y
Triamcinolone *Azmacort*	Adults: 2 inhalations 3 or 4 times a day (maximum, 16 inhalations/day) Children (6–15 y): 1 or 2 inhalations 3 or 4 times a day (maximum, 12 inhalations/day)	Drug disappears rapidly from the lungs; blood levels are maximum in 1–2 h; the major route of elimination is the feces; *not* recommended in children younger than 6 y; improvement is usually noted within 1–2 wk

observed for signs of adrenal insufficiency. The importance of a slow rate of withdrawal cannot be overemphasized.

Nursing Management

Pretherapy Assessment

Assess and record baseline data necessary for detection of adverse effects of inhaled corticosteroids: General: VS, body weight, skin color and temperature; CNS: orientation, reflexes, affect, bilateral grip strength.

Review medical history and documents for existing or previous conditions that:

a. require cautious use of inhaled corticosteroids: systemic fungal infections, untreated local infections, nasal septal ulcers

b. contraindicate use of inhaled corticosteroids: allergy to any ingredient; acute asthmatic attack; status asthmaticus; **pregnancy (Category C)**, lactation (excreted in breast milk, mothers should not nurse while taking these agents)

Nursing Interventions

Medication Administration

Monitor patient during, and for at least several months after, withdrawal of systemic corticosteroids for signs (hypotension and weight loss) and symptoms (eg, weakness, fatigue, depression, lightheadedness, muscle or joint discomfort, nausea and vomiting) of adrenal insufficiency, particularly during periods of increased stress, such as trauma, severe infection, or surgery (see explanation above) if patient is being transferred from systemic to inhaled corticosteroid therapy. If these occur, usually the dosage of systemic steroid is temporarily increased and the withdrawal schedule is slowed.

Arrange for decongestant nose drops to facilitate penetration of intranasal steroids if edema or excessive secretions occur.

Surveillance During Therapy

Carefully monitor laboratory studies and patient for indications of adverse reactions.

Interpret results of diagnostic tests and contact practitioner as appropriate.

Monitor for possible drug–drug and drug–nutrient interactions: refer to **Interactions**.

Patient Teaching

Explain importance of inhaling bronchodilator several minutes *before* inhalation of corticosteroid (see explanation above) if an inhaled bronchodilator is also prescribed.

Teach patient correct technique for use of particular inhaler (directions are included with package inserts). Nasal and oral inhalation products are *not* to be used interchangeably.

Explain that proper administration is required to ensure that drug is adequately absorbed.

Explain that regular use at prescribed intervals is essential to therapeutic effectiveness.

Ensure that patient understands that inhaled corticosteroids are not intended to provide immediate relief of acute symptoms. If the patient is not receiving simultaneous systemic steroids, pulmonary function does not usually improve until after 1 to 4 weeks of therapy.

Warn patient not to exceed prescribed dosage. If symptoms do not improve within several weeks, the practitioner should be notified.

Instruct patient to rinse mouth and gargle with warm water after each inhalation to remove residual medication. This may delay or minimize the occurrence of dry mouth, hoarseness, and oral fungal infections.

Teach patient how to recognize and report indications of oral or pharyngeal candidiasis (eg, oropharyngeal soreness, presence of white patches or red splotches on oral membranes).

Reassure patient that oral or pharyngeal fungal infections usually respond promptly to appropriate therapy (discontinuation of inhaled corticosteroid, antifungal medication) when they occur.

Caution patient not to discontinue medication suddenly without appropriate consultation. After prolonged usage, if inhaled corticosteroids need to be discontinued, they should be terminated gradually under medical supervision.

Anticholinergics

Anticholinergic agents are effective bronchodilators, and the naturally occurring belladonna alkaloids (eg, atropine) have been used for many years in treating bronchial asthma. Unfortunately, the wide range of side effects associated with *systemic* anticholingeric drugs greatly limits their usefulness in the management of bronchoconstrictive disorders. However, the clarification of the role played by the parasympathetic nervous system in asthma has brought about a resurgence of interest in cholinergic antagonists as potential therapeutic agents for treating bronchial asthma. The only available inhalational anticholinergic agent is ipratropium, a quaternary amine that is poorly absorbed from the bronchial tree and thus exerts predominately a local effect. It appears to be particularly useful in asthma triggered by irritants, smoking, or emotional stress. Ipratropium has also been employed in treating bronchitis and emphysema.

• Ipratropium

Atrovent

Mechanism

Ipratropium exerts an anticholinergic action in the bronchioles to prevent the increase in cyclic guanosine monophosphate (GMP) resulting from parasympathetic nerve activation. Thus, the drug blocks the contraction of bronchiolar smooth muscle and the increase in mucus secretion resulting from increased vagal (ie, parasympathetic) activity. In addition, it may inhibit acetylcholine-induced release of allergenic mediators from the mast cells; interpatient variation in the bronchial response to ipratropium appears to be substantial.

Uses

Treatment of bronchospasm associated with chronic obstructive lung diseases, such as asthma, chronic bronchitis, or emphysema

Dosage

Two inhalations (delivering 18 μg each) 4 times a day, to a maximum of 12 inhalations within 24 hours

Fate

Much of an inhaled dose is swallowed, and is eliminated in the feces; systemic absorption is minimal because of the quaternary configuration of the drug, which lowers its lipid solubility; bronchodilation begins within minutes and reaches maximum within 30 to 60 minutes; duration is 4 to 6 hours; elimination $T_{1/2}$ is about 2 hours after inhalation

Common Side Effects

Coughing, dryness of the oropharynx, gastric upset, nervousness

Significant Adverse Reactions

Headache, dizziness, palpitations, skin rash, blurred vision

Rarely: Tachycardia, drowsiness, coordination difficulties, itching, constipation, tremor, paresthesias, mucosal ulceration

Contraindications

Treatment of acute bronchospastic episodes. *Cautious use* in patients with narrow-angle glaucoma, prostatic hypertrophy, or bladder neck obstruction, and in pregnant women, nursing mothers, and young children.

Nursing Management

Nursing Interventions

Patient Teaching

Teach patient correct procedure for using inhaler (directions are on package insert). Treatment failure is often due to improper administration. If patient has difficulty mastering technique, extenders are available for metered dose inhalers.

Inform patient that rinsing mouth after each treatment may help to relieve bitter taste and dry mouth.

Asthma Prophylactic Agents

• Cromolyn Sodium

Intal

(CAN) Fivent

An adjunctive agent for the management of severe bronchial asthma, cromolyn may decrease the severity of the clinical symptoms of asthma, reduce the requirements for concomitant drug therapy, or both. It is strictly a prophylactic drug and possesses no intrinsic bronchodilator or antihistaminic activity. It is of no value in the treatment of acute asthmatic attacks. The drug is available for oral inhalation as a solution for nebulization, and an aerosol spray; no significant difference in effectiveness has been demonstrated between these dosage forms, although the aerosol appears to be the most patient-accepted dosage form.

Cromolyn is also marketed as a *nasal* spray (Nasalcrom) for treatment of chronic allergic rhinitis and as oral capsules (Gastrocrom) for relieving the symptoms of mastocytosis (diarrhea, flushing, urticaria, itching, abdominal pain). The latter two dosage forms are considered briefly after the discussion of the orally inhaled form of cromolyn.

Mechanism

Stabilizes the mast cell membrane, thereby inhibiting the release of endogenous allergens such as histamine and leukotrienes from mast cells that normally occurs after exposure to specific antigens; may also increase cyclic AMP levels in the bronchioles.

Uses

Prophylactic management of severe, perennial bronchial asthma (reduces severity of symptoms or bronchodilator drug dosage requirements). Improvement is usually noted within 4 weeks.

Prevention of exercise-induced bronchospasm

Symptomatic control of chronic allergic rhinitis (Nasalcrom)

Symptomatic treatment of systemic mastocytosis (Gastrocrom)

Investigational uses include treatment of food allergies, eczema, dermatitis, urticaria pigmentosa, chronic urticaria, hay fever, and postexercise bronchospasm.

Dosage

Nebulizer solution: 20 mg inhaled 4 times a day; solution is administered using a power-assisted nebulizer equipped with a suitable face mask (*Note*: hand-operated nebulizers are not suitable).

Metered-dose spray: 2 sprays (800 μg/actuation) 4 times a day

Prevention of exercise-induced bronchospasm: 20 mg inhaled 30 minutes to 60 minutes before exercise

Fate

Approximately 8% to 10% of dose is absorbed by the lungs after inhalation, then rapidly excreted unchanged in the bile and urine; remainder of dose is either exhaled or swallowed and then excreted in the feces (GI absorption is poor); elimination $T_{1/2}$ is 80 to 90 minutes

Common Side Effects

Cough, nasal congestion, pharyngeal irritation

Significant Adverse Reactions

Lacrimation, parotid gland swelling, wheezing, rash, urticaria, angioedema, dysuria, urinary frequency, joint swelling, dizziness

Rarely: Hoarseness, myalgia, vertigo, photosensitivity, peripheral neuritis, nephrosis, anemia, exfoliative dermatitis, vasculitis, pericarditis, eosinophilia, anaphylactic reactions

Contraindications

Children younger than 5 years; to abort an acute asthmatic attack. *Cautious use* in persons with impaired renal or hepatic function, and in pregnancy or lactation.

Nursing Management

Nursing Interventions

Medication Administration

Observe for abatement of an acute attack, clearance of the airway, and ability of patient to inhale adequately. Cromolyn therapy should be initiated only after these conditions have been met. An inhaled bronchodilator may be prescribed for use before each dose of cromolyn to aid penetration into lungs.

Administer inhalant solution only with a power-operated nebulizer with an adequate flow rate and suitable face mask to ensure sufficient penetration. Do *not* use a hand-operated nebulizer.

Surveillance During Therapy

Be alert for worsening of symptoms as attempts are made to reduce dosage to lowest effective level once patient is stabilized on cromolyn. Symptomatic therapy should be provided as necessary.

Closely observe patient for deterioration of condition or symptoms of adrenal insufficiency (refer to **Inhaled Corticosteroids**, above) if a steroid-dependent asthmatic patient improves with cromolyn, and appropriate gradual reduction of the corticosteroid dosage is undertaken. Steroid therapy may need to be reinstituted during periods of stress or loss of respiratory control.

Assist with evaluation of drug efficacy. Patient's drug regimen should be reevaluated if no improvement is noted after 4 weeks of cromolyn therapy.

Patient Teaching

Instruct patient to clear airway of as much mucus as possible before inhalation.

Instruct patient to avoid inhaling drug during acute asthmatic attacks because it may be irritating to respiratory passages, thus worsening symptoms.

Inform patient that cromolyn therapy should not be abruptly discontinued except under professional care because asthma may be exacerbated.

• Cromolyn Intranasal

Nasalcrom

(CAN) Nalcrom

Cromolyn is also available as a nasal spray for the management of symptoms of allergic rhinitis. Repeated inhalation of the drug is believed to decrease the occurrence and severity of attacks of allergic rhinitis. One spray is administered into each nostril 3 to 6 times a day using the inhaler supplied with the drug cartridge. Side effects are rare and the drug is well tolerated, although there are occasional reports of sneezing and nasal stinging or burning. Headaches, bad taste in the mouth, and epistaxis occur rarely. Nasal passages should be cleared by blowing before inhalation. Effects should become apparent within several weeks; however, antihistamines or decongestants will probably be required during this initial period. The need for these drugs should diminish with continued use of intranasal cromolyn.

• Nedocromil

Tilade

Nedocromil is an inhaled anti-inflammatory agent similar to cromolyn that is used for maintenance therapy in mild to moderate cases of bronchial asthma. It inhibits the bronchoconstrictor response to several types of challenges, but has no intrinsic bronchodilator action. The recommended dosage is two oral inhalations (1.75 mg per actuation) 4 times a day at regular intervals, even during symptom-free periods. Refer to the discussion of cromolyn for additional information and nursing considerations.

Selected Bibliography

Anderson B: An overview of drug therapy for chronic adult asthma. Nurs Pract 16(12):39, 1991

Barnes PJ: Asthma: New therapeutic approaches. Br Med Bull 48(1):231, 1992

Bone RC: Step care therapy: A logical approach to asthma management. J Asthma 29(1):13, 1992

Breslin AB: New developments in anti-asthma drugs. Med J Aust 158(11):779, 1993

Clark TJ: Beta-receptor agonists in respiratory disease: A summary. Life Sci 52(26):2193, 1993

Hendeles L, Weinberger M, Szefler S, Ellis E: Safety and efficacy of theophylline in children with asthma. J Pediatr 120(2 Pt 1):177, 1992

Hoag JE, McFadden ER Jr: Long-term effect of cromolyn sodium on nonspecific bronchial hyperresponsiveness: A review. Ann Allergy 66(1):53, 1991

Milgrom H, Bender B: Current issues in the use of theophylline. Am Rev Respir Dis 147(6 Pt 2):533, 1993

Pauwels R: The clinical use of beta-receptor agonists: For and against. Life Sci 52(26):2171, 1993

Snider GL: Theophylline in the ambulatory treatment of chronic obstructive lung disease: Resolving a controversy. Cleveland Clin J Med 60(3):197, 1993

Stempel DA, Szefler SJ: Management of chronic asthma. Pediatr Clin North Am 39(6):1293, 1992

Tashkin DP: New trends in treating chronic persistent asthma in adults. West J Med 156(1):66, 1992

Welch MJ et al: A comparative study of a new once-a-day theophylline preparation with Theo-Dur give twice daily. J Asthma 30(3):211, 1993

Nursing Bibliography

Idris A, et al: Emergency department treatment of severe asthma. Chest 103:665, 1993

Kaliner M, Martin R, O'Byrne R, Wiedeman H: Asthma therapy: Into the 1990's. Patient Care 69, 1992

Lesage J: Advances in pediatric drug therapies of asthma. Nurs Clin North Am 28(4):L263, 1993

Reading P, St. John R: Aerosolized therapy for ventilator-assisted patients. Critical Care Nursing Clinics of North America 5(2):27, 1993

VIII

Anti-infective and Chemotherapeutic Agents

58

Anti-infective Therapy: General Considerations

Drugs used for the treatment of infectious diseases may be termed *antibiotics, anti-infectives, antimicrobials*, or *chemotherapeutic agents*. Although these terms are often used interchangeably, the first three, that is, antibiotics, anti-infectives, and antimicrobials, are properly used to describe those drugs commonly employed for the treatment of infections. The designation *chemotherapeutic agent* has come to be more closely associated with those drugs used in the treatment of cancer.

Antibiotics are strictly defined as *natural* substances produced by microorganisms and capable of inhibiting the growth of other microorganisms. Little distinction is made, however, between those substances having a natural origin and those with a synthetic origin. In fact, the term *semisynthetic* is often applied to the product of a chemical alteration of a naturally derived anti-infective compound.

Although the use of substances extracted from soil, plants, or living organisms to kill other organisms has been described for centuries, the modern age of chemotherapy had its origin in the late 1930s and early 1940s with the introduction of sulfonamides and penicillins, respectively. Since that time, a variety of antimicrobial agents with differing mechanisms of action, spectrum, and profile of side effects have become available. Consequently, overall morbidity and mortality caused by most infectious diseases has diminished over the last 40 years. Nevertheless, the search for newer anti-infective drugs continues unabated, because some infectious diseases still have not been completely eradicated, and other newer diseases are just beginning to appear. In addition, and perhaps most ominously, the treatment of some previously susceptible microorganisms by currently available antimicrobial drugs is becoming more difficult because increasing numbers of resistant strains are emerging. Even such "common" microorganisms as *Streptococcus pneumoniae, Haemophilus influenzae*, and *Shigella dysenteriae* have become resistant to many of the anti-infective agents that previously were successful in their eradication. Multiple-drug–resistant *Mycobacterium tuberculosis* has become a major health threat throughout the country, particularly among poorer populations. Although many different antibiotics are now available to the clinician, enabling a wide range of bacterial infections to be treated successfully, the increase in drug-resistant microorganisms has reached unparalleled proportions and presents a critical challenge to our healthcare system.

Classification

Several different characteristics may be used to classify the currently available antimicrobial drugs. However, no single classification is sufficient to completely categorize a particular drug; rather, complete description of any agent requires reference to a number of these characteristics. The most commonly used classifying characteristics are spectrum of activity, antimicrobial activity, and mechanism of action.

Spectrum of Activity

A broad classification of antibiotics divides them according to the range of their antimicrobial activity into broad spectrum and narrow spectrum. Broad-spectrum antibiotics exert their effects against a number of different types of bacteria and other microorganisms. Tetracyclines are, for example, active against a wide range of both gram-positive and gram-negative bacteria, as well as several other categories of microorganisms, such as *Rickettsia, Chlamydia*, and *Mycoplasma* species. Generally, if an agent is effective against both gram-positive and gram-negative organisms, it is referred to as *broad spectrum*, although some broad-spectrum antibiotics are active against a much wider range of organisms than others.

Antibacterial drugs that primarily affect only one group of microorganisms are termed *narrow-spectrum* antibiotics. For example, penicillin G affects only gram-positive bacteria and *Neisseria* at normal therapeutic dosages and therefore is considered narrow spectrum. It is worth noting here, however, that spectrum of activity does *not* necessarily correlate with antimicrobial effectiveness. In fact, because of excessive use and subsequent emergence of resistant strains, many broad-spectrum antibiotics are much less active against many microorganisms than the more selective narrow-spectrum drugs.

Antimicrobial Activity

Antimicrobial agents may also be categorized on the basis of their antibacterial activity as either bacteriostatic or bactericidal. *Bacteriostatic* drugs (eg, tetracyclines, sulfonamides) suppress the growth of microorganisms without actually killing existing microbes. The invading microorganisms are removed by the host defense mechanisms. *Bactericidal* drugs (such as the penicillins), however, are capable of directly destroying organisms, especially those in an active state of replication. Theoretically, bactericidal drugs are more desirable from a therapeutic standpoint, but it is important to recognize that their lethal action on microorganisms is dependent on their being present in sufficient concentrations. In subtherapeutic doses, bactericidal drugs are merely bacteriostatic, and conversely, at very high doses some bacteriostatic drugs may exert a bactericidal action. Nevertheless, even the most potent bactericidal drug is usually incapable of totally eliminating an infection without intervention of the patient's own natural defense mechanisms, such as antibody production, phagocytosis, and leukocyte proliferation. Impaired defense mechanisms can result from disease states (neoplasms, diabetes, hematologic disorders) or drugs (eg, antineoplastics, corticosteroids) and can severely compromise the action of antimicrobial drugs.

Mechanism of Action

Antimicrobial agents exhibit several different mechanisms of action and may also be categorized on this basis. Most antibiotics exert their effects on microorganisms in one of five ways: 1) by inhibiting synthesis of the bacterial cell wall; 2) by altering cell membrane function; 3) by inhibiting protein synthesis; 4) by inhibiting metabolism of nucleic acid; or 5) by interfering with intermediate cell metabolism.

Inhibition of Bacterial Cell Wall Synthesis

Examples of drugs employing this mechanism are the penicillins, cephalosporins, and bacitracin. Unlike animal cells, bacteria possess a *rigid* cell wall composed of macromolecules cross-linked by peptide chains. This arrangement maintains the shape of the cell and prevents cell rupture, because most bacteria have a high internal osmotic pressure. Thus, the viability of these bacterial cells depends on the integrity of the cell wall. Drugs acting by inhibiting cell wall synthesis do so by interfering with different steps in the assembly of the peptide chains that impart rigidity to the wall. The weakened cell wall can then no longer support the internal pressure and the cells undergo lysis and disintegrate. Drugs acting in this manner are bactericidal.

Alteration in Cell Membrane Function

Drugs that alter bacterial cell membrane function include amphotericin, nystatin, and the polymyxins. The semipermeable bacterial cell membrane (located between the cell wall and cytoplasm) helps control the internal environment of the cell by functioning as a selective barrier to extrusion of cell constituents and nutrients. Disruption of this membrane by antibiotics alters its permeability, allowing escape of proteins, nucleotides, sugars, amino acids, and so on, resulting in damage to the cell and ultimately in cellular death. Drugs acting in this manner may be either bacteriostatic or bactericidal, depending on the drug, dosage, and organism.

Inhibition of Protein Synthesis

The aminoglycosides, erythromycin, and the tetracyclines are among the drugs that inhibit protein synthesis. Certain antibiotics can interfere with ribosomal-mediated protein synthesis in bacterial cells without affecting normal mammalian cells. It is believed that this occurs because the composition of the ribosomes in bacterial cells is different. Antibiotics may disrupt bacterial protein synthesis at several stages; for example, by binding to the ribosomes, blocking attachment of transfer RNA, causing a misreading of the genetic code, interfering with attachment of amino acids to the developing peptide chain, or tying up essential cofactors such as calcium, magnesium, or iron. Drugs inhibiting protein synthesis may be either bactericidal or bacteriostatic.

Inhibition of Nucleic Acid Metabolism

Nalidixic acid, rifampin, and trimethoprim are examples of drugs that inhibit metabolism of nucleic acid. Although most agents interfering with nucleic acid metabolism are used as antineoplastic drugs, a few antibacterial compounds act in this manner as well. Nalidixic acid inhibits DNA synthesis, rifampin interferes with DNA-dependent RNA synthesis, and trimethoprim can inhibit dihydrofolate reductase, an enzyme essential for production of tetrahydrofolic acid, an intermediate in the formation of DNA. These drugs are bacteriostatic.

Interference With Intermediate Cell Metabolism

The sulfonamides are a widely used class of drugs that interfere with bacterial cell metabolism. All bacteria require dihydrofolic acid for production of nucleic acids; however, certain bacteria cannot assimilate preformed dihydrofolic acid but must synthesize it themselves from precursors within the cell. An essential precursor is para-aminobenzoic acid (PABA) and, because sulfonamides are close structural analogs of PABA, they compete with it for active sites within bacterial cells, impairing synthesis of dihydrofolic acid and thus cell replication. Sulfonamides are bacteriostatic at normal dose levels.

Selection of Appropriate Drug

Several important considerations go into the choice of a suitable antimicrobial drug for use in a particular patient. The most important of these factors are examined below.

Necessity of Therapy

Even before deciding which antibiotic should be prescribed, the clinician must determine whether antibiotic therapy is necessary at all. Many infectious conditions do not require systemic antimicrobial therapy, and the patient's status and the location and severity of the infection should be carefully assessed before antibiotic therapy is undertaken. Unfortunately, overprescribing of antibiotics, especially in children with "colds" or "flu," occurs to a significant extent and is responsible for an undue number of untoward reactions as well as the increased development of resistant strains of microorganisms that has become so prevalent today. Likewise, indiscriminate medication of children by parents with "refillable" antibiotics has contributed to the reduced effectiveness of these drugs in many infectious conditions. Although antibiotics occupy a deservedly important place in pharmacotherapy, they are indeed frequently misused, usually to the detriment of the patient.

Identification of the Pathogen

Accurate determination of the infecting organism or organisms is the cornerstone of safe and effective antimicrobial therapy. Appropriate anti-infective therapy is best accomplished by bacteriologic culture of the infected material (sputum, pus, urine), subsequent isolation and identification of the pathogen, and selection of an antibiotic known to be effective against the offending organism. It is always desirable to have the results of bacterial culturing before initiating antimicrobial treatment, but this is not always practical or feasible. For example, in acute, life-threatening infections (such as septicemia, peritonitis, pneumonia), a delay in initiating treatment of 24 to 48 hours while awaiting results of culture testing can prove fatal and cannot be justified. In these situations, as well as others requiring immediate antibiotic therapy, the initial choice of an antibiotic should be made on the basis of a patient history, physical examination, clinical symptoms, and, most especially, an awareness on the part of the clinician as to what microorganisms are *likely* to be present considering the site of infection and the circumstances under which it developed. In some cases, the probable organism can be determined by the attending physician by performing a simple Gram stain on smears of exudate from the infected area. However, proper bacteriologic culturing is essential for *accurate* diagnosis of the infecting pathogen, and it should be ordered as soon as possible. Once the microbiologic information has been obtained, definitive antimicrobial therapy can be initiated. The physician will either continue with the antibiotic prescribed initially if appropriate or change to one that is more active or more selective against the bacterial species shown to be present.

Sensitivity Testing

Because many common microorganisms exhibit varying degrees of antibacterial resistance, once a pathogen has been identified by bacteriologic culturing, the *sensitivity* of the infecting organism to different antimicrobial drugs is often determined. Sensitivity testing, however, is not always necessary, because some microorganisms are uniformly susceptible to certain antibiotics. For example, *Pneumococcus*, group A beta-hemolytic *Streptococcus, Clostridia*, and *Treponema pallidum* respond predictably to penicillin G. Conversely, *Staphylococcus aureus, Streptococcus viridans*, and several gram-negative bacilli (such as *Escherichia coli, Pseudomonas aeruginosa, Klebsiella pneumoniae, Salmonella, Shigella*, and *Haemophilus influenzae*) exhibit varying degrees of resistance to different antibiotics and should be tested for susceptibility in vitro.

The most widely used procedure for sensitivity testing is the Kirby-Bauer or disk diffusion method, in which paper disks containing known amounts of different antibiotics are placed on an agar surface that has been swabbed with bacteria isolated from the patient. After an 18-hour incubation, the size of the clear zone of inhibition around each disk is a measure of the activity of each antibiotic to inhibit the growth of the particular microorganism. Although useful as an index of microbial susceptibility to various antibiotics, the disk method of sensitivity testing measures only growth inhibition and thus is an indication of bacteriostatic activity only. In addition, there are several false-positive reactions to cephalosporins with this method, including enterococci, *Shigella*, and methicillin-resistant *Staphylococcus*.

If *bactericidal* action is essential (as for bacterial endocarditis), demonstration of sensitivity by the disk method is meaningless. In these situations, more reliable tube dilution sensitivity testing may be employed to determine both the minimum inhibitory concentration (ie, lowest concentration of drug that prevents visible growth after 24 hours) and the minimum bactericidal concentration (ie, lowest concentration that sterilizes the medium) of an antibiotic against a particular organism. There is frequently a discrepancy between in vitro results and clinical response, because of a number of factors such as pH, temperature, and the ability of the drug to reach the site of infection. Demonstration of in vitro bacterial susceptibility does not guarantee clinical success but merely provides another parameter on which to base selection of an antimicrobial agent.

Location of the Infection

Generally, once the offending pathogen has been identified and its susceptibility ascertained, an appropriate choice of an antimicrobial agent can be made. However, consideration must also be given to the location of the infection when choosing an antibiotic. The distribution of an antibacterial drug in the body is an important determinant of its ultimate efficacy. Although the concentration of an antimicrobial agent in the body is usually defined in terms of blood or plasma levels, the critical concentration is that which is achieved in the infected tissues themselves. Plasma levels often do *not* accurately reflect tissue levels, and in spite of high plasma concentrations, some drugs may not attain sufficient tissue concentrations at the desired site of action. It is difficult to generalize about the distribution of antibiotics, because the attainment of adequate levels in infected tissue is dependent on a multitude of factors such as dosage and route of administration, protein binding, lipid solubility, presence of tissue fluid or abscesses, pH, site of infection, causative organism, and others. For example, drugs used in meningitis must be able to readily penetrate the central nervous system (CNS) (meninges). Drugs excreted largely unchanged in the urine are quite effective in urinary tract infections (provided they are active at a pH of 5 to 6) even though they may exhibit very low plasma levels.

There are, of course, other factors that can influence the choice of an antibiotic; these include severity of the infection, a previous hypersensitivity or serious adverse reaction to a particular drug, patient acceptance of parenteral administration, and cost of the drug. Although proper selection of antimicrobial agents can lead to quick eradication of most infections with minimal adverse effects or complications, injudicious use of antibiotics may ultimately prove harmful to the patient. The decision to initiate antibacterial therapy must be based on careful assessment of the patient and the choice of drugs determined by accurate bacteriologic and sensitivity testing whenever possible. Antibiotic therapy in the absence of proper culturing should be undertaken only with those drugs most likely to be effective against the *suspected* pathogen. It should then be modified if necessary as soon as the culture and sensitivity test results are known. Further, adequate dosage and duration of therapy are essential to ensuring complete drug efficacy. These factors are considered next.

Dosage and Duration of Therapy

The dosage of an anti-infective drug should always be high enough and duration of treatment long enough to provide effective drug concentrations in infected tissues for a suitable period. As indicated earlier, blood levels of the antibiotic do not always reflect tissue concentrations at the infection site; nonetheless, they are frequently used as a guide to determine if proper dosage is being administered. Despite the importance of maintaining treatment long enough to completely eradicate the microorganism, antibiotics are sometimes discontinued too early. The consequence may be either reinfection with the same organism or emergence of mutant strains resistant to the drug being used.

Although different infections require different treatment durations, oral antimicrobial therapy of most common respiratory and urinary infections should be continued for a minimum of 7 to 10 days. Patients may decide to discontinue antimicrobial drugs as soon as the overt symptoms (eg, fever, sore throat, painful urination) of their disease subside. For this reason, they should be carefully instructed to continue the drugs for at least 48 to 72 hours after symptoms disappear to ensure that the pathogen is completely eliminated. Follow-up cultures are also desirable to confirm the effectiveness of therapy.

More severe infections, such as endocarditis and staphylococcal pneumonia, generally require parenteral administration of higher doses of antibiotics and for longer periods than the more common infections, which can be treated orally. Large doses of antimicrobial drugs may also be necessary in debilitated patients or in patients with disease- or drug-impaired defense mechanisms.

In infections characterized by the presence of purulent exudates or large abscesses, drainage of these areas is often necessary; antibiotics frequently are unable to penetrate these infected lesions sufficiently to eradicate the large quantity of pathogens at these sites. Similarly, patients with urinary infections associated with the presence of renal stones will continue to suffer recurrent infections despite the use of antibiotics unless the stones are removed. It is important to recognize that no antibiotic alone can be expected to completely control every infection, and appropriate adjunctive measures are frequently necessary to treat certain types of infections. Additional supportive measures that may be undertaken to facilitate recovery from severe infections include correction of electrolyte or acid–base disturbances, support of respiration, use of antipyretic drugs such as acetaminophen to reduce elevated temperature, and maintenance of an adequate nutritional status.

Prophylactic Use of Antibiotics

The use of antimicrobial drugs to prevent rather than treat infections is a controversial area of anti-infective therapy. Although doubtless effective in certain situations, anti-infective prophylaxis is without proven value in many conditions and may in fact be detrimental in certain instances. There is general agreement that successful chemoprophylaxis is most often attained when a *single* drug known to be effective against a specific pathogen is used to prevent invasion of that pathogen before it has a chance to become established. Some generally accepted indications for antimicrobial prophylaxis are as follows:

Penicillin G: for prophylaxis of group A streptococcal infection in patients with rheumatic heart disease, recurrent cellulitis in lymphedema, and subacute bacterial endocarditis
Rifampin or minocycline: prophylaxis of meningococcal meningitis
Isoniazid: prophylaxis of tuberculosis
Doxycycline: prevention of "traveler's diarrhea"
Chloroquine: prevention of malaria
Amantadine: prevention of influenza A
Trimethoprim plus sulfamethoxazole: prophylaxis of recurrent urinary tract infections and *Pneumocystis carinii* pneumonia
Cefazolin or metronidazole: perioperatively for surgical prophylaxis in "contaminated surgery" such as colonic resection or vaginal hysterectomy

In contrast, conclusive evidence is lacking on the effectiveness of antibiotics used prophylactically in patients with chronic obstructive pulmonary disease; in patients undergoing urologic, dental, or neurologic surgical procedures; and in patients with acute pancreatitis. Finally, chemoprophylaxis is considered to be ineffective in preventing 1) secondary bacterial infection in "common colds," influenza, or other viral diseases; 2) urinary infections in the presence of stones, obstruction, or indwelling urinary catheters; 3) recurring herpes simplex ulcers of the mouth; 4) secondary infections in burn patients; and 5) infections associated with prolonged use of corticosteroids, immunosuppressants, or antineoplastic drugs.

A major danger of chemoprophylaxis is the development of superinfections with drug-resistant strains, the incidence of which is closely related to the duration of exposure to the antibiotic. Therefore, short-term prophylaxis is preferred wherever possible, and antimicrobial drugs used for surgical prophylaxis generally should be given no more than 48 hours preoperatively and 4 to 6 hours postoperatively. Prolonged use of prophylactic antibiotics, as in rheumatic fever, endocarditis, or chronic bronchitis, must be continually monitored and patients closely observed for signs of a developing superinfection (diarrhea, glossitis, perianal or vaginal itching).

Other disadvantages to antimicrobial chemoprophylaxis include an increased incidence of allergic reactions and diarrhea, and frequently a substantially higher cost to the patient.

Combined Antimicrobial Therapy

Although most infections can be treated adequately with a single anti-infective agent, simultaneous administration of two or more antimicrobial agents is justifiable under certain circumstances. When combination antimicrobial therapy is indicated, it should be accomplished by administration of two or more *individual* drugs whose doses can be titrated independently to provide an optimal effect. The once widespread use of "fixed-dose" antibiotic combinations has essentially been eliminated by the removal of most of these combinations from the market, on the grounds that many contained subtherapeutic amounts of antibiotic drugs, were often ineffective, and favored emergence of resistant bacterial populations.

The primary indications for combination anti-infective therapy are described below.

Treatment of Mixed Bacterial Infections

Some infections (eg, peritonitis, urinary infections, otitis media) may be complicated by the presence of two, or possibly more, microorganisms possessing different antimicrobial susceptibility. Although broad-spectrum antibiotics are occasionally successful when used alone in such infections, combination therapy is frequently necessary to ensure complete eradication of all pathogens present in mixed infections. Sensitivity testing is essential in such cases.

Initial Treatment of Severe Infections Whose Causative Agent Is Unknown

Before the results of bacteriologic culturing in an unknown infection are obtained, combination therapy is occasionally undertaken to ensure that the widest range of possible organisms is covered. Such treatment, of course, should be modified as necessary as soon as culture and sensitivity data are available.

Postponement of the Emergence of Resistant Strains

Development of resistance to antibiotic agents is often delayed (but not necessarily prevented) when a sensitive pathogen is exposed to two drugs simultaneously. This is particularly apparent with the combined use of two or more antitubercular drugs (eg, isoniazid, rifampin) or combinations of carbenicillin and gentamicin or tobramycin for severe pseudomonal infections.

Enhancement of Antibacterial Activity

Increased antibacterial activity compared with that of each drug alone is frequently observed with simultaneous use of two antibiotics. This synergistic effect is noted, for example, with an extended-spectrum penicillin and an aminoglycoside for pseudomonal infections, with isoniazid and ethambutol in treating tuberculosis, with tetracycline and streptomycin in treating brucellosis or glanders, and with amphotericin B and flucytosine in treating certain systemic fungal infections.

A relatively new combination is the use of a penicillin such as ampicillin or ticarcillin with clavulanic acid, an inhibitor of beta-lactamase enzyme (refer to **Resistance**). Clavulanic acid prevents the destruction of the penicillin by the beta-lactamase enzymes secreted by certain microorganisms (eg, staphylococci, *H. influenzae*), thus allowing successful eradication of the microbe by the penicillin drug. Preventing enzymatic destruction can expand the usefulness of certain antibiotics previously ineffective against beta-lactamase–producing organisms.

Reduction of Toxicity

In certain instances, combined antimicrobial therapy is used to reduce the untoward effects of one or more antibacterial agents, especially in cases where the individual drugs are each administered in reduced doses. Conversely, the addition of a second drug to the regimen, especially at full dosage, can *increase* the likelihood of adverse effects compared with that seen with a single drug. Again, a knowledge of the potential toxicities of the anti-infective drugs is essential in maximizing the therapeutic effects while minimizing the potential for untoward reactions.

As indicated, combination anti-infective drug therapy can result in undesirable effects, reduced clinical effectiveness, and superinfections. For example, combined use of two or more aminoglycosides can increase the incidence of ototoxicity and nephrotoxicity above that observed with each drug alone. Therefore, other than those circumstances outlined above where combination antimicrobial therapy has proved beneficial, use of more than one carefully selected anti-infective drug to treat a particular infectious condition should be avoided.

Adverse Effects of Antimicrobial Drugs

A wide range of adverse reactions have been reported with the several classes of drugs used in the treatment of infections, and these are reviewed in detail in the individual chapters dealing with each group of drugs. The most frequently encountered untoward reactions with antibiotics are considered briefly here.

Hypersensitivity Reactions

Both acute and delayed allergic responses have occurred with a number of antimicrobial drugs, most frequently with the penicillins and sulfonamides. These may range from mild dermatologic manifestations such as skin rash, itching, and urticaria, to severe anaphylactic reactions, which have proved fatal in a number of instances. The importance of obtaining a careful patient history before administration of an antimicrobial agent known to be associated with hypersensitivity reactions cannot be overemphasized.

Organ Toxicity

Several classes of antibiotics are known to exert selective toxic effects on certain structures or organs of the body. For example, aminoglycosides and vancomycin cause both renal and eighth cranial nerve damage. Amphotericin B and polymyxins, among others, impair kidney function, and lincomycin and clindamycin often induce severe diarrhea and colitis. Tetracyclines may damage teeth, nails, or bones, and rifampin and the estolate salt of erythromycin can be hepatotoxic.

Superinfection

Development of secondary infections is a potentially serious problem connected with antibiotic usage. It is most often associated with prolonged anti-infective therapy, insufficient drug dosage, impaired host defense mechanisms, concurrent therapy with immunosuppressive drugs, or a combination of these factors. Pathogens frequently responsible for secondary infections include *Pseudomonas, Proteus, Candida*, and drug-resistant staphylococci and fungi. These organisms may be especially difficult to eradicate because they often represent strains resistant to conventional antimicrobial agents. Although superinfection can theoretically occur anywhere in the body, it is found most commonly in the GI tract and may be manifested by diarrhea, glossitis, stomatitis, "furry" tongue, and perineal irritation. Prompt recognition of a secondary infection is critical to its effective management. Therapy is best accomplished by discontinuing the initial antibiotic, culturing the infected area, and administering an antimicrobial drug shown by sensitivity testing to be effective against the new organism.

Resistance

Bacteria are susceptible to eradication by some anti-infective drugs but not others. The phenomenon whereby certain organisms are unaffected by a particular antimicrobial agent is called *resistance*. Bacterial resistance may be broadly categorized as either natural or acquired. *Natural resistance* is genetically determined and may be characteristic of either an entire species or only certain strains within a species. It is not a significant therapeutic problem, inasmuch as the resistance is usually to a particular mechanism of antimicrobial action, and there are usually other antibiotics with different mechanisms of action to which the organism is susceptible. *Acquired resistance*, however, can develop in previously susceptible pathogens for a number of reasons and is a major clinical problem with many anti-infective drugs. Development of bacterial resistance has severely limited the usefulness of many antibiotics in certain infections.

Unfortunately, the more an antimicrobial agent is employed in clinical practice, the greater the likelihood that resistant strains of once-susceptible bacteria will develop. This further underscores the importance of sensitivity testing whenever there is doubt about the susceptibility of an infecting microorga-

(text continues on page 593)

Table 58-1. **Antimicrobial Drugs of Choice for Common Infections**

Organism	***Classification***	***Representative Clinical Illnesses***	***Drugs of First Choice***	***Alternative Drugs***
Acinetobacter (Mima, Herellea) species	Gram-negative bacilli	Bacteremia, endocarditis, meningitis, urethritis	imipenem	amikacin, gentamicin, tobramycin, netilmicin, doxycycline, minocycline, carbenicillin, ticarcillin, mezlocillin, piperacillin, azlocillin
Actinomyces israelli	Actinomycetes	Actinomycosis	penicillin G	tetracycline, erythromycin
Alcaligenes faecalis	Gram-negative bacilli	Urinary infections, wound infections	chloramphenicol, tetracycline	colistimethate, polymyxin B, gentamicin, kanamycin
Aspergillus	Fungi	Systemic fungal infections (eg, skin, lung, bone)	amphotericin B	itraconazole
Bacillus anthracis	Gram-positive bacilli	Anthrax, pneumonia, meningitis	penicillin G	erythromycin, tetracycline, cephalosporins (first-generation)
Bacteroides (several strains)	Gram-negative bacilli	Bacteremia, brain and lung abscesses, genital infections, pulmonary infections, endocarditis	penicillin G (oropharyngeal strains) clindamycin, metronidazole (GI strains, endocarditis)	tetracycline, piperacillin, mezlocillin, azlocillin, chloramphenicol, cefoxitin, cefotetan, metronidazole, imipenem
Blastomyces dermatidis	Fungi	Blastomycosis	ketoconazole *or* amphotericin B	itraconazole
Bordetella pertussis	Gram-negative bacilli	Whooping cough	erythromycin	ampicillin, tetracycline, trimethoprim–sulfamethoxazole
Borrelia recurrentis	Spirochetes	Relapsing fever	tetracycline	penicillin G
Branhamella catarrhalis	Gram-negative cocci	Respiratory infections, sinusitis, otitis media	trimethoprim–sulfamethoxazole	cefuroxime, cefotaxime, ceftizoxime, tetracycline, amoxicillin–clavulanic acid
Brucella	Gram-negative bacilli	Brucellosis	tetracycline with gentamicin	chloramphenicol (with or without streptomycin), trimethoprim–sulfamethoxazole, rifampin with a tetracycline
Calymmato-bacterium granulomatis	Gram-negative bacilli	Granuloma inguinale	tetracycline	streptomycin, trimethoprim-sulfamethoxazole
Candida (several species)	Fungi	Local and systemic fungal infections	Systemic: amphotericin B (with or without flucytosine) Gastrointestinal: oral nystatin, ketoconazole Local: miconazole, clotrimazole, nystatin	fluconazole fluconazole
Chlamydia psittaci	Chlamydiae	Psittacosis, ornithosis	tetracycline	chloramphenicol
Chlamydia trachomatis	Chlamydiae	Inclusion conjunctivitis Pneumonia Trachoma Urethritis Lymphogranuloma venereum	erythromycin erythromycin tetracycline tetracycline tetracycline	tetracycline, sulfonamide sulfonamide sulfonamide erythromycin erythromycin, sulfonamide
Clostridium difficile	Gram-positive bacilli	Pseudomembranous colitis (antibiotic associated)	vancomycin	metronidazole

Clostridium perfringens	Gram-positive bacilli	Gas gangrene	penicillin G	chloramphenicol, metronidazole, clindamycin, tetracycline
Clostridium tetani	Gram-positive bacilli	Tetanus	penicillin G	tetracycline, cephalosporins
Coccidioides immitis	Fungi	Systemic fungal infections	amphotericin B or ketoconazole	itraconazole, fluconazole
Corynebacterium diphtheriae	Gram-positive bacilli	Laryngitis, pharyngitis, pneumonia, tracheitis	erythromycin	cephalosporin (first-generation), penicillin G
Cryptococcus neoformans	Fungi	Systemic fungal infections	amphotericin B (with or without flucytosine)	fluconazole, itraconazole
Dermatophytes (tinea)	Fungi	Infections of the skin, hair, and nails	clotrimazole, miconazole, ketoconazole	Oral: griseofulvin Topical: tolnaftate, haloprogin
Enterobacteriaceae *(Aerobacter aerogenes)*	Gram-negative bacilli	Urinary infections, bacteremia, wound infections	third-generation cephalosporins	amikacin, gentamicin, tobramycin, mezlocillin, piperacillin, azlocillin, aztreonam, netilmicin, imipenem, carbenicillin, ciprofloxacin, ticarcillin
Escherichia coli	Gram-negative bacilli	Urinary infections, bacteremia, meningitis, gastroenteritis	third-generation cephalosporins	ampicillin (with or without gentamicin, tobramycin *or* amikacin) aztreonam, mezlocillin, piperacillin, azlocillin, norfloxacin, ticarcillin, netilmicin, kanamycin, imipenem, trimethoprim-sulfamethoxazole, ciprofloxacin
Francisella tularensis	Gram-negative bacilli	Tularemia	streptomycin, gentamicin	tetracycline, chloramphenicol
Haemophilus ducreyi	Gram-negative bacilli	Chancroid	ceftriaxone, erythromycin	trimethoprim–sulfamethoxazole, ciprofloxacin
Haemophilus influenzae	Gram-negative bacilli	Pharyngitis, pneumonia, meningitis, otitis media, tracheobronchitis, epiglottiditis	Life-threatening— cefotaxime, ceftriaxone Other infections— trimethoprim–sulfamethoxazole	aztreonam, ampicillin, amoxicillin, cefuroxime, amoxicillin, clavulanic acid, tetracycline, cefuroxime, cefaclor, sulfonamide
Haemophilus vaginalis (Gardnerella)	Gram-negative bacilli	Vaginal infections	metronidazole	ampicillin
Herpes simplex	Virus	Keratitis	Topical: acyclovir, trifluridine	Topical: idoxuridine, vidarabine
		Encephalitis	acyclovir	vidarabine
Histoplasma capsulatum	Fungi	Pneumonia, meningitis, skin, lung, and bone lesions	amphotericin B or ketoconazole	itraconazole
Influenza A	Virus	Influenza	amantadine (prophylaxis)	
Klebsiella pneumoniae	Gram-negative bacilli	Pneumonia, urinary and biliary infections, osteomyelitis	cephalosporin (with or without an aminoglycoside)	gentamicin, tobramycin, aztreonam, imipenem, mezlocillin, piperacillin, azlocillin, amikacin, netilmicin, tetracycline, trimethoprim–sulfamethoxazole, chloramphenicol, ciprofloxacin, norfloxacin
Legionella pneumophila	Gram-negative bacilli	Legionnaires' disease	erythromycin (with or without rifampin)	trimethoprim–sulfamethoxazole, azithromycin, clarithromycin, ciprofloxacin

(continued)

Table 58-1. **Antimicrobial Drugs of Choice for Common Infections (Continued)**

Organism	***Classification***	***Representative Clinical Illnesses***	***Drugs of First Choice***	***Alternative Drugs***
Leptospira	Spirochetes	Meningitis, Weil's disease	penicillin G	tetracycline
Leptotrichia buccalis	Gram-negative bacilli	Vincent's infection	penicillin G	tetracycline, clindamycin, an erythromycin
Listeria monocytogenes	Gram-positive bacilli	Bacteremia, meningitis, endocarditis, recurrent abortion	ampicillin (with or without gentamicin)	erythromycin, trimethoprim–sulfamethoxazole
Mucor	Fungi	Systemic fungal infections	amphotericin B	
Mycobacterium (atypical)	Acid-fast bacilli	Lymphadenitis, pulmonary lesions	isoniazid with rifampin (with or without ethambutol)	erythromycin, cycloserine, ethionamide
Mycobacterium leprae	Acid-fast bacilli	Leprosy	dapsone with rifampin	ethionamide, clofazimine, ofloxacin
Mycobacterium tuberculosis	Acid-fast bacilli	Pulmonary, renal, meningeal, or other tuberculosis infections	isoniazid with rifampin and pyrazinamide with or without ethambutol	streptomycin, ethambutol, cycloserine, ethionamide, kanamycin, ciprofloxacin
Mycoplasma hominis	Mycoplasmas	Nonspecific urethritis, septicemia	clindamycin, tetracycline	erythromycin, chloramphenicol, gentamicin
Mycoplasma pneumoniae	Mycoplasmas	Atypical viral pneumonia	erythromycin, tetracycline	clarithromycin
Neisseria gonorrhoeae	Gram-negative cocci	Gonorrhea, meningitis, urethritis, vaginitis, endocarditis, arthritis	ceftriaxone	penicillin G, amoxicillin, spectinomycin, cefoxitin, trimethoprim–sulfamethoxazole, ciprofloxacin
Neisseria meningitidis	Gram-negative cocci	Meningitis, bacteremia	penicillin G, rifampin (carrier state)	chloramphenicol, cefuroxime, cefotaxime, ceftizoxime, trimethoprim–sulfamethoxazole
Nocardia	Actinomycetes	Pulmonary lesions, brain abscess	trimethoprim–sulfamethoxazole	imipenem, minocycline, amikacin, cycloserine
Pasteurella multocida	Gram-negative bacilli	Bacteremia, meningitis	penicillin G	tetracycline, cephalosporin, amoxicillin–clavulanic acid
Pneumocystis carinii	Protozoan	Pneumonia in immunologically compromised patients	trimethoprim–sulfamethoxazole	pentamidine, dapsone
Proteus mirabilis	Gram-negative bacilli	Urinary and other infections	ampicillin	aztreonam, carbenicillin, ticarcillin, amikacin, gentamicin, tobramycin, mezlocillin, azlocillin, piperacillin, norfloxacin, ciprofloxacin, cephalosporin
Proteus (other species, indole positive)	Gram-negative bacilli	Urinary and other infections	cefotaxime, ceftizoxime, ceftriaxone, ceftazidime	carbenicillin, ticarcillin, mezlocillin, azlocillin, piperacillin, gentamicin, tobramycin, amikacin, norfloxacin, ciprofloxacin, aztreonam, tetracycline, imipenem, chloramphenicol
Providencia stuartii	Gram-negative bacilli	Urinary and other infections	cefotaxime, ceftizoxime, ceftriaxone, ceftazidime	gentamycin, tobramycin, amikacin, carbenicillin, ticarcillin, mezlocillin, azlocillin, imipenem, chloramphenicol, aztreonam, trimethoprim–sulfamethoxazole

Pseudomonas aeruginosa	Gram-negative bacilli	Urinary infections	ciprofloxacin	Aminoglycoside (eg, amikacin, gentamicin, tobramycin, netilmicin) with a third-generation cephalosporin (eg, cefoperazone, cefotaxime, ceftizoxime), aztreonam, norfloxacin, ciprofloxacin, imipenem
		Other infections (eg, respiratory, skin)	Antipseudomonal penicillins (eg, mezlocillin, azlocillin, piperacillin) with an aminoglycoside (such as gentamicin, amikacin, or tobramycin)	
Pseudomonas mallei	Gram-negative bacilli	Glanders	streptomycin with tetracycline	streptomycin with chloramphenicol
Pseudomonas pseudomallei	Gram-negative bacilli	Melioidosis	trimethoprim–sulfamethoxazole, ceftazidime	sulfonamide, tetracycline (with or without chloramphenicol)
Rickettsia (several species)	Rickettsiae	Rocky Mountain spotted fever, typhus, Q fever, tick-bite fever	tetracycline	chloramphenicol, a fluroquinolone
Salmonella typhi	Gram-negative bacilli	Typhoid fever	ceftriaxone	ampicillin, amoxicillin, ciprofloxacin, trimethoprim–sulfamethoxazole, chloramphenicol
Salmonella (other species)	Gram-negative bacilli	Paratyphoid fever, gastroenteritis, bacteremia	cefotaxime or ceftriaxone	chloramphenicol, trimethoprim–sulfamethoxazole, ciprofloxacin, ampicillin, amoxicillin
Serratia	Gram-negative bacilli	Several systemic infections (usually secondary to immunosuppressive therapy)	cefotaxime, ceftizoxime, ceftriaxone, ceftazidime	aztreonam, imipenem, trimethoprim–sulfamethoxazole, ciprofloxacin, ticarcillin, mezlocillin, piperacillin, gentamicin, amikacin
Shigella	Gram-negative bacilli	Acute gastroenteritis	a fluroquinolone	trimethoprim–sulfamethoxazole, ampicillin, ceftriaxone
Spirillum minus	Gram-negative bacilli	Rat-bite fever	penicillin G	tetracycline, streptomycin
Sporothrix schenckii	Fungi	Sporotrichosis	amphotericin B	potassium iodide (for cutaneous form *only*), itraconazole
Staphylococcus aureus	Gram-positive cocci	Pneumonia, meningitis, endocarditis, bacteremia, abscesses, osteomyelitis	*Nonpenicillinase-producing*: penicillin G or V	cephalosporin, clindamycin, vancomycin, imipenem, a fluroquinolone
			Penicillinase-producing: penicillinase-resistant penicillin	amoxicillin–clavulanic acid, a fluroquinolone cephalosporin, vancomycin, imipenem, clindamycin
			Methicillin-resistant: vancomycin (with or without gentamycin or rifampin)	trimethoprim–sulfamethoxazole, minocycline
Streptobacillus moniliformis	Gram-negative bacilli	Rat-bite fever, Haverhill fever, bacteremia	penicillin G	tetracycline, streptomycin
Streptococcus (anaerobic species)	Gram-positive cocci	Bacteremia, endocarditis, peritonitis, brain abscess	penicillin G	clindamycin, vancomycin, cephalosporins
Streptococcus bovis	Gram-positive cocci	Urinary infections, endocarditis, bacteremia, meningitis	penicillin G	cephalosporin, vancomycin
Streptococcus faecalis (enterococcus group)	Gram-positive cocci	Endocarditis, septicemia, meningitis, severe systemic infection	ampicillin or penicillin G with gentamicin or amikacin	vancomycin with gentamicin or amikacin

(continued)

Table 58-1. **Antimicrobial Drugs of Choice for Common Infections (Continued)**

Organism	***Classification***	***Representative Clinical Illnesses***	***Drugs of First Choice***	***Alternative Drugs***
Streptococcus (Diplococcus) pneumoniae	Gram-positive cocci	Pneumonia, meningitis, endocarditis, arthritis	penicillin G or V	erythromycin, cephalosporin (first-generation), chloramphenicol, vancomycin with or without rifampin
Streptococcus pyogenes (Groups A, C, G)	Gram-positive cocci	Several infections	penicillin G or V	erythromycin, cephalosporin, vancomycin, clindamycin, clarithromycin, azithromycin
Streptococcus pyogenes (Group B)	Gram-positive cocci	Several infections	penicillin G or V	erythromycin, clarithromycin, azithromycin, clindamycin, vancomycin
Streptococcus (viridans group)	Gram-positive cocci	Urinary infections, dental infections, endocarditis, meningitis, bacteremia	penicillin G (with or without gentamicin)	cephalosporin, vancomycin
Treponema pallidum	Spirochetes	Syphilis	penicillin G	tetracycline, ceftriaxone
Treponema pertenue	Spirochetes	Yaws	penicillin G	tetracycline
Vibrio cholerae	Gram-negative bacilli	Cholera	tetracycline	trimethoprim–sulfamethoxazole, a fluroquinolone
Yersinia (pasteurella) pestis	Gram-negative bacilli	Plague	streptomycin (with or without tetracycline)	tetracycline, chloramphenicol, gentamicin

nism to a chosen antibiotic. Complicating the picture is the problem of *cross-resistance*, that is, not only the resistance of a certain bacteria to all members of a particular antibiotic group (eg, penicillins, tetracyclines, sulfonamides) but resistance to other chemically related drugs (eg, penicillins and cephalosporins) or in some cases to chemically unrelated drugs (eg, erythromycin and lincomycin). Microbial resistance has presented a serious dilemma in many hospitals where a variety of anti-infective agents must be used to control the many types of infections frequently encountered in this setting. Hospital-acquired infections are referred to as *nosocomial* infections. In these situations, secondary infections occur to a significant extent, and these are often caused, as already indicated, by strains or mutants of pathogens resistant to conventional therapy. Control of these nosocomial infections is therefore often difficult. Of particular concern in this regard are infections caused by methicillin-resistant *Staphylococcus aureus* (MRSA), an extremely difficult infection to control. Microorganisms can develop resistance to anti-infective drugs in a number of ways, the most important of which are:

- Elaboration of enzymes (eg, beta-lactamases such as penicillinases or cephalosporinases) that destroy the drug
- Decreased permeability of the microbial cell membrane to certain antibiotics (eg, tetracyclines, aminoglycosides, chloramphenicol) that depend on penetration into the bacteria for their effectiveness
- Development of altered binding sites (eg, loss of specific ribosomal proteins) within the bacterial cell for certain antibiotic drugs (eg, aminoglycosides, erythromycins) that normally interrupt ribosomal function by chemically binding to ribosomal proteins
- Development of altered enzymatic or metabolic pathways that either entirely bypass the reaction inhibited by the antimicrobial drug or that become less susceptible to interruption by antibiotic drugs such as sulfonamides
- Production by bacteria of a direct antibiotic drug antagonist (eg, PABA versus sulfonamides)

In many cases, the emergence of resistant bacterial strains has necessitated the use of less effective and more toxic antimicrobial agents to treat an infection formerly controlled by a more desirable drug. Moreover, the increasing numbers of anti-infective drugs proving ineffective against certain infectious organisms (eg, staphylococci, gram-negative bacilli) have raised the specter of some diseases eventually becoming largely uncontrollable by the currently available antibiotic drugs. To minimize this possibility, it is essential that antimicrobial drugs be used sensibly and that only those drugs necessary to eliminate the organisms known to be present should be prescribed.

Antibiotics in Renal Failure

Kidney function is a major determinant of the response to many antimicrobial drugs. Drugs eliminated principally by the kidney are potentially more hazardous when employed at normal doses in the patient with renal impairment, because the slowed elimination leads to serum levels being more elevated for longer periods. Therefore, clinicians should be aware of the mode of excretion of any anti-infective agent they administer. Further, renal function should be determined not only before administration of an anti-infective agent that is cleared by the kidney but throughout the course of therapy as well, particularly if the course of treatment is prolonged. Antibiotics eliminated largely by the kidneys include the penicillins, cephalosporins, aminoglycosides, polymyxins, vancomycin, trimethoprim–sulfamethoxazole, and most tetracyclines. The penicillins and cephalosporins are relatively nontoxic even at high plasma levels and therefore can be used safely in the presence of limited renal dysfunction. The tetracyclines are cleared by the kidney at varying rates, and those derivatives with extended half-lives (except doxycycline) should not be used when renal function is impaired. The aminoglycosides, polymyxins, and vancomycin will accumulate rapidly when kidney function is reduced; thus, the dosage or frequency of administration of these drugs must be reduced in the patient with renal impairment. Moreover, these latter drugs are themselves nephrotoxic and thus can elicit or aggravate renal failure, further reducing their own excretion. It is unfortunate that patients with renal failure are often subject to precisely those infections (eg, gram-negative bacilli) that are usually most responsive to nephrotoxic drugs such as aminoglycosides, thus setting up a potentially vicious cycle. Nevertheless, there are a number of effective antimicrobial agents that may be employed with reasonable safety in patients with kidney impairment, provided that the appropriate dosage adjustments are made. The excretion patterns and related cautions to be observed with the use of each class of antibiotic drugs are noted in the discussions of individual drugs in succeeding chapters.

Drugs of Choice for Specific Infections

The selection of an individual antimicrobial agent as a drug of choice for a particular infection is sometimes subject to debate, and opinions often change as new drugs become available or resistant strains of previously susceptible organisms emerge. Nevertheless, some agreement does exist on the first-line drugs for a number of common infections, providing sensitivity tests have confirmed pathogen susceptibility. Although it is by no means definitive, Table 58-1 outlines recommended drugs of choice as well as alternative drugs for the treatment of infections resulting from a number of microorganisms. It also lists the type of organism and the most common illnesses associated with it. The recommendations made in Table 58-1 represent a distillate of several sources and are presented *only as a guide* to aid the clinician in choosing an appropriate antibiotic. They are *not* intended as a substitute for careful sensitivity testing, and the drug ultimately used to treat a specific infectious state should be chosen on the basis of as much laboratory and clinical data as can be obtained.

Selected Bibliography

Choice of antimicrobial drugs. Med Lett Drugs Ther 34:49, 1992

Dever LA, Dermody TS: Mechanisms of bacterial resistance to antibiotics Arch Intern Med 151(5):886, 1991

Drugs for viral infections. Med Lett Drugs Ther 34:31, 1992

Finch RG: Antibacterial chemotherapy. Med Int 104:4374, 1992

Liu C: An overview of antimicrobial therapy. Compr Ther 18(11):35, 1992

Ludwig KA, Carlson MA, Condon RE: Prophylactic antibiotics in surgery. Annu Rev Med 44:385, 1993

Mandell GL, Douglas RG, Bennett JE (eds): Principles and Practice of Infectious Diseases, 3rd ed. New York, John Wiley & Sons, 1989

Sanders CC: Beta-Lactamases of gram-negative bacteria: New challenges for new drugs. Clin Infect Dis 14:1089, 1992

Nursing Bibliography

Carr G: Opportunist infections and pharmacology. Critical Care Nursing Clinics of North America 4(3):395, 1992

Littleton M: Trends in agents used for the management of sepsis. Critical Care Nursing Quarterly 15(4):33, 1993

Levy S: Confronting multidrug resistances: A role for each of us. Journal of American Medical Academy 14(269):1840, 1993

Messner R: Nosocomial pneumonia: Combating a hospital menace. RN 55(60):486, 1992

Meyer C: Four against infection. Am J Nurs 4:68, 1993

Schell K: Trends in agents used for the management of sepsis. Critical Care Nursing Quarterly 15(4):23, 1993

Walsh B: Meeting the challenge of infection: A case study. Pediat Oncol Nurs 9(4):146, 1992

59 Sulfonamides

Sulfacetamide	Sulfisoxazole
Sulfacytine	Multiple sulfonamides
Sulfadiazine	Mafenide
Sulfamethizole	Silver sulfadiazine
Sulfamethoxazole	Trimethoprim-sulfamethoxazole
Sulfapyridine	
Sulfasalazine	

Sulfonamides were the first group of systemic antimicrobial agents to be effective when used clinically and were the mainstay of anti-infective therapy before the introduction of the penicillins in the 1940s. Sulfonamides are bacteriostatic against a broad spectrum of both gram-positive and gram-negative organisms, but their use has declined somewhat in recent years with the introduction of more potent and, in some cases, more specific antibacterial drugs. Nonetheless, they remain valuable therapeutic agents in certain infectious conditions, most notably acute urinary tract infections, because the high solubility in urine of certain derivatives allows them to reach effective concentrations without danger of kidney damage.

Significant differences exist among the sulfonamide drugs in their rates of absorption, metabolism, and excretion, and these differences are important with regard to the indications, efficacy, and toxicity of the different compounds. Based on such differences, the sulfonamides may be categorized into several groups; such a classification is presented in Table 59-1, although it should be recognized that not all of the drugs listed here are available as individual drugs. Among the systemic agents, the short-acting compounds are rapidly absorbed and quickly eliminated by the kidney. Sulfamethoxazole, an intermediate-acting sulfonamide, is somewhat more slowly absorbed and excreted than the short-acting drugs, and thus it may be used twice a day rather than 4 to 6 times a day, possibly improving dosing compliance.

Although most systemic sulfonamide use is by oral ingestion, sulfisoxazole is also available for injection. Parenteral use of sulfonamides should be undertaken only where oral administration is impractical (as in a comatose patient) and is best accomplished by slow IV injection. The solutions are highly alkaline and irritating, and the drug may precipitate out of solution.

Locally acting sulfonamides may be employed in several ways. Sulfasalazine is administered orally for the treatment of ulcerative colitis. The compound is split by the action of intestinal microflora into sulfapyridine and 5-aminosalicylate, the latter agent accumulating in significant amounts in the colon, where it may exert an anti-inflammatory action. Other indications for use of locally acting sulfonamides are eye and vaginal infections (sulfacetamide, sulfathiazole, sulfisoxazole) and prevention and treatment of sepsis in second and third-degree burns (mafenide, silver sulfadiazine). Topical application of sulfonamides occasionally elicits allergic hypersensitivity reactions and local ocular irritation.

A major deterrent to the continuing use of sulfonamides has been the emergence of resistant strains of microorganisms that were once sensitive to the action of these drugs (eg, gonococci, beta-hemolytic streptococci, meningococci, coliform organisms). Development of sulfonamide resistance in these organisms has been greatly abetted by the previous widespread prophylactic use of the drugs in subtherapeutic doses for the attempted control of gonorrhea, upper respiratory infections, and urinary infections. Among the major causes of increased sulfonamide resistance among microorganisms are production of excessive amounts of para-aminobenzoic acid (PABA) by the bacteria (PABA is an essential component of folic acid synthesis necessary for cell growth and is competitively antagonized by sulfonamides); enhanced destruction of the sulfonamide molecule by the microorganism; or development of alternative metabolic pathways for handling essential amino acids (see Chapter 58). Acquired bacterial resistance plays a major role in therapeutic failures with sulfonamides, and the clinical usefulness of these agents, despite their relatively low cost, is rather limited. Cross-resistance between sulfonamides is very common as well. The principal indications for sulfonamides are listed under **Uses** in the discussion that follows, and their usefulness in certain infections is also documented in Chapter 58, Table 58-1.

Sulfonamides

The sulfonamides, with the exception of those drugs used in the treatment of severe burns, are reviewed as a group and then are listed in Table 59-2. Mafenide and silver sulfadiazine are then discussed individually, as is trimethoprim-sulfamethoxazole, a synergistic combination of two antibacterial agents, one a sulfonamide, used in both acute and chronic urinary tract infections as well as for several other indications including treatment of *Pneumocystis carinii* pneumonia in AIDS patients. Resistance has been shown to develop more slowly to this combination than to either drug alone. The sulfonamide discussion focuses principally on the systemic effects of the drugs, with mention being made of specific points pertaining to their local application wherever necessary.

Mechanism

Bacteriostatic at normal doses; interfere with bacterial cell synthesis of folic acid, an essential precursor of nucleic acids, by competitively antagonizing PABA; by preventing PABA utilization, bacterial cell replication is halted

Table 59-1. **Sulfonamides**

Systemic	***Local***
Short-Acting	*Intestinal*
sulfacytine	sulfasalazine
sulfadiazine	*Ophthalmic*
sulfamerazine	sulfacetamide
sulfamethazine	sulfisoxazole
sulfamethizole	*Vaginal*
sulfisoxazole	sulfabenzamide
Intermediate-Acting	sulfacetamide
sulfamethoxazole	sulfathiazole
sulfapyridine	sulfisoxazole
	Topical
	mafenide
	silver sulfadiazine

Uses

Refer to Table 59-2 for specific indications for each drug.

- Acute, recurrent, or chronic urinary tract infections in the absence of obstruction. Acute infections generally respond to a single sulfonamide drug, usually sulfisoxazole or sulfamethoxazole; recurrent infections or infections complicated by obstruction or bacteremia are less effectively controlled by a sulfonamide alone and usually require adjunctive therapy.
- Chancroid
- Trachoma
- Nocardiosis
- Toxoplasmosis (with pyrimethamine)
- Acute otitis media due to *Haemophilus influenzae* (with penicillin or erythromycin); also, prophylaxis of recurrent otitis media (sulfisoxazole)
- Adjunctive therapy of malaria (chloroquine-resistant strains of *Plasmodium falciparum*)
- Prophylaxis and treatment of sulfonamide-sensitive group A strains of meningococcal meningitis or haemophilus meningitis (with streptomycin)
- Prophylaxis of recurrent rheumatic fever (sulfadiazine *only*)
- Conjunctivitis and superficial eye infections (sulfacetamide, sulfisoxazole)
- *Haemophilus vaginalis* vaginitis (sulfabenzamide, sulfacetamide, sulfathiazole, sulfisoxazole)
- Ulcerative colitis (sulfasalazine)
- Dermatitis herpetiformis (sulfapyridine only)

Dosage

Refer to Table 59-2.

Fate

Orally administered sulfonamides, except for those designed for their local effects in the bowel, are readily absorbed from the GI tract; absorption from other sites, such as the skin or vagina, is more variable and unreliable. Drugs distribute widely in the body and may be found in cerebrospinal, pleural, peritoneal, synovial, ocular, and placental as well as other body fluids. Protein binding is variable (20%–90%). Duration of action is largely dependent on the rate of metabolism and renal excretion; drugs are metabolized in the liver by several pathways, one of which, acetylation, can occur at varying rates. "Slow acetylators" have an increased risk of drug accumulation and subsequent toxicity. Eliminated in the urine as both unchanged drug and metabolic products, glomerular filtration playing the major role in excretion. Urinary solubility of sulfonamides is pH dependent; alkalinization of the urine favors excretion (increases ionization of molecule and solubility of drug) and reduces danger of crystallization in the urinary fluid.

Some derivatives (eg, sulfacytine, sulfadiazine, sulfisoxazole) are readily absorbed and quickly excreted and must be given up to 6 times a day to maintain adequate plasma concentrations. Sulfamethoxazole is somewhat more slowly absorbed and excreted and is given less frequently (2–3 times a day). Sulfasalazine, an orally administered drug, is only very slightly absorbed and is excreted largely in the feces.

Common Side Effects

GI distress (nausea, abdominal discomfort)

Significant Adverse Reactions

(Incidence differs depending on drug)

CAUTION

Sulfonamides given to pregnant women near term or to neonates may cause a serious disorder known as kernicterus (refer to **Interactions**).

GI: vomiting, diarrhea, anorexia, stomatitis, pancreatitis, jaundice, hepatitis, impaired folic acid absorption
CNS: headache, drowsiness, dizziness, insomnia, vertigo, tinnitus, ataxia, depression, convulsions, hallucinations, peripheral neuritis, hearing loss, psychosis
Renal: proteinuria, albuminuria, hematuria, oliguria, anuria, crystalluria, nephrotic syndrome
Hematologic: petechiae, hemolytic or macrocytic anemia, blood dyscrasias, hypoprothrombinemia, methemoglobinemia, purpura
Allergic hypersensitivity: pruritus, urticaria, photosensitivity, arthralgia, periorbital edema, erythema multiforme, exfoliative dermatitis, serum sickness, anaphylactic reactions, myocarditis
Other: fever, chills, malaise, alopecia, cyanosis, goiter, diuresis, hypoglycemia, reduction in sperm count, periarteritis nodosum, lupuslike syndrome

Contraindications

Advanced kidney disease, near term of pregnancy or during the nursing period, porphyria, in infants younger than 2 months of age (except for treating congenital toxoplasmosis), group A beta-hemolytic streptococcal infections (drugs will not eradicate organisms), hypersensitivity to sulfonylurea antidiabetics or thiazide diuretics

In addition, sulfasalazine is contraindicated in intestinal or urinary obstruction, in children younger than 2 years, and in patients with salicylate allergy. *Cautious use* in persons with liver or kidney dysfunction, blood dyscrasias, a history of allergic reactions, bronchial asthma, or a glucose-6-phosphate dehydrogenase deficiency (hemolytic anemia can occur); also in

Table 59-2. **Sulfonamides**

Drug	Usual Dosage Range	Nursing Considerations
Sulfacetamide *Ak-Sulf, Bleph-10, Cetamide, Isopto Cetamide, Ocusulf 10, Sebizon Lotion, Sodium Sulamyd, Sulf-10, (CAN) Minims, Sulfex, Ophtho-sulf*	Drops: 1 to 2 drops every 1 to 4 h as condition dictates Ointment: small amount in conjunctival sac 2 to 4 times/day Lotion: apply 2 to 4 times/day for bacterial infections or at bedtime for seborrheic dermatitis	Ophthalmic drops or ointment are indicated for treatment of conjunctivitis, corneal ulcers, superficial ocular infections and as adjunctive therapy with systemic sulfonamides for trachoma; lotion is used for seborrheic dermatitis and cutaneous bacterial infections with susceptible organisms; solutions are incompatible with silver preparations; nonsusceptible organisms may proliferate with use of sulfacetamide; drug may be inactivated by PABA produced by purulent exudates; ophthalmic ointment may impair corneal healing; 30% drops may be irritating upon application; do *not* use if ophthalmic solution is dark brown; discontinue drug is signs of hypersensitivity develop; apply topical lotion cautiously to abraded or denuded skin areas; available with phenylephrine as ophthalmic solution (Vasosulf) and combined with sulfathiazole and sulfabenzamide as vaginal creme and vaginal tablets (Sultrin, Triple Sulfa, Trysul)
Sulfacytine	Adults: 500 mg initially, then 250 mg 4 times/day for 10 days	Short-acting sulfonamide not recommended in children younger than 14 years of age; used *only* for treatment of urinary tract infections
Sulfadiazine	Adults: 2–4 g initially, then 2–4 g/day in 3–6 divided doses Children: 75 mg/kg initially, followed by 150 mg/kg/day in 4–6 divided doses (maximum, 6 g/day) Rheumatic fever prophylaxis: 0.5–1 g once daily	Short-acting sulfonamide infrequently used, as drug is poorly soluble in acid urine and danger of nephrotoxicity exists; high urine volume must be maintained; component of triple sulfa formulations with sulfamerazine and sulfamethazine; combination claimed to reduce chance of crystalluria; alkalinization of urine is also recommended when drug is used
Sulfamethizole *Thiosulfil Forte*	Adults: 0.5–1 g 3 or 4 times/day Children: 30–45 mg/kg/day in 4 divided doses	Short-acting sulfonamide principally used for acute and chronic urinary infections; highly bound to plasma proteins; use with caution with other protein-bound drugs; rapidly excreted in urine, mostly in active form; drug may impart an orange-yellow color to urine or skin; available in combination with phenazopyridine and oxytetracycline (Urobiotic)
Sulfamethoxazole *Gantanol, Urobak (CAN) Apo-Sulfamethoxazole*	Adults: 2 g initially, followed by 1 g 2 or 3 times/day Children: 50–60 mg/kg initially, then 25–30 mg/kg morning and night (maximum, 75 mg/kg/day)	Intermediate-acting sulfonamide similar to sulfisoxazole but with somewhat slower oral absorption and urinary excretion; used twice a day in most cases to prevent accumulation; available in combination with trimethoprim (Bactrim, Septra; *see* separate discussion) and phenazopyridine (Azo Gantanol), the latter drug serving as a urinary analgesic for relief of dysuria associated with urinary tract infection
Sulfapyridine *(CAN) Dagenan*	Adults: 500 mg 4 times/day until improvement is noted, then reduce by 500 mg/day at 3-day intervals to effective maintenance level	Intermediate-acting agent used in the treatment of dermatitis herpetiformis (recurrent, inflammatory skin disease, herpetic in nature, characterized by erythema, vesicles, and pustules); slowly absorbed from GI tract (peak levels in 6–8 h); excreted both as intact drug and conjugated metabolites, largely within 3–4 days; administer with sufficient fluids to prevent crystalluria
Sulfasalazine *Azulfidine (CAN) PMS Sulfasalazine, Salazopyrin, SAS-Enema, SAS-500*	Adults: 1–2 g/day in divided doses initially; usual maintenance dosage is 500 mg 4 times/day Children: 40–60 mg/kg/day in 3–6 divided doses initially, followed by 30 mg/kg/day in 4 divided doses	Locally acting sulfonamide used orally in the treatment of mild to moderate ulcerative colitis; hydrolyzed in intestinal tract to sulfapyridine (antibacterial) and 5-aminosalicylic acid (anti-inflammatory); systemic absorption of parent drug and hydrolysis products are variable (increased in the presence of severe ulceration); frequently induces GI intolerance; if noted early in therapy, space daily dosage more evenly or use enteric-coated tablets; note that enteric-coated tablets have passed through GI tract without disintegrating, if this occurs, discontinue therapy; if GI distress is observed after several days of therapy, reduce dosage or stop drug for 5–7 days, then resume at a lower dosage; drug is often continued at reduced levels even when clinical symptoms, including diarrhea, are controlled; dosage and duration of therapy are primarily governed by endoscopic evaluation; if diarrhea recurs, increase dosage to previously effective level; infertility has been reported in men; withdrawal of drug reverses this effect; advise patient that drug may impart an orange-yellow color to skin and to alkaline urine; sulfasalazine may impair absorption of folic acid

(*continued*)

Table 59-2. **Sulfonamides (Continued)**

Drug	Usual Dosage Range	Nursing Considerations
Sulfisoxazole *Gantrisin* *(CAN) Apo-Sulfisoxazole, Novosoxazole*	Adults: 2–4 g initially, then 4–8 g/day in 4–6 divided doses Children: 150 mg/kg/day in 4–6 divided doses (initial dose is 1/2 the 24-h dose) *Ophthalmic* 1–2 drops every 1–4 h as condition warrants or small amount of ointment 3 or 4 times/day	Short-acting sulfonamide used orally, and locally (eye) for a number of bacterial infections; peak blood levels occur within 3–4 h after oral administration; highly protein bound but rapidly excreted in the urine (95% within 24 h); *see* sulfacetamide for remarks concerning ophthalmic and vaginal application; available in combination with phenazopyridine (as Azo Gantrisin), which provides an analgesic effect for relief of dysuria associated with urinary infections, or with erythromycin (as Pediazole), for acute otitis media in children
Multiple Sulfonamides *Triple Sulfa No. 2*	Adults: 2–4 g initially, then 2–4 g/day in 4–6 divided doses Children: 75 mg/kg initially, then 150 mg/kg/day in 4–6 divided doses	A combination of three short-acting sulfonamides that provides the therapeutic effect of the total sulfonamide content, but reduces the risk of precipitation in the kidneys because the solubility of each sulfonamide is independent of the others; *infrequently used preparation orally*, because other equally effective and more soluble sulfonamides are available (eg, sulfisoxazole)
Triple Sulfa *Sultrin, Trysul, and other manufacturers*	1 tablet or 1 applicatorful intravaginally twice a day	Used for treatment of *Haemophilus vaginalis* vaginitis; insert high into vagina; discontinue if local irritation develops

persons receiving anticoagulant or antiplatelet drugs, because increased bleeding can occur.

Interactions

Because of competition for protein-binding sites, sulfonamides may potentiate or be potentiated by other protein-bound drugs (eg, oral anticoagulants, oral hypoglycemics, methotrexate, phenytoin, salicylates, anti-inflammatory agents, sulfinpyrazone, probenecid, and barbiturates).

Effects of sulfonamides may be impaired by local anesthetics that are metabolized to PABA, for example, chloroprocaine, procaine, and tetracaine.

Sulfonamides can displace bilirubin from plasma protein binding sites, possibly resulting in kernicterus (abnormal pigmentation of gray matter of CNS by bilirubin, leading to neuronal degeneration and frequently, death) in premature and newborn infants.

Incidence of crystalluria with sulfonamides can be increased by paraldehyde, methenamine, or urinary acidifiers (eg, ammonium chloride).

Antacids and possibly mineral oil may decrease the effects of sulfonamides by impairing absorption.

Sulfasalazine can reduce the bioavailability of digoxin and can retard the absorption of folic acid.

Concurrent use of sulfonamides may reduce oral contraceptive efficacy and increase the incidence of breakthrough bleeding.

Tolbutamide and methotrexate may increase sulfonamide plasma levels by competing for renal tubular excretory mechanisms.

The effects of tolbutamide, chlorpropamide, and phenytoin may be potentiated by sulfonamides through inhibition of their hepatic metabolism.

Nursing Management

Pretherapy Assessment

Assess and record baseline data necessary for detection of adverse effects of sulfonamides: General: vital signs (VS), body weight, skin color, temperature, and integrity; GI: biliary; genitourinary (GU): renal; cardiovascular (CVS): hematologic; CNS: neurologic function; Lab: culture of infected site.

Review medical history and documents for existing or previous conditions that:

a. require cautious use of sulfonamides: impaired renal or hepatic function; G-6PD deficiency (risk of hemolytic anemia); porphyria
b. contraindicate use of sulfonamides: allergy to sulfonamides, sulfonylureas, thiazide diuretics; **pregnancy (Category C)**, **pregnancy (Category D)** at term (displaces bilirubin from plasma protein binding sites, increasing the risk of kernicterus), lactation (significant concentrations appear in breast milk, producing an increased neonatal risk for kernicterus, diarrhea, and rash).

Nursing Interventions

Medication Administration

Administer oral form of drug on an empty stomach (1 hour before or 2 hours after meals, with a full glass of water).

Assure adequate fluid intake because some sulfonamides are poorly soluble in urine and may cause cystalluria in high concentrations.

Administer sulfonamides on schedule to ensure stable steady-state concentrations for the duration of therapy.

Cleanse wound thoroughly before applying a topical sulfonamide because the drug may be inactivated in the presence of pus, blood, or cell breakdown products.
Provide ready access to bathroom and interventions directed at symptom relief if diarrhea occurs.
Reduce the risk of stomatitis through frequent mouth care.
Initiate a meal schedule that provides small, frequent meals if GI upset occurs.
Protect patient from exposure to sunlight and ultraviolet light. Use sunscreen (not containing PABA) or protective clothing.

Surveillance During Therapy

Monitor complete blood count (CBC), urinalysis, and liver and kidney function tests results obtained over the course of therapy.
NOTE: Renal complications occur much less frequently with the more soluble sulfonamides (sulfisoxazole, sulfamethiazole).
Monitor intake–output, observing for signs and symptoms of possible renal impairment (renal colic, oliguria, hematuria) or dehydration secondary to GI side effects (vomiting, diarrhea).
Monitor for presence of severe headache, rhinitis, urticaria, conjunctivitis, stomatitis, or rash because these may signal early development of Stevens-Johnson syndrome (*severe* erythema multiforme), which may be fatal. If symptoms occur, drug should be discontinued immediately.
Monitor for signs of hypersensitivity (including photosensitivity), which may require discontinuation of drug.
Monitor for signs and symptoms of systemic absorption of the "insoluble" sulfonamides (sulfasalazine) after oral administration in patient with extensive ulceration of the colon.
Interpret results of diagnostic tests and contact practitioner as appropriate.
Monitor for possible drug–laboratory test interactions: false-positive elevated urinary glucose concentrations.
Monitor for possible drug–drug and drug–nutrient interactions: increased risk of hypoglycemia with sulfonylurea antihyperglycemics—tolbutamide, tolazamide, glyburide, glipizide, acetohexamide, and chlorpropamide; diminished response in the presence of PABA dietary supplements.
Provide for patient safety needs to minimize environmental hazards and risk of injury if CNS side effects develop.

Patient Teaching

Instruct patient regarding the importance of completing the full course of therapy as prescribed; that is, not to discontinue the drug once signs and symptoms of the infection being treated subside.
Inform patient of the consequences of not taking or abruptly discontinuing the sulfonamide.
Instruct patient that the prescribed drug is to be taken for the condition for which it is prescribed and not to be used to treat any other infections.
Instruct patient on possible adverse side effects with sulfonamides; sensitivity to sunlight, dizziness, drowsiness, difficulty walking, loss of sensation, nausea, vomiting, diarrhea.
Instruct patient on appropriate action to take if side effects occur:
- Notify practitioner if early signs of hematologic or hepatic toxicity (sore throat, fever, mucosal ulceration, malaise, pallor, jaundice) occur.
- Notify practitioner of any unusual bleeding. Rationale: hypoprothrombinemia and bleeding tendencies caused by decreased synthesis of vitamin K by intestinal microflora may occur.
- Discontinue topically applied sulfonamide at first sign of local irritation or other allergic reaction and notify practitioner.
- Instruct patient to use sunscreens (not containing PABA) or protective clothing.

Instruct patient to minimize use of over-the-counter (OTC) preparations during sulfonamide therapy because some vitamin combinations and analgesic mixtures contain PABA, which can reduce sulfonamide effectiveness.
Inform diabetic patient that dosage of antidiabetic agent (oral sulfonylureas) may need to be adjusted. Serum glucose level should be monitored, and patient should be aware that sulfonamides can produce false-positive urinary glucose tests using Benedict's method.
Teach patient measures that help prevent recurrence of urinary tract infections.

• Mafenide

Sulfamylon

A topical sulfonamide used to retard invasion of avascular burn sites by a variety of gram-positive and gram-negative organisms, mafenide is effective against proliferation of *Pseudomonas aeruginosa* and certain strains of anaerobes, even in the presence of pus and serum, and its activity is not altered by changes in pH. It facilitates spontaneous healing of deep, partial-thickness burns.

Mechanism

Refer to general discussion of sulfonamides.

Uses

Adjunctive therapy to prevent sepsis in second- and third-degree burns

Dosage

Applied aseptically twice a day over burned surface to a depth of 1 to 2 mm; should be reapplied whenever necessary to maintain continuous covering of area; continue application until healing is well along or skin is ready for grafting

Fate

Diffuses through devascularized areas and is quickly absorbed from burn surface, with peak plasma concentrations in 2 to 4 hours; rapidly metabolized and eliminated by the kidney

Common Side Effects

Pain, burning, or stinging at application site

Significant Adverse Reactions

(Often difficult to distinguish between adverse drug reactions and secondary effects of burn)

Bleeding of skin, allergic reactions (rash, itching, surface edema, urticaria, erythema, eosinophilia)
Rarely:
Hyperventilation, acidosis, excoriation of new skin, fungal colonization of wound area, superinfections

Contraindications

No absolute contraindications. *Cautious use* in patients with acute renal failure, pulmonary infection, or impaired respiratory function, history of sulfonamide allergy (cross-sensitivity has *not* been demonstrated), and in pregnant women.

Nursing Management

Pretherapy Assessment

Assess and record baseline data necessary for detection of adverse effects of mafenide: General: VS, body weight, skin color, temperature, and integrity; GI: biliary; GU: renal; CVS: hematologic; CNS: neurologic function; Lab: culture of infected site.

Review medical history and documents for existing or previous conditions that:

a. require cautious use of mafenide: impaired renal or hepatic function; G-6PD deficiency (risk of hemolytic anemia); porphyria
b. contraindicate use of mafenide: allergy to sulfonamides, sulfonylureas, thiazide diuretics; **pregnancy (Category C)**.

Nursing Interventions

Medication Administration

Cleanse wound before applying mafenide. Although a dressing is not required, if needed, use only a thin layer.

Advocate and initiate appropriate multimodality pain management strategies (pharmacologic and nonpharmacologic) during dressing change, wound debridement, and sulfonamide application for patients in whom pain is a factor. Administer analgesics sufficiently in advance of procedure to ensure maximum comfort.

Surveillance During Therapy

Monitor acid–base balance, especially in patient with extensive burns or one who exhibits pulmonary or renal dysfunction. Rationale: the drug and its metabolite inhibit carbonic anhydrase and may cause metabolic acidosis.

Assess patient for early signs of developing acidosis (eg, nausea, vomiting, abdominal pain, weakness, diarrhea, disorientation). If present, inform practitioner.

Identify early signs and symptoms of allergic reaction (rash, itching, urticaria). If present, it may be necessary to discontinue drug temporarily.

Interpret results of diagnostic tests and contact practitioner as appropriate.

Monitor for possible drug–laboratory test interactions: false-positive elevated urinary glucose concentrations.

Monitor for possible drug–drug and drug–nutrient interactions: increased risk of hypoglycemia with sulfonylurea antihyperglycemics-tolbutamide, tolazamide, glyburide, glipizide, acetohexamide, and chlorpropamide; diminished response in the presence of PABA dietary supplements.

Patient Teaching

Instruct patient regarding the importance of completing the full course of therapy as prescribed.

Instruct patient applying sulfonamide topically to discontinue drug at first sign of local irritation or other allergic reaction and notify practitioner.

• Silver sulfadiazine

Silvadene

A condensation product of silver nitrate with sulfadiazine, silver sulfadiazine possesses broad antimicrobial activity and is bactericidal against a number of both gram-positive and gram-negative bacteria as well as yeasts. It is used topically to prevent invasion as well as to eradicate sensitive microorganisms from burns. Does not affect electrolyte or acid–base balance, and application is less painful than mafenide.

Mechanism

Not completely established; appears to exert its bactericidal effect on bacterial cell membranes and cell wall; sulfadiazine is released in body tissues, and may produce a bacteriostatic action by usual means, that is, antagonism of PABA

Uses

Prevention and treatment of sepsis in second- and third-degree burns

Dosage

Apply aseptically 1 or 2 times a day to a thickness of 1 to 2 mm; reapply as necessary to maintain continuous covering until healing has occurred.

Fate

Hydrolyzed to a silver salt, which is poorly absorbed systemically, and sulfadiazine, which may attain significant plasma levels

Common Side Effects

Burning at application site

Significant Adverse Reactions

Rash, itching, pain, interstitial nephritis (rare)

Also, because sulfadiazine may be absorbed in significant amounts, refer to general discussion of sulfonamides for possible systemic adverse effects.

Contraindications

Pregnancy at term, premature infants, and infants younger than 2 months of age. *Cautious use* in patients with a history of sulfonamide hypersensitivity, impaired renal or hepatic function, or glucose-6-phosphate dehydrogenase deficiency (danger of hemolysis), and during pregnancy.

Interaction

Silver may inactivate topically applied proteolytic enzymes.

Nursing Management

Pretherapy Assessment

Assess and record baseline data necessary for detection of adverse effects of silver sulfadiazine: General: VS, body weight, skin color, temperature, and integrity; GI: biliary; GU: renal; CVS: hematologic; CNS: neurologic function; Lab: culture of infected site.

Review medical history and documents for existing or previous conditions that:

a. require cautious use of silver sulfadiazine: impaired renal or hepatic function; G-6PD deficiency (risk of hemolytic anemia); porphyria

b. contraindicate use of silver sulfadiazine: allergy to sulfonamides, sulfonylureas, thiazide diuretics; **pregnancy (Category C)**, not recommended unless >20% of total body surface is burned and potential benefit is greater potential risk to fetus; **pregnancy (Category D)**, at term (displaces bilirubin from plasma protein binding sites, increasing the risk of kernicterus), lactation (significant concentrations appear in breast milk, producing an increased neonatal risk for kernicterus, diarrhea, and rash).

Nursing Interventions

Medication Administration

Use cream only if it retains its white color. Discard if darkened.

Note that silver sulfadiazine, unlike mafenide, is bactericidal as well as bacteriostatic, and it does not appear to alter acid–base balance significantly.

Surveillance During Therapy

Monitor for toxicity. Only 1% of the silver is absorbed, but up to 10% of the sulfadiazine may be absorbed after dermal application.

Monitor CBC, urinalysis, and liver and kidney function tests results obtained over the course of therapy. Sulfadiazine is very insoluble and may cause cystalluria.

Monitor intake–output, observing for signs and symptoms of possible renal impairment (renal colic, oliguria, hematuria).

Monitor for presence of severe headache, rhinitis, urticaria, conjunctivitis, stomatitis, or rash because these may signal early development of Stevens-Johnson syndrome (*severe* erythema multiforme), which is may be fatal. If symptoms occur, drug should be discontinued immediately.

Monitor for signs of hypersensitivity (including photosensitivity), which may require discontinuation of drug.

If photosensitivity occurs, protect patient from exposure to light (eg, use of sunscreens [not containing PABA], protective clothing).

Monitor for fungal infections in and below eschar.

Monitor results of determinations of serum and urine sulfonamide levels (if available), and check results of kidney function tests, all of which should be obtained during long-term treatment of burns involving large areas because continuous silver sulfadiazine absorption may cause the systemic sulfonamide concentration to approach toxic level.

Interpret results of diagnostic tests and contact practitioner as appropriate.

Monitor for possible drug–laboratory test interactions: false-positive elevated urinary glucose concentrations.

Monitor for possible drug–drug and drug–nutrient interactions: increased risk of hypoglycemia with sulfonylurea antihyperglycemics-tolbutamide, tolazamide, glyburide, glipizide, acetohexamide, and chlorpropamide; diminished response in the presence of PABA dietary supplements; inactivation of proteolytic enzymes.

Patient Teaching

Instruct the patient regarding the importance of completing the full course of therapy as prescribed.

Instruct patient applying sulfonamide topically to discontinue drug at first sign of local irritation or other allergic reaction and notify practitioner.

• Trimethoprim–Sulfamethoxazole (Co-Trimoxazole)

Bactrim, Septra, and other manufacturers

(CAN) Apo-Sulfatrim, Novo-Trimel, Nu-Cotrimix, Roubac

A synergistic combination of antimicrobial drugs that interfere with two sequential steps in an essential enzymatic reaction necessary for bacterial multiplication. Consequently, clinical efficacy is enhanced and development of resistance is significantly reduced when compared with the use of either agent alone. Its antibacterial spectrum includes common urinary pathogens (except *Pseudomonas aeruginosa*) and middle ear pathogens, as well as several organisms associated with respiratory conditions such as acute bronchitis and pneumonitis.

A severe form of pneumonitis due to *Pneumocystis carinii* can occur in immunocompromised persons such as those receiving cancer chemotherapy, other immunosuppressant drugs, or those afflicted with AIDS. This opportunistic infection is difficult to eradicate, and trimethoprim–sulfamethoxazole is one of the most effective drugs in treating this serious disease.

Mechanism

Sulfamethoxazole inhibits synthesis of dihydrofolic acid by competitive antagonism of PABA; trimethoprim inhibits the dihydrofolate reductase enzyme, thus blocking production of tetrahydrofolic acid from folic acid; thus, two consecutive steps in the synthesis of essential proteins and nucleic acids in many bacteria are impaired.

Uses

Recurrent or chronic urinary tract infections due to susceptible organisms (ie, *Escherichia coli, Klebsiella-Enterobacter, Proteus mirabilis, Proteus vulgaris, Proteus morgani*)

NOTE: Initial episodes of uncomplicated acute urinary tract infections should be treated with a *single* agent (eg, a sulfonamide or cephalosporin) rather than this combination.

Acute otitis media in children older than 2 years of age caused by susceptible strains of *Haemophilus influenzae* (including ampicillin- and amoxicillin-resistant strains) or *Streptococcus pneumoniae*

Acute exacerbations of chronic bronchitis in adults caused by susceptible strains of *H. influenzae* or *S. pneumoniae*

Enteritis caused by susceptible strains of *Shigella*

Pneumocystis carinii pneumonitis in children and adults immunosuppressed by cancer chemotherapy or other immunosuppressive therapy or suffering from AIDS (drug of choice)

Treatment of *Nocardia asteroides* infections (usually for 6–12 months)

Other uses include treatment of cholera, salmonella-type infections, melioidosis, brucellosis, chancroid, and prophylaxis of traveler's diarrhea

Dosage

(Dosage ratios given refer to the amount of trimethoprim/sulfamethoxazole [TMP/SMZ] in the preparation)

Urinary infections, bronchitis, shigellosis, otitis media; prostatitis

Adults and children weighing 40 kg or more: 160 mg TMP/800 mg SMZ every 12 hours for 10 to 14 days (7 days in shigellosis)

Children under 40 kg: 8 mg TMP/kg/day and 40 mg SMZ/kg/day in two divided doses every 12 hours for 10 days (5 days in shigellosis)

Severe urinary infections or shigellosis

8 mg to 10 mg/kg/day (trimethoprim equivalent) by IV infusion in two to four divided doses for up to 14 days in urinary infections and 5 days in shigellosis

Prevention of recurrent urinary infections in females:

40 mg TMP/200 mg SMZ daily at bedtime or 80 mg/400 mg 2 to 3 times a week

Pneumocystis carinii pneumonitis:

Adults and children: 20 mg TMP/kg/day and 100 mg SMZ/kg/day, orally or by IV infusion in equally divided doses every 6 hours for 14 days

Chancroid:

160 mg TMP/800 mg SMZ orally twice daily for a minimum of 7 days

When administering IV, give slowly over 60 to 90 minutes. Do *not* give IM. Infusion solution (5-mL ampule) is diluted with 125 mL 5% dextrose in water, and the dilution should not be mixed with other drugs or solutions.

Fate

Rapidly absorbed when taken orally; peak serum levels occur in 1 hour with trimethoprim and 4 hours with sulfamethoxazole; half-lives for both drugs are 10 hours with oral administration and 11 to 13 hours with IV infusion; ratio for trimethoprim to sulfamethoxazole in the blood is 1:20; approximately 45% of trimethoprim and 70% of sulfamethoxazole are protein bound; widely distributed in the body, including cerebrospinal fluid; excreted primarily by kidneys; urine concentrations are significantly higher than serum concentrations

Common Side Effects

Nausea, diarrhea, rash, mild thrombocytopenia

Significant Adverse Reactions

GI: vomiting, abdominal pain, glossitis, stomatitis, pancreatitis

CNS: headache, tinnitus, vertigo, fatigue, insomnia, muscle weakness, ataxia, convulsions, peripheral neuritis, depression, hallucinations

Allergic/hypersensitivity: pruritus, urticaria, periorbital edema, generalized skin eruptions, photosensitivity, arthralgia, myocarditis, anaphylactic reactions, serum sickness, erythema multiforme, Stevens-Johnson syndrome, epidermal necrolysis

Hematologic: blood dyscrasias, purpura, hemolytic anemia, hypoprothrombinemia, methemoglobinemia

Other: chills, fever, oliguria, anuria, lupuslike syndrome, goiter, diuresis, hypoglycemia, periarteritis nodosa, jaundice, hepatitis

Intravenous use at high doses or for prolonged periods may result in bone marrow depression.

CAUTION

Patients with AIDS frequently react adversely when trimethoprim–sulfamethoxazole is administered to treat pneumocystis pneumonia. Fever, rash, malaise, and pancytopenia are common occurrences.

Contraindications

Pregnancy, in nursing mothers or infants younger than 2 months of age, streptococcal pharyngitis, megaloblastic anemia caused by folate deficiency. *Cautious use* in patients with reduced hepatic function, folate deficiency, bronchial asthma, severe allergy, or glucose-6-phosphate dehydrogenase deficiency; the drug should *not* be used to treat streptococcal pharyngitis because it will neither eradicate the organism nor prevent complications.

Interactions

Refer to **Interactions** under general sulfonamide monograph earlier in this chapter and under trimethoprim in Chapter 66.

Nursing Management

Pretherapy Assessment

Assess and record baseline data necessary for detection of adverse effects of trimethoprim/sulfamethoxazole (TMP-SMX): General: VS, body weight, skin color, temperature, and integrity; GI: biliary; GU: renal; CVS: hematologic; CNS: neurologic function; Lab: culture of infected site.

Review medical history and documents for existing or previous conditions that:

a. require cautious use of (TMP-SMX): impaired renal or hepatic function; G-6PD deficiency (risk of hemolytic anemia); porphyria
b. contraindicate use of (TMP-SMX): allergy to trimethoprim, megaloblastic anemia secondary to folate deficiency; hepatic dysfunction; renal dysfunction; during pregnancy at term; **pregnancy (Category C)**, lactation (secreted in breast milk; may interfere with folate metabolism in the neonate).

Nursing Interventions

Medication Administration

Administer oral form on an empty stomach (1 hour before or 2 hours after meals).

Assure adequate fluid intake because sulfamethoxazole is poorly soluble in urine and may cause crystalluria in high concentrations.

Administer sulfonamides on schedule to ensure stable steady-state concentrations for the duration of therapy.

Provide ready access to bathroom and interventions directed at symptom relief, if diarrhea occurs.

Reduce the risk of stomatitis through frequent mouth care.

Initiate a meal schedule that provides small, frequent meals if GI upset occurs.

Protect patient from exposure to sunlight and ultraviolet light. Use sunscreen (not containing PABA) or protective clothing.

Surveillance During Therapy

Monitor CBC, urinalysis, and liver and kidney function tests results obtained over the course of therapy.

Monitor intake–output, observing for signs and symptoms of possible renal impairment (renal colic, oliguria, hematuria) or dehydration secondary to gastrointestinal side effects (vomiting, diarrhea).

Monitor for presence of severe headache, rhinitis, urticaria, conjunctivitis, stomatitis, or rash because these may signal early development of Stevens-Johnson syndrome (*severe* erythema multiforme), which may be fatal. If symptoms occur, drug should be discontinued immediately.

Monitor for signs of hypersensitivity (including photosensitivity), which may require discontinuation of drug.

Monitor acid–base balance, especially in patient with extensive burns or one who exhibits pulmonary or renal dysfunction. Rationale: the drug and its metabolite inhibit carbonic anhydrase and may cause metabolic acidosis.

Interpret results of diagnostic tests and contact practitioner as appropriate.

Monitor for possible drug–laboratory test interactions: false-positive elevated urinary glucose concentrations.

Monitor for possible drug–drug and drug–nutrient interactions: increased risk of hypoglycemia with sulfonylurea antihyperglycemics-tolbutamide, tolazamide, glyburide, glipizide, acetohexamide, and chlorpropamide; diminished response in the presence of PABA dietary supplements.

Observe for development of fever, rash, malaise, and other common adverse reactions if patient is immunocompromised (eg, immunosuppression secondary to cancer chemotherapy, AIDS)

If patient is immunocompromised, monitor results of complete blood counts and observe patient for development of symptoms of pancytopenia.

Provide for patient safety needs to minimize environmental hazards and risk of injury if CNS side effects develop.

Patient Teaching

Instruct patient regarding the importance of completing the full course of therapy as prescribed; that is, not to discontinue the drug once signs and symptoms of the infection being treated subside.

Inform patient of the consequences of not taking or abruptly discontinuing the drug.

Instruct patient that the prescribed drug is to be taken for the condition for which it is prescribed and is not to be be used to treat any other infections.

Instruct patient on possible adverse side effects with TMP/SMX; sensitivity to sunlight, dizziness, drowsiness, difficulty walking, loss of sensation, nausea, vomiting, diarrhea.

Instruct patient on appropriate action to take if side effects occur:

- Notify practitioner if early signs of hematologic or hepatic toxicity (sore throat, fever, mucosal ulceration, malaise, pallor, jaundice) occur.
- Notify practitioner of any unusual bleeding. Rationale: hypoprothrombinemia and bleeding tendencies caused by decreased synthesis of vitamin K by intestinal microflora may occur.
- Instruct patient to use sunscreens (not containing PABA) or protective clothing.

Instruct patient to minimize use of OTC preparations during sulfonamide therapy because some vitamin combinations and analgesic mixtures contain PABA, which can reduce sulfonamide effectiveness.

Inform diabetic patient that dosage of antidiabetic agent (oral sulfonylureas) may need to be adjusted. Serum glucose level should be monitored, and patient should be aware that sulfonamides can produce false-positive urinary glucose tests using Benedict's method.

Teach patient measures that help prevent recurrence of urinary tract infections.

Selected Bibliography

Elder NC: Acute urinary tract infection in women. What kind of antibiotic therapy is optimal? Postgrad Med 92(6):159, 1992.

Kovacs JA, Masur H: Prophylaxis for *Pneumocystis carinii* pneumonia in patients infected with human immunodeficiency virus. Clin Infect Dis 14:1005, 1992

Lee BL et al: Dapsone, trimethoprim-sulfamethoxazole plasma levels during treatment of *Pneumocystis* pneumonia in patients with AIDS. Ann Intern Med 110:606, 1989.

Stamm WE, Hooton TM: Management of urinary tract infections in adults. N Engl J Med 329:1328, 1993

Walzer PD et al: Treatment of experimental pneumocystosis. Antimicrob Agents Chemother 36(9):1943, 1992

60
Penicillins, Carbapenems, and Monobactams

Penicillin G
Penicillin V

Penicillinase-resistant penicillins

- Cloxacillin
- Dicloxacillin
- Methicillin
- Nafcillin
- Oxacillin

Broad-spectrum penicillins

- Amoxicillin
- Ampicillin
- Bacampicillin

Extended-spectrum penicillins

- Carbenicillin
- Mezlocillin
- Piperacillin
- Ticarcillin

Imipenem-Cilastatin
Aztreonam

Several groups of anti-infective agents possessing a similar beta-lactam ring structure are considered in this chapter. The penicillin group of antibiotics includes natural extracts from several strains of the *Penicillium* mold and a number of semisynthetic derivatives. The carbapenems are represented by imipenem, a thienamycin antibiotic produced by *Streptomyces cattleya*, whereas the monobactams are represented by aztreonam, a monocyclic beta-lactam isolated from *Chromobacterium violaceum*.

Penicillins

Of the many natural products isolated from the fermentation medium used to culture *Penicillium*, penicillin G exhibits the greatest antimicrobial activity and is the only natural penicillin in current use. Penicillin G, however, possesses several undesirable characteristics, such as instability in gastric acid, susceptibility to inactivation by penicillinase enzyme, rapid renal excretion, and a relatively narrow antimicrobial spectrum of action. Some of these problems have been at least partially eliminated in many of the newer semisynthetic penicillin derivatives. These drugs have been prepared by incorporating specific precursors into the mold cultures (eg, penicillin V) or, more commonly, by chemically replacing a side chain on the 6-aminopenicillanic nucleus, as in ampicillin. Although these chemically modified derivatives of penicillin G each possess distinct advantages in certain aspects, it must be recognized that none of these agents represents the "ideal" penicillin in terms of activity and toxicity. In fact, penicillin G, by virtue of its good antibacterial activity, minimal toxicity, and low cost, is still the preferred drug for a number of infections caused by susceptible organisms, especially the more common gram-positive cocci such as streptococci, gonococci, and meningococci.

Many penicillin derivatives are available, differing principally in stability in gastric acid, resistance to inactivation by penicillinase (a beta-lactamase enzyme produced by many bacteria, which can destroy the activity of penicillin), degree of protein binding, and spectrum of antimicrobial activity. The important pharmacokinetic characteristics of the various penicillins, as well as a general overview of their spectrum of action, are outlined in Table 60-1. In addition, the usefulness of the penicillins in treating *specific* bacterial infections may be ascertained by reference to Chapter 58, Table 58-1, which presents a listing of the preferred antimicrobial drugs for treating a number of bacterial infections.

Penicillins exert their antibacterial effects by blocking biosynthesis of cell wall mucopeptide, rendering the bacteria osmotically unstable and thus unable to survive. Penicillins, in adequate concentrations, are bactericidal, and are most effective when active bacterial cell multiplication is occurring. Moreover, the penicillins are virtually nontoxic toward human cells, inasmuch as these cells do not have rigid walls like those of bacteria but merely a limiting cytoplasmic membrane. The greater activity of most penicillins toward gram-positive organisms than toward gram-negative organisms is due to the higher proportion of mucopeptide in the cell walls of gram-positive bacteria and their higher internal osmotic pressure. Unlike the activity of some other antibiotics, such as sulfonamides, that of the penicillins is not inhibited by blood, pus, or other tissue breakdown products.

The major untoward reaction associated with use of the penicillins is hypersensitivity. This can range from mild skin rash and contact dermatitis to severe allergic reactions, including exfoliative dermatitis, serum sickness, and anaphylaxis. The incidence of allergic reactions to penicillin is higher in patients with previously demonstrated hypersensitivity to multiple allergens or a history of hay fever or asthma, and the drugs should be used with extreme caution in such persons. No single penicillin derivative is safer in this respect than any other. Penicillin-sensitive patients can also exhibit *cross*-sensitivity to certain other antibacterial agents, notably cephalosporins, and caution must be exercised in using any of these drugs in patients sensitive to any of the others.

Bacterial resistance to the penicillins is variable. Despite extensive clinical use of penicillin for more than 40 years, some species of bacteria have remained uniformly susceptible (eg, *Diplococcus pneumoniae, Neisseria meningitidis*), whereas other species have developed progressively increasing resistance. This variability in development of resistance may be explained in part by the fact that there are several mechanisms responsible for resistance to penicillins. Most commonly, resistance occurs because some bacteria (such as staphylococci) can synthesize beta-lactamase enzymes, such as penicillinase, which convert the drugs to inactive products. Such bacteria would display resistance to penicillins susceptible to enzyme activity, but not to penicillinase-resistant derivatives (see Table 60-1). Conversely, certain bacteria may develop resistance to all

(text continues on page 611)

Table 60-1. **Penicillins**

Drug	*Pharmacokinetics/ Antibacterial Spectrum*	*Usual Dosage Range*	*Nursing Considerations*
NARROW-SPECTRUM PENICILLINS			
Penicillin G, Potassium or Sodium *Pfizerpen G, and other manufacturers (CAN) Crystapen, Megacillin, Novopen G*	Adm: Oral (unreliable), IM, IV; $T_{1/2}$ 30–60 min; 60% protein binding; renal excretion 60%–90% unchanged Antibacterial spectrum: Highly active against *Streptococcus*, non–penicillinase-producing *Staphylococcus* and *Neisseria*, and many anaerobic organisms; not clinically effective against most gram-negative organisms	Adults and children older than 12 Oral: 200,000–500,000 U every 6–8 h for at least 10 days IM, IV: 300,000–8 million U daily (some severe infections, eg, meningococcal meningitis, gram-negative bacteremia, clostridial infections may require up to 20–30 million U/day) Children younger than 12 Oral: 25,000–90,000 U/kg/day in 3–6 divided doses IM, IV: 300,000–1.2 million U/day in divided doses (up to 10 million U/day may be required)	Natural penicillin preparation derived from the *Penicillium* mold; considered drug of choice for treating infections due to susceptible organisms (see Chap. 58); rapid-acting, inexpensive, and very effective against many gram-positive cocci and anaerobes, but destroyed by gastric acid and penicillinase—administer orally on an empty stomach; refrigerate reconstituted oral solution and discard within 14 days; do *not* use oral penicillin G as prophylaxis for genitourinary instrumentation or surgery, lower intestinal surgery, sigmoidoscopy, or childbirth; IM is the preferred parenteral route; keep injection volume small and inject deeply into a large muscle mass; maximal plasma concentrations are attained within 30–60 min; doses exceeding 10 million U/day must be given by IV infusion *only*; administer large doses slowly because electrolyte overload may occur depending on which salt is used; use extreme caution in renal insufficiency—half-life (normally 30 min) increases to 10 h in patients with anuria; perform periodic serum electrolyte determinations during high-dosage therapy and be alert for symptoms of hyperkalemia (hyperreflexia, convulsions, arrhythmias) when using potassium salts
Penicillin G, Benzathine *Bicillin, Permapen (CAN) Megacillin Suspension*	Adm: IM repository; $T_{1/2}$ 14 days; pharmacokinetics the same as penicillin G once it is released into the bloodstream Antibacterial spectrum: same as penicillin G	Adults and children older than 12 Oral: 400,000–600,000 U every 4–6 h IM: 1,200,000 U as a single injection *Syphilis (early)*: 2.4 million U as a single dose *Syphilis (of more than 1 yr duration)*: 2.4 million U IM/wk for 3 wk Children younger than 12 Oral: 25,000–90,000 U/kg/day in 3–6 divided doses IM: 600,000–1,200,000 U depending on weight *Prophylaxis of rheumatic fever*: 200,000 U orally twice a day, 1.2 million U IM once a month, *or* 600,000 U IM every 2 wk	Benzathine salt of penicillin G providing a slowly absorbed and hence long-acting dosage form; oral preparations are less effective than IM forms owing to unpredictable GI absorption; use a large-gauge needle for administration, inject deeply into a large muscle, and do *not* massage injection site; not for IV or SC use; when high sustained serum levels of penicillin are desired, use aqueous penicillin G, because benzathine salt provides fairly low serum concentrations; in small children, divide dose between two injection sites if necessary
Penicillin G, Procaine *Crysticillin A.S. Pfizerpen-A.S., Wycillin (CAN) Ayercillin*	Adm: IM repository; $T_{1/2}$ 12 h; pharmacokinetics same as penicillin G once it is released into the bloodstream Antibacterial spectrum: same as penicillin G	600,000–1.2 million U every 1–3 days *Gonorrheal infections*: 1 g probenecid followed in 30 minutes by 4.8 million U divided into 2 doses and injected at different sites	Long-acting form of penicillin G, similar to benzathine penicillin G in most respects; indicated in moderately severe infections due to organisms (eg, pneumococci, streptococci) sensitive to persistent low serum levels of penicillin G; may also be effective in treating syphilis, acute pelvic inflammatory disease, diphtheria, anthrax, Vincent's gingivitis, and for perioperative prophylaxis against bacterial endocarditis; given only IM; contains procaine, which pro-

(*continued*)

Table 60-1. **Penicillins (Continued)**

Drug	*Pharmacokinetics/ Antibacterial Spectrum*	*Usual Dosage Range*	*Nursing Considerations*
			vides for slow release and absorption of penicillin; may be allergenic; procaine may impart a local anesthetic effect, making injections less painful than benzathine preparations; single-dose therapy for gonorrhea has elicited anxiety, confusion, depression, hallucinations, seizures, and extreme weakness; also available in a combination package with probenecid tablets, which delay the excretion of penicillin G
Penicillin G, Benzathine and Procaine *Bicillin C-R*	Adm: IM repository; $T_{1/2}$ see penicillin G procaine and benzathine Antibacterial spectrum: same as penicillin G	*Streptococcal infections* Adults: 2.4 million U IM Children 30–60 lb: 900,000–1.2 million U IM Children under 30 lb: 600,000 U IM *Pneumococcal infections*: 600,000 U in children *or* 1.2 million U in adults every 2–3 days until patient is afebrile for 48 h	Combination of long-acting forms of penicillin G, used to treat moderate to severe streptococcal and pneumococcal infections of the upper respiratory tract, skin and soft tissues and also erysipelas; only administered IM; not effective against streptococcal group D; do *not* use in sexually transmitted diseases; *see* benzathine penicillin G and procaine penicillin G
Penicillin V; Penicillin V, Potassium *Pen-Vee K, V-Cillin K, and other manufacturers (CAN) Apo-Pen-VK, Nadopen-V, Novopen VK, Nu-Pen-VK, PVF-K*	Adm: Oral; $T_{1/2}$ 60 min; 80% protein binding; renal excretion 60%–90% unchanged Antibacterial spectrum: Gram-positive *streptococcus* and non–penicillinase-producing *Staphylococcus*	Adults: 125–500 mg every 6–8 h depending on severity of infection Children: 25–50 mg/kg/day in 3–6 divided doses *Prevention of bacterial endocarditis* Adults: 2 g, 30–60 min before procedure, then 500 mg every 6 h for 8 doses Children: 1 g, 30–60 min before procedure, then 250 mg every 6 h for 8 doses	Phenoxymethyl derivative of penicillin G, with identical range of activity but more resistant to inactivation by gastric acid, hence better absorbed, yielding 2–5 times higher blood levels; potassium salt is preferred owing to better overall GI absorption; used orally only for mild infections of the throat, respiratory tract or soft tissues; also useful to prevent bacterial endocarditis in patients with rheumatic or acquired valvular heart disease about to undergo surgery or dental procedures; not indicated as initial therapy when parenteral penicillins are necessary (eg, in severe infections); highly bound to plasma proteins; rapidly excreted in the urine; effective when given with food, but blood levels are higher if administered on an empty stomach
PENICILLINASE-RESISTANT PENICILLINS			
Cloxacillin *Cloxapen, Tegopen (CAN) Apo-Cloxi, Novocloxin, Nu-Cloxi, Orbenin*	Adm: Oral; $T_{1/2}$ 30–60 min; 95% protein binding; renal excretion mostly unchanged Antibacterial spectrum: Penicillinase-producing *Staphylococcus*	Adults: 250 mg–1 g every 6 h Children: 50 mg–100 mg/kg/day in divided doses every 6 h	Penicillinase-resistant penicillin principally used to treat infections caused by penicillinase-producing staphylococci; may also be used to initiate therapy in patients in whom a staphylococcal infection is suspected; somewhat less effective than penicillin G against most other gram-positive cocci; best absorbed from an empty stomach; highly protein-bound
Dicloxacillin *Dycill, Dynapen, Pathocil*	Adm: Oral; $T_{1/2}$ 30–60 min; 95%–98% protein binding; renal excretion mostly unchanged Antibacterial spectrum: same as cloxacillin	Adults and children over 40 kg: 125–250 mg every 6 h, up to 4 g/day Children under 40 kg: 12.5–25 mg/kg/day in divided doses every 6 h	Penicillinase-resistant penicillin similar to cloxacillin and oxacillin, but producing slightly higher plasma levels than equivalent doses of other related penicillins; do *not* use in neonates; *see* Cloxacillin
Methicillin *Staphcillin*	Adm: IM, IV; $T_{1/2}$ 30–60 min; 40% protein binding;	Adults: IM or IV infusion 4–12 g/day in divided doses every 4–6 h Children: 100–300 mg/kg/day in di-	Penicillinase-resistant penicillin with same uses as cloxacillin but used by injection *only*; considerably less active

(*continued*)

Table 60-1. **Penicillins (Continued)**

Drug	Pharmacokinetics/ Antibacterial Spectrum	Usual Dosage Range	Nursing Considerations
	renal excretion mostly unchanged Antibacterial spectrum: same as cloxacillin *Note*: Penicillinase-producing *Staphylococcus* is the only indication for all the penicillinase-resistant penicillins	vided doses every 4–6 h Infants: 50–150 mg/kg/day in divided doses every 6–12 h	than penicillin G against streptococci and pneumococci; well tolerated by deep IM injection, slow IV injection, or continuous IV infusion; observe injection sites for signs of irritation, inflammation, or hypersensitivity; be alert for development of drug-induced febrile reactions with IV administration; drug has produced interstitial nephritis within 2–4 wk of start of therapy—observe for early indications (eg, cloudy urine, oliguria, spiking fever) and discontinue drug; methicillin is *incompatible* in solution with a wide range of drugs—do *not* mix with other drugs, including antibiotics but administer separately; carefully follow instructions on container when diluting powder for injection; higher concentrations (10–30 mg/mL) are stable for 8 h at room temperature, but weaker dilutions (2 mg/mL) are only stable for 4 h
Nafcillin *Nafcil, Nalipen, Unipen*	Adm: Oral, IM, IV; $T_{1/2}$ 30–60 min; 87%–90% protein binding; excretion is mainly via the biliary route	Adults *Oral*: 250–1000 mg every 4–6 h depending on severity of infection IM: 500 mg every 4–6 h IV: 500–1,000 mg every 4 h Children *Oral*: 50 mg/kg/day in 4 divided doses *Scarlet fever/pneumonia*: 25 mg/kg/day in 4 divided doses Neonates IM: 10 mg/kg twice a day	Penicillinase-resistant penicillin with same indications as cloxacillin; oral absorption is inferior to that of other similar penicillins; major route of elimination is by way of the bile; parenteral therapy is indicated initially in severe infections—change to oral therapy should be made as condition warrants; not as active as penicillin G against non–penicillin-producing organisms; for IV use, dilute powder in 15–30 mL sterile water for injection or sodium chloride injection and inject over 5–10 min; avoid extravasation because tissue necrosis can occur; reconstitute solution for IM injection with sterile or bacteriostatic water for injection; administer immediately by deep intragluteal injection; solution may be kept refrigerated for up to 48 h
Oxacillin *Bactocil, Prostaphlin*	Adm: Oral, IM, IV; $T_{1/2}$ 30–60 min; 90%–95% protein binding; renal excretion mostly unchanged	Adults and children over 40 kg Oral: 500–1,000 mg every 4–6 h for a minimum of 7 days depending on severity of infection IM, IV: 250–1,000 mg every 4–6 h depending on severity of infection Children under 40 kg Oral: 50–100 mg/kg/day in divided doses IM, IV: 50–100 mg/kg/day in divided doses	Penicillinase-resistant drug similar in most respects to cloxacillin and dicloxacillin but slightly less potent orally; in serious infections, parenteral therapy is indicated, because oral absorption may be unreliable; following initial control of infection, oral therapy may then be substituted; drug should be taken on an empty stomach; solutions for IM or IV use should be prepared by diluting powder with sterile water for injection or sodium chloride injection; discard unused IM injection after 3 days at room temperature or 7 days with refrigeration; consult package for suitable diluents for IV infusion solutions; at concentrations of 0.5–40-mg/mL dilutions are stable for approximately 6–8 h at room temperature—adjust rate of infusion to deliver intended drug dose within this time; transient elevations in serum enzymes (ALT, AST, LDH) may occur with oxacillin *(continued)*

Table 60-1. **Penicillins (Continued)**

Drug	*Pharmacokinetics/ Antibacterial Spectrum*	*Usual Dosage Range*	*Nursing Considerations*
BROAD-SPECTRUM PENICILLINS			
Amoxicillin *Amoxil, and other manufacturers* *(CAN) Apo-Amoxi, Novamoxin, Nu-Amoxi*	Adm: Oral; $T_{1/2}$ 60 min; 20% protein binding; renal excretion mostly unchanged Antibacterial spectrum: Gram-positive same as penicillin G; Gram-negative includes non–penicillinase-producing *E. coli, Haemophilus influenzae, Proteus mirabilis, Neisseria*, and some *Shigella*	*General indications* Adults and children over 20 kg: 250–500 mg every 8 h Children under 20 kg: 20–40 mg/kg/day in divided doses every 8 h *Uncomplicated gonorrhea (adults)* 3 g with 1 g oral probenecid as a single dose *Disseminated gonococcal infection* As above, followed by 500 mg oral amoxicillin 4 times/day for 7–10 days *Pelvic inflammatory disease* As above, followed by 100 mg oral doxycycline twice daily for 14 days	Broad-spectrum acid-stable penicillin rapidly and completely absorbed from the GI tract; absorption is not significantly affected by food; activity similar to ampicillin but less effective against *Shigella*; widely used in acute otitis media due to *Haemophilus*, although resistant strains are emerging; also effective against *E. coli, Proteus, Neisseria gonorrhoeae*, streptococci, pneumococci, and non–penicillinase-producing staphylococci; less likely to disturb GI flora than ampicillin; often used as initial therapy before culture and sensitivity tests because of broad spectrum of action; no more effective than penicillin G or V against susceptible gram-positive organisms; available in combination with potassium clavulanate as Augmentin (see below)
Amoxicillin and Potassium Clavulanate *Augmentin*	Adm: Oral; pharmacokinetics similar to amoxicillin; antibacterial spectrum similar to amoxicillin but addition of clavulanate confers penicillinase resistance	Dosage is given as amoxicillin equivalent Adults: 250–500 mg every 8 h Children: 20–40 mg/kg/day in divided doses every 8 h *Pelvic inflammatory disease*: 500 mg 3 times a day for 10 days with doxycycline, 100 mg twice a day	Contains the potassium salt of clavulanic acid, a beta-lactam that inactivates beta-lactamase enzymes that destroy amoxicillin; combination serves to protect amoxicillin from degradation by beta-lactamase enzymes produced by certain bacteria, thereby extending the spectrum of action of amoxicillin to include organisms normally resistant to the drug (eg, *Klebsiella*, beta-lactamase-producing strains of *Haemophilus, E. coli*, and staphylococci)
Ampicillin *Omnipen, Polycillin, Principen and other manufacturers* *(CAN) Ampicin, Apo-Ampi, Novo-Ampicillin, Nu-Ampi, Penbritin*	Adm: Oral, IM, IV; $T_{1/2}$ 60 min; 20% protein binding; excretion both renal and biliary Antibacterial spectrum: same as amoxicillin without clavulanate	*Respiratory and soft tissue infections* Adults and children over 40 kg Oral: 250 mg every 6 h IM, IV: 250–500 mg every 6 h Children under 40 kg Oral: 50 mg/kg/day in divided doses IM, IV: 25–50 mg/kg/day in divided doses *GI and urinary infections* Adults and children over 40 kg Oral, IM, IV: 500 mg every 6 h Children under 40 kg Oral: 100 mg/kg/day in divided doses IM, IV: 50 mg/kg/day in divided doses *Bacterial meningitis and septicemia* Adults and children: 150–200 mg/kg/day in divided doses every 3–4 h; begin with IV administration, then continue with IM *Gonorrheal urethritis* 3.5 g with 1 g probenecid orally or 500 mg IM every 8–12 h *Gonorrhea* 3.5 g with 1 g probenecid orally as single dose *Disseminated gonococcal infection* As above, followed by 500 mg oral ampicillin 4 times/day for 7 days	Broad-spectrum penicillin widely used in respiratory, GI, urinary, and soft tissue infections including otitis media, septicemia, and bacterial meningitis; skin rash can occur, especially in patients with mononucleosis or hyperuricemia; parenteral form should be used only for severe infections or in patients unable to take oral medications; treatment should be continued 48–72 h after symptoms have disappeared; administer on an empty stomach to enhance GI absorption; during extended therapy (eg, chronic urinary infections), frequent bacteriologic tests should be performed and sufficient doses must be given; clinical and bacteriologic follow-up should be maintained for several months after cessation of therapy; use only freshly prepared solutions for parenteral administration, dilute according to package directions with suitable diluent, and use within 1 h after preparation; available with sulbactam sodium as Unasyn (see below)

(*continued*)

Table 60-1. **Penicillins (Continued)**

Drug	*Pharmacokinetics/ Antibacterial Spectrum*	*Usual Dosage Range*	*Nursing Considerations*
		Pelvic inflammatory disease As above, followed by 100 mg oral doxycycline twice a day for 14 days *Prevention of bacterial endocarditis* 1 g IM or IV plus gentamicin 1.5 mg/kg; give initial doses 30–60 min before procedure and then 2 additional doses every 8 h thereafter	
Ampicillin and Sulbactam Sodium *Unasyn*	Adm: IM, IV; pharmacokinetics similar to ampicillin Antibacterial spectrum: similar to amoxicillin/clavulanate; addition of sulbactam confers penicillinase resistance	(Dosage given in ampicillin equivalents) 1–2 g ampicillin IV or IM every 6 h (maximum, 4 g/day); reduce frequency of dosing in patients with renal impairment	Sulbactam inhibits a wide range of beta-lactamases found in many microorganisms, thereby extending the spectrum of action of ampicillin to include many bacteria normally resistant to it (eg, beta-lactamase–producing strains of *E. coli, Klebsiella, Enterobacter, Proteus, Bacteroides*, and *Staphylococcus aureus*); pain at injection site occurs frequently; both drugs are eliminated largely unchanged in the urine—*caution* in renal impairment
Bacampicillin *Spectrobid* *(CAN) Penglobe*	Rapidly hydrolyzed to ampicillin during GI absorption; peak ampicillin blood levels 3 times those obtained with ampicillin; $T_{1/2}$ 60 min; 20% protein binding; excretion same as ampicillin Antibacterial spectrum: same as ampicillin	*Upper respiratory, urinary and skin infections* Adults: 400–800 mg every 12 h Children: 25–50 mg/kg/day in 2 equally divided doses *Lower respiratory infections* 800 mg every 12 h *Gonorrhea* 1.6 g with 1 g probenecid as a single dose	Rapidly hydrolyzed to ampicillin during GI absorption; each tablet equivalent to 280 mg ampicillin; more completely absorbed than ampicillin, yielding effective serum levels for up to 12 h; much more costly than ampicillin; *see* ampicillin for additional remarks; do *not* administer with disulfiram (see Chap. 81)
EXTENDED-SPECTRUM PENICILLINS			
Carbenicillin Indanyl Sodium *Geocillin*	Adm: Oral, for urinary tract infections only; $T_{1/2}$ 60–80 min; 50% protein binding; renal excretion mostly unchanged Antibacterial spectrum: similar to ampicillin with greater gram-negative activity to include *Enterobacter, Proteus*, and *Pseudomonas*	382–764 mg 4 times a day	Indanyl ester of carbenicillin, suitable for oral use; indicated mainly for acute and chronic upper and lower urinary tract infections and prostatitis due to *Escherichia coli, Proteus, Pseudomonas, Enterobacter*, and *Enterococcus*; readily absorbed orally and hydrolyzed to carbenicillin, which is rapidly excreted in the urine, attaining high levels
Mezlocillin *Mezlin*	Adm: IM, IV; $T_{1/2}$ 60 min; 40%–50% protein binding; renal excretion mostly unchanged Antibacterial spectrum: similar to carbenicillin with higher activity against *Enterobacter, Pseudomonas*, and most other gram-negative organisms	Adults IV: 1.5–4 g every 4–6 h, depending on the severity of infection (life-threatening infections—4 g every 4 h) IM: 1.5–2 g every 6 h *Acute gonococcal urethritis* 1–2 g, as a single IV or IM injection, together with 1 g probenecid orally *Prevention of postoperative infection in contaminated surgery*: 4 g IV 1 h before surgery, and again 6 and 12 h after surgery Children IV, IM: 75 mg/kg every 6–8 h (neonates, every 12 h)	Extended-spectrum penicillin similar in activity to piperacillin but somewhat less effective against *Pseudomonas*; may be used with an aminoglycoside or cephalosporin in severe infections for which the causative agent is unknown; do *not* inject more than 2 g IM and give slowly (15 sec) well into the body of a large muscle mass; inject IV over a period of 3–5 min (concentration of drug in solution should not exceed 10% to minimize venous irritation); IV infusion should be given over 30 min; follow package directions for mixing and diluting, for dosage reductions in patients with impaired renal function (based on creatinine clearance), and for compatibility and stability data; low sodium content (1.85 mEq/g) *(continued)*

Table 60-1. **Penicillins (Continued)**

Drug	Pharmacokinetics/ Antibacterial Spectrum	Usual Dosage Range	Nursing Considerations
Piperacillin *Pipracil*	Adm: IM, IV; $T_{1/2}$ 60–90 min; 40%–50% protein binding; renal excretion mostly unchanged Antibacterial spectrum: similar to mezocillin with the highest activity of this group against *Enterobacter* and *Pseudomonas*	Adults: 3–4 g every 4–6 h over 20–30 min (maximum, 24 g/day) *Uncomplicated gonorrheal infection*: 2 g IM in a single dose with 1 g probenecid ½ h before injection *Prophylaxis during surgery*: 2 g IV just before surgery, 2 g during or immediately after surgery and 2 g 6–12 h after surgery	Extended-spectrum penicillin, used IM or IV for treatment of a variety of gram-positive and gram-negative infections; similar to mezlocillin in spectrum of activity and efficacy; synergistic with aminoglycosides against *Pseudomonas aeruginosa* but do *not* mix in the same bottle; sodium content (1.88 mEq/g) is lower than that of carbenicillin or ticarcillin; reduce dosage in patients with renal impairment according to creatinine clearance values; *not* recommended for use in children under 12; maximum adult daily dosage is 24 g; do not inject more than 2 g at any one IM injection site; refer to package insert for mixing, diluting, and storage instructions; solutions are stable for 24 h at room temperature, and up to 1 wk refrigerated
Piperacillin and Tazobactam *Zosyn*	Similar to piperacillin; tazobactam confers pencillinase resistance and extends the spectrum of action of piperacillin	Adults: 3.375 g by IV infusion every 6 h (reduce dosage in renal impairment to 2.25 g every 6–8 h)	Combination of an extended-spectrum penicillin (see above) and tazobactam, an inhibitor of beta-lactamase; most common side effects are diarrhea, headache, constipation, nausea and insomnia; do not give IM; therapy should be continued 7–10 days; if given together with an aminoglycoside (see Chap. 64), administer separately
Ticarcillin *Ticar*	Adm: IM, IV; $T_{1/2}$ 60–80 min; 50% protein binding; renal excretion mostly unchanged Antibacterial spectrum: similar to mezocillin and piperacillin but with less activity against *Pseudomonas* and other gram-negative organisms	Adults and children over 40 kg IV infusion: 150–300 mg/kg/day in divided doses every 3–6 h IV, IM injection: 1 g every 6 h Children under 40 kg IV infusion: 150–300 mg/kg/day in divided doses every 4–6 h IV, IM injection: 50–100 mg/kg/day in divided doses every 6–8 h Neonates younger than 7 days: 150–225 mg/kg/day in divided doses every 8–12 h by IM injection or IV infusion for 7 days Neonates older than 7 days: 225–300 mg/kg/day in divided doses every 8 h by IM injection or IV infusion	Extended-spectrum penicillin, not absorbed when taken orally; similar in activity to carbenicillin but more active against most strains of *Pseudomonas*; synergistic with gentamicin and tobramycin against *Pseudomonas* organisms; high in sodium content, therefore monitor serum electrolytes during prolonged therapy and use with *caution* in sodium-restricted patients; IM injections should not exceed 2 g/dose; children weighing more than 40 kg should receive the adult dose; administer IM deeply into large muscle mass; discard IM solutions after 24 h at room temperature or 72 h if refrigerated; inject slowly IV to avoid vein irritation; reduce dosage according to package instructions in patients with renal insufficiency based on creatinine clearance; do *not* mix ticarcillin and gentamicin or tobramycin in same solution because latter drugs may be inactivated
Ticarcillin and potassium clavulanate *Timentin*	Similar to ticarcillin; addition of clavulanate confers penicillinase resistance against penicillinase-producers of the same species	Adults: 3.1 g ticarcillin/0.1 g clavulanic acid every 4–6 h by IV infusion Children (older than 12): 200 mg/kg/day to 300 mg/kg/day (ticarcillin content) in divided doses every 4–6 h	Combination of ticarcillin and potassium salt of clavulanic acid which protects ticarcillin from destruction by beta-lactamase enzymes produced by certain bacteria, thereby extending its spectrum of action; use in children younger than 12 has not been established; dosage must be reduced in presence of renal impairment; solutions are stable up to 6 h at room temperature and up to 72 h if refrigerated; drug is reconstituted for infusion with either sterile water for injection or sodium chloride injection

penicillins, possibly because their cell surfaces have become impermeable to the drugs or because they have developed alternative metabolic pathways that avoid steps sensitive to the action of the drugs.

The penicillin drugs may be categorized into several classes based on their respective characteristics, such as spectrum of activity, resistance to penicillinase, and source (see Chapter 58). The major groups of penicillin drugs are briefly described below.

Natural Products

Penicillin G

First penicillin in extensive clinical use; still considered a first-line drug against most gram-positive bacteria (except penicillinase-producing staphylococci) when given by parenteral (IM, IV) injection. Virtually nontoxic to human cells, thus can be given safely in large amounts. Widely distributed in the body, especially after parenteral injections, and rapidly bactericidal. Low cost. Major disadvantages are irregular oral absorption, destruction by gastric acid, inactivation by penicillinase enzyme, and rather narrow antimicrobial spectrum of action. Effects may be prolonged by parenteral (IM) use of benzathine or procaine salts of penicillin G, repository forms of the drug producing lower serum blood levels but longer duration of action.

Semisynthetic Derivatives

Penicillin V

Semisynthetic analogue of penicillin G with similar spectrum of activity. More completely absorbed orally than penicillin G and not destroyed by gastric acid, thus yielding 3 to 5 times higher blood levels. Preferred over penicillin G for oral therapy of mild infections of the throat, upper respiratory tract, or soft tissues caused by non–penicillinase-producing staphylococci and other gram-positive cocci, but ineffective for gonorrhea. Used only orally, therefore not indicated during *acute* stages of serious infections with susceptible organisms, because these usually require parenteral penicillin G. Potassium salt is the preferred form, because it is better absorbed than plain penicillin V.

Penicillinase-Resistant Penicillins (Cloxacillin, Dicloxacillin, Methicillin, Nafcillin, Oxacillin)

Resistant to inactivation by penicillinase and used in the treatment of infections due to penicillinase-producing *Staphylococcus aureus*. Cloxacillin or dicloxacillin is indicated for oral use, because these drugs are acid stable and well absorbed, although their GI absorption is reduced by food. Parenteral methicillin, nafcillin, or oxacillin should be employed in serious infections. Less effective than penicillin G against *non*–penicillinase-producing staphylococci and other gram-positive organisms. Inactive against gram-negative organisms.

Broad-Spectrum Penicillins (Amoxicillin, Ampicillin, Bacampicillin)

Effective against a range of both gram-positive and gram-negative organisms. No real advantage over the less costly penicillin G or V in treating most gram-positive infections, but significantly more active against many gram-negative organisms, especially *Haemophilus influenzae, Escherichia coli, Proteus mirabilis, Salmonella*, and *Shigella*. Thus, frequently employed as initial drugs where the identity of the microorganism has not been determined, for example, urinary infections, respiratory infections such as sinusitis or bronchitis, and otitis media. Drugs are not resistant to penicillinase enzyme, but are acid stable.

Extended-Spectrum (Antipseudomonal) Penicillins (Carbenicillin, Mezlocillin, Piperacillin, Ticarcillin)

Wide antimicrobial spectrum, including *Pseudomonas* and many other gram-negative bacilli resistant to the broad-spectrum penicillins. In addition to the organisms listed under Broad-Spectrum Penicillins, above, these agents are *also* effective against *Pseudomonas*, several *Proteus* species, *Acinetobacter, Enterobacter*, and *Serratia*. In addition, mezlocillin, and piperacillin also demonstrate in vitro activity against *Klebsiella* and *Citrobacter* and contain less than one half the sodium content of carbenicillin and ticarcillin. Their activity is nearly comparable to that of the aminoglycosides, but they are considerably less toxic. Extended-spectrum penicillins are not penicillinase-resistant.

Discussion of the penicillins focuses on these agents as a group, inasmuch as the basic pharmacology and toxicology of all derivatives are identical. Drugs are listed in Table 60-1, where appropriate dosages and individual characteristics are given.

Mechanism

Bind to cellular receptor proteins (penicillin-binding proteins, PBPs) and inhibit the action of enzymes necessary for formation of cell wall peptidoglycans, substances necessary for rigidity of the bacterial cell wall; thus, cells become osmotically unstable and the high internal pressure causes swelling and lysis of the bacterial cells; most penicillins bind to PBP $1B_S$ and 3; gram-positive microorganisms possess much larger amounts of peptidoglycan in their cell walls than gram-negative organisms, and these walls are up to 50 times thicker. The greater susceptibility of some gram-positive organisms to penicillins compared with gram-negative organisms is related to several factors, including the relative amounts of cell wall peptidoglycans, increased affinity of cellular receptors for the drugs, and higher internal osmotic pressure, which causes rupture of the cells as the cell wall is weakened; in adequate concentrations, penicillins are bactericidal and most effective during active cellular multiplication; lower concentrations may produce only bacteriostatic activity

Uses

(See Chapter 58, Table 58-1, for specific indications for different penicillins in various infections; see also Table 60-1)

Treatment of infections due to organisms sensitive to normal serum levels of the drugs

Dosage

See Table 60-1.

Fate

Oral absorption ranges from excellent (amoxicillin, bacampicillin) to fair-to-poor (nafcillin, penicillin G); most other orally effective derivatives are reasonably well absorbed. Peak serum levels occur within 1 to 2 hours after oral administration. After IM injection, most drugs yield rapid and high serum levels, except for the procaine and benzathine salts of penicillin G, which provide lower blood levels but more prolonged effects. Drugs diffuse readily into most body tissues, and tissue levels equal serum levels at most sites except the CNS and the eye, where significant penetration occurs only when the meninges are inflamed. All derivatives are protein bound to varying degrees (15% with piperacillin and mezlocillin to 98% with dicloxacillin). Penicillin V and oxacillin are the only derivatives metabolized to any extent; others are rapidly excreted largely unchanged in the urine. Elimination half-life is less than 1 hour for most drugs, slightly longer for ampicillin and amoxicillin. Also secreted into the bile, which is only a minor route of elimination for all drugs except nafcillin and oxacillin, which are excreted in significant amounts in the bile

Common Side Effects

Allergic reactions (eg, skin rash, urticaria, itching), especially in patients with a history of allergies

Significant Adverse Reactions

NOTE: Most adverse reactions are rare and are usually only seen with large doses. Hypersensitivity reactions, however, can occur with small doses of any penicillin derivative.

Hypersensitivity: severe reactions (wheezing, laryngeal edema, macropapular rash, serum sickness, exfoliative dermatitis, erythema multiforme, arthralgia, prostration, anaphylaxis)

GI: nausea, vomiting, epigastric distress, glossitis, stomatitis, dry mouth, abnormal taste, "hairy" tongue, diarrhea, flatulence, enterocolitis (due to secondary microbial overgrowth), abdominal pain, GI bleeding

Electrolyte: hypokalemia (extended-spectrum penicillins), hypernatremia (especially carbenicillin, ticarcillin)

Renal-hepatic: interstitial nephritis (most frequently with methicillin), glomerulonephritis, cholestatic hepatitis

CNS: neurotoxicity (irritability, lethargy, hallucinations, seizures), anxiety, confusion, agitation, depression

Hematologic: blood dyscrasias, bone marrow depression, hemolytic anemia, hemorrhagic manifestations associated with abnormalities of coagulation tests

Other: pain and irritation at injection site, phlebitis, oral and rectal candidiasis, overgrowth of nonsusceptible organisms, vaginitis, neuropathy, sciatic neuritis

Contraindications

History of previous hypersensitivity to any penicillin. *Cautious use* in nursing mothers and in patients with asthma, hay fever, history of any allergy, or renal impairment; always skin test for allergenicity if doubt exists.

CAUTION

Care must be taken to avoid inadvertent intravascular injection because severe neurovascular damage has occurred, including necrosis and sloughing at the injection site, and gangrene. Repeated IM injections into the anterolateral thigh have resulted in development of fibrosis and localized tissue atrophy. IV injection can result in thrombophlebitis, neuromuscular excitability, and convulsions.

Interactions

Concurrent use of *bacteriostatic* antibiotics (eg, tetracyclines, erythromycin) may diminish the effectiveness of penicillins by slowing the rate of bacterial growth, because penicillins are most effective during rapid multiplication.

Probenecid prolongs blood levels of penicillins by blocking their elimination by renal tubular secretion.

Highly protein-bound penicillins, for example, cloxacillin, dicloxacillin, nafcillin, and oxacillin, can be potentiated by other highly protein-bound drugs (eg, oral anticoagulants, anti-inflammatory agents).

Antacids and other alkalinizing agents as well as colestipol and cholestyramine can inhibit the action of oral penicillins by impairing absorption.

Increased incidence of skin rash can occur with combined use of ampicillin and allopurinol.

The effectiveness of oral contraceptives may be reduced by ampicillin or penicillin V.

Penicillins mixed in solution with an aminoglycoside may inactivate the aminoglycoside.

High doses of IV penicillins (especially carbenicillin) may increase the risk of bleeding in patients receiving heparin or oral anticoagulants.

Use of penicillin and chloramphenicol together may reduce the effectiveness of penicillin and slow the elimination of chloramphenicol.

Extended-spectrum penicillins may be synergistic with aminoglycosides against certain gram-negative organisms, such as *Pseudomonas, Providencia*, and enterococci.

Nursing Management

Refer to Table 60-1. In addition:

Pretherapy Assessment

Assess and record baseline data necessary for detection of adverse effects of penicillin derivatives: General: vital signs (VS), body weight, skin color, temperature, and integrity; GI: biliary; genitourinary (GU): renal; cardiovascular system (CVS): hematologic; CNS: neurologic function; Lab: culture of infected site, skin test with benzylpenicyllolyl-polylysine if hypersensitivity reactions to penicillins are suspected to have occurred in the past.

Review medical history and documents for existing or previous conditions that:

a. require cautious use of penicillins: impaired renal function
b. contraindicate use of penicillins: allergy to penicillins, cephalosporins, other allergens; **pregnancy (Category B)**

In suspected staphylococcal infections, because there are a number of resistant strains, be sure that appropriate, correctly timed culture and sensitivity tests are performed to ensure that the proper antibiotic is prescribed. Penicillinase-resistant penicillins are commonly used as *initial* therapy for any suspected staphylococcal infection until culture and sensitivity results are known. However, some strains of staphylococci capable of producing serious disease and death are resistant to penicillinase-resistant penicillins.

Nursing Interventions

Medication Administration

Administer oral form of drug on an empty stomach (1 hour before or 2 hours after meals, with a full glass of water).

Administer penicillins on schedule to ensure stable steady-state concentrations for the duration of therapy.

Avoid oral administration of penicillins with milk, fruit juices, or soft drinks.

Provide ready access to bathroom and interventions directed at symptom relief if diarrhea occurs.

Reduce the risk of stomatitis through frequent mouth care.

Initiate a meal schedule that provides small, frequent meals if GI upset occurs.

Have emergency drugs and measures for life support available in the event of serious allergic reaction.

With parenteral dosage forms:

- Use appropriate volume of medication for IM injection to avoid pain and discomfort and administer into large muscles (gluteal, vastus lateralis).
- Prepare parenteral solutions for injection with Sterile Water for Injection, Isotonic Sodium Chloride Injection, or Dextrose Injection. Avoid carbohydrate solutions at alkaline pH.

Use particular care in aspirating syringe before injecting a penicillin IM because intravascular administration may result in severe neurovascular damage, including gangrene and paralysis (see *Caution* above). Injection into or near a nerve may cause permanent neurologic damage.

Surveillance During Therapy

Monitor parenteral administration site (IM, IV) for signs of phlebitis, thrombosis, or local drug reaction.

Monitor CBC, urinalysis, and liver and kidney function tests results obtained over the course of therapy.

Monitor for signs of hypersensitivity which require discontinuation of therapy and notification of practitioner.

Interpret results of diagnostic tests and contact practitioner as appropriate.

Monitor for possible drug–drug and drug–nutrient interactions: decreased effectiveness when used with tetracyclines; inactivation of parenteral aminoglycosides (gentamicin, tobramycin, amikacin, kanamycin, netilmicin, streptomycin).

Monitor for possible drug–laboratory test interactions: false-positive Coombs' test with IV penicillins.

Interpret results of the following laboratory tests cautiously because penicillins may cause the following alterations: urine glucose using Clinitest (false-positive with ampicillin), serum proteins (false-positive with mezlocillin), plasma estrogens (decreased with ampicillin), Coombs' test (positive with IV piperacillin).

Be alert for possible development of coagulation test abnormalities associated with bleeding tendencies when large doses of nafcillin or one of the extended-spectrum penicillins are administered. On drug withdrawal, bleeding should cease, and test results should revert to normal.

Monitor results of serum electrolyte determinations during prolonged infusion or repeated IV administration of the sodium or potassium salts of penicillins. Rationale: high-dose IV therapy with these salts can produce electrolyte imbalance.

Patient Teaching

Instruct patient regarding the importance of completing the full course of therapy as prescribed; that is, not to discontinue the drug once signs and symptoms of the infection being treated subside.

Inform patient of the consequences of not taking or of abruptly discontinuing penicillin therapy.

Instruct patient that the prescribed drug is to be taken for the condition for which it is prescribed and not to be used to treat any other infections.

Instruct patient on appropriate action to take if side effects occur:

- Notify practitioner if early signs of hematologic or hepatic toxicity (sore throat, fever, mucosal ulceration, malaise, pallor, jaundice) occur.
- Notify practitioner if symptoms such as difficulty breathing, rashes, severe diarrhea, mouth sores, unusual bleeding, or unusual bruising occur.

Inform patient that stomatitis, upset stomach, nausea, vomiting, diarrhea, and discomfort at injection sites are typical side effects associated with penicillin therapy.

Inform patient for whom either penicillin V, bacampicillin, or amoxicillin has been prescribed that the oral form of the drug may be taken with meals to reduce GI distress.

Carbapenems

• Imipenem-Cilastatin

Primaxin

Imipenem is a beta-lactam that is structurally different from the penicillins and cephalosporins but possesses a similar mechanism of action. It is effective against a wide range of gram-positive, gram-negative, and anaerobic microorganisms and is useful in treating serious infections caused by a variety of bacteria resistant to many other antimicrobial drugs. It may be useful as a *single agent* in infections that would ordinarily require multiple anti-infective drug therapy. The drug is as effective as aminoglycosides or third-generation cephalosporins for severe gram-negative infections. Imipenem is rapidly hydrolyzed by an enzyme in the proximal renal tubules resulting in urinary drug levels that are very low and are probably inadequate for an antibacterial action. This problem has been overcome by the addition to the formulation of cilastatin, which is an inhibitor of the renal enzyme that destroys imipenem.

Mechanism

Penetrates gram-positive and gram-negative bacterial cells and binds avidly to penicillin-binding proteins 1B and 2, thus interfering with synthesis of peptidoglycan and subsequent cell wall formation; highly resistant to destruction by beta-lactamase enzymes; inhibits more than 90% of the clinically important pathogens, the notable exceptions being *Pseudomonas maltophilia; Streptococcus faecium*; groups A, C, and G streptococci; and methicillin-resistant staphylococci

Uses

Treatment of serious infections caused by most common pathogens, except those mentioned under Mechanism above

NOTE: Many infections resistant to antibiotics such as penicillins, cephalosporins, or aminoglycosides have responded to treatment with imipenem.

Dosage

250 mg to 1 g every 6 to 8 hours by IV infusion (30 minutes), depending on severity of infection; maximum daily dose is 4 g

Fate

Plasma half-life is about 1 hour and plasma levels decline to 1 μg/mL or less within 4 to 6 hours; about 20% protein bound. If administered alone, is rapidly metabolized in the kidneys by a dihydropeptidase enzyme; this metabolism is markedly slowed by cilastatin. Approximately 75% of a dose appears in the urine within 10 hours after administration.

Common Side Effects

Nausea, diarrhea, thrombophlebitis (approximately 3%)

Significant Adverse Reactions

GI: vomiting, colitis, abdominal pain, glossitis, gastroenteritis

CNS: fever, dizziness, fatigue, confusion, headache, paresthesia, seizures, somnolence, myoclonus, vertigo, encephalopathy

CV: tachycardia, palpitations, hypotension

Allergic/dermatologic: skin rash, pruritus, urticaria, flushing, candidiasis, erythema multiforme

Respiratory: dyspnea, chest discomfort, hyperventilation, cyanosis

Other: tinnitus, transient hearing loss, polyarthralgia, weakness, oliguria, polyuria, sweating, pain at injection site, venous induration

Altered laboratory values include:

Increased: serum alanine aminotransferase (ALT), aspartate aminotransferase, alkaline phosphatase, lactate dehydrogenase (LDH), bilirubin, blood urea nitrogen (BUN), creatinine, potassium, chloride, eosinophils, basophils, lymphocytes, monocytes

Decreased: sodium, platelets, hemoglobin, hematocrit, neutrophils

Contraindications

No absolute contraindications. *Cautious use* in patients with a history of seizure disorders, thrombophlebitis, renal impairment, or allergic reactions, and in pregnant women or nursing mothers.

Interactions

Refer to the Interactions under Penicillins (this chapter) and Cephalosporins (Chapter 61) for *possible* interactions, because the drug is also a beta-lactam.

Concurrent use with ganciclovir may cause generalized seizures; the mechanism has not been established.

Nursing Management

Pretherapy Assessment

Assess and record baseline data necessary for detection of adverse effects of imipenem-cilastatin: General: VS, body weight, skin color, temperature, and integrity; GI: biliary; GU: renal; CVS: hematologic; CNS: neurologic function; Lab: culture of infected site.

Review medical history and documents for existing or previous conditions that:

a. require cautious use of imipenem-cilastatin: CNS disorders (eg, seizures); impaired renal function; safe use is not established in children.
b. contraindicate use of imipenem-cilastatin: allergy to beta-lactams, cephalosporins, other allergens; **pregnancy (Category B)**.

Nursing Interventions

Medication Administration

Administer imipenem-cilastatin on schedule to ensure stable steady-state concentrations for the duration of therapy.

Have emergency drugs and measures for life support available in the event of serious allergic reaction.

Initiate interventions to relieve symptoms of nausea, vomiting, or diarrhea.

Use appropriate volume of drug for IM injection to avoid pain and discomfort and administer into a large muscle mass (gluteus, vastus lateralis).

Administer IV piggyback over 30 minutes.

Surveillance During Therapy

Monitor parenteral administration site (IM, IV) for signs and symptoms of phlebitis, thrombosis, or local drug reaction.

Monitor CBC, urinalysis, and liver and kidney function tests results obtained over the course of therapy.

Monitor for signs of hypersensitivity that require discontinuation of therapy and notification of practitioner.

Interpret results of diagnostic tests and contact practitioner as appropriate.

Monitor for possible drug–laboratory test interactions: false-positive Coombs' test with IV penicillins.

Do not mix imipenem-cilastatin with other parenteral antibiotics, to prevent drug–drug interactions.

Provide for patient safety needs in the event that seizures occur.

Patient Teaching

Inform patient that stomatitis, nausea, upset stomach, vomiting, diarrhea, and discomfort at injection sites are typical side effects associated with imipenem-cilastatin.

Monobactams

• Aztreonam

Azactam

The monobactam group of anti-infective agents are a relatively new class of drugs that differ from other beta-lactams in that they have a monocyclic rather than a bicyclic nucleus. Aztreonam is the first of the clinically available monobactams. It possesses a wide spectrum of action against gram-negative aerobic pathogens but is inactive against gram-positive organisms or anaerobes.

Mechanism

Binds to penicillin-binding protein 3, thus inhibiting bacterial cell wall synthesis; highly resistant to beta-lactamase enzymes; bactericidal toward gram-negative aerobic pathogens, including *Pseudomonas aeruginosa, E. coli, Enterobacter, Klebsiella, Proteus mirabilis, Serratia*, and *Haemophilus*; antibacterial efficacy is maintained over a pH range of 6 to 8; synergistic with aminoglycosides against many gram-negative aerobic bacilli

Uses

Treatment of infections resulting from susceptible strains of the above-named organisms; responsive diseases include urinary tract, lower respiratory tract, intra-abdominal, gynecologic, skin and soft tissue infections, and septicemia

CAUTION

Aztreonam is usually given initially with another antimicrobial agent in seriously ill patients because it is largely ineffective against gram-positive organisms and anaerobic organisms.

Dosage

Urinary tract infections: 500 mg to 1 g IV or IM every 8 to 12 hours

Other infections: 1 g to 2 g IV or IM every 6 to 12 hours

NOTE: In patients with impaired renal function (ie, creatinine clearance between 10 and 30 mL/min), administer an initial loading dose of 1 to 2 g, then reduce subsequent doses by one half.

Fate

After IM injection, peak serum levels occur within 1 hour; serum half-life ($T_{1/2}$) is 1.5 to 2 hours in patients with normal renal function; approximately 70% of an IV or IM dose is recovered in the urine within 8 hours; smaller amounts are found in the feces; serum protein binding is approximately 50%, and single doses given 8 hours apart do not appear to result in cumulation of drug in the body.

Common Side Effects

Swelling or discomfort at IM injection site, phlebitis with IV administration, nausea, diarrhea, mild skin rash

Significant Adverse Reactions

Vomiting, confusion, headache, weakness, paresthesia, insomnia, abdominal cramping, hypotension, tinnitus, altered taste, nasal congestion, urticaria, petechiae, muscular aching, fever, malaise, breast tenderness, blood dyscrasias, jaundice, hepatitis

Alterations in liver function enzymes, prothrombin and partial thromboplastin times, serum creatinine, and a positive direct Coombs' test have also been reported during aztreonam treatment.

Contraindications

No absolute contraindications. *Cautious use* in patients with liver or kidney dysfunction or previous hypersensitivity to beta-lactam anti-infectives and in pregnant or nursing women.

Interactions

Beta-lactamase–inducing antibiotics (eg, cefoxitin, imipenem) should not be used concurrently with aztreonam, because they may reduce its effectiveness against beta-lactamase–secreting gram-negative aerobes.

Aztreonam is incompatible in solution with nafcillin, cephradine, and metronidazole.

Nursing Management

Pretherapy Assessment

Assess and record baseline data necessary for detection of adverse effects of aztreonam: General: VS, body weight, skin color, temperature, and integrity; GI: biliary; GU: renal; CVS: hematologic; CNS: neurologic function; Lab: culture of infected site.

Review medical history and documents for existing or previous conditions that:

a. require cautious use of aztreonam: impaired renal and hepatic function; immediate hypersensitivity to penicillins or cephalosporins.

b. contraindicate use of aztreonam: allergy to aztreonam; **pregnancy (Category B)**, lactation (secreted in breast milk; advisable to employ alternative method of infant feeding while on aztreonam therapy).

Nursing Interventions

Medication Administration

With parenteral dosage form:

Reconstitute with Sterile Water for Injection, for IV injection, and immediately shake vigorously; inject slowly over several minutes into vein or tubing of compatible IV infusion.

Reconstitute according to manufacturers' directions for IV infusion and immediately shake vigorously; administer over 20 to 60 minutes; flush tubing with delivery solution before and after aztreonam administration.

Reconstitute with appropriate diluent (Sterile Water for Injection, Bacteriostatic Water for Injection, 0.9% Sodium Chloride, Bacteriostatic Sodium Chloride Injection), for IM administration, and immediately shake vigorously. Do not mix with local anesthetic. Inject deeply into a large muscle mass (gluteus, vastus lateralis).

Initiate interventions to relieve symptoms of nausea, vomiting, or diarrhea.

Have emergency drugs and measures for life support available in the event of serious allergic reaction.

Surveillance During Therapy

Monitor parenteral administration site (IM, IV) for signs and symptoms of phlebitis, thrombosis, or local drug reaction.

Monitor for adverse effects and toxicity.

Monitor CBC, urinalysis, and liver and kidney function tests results obtained over the course of therapy.

Monitor for signs of hypersensitivity, which requires discontinuation of drug and notification of practitioner.

Interpret results of diagnostic tests and contact practitioner as appropriate.

Monitor for possible drug–drug interactions: incompatible in solution with nafcillin sodium, cephradine, metronidazole.

Patient Teaching

Inform patient that stomatitis, nausea, upset stomach, vomiting, diarrhea, and discomfort at injection sites are typical side effects associated with aztreonam.

Selected Bibliography

Donowitz GR, Mandel GL: Beta-lactam antibiotics. N Engl J Med 318(7): 419, 1988

Gentry LO: Therapy with newer oral β-lactam and quinolone agents for infections of the skin and skin structures. Clin Infect Dis 14:285, 1992

Sanders CC, Sanders EW: β-lactam resistance in gram-negative bacteria: global trends and clinical impact. Clin Infect Dis 15:824, 1992

Shepherd GM: Allergy to β-lactam antibiotics. Immunol Allergy Clin North Am 611, 1991

Wright AL, Wilkowske CL: The penicillins. Mayo Clin Proc 66:1047, 1991.

Nursing Bibliography

Fulton B, et al: Antiinfectives in breast milk: Penicillins and cephalosporins. Journal of Human Lactation 8(3):157, 1992

Gray M: Penicillin and pharmacokinetics. Orthopedic Nursing 11(2):93, 1992

61
Cephalosporins

First Generation

- Cefadroxil
- Cefazolin
- Cephalexin
- Cephalothin
- Cephapirin
- Cephradine

Second Generation

- Cefaclor
- Cefamandole
- Cefmetazole
- Cefonicid
- Ceforanide
- Cefotetan
- Cefoxitin
- Cefprozil
- Cefuroxime
- Loracarbef

Third Generation

- Cefixime
- Cefoperazone
- Cefotaxime
- Cefpodoxime
- Ceftazidime
- Ceftizoxime
- Ceftriaxone

The cephalosporins are a large group of semisynthetic antibiotics mostly derived from cephalosporin C, a natural product of the fungus *Cephalosporium acremonium*. In addition to the several cephalosporin C derivatives, cefoxitin and cefotetan (semisynthetic derivatives of cephamycin C) are also viewed as cephalosporins because of their structural and pharmacologic similarities to the other derivatives. Loracarbef, a carbacephem chemically related to cefaclor, is also included with the cephalosporins.

Cephalosporins are divided into first-, second-, and third-generation drugs. As outlined in Table 61-1, differences among the three groups are noted primarily in their antibacterial spectrum of action. Activity against gram-negative bacilli *increases* from first- to third-generation drugs, as does efficacy against resistant organisms as well as drug cost. Conversely, efficacy against gram-positive organisms is greatest with the first-generation drugs and progressively *decreases* through the second- and third-generation compounds. The organisms most susceptible to each of the cephalosporins are also indicated in Table 61-1. Within each group of drugs, the individual agents differ primarily in their pharmacokinetic properties, such as oral versus parenteral efficacy, half-life, protein binding, and principal route of excretion. Some of these differences also are presented in Table 61-1.

Cephalosporin antibiotics are usually bactericidal against most gram-positive cocci (except enterococci, which are unaffected by any drug except possibly cefoperazone) and many gram-negative bacilli. In general, the older, first-generation drugs are the most effective against staphylococci and streptococci, whereas the newer, second- and third-generation drugs display increased activity against the gram-negative enterobacteria. Although widely prescribed, cephalosporins are recognized as drugs of choice for only a few infections, owing primarily to the availability of more specific, more effective, or less costly alternatives.

Cephalosporins (especially cefazolin) are indicated for surgical prophylaxis, and for treatment of gram-positive infections (except enterococci) in patients allergic to penicillin. Cross-allergenicity exists between the penicillins and the cephalosporins (estimated incidence is 5%–15%), however, so caution is indicated when cephalosporins are given to patients with a history of penicillin allergy.

Second- and third-generation drugs should be viewed as alternative choices *only* for treating common gram-positive infections, because they are less effective than first-generation agents and also significantly more expensive. More specific, more active, and less costly alternatives (eg, penicillins, erythromycins) should be considered.

Many gram-negative bacilli are susceptible to the second- and third-generation cephalosporins (see Table 61-1), so these drugs are used frequently in respiratory, genitourinary, skin, and soft tissue infections caused by a variety of gram-negative microorganisms. In addition, the third-generation drugs display differing degrees of activity against *Pseudomonas*, *Serratia*, and possibly *Salmonella* and *Acinetobacter*, and are often used in combination with or as alternatives to the more toxic (although more effective) aminoglycosides. Cefoxitin, as well as the third-generation drugs, is variably active against *Bacteroides fragilis*, but this activity is not as great or as predictable as with other noncephalosporin drugs. Moreover, many gram-negative bacilli develop resistance to the cephalosporins, greatly restricting their usefulness in many infections.

Most first-generation drugs are susceptible to inactivation by beta-lactamase (ie, cephalosporinase) enzymes. Second-generation agents (except cefamandole) and all third-generation cephalosporins display greater resistance to enzymatic inactivation, including that of the cephalosporinases produced by many gram-negative pathogens, such as *Pseudomonas*, *Haemophilus*, *Acinetobacter*, *Neisseria*, and some strains of *Bacteroides*.

Compared to many other antibacterial drugs, cephalosporins are relatively nontoxic. The most commonly occurring adverse reactions are allergic, and include rash, urticaria, fever, angioedema, and occasionally serum sickness, eosinophilia, and anaphylaxis (for additional untoward reactions, refer to the general discussion of cephalosporins that follows).

A major factor in the selection of cephalosporins is their cost. Parenterally administered cephalosporins are among the most expensive antibiotics in use today, and their cost increases substantially as their spectrum broadens. Thus, second-generation drugs are approximately twice as expensive as first-generation drugs, whereas third-generation drugs can exceed the cost of first-generation drugs by a factor of four or five. It becomes cost imperative, then, to use the least expensive cephalosporin that is effective against the microorganisms shown to be present. Empiric therapy with third-generation cephalosporins is a

(*text continues on page 624*)

Table 61-1. **Cephalosporins**

Drug	Pharmacokinetics/ Antibacterial Spectrum	Usual Dosage Range	Nursing Considerations
FIRST GENERATION			
Cefadroxil *Duricef, Ultracef, and other manufacturers*	Adm: oral; $T_{1/2}$ 70–80 min; 20% protein binding; renal excretion 90%–95% unchanged Gram-positive spectrum: includes most staphylococci and nonenterococcal streptococci Gram-negative spectrum: *Escherichia coli, Proteus mirabilis, Klebsiella pneumoniae* NOTE: Antibacterial spectrum of all first-generation drugs is essentially the same	Adults: 1–2 g/d in a single or divided doses Children: 30 mg/kg/d in divided doses every 12 h	Orally effective drug used principally to treat urinary tract infections due to *Escherichia coli, Proteus mirabilis*, or *Klebsiella*; also used in staphylococcal and streptococcal infections of skin, pharynx, and tonsils; not metabolized to any extent and excreted essentially intact in the urine; oral absorption is not significantly affected by food; adjust dosage according to package instructions in patients with renal impairment
Cefazolin *Ancef, Kefzol, Zolicef*	Adm: IM, IV; $T_{1/2}$ 90–120 min; 75%–85% protein binding; renal excretion 75%–100% unchanged	Adults: 250 mg–1.5 g IV *or* IM every 6–12 h depending on severity of infection (maximum 12 g/d) Children: 25–100 mg/kg/d in 3 or 4 divided doses *Acute uncomplicated urinary tract infections*: 1 g/12 h *Perioperative prophylaxis*: 1 g 0.5–1 h before surgery, 0.5–1 g during surgery of 2 h or longer, then 0.5–1 g every 6–8 h for 24 h after surgery	Parenteral cephalosporin similar to cephalothin but claimed to be less irritating and less nephrotoxic; used in treatment of respiratory, urinary, and biliary tract infections, skin and soft tissue infections, septicemia, bone and joint infections, and endocarditis; also indicated as alternative therapy for gonorrhea in pregnant patients allergic to penicillin; widely used perioperatively to reduce risk of infection after certain surgical procedures; highly protein bound; do *not* use in children younger than 1 mo; follow manufacturer's recommendations for dosing in renal impairment; pain on injection is infrequent; diluted solutions are stable for 24 h at room temperature and 96 h under refrigeration; hemiparesis has occurred after large doses
Cephalexin *Keflex, Keftab, and other manufacturers* *(CAN) Apo-Cephalex, Novo-Lexin, Nu-Cephalex*	Adm: oral; $T_{1/2}$ 30–50 min; 10%–15% protein binding; renal excretion 80%–100% unchanged	Adults: 250–500 mg every 6 h (maximum dose is 4 g/d) Children: 25–100 mg/kg/d in 4 divided doses depending on severity of infection	Orally effective cephalosporin indicated for respiratory, urinary, skin, bone, and soft-tissue infections, and otitis media in penicillin-sensitive patients, due to susceptible organisms (see Table 58-1); some staphylococci are resistant; stable in gastric acid, well absorbed, and only slightly protein bound; if doses greater than 4 g/d are necessary, parenteral cephalosporins should be used; refrigerate oral suspension and discard unused portion in 14 days
Cephalothin *Keflin* *(CAN) Ceporacin*	Adm: IM, IV; $T_{1/2}$ 30–60 min; 65%–75% protein binding; renal excretion 50%–75% unchanged	Adults: 500–1000 mg IM *or* IV injection every 4–6 h (up to 2 g every 4 h IV in life-threatening infections) Children: 80–160 mg/kg/d IM in divided doses *Perioperative prophylaxis*: Adults: 1–2 g IM *or* IV 0.5–1 h before surgery, during surgery as needed, and every 6 h following surgery for 24 h Children: 20–30 mg/kg following the above schedule	Prototype cephalosporin used to treat respiratory, GI, urinary, skin, bone, joint, and soft tissue infections as well as septicemia and meningitis (see Table 58-1); not effective against *Pseudomonas, Serratia*, indole-positive *Proteus* or *Enterococcus*; may be used perioperatively to reduce incidence of certain infections in high-risk situations (eg, vaginal hysterectomy, intestinal or colorectal surgery, open heart surgery, cholecystectomy, prosthetic arthroplasty); IM injection often elicits pain, induration, and sloughing; IV administration may lead to phlebitis or other inflammatory reactions; may be added to peritoneal dialysis fluid in concentrations up to 6 mg/100 mL and instilled throughout

(*continued*)

Table 61-1. **Cephalosporins (Continued)**

Drug	Pharmacokinetics/ Antibacterial Spectrum	Usual Dosage Range	Nursing Considerations
			the dialysis procedure; owing to short half-life (30–45 min), initial perioperative dose should be given just before start of surgery and readministered at appropriate intervals throughout procedure to maintain sufficient blood levels; prophylactic use should be discontinued within 24 h after surgery; maintenance dose must be reduced according to creatinine clearance in patients with impaired renal function; solutions are stable for 12–24 h at room temperature and 96 h under refrigeration; slight darkening does not affect potency
Cephapirin *Cefadyl*	Adm: IM, IV; $T_{1/2}$ 20–40 min; 40%–50% protein binding; renal excretion 50%–75% unchanged	Adults: 500–1000 mg IM *or* IV every 4–6 h (up to 12 g/d IV in serious infections) Children: 40–80 mg/kg/d IM in divided doses *Perioperative prophylaxis*: 1–2 g IM *or* IV 0.5–1 h before surgery, during surgery if needed, and every 6 h after surgery for 24 h	Parenteral cephalosporin similar to cephalothin in action but causing less tissue irritation; clinical evidence of renal damage has not been reported; jaundice has occurred; do *not* use in children younger than 3 mo; dilutions are stable for 24 h at room temperature and up to 10 days with refrigeration; check package instructions for compatibility with other infusion solutions
Cephradine *Velosef and other manufacturers*	Adm: oral, IM, IV; $T_{1/2}$ 45–60 min; 10%–15% protein binding; renal excretion 80%–90% unchanged; high sodium content (6.0 mEq/g)	*Oral* Adults: 250–500 mg every 6 h *or* 1 g every 12 h Children (> 9 mo): 25–100 mg/kg/d in divided doses every 6–12 h (maximum 4 g/d) *IV, IM* Adults: 500–1000 mg 4 times/day (maximum 8 g/d) Children (> 12 mo): 50–100 mg/kg/d in 4 divided doses *Perioperative prophylaxis*: 1 g IV *or* IM 30–40 min before surgery, then 1 g every 4–6 h thereafter up to 24 h *Cesarean section* 1 g IV when cord is clamped, then again at 6 and 12 h	Available in both oral and parenteral dosage forms; oral preparations are primarily used as follow-up therapy to parenteral treatment; may be given without regard to meals because drug is acid stable; excreted largely unchanged in urine, mostly within 6 h, thus is effective in urinary infections due to susceptible organisms; very slightly protein bound; after reconstitution, IM or direct IV solutions should be used within 2 h at room temperature; continuous IV solutions retain potency for 10 h at room temperature, infusion solution should be replaced at that time; do *not* combine cephradine solutions with those of other antibiotics; doses smaller than those indicated should not be used; persistent infections may require several weeks of therapy
SECOND GENERATION			
Cefaclor *Ceclor*	Adm: oral; $T_{1/2}$ 40–50 min; 25% protein binding; renal excretion 60%–80% unchanged Antibacterial spectrum: Similar to first-generation drugs (see cefadroxil) plus *Haemophilus influenzae* for sinusitis and otitis media infections, and *Moraxella catarrhalis*	Adults: 250–500 mg every 8 h (maximum 4 g/d) Children: 20–40 mg/kg/d in divided doses every 8 h (maximum 1 g/d)	Orally effective, short-acting cephalosporin used in respiratory, urinary, skin, and soft tissue infections and otitis media; classified as second generation but spectrum resembles first generation; a single 2-g dose has been used in acute, uncomplicated urinary tract infections; be alert for onset of skin rash, fever, polyarthritis, and erythema multiforme within 1–2 wk—corticosteroids and antihistamines may be used to treat symptoms, which usually resolve within several days

(*continued*)

Table 61-1. **Cephalosporins (Continued)**

Drug	*Pharmacokinetics/ Antibacterial Spectrum*	*Usual Dosage Range*	*Nursing Considerations*
Cefamandole *Mandol*	Adm: IM, IV; $T_{1/2}$ 30–60 min; 65%–75% protein binding; renal excretion 60%–80% unchanged Possession of a methylthiotetrazole side chain is associated with bleeding problems and a disulfiram-like reaction when taken with alcohol Antibacterial spectrum: similar to first generation plus *Proteus vulgaris, Haemophilus influenzae, Morganella morganii, Enterobacter*, and some anaerobes	Adults: 500–1000 mg IM *or* IV every 4–8 h (up to 2 g/4 h in severe infections) Children: 50–100 mg/kg/d in divided doses every 4–8 h *Perioperative prophylaxis*: Adults: 1–2 g IM *or* IV 1 h prior to incision, then 1–2 g every 6 h for 24–48 h Children: 50–100 mg/kg/d in equally divided doses according to above schedule	Parenteral cephalosporin indicated for infections of the respiratory or urinary tracts and skin, for surgical prophylaxis, and for septicemia and peritonitis caused by susceptible organisms; effective against anaerobic organisms (*Clostridium, Peptococcus*), indole-positive *Proteus* and some strains of *Bacteroides fragilis*; also used in combination with an aminoglycoside for gram-positive or gram-negative sepsis (danger of nephrotoxicity, see Interactions); reduce dosage as indicated in package insert in patients with renal impairment—may cause acute tubular necrosis; bleeding episodes have occurred—monitor prothrombin time and platelet count; jaundice has been noted in some patients; do *not* mix with aminoglycoside in same container; dilute drug solution as instructed with appropriate diluent; reconstituted cefamandole is stable for 24 h at room temperature and 96 h under refrigeration; IV dosage can be up to 12 g/d depending on severity of infection (eg, bacterial septicemia)
Cefmetazole *Zefazone*	Adm: IM, IV; $T_{1/2}$ 90 min; 65% protein binding; renal excretion 80%–85% unchanged Possesses methylthiotetrazole side chain (see cefamandole) Antibacterial spectrum: similar to cefamandole	Adults: 1–8 g IM *or* IV daily dose divided every 6–12 h *Perioperative prophylaxis*: Adults: 2 g IV 30–90 min before incision	A second-generation bactericidal cephalosporin similar to cefamandole used to treat dermatologic and intraabdominal infections caused by gram-positive and gram-negative organisms; also used for perioperative prophylaxis for cesarean section, hysterectomy, cholecystectomy, and colorectal surgery; reduce dosage as indicated in package insert in patients with renal impairment or in geriatric patients; may cause nephrotoxicity when used with aminoglycosides, bleeding episodes with oral anticoagulants requiring monitoring of prothrombin times and platelet counts; disulfiram-like reaction seen with alcohol consumption up to 72 h after cefmetazole administration; reconstituted solution is stable for 24 h, 7 days if refrigerated or 6 wk if frozen; do not refreeze thawed solutions; discard any unused solution; have vitamin K available in case of hypoprothrombinemia
Cefonicid *Monocid*	Adm: IM, IV; $T_{1/2}$ 4–5 h; 95%–98% protein binding; renal excretion 99% unchanged Antibacterial spectrum: similar to cefamandole	Adults: 0.5–1 g IM *or* slow IV injection once every 24 h (maximum dose is 2 g once daily) *Perioperative prophylaxis*: Adults: 1 g given 1 h before incision, then 1 g once daily for 48 h	Long-acting cephalosporin given once daily for respiratory, urinary, skin, bone, and joint infections, and septicemia; not active against *Pseudomonas, Serratia, Enterococcus, Acinetobacter*, and most strains of *B fragilis*; may cause pain on injection; doses larger than 1 g should be divided and given at two different IM sites; reduce dosage in patients with impaired renal function according to package directions; dilutions are stable for 24 h at room temperature and 72 h if refrigerated
Ceforanide *Precef*	Adm: IM, IV; $T_{1/2}$ 150–180 min; 80% protein binding; renal excretion 80%–95% unchanged Antibacterial spectrum: similar to cefamandole,	Adults: 0.5–1 g IM *or* IV every 12 h Children: 20–40 mg/kg/d in equally divided doses every 12 h	Long-acting parenteral cephalosporin given twice a day for respiratory, urinary, and skin and soft tissue infections due to staphylococci, streptococci, *Klebsiella, Haemophilus, E coli, Proteus mirabilis*, also effective in bone and joint infections and endocarditis

(*continued*)

Table 61-1. **Cephalosporins (Continued)**

Drug	Pharmacokinetics/ Antibacterial Spectrum	Usual Dosage Range	Nursing Considerations
	plus *Neisseria gonorrhoeae, Citrobacter*, and *Providencia*	*Perioperative prophylaxis*: 0.5–1 g IM or IV 1 h before start of surgery; intraoperative administration is not necessary	caused by staphylococci, septicemia due to staphylococci, streptococci, or *E coli*, and for perioperative prophylaxis, active against *Enterobacter, Citrobacter*, and *Providencia*; reduce dosage in renal impairment; elevated creatinine phosphokinase has occurred after IM injection; contains no sodium
Cefotetan *Cefotan*	Adm: IM, IV; $T_{1/2}$ 3–4 h; 75%–90% protein binding; renal excretion 90%–100% unchanged Possesses methylthiotetrazole side chain (see cefamandole) Antibacterial spectrum: similar to cefamandole, plus *Neisseria gonorrhoeae, Bacteroides*, including *Bacteroides fragilis*, and *Serratia marcescens*	Adults: 1–2 g IV *or* IM every 12 h for 5–10 d (maximum 3 g every 12 h in life-threatening infections) *Perioperative prophylaxis*: 1–2 g IV 30–60 min before surgery	Long-acting parenteral cephamycin effective against most common organisms *except Pseudomonas* and *Acinetobacter*; highly resistant to beta-lactamases; use cautiously in patients with bleeding tendencies because drug may interfere with hemostasis; may produce acute alcohol intolerance; reconstituted solutions retain potency for 24 h at room temperature, 96 h refrigerated, and at least 1 wk frozen; do not refreeze; reduce dosage in patients with renal failures based on creatinine clearance
Cefoxitin *Mefoxin*	Adm: IM, IV; $T_{1/2}$ 30–60 min; 65%–75% protein binding; renal excretion 90%–100% unchanged Antibacterial spectrum: similar to cefamandole, plus *Neisseria gonorrhoeae* and *Bacteroides fragilis*	Adults: 1–2 g every 6–8 h IV *or* IM (maximum is 12 g/d) Children: 80–160 mg/kg/d in 4–6 divided doses; maximum 12 g/d *Gonorrhea* (see Nursing Considerations): 2 g IM with 1 g probenecid *Disseminated gonorrhea*: 1 g IV 4 times/d for at least 7 d *Acute pelvic inflammatory disease*: 2 g IV 4 times/d with 100 mg doxycycline IV twice a day for at least 4 d; continue 100 mg doxycycline, orally, twice a day for an additional 10–14 d *Perioperative prophylaxis*: 2 g IV *or* IM 0.5–1 h before surgery and every 6 h thereafter for up to 24 h	Effective against a variety of organisms susceptible to first-generation cephalosporins as well as anaerobic organisms, indole-positive *Proteus, Bacteroides fragilis*, and some gram-negative bacteria resistant to other cephalosporins and broad-spectrum penicillins; may reduce incidence of postoperative infections in patients undergoing surgical procedures that are classified as potentially contaminated (eg, GI surgery, vaginal hysterectomy); also indicated for penicillinase-producing *Neisseria gonorrheae* resistant to spectinomycin and for acute pelvic inflammatory disease; highly resistant to beta-lactamase; reconstituted solutions maintain potency for 24 h at room temperature, 1 wk under refrigeration, and up to 26 wk frozen; dry material may darken with time but potency is not affected; frequently painful on IM injection; follow package directions for dosing patients with renal impairment
Cefprozil *Cefzil*	Adm: oral; $T_{1/2}$ 70–90 min; 36% protein binding; renal excretion 60% unchanged Antibacterial spectrum: similar to cefamandole, plus *Neisseria gonorrhoeae, Salmonella, Shigella, Vibrio*, and a number of anaerobes, but not *Bacteroides fragilis*	Adults: 250–500 mg every 12–24 h Children: 7.5 mg/kg every 12 h for pharyngitis and tonsilitis Infants: 15 mg/kg every 12 h for otitis media	Effective orally against a variety of organisms, including gram-negative bacteria and possibly anaerobes; decrease dose by 50% if creatinine clearance is less than 30 mL/min; see cefamandole
Cefuroxime *Kefurox, Zinacef* **Cefuroxime axetil** *Ceftin*	Adm: oral, IM, IV; $T_{1/2}$ 60–120 min; 40%–50% protein binding; renal excretion 70%–95% unchanged	*Oral* Adults and children older than 12 mo: 125–500 mg every 12 h depending on severity of infection	Unlike other first- and second-generation drugs, attains significant concentrations in the CSF, especially if the meninges are inflamed; effective against many gram-negative bacilli, including *Enterobacter* and *Citrobac-*

(continued)

Table 61-1. **Cephalosporins (Continued)**

Drug	Pharmacokinetics/ Antibacterial Spectrum	Usual Dosage Range	Nursing Considerations
	Antibacterial spectrum: similar to cefamandole, plus *Neisseria, Citrobacter, Morganella morganii*, and *Providencia*	Children (< 12 mo): 125 mg every 12 h *Parenteral* Adults: 2.25–6 g/d IM *or* IV in divided doses every 6–8 h (maximum dose is 9 g/d in bacterial meningitis) Children (> 3 mo): 50–100 mg/kg/d in divided doses every 6–8 h *Uncomplicated gonorrhea*: 1.5 g IM as a single dose with 1 g oral probenecid *Perioperative prophylaxis*: 1.5 g IV just before surgery, then 750 mg IV *or* IM every 8 h for 24 h *Bacterial meningitis (children)*: 200–240 mg/kg/d IV in divided doses every 6–8 h; reduce to 100 mg/kg/d IV on improvement	*ter* (some strains, however, are resistant); oral treatment indicated for upper and lower respiratory tract, urinary, skin and soft tissue infections, and otitis media due to susceptible organisms (see Table 58-1); administer single 1.5-g IM dose for gonorrhea at two different sites; dosage is reduced according to package instructions in patients with renal dysfunction; inject slowly (3–5 min) IV or infuse either intermittently or continuously; do *not* mix with aminoglycosides; powder and solutions may darken with time, but potency of solution is unaffected for 24 h at room temperature and 48 h refrigerated
Loracarbef *Lorabid*	Adm: oral; $T_{1/2}$ 60 min; 25% protein binding; renal excretion 90% unchanged Antibacterial spectrum: similar to cefaclor	Adults: 200–400 mg every 12 h Children: 7.5–15 mg/kg every 12 h	Administer at least 1 h before or 2 h after meals; use of the *suspension* results in higher peak plasma levels than the capsules; give one half the recommended dose if creatinine clearance is between 10 and 49 mL/min; see cefaclor
THIRD GENERATION			
Cefixime *Suprax*	Adm: Oral; $T_{1/2}$ 3–4 h; 65% protein binding; renal excretion 40%–50% unchanged Antibacterial spectrum: third-generation drugs are usually less effective against gram-positive organisms than first-generation drugs; gram-negative spectrum includes *E coli, Klebsiella pneumoniae, Haemophilus influenzae, Moraxella catarrhalis*, and *Proteus mirabilis*	Adults: 400 mg/d in a single or 2 divided doses Children younger than 12: 4 mg/kg every 12 h	Orally effective drug used in urinary tract infections, otitis media, pharyngitis, and acute and chronic bronchitis; *not* active against staphylococci, *Proteus morganii, Pseudomonas aeruginosa, Acinetobacter* sp, or *Salmonella* typhi; suspension yields higher peak blood levels than tablet; reduce dose if creatinine clearance is less than 60 mL/min
Cefoperazone *Cefobid*	Adm: IM, IV; $T_{1/2}$ 100–150 min; 80%–90% protein binding; renal excretion 20%–25% unchanged Possesses methylthiotetrazole side chain (see cefamandole) Antibacterial spectrum: similar to second-generation drugs but with increased activity against *E coli, Enterobacter, Haemophilus influenzae, Pseudomonas, Serratia, Citrobacter, Providencia*, and *Bacteroides fragilis*	Adults: 2–4 g/d IM *or* IV in equally divided doses every 12 h; up to 16 g/d has been given by constant infusion in severe infections	Cephalosporin with an extensive spectrum of action; used in respiratory, intraabdominal, and urogenital infections, bacterial septicemia, and infections of the skin and associated structures; highly protein bound; extensively excreted in the bile, do *not* exceed 4 g/d in patients with hepatic disease or biliary obstruction; no dosage adjustment is required in the presence of renal failure; long half-life requires only twice-a-day dosing, although more frequent administration can be used in severe infections; highly resistant to beta-lactamase enzymes produced by most gram-negative pathogens; pseudomembranous colitis has occurred—be alert for development of diarrhea; symptoms of hepatitis have been reported; may interfere with hemostasis resulting in bleeding—supplemental vitamin K (10 mg/wk) reduces likelihood of bleeding

(*continued*)

Table 61-1. **Cephalosporins (Continued)**

Drug	*Pharmacokinetics/ Antibacterial Spectrum*	*Usual Dosage Range*	*Nursing Considerations*
Cefotaxime *Claforan*	Adm: IM, IV; $T_{1/2}$ 60–70 min; 30%–50% protein binding; renal excretion 50%–60% unchanged; good CSF penetration Antibacterial spectrum: similar to cefoperazone plus *Neisseria* (including beta-lactamase producers)	Adults: 1–2 g every 6–12 h IV *or* IM (maximum dose 12 g/d) Children: 50–180 mg/kg/d in 4–6 divided doses *Perioperative prophylaxis:* 1 g IV *or* IM 30–90 min before surgery, then 1 g within 2 h after surgery *Gonorrhea*: 1 g IM as a single injection *Disseminated gonorrhea*: 500 mg IV 4 times/d for at least 7 d	Parenteral cephalosporin used in the treatment of serious infections of the abdomen, lower respiratory tract, urinary tract, skin, and genital tract; also indicated as a surgical prophylactic agent and for penicillinase-producing *Neisseria gonorrhoeae* infections resistant to spectinomycin; many strains of *Pseudomonas* and enterococci are resistant; most common adverse reactions are pain, tenderness, and inflammation at injection site; reduce dosage according to package instructions in patients with renal impairment; does not appear to be nephrotoxic; may be used concurrently with an aminoglycoside, but *do not* mix in same syringe; drug and metabolite attain high concentration in the bile
Cefpodoxime proxetil *Vantin*	Adm: oral; $T_{1/2}$ 120–150 min; renal excretion 50%–80% unchanged Antibacterial spectrum: gram-positive activity against *Streptococcus* and *Staphylococcus*, gram-negative activity includes *Neisseria, Haemophilus influenzae, Moraxella catarrhalis*, and many *Enterobacteriaceae*	Adults: 100–400 mg every 12 h Children: 5 mg/kg every 12 h	An extended spectrum cephalosporin administered as a prodrug; should be administered with food to improve absorption (by 21%–33%); active form (cefpodoxime metabolite) is active against a wide range of gram-positive and gram-negative organisms as well as being resistant to beta-lactamase activity; inactive against most strains of *Pseudomonas, Enterobacteriaceae*, methicillin-resistant staphylococci, and enterococci; useful in the treatment of infection of the lower respiratory tract, urinary tract, the skin, and in sexually transmitted infection
Ceftazidime *Fortaz, Tazicef, Tazidime (CAN) Magnacef*	Adm: IM, IV; $T_{1/2}$ 100–120 min; 5%–15% protein binding; renal excretion 80%–90% unchanged Antibacterial spectrum: similar to cefoperazone, plus *Neisseria* and *Pseudomonas*	Adults: usually 1–2 g IV *or* IM every 8–12 h Children: 30–50 mg/kg IV every 8 h (neonates every 12 h) *Urinary infections*: 250–500 mg every 8–12 h *Pseudomonal lung infection in cystic fibrosis patients*: 30–50 mg/kg IV every 8 h to a maximum of 6 g/d *Dialysis*: 1-g loading dose followed by 1 g after each hemodialysis period	Very broad-spectrum cephalosporin used for a variety of infections (respiratory, urinary, bone, skin, gynecologic, intraabdominal, central nervous system, septicemia); good activity against *Pseudomonas* but poorly active against *Bacteroides fragilis*; protein binding is minimal; very stable in the presence of beta-lactamases; administer separately from aminoglycosides
Ceftizoxime *Cefizox*	Adm: IM, IV; $T_{1/2}$ 100–120 min; 30% protein binding; renal excretion 75%–80% unchanged Antibacterial spectrum: similar to cefotaxime	Adults: 1–2 g IM *or* IV every 8–12 h (maximum dose is 12 g/d) Children: 50 mg/kg every 6–8 h (see Nursing Considerations) *Uncomplicated gonorrhea*: 1 g IM as a single dose	Broad-spectrum drug used in a variety of infections due to both gram-positive and gram-negative organisms; long half-life allows twice-daily dosing in less severe infections, but serious infections require administration every 8 h; stable *against* beta-lactamase enzymes and only slightly (30%) protein-bound; may be active against some microorganisms that have developed resistance to other cephalosporins; dosage must be reduced in patients with impaired renal function; may be injected directly IV (3–5 min) *or* given by intermittent or continuous infusion; reconstitute powder in sterile water for injection; stable for 8 h at room temperature and 48 h if refrigerated; may result in elevations in ALT, AST, CPK in children

(*continued*)

Table 61-1. **Cephalosporins (Continued)**

Drug	Pharmacokinetics/ Antibacterial Spectrum	Usual Dosage Range	Nursing Considerations
Ceftriaxone *Rocephin*	Adm: IM, IV; $T_{1/2}$ 350–500 min; 85%–95% protein binding; renal excretion 30%–60% unchanged Antibacterial spectrum: similar to cefotaxime, highly active against *Neisseria gonorrhoeae*, including penicillinase-producing organisms	Adults: 1–2 g daily in a single or two divided doses IM *or* IV (maximum 4 g/d) Children: 50–75 mg/kg/d in divided doses every 12 h *Meningitis*: 100 mg/kg/d in divided doses IV every 12 h after a loading dose of 75 mg/kg *Uncomplicated gonorrhea*: 250 mg as a single IM dose *Surgical prophylaxis*: 1 g IM *or* IV 0.5–2 h before surgery	Very long-acting cephalosporin usually given once daily (except for meningitis); stable against beta-lactamase enzymes; highly protein-bound; excreted in both the urine and the bile; may alter prothrombin time; casts in urine have occurred during therapy; dosage adjustment is seldom necessary in patients with renal or hepatic impairment; solutions should *not* be mixed with other antimicrobial drugs owing to incompatibility

frightfully expensive undertaking, and considerable justification should be established for this procedure, such as the presence of severe ototoxicity or nephrotoxicity that would contradict the use of aminoglycosides.

The cephalosporins are considered here as a group. Individual drugs are listed in Table 61-1, together with specific information pertaining to each drug. In addition, reference should be made to Table 58-1 (Chapter 58) for recommended indications for the cephalosporins.

Cephalosporins

Mechanism

Inhibit mucopeptide synthesis in the bacterial cell wall, resulting in a defective, osmotically unstable wall; may be bactericidal or bacteriostatic depending on dosage, tissue concentrations of drug, organism susceptibility, and rate of bacterial replication; most effective against rapidly growing organisms.

Uses

- Alternatives to penicillins for treatment of infections of the respiratory tract, skin and soft tissues, genitourinary tract, middle ear, and bloodstream caused by susceptible organisms (see Chapter 58, Table 58-1, and Table 61-1 for principal indications)
- Surgical prophylaxis when expanded gram-negative activity is desired, in procedures in which there is a significant risk of contamination (eg, GI surgery, cholecystectomy, vaginal hysterectomy); usually first-generation drugs (eg, cefazolin) are used
- Treatment of serious *Klebsiella* infections, frequently in conjunction with an aminoglycoside
- Treatment of meningitis caused by gram-negative enteric bacteria
- Adjunctive treatment (with an aminoglycoside) of bacteremia of unknown origin in debilitated or immunosuppressed patients
- Adjunctive therapy in septicemia, acute endocarditis, meningitis, and bone and joint infections

Dosage

See Table 61-1.

Fate

Oral drugs are well absorbed from GI tract, but absorption may be delayed by food. Absorption from IM sites is good. Peak blood levels are attained rapidly (usually 30–60 min). Half-lives are given in Table 61-1. Cephalosporins are distributed extensively, but only cefuroxime and the third-generation drugs diffuse into the cerebrospinal fluid, especially when the meninges are inflamed. Penetration into bone is variable. Drugs readily cross placental barrier and are secreted into milk of nursing mothers. Most derivatives (except cefotaxime, cephalothin, ceftriaxone, and cephapirin) are not appreciably metabolized and are excreted largely unchanged in the urine. Cefoperazone, however, is eliminated predominantly in the bile; ceftriaxone and cefotaxime are also found in appreciable amounts in the bile.

Common Side Effects

Nausea and diarrhea with oral administration, hypersensitivity reactions in people with a history of allergy.

Significant Adverse Reactions

Most reactions occur more commonly with large doses or during prolonged therapy.

- *GI*: anorexia, abdominal pain, dyspepsia, heartburn, vomiting, severe diarrhea, oral candidiasis, glossitis, GI bleeding, enterocolitis
- *Allergic/hypersensitivity*: urticaria, pruritus, skin rash, fever, chills, serum sickness, eosinophilia, angioedema, exfoliative dermatitis, anaphylactic reactions

Hematologic: neutropenia, leukopenia, thrombocytopenia, agranulocytosis, hemolytic anemia, bleeding due to hypoprothrombinemia, positive direct Coombs' test
Genitourinary: dysuria, elevated blood urea nitrogen, proteinuria, hematuria, vaginal discharge, candidal vaginitis, genitoanal pruritus, genital candidiasis
Hepatic: elevated alanine and aspartate aminotransferase, bilirubin, alkaline phosphatase, and lactate dehydrogenase levels; hepatitis (rare)
Other: headache, weakness, dizziness, dyspnea, paresthesia, candidal overgrowth, hepatomegaly; IM administration may cause pain, induration, tenderness, fever, and tissue sloughing

CAUTION

Coagulation abnormalities associated with bleeding episodes, some of a severe nature, have occurred with use of several cephalosporins, including cefamandole and cefoperazone.

Contraindications

No absolute contraindications. *Cautious use* in patients with a history of allergies, asthma, hay fever, penicillin sensitivity (see introductory comments), or impaired renal function, and in small children, during pregnancy, and in nursing mothers.

In addition, cefoperazone, ceftriaxone, and cefotaxime should be given cautiously to patients with impaired liver function, because they are excreted in the bile.

Interactions

Use of bacteriostatic antibiotics (eg, tetracyclines, erythromycins) may reduce cephalosporin effectiveness, especially in acute infections in which the organisms are proliferating rapidly
The nephrotoxic effects of cephalosporins may be augmented by aminoglycosides, colistin, vancomycin, polymyxin B, ethacrynic acid, furosemide, bumetanide, probenecid, and sulfinpyrazone
Cephalosporins are incompatible in parenteral mixtures with tetracyclines, erythromycins, calcium chloride, and magnesium salts
Probenecid may increase and prolong cephalosporin plasma levels by inhibiting renal tubular secretion of the drugs
Alcohol may elicit a disulfiram-like reaction (see Chapter 81) with cefamandole, cefoperazone, or cefotetan

Nursing Management

See Table 61-1 for specific information on each drug. In addition:

Pretherapy Assessment

Assess and record baseline data necessary for detection of adverse effects of cephalosporin derivatives: General: vital signs, body weight, skin color, temperature, and integrity; GI: biliary; Genitourinary: renal; Cardiovascular system: hematologic; Central nervous system: neurologic function; Laboratory: culture of infected site.
Review medical history and documents for existing or previous conditions that:

a. require cautious use of cephalosporins: impaired renal function; immediate hypersensitivity to penicillins or cephalosporins.
b. contraindicate use of cephalosporins: allergy to cephalosporins; **pregnancy (Category B)**; lactation (secreted in breast milk; may alter infant bowel flora or infant culture and sensitivity tests).

Nursing Interventions

Medication Administration

Refrigerate oral dosage form (suspensions); discard unused portion after 14 days.
Administer oral dosage forms with meals to reduce occurrence of GI symptoms (nausea, upset stomach, vomiting).
Administer IM dosage form deeply into large muscle (gluteus, vastus lateralis).
Administer cephalosporins and aminoglycoside solutions separately, do not mix.
Provide ready access to bathroom and interventions directed at symptom relief if diarrhea occurs.

Surveillance During Therapy

Monitor for signs and symptoms of hypersensitivity, which require discontinuation of therapy.
Observe for signs and symptoms of diminished renal function (eg, decreased urine output, proteinuria, elevated blood urea nitrogen, or serum creatinine). Rationale: nephrotoxicity may occur.
Monitor results of electrolyte determinations during prolonged therapy. Rationale: sodium excess can occur with cephalosporins that contain significant amounts of sodium.
Monitor complete blood count, urinalysis, and liver and kidney function test results obtained over the course of therapy.
Monitor results of prothrombin times. Rationale: cephalosporins (especially cefamandole and cefoperazone) can interfere with hemostasis by decreasing availability of vitamin K and interfering with normal platelet function.
Administer supplemental vitamin K (10 mg/wk) if prescribed.
Interpret results of diagnostic tests and contact practitioner as appropriate.
Monitor for possible drug–drug interactions (see Interactions).
Interpret results of the following laboratory tests cautiously because cephalosporins may cause false readings: urinary glucose using Benedict or Fehling solution or Clinitest tablets, urinary protein with acid and denaturization–precipitation tests, urinary 17-ketosteroids, positive direct Coombs' test, and creatinine concentrations (may be falsely elevated when high doses of cephalosporins are administered).

Patient Teaching

Instruct patient regarding the importance of completing the full course of therapy as prescribed; that is, not to discontinue the drug once signs and symptoms of the infection being treated subside. Inform patient of the consequences of not taking or abruptly discontinuing the cephalosporin.

Instruct patient that the prescribed drug is to be taken for the condition for which it is prescribed and is not to be used to treat any other infections.

Instruct patient regarding possible adverse side effects with cephalosporins: stomach upset, loss of appetite, nausea, vomiting, diarrhea, headache, and dizziness.

Instruct patient on appropriate action to take if side effects occur: Notify practitioner regarding severe diarrhea with blood, pus, or mucus; rash or hives; difficulty breathing; unusual fatigue; and unusual bleeding or bruising.

Selected Bibliography

Cunha BA: Oral cephalosporins for common infections. Emergency Medicine 22(5):89, 1990

Donowitz GR, Mandell GL: Drug therapy: Beta-lactam antibiotics. N Engl J Med 318:490, 1988

Frampton JE, et al: Cepodoxime proxetil: A review of its antibacterial action. Drugs 44:889, 1992

Goldstein E, Lipman M: Appropriate use of the newer penicillins and cephalosporins. Modern Medicine 56:102, 1988

LeFrock JL: A new oral cephalosporin (cefprozil). Infect Med 9(Suppl C):7, 1992

Loracarbef. Med Lett Drugs Ther 34:87, 1992

Nursing Bibliography

Francioli P: Ceftriaxone and outpatient treatment of infective endocarditis. Infectious Disease Clinics of North America 7(1):97, 1993

Holdcroft C: An update on cephalosporins. Nurse Practitioner 17(9):66, 1992

Hussar D: New drugs. Nursing '93 23(5):57, 1993

Remington J: Current clinical management of infections: Use of third generation cephalosporins. Part 1. Hosp Pract 26(Suppl 4):5, 1991

62

Tetracyclines and Quinolones

Tetracyclines	***Quinolones***
Chlortetracycline	Cinoxacin
Demeclocycline	Ciprofloxacin
Doxycycline	Enoxacin
Meclocycline	Lomefloxacin
Minocycline	Nalidixic Acid
Oxytetracycline	Norfloxacin
Tetracycline	Ofloxacin

The *tetracycline* group of antibiotics is composed of a number of naturally derived and semisynthetic compounds possessing similar pharmacologic properties. The *quinolone* derivatives encompass several agents that are selectively used for urinary tract infections as well as newer fluorinated derivatives (fluoroquinolones) that possess a very broad spectrum of action in treating systemic infections.

Tetracyclines *(Pregnancy Category D)*

Tetracyclines are bacteriostatic antiinfective agents that exhibit a broad spectrum of activity, but because of their extensive and often indiscriminate use in past years, their clinical usefulness has been restricted by the emergence of a number of resistant bacterial strains. Many previously sensitive staphylococcal, streptococcal, pneumococcal, and other gram-positive organisms are now largely resistant to the tetracyclines, and in vitro laboratory susceptibility tests are necessary to determine the usefulness of a given tetracycline in a particular patient.

Although essentially alike in their antimicrobial activity, the tetracyclines differ in some of their pharmacokinetic properties, and these differences are indicated in Table 62-1. Oral absorption is variable and erratic, and, except for doxycycline and minocycline, may be reduced by elevated gastric pH and/or the presence of food or polyvalent cations such as iron, calcium, magnesium, and aluminum. Plasma protein binding varies among the derivatives. Tetracyclines diffuse readily into most body tissues, attaining highest concentrations in the lungs, liver, kidney, spleen, bone marrow, and lymph. Penetration of the drugs into the CNS is largely determined by their lipid solubility, with minocycline and doxycycline being the most lipophilic derivatives and thus best able to enter the CNS. In addition, minocycline attains high levels in saliva, making it useful in eliminating meningococci from the nasopharynx of carriers (see Uses).

The drugs cross the placental barrier, and concentrations in the fetal circulation may reach 70% of the concentration in the maternal circulation. Owing to the high affinity of tetracyclines for calcium, the development of any fetal tissue undergoing active calcification (eg, bone, teeth) may be impaired by the presence of tetracyclines. Likewise, prolonged use of tetracyclines during the entire period of tooth development (fourth fetal month through the eighth year of life) may cause inadequate calcium deposition and discoloration of both deciduous and permanent teeth. Therefore, these drugs should be avoided if possible during pregnancy and lactation (because they are secreted in breast milk), and in children younger than 8 years of age.

With the exception of minocycline, the other tetracyclines are not metabolized to an appreciable extent. Except for minocycline and doxycycline, these drugs are excreted largely in the urine. Doxycycline is secreted into the intestinal lumen and is eliminated in the feces. Minocycline and its metabolites are found in both the urine and feces, but renal clearance is quite low. The percentage of unchanged drug eliminated by the kidneys varies widely among the different derivatives (see Table 62-1). Drugs having a high renal clearance (eg, oxytetracycline, tetracycline) are more effective in treating urinary tract infections than drugs with low renal clearances, but they may be more dangerous in the presence of renal impairment because of accumulation of drug in the body.

The systemic tetracyclines can be divided arbitrarily into two broad groups on the basis of their serum half-lives. Tetracycline and oxytetracycline are considered short-acting drugs, having half-lives of 6 to 10 hours. The remaining derivatives possess half-lives of approximately 10 to 20 hours and thus exhibit a longer duration of action. There is no convincing evidence, however, that one derivative is significantly more effective than any other for most susceptible infections. The more completely absorbed, longer-acting drugs (ie, doxycycline, minocycline) require less frequent administration (twice a day vs. three or four times a day) than the other derivatives, and thus may improve patient compliance; however, they are considerably more expensive, and minocycline is associated with a high incidence of vestibular disturbances (eg, dizziness, ataxia, lightheadedness). Because doxycycline and minocycline are not appreciably excreted by the kidney, they are the preferred tetracyclines for use in patients with renal impairment.

As noted, the emergence of resistant strains has severely limited the clinical application of the tetracyclines. They are considered first-choice drugs for the following infections only: cholera, brucellosis, granuloma inguinale, melioidosis, chlamydial infections (ornithosis, psittacosis, trachoma, urethritis, cervicitis, lymphogranuloma venereum), *Mycoplasma pneumoniae* infections, rickettsial infections (Rocky Mountain spotted fever, endemic typhus, tick-bite fever, typhus, Q fever), relapsing fever, Lyme disease, and gonorrhea and syphilis in penicillin-sensitive patients. Tetracyclines are also indicated as alternative drugs for a number of gram-positive and gram-negative infections (see Chapter 58, Table 58-1), although sensitivity tests are necessary to confirm susceptibility. Although active in vitro against many gram-positive cocci, tetracyclines should not be used to treat staphylococcal, group A beta-hemolytic strep-

(text continues on page 630)

Table 62-1. **Tetracyclines**

Drug	Pharmacokinetics	Usual Dosage Range	Nursing Considerations
Chlortetracycline *Aureomycin*	Topical administration, ophthalmic	Ophthalmic: place small amount of ointment into lower conjunctival sac every 3 h as needed Topical: apply small amount every 3–6 h as needed	Tetracycline derivative not given systemically and infrequently used topically owing to risk of sensitization; be alert for appearance of allergic reactions and discontinue drug; ophthalmic ointment may retard corneal healing; topical use should be supplemented by appropriate systemic antibiotics
Demeclocycline *Declomycin*	Administration: oral; bioavailability 60%–70%; $T_{1/2}$ 10–16 h; 50%–80% protein binding; renal excretion 40%–50% unchanged	Adults: 150 mg 4 times a day or 300 mg twice a day Children: 6.6–13.2 mg/kg divided into 2–4 daily doses *Gonorrhea in penicillin-sensitive patients*: 600 mg initially, followed by 300 mg every 12 h for 5 d *Uncomplicated chlamydial infections*: 300 mg 4 times/d for at least 7 d	Orally effective tetracycline that is slowly excreted in part because of enterohepatic circulation; among tetracyclines, produces highest incidence of photosensitivity reactions; may precipitate diabetes insipidus-like syndrome (polyuria, polydipsia, weakness) on prolonged therapy—syndrome is caused by interference with action of vasopressin (antidiuretic hormone) on the kidneys, is dose dependent, and is reversible on discontinuation of drug; intake–output ratio should be monitored routinely
Doxycycline *Doxychel, Vibramycin, Vibra-Tabs and other manufacturers* *(CAN) Apo-Doxy, Doxycin, Novo-Doxylin*	Administration: oral, IV; oral bioavailability 90%–95%; $T_{1/2}$ 12–24 h; 60%–90% protein binding; main excretion route is intestinal, renal excretion 30%–40% unchanged	*Oral* Adults: 200 mg in 2 divided doses initially, followed by 100 mg/d in single *or* 2 divided doses; severe infections require 100 mg every 12 h Children: 4.4 mg/kg in divided doses the first day; then 2.2–4.4 mg/kg as a single dose or 2 divided doses each day. *Gonococcal infections*: After a single dose of penicillin or cephalosporin, 100 mg twice a day for 7 d; for patients allergic to penicillin and cephalosporins—100 mg twice a day for 7 d *Syphilis*: 300 mg/d orally or IV for at least 10 d *Uncomplicated chlamydial infections*: 100 mg twice a day for at least 7 d *Acute pelvic inflammatory disease*: 100 mg twice a day for 10–14 d after a single dose of a third-generation cephalosporin *Prevention of "travelers' diarrhea"*: 100 mg/d as a single dose *IV infusion* Adults: 200 mg the first day; then 100–200 mg/d in 1–2 infusions Children 8 y and older: 4.4 mg/kg first day in 1–2 infusions; then 2.2–4.4 mg/kg in 1–2 infusions each day	Semisynthetic tetracycline that is well absorbed orally, exhibits a prolonged duration of action, and is slowly excreted, primarily in the feces; may be used safely in patients with renal impairment; IV infusion is *not* recommended in children younger than 8 y of age; oral absorption is not significantly affected by food or milk—drug has low affinity for calcium; low incidence of photosensitivity; duration of IV infusion varies with the dose, and ranges from 1–4 h; minimum infusion time for 100 mg of a 0.5 mg/mL solution is 1 h; therapy should be continued for at least 24–48 h after symptoms have subsided; follow package instructions for preparation and storage of IV infusion solutions; do *not* inject solutions IM or SC, and avoid extravasation, because solutions are irritating
Oxytetracycline *Terramycin, Uri-Tet*	Administration: oral, IM, IV; oral bioavailability 50%–60%; $T_{1/2}$ 6–10 h; 20%–30% protein binding; renal excretion 50%–70% unchanged	*Oral* Adults: 1–2 g/d in 2–4 equally divided doses Children: 22–44 mg/kg/d in 2–4 equally divided doses	Naturally derived tetracycline with actions similar to tetracycline itself; oral absorption is incomplete, half-life is 6–10 h, and protein binding is minimal; renal clearance is highest of all tetracyclines, thus drug may be more effective than other derivatives

(*continued*)

Table 62-1. **Tetracyclines** **(Continued)**

Drug	Pharmacokinetics	Usual Dosage Range	Nursing Considerations
		IM Adults: 250 mg/d in a single dose *or* 300 mg/d in divided doses every 8–12 h Children: 15–25 mg/kg/d in divided doses every 8–12 h (maximum 250 mg/d) *IV* Adults: 250–500 mg every 12 h (maximum 2 g/d) Children: 12 mg/kg/d in 2 divided doses (range 10–20 mg/kg/d)	in urinary infections; use with *caution* in presence of renal impairment, because drug may accumulate rapidly; IM solution contains 2% lidocaine—do *not* inject IV; use only injection marked "IV" for IV administration; reconstituted solutions for injection are stable for 48 h with refrigeration
Tetracycline *Achromycin, Panmycin, Sumycin, and other manufacturers* *(CAN) Apo-Tetra, Neo-Tetrine, Novotetra*	Administration: oral, IM, IV, topical, ophthalmic; oral bioavailability 70%–80%; $T_{1/2}$ 6–10 h; 20%–60% protein binding; renal excretion 60%–70% unchanged	*Oral* Adults: 1–2 g/d in 2–4 equal doses Children: 25–50 mg/kg/d in 2–4 equal doses *Gonorrhea*: 1.5 g initially; then 0.5 g every 6 h for 5–7 d *Syphilis*: 30–40 g in equally divided doses over 10–15 d *Chlamydial infections*: 500 mg 4 times/d for at least 7 d *Acne*: 1 g/d initially (maintenance 125–500 mg/d) *IM* Adults: 250 mg/d in a single dose *or* 300 mg/d in divided doses every 8–12 h (maximum 800 mg/d) Children: 15–25 mg/kg/d in divided doses every 8–12 h *IV* Adults: 250–500 mg every 12 h (maximum 2 g/d) Children: 10–20 mg/kg/d in 2 divided doses *Ophthalmic* 1–2 drops or small amount of ointment in affected eye 2–4 times a day *Topical* Apply 2–4 times a day	Most widely used and least expensive of the tetracyclines; used orally, parenterally, or locally; topical application may result in hypersensitivity reactions—discontinue drug at first sign of allergic response; ophthalmic use may retard corneal healing; IM injections contain procaine and are *not* suitable for IV administration; injection of IM solution into subcutaneous layer may cause pain and induration; do *not* dilute injectable solutions with calcium-containing diluents because precipitate can form; reconstituted solutions stable for 12 h at room temperature
Meclocycline *Meclan*	Topical administration to skin	Apply twice a day in generous amounts until skin is thoroughly wet	Locally acting tetracycline that is not absorbed to a significant extent; used in the treatment of mild to moderate acne vulgaris; avoid contact with eyes, nose, or mouth; may produce skin irritation; slight yellowing of the skin can occur but may be removed by washing; cosmetics may be applied in the usual manner during treatment; formaldehyde is a component of the vehicle—*caution* in people allergic to this substance
Minocycline *Minocin*	Administration: oral, IV; oral bioavailability 95%–100%; $T_{1/2}$ 12–20 h; 60%–75% protein binding; excretion intestinal and renal; renal excretion 5%–10% unchanged	*Oral* Adults: 200 mg initially, then 100 mg every 12 h *or* 50 mg 4 times a day Children (> 8 y): 4 mg/kg initially; then 2 mg/kg every 12 h *Gonorrhea*: 200 mg initially then 100 mg every 12 h for a minimum of 5 d *Syphilis*: 100 mg every 12 h for 10–15 d	Semisynthetic tetracycline that is almost completely absorbed orally; very lipid soluble and possesses a long half-life (up to 20 h); low renal clearance; oral absorption is not appreciably altered by food or dairy products; only tetracycline drug metabolized to any extent; photosensitivity occurs rarely; vestibular side effects are *very common* (light-

(*continued*)

Table 62-1. **Tetracyclines (Continued)**

Drug	Pharmacokinetics	Usual Dosage Range	Nursing Considerations
		Meningococcal carrier state: 100 mg every 12 h for 5 d *Chlamydial infections*: 100 mg twice a day for at least 7 d *IV injection* Adults: 200 mg initially then 100 mg every 12 h (maximum 400 mg/d) Children: 4 mg/kg initially, then 2 mg/kg every 12 h	headedness, dizziness, vertigo)—therefore, urge caution in driving or operating machinery; indicated in treatment of asymptomatic carriers of *Neisseria meningitidis* to eliminate organism from nasopharynx; *not* recommended for treatment of meningococcal infection; also used in treatment of nocardiosis; IV solutions are stable at room temperature for 24 h; may result in blue-gray skin pigmentation

tococcal or *Streptococcus pneumoniae* infections because of the occurrence of many resistant strains. Oral tetracyclines have been used as adjunctive therapy for severe acne because they reduce the amount of free fatty acids in acne lesions as well as decreasing the population of *Proprionibacterium acnes* in sebaceous glands. Topical application of tetracycline solution or meclocycline cream is also effective in the treatment of acne vulgaris lesions, although the mechanism is not well established. Both oral and topical tetracyclines may be used for treatment of inclusion conjunctivitis. Finally, doxycycline appears to be useful in preventing "travelers' diarrhea" caused by *Escherichia coli*, and minocycline can be used to treat asymptomatic carriers of *Neisseria meningitidis*.

The following discussion considers the tetracyclines as a group. Individual members of the class are listed in Table 62-1.

Mechanism

Bacteriostatic at recommended doses against a range of gram-positive and gram-negative organisms; inhibit protein synthesis in microbial cells by binding to 30S ribosomes, thereby blocking binding of transfer RNA to the messenger RNA–ribosome complex; may also inhibit replication of DNA on the cell membrane at high doses.

Uses

Treatment of infections due to susceptible organisms (see introduction, and also Chapter 58, Table 58-1)
Adjunctive therapy for severe acne or inclusion conjunctivitis (oral or topical tetracycline)
Adjunctive therapy (with amebicides) in the treatment of acute intestinal amebiasis
Treatment of uncomplicated urethral, endocervical, or rectal infections in adults caused by *Chlamydia trachomatis*
Alternative therapy for gonorrhea or syphilis in penicillin-sensitive patients
Treatment of early (stage I and II) Lyme disease
Elimination of meningococci from the nasopharynx of asymptomatic carriers of *Neisseria meningitidis* (oral minocycline only)
Investigational uses include:
- Prevention of travelers' diarrhea due to enterotoxic *E coli* infection (doxycycline)
- Management of chronic inappropriate antidiuretic hormone secretion (demeclocycline)
- Alternative to sulfonamides in treatment of nocardiosis (minocycline)
- Sclerosing agent (by chest tube) in malignant pleural effusion (tetracycline)

Dosage

See Table 62-1.

Fate

Oral absorption of the tetracyclines is variable, being greatest for doxycycline and minocycline and intermediate for the other derivatives; absorption is greater in the fasting state, except for doxycycline and minocycline, which should be taken with food. Oral absorption of tetracyclines is reduced in the presence of milk or dairy products, calcium, magnesium, aluminum, and iron, probably owing to chelation (see Interactions). Distribution of tetracyclines is variable; most derivatives are widely distributed in the body, except for the CNS, where only highly lipophilic derivatives (eg, doxycycline, minocycline) attain appreciable levels. Minocycline is also highly concentrated in saliva and tears. Plasma half-lives vary from 6 to 24 hours (see Table 62-1), and extent of protein binding differs considerably among the different drugs. Other than minocycline, the drugs are not metabolized to a significant extent. Doxycycline and minocycline and its metabolites are excreted largely in the feces, whereas other derivatives are eliminated primarily by the kidneys, a considerable amount as unchanged drug. Thus, dosage reduction may be necessary in patients with renal impairment.

Common Side Effects

Diarrhea, nausea, anorexia, vestibular disturbances (minocycline only), photosensitivity (especially with demeclocycline).

Significant Adverse Reactions

GI: stomatitis, glossitis, sore throat, dysphagia, vomiting, enterocolitis, steatorrhea, inflammation in the anogenital region, esophageal ulceration
Dermatologic: macropapular and erythematous rash, exfoliative dermatitis
Hypersensitivity: fever, urticaria, angioedema, headache,

impaired vision, papilledema, pericarditis, anaphylaxis, exacerbation of systemic lupus erythematosus

Hematologic: hemolytic anemia, eosinophilia, neutropenia, thrombocytopenia, leukopenia, leukocytosis

Other: increased blood urea nitrogen (BUN), hepatic toxicity (large doses), permanent discoloration of teeth, enamel hypoplasia, impaired calcification of bony structures, increased intracranial pressure and bulging fontanels in young infants, nephrogenic diabetes insipidus (demeclocycline only), irritation at IM injection sites, thrombophlebitis with IV administration, overgrowth of nonsusceptible organisms

CAUTION

Outdated tetracycline products are potentially nephrotoxic, and use has resulted in development of the Fanconi syndrome, characterized by nausea, vomiting, polyuria, polydipsia, proteinuria, glycosuria, and acidosis. Symptoms disappear within several weeks after cessation of therapy.

Contraindications

Severe renal or liver impairment (except doxycycline), pregnancy, in nursing mothers, and in children younger than 8 years of age (unless no other drugs are effective for a particular infection). *Cautious use* in the presence of renal dysfunction.

Interactions

Oral absorption of tetracyclines (except doxycycline and minocycline) may be impaired by the presence of food, dairy products, antacids, iron, or other polyvalent cations (eg, calcium, magnesium, aluminum), and alkali (eg, sodium bicarbonate).

Because they are bacteriostatic, tetracyclines can reduce the effectiveness of penicillins and other bactericidal antibiotics if used concurrently.

The action of doxycycline may be shortened by barbiturates, other sedative–hypnotics, phenytoin, and carbamazepine because of increased hepatic enzymatic breakdown.

Elevation of BUN can occur with combined tetracycline–diuretic use.

Tetracycline may enhance the effects of oral anticoagulants by interfering with synthesis of vitamin K by intestinal microorganisms.

Plasma levels of digoxin and lithium can be increased by tetracyclines.

Tetracyclines may enhance methoxyflurane-induced nephrotoxicity.

The effects of oral contraceptives may be reduced by tetracyclines, possibly resulting in breakthrough bleeding or pregnancy.

Theophylline and tetracyclines can result in increased GI side effects.

Cimetidine may decrease the oral absorption of tetracyclines.

Nursing Management

See Table 62-1 for specific information on each drug. In addition:

Pretherapy Assessment

Assess and record baseline data necessary for detection of adverse effects of tetracyclines: General: vital signs (VS), body weight, skin color, temperature, and integrity; GI: biliary; Genitourinary (GU): renal; Cardiovascular system (CVS): hematologic; CNS: neurologic function; Laboratory: culture of infected site.

Review medical history and documents for existing or previous conditions that:

a. require cautious use of tetracyclines: impaired renal or hepatic function.
b. contraindicate use of tetracyclines: allergy to tetracyclines, severe renal or liver impairment, children younger than 8 years of age; **pregnancy (Category D)**; lactation (significant concentrations appear in breast milk, deposited in neonatal teeth and bones, damaging to teeth).

Nursing Interventions

Medication Administration

Administer oral form of drug on an empty stomach (1 h before or 2 h after meals), with a full glass of water.

Do not use outdated drugs; degraded drugs are highly nephrotoxic.

Administer tetracyclines on schedule to ensure stable steady-state concentrations for the duration of therapy.

Reduce the risk of stomatitis through frequent mouth care.

Initiate a meal schedule that provides small, frequent meals if GI upset occurs.

Administer antacids, if ordered, 3 hours after tetracycline administration.

Provide ready access to bathroom and interventions directed at symptom relief if diarrhea occurs.

Question patient about lidocaine or procaine allergy (IM preparations of oxytetracycline contain lidocaine and IM preparations of tetracycline contain procaine) when giving IM. Inject deeply into body of large muscle.

Administer IV at a slow rate, and observe infusion site for redness or swelling because prolonged IV administration can cause thrombophlebitis.

Protect patient from exposure to sunlight and ultraviolet light. Use sunscreen (*not* one containing para-aminobenzoic acid [PABA]) and protective clothing.

Surveillance During Therapy

Monitor complete blood count, urinalysis, and liver and kidney function tests results obtained over the course of therapy.

Monitor intake–output, observing for signs and symptoms of possible renal impairment (renal colic, oliguria, hematuria) and dehydration secondary to gastrointestinal side effects (vomiting, diarrhea).

Monitor for signs of hypersensitivity (including photosensitivity), which may require discontinuation of drug.

Monitor hematologic laboratory findings and patient symptoms for signs of hemolytic anemia and thrombocytopenia.

Interpret results of diagnostic tests and contact practitioner as appropriate.

Interpret results of laboratory tests cautiously because tetracyclines may increase serum levels of creatinine, BUN, bilirubin, alkaline phosphatase, alanine and aspartate aminotransferases, and urinary levels of catecholamines and protein. Hemoglobin and platelet values may be decreased, and urine glucose results may be false positive with Clinitest or false negative with Clinistix or TesTape.

Monitor results of liver and kidney function tests, which should be obtained frequently, when drug is administered IV. IV administration should be prescribed very cautiously in the presence of renal dysfunction or pregnancy, and dosage should not exceed 2 g/d. Rationale: high-dosage IV tetracycline therapy has been associated with liver failure and death.

Assess indicators of renal, hepatic, and hematopoietic function at regular intervals.

Determine whether diarrhea, if it occurs, is related to the drug (first few days of therapy) or an intestinal superinfection (later in therapy and often more intense).

Monitor for possible drug–drug and drug–nutrient interactions: decreased absorption of tetracyclines if taken with antacids (calcium, magnesium, aluminum salts), foods, dairy products, urinary alkalinizers; enhances risk of digitalis glycoside toxicity; increased risk of nephrotoxicity with methoxyflurane; decreased tetracycline activity with penicillins; decreased effectiveness of oral contraceptives, leading to increased risk of breakthrough bleeding or pregnancy.

Provide for patient safety needs to minimize environmental hazards and risk of injury if CNS side effects develop.

Patient Teaching

Instruct patient regarding the importance of completing the full course of therapy as prescribed; that is, not to discontinue the drug once signs and symptoms of the infection being treated subside.

Inform patient of the consequences of not taking or abruptly discontinuing the tetracycline.

Inform patient never to take outdated tetracycline products; to finish the complete prescription; and to immediately discard any leftover tetracyclines once therapy is complete.

Instruct patient that the prescribed drug is to be taken for the condition for which it is prescribed and not to be used to treat any other infections.

Instruct patient about possible adverse side effects of tetracyclines: upset stomach, nausea, diarrhea, superinfection of the oral or vaginal mucosa, sensitivity of the skin to ultraviolet (sun) light.

Inform patient about the ability of tetracyclines to diminish the effectiveness of oral contraceptives and the need for additional measures of conceptive control.

Instruct patient on appropriate action to take if side effects occur:

Notify practitioner if early signs of hematologic or hepatic toxicity (sore throat, fever, mucosal ulceration, malaise, pallor, jaundice) occur.

Notify practitioner of any unusual bleeding. Rationale: hypoprothrombinemia and bleeding tendencies due to decreased synthesis of vitamin K by intestinal microflora may occur.

Notify practitioner if symptoms such as severe cramps, watery stools, dark-colored urine, light-colored stools, rash or itching, difficulty breathing, yellowing of skin or eyes occur.

Instruct patient to use sunscreens (not containing PABA) or protective clothing.

Suggest that patient take drug with small quantities of food (except those that are high in calcium) if nausea, GI distress, or diarrhea occur, because this should not significantly impair efficacy. Food does not appreciably alter absorption of doxycycline or minocycline.

Instruct patient to avoid using antacids, antidiarrheals, milk or other dairy products, and calcium-containing foods while taking a tetracycline because these substances significantly impair oral tetracycline absorption.

Quinolones

The quinolones are a group of structurally similar antiinfectives that exhibit a variety of actions against many different microorganisms. The older derivatives, nalidixic acid and cinoxacin, are primarily used in treating acute urinary tract infections due to common gram-negative pathogens. The addition of a fluoride molecule to the basic quinoline structure provides increased potency against gram-negative organisms. Fluoroquinolone derivatives, which include ciprofloxacin, enoxacin, lomefloxacin, norfloxacin, and ofloxacin, have an extended spectrum of action that includes some gram-positive organisms as well as the more serious gram-negative organisms such as *Pseudomonas* sp and gram-negative aerobic bacteria. The quinolone drugs are more active at acidic than at alkaline pHs (eg, in blood, pH 7.4). Norfloxacin and enoxacin are mainly used to treat severe or resistant urinary tract infections and diarrheal illnesses because of their favorable pharmacokinetics relative to these indications. Ciprofloxacin, ofloxacin, and lomefloxacin may be used for these indications, and also are used for serious systemic infections.

The fluoroquinolones possess several favorable features, especially in the context of the treatment of serious gram-negative infections. Unlike the wider spectrum penicillins and cephalosporins, which must be administered parenterally, the fluoroquinolones can be taken orally and they provide excellent bioavailability. This may eliminate the need for hospitalization. These drugs also have relatively long half-lives compared to most penicillins and cephalosporins. In addition, the fluoroquinolones readily penetrate most body fluids and tissues. Their broad spectrum of activity is useful in a wide variety of infections.

These broad-spectrum drugs are most active against aerobic gram-negative bacilli, including species of *Escherichia*, *Klebsiella*, *Proteus*, *Salmonella*, *Shigella*, *Serratia*, *Haemophilus*, and *Pseudomonas*. Ciprofloxacin is the most active of the available fluoroquinolones, especially against *Pseudomonas aeruginosa*. Ciprofloxacin and ofloxacin are also active against *Chlamydia trachomatis* and *Mycobacterium tuberculosis*. The fluoroquinolones usually do not have activity against anaerobic organisms, although ofloxacin does demonstrate some activity against *Clostridium* sp.

The activity of the fluoroquinolones against gram-positive

organisms is more variable. Ciprofloxacin is the most widely used drug, and has moderate activity against staphylococci, including methicillin-resistant strains of *Staphylococcus aureus*. Unfortunately, the resistance of these organisms to ciprofloxacin is increasing. The activity of fluoroquinolones against streptococci is even more variable, and other antimicrobial drugs usually are preferred. The following discussion considers the quinolones as a group. Individual drug characteristics and dosages are presented in Table 62-2.

Mechanism

Inhibits bacterial DNA gyrase (topoisomerase II), an enzyme essential for bacterial DNA synthesis; rapidly bactericidal for susceptible bacteria; broad spectrum of activity against many gram-negative and some gram-positive organisms.

NOTE: Bacterial resistance to the fluoroquinolones is the result of alterations in both the A subunit of DNA gyrase and the outer bacterial membrane. Resistance to the fluoroquinolones is increasing, particularly in two organisms, *P aeruginosa* and *S aureus*.

Uses

Treatment of uncomplicated urinary tract infections (main use of cinoxacin and nalidixic acid), and severe or resistant urinary tract infections (fluoroquinolones, especially norfloxacin and enoxacin)
Treatment of gastrointestinal infections, including travelers' diarrhea
Treatment of bone and joint infections, especially those caused by *Pseudomonas* and *Staphylococcus* (mainly ciprofloxacin)
Treatment of skin and soft tissue infections
Treatment of lower respiratory tract infections, especially those caused by *Haemophilus influenzae* and *Pseudomonas*
Treatment of malignant external otitis, primarily seen in elderly diabetics and usually caused by *P aeruginosa*
Alternative therapy of uncomplicated urethritis and cervicitis due to *Neisseria gonorrhoeae* infection
Prophylactic use before procedures involving urinary, intestinal, orthopedic, and vascular surgery

Dosage

See Table 62-2.

Fate

All quinolones are rapidly absorbed from the GI tract, with bioavailability ranging from 40% to 95%; peak serum concentrations occur within 1 to 2 hours after ingestion and are slightly delayed by food. Bioavailability is reduced by antacids containing aluminum, magnesium, or calcium, and by other drugs containing iron or zinc. Quinolones are widely distributed; protein binding is relatively low for the fluoroquinolones and higher for cinoxacin and nalidixic acid. Cinoxacin, nalidixic acid, lomefloxacin, and ofloxacin are primarily excreted by the the urinary tract both as unchanged drug and as metabolites; ciprofloxacin, norfloxacin, and enoxacin are partially metabolized in the liver and excreted by both the intestinal and urinary routes. All quinolones attain urinary concentrations that exceed inhibitory levels for most urinary pathogens. Specific pharmacokinetic data for each drug are presented in Table 62-2.

Common Side Effects

Nausea, vomiting, abdominal cramping and diarrhea, headache, dizziness, skin rash.

Significant Adverse Reactions

GI: dysphagia, oral candidiasis, intestinal bleeding
CNS: headache, tinnitus, photophobia, visual disturbances, insomnia, dizziness, tingling sensation, nervousness, tremors, confusion, mania, toxic psychosis, convulsions
Hypersensitivity: rash, pruritus, urticaria, edema, photosensitivity, hyperpigmentation
CV: palpitations, ventricular ectopy, hypertension, angina
Respiratory: epistaxis, laryngeal edema, hiccoughs, dyspnea, bronchospasm
Genitourinary: crystalluria (especially in alkaline urine), dysuria, polyuria, urinary retention, vaginitis
Other: altered BUN, alanine and aspartate aminotransferases, serum creatinine, and alkaline phosphatase; joint or back pain

Contraindications

Anuria, pregnant women and prepubertal children (cartilage erosion has been reported in developing laboratory animals). *Cautious use* in people with reduced renal or hepatic function and in nursing mothers.

Interactions

Antacids and other drugs containing aluminum (sucralfate), magnesium, calcium, iron, or zinc may decrease oral absorption of the quinolones.
Probenecid blocks tubular secretion of quinolones and may increase serum levels.
Plasma concentrations of theophylline may be elevated if given together with the quinolones (except lomefloxacin).
Quinolones may interfere with the metabolism of caffeine and prolong its serum half-life.
Fluoroquinolones can increase the effects of digoxin, oral anticoagulants, and cyclosporine.

Nursing Management

See Table 62-1 for specific information on each drug. In addition:

Pretherapy Assessment

Assess and record baseline data necessary for detection of adverse effects of quinolone-type antiinfectives: General: VS, body weight, skin color, temperature, and integrity; GI: biliary; GU: renal; CVS: hematologic; CNS: neurologic function; Laboratory: culture of infected site.
Review medical history and documents for existing or previous conditions that:
a. require cautious use of quinolones: impaired renal or hepatic function.
b. contraindicate use of quinolones: allergy to quinolones, severe renal impairment (anuria), prepubertal children (possibility of cartilage erosion), seizures (epilepsy), cerebral arteriosclerosis; **pregnancy (Category C)**; lactation (significant concen-

Table 62-2. Quinolones

Drug	Pharmacokinetics	Usual Dosage Range	Nursing Considerations
FLUOROQUINOLONES			
Ciprofloxacin *Ciloxin Ophthalmic, Cipro, Cipro IV*	Administration: oral, IV; bioavailability 70%–80%; $T_{1/2}$ 4 h; 20%–40% protein binding; renal excretion 30%–50% unchanged	*Urinary tract infections*: Oral: 250–500 mg every 12 h for 7–14 d IV infusion: 200–400 mg every 12 h for 7–14 d *Respiratory, bone, joint, and skin infections*: Oral: 500–750 mg every 12 h IV infusion: 400 mg every 12 h *Infectious diarrhea*: Oral: 500 mg every 12 h *Ophthalmic*: 1–2 drops in affected eye every 15–30 min for severe infections; reduce frequency as infection improves	Broad-spectrum antimicrobial action against gram-negative bacteria; primary use in treatment of serious gram-negative infections; unlike many penicillins and cephalosporins, this drug may be administered orally (with excellent bioavailability) as well as parenterally; it has a relatively long $T_{1/2}$ and readily penetrates most body fluids and tissues; not recommended for use in children; use with *caution* in renal dysfunction, seizure disorders; *contraindicated* in ciprofloxacin or norfloxacin allergy
Enoxacin *Penetrex*	Administration: oral; bioavailability 90%; $T_{1/2}$ 3–6 h; 40% protein binding; renal excretion greater than 40% unchanged	*Oral* *Urinary tract infections*: 200–400 mg every 12 h for 7–14 d *Uncomplicated gonorrhea*: 400 mg single dose for 1 d	Excellent oral availability; primarily used for uncomplicated urinary tract infections and urethral and cervical gonorrhea; not indicated in children under 18 y of age
Lomefloxacin *Maxaquin*	Administration: oral; bioavailability 95%–98%; $T_{1/2}$ 8 h; 10% protein binding; renal excretion 65% unchanged	*Oral* *Urinary tract infections*: 400 mg once a day for 10–14 d *Lower respiratory tract infections*: 400 mg once daily for 10 d	Used orally for lower respiratory or urinary tract infections; once daily administration, without regard to meals
Norfloxacin *Chibroxin, Noroxin*	Administration: oral; bioavailability 30%–55%; $T_{1/2}$ 3–4.5 h; 10%–15% protein binding; renal excretion 26%–32% unchanged	*Oral* *Urinary tract infections*: 400 mg every 12 h for 3–10 d *Uncomplicated gonorrhea*: 800 mg single dose for 1 d *Ophthalmic*: 1–2 drops every 15–30 min for severe infections; reduce frequency as infection improves	Indicated for uncomplicated gonorrheal infections and resistant urinary tract infections; also available as an eye drop; patients should be well hydrated; do *not* take with meals
Ofloxacin *Ocuflox, Floxin*	Administration: oral, IV; bioavailability 98%; $T_{1/2}$ 5–7 h; 32% protein binding; renal excretion 70%–80% unchanged	*Oral* *Urinary tract infections*: 200 mg every 12 h for 3–10 d *Uncomplicated gonorrhea*: 400 mg single dose, 1 d *Cervicitis/urethritis infections*: 300 mg every 12 h for 7 d *Skin infections*: 400 mg every 12 h for 10 d *Lower respiratory infections*: 400 mg every 12 h for 10 d *Prostatitis*: 300 mg every 12 h for 6 wk *IV infusion* All doses 200–400 mg every 12 h *Ophthalmic*: 1–2 drops every 15–30 min for severe infections; reduce frequency as infection improves	Broad-spectrum antimicrobial; similar to ciprofloxacin; do not use IV formulation longer than 10 days; do not give SC, IM, or intrathecally; oral dose is given every 12 h; has been used in INH-resistant tuberculosis with ethambutol and pyrizamide; also available as an eye drop
NONFLUORINATED QUINOLONES			
Cinoxacin *Cinobac Pulvules*	Administration: oral; bioavailability 60%–80%; $T_{1/2}$ 1–2 h; 60%–80% protein binding; renal excretion 60% unchanged	*Oral* *Urinary tract infections*: 1 g daily in 2 to 4 divided doses for 7–14 d	Same as for nalidixic acid; also, use with *caution* in hepatic or renal dysfunction; *contraindicated* in cinoxacin allergy, pregnancy (Category B), do not use in children under 12 y of age

(*continued*)

Table 62-2. **Quinolones (Continued)**

Drug	*Pharmacokinetics*	*Usual Dosage Range*	*Nursing Considerations*
Nalidixic acid *Neg Gram*	Administration: oral; bioavailability greater than 90%; $T_{1/2}$ 1–3 h; 90%–95% protein binding; renal excretion of unchanged drug, active metabolites, and inactive metabolites accounts for most of dosage	*Oral* *Urinary tract infections*: Adults: 1 g 4 times/d for 2 wk, then 2 g/d in divided doses Children: 55 mg/kg/d in 4 divided doses for 2 weeks, then 33 mg/kg/d	Broad-spectrum antimicrobial action against gram-negative bacteria; primary use in treatment of urinary tract infection; oral route of administration; use with *caution* in hepatic or renal dysfunction, seizure disorders, lactation (secreted in breast milk); *contraindicated* in nalidixic acid allergy, G-6-phosphate dehydrogenase deficiency, pregnancy (Category C), children younger than 3 mo of age

trations appear in breast milk, safety not established, avoid use in nursing mothers).

Nursing Interventions

Medication Administration

Administer oral form of drug with meals, with a full glass of water.

Administer quinolones on schedule to ensure stable steady-state concentrations for the duration of therapy.

Provide ready access to bathroom and interventions directed at symptom relief if diarrhea occurs.

Reduce the risk of stomatitis through frequent mouth care.

Initiate a meal schedule that provides small, frequent meals if GI upset occurs.

Surveillance During Therapy

Monitor complete blood count, urinalysis, and liver and kidney function tests results obtained over the course of therapy.

Monitor intake–output, observing for signs and symptoms of possible renal impairment (renal colic, oliguria, hematuria) and dehydration secondary to gastrointestinal side effects (vomiting, diarrhea).

Monitor for signs of hypersensitivity (including photosensitivity), which may require discontinuation of drug.

Monitor CNS function for drowsiness, weakness, dizziness, visual disturbances, photophobia, diplopia.

Monitor hematologic laboratory data and patient for signs of thrombocytopenia, leukopenia, or hemolytic anemia.

Interpret results of diagnostic tests and contact practitioner as appropriate.

Assess indicators of renal, hepatic, and hematopoietic function at regular intervals.

Determine whether diarrhea, if it occurs, is related to the drug (first few days of therapy) or an intestinal superinfection (later in therapy and often more intense).

Monitor for possible drug–laboratory tests interactions: false-positive urinary glucose result with Benedict and Fehling tests, or Clinitest tabs; false elevation of urinary 17-keto and ketogenic steroids.

Monitor for possible drug–drug and drug–nutrient interactions: increased bleeding risk with oral anticoagulants, requiring a decrease in oral anticoagulant dosage; actions of other highly protein-bound drugs may be increased; *with norfloxacin*—decreased therapeutic effect when taken with iron salts and sucralfate; decreased absorption if taken with antacids; increased serum concentration and risk of toxicity with theophylline.

Provide for patient safety needs to minimize environmental hazards and risk of injury if CNS side effects occur.

Patient Teaching

Instruct patient regarding the importance of completing the full course of therapy as prescribed; that is, not to discontinue the drug once signs and symptoms of the infection being treated subside.

Inform patient of the consequences of not taking or abruptly discontinuing the quinolone agents.

Instruct patient that the prescribed drug is to be taken for the condition for which it is prescribed and not to be used to treat any other infections.

Instruct patient about possible adverse side effects of quinolones: upset stomach, nausea, diarrhea, superinfection of the oral or vaginal mucosa, sensitivity of the skin to ultraviolet (sun) light.

Inform patient that drug may be taken with a small amount of nondairy food if GI distress occurs. Although food delays rate of drug absorption, it does not affect total amount absorbed.

Instruct patient taking antacid to take it 2 or more hours after the quinolone to avoid interfering with absorption.

Encourage patient to maintain high fluid intake during therapy to minimize the risk of crystalluria.

Warn patient to exercise caution in driving or performing tasks requiring mental alertness until response to drug is known, because dizziness may occur.

Instruct patient and family to observe for and report signs of CNS stimulation (see Significant Adverse Reactions) and reassure them that if any of these infrequent effects occur, they are reversible.

Instruct patient on appropriate action to take if side effects occur:

Notify practitioner if early signs of hematologic or hepatic toxicity (sore throat, fever, mucosal ulceration, malaise, pallor, jaundice) occur.

Notify practitioner of any unusual bleeding. Rationale: hypoprothrombinemia and bleeding tendencies due to decreased synthesis of vitamin K by intestinal microflora may occur.

Notify practitioner if symptoms such as severe rash, visual changes, or weakness and tremors occur.

Instruct patient to use sunscreens (*not* one containing PABA) or protective clothing.

Selected Bibliography

Gentry LO: Therapy with newer oral beta-lactam and quinolone agents for infections of the skin and skin structures: A review. Clin Infect Dis 14:285, 1992

Gootz TD, McGuirk PR, Moynihan MS, Haskell SL: Placement of alkyl substituents on the C-7 piperazine ring of fluoroquinolones: Dramatic differential effects on mammalian topoisomerase II and DNA gyrase. Antimicrob Agents Chemother 38:130, 1994

Hooper DC, Wolfson JS: Fluoroquinolone antimicrobial agents. N Engl J Med 324:384, 1991

Neu HC: Quinolone antimicrobial agents. Annu Rev Med 43:465, 1992

Sable CA, Scheld WM: Fluoroquinolones: How to use (but not overuse) these antibiotics. Geriatrics 48(6):41, 1993

Standiford HC: Tetracyclines and chloramphenicol. In Mandell GL, Douglas RG, Bennett JE (eds): Principles and Practice of Infectious Diseases, 3rd ed, p 284. New York, Churchill-Livingstone, 1990

Stein G: Drug interactions with fluoroquinolones. Am J Med 91(Suppl 6A):81S, 1991

Nursing Bibliography

Fluoroquinolones: Resistance on the rise. Patient Care 25(11):41, 1991

Gerding G: Oxyquinolone-containing ointment vs standard therapy for stage 1 and stage 2 skin lesions. Dermatology Nursing 4:389, 1992

Long K: Fluoroquinolones: Great expectations. Nurse Practitioner Forum 1(3):128, 1990

Ofloxacin related psychopathologic reaction. Nurses Drug Alert 16(6): 41, 1992

Tunkel A, Scheld W: Ofloxacin. Infection Control and Hospital Epidemiology. 12:549, 1991

63 Macrolide Antibiotics

Erythromycin
Azithromycin
Clarithromycin
Troleandomycin

The macrolide group of antibiotics is so named because the chemical structure of the compounds consists of a large lactone ring to which one or more sugars are attached. *Erythromycin* was introduced in the 1950s and has since gained widespread use in treating a variety of infections. *Azithromycin* and *clarithromycin* are chemical derivatives of erythromycin that were developed to improve the efficacy and safety of erythromycin. The other clinically available macrolide antibiotic is *troleandomycin*, an agent resembling erythromycin in both structure and pharmacologic activity, but somewhat less effective and more toxic and hence infrequently used. It is discussed briefly at the end of the chapter.

The macrolides inhibit protein synthesis and are bacteriostatic at normal therapeutic doses, although they may be bactericidal against certain organisms at high concentrations. Despite their differing structures, the macrolides demonstrate similar antibacterial spectrums, mechanisms of action, and bacterial resistance. These drugs differ primarily in their pharmacokinetics and potency against certain organisms. The antibacterial spectrum includes gram-positive cocci, such as staphylococci, streptococci, enterococci, and pneumococci. The macrolides are used principally as *alternatives* to penicillin in treating susceptible gram-positive coccal infections; however, erythromycin is considered the drug of choice against the following organisms: *Bordetella pertussis* (whooping cough), *Corynebacterium diphtheriae*, *Legionella pneumophila* (Legionnaires' disease), *Mycoplasma pneumoniae* (atypical viral pneumonia), and strains of *Chlamydia trachomatis* causing pneumonia and inclusion conjunctivitis. The role of azithromycin and clarithromycin in therapy is still being evaluated, but these drugs may replace erythromycin for treatment of specific infections in the future (see Chapter 58, Table 58-1, for a listing of the organisms for which erythromycin and the other macrolides are indicated).

Over the years, microbial resistance has become a problem with the use of erythromycin, and is especially prevalent in staphylococci. Prolonged use of erythromycin in staphylococcal infections is almost invariably associated with the emergence of resistance, and alternative drugs should be used in treating severe staphylococcal infections. Erythromycin-resistant streptococci and pneumococci are likewise developing with increasing frequency. Although cross-resistance is not a significant problem between erythromycin and most other antibiotics, it has been reported with lincomycin and clindamycin and is virtually complete among all the members of the macrolides. Most gram-negative organisms are largely impermeable to erythromycin and are usually resistant to the drug unless their cell walls are altered. One feature of azithromycin is that it has increased activity against gram-negative organisms.

• Erythromycins

Erythromycin base
Erythromycin estolate
Erythromycin ethylsuccinate
Erythromycin gluceptate
Erythromycin lactobionate
Erythromycin stearate

Erythromycin itself as a base is an orally effective antibiotic originally isolated from a strain of *Streptomyces erythreus*. Although erythromycin base is a biologically active form, it is unstable in gastric acid and thus must be formulated in an enteric-coated preparation for oral administration. Absorption of enteric-coated products is occasionally less than adequate, however, and blood levels may not reach sufficient concentrations. Therefore, to avoid destruction of the drug by gastric juices while maintaining good oral absorption, erythromycin has also been formulated in several salts (estolate, ethylsuccinate, stearate), all of which are largely acid stable and yield biologically effective plasma levels of free erythromycin base. The strength of erythromycin products is expressed in terms of base equivalents. Thus, 400 mg of the ethylsuccinate salt provides serum levels of free erythromycin equivalent to those resulting from administration of 250 mg of erythromycin base or the stearate or estolate salts. Two other soluble salts of erythromycin (gluceptate, lactobionate) are available for IV use and are indicated mainly in severe infections in which high serum levels of the drug are required immediately.

As noted, erythromycin is used in the free-base form as well as as several salts, and the several preparations are available for oral, IV, topical, and ophthalmic administration. Absorption of the base and the stearate preparations is impaired by the presence of food, and these drugs should be administered on an empty stomach, if possible. Conversely, absorption of the estolate and ethylsuccinate salts is unaffected or enhanced by the presence of food. The estolate and ethylsuccinate salts, however, have been associated with cholestatic hepatitis, especially in adults, and must be used with caution in the presence of liver disease. Still, erythromycins are relatively safe antibiotics, the most frequently reported side effects being GI distress such as nausea, diarrhea, and abdominal cramping.

Mechanism

Inhibit bacterial protein synthesis by attaching to 50S ribosomal subunits of sensitive microorganisms, thereby blocking binding of tRNA to donor site; do not affect nucleic acid synthesis nor act on the cell wall; the nonionized form of the drug penetrates bacterial cells most efficiently, and thus the antimicrobial activity of macrolides is increased in an alkaline pH, because the drug exists predominantly in the nonionized form in such an environment.

Uses

Treatment of respiratory infections caused by susceptible organisms, such as the following: *Mycoplasma pneumoniae* (drug of choice), *Legionella pneumophila* (drug of choice), *Streptococcus pneumoniae*, group A beta-hemolytic streptococci (in penicillin-sensitive patients), and *Bordetella pertussis*
Treatment of acute skin and soft tissue infections due to *Staphylococcus aureus* (resistance is commonly encountered)
Prophylaxis of subacute bacterial endocarditis and recurrence of acute rheumatic fever in penicillin-sensitive patients
Treatment of *Neisseria gonorrhoeae* (gonorrhea) and *Treponema pallidum* (syphilis) infections in penicillin- and tetracycline-sensitive patients
Treatment of chlamydial infections (eg, uncomplicated urethritis, endocervicitis, conjunctivitis, pneumonia) in tetracycline-sensitive patients
Treatment of *Campylobacter jejuni* gastroenteritis
Treatment of respiratory and middle ear infections due to *Haemophilus influenzae* (in conjunction with sulfonamides)
Adjunctive treatment of *Corynebacterium* infections (with antitoxin)
Topical control of mild to moderate acne vulgaris
Reduction of wound complications when given with neomycin before colorectal surgery

Dosage

See Table 63-1.

Fate

Oral absorption usually is good, but base and stearate absorption may be impaired by food, and these preparations should be given on an empty stomach; base is destroyed by gastric acid, and thus is formulated in enteric-coated tablets or capsules; drug diffuses readily into most body tissues (except CNS, unless meninges are inflamed) and passes through the placental barrier, although fetal blood levels remain rather low; one of only a few antibiotics to attain high levels in prostatic fluid; peak serum levels occur in 1 to 4 hours with oral use; drug is approximately 70% protein bound; concentrated in the liver and excreted in active form primarily in the bile; less than 5% of an oral dose and 15% of an IV dose is excreted in the urine.

Common Side Effects

Abdominal discomfort (cramping, nausea, diarrhea, and anorexia).

Significant Adverse Reactions

Vomiting, allergic reactions (rash, urticaria, fever, eosinophilia, anaphylaxis); reversible hearing loss; superinfections by nonsusceptible organisms; cholestatic hepatitis (primarily from estolate and ethylsuccinate salt); pain, irritation, or phlebitis with IV injection; impaired hearing with IV infusion of lactobionate or gluceptate salts (4 g/day or more).

Contraindications

Estolate and ethylsuccinate salt in preexisting liver disease. *Cautious use* in patients with impaired liver function or history of allergic disorders, and in pregnant or nursing women.

Interactions

The activity of erythromycins may be enhanced by urinary alkalinizers (eg, sodium bicarbonate, acetazolamide) and decreased by urinary acidifiers (eg, ammonium chloride, citric acid beverages).
The effects of lincomycin and clindamycin may be antagonized by erythromycin, which competes for ribosomal binding sites.
Tetracyclines and cephalothin are incompatible with erythromycin in parenteral mixtures.
Erythromycin can elevate serum digoxin levels in a small percentage of patients who metabolize digoxin in the GI tract by slowing its metabolism in the gut.
Erythromycins can increase serum levels of theophylline, carbamazepine, and cyclosporine by reducing their clearance.
Erythromycin, being primarily bacteriostatic, may impair the antimicrobial activity of penicillins or other bactericidal antibiotics.
The effects of oral anticoagulants may be increased by erythromycins.

Nursing Management

See Table 63-1 for information on specific drugs. In addition:

Pretherapy Assessment

Assess and record baseline data necessary for detection of adverse effects of erythromycin: General: vital signs (VS), body weight, skin color, temperature, and integrity; GI: biliary function; Genitourinary (GU): renal function; Cardiovascular system (CVS): hematologic function; CNS: neurologic function; Laboratory: culture of infected site.
Review medical history and documents for existing or previous conditions that:
a. require cautious use of erythromycin: impaired hepatic function (elimination depends on biliary function).
b. contraindicate use of erythromycin: allergy to erythromycin; **pregnancy (Category B)**; lactation (significant concentrations appear in breast milk, safety not established).

Nursing Interventions

Medication Administration

Administer oral form of drug on an empty stomach (1 hour before or 2 hours after meals), with a full glass of water.
Administer erythromycin on schedule to ensure stable steady-state concentrations for the duration of therapy.
Clean affected area of skin before application of topical solution or ointment unless directed otherwise. Keep topical preparations away from eyes, nose, mouth, and other mucous membranes.

Table 63-1. **Macrolide Antibiotics**

Drug	*Usual Dosage Range*	*Nursing Considerations*
Erythromycin Base *Ak-Mycin, E-Mycin, Ery-Tab, Eryc Ilotycin, PCE, Robimycin* *(CAN) Apo-Erythro Base, Erybid, Erythromid, Novorythro Base*	*Oral* Adults: 250–500 mg every 6–12 h up to 4 g/d for severe infections Children: 30–50 mg/kg/d in 3–4 divided doses, up to 100 mg/kg/d *Legionnaires' disease*: 1–4 g daily in divided doses *Pertussis*: 40–50 mg/kg/d in divided doses for 5–15 d *Sexually transmitted diseases* (syphilis, gonorrhea, nongonococcal urethritis, chancroid, lymphogranuloma): 500 mg 4 times a day for at least 7–10 d (up to 30 d for syphilis) *Ophthalmic* Prevention of neonatal conjunctivitis: Apply 2–3 times a day, 0.5% ointment *Topical* Apply to skin or eye 2–4 times/day as necessary, 2% ointment	Free-base form of erythromycin, which is acid labile and thus administered orally in enteric-coated form; absorption is variable depending on product used; should be administered on an empty stomach if possible; do not break or crush enteric-coated tablets; ophthalmic ointment may retard corneal healing; be alert for hypersensitivity reactions with topical application
Erythromycin Base, Topical Solution *Akne-Mycin, A/T/S, C-Solve, Erycette, Eryderm, Erymax, E-Solve-2, ETS-2%, Staticin*	Apply morning and evening to areas usually affected by acne, 1.5% and 2% topical solution	Alcohol solution of erythromycin base used in the treatment of acne vulgaris; avoid contact with eyes, nose, mouth, or other mucous membranes; use *cautiously* with other topical acne treatment, because severe irritation can occur; most common side effect is excessive drying of treated area; erythema, pruritus, burning, and desquamation have also been reported; wash, rinse, and dry area to be treated before application; also available as a gel in combination with benzoyl peroxide as Benzamycin
Erythromycin Estolate *Ilosone* *(CAN) Novorythro estolate*	Adults: 250 mg every 6 h (*or* 500 mg every 12 h) up to 4 g/d Children: 30–50 mg/kg/d orally in divided doses, up to 100 mg/kg/d *Syphilis*: 20 g over 10 days in divided doses	Ester salt of erythromycin that is acid-stable, well absorbed in the presence of food, and yields higher and more sustained blood levels than other derivatives; may produce hepatotoxicity—thus be alert for early signs of liver dysfunction (vomiting, malaise, cramping, right upper quadrant pain, fever, jaundice), and discontinue drug; symptoms usually occur with 1–2 wk of continuous therapy and are reversible on discontinuation of medication; not indicated for prolonged administration (eg, acne, prophylaxis or rheumatic fever) or for treatment of syphilitic infections in pregnant women; regular tablets should be swallowed whole; liquid should be kept refrigerated and unused portion discarded after 14 days
Erythromycin Ethylsuccinate *E.E.S., EryPed* *(CAN) Apo-Erythro-ES*	Adults: 400 mg every 6 h, up to 4 g/d for severe infections Children: 30–50 mg/kg/d, up to 100 mg/kg/d *Syphilis*: 48–64 g over 10 days in divided doses	Acid-stable salt of erythromycin that is reliably absorbed from the GI tract; requires a higher dose (ie, 400 mg vs 250 mg) than other oral salts to yield comparable blood levels of erythromycin base, the active form; oral liquids are stable for 14 days with refrigeration; reconstituted powder is stable for 10 days
Erythromycin Gluceptate *Ilotycin Gluceptate*	Adults and children: 15–20 mg/kg/d by continuous (preferred) *or* intermittent infusion; up to 4 g/d can be used in severe infections *Acute pelvic inflammatory disease due to* Neisseria gonorrhoeae: 500 mg every 6 h for 3 days, followed by 250 mg oral erythromycin every 6 h for 7 days	Soluble salt of erythromycin indicated in severe infections requiring immediate high serum levels or when oral administration is not possible or feasible; may produce pain, irritation, and possibly phlebitis on administration; solution is prepared initially by adding sterile water for injection to the vial according to package directions and shaking until dissolved; *no* preservatives should be used; reconstituted solution should be stored in refrigerator and used within 7 days; intermittent infusion is performed by administering 250–500 mg in 100–250 mL of sodium chloride injection or 5% dextrose over 30–60

(continued)

Table 63-1. **Macrolide Antibiotics (Continued)**

Drug	***Usual Dosage Range***	***Nursing Considerations***
		min 4 times a day; initial solution may be added to sodium chloride injection or 5% dextrose in water to give 1 g/L for slow IV infusion; pH of diluted solution should be kept between 6 and 8; do *not* give by IV push because irritation is common; high dosages have resulted in alterations in liver function—periodic hepatic function tests are required during prolonged therapy
Erythromycin Lactobionate *Erythrocin Lactobionate-IV*	Adults and children: 15–20 mg/kg/d by continuous (preferred) *or* intermittent infusion; up to 4 g/d may be given in severe infections *Acute pelvic inflammatory disease*: See erythromycin gluceptate, above	Soluble salt of erythromycin used in a manner similar to the gluceptate salt; see gluceptate for mixing and diluting instructions; IV infusion of 4 g/d or more has caused reversible hearing loss; *do not exceed this dosage*; intermittent IV administration is accomplished by giving one quarter the daily dose over 30–60 min every 6 h by slow injection of 250–500 mg in 100–250 mL of sodium chloride or 5% dextrose; IV therapy should be replaced by oral therapy as soon as is feasible
Erythromycin Stearate *Eramycin, Erythrocin* *(CAN) Apo-Erythro-S, Novorythro Stearate*	Adults: 250 mg every 6 h (*or* 500 mg every 12 h) up to 4 g/d in divided doses Children: 30–50 mg/kg/d in divided doses 4 times a day, up to 100 mg/kg/d *Syphilis*: 30–40 g in divided doses over 10–15 days	Acid-stable salt of erythromycin claimed to be the most completely and reliably absorbed of all the derivatives when taken on an empty stomach; may be associated with a slightly higher incidence of allergic reactions than other forms of erythromycin

Reduce the risk of stomatitis through frequent mouth care.

Initiate a meal schedule that provides small, frequent meals if GI upset occurs.

Provide ready access to bathroom and interventions directed at symptom relief if diarrhea occurs.

Inject deeply into large muscle mass, when giving IM, because injection can cause considerable pain. Rotate injection sites, and administer no more than 600 mg at a single site.

Use only dilute solutions when administering IV, and closely observe patient for signs of phlebitis.

Surveillance During Therapy

Monitor complete blood count (CBC), urinalysis, and liver and kidney function test results obtained over the course of therapy, especially with long-term therapy.

Monitor for early signs of hepatic dysfunction (malaise, nausea, vomiting, cramping, fever). Jaundice (dark urine, pale stools, pruritus, yellow skin or sclerae) may occur. Withhold drug and notify prescriber immediately if these signs occur.

Interpret results of diagnostic tests and contact practitioner as appropriate.

Monitor for possible drug–laboratory test interactions: interferes with fluorometric determination of urinary catecholamines; decreased urinary estriol levels due to inhibition of hydrolysis in gut; erythromycins also can elevate serum levels of alanine and aspartate aminotransferases and alkaline phosphatase, and decrease serum levels of glucose and cholesterol.

Monitor for possible drug–drug and drug–nutrient interactions: activity enhanced by urinary alkalinizers and decreased by urinary acidifiers; effects of other macrolides impaired by erythromycin; incompatible with tetracyclines and cephalothin; increases digoxin, theophylline, carbamazepine, and oral anticoagulant serum concentrations; increases therapeutic and toxic effects of corticosteroids; and increases cyclosporine concentrations and risk of renal toxicity.

Note that 400 mg of erythromycin ethylsuccinate produces the same free erythromycin serum levels as 250 mg of the base, stearate, or estolate.

Patient Teaching

Instruct patient regarding the importance of completing the full course of therapy as prescribed; that is, not to discontinue the drug once signs and symptoms of the infection being treated subside.

Inform patient of the consequences of not taking or abruptly discontinuing the erythromycin agent.

Instruct patient that the prescribed drug is to be taken for the condition for which it is prescribed, and not to be used to treat any other infections.

Instruct patient to avoid fruit juice or other acidic beverages when taking drug. Estolate and ethylsuccinate salts may be taken without regard for meals.

Instruct patient to swallow enteric-coated tablets whole.

Instruct patient about possible adverse side effects with erythromycin: nausea, vomiting, diarrhea; uncontrollable emotions.

Instruct patient on appropriate action to take if side effects occur:

Notify practitioner if severe or watery diarrhea, severe

nausea or vomiting, dark-colored urine, yellowing of the skin or eyes, loss of hearing, skin rash, or itching occur.

Notify practitioner of any unusual bleeding. Rationale: hypoprothrombinemia and bleeding tendencies due to decreased synthesis of vitamin K by intestinal microflora may occur.

Discontinue topically applied erythromycin at first sign of local irritation or other allergic reaction and notify practitioner.

Azithromycin

Zithromax

Azithromycin differs chemically from erythromycin in that a methyl-substituted nitrogen is incorporated into the lactone ring. This chemical addition prevents gastric acid destruction of the drug during absorption and therefore results in less gastric irritation. Although azithromycin is less active than erythromycin against gram-positive staphylococci and streptococci, it has a broader spectrum of activity than erythromycin against gram-negative organisms—in particular, *Haemophilus influenzae*, *Borrelia burgdorferi*, and anaerobic organisms.

Uses

Treatment of lower respiratory infections caused by susceptible organisms, such as the following: *Haemophilus influenzae*, *Moraxella catarrhalis*, or *Streptococcus pneumoniae*; and upper respiratory infections due to *Streptococcus pyogenes*

Treatment of uncomplicated skin and skin structure infections caused by common staphylococcal and streptococcal organisms

Treatment of nongonococcal urethritis and cervicitis due to *Chlamydia trachomatis* infection

Dosage

Adults: 500 mg the first day, followed by 250 mg once daily on days 2 through 5.

Chlamydia urethritis/cervicitis: a single 1-g dose

Fate

Azithromycin is rapidly absorbed after oral administration, but bioavailability is reduced by food; the drug is widely distributed throughout the body; concentrations are attained within tissues and cells that are greater than those in plasma; plasma protein binding is variable, about 50%, but this decreases with increased dosage; half-life averages 68 hours and loading doses are usually recommended; drug undergoes little metabolism and is eliminated primarily through the biliary–intestinal route, with only small amounts of drug recovered in the urine.

Common Side Effects

Mild abdominal discomfort (nausea, diarrhea).

Significant Adverse Effects

Vomiting, allergic reactions (rash, photosensitivity, angioedema), cardiac palpitations and chest pain, dizziness, headache, vertigo, hearing loss (possible at high doses), somnolence, fatigue, monilial vaginitis, nephritis.

Contraindications

Hypersensitivity to any of the macrolides. *Cautious use* in patients with impaired liver function and cardiac arrhythmias; the safety of azithromycin has not been established in pregnancy, nursing mothers, or children younger than 16 years of age.

Interactions

(Also see erythromycin.) Antacids containing aluminum and magnesium reduce peak blood levels of azithromycin but do not affect the extent of absorption.

Nursing Management

Pretherapy Assessment

Assess and record baseline data necessary for detection of adverse effects of azithromycin: General: VS, body weight, skin color, temperature, and integrity; GI: biliary function; GU: renal function; CVS: hematologic function; CNS: neurologic function; Laboratory: culture of infected site.

Review medical history and documents for existing or previous conditions that:

a. require cautious use of azithromycin: impaired hepatic function; cardiac arrhythmias; children younger than 16 years of age.
b. contraindicate use of azithromycin: allergy to any macrolide antiinfective; **pregnancy (Category B)**; lactation (significant concentrations appear in breast milk, safety not established, avoid use in nursing mothers).

Nursing Interventions

Medication Administration

Administer oral form of drug on an empty stomach (1 hour before or 2 hours after meals), with a full glass of water.

Administer azithromycin on schedule to ensure stable steady-state concentrations for the duration of therapy.

Reduce the risk of stomatitis through frequent mouth care.

Initiate a meal schedule that provides small, frequent meals if GI upset occurs.

Surveillance During Therapy

Monitor CBC, urinalysis, and liver and kidney function test results obtained over the course of therapy.

Monitor intake–output, observing for dehydration secondary to GI side effects (vomiting, diarrhea).

Monitor for signs of fungal superinfection involving the oral or vaginal mucous membranes.

Monitor for signs and symptoms of hypersensitivity (including photosensitivity), which may require discontinuation of drug.

Interpret results of diagnostic tests and contact practitioner as appropriate.

Monitor for possible drug–drug and drug–nutrient interactions: antacids containing aluminum and magnesium reduce blood levels of azithromycin but do not affect the extent of absorption; consider interactions listed with erythromycin as applicable.

Provide for patient safety needs to minimize environmental hazards and risk of injury if CNS side effects develop.

Patient Teaching

Instruct patient regarding the importance of completing the full course of therapy as prescribed; that is, not to discontinue the drug once signs and symptoms of the infection being treated subside.

Inform patient of the consequences of not taking or abruptly discontinuing azithromycin.

Instruct patient that the prescribed drug is to be taken for the condition for which it is prescribed, and not to be used to treat any other infections.

Instruct patient about possible adverse side effects with azithromycin: sensitivity to sunlight; dizziness, drowsiness, nausea, vomiting, diarrhea; allergic reactions (rash, photosensitivity, angioedema); vaginitis, nephritis.

Instruct patient on appropriate action to take if side effects occur:

Notify practitioner if early signs of hematologic or hepatic toxicity (sore throat, fever, mucosal ulceration, malaise, pallor, jaundice) occur.

Notify practitioner of any unusual bleeding. Rationale: hypoprothrombinemia and bleeding tendencies due to decreased synthesis of vitamin K by intestinal microflora may occur.

Instruct patient to use sunscreens (not one containing paraaminobenzoic acid) or protective clothing.

Teach patient measures that help prevent recurrence of urinary tract infections.

• Clarithromycin

Biaxin

Clarithromycin is the 6-methoxy derivative of erythromycin; this change prevents rearrangement of the lactone ring that readily occurs in gastric acid and accounts for the reduced gastrointestinal toxicity of clarithromycin compared to erythromycin. Clarithromycin exhibits the same spectrum of antimicrobial activity as erythromycin, but demonstrates increased potency against the following organisms: *Haemophilus influenzae*, *Legionella pneumophila*, and *Chlamydia trachomatis*.

Uses

Treatment of upper respiratory infections due to *Streptococcus pyogenes* and *Streptococcus pneumoniae*; and lower respiratory infections caused by *Haemophilus influenzae*, *Moraxella catarrhalis*, or *Streptococcus pneumoniae*; and pneumonia due to *Mycoplasma pneumoniae* or *Streptococcus pneumoniae*

Treatment of uncomplicated skin and skin structure infections due to common staphylococcal and streptococcal organisms

Dosage

Adults/children older than 12 years: 250 mg every 12 hours for 7 to 14 days

Haemophilus influenzae infection: 500 mg every 12 hours for 10 to 14 days

Fate

Clarithromycin is well absorbed from the GI tract and absorption is not significantly affected by food; half-life ranges from 3 to 7 hours; an active metabolite, 14-OH clarithromycin, formed in the liver (during first-pass metabolism), has a half-life of 5 to 6 hours and accounts for significant antimicrobial activity; drug is 65% to 70% bound to plasma proteins and, like azithromycin, attains concentrations in tissues and cells that are greater than plasma concentrations; additional liver metabolism forms several inactive metabolites that together with 14-OH clarithromycin and small amounts of the parent drug are eliminated by both urinary and intestinal routes.

Common Side Effects

Mild gastrointestinal discomfort (nausea, diarrhea), headache.

Significant Adverse Effects

Increased abdominal discomfort and pain, dizziness, possible hearing loss at high dosages, rash and other allergic reactions.

Contraindications

Hypersensitivity to any of the macrolide antibiotics. *Cautious use* in patients with renal or hepatic impairment; safety during pregnancy, lactation, and in children younger than the age of 12 years has not been established.

Interactions

(Also see erythromycin.) Blood levels of carbamazepine or theophylline may be increased by clarithromycin.

Nursing Management

Pretherapy Assessment

Assess and record baseline data necessary for detection of adverse effects of clarithromycin: General: VS, body weight, skin color, temperature, and integrity; GI: biliary function; GU: renal function; CVS: hematologic function; CNS: neurologic function; Laboratory: culture of infected site.

Review medical history and documents for existing or previous conditions that:

a. require cautious use of clarithromycin: impaired hepatic function; children younger than 12 years of age.

b. contraindicate use of clarithromycin: allergy to any macrolide antiinfective; **pregnancy (Category B)**; lactation (significant concentrations appear in breast milk, safety not established, avoid use in nursing mothers).

Nursing Interventions

Medication Administration

Administer oral form of drug with meals, with a full glass of water.

Administer clarithromycin on schedule to ensure stable steady-state concentrations for the duration of therapy.

Reduce the risk of stomatitis through frequent mouth care.

Initiate a meal schedule that provides small, frequent meals if GI upset occurs.

Surveillance During Therapy

Monitor CBC, urinalysis, and liver function test results obtained over the course of therapy.
Monitor intake–output, observing for dehydration secondary to GI side effects (vomiting, diarrhea).
Monitor for signs of superinfection involving the oral and vaginal mucous membranes and fungal organisms.
Monitor for signs of hypersensitivity, which may require discontinuation of drug.
Interpret results of diagnostic tests and contact practitioner as appropriate.
Monitor for possible drug–drug and drug–nutrient interactions: blood levels of carbamazepine may be elevated with clarithromycin; consider interactions listed with erythromycin as applicable.
Provide for patient safety needs to minimize environmental hazards and risk of injury if CNS side effects develop.

Patient Teaching

Instruct patient regarding the importance of completing the full course of therapy as prescribed; that is, not to discontinue the drug once signs and symptoms of the infection being treated subside.
Inform patient of the consequences of not taking or abruptly discontinuing the clarithromycin.
Instruct patient that the prescribed drug is to be taken for the condition for which it is prescribed, and not to be used to treat any other infections.
Instruct patient about possible adverse side effects of clarithromycin: dizziness, drowsiness, nausea, vomiting, diarrhea; allergic reactions (rash, photosensitivity, angioedema); vaginitis, nephritis.
Instruct patient on appropriate action to take if side effects occur:
- Notify practitioner if early signs of hematologic or hepatic toxicity (sore throat, fever, mucosal ulceration, malaise, pallor, jaundice) occur.
- Notify practitioner of any unusual bleeding. Rationale: hypoprothrombinemia and bleeding tendencies due to decreased synthesis of vitamin K by intestinal microflora may occur.
- Notify practitioner if hearing loss, rash, or other allergic reactions occur.

• Troleandomycin

Tao

A semisynthetic derivative of oleandomycin, troleandomycin is a macrolide antibiotic obtained from *Streptomyces antibioticus*. It is similar to erythromycin in activity but somewhat less effective and more toxic, hence its clinical usefulness is limited. Troleandomycin usually is effective in eradicating streptococci from the nasopharynx.

Mechanism

Inhibits protein synthesis in susceptible bacteria.

Uses

Treatment of upper respiratory infections due to susceptible strains of *Diplococcus pneumoniae* and *Streptococcus pyogenes* (alternative therapy *only*).

Dosage

Adults: 250–500 mg 4 times/day
Children: 125–250 mg every 6 hours

Fate

Well absorbed orally; widely distributed in the body, including the CNS; metabolized in the liver and excreted in the bile and urine.

Common Side Effects

Abdominal discomfort and cramping.

Significant Adverse Reactions

Nausea, vomiting, diarrhea, allergic reactions (rash, fever, pruritus, urticaria, anaphylaxis), overgrowth of nonsusceptible organisms, and cholestatic hepatitis.

Contraindications

Liver impairment.

Interactions

Combined use of ergotamine and troleandomycin can induce ischemic reactions.
Troleandomycin may elevate serum levels of theophylline, carbamazepine, and corticosteroids if used concurrently.
Concomitant use of troleandomycin and oral contraceptives can cause cholestatic jaundice.

Nursing Management

Pretherapy Assessment

See **erythromycin**.

Nursing Interventions

Medication Administration

See **erythromycin**.

Surveillance During Therapy

See **erythromycin**.

Patient Teaching

See **erythromycin**.

Selected Bibliography

Bahal N, Nahata MC: The new macrolide antibiotics: Azithromycin, clarithromycin, dirithromycin, and roxithromycin. Ann Pharmacother 26:46, 1992
Chu SY, et al: Pharmacokinetics of clarithromycin, a new macrolide, after single ascending oral doses. Antimicrob Agents Chemother 36:2447, 1992
Clarithromycin and azithromycin. Med Lett Drugs Ther 34:45, 1992
Hammerschlag MR, Qumei KK, Roblin PM: In vitro activities of azithromycin, clarithromycin, L-ofloxacin, and other antibiotics against *Chlamydia pneumoniae*. Antimicrob Agents Chemother 36:1573, 1992
Peters DH, Clissold SP: Clarithromycin: A review of its antimicrobial activity, pharmacokinetic properties and therapeutic potential. Drugs 44:117, 1992
Spiritus EM: Diagnosis and treatment of acute lower respiratory tract infections. Res Staff Phys 40(1):28, 1994

Nursing Bibliography

Bartolo G: The effect of IV erythromycin on gastric volume in post partum patients undergoing tubal sterilization under general anesthesia. American Association of Nurse Anesthetists 60:360, 1992

Countering IV erythromycin: Ill effects. Emergency Medicine 24(9):49, 1992

Erythromycin-related hearing loss. Nurses Drug Alert 17(5):34, 1993

Fighting chlamydia during pregnancy. Emergency Medicine 24(3):151, 1992

64

Aminoglycosides

Amikacin
Gentamicin
Kanamycin
Neomycin
Netilmicin
Streptomycin
Tobramycin

The aminoglycosides are a group of broad-spectrum bactericidal antibiotics that exhibit similar pharmacologic, antimicrobial, and toxicologic properties. Their principal use is in the treatment of serious systemic gram-negative infections caused by *Pseudomonas*, *Proteus*, *Klebsiella*, *Enterobacter*, *Serratia*, and *Escherichia* species. Aminoglycoside treatment of infections due to other organisms, both gram negative and gram positive, usually is reserved for those instances in which less toxic agents have failed. The major limitation to the routine use of aminoglycoside antibiotics is their potential for eliciting serious untoward reactions, most notably ototoxicity (both auditory and vestibular) and nephrotoxicity. Toxicity can develop even with conventional therapeutic doses, especially in patients with impaired renal function. It is also commonly encountered with prolonged or high-dosage therapy. Adverse effects are considered in more detail later. Because of the narrow margin between efficacy and toxicity with aminoglycosides, serum concentrations should be monitored frequently in critically ill patients and in people with renal impairment. Peak serum concentrations are determined 30 minutes after completion of IV infusion or 1 hour after IM injection. Minimum (ie, trough) levels are taken immediately before the next dosing. Peak levels are used as an indication of drug activity, whereas excessive trough levels serve to indicate drug accumulation and possible toxicity (Table 64-1).

Absorption of aminoglycosides from the GI tract is negligible, and the drugs must be administered parenterally for treatment of systemic infections. Several aminoglycosides may also be given orally for localized intraintestinal infections or as adjunctive therapy in the treatment of hepatic coma. Some drugs are also applied topically to the eye, skin, or mucous membranes for treatment of superficial infections due to susceptible organisms. Thus, despite similar chemical and pharmacologic properties, the aminoglycosides do *not* share similar modes of administration or clinical indications. Table 64-1 lists the routes of administration for each of the aminoglycosides, as well as their major antimicrobial spectrum of action. Although the aminoglycosides are active against a variety of gram-positive organisms, they are rarely used clinically against these organisms because more effective, less toxic antibacterial agents are available. As indicated, their principal application is in treating severe systemic infections caused by a number of gram-negative aerobic bacilli (see Table 64-1).

Of the available aminoglycosides, gentamicin, tobramycin, amikacin, and netilmicin are the most often used derivatives and are virtually interchangeable in the treatment of most infections caused by *Acinetobacter* sp, *Enterobacter* sp, *Escherichia coli*, *Klebsiella pneumoniae*, *Proteus* sp, *Pseudomonas aeruginosa*, *Providencia* sp, and *Serratia* sp. In many instances, a synergistic action is obtained against these organisms when an extended-spectrum penicillin (such as ticarcillin) or a third-generation cephalosporin (such as cefoperazone or ceftizoxime) is used in conjunction with one of these aminoglycosides. Streptomycin is the agent of choice for treating infections due to *Francisella tularensis* (tularemia), *Pseudomonas mallei* (melioidosis), and *Yersinia pestis* (plague), and also may be useful in treating tuberculosis (see Chapter 68). Orally administered neomycin has been used for preoperative bowel sterilization, relief of *E coli*-induced diarrhea, and as adjunctive therapy for hepatic coma. Kanamycin has a somewhat more limited spectrum of action than other aminoglycosides, and its use has declined.

The aminoglycosides are also used as alternative agents against a wide variety of organisms, as outlined in Chapter 58, Table 58-1.

Resistance to aminoglycosides is becoming more prevalent as their use increases. Resistant strains of *Enterobacter*, *Klebsiella*, *Proteus*, *Pseudomonas*, and *Serratia* have appeared in many hospitals in which the aminoglycosides are widely used. This resistance can occur in a number of ways, the most common being decreased penetration of the drug into the bacterial cell, a deficiency of the ribosomal receptor (see Mechanism), or increased enzymatic destruction of the drug. The newer derivatives (amikacin, netilmicin) may still be effective, however, against certain organisms that have become resistant to the action of the older agents such as kanamycin, tobramycin, and gentamicin. In addition, amikacin is not degraded by most aminoglycoside-inactivating enzymes that affect other derivatives, and hence it may be useful against enzyme-producing organisms resistant to the other systemic aminoglycosides. Nevertheless, culture and sensitivity tests should be performed to determine the susceptibility of an infecting organism to a particular aminoglycoside.

The possibility of serious adverse reactions is a major limitation to the routine use of the aminoglycosides. All derivatives exhibit essentially the same range of toxic effects, although some effects occur less frequently with some of the newer agents. Foremost among the untoward reactions seen with aminoglycoside use is ototoxicity, which can involve both the auditory and vestibular functions of the eighth cranial nerve. The risk is greatest in patients with renal impairment or preexisting hearing loss, and although the incidence of ototoxicity usually is related to the dosage and duration of treatment, it has occasionally occurred with normal therapeutic dosages. Patients should be observed closely for early signs of impending toxicity (tinnitus, vertigo, high-frequency deafness), and the dosage lowered or the drug discontinued to prevent irreversible deafness. Vestibular toxicity is more common with gentamicin and streptomycin, whereas auditory toxicity is more prevalent with kanamycin, neomycin, amikacin, and netilmicin. The relative

Table 64-1. **Administration, Antimicrobial Spectrum, and Toxic Serum Levels of Aminoglycosides**

Drug	*Routes of Administration*	*Plasma Half-Life (h)*	*Toxic Serum Levels (μg/mL)*		*Principal Antimicrobial Spectrum of Action**
			Peak	*Trough*	
Amikacin	IM, IV	2–3	>35	>10	1, 2, 3, 7, 10, 11, 12, 15
Gentamicin	IM, IV, intrathecal, ophthalmic, topical	1–4	>12	>2	2, 3, 7, 10, 12, 13, 14, 15
Kanamycin	IM, IV, intraperitoneal, aerosol, oral	2–4	>35	>10	1, 3, 6, 7, 9, 10, 13, 14, 15
Neomycin	Ophthalmic, topical, oral	2–3	—	—	3, 7, 10, 12
Netilmicin	IM, IV	2–3	>16	>4	1, 2, 3, 7, 10, 12, 13, 14, 15
Streptomycin	IM	2–3	>50	—	3, 4, 5, 6, 7, 8, 10, 16, 17
Tobramycin	IM, IV, ophthalmic	2–3	>12	>2	2, 3, 7, 10, 11, 12, 15

Organisms
1. *Acinetobacter* sp
2. *Citrobacter freundii*
3. *Escherichia coli*
4. *Francisella tularensis*
5. *Haemophilus ducreyi*
6. *Haemophilus influenzae*
7. *Klebsiella–Enterobacter–Serratia* sp
8. *Mycobacterium tuberculosis*
9. *Neisseria gonorrhoeae*
10. *Proteus* sp
11. *Providencia* sp
12. *Pseudomonas aeruginosa*
13. *Salmonella* sp
14. *Shigella* sp
15. *Staphylococcus* sp
16. *Streptococcus* (group D)
17. *Yersinia pestis*

* Does *not* necessarily indicate drug of choice; see Chapter 58, Table 58-1.

ototoxicity of aminoglycosides is neomycin > streptomycin, kanamycin > amikacin, gentamicin, tobramycin, netilmicin.

Because aminoglycosides are eliminated almost entirely by the kidneys, they may accumulate in patients with compromised renal function. Moreover, the drug's own toxic effects may further reduce the organ's ability to excrete nitrogenous wastes. The result is increased nitrogen retention (ie, elevated blood urea nitrogen [BUN] or serum creatinine), frequently accompanied by oliguria, proteinuria, azotemia, and the presence of red and white cell casts in the urine. Because renal tubular damage is usually reversible if detected early enough, careful monitoring of renal function and serum creatinine levels is essential during prolonged aminoglycoside therapy, especially in the patient with preexisting renal dysfunction. Decreased creatinine clearance necessitates a reduction in drug dosage or an increase in dosing intervals, or both; the presence of casts in the urine suggests that hydration of the patient should be increased; the appearance of symptomatic azotemia or a progressive decrease in urine output is usually an indication to discontinue the drug. When patients are well hydrated and kidney function is normal, however, the risk of nephrotoxicity with aminoglycosides is *comparatively low*, provided dosage limits are not exceeded. The relative nephrotoxicity of these agents is approximately neomycin > amikacin, gentamicin, kanamycin, netilmicin > tobramycin > streptomycin.

Interference with neuromuscular transmission, possibly leading to respiratory depression or paralysis, has occurred with the aminoglycosides, especially when given simultaneously with or shortly after general anesthetics or muscle relaxants. Reversal of aminoglycoside-induced neuromuscular blockade, characterized by apnea and muscle paralysis, may be accomplished with either neostigmine or calcium salts.

Inasmuch as the different aminoglycosides share the same properties, they are considered as a group. Characteristics of individual drugs are presented in Table 64-2. The discussion focuses primarily on the parenteral use of the drugs, with references to their oral and topical application where appropriate.

Mechanism

Inhibit protein synthesis in the bacterial cell; bind to the 30S ribosomal subunit, causing a misreading of the genetic code and thus formation of improper peptide sequences in the protein chain. Drugs are more active in an alkaline medium; thus, their efficacy against urinary pathogens can be increased by alkalinization of the urine.

Uses

See Tables 58-1 and 64-1 for susceptible organisms.

Treatment of severe gram-negative infections of the GI, respiratory, or urinary tracts, CNS, skin, bone, and soft tissues due to susceptible organisms (parenteral use only)

Suppression of intestinal bacteria (kanamycin or neomycin orally)

Adjunctive therapy of hepatic coma to reduce concentra-

Table 64-2. **Aminoglycosides**

Drug	Usual Dosage Range	Nursing Considerations
Amikacin *Amikin*	*IM, IV* Adults and older children: 15 mg/kg/d in 2–3 divided doses (maximum 1.5 g/d) *Urinary tract infections*: 250 mg IM twice a day *Neonatal sepsis*: Initially 10 mg/kg, followed by 7.5 mg/kg every 12 h	Semisynthetic aminoglycoside derived from kanamycin, exhibiting a similar spectrum of action; *not* degraded by most aminoglycoside-inactivating enzymes, therefore may be effective against organisms resistant to other derivatives; amikacin resistance is emerging, however, as its use increases; duration of treatment should be 7–10 days—longer therapy necessitates daily monitoring of renal and auditory function; if a clinical response does *not* occur within 5 days, stop drug and reevaluate; may be used in uncomplicated urinary tract infections (dose: 250 mg IM twice a day) due to organisms not susceptible to other, less toxic agents; urine should be examined during treatment for the presence of protein, blood cells, or casts; maintain high degree of hydration to minimize renal irritation; solution for IV use is prepared by adding contents of 500-mg vial to 200 mL of appropriate diluent (see package instructions) and administered over a 30–60-min period (1–2 h for neonates); do *not* premix with other drugs; stable for extended period at room temperature
Gentamicin *Garamycin, Genoptic, Gentacidin, GentAK, Jenamicin* *(CAN) Alcomicin, Cidomycin, PMS Gentamicin*	*IM, IV* Adults: 3–5 mg/kg/d in 3–4 divided doses Children: 6–7.5 mg/kg/d in 3 divided doses Infants and neonates: 7.5 mg/kg/d in 3 divided doses Premature infants and neonates (< 1 wk): 5 mg/kg/d in 2 equal doses *Intrathecal* Adults: 4–8 mg/d in a single dose Children and infants (>3 mo): 1–2 mg once/day *Ophthalmic* 1 or 2 drops or small amount of ophthalmic ointment 2–4 times/day *Topical* Apply sparingly to affected area 3–4 times/day	Broad-spectrum aminoglycoside obtained from an *Actinomyces* organism; drug of choice against several gram-negative organisms (see Chapter 58, Table 58-1), synergistic with extended-spectrum penicillins against *Pseudomonas* infections, may be used in combination with a penicillin or cephalosporin in treating serious unknown infections before sensitivity testing; also used with antistaphylococcal penicillins for treatment of staphylococcal endocarditis; usually given IM but may be used IV in patients with septicemia, shock, congestive heart failure, severe burns, or hematologic disorders; do *not* mix with other drugs before injection; intrathecal administration is used as an adjunct to systemic administration in serious CNS infections (eg, meningitis, ventriculitis) due to *Pseudomonas* species; topical application is used to treat superficial infections of the skin and mucous membranes due to susceptible organisms; photosensitivity reactions have occurred after topical use; systemic toxicity can result from application to large abraded areas of skin; use *cautiously* on burns or large wounds
Kanamycin *Kantrex* *(CAN) Anamid*	*IM* Adults and children: 7.5 mg/kg every 12 h (maximum 1.5 g/d) *IV* Up to 15 mg/kg/d in 2–3 divided doses infused over a 30–60-min period *Intraperitoneal* 500 mg/20 mL sterile distilled water instilled into peritoneal cavity through a wound catheter *Aerosol* 250 mg (1 mL) diluted with 3 mL saline 2 to 4 times/day, using a nebulizer *Oral* *Suppression of intestinal bacteria*: 1 g every hour for 4 h, then 1 g every 6 h for 36–72 h *Hepatic coma*: 8–12 g/d in divided doses	Aminoglycoside derived from a species of *Streptomyces*; similar in activity to neomycin but not as toxic; effective against many common gram-negative organisms except *Pseudomonas* but not considered drug of choice for any infection; occasionally used as adjunctive therapy of *Mycobacterium tuberculosis*; inject deeply IM and rotate sites; discontinue drug if a clinical response does not occur within 5 days; prepare IV solutions by adding 500 mg to 200 mL, *or* 1 g to 400 mL of sterile diluent, and infuse over 30–60 min 2–3 times a day; do *not* mix dilution with other drug solutions; solution in vials may darken on shelf with no loss of potency, intraperitoneal instillation should be postponed until patient has recovered from effects of anesthesia and muscle relaxants (danger of respiratory depression and muscle paralysis); may be used as an irrigating solution (0.25%) in abscess cavities, peritoneal, ventricular, or pleural spaces; when used orally, be alert for malabsorption syndrome (eg, increased fecal fat) or secondary bacterial or fungal infections (eg, diarrhea, stomatitis); use with caution orally in patients with gastrointestinal ulceration, because enhanced systemic absorption can occur; nausea, vomiting, and diarrhea are common with oral ingestion

(*continued*)

Table 64-2. **Aminoglycosides (Continued)**

Drug	Usual Dosage Range	Nursing Considerations
Neomycin *Mycifradin, Myciguent*	*Oral* *Preoperative bowel preparation*: 88 mg/kg in 6 equally divided doses every 4 h before surgery or 1 g every hour for 4 doses, then 1 g every 4 h for the next 20 h *Hepatic coma* Adults: 4–12 g/d in divided doses Children: 50–100 mg/kg/d in divided doses *Infectious diarrhea*: 50 mg/kg/d in divided doses for 2–3 days *Topical* Apply 2–4 times a day	Broad-spectrum antibiotic obtained from a species of *Streptomyces*; similar in action to kanamycin but is the more potent neuromuscular blocker and reportedly the most toxic of all aminoglycosides; many organisms exhibit moderate to marked resistance against neomycin; principal indications for oral neomycin are severe diarrhea due to *Escherichia coli* and preoperative bowel sterilization in conjunction with a low-residue diet; a saline cathartic is administered before first dose of neomycin; may interfere with absorption of other drugs (eg, digitalis glycosides, methotrexate, penicillins; see Interactions); nausea and diarrhea are fairly common with oral administration; widest application is topically, either alone or more commonly with bacitracin and polymyxin (eg, Neosporin, Mycitracin, Neo-Polycin) for superficial infections of eye, skin, and mucous membranes; hypersensitivity reactions are common with topical application; discontinue drug if irritation, redness, or itching occurs; do *not* use over large body surface areas or if skin is broken or abraded, because increased systemic absorption and toxicity can occur
Netilmicin *Netromycin*	*IM, IV* Adults: 3–6.5 mg/kg/d in divided doses every 8–12 h Children: 5.5–8 mg/kg/d in divided doses every 8–12 h Neonates: 4–6 mg/kg/d in divided doses every 12 h	Semisynthetic derivative similar to gentamicin in activity but somewhat less effective against *Pseudomonas*; may be slightly less nephrotoxic and ototoxic than other aminoglycosides; used in serious staphylococcal infections where penicillins are contraindicated and in suspected or confirmed gram-negative infections; usual duration of treatment is 7–14 days—for longer therapy, carefully monitor renal, auditory, and vestibular functions; follow package instructions for dosage adjustment in the presence of impaired renal function
Streptomycin *Streptomycin*	*IM use only* *Tuberculosis*: 1 g/d, together with other antitubercular drugs (eg, isoniazid, ethambutol, rifampin); may reduce to 1 g 2–3 times a week as condition improves *Tularemia*: 1–2 g/d in divided doses for 7–10 days *Plague*: 2–4 g/d in divided doses *Bacterial endocarditis*: 0.5–1 g twice a day for 2 wk with a penicillin *Prophylaxis of bacterial endocarditis in patients undergoing intestinal or urinary tract surgery*: 1 g IM 0.5–1 h before surgery in combination with 2 million U penicillin G *or* 1 g ampicillin IM *or* IV *Other infections*: 1–4 g/d in divided doses depending on severity of infection *Children*: 20–40 mg/kg/d in divided doses every 6–12 h	Aminoglycoside isolated from a species of *Streptomyces*; fairly high toxicity and rapid development of resistance limits its usefulness to those infections not controlled by other, less toxic drugs, except in tularemia, plague, and meliodosis, where it is the drug of choice, and tuberculosis, where it is commonly used in combination with several other tuberculostatic agents (see Chapter 68); total treatment period for tuberculosis is a minimum of 1 y; also indicated for prophylaxis of bacterial endocarditis in high-risk patients undergoing respiratory, gastrointestinal, or genitourinary surgery or instrumentation, in combination with penicillin G or ampicillin; most frequent adverse effect is vestibular toxicity; observe for headache, vomiting, dizziness, difficulty in reading, or ataxia, and consult physician; incidence of nephrotoxicity is lowest of all aminoglycosides, but use with caution in renal impairment and perform frequent determinations of serum drug concentration; adequate hydration is important, especially during prolonged therapy (eg, tuberculosis therapy); commercially available IM solutions contain a preservative and should *not* be injected IV or SC; solution may darken during storage but potency is not affected
Tobramycin *Nebcin, Tobrex*	*IM, IV* Adults: 3–5 mg/kg/d in 3–4 equally divided doses, depending on severity of infection Children: 6–7.5 mg/kg/d in 3–4 equally divided doses Neonates (1 wk or less): up to 4 mg/kg/d in 2 equal doses every 12 h	Aminoglycoside antibiotic with pharmacologic properties, indications, and overall toxicity similar to gentamicin; somewhat lower incidence of vestibular toxicity has been reported; do *not* exceed 5 mg/kg/d unless serum levels are monitored; prolonged serum concentrations above 12 μg/mL should be avoided; urine should be observed for presence of protein, cells, and casts; follow package directions for dosage reduction in patients with renal impairment—reduced doses may be based on creatinine clearance or serum cre-

(*continued*)

Table 64-2. **Aminoglycosides (Continued)**

Drug	Usual Dosage Range	Nursing Considerations
	Ophthalmic 1–2 drops or 0.5-inch ribbon of ointment every 4 h; in severe infections, 2 drops every hour until improvement is noted	atinine; IV dose should be diluted to 50–100 mL for adults (and proportionately less for children) with sodium chloride or 5% dextrose injection and infused over 20–60 min; do *not* premix with other drugs but administer separately; usual duration of treatment is 7–10 days; in severe or complicated infections, a longer course of therapy may be necessary; auditory, vestibular, and renal function should be monitored frequently during prolonged therapy; local allergic reactions have occurred with eye drops or eye ointment

tion of ammonia-forming bacteria in the GI tract (kanamycin, neomycin, or paromomycin orally)

Treatment of superficial infections of the eye, skin, or mucous membranes due to susceptible organisms (gentamicin or tobramycin)

Treatment of severe diarrhea due to *E coli* (neomycin orally)

Dosage

See Table 64-2.

Fate

Not appreciably absorbed from the GI tract; absorption after IM injection is rapid; peak blood levels occur in 1 to 2 hours; plasma half-life is 1 to 4 hours with normal kidney function but may be longer in infants (5–8 h), in elderly people, or in patients with renal impairment (up to 96 h); widely distributed in the body, except for the CNS (unless meninges are inflamed); drugs are not significantly protein bound; serum levels in febrile patients usually are lower than those in afebrile patients given the same dosage, and half-lives are shorter; not metabolized to a significant extent, but eliminated largely unchanged by the kidneys after parenteral injection (up to 98% of a single IV dose is excreted within 24 h); orally administered drugs are excreted almost completely in the feces; drugs have a narrow margin between the therapeutic and toxic serum levels.

Common Side Effects

Oral: nausea, diarrhea

Parenteral: headache, tinnitus, dizziness (especially at high doses)

Topical: hypersensitivity reactions (especially with neomycin)

Significant Adverse Reactions

Oral

Malabsorption syndrome (ie, decreased absorption of vitamins, minerals, electrolytes, fats), steatorrhea, anorexia, stomatitis, salivation

Parenteral

CNS: ototoxicity (vertigo, ataxia, impaired hearing, irreversible deafness), confusion, disorientation, lethargy, depression, visual disturbances, amblyopia, nystagmus, optic neuritis, numbness and paresthesias, muscle twitching, tremor, convulsions

Renal: proteinuria, oliguria, azotemia, red and white cell casts in urine, elevated BUN and serum creatinine

Allergic–hypersensitivity: rash, pruritus, urticaria, alopecia, laryngeal edema, fever, exfoliative dermatitis, anaphylaxis

Hematologic: agranulocytosis, leukopenia, thrombocytopenia, eosinophilia, pancytopenia, anemia

Hepatic: increased serum transaminase and bilirubin, hepatomegaly, hepatic necrosis

Other: palpitations, myocarditis, splenomegaly, arthralgia, hypotension, pulmonary fibrosis, superinfections, muscle weakness, respiratory depression, pain and irritation with IM injection

Topical

Burning, itching, urticaria, erythema, photosensitivity, maculopapular dermatitis

Contraindications

Oral use in patients with bowel obstruction, long-term parenteral therapy in patients with renal impairment, and concurrent administration with other ototoxic or nephrotoxic drugs (see Interactions). *Cautious use* in people with neuromuscular disorders or those taking skeletal muscle relaxants and in children, elderly patients, and pregnant or nursing women.

Interactions

Concurrent use of aminoglycosides and amphotericin, bacitracin, cephalothin, cisplatin, colistimethate, cyclosporine, polymyxin, or vancomycin can increase the incidence of nephrotoxicity.

The ototoxic effects of the aminoglycosides can be enhanced by potent diuretics such as ethacrynic acid, bumetanide, furosemide, torsemide, and mannitol.

Dimenhydrinate, meclizine, cyclizine, and other antivertigo drugs may mask the ototoxic effects of aminoglycosides.

Aminoglycosides can enhance the muscle-relaxing effects of neuromuscular blocking agents and general anesthetics, possibly leading to respiratory depression.

Aminoglycosides exert a synergistic effect with antipseudomonal penicillins (eg, carbenicillin, ticarcillin, piperacillin, mezlocillin, azlocillin) against *Pseudomonas* infections at normal concentrations; however, high concentrations of the penicillins may inhibit the antibacterial activity of aminoglycosides.

Orally administered neomycin and possibly other aminoglycosides may decrease the absorption of digoxin, penicillin V, and vitamin B_{12}.

Nursing Management

See Table 64-2 for information on specific drugs. In addition:

Pretherapy Assessment

Assess and record baseline data necessary for detection of adverse effects of aminoglycosides: General: vital signs, body weight, skin color, temperature, and integrity; GI: biliary function; Genitourinary: renal function (urinalysis, BUN, creatinine); Cardiovascular system: hematologic function; CNS: neurologic function (vestibular and auditory); Laboratory: culture of infected site.

Review medical history and documents for existing or previous conditions that:

a. require cautious use of aminoglycosides: advanced patient age; decreased renal function; preexisting hearing loss; active herpes, varicella, fungal, or mycobacterial infection; neuromuscular disorders (myasthenia gravis; Parkinson disease, infant botulism).
b. contraindicate use of aminoglycosides: allergy to aminoglycosides; renal disease; hepatic disease; **pregnancy (Category C)**; **pregnancy (Category D)** at term (crosses the placenta; produces deafness); lactation (significant concentrations appear in breast milk, affect on infant unknown).

Nursing Interventions

Medication Administration

Administer aminoglycosides on schedule to ensure stable steady-state concentrations for the duration of therapy.

Ensure adequate hydration (fluid intake 2000–3000 mL/day) during aminoglycoside therapy. Rationale: facilitate renal perfusion and minimize nephrotoxicity.

Administer parenteral (IM, IV), topical, and ophthalmic dosage forms using appropriate technique:

- Use only ophthalmic preparations (ophthalmic ointment or drops) in the eye. Do not apply topical neomycin or gentamicin ointment to the eyes or to external ear canal if eardrum is perforated.
- Clean wound thoroughly before applying a topical aminoglycoside. Rationale: the drug may be inactivated in the presence of pus, blood, or cell breakdown products.
- Administer IM deeply into large muscle (gluteal, vastus lateralis), observe for signs of irritation, and rotate injection sites.
- Administer IV slowly to minimize possibility of severe neuromuscular blockade with subsequent development of apnea.
- Use solutions as soon as possible after reconstituting.
- Consult package instructions for appropriate dosage modification if renal function is impaired.

Reduce the risk of stomatitis through frequent mouth care.

Initiate a meal schedule that provides small, frequent meals if GI upset occurs.

Provide ready access to bathroom and interventions directed at symptom relief if diarrhea occurs.

Surveillance During Therapy

Monitor complete blood count, urinalysis, liver and kidney function test results, and peak and trough serum levels of aminoglycoside and creatinine clearance.

Interpret results of diagnostic tests and contact practitioner as appropriate.

Assess vestibular and auditory function (dizziness, tinnitus, vertigo, ataxia, nystagmus, hearing loss at high frequencies) before, at regular intervals during, and for 3 to 4 weeks after therapy (*particularly* if there is impaired kidney function or prolonged treatment). Rationale: aminoglycosides cause ototoxicity, even in normal therapeutic doses.

Monitor intake–output, observing for signs and symptoms of possible nephrotoxicity (decreased urine output, increased serum creatinine, increased BUN). Rationale: signs and symptoms of possible nephrotoxicity are indications for dose reduction or discontinuation of therapy.

Monitor for possible drug–drug interactions and avoid concurrent or sequential administration of other potentially ototoxic or nephrotoxic drugs:

- Increased ototoxicity and/or nephrotoxicity with potent diuretics (furosemide, bumetanide, torsemide, ethacrynic acid).
- Increased risk for neuromuscular blockade and muscle paralysis with general anesthetics, citrated blood, neuromuscular blockers.
- Potential inactivation of mixed beta-lactam antibiotics.
- Increased bactericidal effect with penicillins, cephalosporins.
- Decreased absorption and efficacy of digoxin with neomycin.

Monitor for possible drug–laboratory test interactions:

- With neomycin: falsely low serum aminoglycoside levels.
- With penicillins, cephalosporins: falsely high serum aminoglycoside levels.

Patient Teaching

Instruct patient regarding the importance of completing the full course of therapy as prescribed; that is, not to discontinue the drug once signs and symptoms of the infection being treated subside.

Inform patient of the consequences of not taking the prescribed aminoglycoside.

Instruct patient that the drug is to be taken for the condition for which it is prescribed, and not to be used to treat any other infections.

Instruct patient about possible adverse side effects of aminoglycosides: tinnitus, decreased hearing acuity, dizziness, headache, unsteady gait, nausea, vomiting, anorexia, burning eye–blurred vision (with ophthalmics).

Instruct patient on appropriate action to take if side effects occur:

Notify practitioner if early signs of ototoxicity, nephrotoxicity, or hematologic reactions (sore throat, fever, mucosal ulceration, malaise, pallor) occur.

Explain that treatment may be prolonged if infection is severe or complicated. Bacterial resistance to aminoglycosides develops slowly, with the exception of streptomycin, to which resistance can develop rapidly.

Selected Bibliography

Hansten PD, Horn JR: Aminoglycoside interactions, update. Drug Interactions Newsletter 8:U-11, 1988

Johnson JG: Aminoglycosides, imipenem, and aztreonam. Clin Podiatr Med Surg 9:443, 1992

Manian FA, Stone WJ, Alford RH: Adverse antibiotic effects associated with renal insufficiency. Rev Infect Dis 12:236, 1990

Singh GR, Sachdev HP, Puri RK: Aminoglycosides. Indian Pediatr 29:343, 1992

Winstanley TG, Hastings JG, Synergy between penicillin and gentamicin against enterococci. J Antimicrob Chemother 25:551, 1990

Nursing Bibliography

Dyer J: Drug watch . . . flosequinan . . . gentamicin . . . estrogen. . . streptokinase. Am J Nurs 93(8):47, 1993

Gentamicin dosing regimens compared. Nurses Drug Alert 17(4):26, 1993

Swenson C, Pilkiewicz F, Cynamon M: Liposomal aminoglycosides and TLC G-56: Potential role in the therapy of disseminated mycobacteria aversion–intercellular infections. AIDS Patient Care 5:290, 1991

65 Polypeptides

Bacitracin
Colistimethate
Colistin Sulfate
Polymyxin B Sulfate

The polypeptide group of antibiotics comprises polymyxin B, colistin (polymyxin E), the methanesulfonate salt of colistin (colistimethate), and bacitracin. The first three of these drugs are commonly termed the *polymyxins*, and although certain similarities exist between these agents and bacitracin, significant differences are noted as well.

The polymyxins, a group of strongly basic polypeptides obtained from *Bacillus polymyxa* and variants, are designated as polymyxins A, B, C, D, and E. Of these, only polymyxins B and E are used clinically, because the remaining derivatives are too toxic for human use.

The polymyxins are bactericidal, primarily against gram-negative bacilli such as *Pseudomonas* sp, *Escherichia coli*, *Klebsiella* sp, *Enterobacter* sp, *Salmonella* sp, and Shigella sp. Most strains of *Proteus* and *Neisseria*, however, and virtually all gram-positive organisms are unaffected by the polymyxins. These drugs exert their antibacterial action by disrupting the bacterial cell membrane, thus allowing cell constituents to escape. The drugs are not absorbed orally, and after parenteral administration they do not reach the CNS (unless given intrathecally), the joints, or the eye in appreciable amounts. Excretion is by the kidney (except for orally administered colistin); thus, cumulation toxicity can occur in the presence of renal impairment. The polymyxins are used systemically for severe infections only, especially of the urinary tract, caused by susceptible gram-negative organisms not sensitive to other, less toxic antimicrobial drugs. They find their widest application for topical treatment of skin and mucous membrane infections (including the eye and ear), especially if *Pseudomonas* is the offending pathogen. Principal adverse effects are of two major types, neurotoxicity and nephrotoxicity, and the incidence and severity of these untoward reactions severely limit the systemic usefulness of the polymyxins to all but very severe infections.

Polymyxin B is available as an injection, as a powder for preparing ophthalmic drops, and in several combination products (eg, with neomycin, bacitracin, and corticosteroids) for ophthalmic or otic use. Colistin sulfate (polymyxin E) can be used either as an oral suspension for control of diarrhea and gastroenteritis or in combination with hydrocortisone and neomycin as ear drops (ColyMycin S Otic). Colistimethate, as a powder for injection, may be administered either IV or IM for serious systemic or urinary infections, particularly those caused by *Pseudomonas* sp. Because there are many differences among these three polymyxin preparations, they are considered individually in this chapter.

Bacitracin is a mixture of several polypeptides isolated from a strain of *Bacillus subtilis*, the major constituent being bacitracin A. This antibiotic appears to inhibit bacterial cell wall formation and is bactericidal against a variety of gram-positive bacteria as well as a few gram-negative organisms. The drug is available for IM injection and as a topical and ophthalmic ointment. Because of its potential for serious toxicity, however, it is used parenterally *only* for treatment of staphylococcal pneumonia or empyema in infants. Bacitracin is most often used topically, alone or in combination with neomycin and polymyxin, for treatment of cutaneous or ocular infections, because it is highly effective against susceptible organisms and rarely causes hypersensitivity reactions. Kidney damage is a major danger with parenteral use of bacitracin, and renal function must be closely monitored during therapy.

• Bacitracin

AK-Tracin, Baci-IM, Baciguent

Mechanism

Not completely established; probably acts by inhibiting bacterial cell wall synthesis and may alter cell membrane permeability as well; bactericidal at therapeutic doses; spectrum of action in vitro is similar to that of penicillin G; systemic use is virtually obsolete because parenteral administration is highly nephrotoxic.

Uses

Treatment of superficial infections of the skin, mucous membrane, and eye due to susceptible organisms (topical use *only*)

Treatment of antibiotic-induced pseudomembranous colitis caused by *Clostridium difficile* (investigational use for *orally* administered bacitracin)

Treatment of infants with pneumonia and empyema caused by staphylococci (rarely used)

Dosage

IM:

Infants under 2.5 kg: 900 U/kg/day in two or three divided doses

Infants over 2.5 kg: 1000 U/kg/day in two or three divided doses

Topical: apply two or three times a day to affected area

Ophthalmic: apply to lower conjunctival sac several times a day

Fate

Rapidly absorbed from IM injection site; distributed widely in the body, duration of action is 6 to 8 hours with single IM doses; excreted largely in the urine; absorption from topical sites is minimal.

Common Side Effects

Pain and irritation at IM injection site.

Significant Adverse Reactions

CAUTION

Bacitracin (IM) can result in renal failure due to glomerular injury or tubular necrosis. Use only when indicated (see Uses), monitor renal function daily, and maintain adequate fluid intake.

Renal: proteinuria, azotemia, urinary frequency, oliguria, hematuria, increased blood urea nitrogen (BUN), uremia, renal failure

Other: neuromuscular weakness, hypersensitivity reactions (rash, urticaria, hypotension), nausea, vomiting, tinnitus, diarrhea, altered taste sensations, allergic contact dermatitis (with topical use); with ophthalmic use, ocular burning, stinging, and irritation

Contraindications

Severe renal impairment; intraocular use in patients with viral or fungal infections. *Cautious use* in patients with myasthenia gravis or a history of allergic reactions.

Interactions

Nephrotoxic effects of bacitracin may be additive to those of other antibiotics having similar toxicity, for example, aminoglycosides, polymyxins, vancomycin.

Bacitracin can enhance or prolong the muscle-relaxing effects of neuromuscular blocking agents and anesthetics, or other drugs with neuromuscular blocking actions (ie, aminoglycosides, procainamide, succinylcholine).

Nursing Management

Pretherapy Assessment

Assess and record baseline data necessary for detection of adverse effects of bacitracin: General: vital signs (VS), body weight, skin color, temperature, and integrity; Genitourinary (GU): renal function (urinalysis, BUN, creatinine); CNS: neurologic function; Laboratory: culture of infected site.

Review medical history and documents for existing or previous conditions that:

a. require cautious use of bacitracin: impaired renal function; allergy to bacitracin; patients with myasthenia gravis.
b. contraindicate use of bacitracin: severe renal impairment; opthalmic use in patients with viral or fungal infections; **pregnancy (Category C)**.

Nursing Interventions

Medication Administration

Administer bacitracin on schedule to ensure stable steady-state concentrations for the duration of therapy.

Clean wound thoroughly before applying a topical bacitracin because the drug may be inactivated in the presence of pus, blood, or cell breakdown products.

Provide adequate hydration (2000–3000 mL/day) when drug is administered IM. Rationale: prevent renal toxicity.

Dissolve drug in sodium chloride injection containing 2% procaine hydrochloride because IM injections are painful.

Refrigerate bacitracin solutions (stable up to 1 week) because they are rapidly inactivated at room temperature.

Surveillance During Therapy

Monitor complete blood count, urinalysis, and liver and kidney function test results obtained over the course of therapy.

Monitor intake–output, observing for signs and symptoms of possible renal impairment (hematuria, proteinuria, oliguria, polyuria, elevated BUN). Discontinue drug immediately if signs appear.

Interpret results of diagnostic tests and contact practitioner as appropriate.

Monitor for possible drug–drug interactions:

- Increased neuromuscular blockade and paralysis with anesthetics and drugs with neuromuscular blocking activity.
- Additive nephrotoxic effects when administered along with other antibiotics that are potentially nephrotoxic (eg, aminoglycosides, polymyxins, vancomycin).

Provide for patient safety needs to minimize environmental hazards and risk of injury if neurologic side effects develop.

Patient Teaching

Instruct patient regarding the importance of completing the full course of therapy as prescribed; that is, not to discontinue the drug once signs and symptoms of the infection being treated subside.

Inform patient of the consequences of not taking the bacitracin as prescribed.

Instruct patient that the prescribed drug is to be taken for the condition for which it is prescribed, and not to be used to treat any other infections.

Instruct patient about possible adverse side effects of bacitracin: potential renal damage; neuromuscular weakness; allergic response to topical application; irritation and burning with ocular application.

Instruct patient on appropriate action to take if side effects occur:

- Discontinue topically applied (dermal, optic) bacitracin at first sign of local irritation or other allergic reaction and notify practitioner.
- Notify practitioner if signs and symptoms of renal damage or neuromuscular impairment occur.

• Colistimethate

Coly-Mycin M

Mechanism

Disrupts the bacterial cell membrane, probably through a surface action, thus allowing escape of cell constituents.

Uses

Treatment of acute or chronic infections due to sensitive strains of certain gram-negative organisms, especially *Pseudomonas aeruginosa*, *E coli*, *Klebsiella pneumoniae*, and *Enterobacter aerogenes* (not effective against *Proteus* or *Neisseria* sp).

Dosage

Adults and children: 2.5 to 5 mg/kg/day, IM or IV, in two to four divided doses (maximum 5 mg/kg/day in patients with normal renal function). IV administration may be by direct injection (one half daily dose over 3–5 min every 12 h) or by infusion (one half dose over 3–5 min, then 5–6 mg/h starting 1–2 h after initial injection).

Fate

Absorption from IM sites is good; blood levels are maximum 1 to 2 hours after IM injection; serum half-life is 2 to 3 hours; does not enter CNS, even if meninges are inflamed; excreted primarily in the urine, mostly within 18 to 24 hours.

Common Side Effects

Pain at IM injection site.

Significant Adverse Reactions

Renal: decreased urine output, increased BUN, proteinuria, azotemia, renal failure
Neurologic: paresthesias; numbness in the extremities; visual, auditory, or speech disturbances; dizziness; ataxia
Allergic–hypersensitivity: pruritus, urticaria, drug fever, dermatoses
Other: neuromuscular blockade (muscle weakness, respiratory depression or paralysis), GI upset, agranulocytosis, superinfections

Contraindications

Severe renal failure. *Cautious use* in patients with myasthenia gravis, renal impairment, or in people receiving muscle relaxants or potentially nephrotoxic drugs (eg, aminoglycosides, vancomycin).

Interactions

Additive nephrotoxic effects can result from concurrent use of colistimethate and other drugs that impair renal function (eg, aminoglycosides, vancomycin).
Extreme muscle weakness and muscle paralysis can occur if colistimethate is administered with several anesthetics, neuromuscular blocking agents, aminoglycosides, or other drugs having a neuromuscular blocking action.

Nursing Management

Pretherapy Assessment

Assess and record baseline data necessary for detection of adverse effects of colistimethate: General: VS, body weight, skin color, temperature, and integrity; GI: biliary function; GU: renal function (urinalysis, BUN, creatinine); Cardiovascular system (CVS): hematologic function; CNS: neurologic function (eighth cranial nerve function); Laboratory: culture of infected site.
Review medical history and documents for existing or previous conditions that require cautious use of colistimethate: impaired renal function; patients with myasthenia gravis.

Nursing Interventions

Medication Administration

Have appropriate resuscitative equipment and drugs available, and observe patient closely for signs of respiratory distress (dyspnea, chest pain, restlessness). Rationale: respiratory arrest has occurred after injection.
Seek clarification if dosage exceeds 5 mg/kg/day, even if patient's renal function is normal. Rationale: overdose can result in neuromuscular blockade and renal insufficiency (see Significant Adverse Reactions).
Inject deeply into large muscle and rotate injection sites when giving IM. Injection may be painful.
Discard unused portion of IM drug solution 7 days after reconstitution. Solution may be stored at room temperature.
Prepare IV infusion solution with appropriate diluent according to package instructions; use within 24 hours.

Surveillance During Therapy

Assess patient for changes in visual, auditory, or verbal function or development of drowsiness, dizziness, or paresthesias, early signs of possible neurologic toxicity.
Ensure that prescribed baseline renal function tests are obtained before therapy is initiated. During therapy, be alert for changes in urinary output or elevations in BUN, serum creatinine, or plasma drug levels because they may indicate renal toxicity.

• Colistin Sulfate

Coly-Mycin S

Mechanism

Disrupts bacterial cell membrane, causing loss of cellular constituents; bactericidal against most gram-negative enteric pathogens, except *Proteus* sp.

Uses

Control of diarrhea in infants and children due to infection with susceptible strains of enteropathogenic *E coli* (oral suspension)
Treatment of gastroenteritis due to infection with *Shigella* organisms (oral suspension)
Treatment of superficial infections of the ear canal (combination with neomycin and hydrocortisone as Coly-Mycin S Otic)

Dosage

Oral: adults and children—5 to 15 mg/kg/day in three divided doses; higher doses may be required in severe infections
Otic: 3 or 4 drops into external ear canal three or four times a day

Fate

Not absorbed to a significant extent from the GI tract; excreted in the feces.

Significant Adverse Reactions

Rare at recommended doses; intestinal superinfection can occur with prolonged oral use.

Contraindications

Topical use: fungal or viral infections of the ear (prolonged use may result in overgrowth of nonsusceptible organisms, eg, herpes simplex, vaccinia, varicella). *Cautious use* orally in patients with preexisting renal damage.

Interactions

See Bacitracin for *potential* drug interactions; actual incidence is minimal, because drug is not absorbed systemically.

Nursing Management

Pretherapy Assessment

Assess and record baseline data necessary for the detection of adverse effects that may occur with an antiinfective otic agent: General: VS, body weight, skin color and temperature, integrity of tympanic membranes; GU: renal function; CVS: hematologic function; CNS: neurologic function; Laboratory: culture of infected site.

Review medical history and documents for existing or previous conditions that:
- a. require cautious use of colistin: preexisting renal damage.
- b. contraindicate use of colistin: fungal or viral infections of the ear; herpes simplex, vaccinia, or varicella infections; known allergy.

Nursing Interventions

Medication Administration

Reconstitute powder for oral suspension with distilled water. Store in refrigerator; discard unused portion after 2 weeks.

Clean and dry external ear canal before instillation of drops.

Question use of otic solution if patient has perforated eardrum or chronic otitis media. It should be used very cautiously with such patients because it contains neomycin, which is ototoxic.

Surveillance During Therapy

Be alert for signs of possible renal toxicity, especially if large doses are used or azotemia is present, because slight systemic absorption may occur in some instances.

Monitor patient closely for adverse reactions during therapy.

Monitor for evidence of superinfection: continued ear pain, inflammation, or fever.

Monitor for signs of nephrotoxicity: abnormal urinalysis results, increased creatinine and BUN, altered urinary void patterns.

Monitor the patient for evidence of developing hypersensitivity to colistin: pruritus, urticaria, vesicular or maculopapular dermatitis.

Patient Teaching

Teach the patient the name, dose, action, and adverse effects of colistin.

Advise the patient to discontinue the colistin and contact practitioner if an allergic reaction occurs.

• Polymyxin B Sulfate

Aerosporin

Mechanism

Disrupts the lipoprotein cell membrane of susceptible bacteria, resulting in leakage of cellular constituents and cell death; bactericidal against most gram-negative bacilli, except *Proteus* sp; gram-positive bacteria and gram-negative cocci are resistant.

Uses

Treatment of acute infections due to susceptible strains of *Pseudomonas aeruginosa* (IM, IV)

CAUTION

Parenteral administration is no longer recommended; used only when less toxic drugs are ineffective.

Alternative treatment of severe infections of the blood, meninges, or urinary tract due to *E coli*, *Klebsiella pneumoniae*, *Enterobacter aerogenes*, or *Haemophilus influenzae*, used only when less toxic drugs are ineffective (IM, IV)

Treatment of superficial infections of the eye, ear, mucous membranes, or skin due to susceptible organisms (topical combination products containing polymyxin B)

Dosage

IV Infusion

Adults and children: 15,000 to 25,000 U/kg/day; infusions may be given every 12 hours

Infants: up to 40,000 U/kg/day

IM

Adults and children: 25,000 to 30,000 U/kg/day, divided and given at 4- to 6-hour intervals

Infants: up to 40,000 U/kg/day

Intrathecal (eg, in pseudomonal meningitis)

Adults and children older than 2 years: 50,000 U once daily for 3 to 4 days; then 50,000 U every other day for at least 2 weeks after cultures of the cerebrospinal fluid are negative and its glucose content has returned to normal

Children younger than 2 years: 20,000 U once daily for 3 to 4 days; then 25,000 U every other day

Bladder Irrigation (Neosporin G.U. Irrigant—Polymyxin Plus Neomycin)

Add 1 mL irrigant to 1 L isotonic saline solution; infuse by catheter at a rate of 1 L/24 h *continuously*; if urine output exceeds 2 L/day, increase flow rate to 2 L/24 h

Ophthalmic

1 or 2 drops in affected eye several times a day, as necessary

Topical

Apply several times a day to affected area

Fate

Not significantly absorbed from the GI tract or mucous membranes; peak plasma concentrations are reached within 2 hours after IM injection; plasma half-life is 4 to 6 hours; active blood levels are low, because drug loses up to half its activity in the serum; activity levels are higher in infants and children than in adults; diffusion into many tissues is poor, and drug does not enter CNS unless given intrathecally; slowly excreted by the kidneys, largely in unchanged form.

Common Side Effects

Pain on IM injection.

Significant Adverse Reactions

CAUTION

Nephrotoxicity and neurotoxicity can occur, especially with IM or intrathecal administration. Administer only to hospitalized patients and provide constant supervision.

Renal: proteinuria, hematuria, azotemia, cellular casts, increasing blood levels of drug without increases in dosage
Neurologic: flushing, paresthesias, drowsiness, dizziness, neuromuscular blockade (muscle weakness, respiratory depression, apnea)
Hypersensitivity–allergic: pruritus, dermatoses, urticaria, drug fever, local burning or irritation with topical application
Other: meningeal irritation (headache, stiff neck, fever) with intrathecal administration, thrombophlebitis with IV infusion, GI disturbances, overgrowth of nonsusceptible organisms

Contraindications

Severe renal impairment, concurrent use of other nephrotoxic or neurotoxic drugs (eg, bacitracin, aminoglycosides, colistimethate). *Cautious use* in people with neurologic disorders and in pregnant or nursing women.

Interactions

Concurrent use of polymyxin and other nephrotoxic drugs (eg, aminoglycosides, vancomycin, bacitracin, colistimethate) may increase the danger of kidney damage.
Use of polymyxin with neuromuscular blocking agents, general anesthetics, or aminoglycosides can lead to extreme muscle weakness and respiratory paralysis.

Nursing Management

Pretherapy Assessment

Assess and record baseline data necessary for detection of adverse effects of polymyxin B: General: VS, body weight, skin color, temperature, and integrity; GU: renal function; CNS: neurologic function; Laboratory: culture of infected site.
Review medical history and documents for existing or previous conditions that:
a. require cautious use of polymyxin B: impaired renal function.
b. contraindicate use of polymyxin B: allergy to polymyxin B; **pregnancy (Category B)**; lactation (effects and safety unknown).

Nursing Interventions

Medication Administration

Ensure that patient receiving drug IM or intrathecally is under constant professional supervision. The drug should be administered IM or intrathecally *only* to patients who are hospitalized (see Significant Adverse Reactions).
Have appropriate resuscitative equipment and drugs available, and observe patient closely for signs of neuromuscular blockade (dyspnea, shortness of breath, muscle weakness). If these occur, the drug should be discontinued and symptoms treated as necessary.
Ensure adequate fluid intake (to produce urine output of at least 1500 mL/day).
Refrigerate reconstituted parenteral solution. Discard unused portion after 72 hours.
Note that polymyxin is available as an ophthalmic solution or ointment with bacitracin (Polysporin), oxytetracycline (Terramycin), neomycin plus bacitracin (Neosporin Ophthalmic, Ak-Spore), and neomycin plus a corticosteroid (Cortisporin Ophthalmic, Maxitrol).
Note that polymyxin is available as an otic solution or suspension with hydrocortisone plus neomycin (Cortisporin Otic, Otocort) for treatment of superficial ear infections.
Note that polymyxin is not available *alone* for topical application, but is found in combination with several other antibiotics in many different ointments, aerosols, and powders.
Note that polymyxin and neomycin are available as a genitourinary irrigant solution (Neosporin G.U. Irrigant) for use with catheter systems, permitting continuous irrigation of the urinary bladder. The solution contains 40 mg of neomycin and 200,000 U of polymyxin B sulfate per mL.

Surveillance During Therapy

Notify practitioner if signs and symptoms of renal toxicity (reduced urine output; elevated BUN and serum creatinine, plasma drug levels, and urinary proteins) occur because these may necessitate discontinuing polymyxin B.
Monitor for signs of hypersensitivity, which may require discontinuation of drug.
Monitor urinalysis and kidney function test results obtained over the course of therapy.
Monitor patient's neurologic status frequently for symptoms of neurotoxicity (irritability, dizziness, paresthesias, numbness, blurred vision). These usually can be eliminated by a dosage reduction.

Interpret results of diagnostic tests and contact practitioner as appropriate.
Monitor for possible drug–drug and drug–nutrient interactions: use of polymyxin and other nephrotoxic agents may increase the danger of kidney damage; use of polymyxin with neuromuscular blockers can lead to extreme muscle weakness and respiratory paralysis.
Monitor intake–output, observing for signs and symptoms of possible renal impairment (renal colic, oliguria, hematuria).

Patient Teaching

Instruct patient regarding the importance of completing the full course of therapy as prescribed; that is, not to discontinue the drug once signs and symptoms of the infection being treated subside.
Inform patient of the consequences of not taking or abruptly discontinuing the polymyxin therapy.
Instruct patient that the prescribed drug is to be taken for the condition for which it is prescribed, and not to be used to treat any other infections.
Instruct patient about possible adverse side effects of polymyxin: vertigo, dizziness, drowsiness and slurring of speech; numbness, tingling of extremities, tongue; superinfection; burning and stinging; blurring of vision (transient).
Instruct patient on appropriate action to take if side effects occur: notify practitioner if the following signs or symptoms occur: difficulty breathing, rash or skin lesions, pain at injection site, change in urinary voiding pattern, fever, flu-like symptoms, changes in vision, severe stinging or itching.

Selected Bibliography

Drapeau G, Toulouse A, Marceau F: Dissociation of the antimicrobial activity of bacitracin USP from its renovascular effects. Antimicrob Agents Chemother 36:955, 1992
Eedy DJ, McMillan JC, Bingham EA: Anaphylactic reactions to topical antibiotic combinations. Postgrad Med J 66:858, 1990
Garcia-Patrone M: Bacitracin-induced proteins in *Bacillus subtilis* and *Bacillus thuringiensis* and their relationship with resistance. Antimicrob Agents Chemother 34:796, 1990
Quinlan GJ, Gutteridge JM: DNA base damage by beta-lactam, tetracycline, bacitracin and rifamycin antibacterial antibiotics. Biochem Pharmacol 42:1595, 1991
Walton MA, et al: The efficacy of polysporin first aid antibiotic spray (polymyxin B sulfate and bacitracin zinc) against clinical burn wound isolates. J Burn Care Rehabil 12:116, 1991

Nursing Bibliography

Lindsay C, Every L, Harrison G : Formulation for the use of inhaled colistin. Respiratory Care 37:1446, 1992

66
Urinary Anti-infectives

Methenamine
Methylene Blue
Nitrofurantoin
Trimethoprim

Urinary Analgesic
Phenazopyridine

Urease Inhibitor
Acetohydroxamic acid

Although the term *urinary anti-infective* refers in theory to any drug capable of eradicating pathogens present in the urinary tract, it usually is applied only to those agents specific for urinary infections by virtue of their lack of significant *systemic* antibacterial action. Thus, although other antimicrobial drugs, such as broad-spectrum penicillins, cephalosporins, tetracyclines, sulfonamides, aminoglycosides, and polypeptides all have been used successfully in the treatment of urinary tract infections, they are not considered specific urinary anti-infectives because most attain significant plasma levels throughout the body and can therefore be used to treat a number of systemic infections as well. The drugs considered to be selective urinary anti-infectives are cinoxacin, methenamine, nalidixic acid, nitrofurantoin, norfloxacin, and trimethoprim. Cinoxacin, nalidixic acid, and norfloxacin are members of the quinolone group of anti-infectives and are discussed with other quinolones in Chapter 62. The remaining urinary anti-infectives are considered here.

Although specific for urinary infections by virtue of their rapid elimination in the urine and their lack of significant systemic antimicrobial activity, these agents usually are not considered drugs of choice for acute, uncomplicated urinary tract infections, inasmuch as they often are less effective against many common urinary pathogens than sulfonamides, broad-spectrum penicillins, or cephalosporins. The urinary anti-infectives are most often reserved for those people who are either intolerant of or unresponsive to one of the first-line drugs. Urinary anti-infectives are also of value for the control of *chronic* urinary infections due to organisms that have developed resistance to commonly used antibiotics. For example, low doses of nitrofurantoin, administered once a day at bedtime, have been used successfully for long-term prophylaxis in chronic urinary infections. Likewise, trimethoprim–sulfamethoxazole and methenamine also have been used in treating chronic urinary infections.

Perhaps the most troublesome situation is the chronic urinary infection that often complicates an anatomic or physiologic abnormality such as urinary stones, urethral strictures, or prostate enlargement. Treatment of these conditions requires prolonged therapy with a urinary anti-infective capable of interfering with bacterial growth without favoring emergence of resistant organisms. The drugs most commonly used for chronic urinary conditions are trimethoprim–sulfamethoxazole (see Chapter 59), nitrofurantoin, and methenamine. Of course, surgical intervention is often necessary when a blockage or some other anatomic lesion is present.

The fact that urinary anti-infectives usually do not attain effective antibacterial blood levels does not mean that they are free of systemic toxic effects. On the contrary, with the exception of methenamine, the other agents in this group all have the potential to elicit serious untoward reactions, and their use should be accorded the same respect as any other antimicrobial drug.

Patients receiving a urinary anti-infective drug should be advised to continue taking the prescribed dose for the recommended period (usually 10–14 days), even though the symptoms of the infection, such as low back pain, burning on urination, or fever, have disappeared. *Complete* eradication of the infecting organism, not simply symptomatic relief, is the goal of urinary chemotherapy, because relapses and reinfection are major problems in the treatment of urinary infections. A *relapse*, the result of failure to eliminate completely the original pathogen from the urinary system with the initial course of therapy, is usually the result of insufficient dose or duration of therapy, or both. *Recurring infections* are frequently noted some time after successful recovery from an initial attack and are often caused by microorganisms different from those responsible for the initial infection. These may include resistant forms that have emerged during the first course of therapy.

In addition to the urinary anti-infectives mentioned, several other drugs may be used in urinary infections. Methylene blue, a dye, is a weak germicide and is occasionally used orally as a mild urinary antiseptic. Phenazopyridine, another dye, is excreted in the urine after oral ingestion and exerts a mild analgesic effect. It is used to relieve irritation and pain in conjunction with an appropriate anti-infective. Acetohydroxamic acid (AHA) inhibits the urease-mediated hydrolysis of urea and the subsequent production of ammonia in urine infected with urea-splitting organisms. It is indicated as adjunctive therapy in chronic urea-splitting urinary infections. The foregoing drugs are considered in this chapter along with the urinary anti-infectives.

• Methenamine

Methenamine is a urinary antibacterial agent whose action depends on its hydrolysis to ammonia and formaldehyde in an acidic urine. Formaldehyde is bactericidal against a variety of gram-positive and gram-negative organisms (see Mechanism). Methenamine is used in the form of an acid salt (hippurate or mandelate), which helps maintain a low urinary pH.

Mechanism

In an acid urine (pH 5.5 or lower), drug is hydrolyzed to form ammonia and formaldehyde, the latter being bactericidal; acid liberated from the salt (ie, mandelic or hippuric) may also exert a weak antibacterial action; susceptible organisms include *Escherichia coli*, staphylococci, and enterococci. *Enterobacter aerogenes* is resistant, as are *Pseudomonas* and *Proteus* sp, the latter two being urea-splitting organisms that can raise urinary pH above the effective level; bacteria do *not* appear to develop resistance to formaldehyde, which is therefore well suited for treating chronic infections.

Uses

Treatment of chronic bacteriuria associated with cystitis, pyelonephritis, or other chronic urinary conditions
Adjunctive treatment of patients with anatomic abnormalities of the urinary tract

Dosage

See Table 66-1.

Fate

Readily absorbed orally; excreted largely unchanged (75%–90%) in the urine within 24 hours; formation of formaldehyde depends on urinary pH, level of methenamine, and length of time urine is retained in the bladder; peak formaldehyde concentrations occur at a urine pH of 5.5 or less; a level of 25 μg/mL or greater is necessary for antimicrobial activity; peak urinary formaldehyde levels occur within 2 to 6 hours; steady-state levels are attained within 2 to 3 days with regular dosing.

Common Side Effects

GI upset with large doses.

Significant Adverse Reactions

Cramping, vomiting, diarrhea, stomatitis, anorexia, urinary frequency or urgency, bladder irritation, dysuria, proteinuria, hematuria, hypersensitivity reactions (rash, pruritus), and abdominal pain.

Contraindications

Renal insufficiency, severe hepatic disease (because ammonia is liberated), and severe dehydration. *Cautious use* in pregnant women or nursing mothers, and in patients with gout, because methenamine salts may cause precipitation of urate crystals in the urine.

Interactions

Sulfonamides can form insoluble precipitates with formaldehyde in the urine.
Effectiveness of methenamine can be reduced by drugs that raise urinary pH (eg, sodium bicarbonate, acetazolamide, thiazide diuretics).
Methenamine salts may increase the urinary excretion of amphetamines, lowering their activity.

Nursing Management

Pretherapy Assessment

Assess and record baseline data necessary for detection of adverse effects of methenamine: General: vital signs (VS), body weight, skin color, temperature, and integrity, ear lobes–tophi, joints, state of hydration; GI: biliary function; Genitourinary (GU): renal function; Cardiovascular system (CVS): hematologic function; Central nervous system (CNS): neurologic function; Laboratory: urinalysis, liver function, serum uric acid, culture of infected site.
Review medical history and documents for existing or previous conditions that:
a. require cautious use of methenamine: impaired hepatic and renal function; dehydration; impaired uric acid metabolism and excretion.
b. contraindicate use of methenamine: allergy to methenamine; allergy to tartrazine; allergy to aspirin (cross sensitization to tartrazine); **pregnancy (Category C)**; lactation (significant concentrations appear in breast milk, safety not established, avoid use in nursing mothers).

Nursing Interventions

Medication Administration

Administer oral form of drug with meals, with a full glass of water.
Administer methenamine agents on schedule to ensure stable steady-state concentrations for the duration of therapy.
Initiate a meal schedule that provides small, frequent meals if GI upset occurs.
Note that methenamine is available in combination products with anticholinergics, urinary acidifiers, methylene blue, and salicylates.
Ensure that patient avoids excessive intake of foods or medications that alkalinize the urine.
Ensure adequate hydration.

Table 66-1. **Methenamine Salts**

Drug	*Usual Dosage Range*	*Nursing Considerations*
Methenamine Hippurate *Hiprex, Urex* *(CAN) Hip-Rex*	Adults: 1 g twice a day Children (6–12 y): 0.5–1 g twice a day	Effective in lower daily doses than mandelate salt; safe use in early pregnancy has not been established; may transiently elevate serum transaminase levels; periodic liver function tests are indicated
Methenamine Mandelate *Mandameth, Mandelamine*	Adults: 1 g 4 times a day Children (6–12 y): 0.5 g 4 times a day Children younger than 6 y: 0.25 g/30 lb 4 times a day	Most commonly used methenamine salt; enteric-coated tablets are claimed to lower incidence of GI upset; oral suspensions have a vegetable oil base; use cautiously in elderly or debilitated patients because of danger of aspiration (lipid) pneumonia; granules are orange flavored

Surveillance During Therapy

Monitor intake and output to ensure that normal levels are maintained.
Monitor complete blood count (CBC), urinalysis, and liver and kidney function test results obtained over the course of therapy.
Monitor intake–output, observing for dehydration secondary to gastrointestinal side effects (vomiting, diarrhea).
Interpret results of the following urine tests cautiously because methenamine can interfere with them: catecholamines, estriol, 17-hydroxycorticosteroids, and 5-hydroxyindoleacetic acid, a serotonin metabolite.
Monitor for signs of superinfection involving the oral and vaginal mucous membranes and fungal organisms.
Interpret results of diagnostic tests and contact practitioner as appropriate.
Monitor for possible drug–drug and drug–nutrient interactions: insoluble precipitates formed with sulfonamides and urinary formaldehyde; effectiveness reduced in presence of drugs that increase urinary pH (eg, sodium bicarbonate, acetazolamide, thiazide diuretics).
Note that bacteria and fungi do *not* develop resistance to formaldehyde, making methenamine suitable for long-term prophylaxis in chronic infections. It is *not*, however, suitable for prevention of urinary tract infections in patients with indwelling catheters because the bladder does not retain the drug long enough to form sufficient levels of formaldehyde, and it should not be used alone for acute infections or infections with renal parenchymal involvement associated with systemic symptoms.

Patient Teaching

Instruct patient regarding the importance of completing the full course of therapy as prescribed; that is, not to discontinue the drug once signs and symptoms of the infection being treated subside.
Inform patient of the consequences of not taking or abruptly discontinuing the methenamine.
Instruct patient that the prescribed drug is to be taken for the condition for which it is prescribed, and not to be used to treat any other infections.
Instruct patient to drink adequate fluids (8–10 glasses/day) but to avoid *excessive* hydration because increased urinary flow can reduce the amount of free formaldehyde in urine.
Teach patient how to monitor urinary pH with Nitrazine paper (see Chap. 80). Supplementary acidification (eg, ascorbic acid [vitamin C], 4–12 g/day in divided doses) may be prescribed as needed if urine pH exceeds 5.5.
Inform patient to avoid excessive intake of alkalinizing foods such as milk or citrus fruits.
Inform patient with liver dysfunction who is undergoing prolonged therapy that periodic liver function studies are recommended.
Instruct patient on possible adverse side effects with methenamine: nausea, vomiting, diarrhea, painful urination.
Teach patient measures that help prevent recurrence of urinary tract infections.

• Methylene Blue

Urolene Blue

Mechanism

Exerts a weak germicidal action; is primarily bacteriostatic; high concentrations convert the ferrous iron of reduced hemoglobin to the ferric state, resulting in formation of methemoglobin; this latter action is the basis for its use as an antidote in cyanide poisoning, because methemoglobin competes with cytochrome oxidase, a vital enzyme, for the cyanide ion, leading to formation of cyanmethemoglobin and the resulting preservation of cytochrome oxidase.

Uses

Symptomatic treatment of cystitis and urethritis (infrequent use)
Treatment of idiopathic and drug-induced methemoglobinemia and as an antidote for cyanide poisoning (IV)
Investigational uses include treatment of oxalate urinary tract calculi and diagnostic confirmation of rupture of amniotic membranes

Dosage

Oral: 55 to 130 mg 3 times/day
IV: 1 to 2 mg/kg injected over several minutes

Common Side Effects

Discoloration of the urine.

Significant Adverse Reactions

Nausea, vomiting, diarrhea, bladder irritation; large doses can cause abdominal pain, fever, dizziness, headache, sweating, confusion and cyanosis.

Contraindications

Renal insufficiency, intraspinal injection. *Cautious use* in patients with glucose-6-phosphate dehydrogenase deficiency, anemia, and decreased hemoglobin levels; IV use with caution in people with cardiovascular disease.

Nursing Management

Pretherapy Assessment

Assess and record baseline data necessary for detection of adverse effects of methylene blue: General: VS, body weight, skin color, temperature, and integrity, state of hydration; GI: biliary function; GU: renal function; CVS: hematologic function; CNS: neurologic function; Laboratory: urinalysis, liver function, serum electrolytes, culture of infected site.

Nursing Interventions

Medication Administration

Administer methylene blue on schedule to ensure stable steady-state concentrations for the duration of therapy.

Surveillance During Therapy

Manage GI side effects (nausea, vomiting, diarrhea) symptomatically.
Monitor for adverse effects, toxicity, and interactions.
Monitor intake and output.

Patient Teaching

Instruct patient to take oral drug after meals with a full glass of water.
Inform patient that drug may discolor urine and possibly the stool blue-green.

• Nitrofurantoin

Furadantin, Furanite, Nitrofan

(CAN) Apo-Nitrofurantoin, Nephronex, Novofuran, Nu-Nifed

• Nitrofurantoin Macrocrystals

Macrodantin

A synthetic nitrofuran derivative, nitrofurantoin is a specific urinary antibacterial agent effective against a range of gram-positive and gram-negative organisms. The macrocrystalline dosage form is most often preferred, because it causes less GI distress than the normal oral dosage forms.

Mechanism

Bacteriostatic in low concentrations and bactericidal in higher concentrations; probable mechanism is interference with carbohydrate metabolism by inhibition of acetyl coenzyme A; may also impair bacterial cell wall formation; most effective against *E coli*, *Klebsiella*, *Enterobacter*, and *Citrobacter* sp, group B streptococci, enterococci, and staphylococci; some strains of *Enterobacter* and *Klebsiella* are resistant, as are most strains of *Proteus*, *Serratia*, and *Acinetobacter*; *Pseudomonas* is highly resistant; acquired resistance of susceptible organisms is minimal.

Uses

Treatment of urinary tract infections due to susceptible organisms
Prophylaxis against recurrent bacteriuria (Macrodantin—small dose)

Dosage

Adults: 50 to 100 mg four times a day orally for 10 to 14 days; long-term therapy 50 to 100 mg once daily at bedtime
Children (older than 3 months): 5 to 7 mg/kg/day in 4 divided doses
Prophylaxis of recurrent infections (Macrodantin): 50 mg daily at bedtime for at least 6 months

Fate

Well absorbed orally (macrocrystalline form is absorbed more slowly than other oral forms but causes less GI distress); absorption is *enhanced* by ingestion of food; therapeutic serum and tissue levels are not attained, except in the urinary tract; plasma half-life is 15 to 30 minutes; approximately half of a dose is rapidly inactivated in body tissues and excreted in the urine and bile, the remainder is eliminated unchanged in the urine; activity is increased in an acid urine.

Common Side Effects

Nausea, anorexia, vomiting.

Significant Adverse Reactions

GI: diarrhea, abdominal pain, pancreatitis, parotitis
Pulmonary: chills, cough, chest pain, dyspnea, pulmonary infiltration with consolidation or pleural effusion, diffuse interstitial pneumonitis or fibrosis (with prolonged therapy)
Dermatologic: rash, pruritus, urticaria, angioedema, alopecia; *rarely*, exfoliative dermatitis, erythema multiforme
Hematologic: hemolytic anemia, megaloblastic anemia, leukopenia, granulocytopenia, eosinophilia, thrombocytopenia, agranulocytosis
Allergic: drug fever, asthmatic attack, cholestatic jaundice, arthralgia, anaphylaxis
Neurologic: dizziness, paresthesias, headache, drowsiness, nystagmus, peripheral neuropathy
Other: hypotension, myalgia, superinfections, tooth staining from oral suspension

Contraindications

Anuria, oliguria, significant renal impairment (creatinine clearance less than 40 mL/min) and pregnancy at term; in infants younger than 3 months (possibility of hemolytic anemia due to immature enzyme systems). *Cautious use* in the presence of anemia, chronic lung disease, vitamin B deficiency, electrolyte imbalances, hepatic disease, glucose-6-phosphate dehydrogenase deficiency, and in pregnant or nursing women.

Interactions

Nitrofurantoin can antagonize the action of nalidixic acid.
Acidifying agents (eg, ammonium chloride, ascorbic acid) may potentiate nitrofurantoin, whereas alkalinizing agents (eg, acetazolamide, sodium bicarbonate) can reduce its effectiveness.
Probenecid reduces the renal clearance of nitrofurantoin, and may increase its toxicity.
Antacids can reduce the effectiveness of nitrofurantoin by impairing its GI absorption.
Anticholinergics, other GI antispasmodic drugs, and food may increase GI absorption of nitrofurantoin by prolonging gastric emptying time.

Nursing Management

Pretherapy Assessment

Assess and record baseline data necessary for detection of adverse effects of nitrofurantoin: General: VS, body weight, skin color, temperature, and integrity, state of hydration; GI: biliary function; GU: renal function; CVS: hematologic function; CNS: neurologic function; Laboratory: urinalysis, liver function, serum electrolytes, glucose, culture of infected site.
Review medical history and documents for existing or previous conditions that:

a. require cautious use of nitrofurantoin: anemia, chronic lung disease, vitamin B deficiency, electrolyte imbalances, hepatic disease, glucose-6-phosphate dehydrogenase deficiency.
b. contraindicate use of nitrofurantoin: allergy to nitrofurantoin; anuria; significant renal impairment (creatinine clearance less than 40 mL/min; infants

younger than 3 months; **pregnancy (Category B)**; lactation (significant concentrations appear in breast milk, safety not established, avoid use in nursing mothers).

Nursing Interventions

Medication Administration

Administer oral form of drug with meals, with a full glass of water. Use of macrocrystalline dosage form further minimizes GI upset.

Administer nitrofurantoin on schedule to ensure stable steady-state concentrations for the duration of therapy.

Initiate a meal schedule that provides small, frequent meals if GI upset occurs.

Arrange to continue nitrofurantoin for 3 days after a sterile urine specimen is achieved.

Protect drug from light to prevent darkening and possible loss of potency.

Surveillance During Therapy

Monitor for development of acute pulmonary sensitivity reaction during early days (up to 3 weeks) of therapy. Common symptoms are fever, chills, cough, dyspnea, chest pain, and eosinophilia. Discontinuation of drug usually results in rapid resolution of symptoms.

Monitor during prolonged therapy for insidious development of subacute or chronic pulmonary reactions (cough, malaise, dyspnea on exertion, radiographic findings of diffuse pneumonitis or pulmonary fibrosis). Early recognition is important in preventing serious pulmonary impairment.

Monitor results of hematologic evaluations and liver function tests, which should be performed periodically during extended therapy because hemolytic anemia and hepatitis have occurred.

Monitor intake–output, and assess patient for signs of renal impairment (oliguria, anuria, creatinine clearance below 40 mL/min). If these are present, therapy should be terminated to minimize risk of serious toxicity.

Monitor for signs of urinary tract superinfection, which, during nitrofurantoin therapy, is most commonly caused by *Pseudomonas*.

Monitor intake–output, observing for dehydration secondary to gastrointestinal side effects (vomiting, diarrhea).

Monitor for signs of superinfection involving the oral and vaginal mucous membranes and fungal organisms.

Monitor CBC, urinalysis, and liver and kidney function test results obtained over the course of therapy.

Interpret results of diagnostic tests and contact practitioner as appropriate.

Monitor for possible drug–laboratory test interaction: false-positive elevation of serum glucose, bilirubin, alkaline phosphatase, blood urea nitrogen, urinary creatinine; false-positive urine glucose with Benedict reagent.

Monitor for possible drug–drug and drug–nutrient interactions: delayed or decreased absorption when taken with magnesium trisilicate, magaldrate; nitrofurantoin can antagonize the action of nalidixic acid; acidifying agents (eg, ammonium chloride, ascorbic acid) may potentiate nitrofurantoin, whereas alkalinizing agents (eg, acetazolamide, sodium bicarbonate) can reduce its effectiveness; probenecid reduces the renal clearance of nitrofurantoin, and may increase its toxicity; antacids can reduce the effectiveness of nitrofurantoin by impairing its GI absorption; anticholinergics, other GI antispasmodic drugs, and food may increase GI absorption of nitrofurantoin by prolonging gastric emptying time.

Patient Teaching

Instruct patient regarding the importance of completing the full course of therapy as prescribed; that is, not to discontinue the drug once signs and symptoms of the infection being treated subside.

Inform patient of the consequences of not taking or abruptly discontinuing the nitrofurantoin.

Instruct patient that the prescribed drug is to be taken for the condition for which it is prescribed, and not to be used to treat any other infections.

Instruct patient about possible adverse side effects of nitrofurantoin: nausea, vomiting, diarrhea; drowsiness; blurring of vision; dizziness; brown or yellow-rust discoloration to urine.

Instruct patient on appropriate action to take if side effects occur:

- Notify practitioner if early signs of hematologic or hepatic toxicity (sore throat, fever, mucosal ulceration, malaise, pallor, jaundice) occur.
- Notify practitioner of any unusual bleeding. Rationale: hypoprothrombinemia and bleeding tendencies due to decreased synthesis of vitamin K by intestinal microflora may occur.
- Notify practitioner if fever and chills, cough, chest pain or difficulty breathing, rash, numbness or tingling of fingers or toes occur.

Teach patient measures that help prevent recurrence of urinary tract infections.

Instruct patient to rinse mouth thoroughly after using oral suspension to prevent staining of the teeth.

• Trimethoprim

Proloprim, Trimpex

A synthetic antibacterial agent, trimethoprim has demonstrated activity against common urinary tract pathogens, *except Pseudomonas aeruginosa*.

Mechanism

Blocks production of tetrahydrofolic acid by reversible inhibition of dihydrofolate reductase, thus interfering with synthesis of proteins and nucleic acids in susceptible bacteria; acts synergistically with sulfonamides (see trimethoprim–sulfamethoxazole, Chapter 59).

Use

Treatment of initial episodes of uncomplicated urinary tract infections due to susceptible strains of *E coli*, *Proteus mirabilis*, *Klebsiella pneumoniae*, *Enterobacter* sp, and coagulase-negative *Staphylococcus* sp.

Dosage

Adults and children (> 12 years): 100 mg every 12 hours for 10 days, or 200 mg once daily.

Fate

Rapidly absorbed orally; peak serum levels occur in 1 to 4 hours; half-life is 8 to 10 hours; about half is protein bound in plasma; excreted in the urine, largely as unmetabolized drug, 50% to 60% of an oral dose within 24 hours.

Common Side Effect

Pruritic rash.

Significant Adverse Reactions

GI: epigastric distress, nausea, vomiting, glossitis
Dermatologic: maculopapular or morbilliform rash, exfoliative dermatitis
Hematologic: thrombocytopenia, leukopenia, neutropenia, megaloblastic anemia, methemoglobinemia
Other: fever; elevations in blood urea nitrogen, serum creatinine, serum transaminase, and bilirubin

Contraindications

Megaloblastic anemia due to folate deficiency, severe renal impairment (creatinine clearance below 15 mL/min). *Cautious use* in patients with liver impairment, reduced renal function, folate deficiency, and in pregnant or nursing women.

Interactions

Trimethoprim may potentiate the action of oral anticoagulants and possibly phenytoin owing to impairment of hepatic metabolism.

Nursing Management

Pretherapy Assessment

Assess and record baseline data necessary for detection of adverse effects of trimethoprim: General: VS, body weight, skin color, temperature, and integrity, state of hydration; GI: mucous membranes, biliary function; GU: renal function; CVS: hematologic function; CNS: neurologic function; Laboratory: urinalysis, liver function, culture of infected site.

Review medical history and documents for existing or previous conditions that:

a. require cautious use of trimethoprim: anemia, blood dyscrasias, hepatic disease, folate deficiency, reduced renal function.
b. contraindicate use of trimethoprim: allergy to trimethoprim; megaloblastic anemia; significant renal impairment (creatinine clearance less than 15 mL/min; **pregnancy (Category C)**; lactation (significant concentrations appear in breast milk, safety not established; may interfere with folic acid metabolism in the neonate, avoid use in nursing mothers).

Nursing Interventions

Medication Administration

Administer oral form of drug with meals, with a full glass of water.

Administer trimethoprim on schedule to ensure stable steady-state concentrations for the duration of therapy.

Initiate a meal schedule that provides small, frequent meals if GI upset occurs.

Protect drug (200-mg dosage form) from strong light to prevent darkening and possible loss of potency.

Note that trimethoprim is available in combination with sulfamethoxazole (Bactrim, Septra) for treatment of both acute and chronic urinary infections, acute otitis media, acute exacerbations of chronic bronchitis, and enteritis (see Chapter 59).

Surveillance During Therapy

Monitor results of hematologic evaluations and liver function tests, which should be performed periodically during extended therapy because of the risk of megaloblastic anemia.

Monitor intake–output, and assess patient for signs of renal impairment (oliguria, anuria, creatinine clearance below 15 mL/min). If these are present, therapy should be terminated to minimize risk of serious toxicity.

Monitor intake–output, observing for dehydration secondary to gastrointestinal side effects (vomiting, diarrhea).

Monitor CBC, urinalysis, and liver and kidney function test results obtained over the course of therapy.

Monitor for signs of superinfection involving the oral and vaginal mucous membranes and fungal organisms.

Monitor results of complete blood counts, which should be performed during prolonged therapy. If signs of bone marrow depression are noted (thrombocytopenia, leukopenia, megaloblastic anemia), the drug should be discontinued, and 3 to 6 mg of leucovorin should be administered intramuscularly daily for 3 days to restore normal hematopoiesis.

Interpret results of diagnostic tests and contact practitioner as appropriate.

Monitor for possible drug–drug and drug–nutrient interactions: may potentiate the actions of oral anticoagulants and phenytoin owing to impairment of hepatic metabolism.

Patient Teaching

Instruct patient regarding the importance of completing the full course of therapy as prescribed; that is, not to discontinue the drug once signs and symptoms of the infection being treated subside.

Inform patient of the consequences of not taking or abruptly discontinuing the trimethoprim.

Instruct patient that the prescribed drug is to be taken for the condition for which it is prescribed, and not to be used to treat any other infections.

Instruct patient about possible adverse side effects of trimethoprim: epigastric distress, nausea, vomiting, diarrhea, skin rash.

Instruct patient on appropriate action to take if side effects occur:

Notify practitioner if early signs of hematologic or hepatic toxicity (sore throat, fever, mucosal ulceration, malaise, pallor, jaundice) occur.

Notify practitioner of any unusual bleeding. Rationale: hypoprothrombinemia and bleeding tendencies due

to decreased synthesis of vitamin K by intestinal microflora may occur.
Notify practitioner if fever and chills, cough, sore throat; unusual bleeding or bruising; dizziness, headaches; skin rash occur.
Teach patient measures that help prevent recurrence of urinary tract infections.

Urinary Analgesic

• *Phenazopyridine*

Pyridium, and other manufacturers

(CAN) Phenazo, Pyronium

Phenazopyridine is an azo dye that is excreted in the urine, where it exerts a mild analgesic action. It is usually given in combination with a urinary anti-infective, most often a sulfonamide.

Mechanism

Not established; may exert a local anesthetic effect on mucosal membranes.

Uses

Symptomatic relief of pain, burning, irritation, and urinary urgency or frequency resulting from lower urinary tract infections, trauma, surgery, or endoscopic procedures

Dosage

Adults: 200 mg three times a day
Children 6 to 12 years of age: 100 mg three times a day

Fate

Adequately absorbed orally; partially metabolized, but mainly excreted unchanged in the urine.

Significant Adverse Reactions

Rare—GI distress, hemolytic anemia, methemoglobinemia, renal or hepatic damage.

Contraindications

Renal insufficiency, uremia, and chronic glomerulonephritis.

Nursing Management

Pretherapy Assessment

Assess and record baseline data necessary for detection of adverse effects of phenazopyridine: General: VS, body weight, skin color, temperature, and integrity, state of hydration; GI: mucous membranes, biliary function; GU: renal function; CVS: hematologic function; CNS: neurologic function; Laboratory: urinalysis, liver function, culture of infected site.
Review medical history and documents for existing or previous conditions that:
a. require cautious use of phenazopyridine: anemia, blood dyscrasias, hepatic disease, folate deficiency, reduced renal function.
b. contraindicate use of phenazopyridine: allergy to phenazopyridine; megaloblastic anemia; significant renal impairment (creatinine clearance less than 15 mL/min); uremia; chronic glomerulonephritis; **pregnancy (Category B)**.

Nursing Interventions

Medication Administration

Administer oral form of drug after meals, with a full glass of water to avoid GI upset.
Administer phenazopyridine on schedule to ensure stable steady-state concentrations for the duration of therapy.
Initiate a meal schedule that provides small, frequent meals if GI upset occurs.
Do not administer for longer than 2 days when used in combination with antibacterial in treatment of urinary tract infection.
Note that phenazopyridine is available in fixed combination with sulfamethoxazole (Azo Gantanol), and sulfisoxazole (Azo Gantrisin).

Surveillance During Therapy

Monitor for toxicity and interactions.
Monitor intake–output, observing for dehydration secondary to GI side effects (vomiting, diarrhea).
Monitor intake–output, and assess patient for signs of renal impairment (oliguria, anuria, creatinine clearance below 15 mL/min).
Monitor CBC, urinalysis, and liver and kidney function test results obtained over the course of therapy.
Interpret results of diagnostic tests and contact practitioner as appropriate.
Monitor for signs of superinfection.
Interpret laboratory test results based on urinary colorimetric procedures cautiously because the drug can interfere with them.

Patient Teaching

Instruct patient regarding the importance of completing the full course of therapy as prescribed; that is, not to discontinue the drug once signs and symptoms of the infection being treated subside.
Inform patient of the consequences of not taking or abruptly discontinuing the phenazopyridine.
Instruct patient that the prescribed drug is to be taken for the condition for which it is prescribed, and not to be used to treat any other infections.
Instruct patient about possible adverse side effects of phenazopyridine: red-orange discoloration of urine (which may stain fabrics).
Instruct patient on appropriate action to take if side effects occur:
Notify practitioner if early signs of hematologic or hepatic toxicity (sore throat, fever, mucosal ulceration, malaise, pallor, jaundice) occur.
Notify practitioner of any unusual bleeding. Rationale: hypoprothrombinemia and bleeding tendencies due to decreased synthesis of vitamin K by intestinal microflora may occur.
Notify practitioner if fever, sore throat; unusual bleeding or bruising; dizziness; headaches; skin rash; yellowing of the skin or eyes occur.
Teach patient measures that help prevent recurrence of urinary tract infections.

Urease Inhibitor

• Acetohydroxamic acid

(Pregnancy Category X)

Lithostat

Acetohydroxamic acid is used to enhance the effectiveness of antimicrobial agents used to treat chronic urinary infections resulting from urea-splitting organisms.

Mechanism

Inhibits the bacterial enzyme urease, thus retarding hydrolysis of urea to ammonia in the presence of urea-splitting organisms; decreased ammonia levels and reduced pH enhance the action of antimicrobial agents and improve the cure rate; the drug does not acidify the urine directly, nor does it possess an antibacterial action.

Uses

Adjunctive treatment of urinary infections due to urea-splitting organisms (*not* indicated in place of appropriate antimicrobial therapy).

Dosage

Adults: 250 mg three to four times/day to a maximum of 12 mg/kg/day
Children: 10 mg/kg/day, initially, in divided doses; titrated to desired response

Fate

Well absorbed orally; peak blood levels occur within 1 hour; plasma half-life is approximately 5 to 10 hours in patients with normal renal function and is prolonged in persons with impaired renal function; one third to two thirds of a dose, which constitutes the active fraction of the drug, is excreted unchanged in the urine.

Common Side Effects

Headache (30%); anxiety, nervousness, mild tremor, depression, nausea, vomiting, anorexia, malaise (20%); reticulocytosis (5%).

Significant Adverse Reactions

Hemolytic anemia, superficial phlebitis, palpitations, nonpruritic skin rash, alopecia, teratogenicity.

Contraindications

Decreased renal function (serum creatinine greater than 2.5 mg/dL), urinary infections due to *non*–urease-producing organisms, pregnancy, and women not using contraceptive methods. *Cautious use* in patients with anemia, blood dyscrasias, bone marrow depression, thrombophlebitis, skin rash, depression, and in nursing mothers.

Interactions

Alcohol has produced a rash in the presence of acetohydroxamic acid.
Acetohydroxamic acid can reduce oral absorption of iron by forming a chelate with the metal.

Nursing Management

Pretherapy Assessment

Assess and record baseline data necessary for detection of adverse effects of acetohydroxamic acid: General: VS, body weight, skin color, temperature, and integrity, state of hydration; GI: mucous membranes, biliary function; GU: renal function; CVS: hematologic function; CNS: neurologic function; Laboratory: urinalysis, liver function, culture of infected site (presence of a urease active bacteria).

Review medical history and documents for existing or previous conditions that:

a. require cautious use of acetohydroxamic acid: anemia, blood dyscrasias, bone marrow depression, thrombophlebitis, skin rash, depression.
b. contraindicate use of acetohydroxamic acid: allergy to acetohydroxamic acid; megaloblastic anemia; significant renal impairment (serum creatine less than 2.5 mg/dL); uremia; urinary infections due to *non*–urease-producing organisms; **pregnancy (Category X)**; lactation (safety not established, do not use in nursing mothers).

Nursing Interventions

Medication Administration

Administer oral form of drug 1 or 2 hours after meals, with a full glass of water to avoid GI upset.

Administer acetohydroxamic acid on schedule to ensure stable steady-state concentrations for the duration of therapy.

Initiate a meal schedule that provides small, frequent meals if GI upset occurs.

Surveillance During Therapy

Monitor intake–output, observing for dehydration secondary to GI side effects (vomiting, diarrhea).

Monitor results of CBC, which should be performed 2 weeks after beginning therapy and every 3 months thereafter. If reticulocyte count is greater than 6%, dosage should be reduced. Most patients manifest a *mild* reticulosis, but hemolytic anemia occurs in about 30% of patients, usually accompanied by nausea, vomiting, anorexia, and malaise.

Monitor for renal impairment and signs of overdose because drug is eliminated primarily by the kidneys.

Monitor for signs of superinfection involving the oral and vaginal mucous membranes and fungal organisms.

Monitor CBC, urinalysis, and liver and kidney function test results obtained over the course of therapy.

Interpret results of diagnostic tests and contact practitioner as appropriate.

Monitor for possible drug–drug interactions: rash occurs if taken concurrently with alcohol ingestion; absorption decreased when taken with iron supplements (chelation effect).

Patient Teaching

Instruct patient regarding the importance of completing the full course of therapy as prescribed; that is, not to discontinue the drug once signs and symptoms of the infection being treated subside.

Inform patient of the consequences of not taking or abruptly discontinuing the acetohydroxamic acid.

Instruct patient that the prescribed drug is to be taken for the condition for which it is prescribed, and not to be used to treat any other infections.

Inform women of childbearing potential receiving the drug to use appropriate contraceptive measures because the drug may cause fetal damage.

Inform patient that headache is very common during the first 48 to 72 hours of treatment, but that it usually disappears spontaneously. Mild analgesics may be used if necessary.

Inform patient that alcohol ingestion during therapy often results in development of a nonpruritic macular skin rash, which may range from mild and transient to severe.

Inform patient taking oral iron supplement that iron absorption is impaired by acetohydroxamic acid. If iron is necessary, parenteral iron is recommended.

Prepare patient supportively and with reassurance, as indicated, for the possibility that treatment may be lengthy because it must continue until the urea-splitting organism is eradicated.

Instruct patient on appropriate action to take if side effects occur:

Notify practitioner if early signs of hematologic or hepatic toxicity (sore throat, fever, mucosal ulceration, malaise, pallor, jaundice) occur.

Notify practitioner of any unusual bleeding. Rationale: hypoprothrombinemia and bleeding tendencies due to decreased synthesis of vitamin K by intestinal microflora may occur.

Notify practitioner if unusual bleeding or bruising; malaise; lethargy; leg pain or swelling of lower limbs; severe nausea and vomiting occur.

Teach patient measures that help prevent recurrence of urinary tract infections.

Selected Bibliography

Andriole VT: Urinary tract agents: nitrofurantoin and methenamine. In Mandell GL, Douglas RG, Bennett JE (eds): Principles and Practice of Infectious Diseases, 3rd ed, p 345. New York, Churchill-Livingstone, 1990

Baldassarre JS, Kaye D: Special problems of urinary tract infection in the elderly. Med Clin North Am 75:375, 1991

Norrby SR: Short-term treatment of uncomplicated lower urinary tract infections in women. Rev Infect Dis 12:458, 1990

Rubin RH, Shapiro ED, et al: Evaluation of new anti-infective drugs for the treatment of urinary tract infection. Clin Infect Dis 15(Suppl 1):216, 1992

Stamm WE, Hooton TM: Management of urinary tract infections in adults. N Engl J Med 329:1328, 1993

Nursing Bibliography

Garibaldi R: Catheter associated urinary tract infection. Current Opinion in Infectious Diseases 5:517, 1992

Scheck D: Lower urinary tract infections in women: A pragmatic approach. Hospital Medicine 29(5):41, 1993

The prevention and management of urinary tract infections among people with spinal cord injuries. SCI Nursing 10(2):49, 1993

Tucker M: Recurrent UTI: Who should treat herself. Patient Care 26(12): 259, 1992

67
Miscellaneous Antibiotics

Atovaquone
Chloramphenicol

Lincosamides

- Clindamycin
- Lincomycin

Clofazimine
Dapsone
Eflornithine
Furazolidone
Nitrofurazone
Novobiocin
Pentamidine
Spectinomycin
Trimetrexate
Vancomycin

A number of antimicrobial drugs in clinical use cannot be precisely categorized according to their chemical structure or biologic activity. These drugs are most conveniently grouped under a miscellaneous heading and are reviewed here individually.

• Atovaquone

Mepron

Atovaquone is classified as an antiprotozoal drug and exhibits activity against *Pneumocystis carinii*, the organism that frequently causes pneumonitis in human immunodeficiency virus (HIV)-infected people.

Mechanism

Not completely established; in protozoans such as *Plasmodium* sp, atovaquone inhibits electron transport activity and the function of cytochrome enzymes that are essential for cellular activity.

Uses

Treatment of mild to moderate *Pneumocystis carinii* pneumonia (PCP) in patients who do not tolerate trimethoprim–sulfamethoxazole.

Dosage

Adults: 750 mg orally with food 3 times a day for 21 days. NOTE: Food increases bioavailability significantly; failure to take with food will lower plasma drug levels and the therapeutic effect.

Fate

Atovaquone is highly lipid soluble, administration with food increases bioavailability threefold; drug undergoes enterohepatic cycling, which contributes to a secondary peak plasma concentration between 24 and 96 hours after administration; drug metabolism is minimal; excretion is predominantly in the feces; half-life ranges between 2 and 3 days.

Common Side Effects

Nausea, headache, dizziness, rash, fever.

Significant Adverse Reactions

Vomiting, diarrhea, abdominal pain, insomnia, elevation of liver enzymes and other laboratory values (creatinine, blood urea nitrogen [BUN], amylase), anemia, neutropenia.

Contraindications

No specific contraindications other than the development of allergy.

Interactions

Atovaquone is highly protein bound and caution must be exercised when other highly bound drugs are administered concurrently.

Nursing Management

Pretherapy Assessment

Assess and record baseline data necessary for detection of adverse effects of atovaquone: General: vital signs (VS), body weight, skin color, temperature, and integrity; Gastrointestinal (GI): output, absorption disorders; Genitourinary (GU): renal function (urinalysis, BUN, creatinine); Cardiovascular system (CVS): hematologic function; Laboratory: renal and hepatic function tests, complete blood count (CBC), hematocrit.

Review medical history and documents for existing or previous conditions that:

a. require cautious use of atovaquone: impaired hepatic or biliary function; breast feeding.
b. contraindicate use of atovaquone: allergy to any component of the formulation; **pregnancy (Category C)**.

Nursing Interventions

Medication Administration

Administer oral form of drug with food; food enhances the absorption of this drug threefold; failure to administer with food may limit the patient's response to the drug.

Administer drug three times a day (total daily dose, 2250 mg) for 21 days.

Surveillance During Therapy

Monitor for toxicity and interactions.

Monitor for presence of severe headache, maculopapular rash, diarrhea, vomiting, stomatitis (oral *Candida* infection), or fever.

Monitor for signs of hypersensitivity, which may require discontinuation of drug.

Monitor CBC, urinalysis, and liver and kidney function test results obtained over the course of therapy.

Interpret results of diagnostic tests and contact practitioner as appropriate.
Monitor intake–output, observing for signs and symptoms of possible renal impairment and dehydration secondary to GI side effects (vomiting, diarrhea).
Provide for patient safety needs to minimize risk of injury if CNS side effects develop.
Initiate interventions to minimize environmental hazards.

Patient Teaching

Instruct patient regarding the importance of completing the full course of therapy as prescribed, that is, not to discontinue the drug once signs and symptoms of the infection being treated subside.
Inform patient of the consequences of not taking or abruptly discontinuing the atovaquone.
Instruct patient that the prescribed drug is to be taken for the condition for which it is prescribed, and not to be used to treat any other infections.

• Chloramphenicol

Ak-Chlor, Chloromycetin, Chloroptic

(CAN) Nova Phenicol, Ophtho-Chloram, Sopamycetin

Chloramphenicol is a synthetic, broad-spectrum, bacteriostatic antibiotic effective against a wide range of gram-positive and gram-negative bacteria, rickettsiae, and chlamydiae. Its potential for eliciting serious toxicity, however, largely restricts its systemic use to *severe* infections in which other, less toxic drugs are ineffective or contraindicated. The drug is also commonly used locally in the eye for treating superficial ocular infections and in the ear for infections of the external auditory canal. Currently, it is considered to be the drug of choice for acute *Salmonella typhi* infections (typhoid fever), but it should not be used for routine treatment of the typhoid "carrier state." Other organisms against which it is quite active are *Haemophilus influenzae*, *Bacteroides fragilis*, other *Salmonella* sp, rickettsiae, the lymphogranuloma–psittacosis group, and various gram-negative bacteria causing bacteremia or meningitis. The major danger associated with chloramphenicol is bone marrow depression, and fatal blood dyscrasias have occurred after both short-term and long-term use. Frequent blood studies are therefore essential during its administration. Other untoward reactions noted with chloramphenicol are neurotoxicity and the gray syndrome in newborns (see Adverse Reactions). Although it is a valuable antiinfective for certain severe infections, chloramphenicol should never be used for minor infections (eg, colds, flu, throat infections) or as a prophylactic agent.

Mechanism

Binds to the 50S ribosomal subunits of bacteria, preventing binding of tRNA to the ribosome; inhibits synthesis of bacterial protein by cellular ribosomes; bacteriostatic at normal concentrations.

Uses

Treatment of acute infections caused by *Salmonella typhi* (drug of choice)
Alternative treatment of severe infections due to susceptible organisms for which less toxic drugs are ineffective or contraindicated (see Chapter 58, Table 58-1). Principal indications include *Haemophilus influenzae* meningitis, pneumococcal or meningococcal meningitis in penicillin-sensitive patients, *Bacteroides fragilis* infections, and rickettsial infections in tetracycline-sensitive patients.
Adjunctive therapy in cystic fibrosis regimens
Treatment of superficial infections of the eye and external auditory canal due to susceptible microorganisms (topical application only)

Dosage

Oral, IV

Adults and children: 50 mg/kg/day in divided doses every 6 hours (maximum 100 mg/kg/day)
Newborns and infants with immature metabolic processes: 25 mg/kg/day in four equally divided doses

Ophthalmic

1 or 2 drops or small amount of ointment to infected eye two to four times a day

Otic

2 to 3 drops three times a day

Fate

Rapidly absorbed orally; peak serum levels occur in 1 to 2 hours; distribution is variable—highest concentrations occur in the liver and kidney, whereas lowest amounts are found in the brain and cerebrospinal fluid (about one half the levels in the blood); approximately 50% to 60% protein bound; elimination half-life is 3 to 4 hours; metabolized by the liver and excreted in the urine, largely as glucuronic acid conjugate, with small amounts (8%–12%) of unchanged drug; minor quantities of active drug are found in the bile and feces; readily crosses the placental barrier and appears in breast milk.

Common Side Effects

GI distress.

Significant Adverse Reactions

CAUTION

Serious and potentially fatal blood dyscrasias (eg, aplastic anemia, thrombocytopenia, granulocytopenia) have occurred with both short-term and prolonged use of chloramphenicol. Thus, it should be used only in severe infections unresponsive to other, less hazardous antibiotics, and careful blood studies should be performed at least every 2 days during therapy. A dose-related *reversible* type of bone marrow depression may occur during treatment. It is readily detectable by blood studies, and responds promptly to discontinuation of the drug. An *irreversible* type of bone marrow depression, leading to aplastic anemia that may terminate in leukemia with a high mortality rate has also been reported (1:25,000–40,000), but does not appear to be dose related. It may occur weeks or even months after therapy and is characterized by bone marrow aplasia or hypoplasia. Most importantly, it is not readily predictable by routine blood studies performed *during* treatment. Follow-up blood tests and close observation of the patient are necessary.

Hematologic: blood dyscrasias (leukopenia, reduction in erythrocytes, granulocytopenia, hypoplastic anemia, thrombocytopenia, aplastic anemia)
Neurologic: headache, confusion, depression, delirium, optic and peripheral neuritis
Allergic–hypersensitivity: fever, rash, urticaria, angioedema, anaphylaxis; itching or burning with topical application
GI: vomiting, glossitis, stomatitis, diarrhea, enterocolitis (rare)
Other: jaundice, superinfections, *gray syndrome* in premature infants and newborns (abdominal distention, emesis, pallid cyanosis, vasomotor collapse, irregular respiration, hypothermia; occurs within 3 or 4 days, usually after initiation of high-dosage therapy within the first 48 hours of life and can be fatal)

Contraindications

Treatment of trivial infections (colds, flu, sore throat), prophylactic use, infections other than those indicated as susceptible by testing, and concurrent therapy with other bone marrow-depressive drugs. *Cautious use* in patients with renal or hepatic impairment, glucose-6-phosphate dehydrogenase (G-6-PD) deficiency, acute intermittent porphyria; in infants and in pregnant or nursing women.

Repeated courses of therapy should be avoided; do not extend treatment longer than the time required to effect a cure with little risk of relapse (eg, a normal temperature for 48 hours).

Interactions

Chloramphenicol can inhibit the metabolism of oral anticoagulants, oral hypoglycemics, cyclophosphamide, barbiturates, and phenytoin, thus potentiating their effects.
Chloramphenicol may inhibit the hematinic activity of vitamin B_{12}, folic acid, and iron.
The bactericidal action of other antibiotics (eg, penicillins) may be reduced by chloramphenicol.
Chloramphenicol can interfere with the immune response to diphtheria and tetanus toxoids.
Concomitant administration of acetaminophen may elevate serum levels of chloramphenicol.
A disulfiram-like reaction to alcohol may occur with use of chloramphenicol (see Chapter 81).

Nursing Management

Pretherapy Assessment

Assess and record baseline data necessary for detection of adverse effects of chloramphenicol: General: VS, body weight, skin color, temperature, and integrity; GI: biliary function; GU: renal function (urinalysis, BUN, creatinine); CVS: hematologic; CNS: neurologic function; Laboratory: culture of infected site.
Review medical history and documents for existing or previous conditions that:
a. require cautious use of chloramphenicol: impaired renal or hepatic function; G-6-PD deficiency (risk of hemolytic anemia); acute intermittent porphyria; use in infants.
b. contraindicate use of chloramphenicol: allergy to chloramphenicol; treatment of trivial infections; when used with other bone marrow-suppressive agents; **pregnancy (Category C)**; lactation (significant concentrations appear in breast milk, producing an increased neonatal risk for gray syndrome).

Nursing Interventions

Medication Administration

Administer oral form of drug on an empty stomach (1 hour before or 2 hours after meals), with a full glass of water.
Administer chloramphenicol on schedule to ensure stable steady-state concentrations for the duration of therapy.
Reduce the risk of stomatitis through frequent mouth care.
Initiate a meal schedule that provides small, frequent meals if GI upset occurs.
Provide ready access to bathroom and interventions directed at symptom relief if diarrhea occurs.
Do not give IM because drug is ineffective by this route.
Arrange for dosage reduction in patients with renal or hepatic disease.
Note that chloramphenicol *base* solution is used by IV infusion in adults only, whereas the *sodium succinate salt* may be given by slow (1–2 min) IV injection to both adults and children. Oral dosage should be substituted as soon as possible.

Surveillance During Therapy

Monitor for presence of severe headache, rhinitis, urticaria, conjunctivitis, stomatitis, or rash.
Monitor for signs of hypersensitivity, which may require discontinuation of drug.
Monitor hematologic data, especially with long-term therapy, for signs of bone marrow suppression; monitoring should be performed before initiation of therapy (baseline), at 48-hour intervals during therapy, and periodically for *several months* after termination. The drug should be discontinued immediately if any abnormality is noted.
Periodically monitor serum chloramphenicol concentrations to reduce the risk of blood dyscrasias in the adult and gray syndrome in the neonate; monitoring frequency should be weekly; therapeutic concentrations of chloramphenicol: peak: 10–20 μg/mL; trough: 5–10 μg/mL.
Monitor CBC, urinalysis, and liver and kidney function test results obtained over the course of therapy.
Interpret results of diagnostic tests and contact practitioner as appropriate.
Monitor intake–output, observing for signs and symptoms of possible renal impairment and dehydration secondary to GI side effects (vomiting, diarrhea).
Monitor for possible drug–drug and drug–nutrient interactions: increased serum concentrations and drug effects with oral anticoagulants, phenytoin, oral antihyperglycemics; decreased hematologic responsiveness to iron salts and vitamin B_{12}.
Provide for patient safety needs to minimize risk of injury if CNS side effects develop.
Initiate interventions to minimize environmental hazards.

Patient Teaching

Instruct patient regarding the importance of completing the full course of therapy as prescribed, that is, not to discontinue the drug once signs and symptoms of the infection being treated subside.
Inform patient of the consequences of not taking or abruptly discontinuing the chloramphenicol.
Instruct patient that the prescribed drug is to be taken for the condition for which it is prescribed, and not to be used to treat any other infections.
Instruct patient about possible adverse side effects of chloramphenicol: nausea; vomiting; diarrhea; headache; confusion; superinfection; hematologic disturbances.
Instruct patient on appropriate action to take if side effects occur:
  Notify practitioner if early signs of hematologic or hepatic toxicity (sore throat, fever, mucosal ulceration, malaise, pallor, jaundice) occur.
  Notify practitioner of any unusual bleeding. Rationale: hypoprothrombinemia and bleeding tendencies due to decreased synthesis of vitamin K by intestinal microflora may occur.
  Discontinue topically applied chloramphenicol at first sign of local irritation or other allergic reaction and notify practitioner.
  Notify practitioner of numbness, tingling, or pain in the extremities; pregnancy.
Inform patient with diabetes that dosage of antidiabetic agent (oral sulfonylureas) may need to be adjusted. Serum glucose level should be monitored.

• Lincosamides

Clindamycin
Lincomycin

Clindamycin and lincomycin are two chemically related, primarily bacteriostatic antibiotics frequently termed *lincosamides*. They exhibit antibacterial activity similar to but not identical to that of the erythromycins. Lincomycin and its chlorine-substituted derivative clindamycin are effective against most of the common gram-positive pathogens, particularly *Staphylococcus*, *Streptococcus*, *Corynebacterium*, and *Nocardia* sp, as well as many anaerobic organisms, such as *Bacteroides*, *Actinomyces*, *Propionibacterium*, and *Peptococcus* sp, and most strains of *Clostridium* (except *C difficile*). In contrast, most gram-negative organisms are resistant. Because of their toxic potential, however, lincomycin and clindamycin are usually recommended only for treatment of serious anaerobic infections for which penicillin or erythromycin are ineffective or inappropriate (eg, when penicillin hypersensitivity is present). The major dangers associated with use of clindamycin and lincomycin are related to the GI tract and include persistent, profuse diarrhea, severe abdominal cramping, and pseudomembranous colitis. These effects, although most frequent with systemic use, have occurred on topical application of clindamycin as well. Clindamycin usually is regarded as the preferred drug of the two for systemic use, because it is better absorbed orally, has a somewhat broader spectrum of action, including against *Bacteroides fragilis*, and is reported to elicit fewer GI side effects. In addition, clindamycin is commonly used as a topical solution for the management of acne because it exhibits good activity against *Propionibacterium*, the causative agent found in acne lesions.

Although the two drugs are sufficiently alike in their pharmacologic properties to be discussed together, some important differences do exist, and these are noted whenever appropriate in the following discussion. The two drugs are then listed in Table 67-1.

Mechanism

Interfere with protein synthesis in susceptible organisms by binding to the 50S subunits of bacterial ribosomes; resistance, possibly related to chromosomal alterations develops slowly; possess neuromuscular blocking activity; both drugs are active against most common gram-positive pathogens; clindamycin demonstrates a slightly wider range of action against anaerobic gram-positive organisms (eg, *Actinomyces*, *Peptococcus*, *Clostridium* sp, microaerophilic streptococci) and anaerobic gram-negative bacilli (eg, *Bacteroides*, *Fusobacterium* sp).

Uses

Alternative therapy for serious streptococcal, pneumococcal, or staphylococcal infections in patients in whom penicillins and erythromycins are ineffective or inappropriate
Alternative treatment of serious infections due to anaerobic organisms, such as *Bacteroides*, *Fusobacterium*, *Peptococcus*, or *Actinomyces* sp, in penicillin-sensitive patients (clindamycin is most effective)
Treatment of acne (topical application of clindamycin solution)
Treatment of acute pelvic inflammatory disease (eg, endometritis, pelvic cellulitis, nongonococcal tuboovarian abscess)

Dosage

See Table 67-1.

Fate

Oral absorption is rapid and virtually complete (90%) for clindamycin, whereas only about 20% to 30% of an oral dose of lincomycin is absorbed. Food markedly impairs absorption of lincomycin but not clindamycin. Peak plasma levels occur within 45 minutes with oral clindamycin and 2 to 4 hours with oral lincomycin. IM injection yields peak serum levels within 30 minutes with lincomycin and 1 to 3 hours with clindamycin. Plasma half-lives are 2 to 3 hours for clindamycin and 4 to 6 hours for lincomycin. Both drugs are widely distributed in the body and are approximately 70% protein bound. Effective antibacterial blood levels are maintained for 6 to 8 hours after oral administration, and up to 12 hours after IM injection or IV infusion; excreted in the urine, bile, and feces, primarily (90%) as inactive metabolites. Most of a dose of clindamycin is metabolized in the liver and excreted in the urine and bile. Less than 15% is eliminated unchanged by the kidneys. Lincomycin is partially metabolized in the liver and excreted both in the urine and the feces.

Common Side Effects

Nausea, diarrhea, skin rash.

Table 67-1. **Lincosamides**

Drug	*Usual Dosage Range*	*Nursing Considerations*
Clindamycin *Cleocin* *(CAN) Dalacin C*	*Oral* Adults: 150–450 mg every 6 h depending on severity of infection Children: 8–12 mg/kg/d in 3–4 divided doses (up to 25 mg/kg/d in severe infections) *IM, IV* Adults: 600–2700 mg/d in 2–4 equally divided doses depending on severity of infection Children > 1 mo: 15–40 mg/kg/d in 3–4 equal doses depending on severity of infection *or* 350–450 mg/m²/d *Acute pelvic inflammatory disease* 900 mg IV every 8 h *plus* gentamicin or tobramycin (2 mg/kg initially, followed by 1.5 mg/kg 3 times/d for 4 d). Continue clindamycin orally (450 mg 5 times/d for at least 10–14 d) *Topical (Cleocin-T)* Apply thin film to affected area twice a day	Do *not* use in children younger than 1 mo; minimum recommended oral dose in children weighing 10 kg or less is 37.5 mg 3 times a day; do *not* refrigerate reconstituted granules because mixture may thicken and become difficult to pour; solution is stable for 2 wk at room temperature; use parenteral therapy initially in children to treat anaerobic infections; follow with oral administration when appropriate; in severe infections children should receive no less than 300 mg a day parenterally, regardless of body weight; adults may be given up to 4.8 g a day IV in life-threatening infections; single IM injections of more than 600 mg are *not* recommended; do *not* give more than 1200 mg an hour by IV infusion; physically incompatible with ampicillin, phenytoin, aminophylline, barbiturates, calcium gluconate, and magnesium sulfate; applied topically to acne vulgaris lesions; alcohol base may be irritating to sensitive surfaces (eye, mucous membranes, wounds)
Lincomycin *Lincocin, Lincorex*	*Oral* Adults: 500 mg 3–4 times a day Children > 1 mo: 30–60 mg/kg/d in 3–4 divided doses *IM* Adults: 600 mg every 12–24 h Children > 1 mo: 10 mg/kg every 12–24 h *IV infusion* Adults: 600 mg–1 g every 8–12 h Children > 1 mo: 10–20 mg/kg/d in divided doses *Subconjunctival injection* 0.25 mL (75 mg)	Do *not* use in children younger than 1 mo; administer orally on an empty stomach; IM injections should be made deeply and slowly to minimize pain; severe cardiopulmonary reactions have occurred when drug has been given IV at higher than recommended doses or rates; in life-threatening situations, daily IV doses of up to 8 g have been used; dilute 1 g lincomycin in 100 mL of a compatible infusion solution (see package insert) and infuse over a period of not less than 1 h; repeat as often as needed to a maximum of 8 g a day; subconjunctival injection results in effective ocular fluid levels of antibiotic for 5 h; drug is incompatible with novobiocin and kanamycin, as well as phenytoin sodium and protein hydrolysates

Significant Adverse Reactions

CAUTION

Severe persistent diarrhea and pseudomembranous colitis, occasionally fatal, have occurred with these drugs. The colitis is probably caused by toxins secreted by resistant strains of *Clostridium difficile*. Do *not* use for minor infections, and discontinue drug if diarrhea, bloody stools, severe abdominal pain, or high fever occurs. Vancomycin, 2 g/day administered orally in divided doses, may be effective for *C difficile*-induced colitis (see Vancomycin, this chapter).

GI: vomiting, persistent or severe diarrhea, abdominal pain, glossitis, esophagitis, stomatitis, acute enterocolitis, or pseudomembranous colitis (occasionally fatal)

Hypersensitivity: urticaria, angioedema, serum sickness, erythema multiforme (rare), Stevens-Johnson syndrome (rare), exfoliative dermatitis (rare)

Hematologic: eosinophilia, infrequent blood dyscrasias (neutropenia, leukopenia, thrombocytopenia, agranulocytosis, aplastic anemia)

CV: hypotension (parenteral injection), cardiopulmonary arrest after IV injection

Other: vaginitis, pruritus ani, jaundice, abnormal liver function tests, tinnitus, vertigo, pain or induration on IM injection; topical application of clindamycin can result in contact dermatitis, skin dryness, oily skin, facial swelling, stinging sensation, gram-negative folliculitis

Contraindications

Minor systemic bacterial or viral infections or meningitis, pregnancy, liver disease; in nursing mothers and in neonates. *Cautious use* in patients with mild liver impairment, history of GI disease, asthma or other allergic diseases, or renal dysfunction; and in elderly or debilitated people.

Interactions

The activity of clindamycin and lincomycin may be antagonized by concurrent use of erythromycin or chloramphenicol.

Clindamycin and lincomycin can enhance the action of neuromuscular blocking drugs.

Use of antiperistaltic drugs such as opiates, loperamide,

and diphenoxylate may prolong or aggravate the diarrhea observed with clindamycin and lincomycin.

The oral absorption of clindamycin and lincomycin can be impaired by kaolin, pectin, other antidiarrheal medications, and cyclamates.

Nursing Management

See Table 67-1. In addition:

Pretherapy Assessment

Assess and record baseline data necessary for detection of adverse effects of lincosamides: General: VS, body weight, skin color, temperature, and integrity; GI: biliary function; GU: renal function (urinalysis, BUN, creatinine); CVS: hematologic function; Laboratory: culture of infected site.

Review medical history and documents for existing or previous conditions that:

a. require cautious use of lincosamides: impaired renal or hepatic function; history of GI disease, asthma, or other allergic diseases; use in elderly or debilitated people.

b. contraindicate use of lincosamides: allergy to clindamycin, tartrazine; history of regional enteritis, ulcerative colitis, or antibiotic associated colitis; **pregnancy (Category B)**; lactation (secreted in breast milk, another method of feeding is suggested).

Nursing Interventions

Medication Administration

Administer oral form of drug with a full glass of water or with food to prevent esophageal irritation.

Ensure adequate fluid intake.

Administer drugs on schedule to ensure stable steady-state concentrations for the duration of therapy.

Clean skin thoroughly before applying topical clindamycin.

Reduce the risk of stomatitis through frequent mouth care.

Initiate a meal schedule that provides small, frequent meals if GI upset occurs.

Provide ready access to bathroom and interventions directed at symptom relief if diarrhea occurs.

Question prescription of a systemic antiperistaltic drug such as an opiate, diphenoxylate, or loperamide, for a patient experiencing drug-induced diarrhea because it may aggravate the condition. Fluid and electrolyte supplementation is indicated. Corticosteroids may help relieve colitis.

Expect dosage to be reduced by 50% to 75% in the presence of impaired renal function.

Surveillance During Therapy

Monitor for presence of severe headache, rhinitis, urticaria, conjunctivitis, stomatitis, or rash.

Monitor bowel function. Diarrhea is a common side effect of clindamycin or lincomycin, although it may not indicate GI superinfection with a resistant organism, as it usually does.

Monitor for signs of hypersensitivity, which may require discontinuation of drug.

Monitor CBC, urinalysis, and liver and kidney function test results obtained over the course of therapy.

Interpret results of diagnostic tests and contact practitioner as appropriate.

Monitor intake–output, observing for signs and symptoms of possible renal impairment and dehydration secondary to gastrointestinal side effects (vomiting, diarrhea).

Monitor serum levels of aminotransferases and alkaline phosphatase because these drugs may increase them. Platelet counts may be decreased.

Monitor for possible drug–drug and drug–nutrient interactions; see Interactions.

Patient Teaching

Instruct patient regarding the importance of completing the full course of therapy as prescribed, that is, not to discontinue the drug once signs and symptoms of the infection being treated subside.

Inform patient of the consequences of not taking or abruptly discontinuing the drugs.

Instruct patient that the prescribed drug is to be taken for the condition for which it is prescribed, and not to be used to treat any other infections.

Inform patient that periodic blood studies and liver and kidney function tests are recommended during prolonged therapy.

Instruct patient about possible adverse side effects of lincosamides: nausea; vomiting; superinfections in the mouth, vagina; skin rash.

Instruct patient on appropriate action to take if side effects occur:

Notify practitioner if early signs of hematologic or hepatic toxicity (sore throat, fever, mucosal ulceration, malaise, pallor, jaundice) occur.

Notify practitioner of any unusual bleeding. Rationale: hypoprothrombinemia and bleeding tendencies due to decreased synthesis of vitamin K by intestinal microflora may occur.

Discontinue topically applied clindamycin at first sign of local irritation or other allergic reaction and notify practitioner.

Notify practitioner of severe or watery diarrhea; abdominal pain; inflamed mouth or vagina; skin rash or lesions.

• Clofazimine

Lamprene

Clofazimine is an antibacterial and antiinflammatory leprostatic drug that is slowly bactericidal toward *Mycobacterium leprae* or Hansen's bacillus. The drug is deposited in tissues on systemic absorption, and pigmentation (pink to brownish-black) usually occurs on the skin, conjunctivae, on other tissues, and in urine. Clearing of the discoloration occurs gradually on drug withdrawal.

Mechanism

Not completely established; drug binds preferentially to mycobacterial DNA and can inhibit growth of the organism; its antiinflammatory effects are useful for controlling erythema nodosum leprosum reactions.

Uses

Treatment of leprosy, including dapsone-resistant leprosy and lepromatous leprosy complicated by erythema nodosum leprosum. (Drug usually is administered in combination with one or more other antileprosy drugs, such as dapsone or rifampin.)

Dosage

100 mg daily in combination with one or more other antileprosy drugs for 3 years, followed by 100 mg clofazimine alone thereafter.

Fate

Absorption is variable and can range from about 45% to 65% of an oral dose; highly lipophilic and is deposited primarily in fatty tissue and in the reticuloendothelial system; drug is retained by the body for long periods; half-life with repeated dosage is at least 60 to 70 days; some drug is eliminated in the feces, probably by biliary excretion.

Common Side Effects

Discoloration of the skin, urine, feces, and other bodily fluids; GI distress, dryness of the skin.

Significant Adverse Reactions

GI: bleeding, constipation, weight loss, bowel obstruction, hepatitis, jaundice, enteritis, enlarged liver
CNS: dizziness, drowsiness, fatigue, depression, neuralgia, taste alteration
Skin: rash, pruritus, phototoxicity, acneiform eruptions, monilial cheilosis
Ocular: dryness, itching, or burning of the eyes
Other: cystitis, anemia, edema, fever, bone pain, lymphadenopathy, reduced vision, splenic infarction, thromboembolism, vascular pain, elevated serum albumin, bilirubin, and aspartate aminotransferase, eosinophilia, hypokalemia

Contraindications

No absolute contraindications. *Cautious use* in people with serious GI disorders, and in pregnant or nursing women.

Nursing Management

Pretherapy Assessment

Assess and record baseline data necessary for detection of adverse effects of clofazimine: General: VS, body weight, skin color, temperature, and integrity; GI: biliary function; GU: renal function (urinalysis, BUN, creatinine); CVS: hematologic function; CNS: ocular examination; Laboratory: culture of infected site.

Review medical history and documents for existing or previous conditions that:
a. require cautious use of clofazimine: GI problems.
b. contraindicate use of clofazimine: allergy to clofazimine; **pregnancy (Category C)**; lactation (secreted in breast milk, another method of feeding is suggested).

Nursing Interventions

Medication Administration

Administer oral form of drug with food to minimize GI upset.

Ensure adequate fluid intake.

Administer clofazimine on schedule to ensure stable steady-state concentrations for the duration of therapy.

Reduce the risk of stomatitis through frequent mouth care.

Initiate a meal schedule that provides small, frequent meals if GI upset occurs.

Provide ready access to bathroom and interventions directed at symptom relief if diarrhea occurs.

Arrange to reduce dosage if abdominal pain, diarrhea, or colic occur.

Surveillance During Therapy

Monitor for adverse effects, toxicity, and interactions.

Monitor CBC, urinalysis, and liver and kidney function test results obtained over the course of therapy.

Interpret results of diagnostic tests and contact practitioner as appropriate.

Patient Teaching

Instruct patient regarding the importance of completing the full course of therapy as prescribed, that is, not to discontinue the drug once signs and symptoms of the infection being treated subside.

Inform patient of the consequences of not taking or abruptly discontinuing the clofazimine.

Instruct patient that the prescribed drug is to be taken for the condition for which it is prescribed, and not to be used to treat any other infections.

Instruct patient to take drug with meals to minimize GI distress.

Instruct patient about possible adverse side effects of clofazimine: nausea; vomiting; GI cramping; discoloration of skin, urine, feces, and other body fluids; dryness of the skin.

Explain to patient that, within a few weeks after treatment is initiated, the drug usually causes skin, conjunctivae, tears, sweat, sputum, urine, or feces to turn reddish-brown (incidence is 75%–90%). Skin discoloration may persist for months or even years after therapy is terminated. Provide appropriate support and reassurance.

Inform patient not to operate hazardous equipment until reaction to drug is known because dizziness and drowsiness, which usually are dosage related, may occur.

Teach patient interventions to alleviate dry skin and thickened, scaling scalp. Hydration and lubrication usually are adequate, but patient should also be instructed to use soap sparingly, to avoid applying it directly to dry skin, and to rinse it thoroughly off skin.

Inform patient that artificial tears or other appropriate eye drops may be used if eyes feel dry or burn.

Teach patient to increase fluid and dietary fiber intake to prevent constipation.

Instruct patient to promptly report symptoms suggestive of crystalline drug deposition (eg, bone or joint pain, GI bleeding, reduced vision). Although usually reversible, these reactions may linger (months to years), and they may necessitate long-term corticosteroid therapy.

Instruct patient on appropriate action to take if side effects occur: notify practitioner if symptoms of

Hansen's disease worsen; or severe GI upset or colicky pain, or severe depression occur.

• Dapsone

(CAN) Avlosulfon

Sulfones, of which the sole clinically available representative is dapsone, are chemical analogues of the sulfonamides that are used in the treatment of all forms of leprosy (Hansen's disease). Although clinical benefit is often noted within a few months, the more severe skin lesions characteristic of the disease may require several years for complete resolution. Because of its high potential for toxicity, dapsone is usually used only for the treatment of leprosy, although it has been shown to be effective in the treatment of dermatitis herpetiformis and relapsing polychondritis, and for prophylaxis of malaria.

Mechanism

Not completely established; may interfere with essential components of bacterial nutrition; also possesses immunosuppressant action and may inhibit certain bacterial enzymes.

Uses

Treatment of leprosy (except in cases of proven dapsone resistance)
Treatment of dermatitis herpetiformis
Management of relapsing polychondritis (investigational use only)
Prophylaxis of malaria (investigational use only)

Dosage

Leprosy

Adults: 50 to 100 mg per day
Children: 1/4 to 1/2 adult dose
Therapy is usually continued for many years

Dermatitis Herpetiformis

Initially 50 mg/day; increase gradually until desired effect (usual dosage range, 50–300 mg daily); reduce to maintenance level when skin lesions have cleared

Fate

Slowly and completely absorbed orally; peak plasma concentrations occur in 4 to 8 hours; dapsone is 70% to 90% protein bound; well distributed in the body; metabolized in the liver by acetylation and slowly excreted in the urine (70%–85%) as both unchanged drug and metabolites; plasma half-life averages 25 to 30 hours.

Common Side Effects

Anorexia, pallor, skin rash, back or leg pain; hemolysis is common at dosages above 100 mg/day, "sulfone syndrome" is common during the *first year* of therapy (fever, malaise, joint swelling, epistaxis, orchitis, tender skin).

Significant Adverse Reactions

Dermatologic: dermatitis, phototoxicity, drug-induced lupus erythematosus
Hematologic: hemolytic anemia, leukopenia, granulocytopenia, agranulocytosis
GI: nausea, vomiting
CNS: headache, paresthesias, tinnitus, insomnia, vertigo, psychotic reactions (rare)
Other: muscle weakness, drug fever, methemoglobinemia, blurred vision, hematuria, albuminuria, nephrotic syndrome, renal papillary necrosis, liver damage, motor neuropathy, infertility, infectious mononucleosis-like syndrome

Contraindications

Advanced renal amyloidosis. *Cautious use* in patients with anemia, liver or kidney disease, glucose-6-phosphate dehydrogenase (G-6-PD) deficiency, or hypersensitivity to sulfonamides; and in pregnant or nursing women.

Interactions

Probenecid inhibits the renal tubular secretion of dapsone, thus elevating its plasma level.
Rifampin and barbiturates can reduce the effects of dapsone by increasing hepatic microsomal enzyme activity.
The leprostatic effects of dapsone can be antagonized by para-aminobenzoic acid (PABA).

Nursing Management

Pretherapy Assessment

Assess and record baseline data necessary for detection of adverse effects of dapsone: General: VS, body weight, skin color, temperature, and integrity; GI: biliary function; GI: hepatic function; GU: renal function (urinalysis, BUN, creatinine); CVS: hematologic function; CNS: ocular examination; Laboratory: culture of infected site.
Review medical history and documents for existing or previous conditions that:
a. require cautious use of dapsone: anemia; liver or kidney disease; G-6-PD deficiency; methemoglobin reductase deficiency.
b. contraindicate use of dapsone: allergy to dapsone, sulfonamides; **pregnancy (Category C)**; lactation (secreted in breast milk, drug is carcinogenic, another method of feeding is suggested).

Nursing Interventions

Medication Administration

Administer oral form of drug with food to minimize GI upset.
Ensure adequate fluid intake.
Administer dapsone on schedule to ensure stable steady-state concentrations for the duration of therapy.
Reduce the risk of stomatitis through frequent mouth care.
Initiate a meal schedule that provides small, frequent meals if GI upset occurs.
Provide ready access to bathroom and interventions directed at symptom relief if diarrhea occurs.
Arrange for liver function tests during therapy.
Arrange for regular CBCs during therapy.

Surveillance During Therapy

Monitor for interactions.
Monitor patient for indications of possible blood dyscra-

sias (fever, sore throat, bruising, malaise). Blood counts should be performed at frequent intervals, and the drug should be discontinued if blood picture is abnormal or if signs of severe anemia are present.
Monitor hepatic function at regular intervals, and note early signs of developing hepatotoxicity (anorexia, vomiting, abdominal pain, light-colored stools). Evidence of liver impairment mandates immediate drug withdrawal.
Monitor CBC, urinalysis, and liver and kidney function test results obtained over the course of therapy.
Interpret results of diagnostic tests and contact practitioner as appropriate.
Monitor for signs and symptoms of agranulocytosis, aplastic anemia, and other blood dyscrasias.
Monitor for leprosy reactional episodes indicative of worsening of disease activity related to therapy.

Patient Teaching

Instruct patient regarding the importance of completing the full course of therapy as prescribed, that is, not to discontinue the drug once signs and symptoms of the infection being treated subside.
Inform patient of the consequences of not taking or abruptly discontinuing the dapsone.
Instruct patient that the prescribed drug is to be taken for the condition for which it is prescribed, and not to be used to treat any other infections.
Instruct patient to take drug with meals to minimize GI distress.
Explain that, as appropriate, because bacterial resistance can develop when sulfones are used alone, rifampin or ethionamide is frequently prescribed for concurrent use during initial months of therapy. In most cases, sulfone therapy must be continued for several years, and occasionally for a lifetime in severe, complicated forms of leprosy.
Inform patient that drug needs to be temporarily discontinued if hypersensitivity develops, but that it can be resumed at a low dosage after the reaction has subsided.
Instruct patient about possible adverse side effects of dapsone: nausea, vomiting, loss of appetite; sensitivity to sunlight; numbness, tingling; weakness.
Inform patient not to operate hazardous equipment until reaction to drug is known because dizziness and drowsiness, which usually are dosage related, may occur.
Instruct patient on appropriate action to take if side effects occur: notify practitioner if symptoms of Hansen's disease worsen; or severe GI upset or colicky pain; unusual bleeding or bruising, sore throat, fever or chills, yellowing of skin or eyes occur.

• Eflornithine

Ornidyl

Eflornithine is an antiprotozoal agent used in the treatment of African trypanosomal infection, the cause of sleeping sickness.

Mechanism

Irreversibly inhibits the enzyme ornithine decarboxylase. Decarboxylation of ornithine is essential for synthesis of various polyamines, such as putrescine, spermidine, and spermine that are required for cellular division and differentiation.

Uses

Treatment of the meningoencephalitic stage of *Trypanosoma brucei gambiense* (sleeping sickness) infection.

Dosage

100 mg/kg/dose, administered every 6 hours for 14 days, by slow IV infusion.

Fate

Eflornithine is insignificantly bound to plasma proteins and attains cerebrospinal fluid levels that may reach 50% of plasma concentrations; plasma half-life averages 3 hours with 80% of the dose excreted unchanged in the urine within 24 hours; dosage adjustments are required in patients with impaired renal function.

Common Side Effects

Nausea, headache, dizziness, vomiting.

Significant Adverse Reactions

Anemia, leukopenia, thrombocytopenia, diarrhea, seizures, hearing impairment. NOTE: CBCs should be performed before, during, and after treatment until values return to baseline levels.

Contraindications

No specific contraindications; safety during pregnancy and in children has not been established; teratogenic effects have been observed in animals.

Nursing Management

Pretherapy Assessment

Assess and record baseline data necessary for detection of adverse effects of eflornithine: General: VS, body weight, skin color and temperature; GI: output; GU: renal function, output; CNS: reflexes, orientation, audiologic examination; Laboratory: CBC with differential, hemoglobin, hematocrit, BUN, creatinine, electrolytes.
Review medical history and documents for existing or previous conditions that:
a. require cautious use of eflornithine: breast-feeding; seizure disorders; renal disorders.
b. contraindicate use of eflornithine: allergy to eflornithine; **pregnancy (Category C)**.

Nursing Interventions

Medication Administration

Drug is administered by slow IV infusion (100 mg/kg), every 6 hours for 14 days.
Arrange for CBC with differential before, during, and periodically after treatment until baseline values are reestablished.
Arrange for audiologic evaluation before therapy.
Reduce the risk of stomatitis through frequent mouth care.

Initiate a meal schedule that provides small, frequent meals if GI upset occurs.
Provide ready access to bathroom and interventions directed at symptom relief if diarrhea occurs.

Surveillance During Therapy

Monitor for toxicity and interactions.
Monitor for signs of hypersensitivity, which may require discontinuation of drug.
Monitor CBC, urinalysis, and kidney function test results obtained over the course of therapy.
Interpret results of diagnostic tests and contact practitioner as appropriate.
Monitor intake–output, observing for signs and symptoms of possible renal impairment and dehydration secondary to GI side effects (vomiting, diarrhea).
Provide for patient safety needs in the event of seizures or other CNS side effects.
Initiate interventions to minimize environmental hazards.

Patient Teaching

Instruct patient regarding the importance of completing the full course of therapy as prescribed.

• Furazolidone

Furoxone

Furazolidone is a synthetic nitrofuran with both antibacterial and antiprotozoal activity. It is effective against many common GI pathogens, such as *Escherichia coli*, *Salmonella* sp, *Shigella* sp, *Enterobacter aerogenes*, *Proteus* sp, *Vibrio cholerae*, and staphylococci, as well as the protozoan *Giardia lamblia*. Furazolidone is poorly absorbed orally, and its action is largely restricted to the GI tract.

Mechanism

Interferes with several bacterial enzyme systems; development of resistance is minimal; does not alter normal bowel flora nor lead to fungal overgrowth; possesses a monoamine oxidase (MAO)-inhibitory action if used for longer than 4 to 5 days, which is probably caused by accumulation of a metabolite, 2-hydroxyethylhydrazine.

Uses

Treatment of bacterial or protozoal diarrhea and enteritis due to susceptible organisms.

Dosage

Adults: 100 mg four times a day
Children 5 years and older: 25 to 50 mg four times a day
Children 1 through 4 years: 17 to 25 mg four times a day
Children younger than 1 year: 8 to 17 mg four times a day (maximal daily dose 8.8 mg/kg/day)

Fate

Oral absorption is minimal; drug is metabolized in the intestine and excreted largely in the feces; approximately 5% is eliminated in the urine, along with metabolites, which may color the urine brown.

Common Side Effects

Nausea, anorexia.

Significant Adverse Reactions

Vomiting, headache, malaise, hypersensitivity reactions (fever, skin rash, urticaria, arthralgia), hypotension, hypoglycemia, reversible intravascular hemolysis, disulfiram-like reaction to alcohol (see Chapter 81).

Contraindications

In infants younger than 1 month; concurrent use of alcohol, other drugs having an MAO-inhibitory action, sympathomimetic amines, or tyramine-containing foods (see MAO Inhibitors, Chapter 26). *Cautious use* in people with diabetes or glucose-6-phosphate dehydrogenase deficiency; and in pregnant or nursing women.

Interactions

Alcohol may elicit a mild disulfiram-like reaction (flushing, hyperthermia, sweating, dyspnea, tachycardia, palpitations) in the presence of furazolidone.
Hypertension can result from concurrent use of furazolidone with other MAO inhibitors, sympathomimetic amines, or tyramine-containing foods.
The actions of sedatives, narcotics, and other CNS depressants can be enhanced by furazolidone, leading to hypotension and excessive drowsiness.
A toxic psychosis can result from concurrent use of furazolidone and a tricyclic antidepressant.
The antihypertensive effectiveness of guanethidine or guanadrel may be reduced by furazolidone.
Furazolidone may potentiate the hypoglycemic effect of insulin and sulfonylurea antidiabetic drugs.
Concurrent use of furazolidone and meperidine may lead to sudden development of hypertension, restlessness, agitation, seizures, and coma.

Nursing Management

Pretherapy Assessment

Assess and record baseline data necessary for detection of adverse effects of furazolidone: General: VS, body weight, skin color, temperature, and integrity; GI: biliary function; hepatic function; GU: renal function (urinalysis, BUN, creatinine); CVS: hematologic function; CNS: ocular examination; Laboratory: culture of infected site.
Review medical history and documents for existing or previous conditions that:
a. require cautious use of furazolidone: diabetes; G-6-PD deficiency.
b. contraindicate use of furazolidone: allergy to furazolidone; use in infants younger than 1 month of age; concurrent use of alcohol, MAO inhibitors, sympathomimetic amines, tyramine-containing foods; **pregnancy (Category B)**; lactation (secreted in breast milk, safety not established).

Nursing Interventions

Medication Administration

Administer oral form of drug with food to minimize GI upset.
Ensure adequate fluid intake.

Administer furazolidone on schedule to ensure stable steady-state concentrations for the duration of therapy.
Reduce the risk of stomatitis through frequent mouth care.
Initiate a meal schedule that provides small, frequent meals if GI upset occurs.
Provide ready access to bathroom and interventions directed at symptom relief if diarrhea occurs.

Surveillance During Therapy

Monitor patient for indications of possible blood dyscrasias (fever, sore throat, bruising, malaise). Blood counts should be performed at frequent intervals.
Monitor CBC, urinalysis, and liver and kidney function test results obtained over the course of therapy.
Monitor patient for signs of dehydration or electrolyte depletion (hypotension, "sunken" eyes, irregular pulse, cramping) during episodes of diarrhea. Notify drug prescriber if signs occur.
Interpret results of diagnostic tests and contact practitioner as appropriate.
Monitor for possible drug–drug and drug–nutrient interactions; see Interactions.

Patient Teaching

Caution patient to avoid alcohol during treatment and for at least 4 days after therapy to prevent development of a disulfiram-like reaction.
Instruct patient to limit or avoid foods high in tyramine (eg, unpasteurized cheese, beer, wine, broad beans, yeast, and fermented products) to minimize the danger of a hypertensive reaction secondary to the MAO-inhibitory action of furazolidone.
Warn patient to avoid over-the-counter drugs unless specifically prescribed. Hypertension can occur if furazolidone and products containing vasopressor agents are used concurrently.
Instruct patient regarding the importance of completing the full course of therapy as prescribed, that is, not to discontinue the drug once signs and symptoms of the infection being treated subside.
Inform patient of the consequences of not taking or abruptly discontinuing the furazolidone.
Instruct patient that the prescribed drug is to be taken for the condition for which it is prescribed, and not to be used to treat any other infections.
Instruct patient to take drug with meals to minimize GI distress.
Instruct patient about possible adverse side effects of dapsone: nausea, vomiting, loss of appetite; sensitivity to sunlight; numbness, tingling; weakness.
Inform patient not to operate hazardous equipment until reaction to drug is known because dizziness and drowsiness, which usually are dosage related, may occur.
Inform patient that drug may cause urine to turn brown, a harmless effect.
Instruct patient to report weakness, faintness, or dizziness, possible signs of hypotension or hypoglycemia. Dosage adjustment may be necessary.
Advise patient with diabetes that blood sugar needs to be monitored closely because hypoglycemia may occur, in which case the dosage of antidiabetic medication may need to be adjusted.
Instruct patient on appropriate action to take if side effects occur: notify practitioner if diarrhea persists longer than 5 days; if severe GI upset or colicky pain; or unusual bleeding or bruising, sore throat, fever or chills, yellowing of skin or eyes occur.

• *Nitrofurazone*

Furacin

A synthetic nitrofuran, nitrofurazone exhibits a broad antibacterial spectrum of action. It is used topically to prevent infection in burns or skin grafts.

Mechanism

Inhibits function of enzymes necessary for carbohydrate metabolism in bacteria; bactericidal against both aerobic and anaerobic organisms, although some strains of *Pseudomonas* and *Proteus* are resistant; virtually nontoxic to human cells.

Uses

Adjunctive therapy to prevent bacterial contamination of second- or third-degree burns or skin grafts.

NOTE: Not for treatment of minor burns, wounds, or skin infections, because effectiveness has not been demonstrated in these conditions.

Dosage

Soluble dressing or cream: apply directly to lesion or place on sterile gauze; reapply once daily or every few days as necessary.

Significant Adverse Reactions

Contact dermatitis, irritation, and superinfections.

Contraindications

No absolute contraindications. *Cautious use* in patients with G-6-PD deficiency (danger of hemolytic anemia if significant systemic absorption occurs); marked renal impairment; and in pregnant women.

Nursing Management

Pretherapy Assessment

Assess and record baseline data necessary for detection of adverse effects of nitrofurazone: General: VS, body weight, skin color, temperature, and integrity; Laboratory: culture of infected site.
Review medical history and documents for existing or previous conditions that:

a. require cautious use of nitrofurazone: impaired renal function; G-6-PD deficiency (risk of hemolytic anemia).
b. contraindicate use of nitrofurazone: allergy to nitrofurazone; safety and efficacy has not been established in children; **pregnancy (Category C)**; lactation (safety not established, discontinue drug or discontinue nursing of infant).

Nursing Interventions

Medication Administration

Apply directly to lesion or first place on gauze; impregnated gauze may be used.
Apply only to affected area. Protect surrounding skin with petrolatum or zinc oxide.
Autoclave gauze only once. Solutions used to impregnate gauze may become discolored on autoclaving or exposure to light, but this does not affect drug potency.

Surveillance During Therapy

Monitor for toxicity and interactions.
Monitor for signs of allergic hypersensitivity (itching, burning, swelling, rash), and discontinue drug if these occur.
Interpret results of diagnostic tests and contact practitioner as appropriate.

Patient Teaching

Instruct patient regarding the importance of completing the full course of therapy as prescribed, that is, not to discontinue the drug once signs and symptoms of the infection being treated subside.
Instruct patient that the prescribed drug is to be taken for the condition for which it is prescribed, and not to be used to treat any other infections.

• Novobiocin

Albamycin

A bacteriostatic antibiotic effective against certain gram-positive cocci, especially *Staphylococcus aureus* and some strains of *Proteus vulgaris*, novobiocin is infrequently used because resistance usually develops rapidly and there is a high incidence of hypersensitivity reactions (such as urticaria, dermatitis) associated with it. Blood dyscrasias and hepatic dysfunction have also occurred.

Mechanism

Not completely established; inhibits protein and nucleic acid synthesis and interrupts bacterial cell wall synthesis; may also alter stability of cell membrane by complexing with magnesium within the bacterial cell.

Uses

Treatment of serious infections due to susceptible strains of *Staphylococcus aureus* or *Proteus* sp in patients unresponsive or sensitive to other, less toxic antibiotics, such as penicillins, cephalosporins, tetracyclines, or erythromycin.

Dosage

Adults: 250 mg every 6 hours or 500 mg every 12 hours (maximum 1 g every 12 hours)
Children: 15 to 45 mg/kg/day in divided doses every 6 to 12 hours, depending on severity of infection

Fate

Well absorbed orally; peak plasma levels occur within 2 hours; highly (90%–95%) bound to plasma proteins; diffuses poorly into most body tissues; excreted primarily in the bile and feces.

Common Side Effects

Hypersensitivity reactions (urticarial, erythematous, maculopapular, or scarlatiniform rash).

Significant Adverse Reactions

Erythema multiforme (rare), liver dysfunction, jaundice, nausea, vomiting, diarrhea, intestinal hemorrhage, alopecia, and blood dyscrasias (leukopenia, eosinophilia, anemia, pancytopenia, agranulocytosis, thrombocytopenia).

Contraindications

In newborn or premature infants. *Cautious use* in patients with hepatic disease or history of allergic reactions and in pregnant or nursing women.

Nursing Management

Nursing Interventions

Medication Administration

Expect to administer another antibiotic concurrently. Because resistance to novobiocin emerges rapidly, it is rarely used alone. It may be given with penicillin because cross-resistance has not been demonstrated.
Question use for minor infections or for infections caused by organisms other than those with demonstrated sensitivity to novobiocin.

Surveillance During Therapy

Monitor results of hepatic function studies, which should be performed periodically during treatment. Therapy should be terminated if signs of liver disease are noted (eg, elevated serum bilirubin).

Patient Teaching

Teach patient how to recognize and report hypersensitivity reactions (rash, urticaria, fever). Drug should be discontinued if reactions cannot be managed by usual measures.
Inform patient that routine blood studies are recommended, and teach patient how to recognize and report early signs of possible blood dyscrasias (fever, sore throat, bruising, or bleeding). Patient should discontinue therapy if signs occur.
Instruct patient to note and report any yellowing of skin or eyes or abdominal pain, signs of possible liver disease.

• Pentamidine

Pentam 300, NebuPent

Pentamidine is a diamidine antiprotozoal agent that is effective against several protozoa and fungi. It is used for both the prevention and treatment of pneumocystis pneumonia due to *Pneumocystis carinii* infection, a serious, opportunistic respiratory infection occurring frequently in immunocompromised patients, such as patients with acquired immunodeficiency syndrome (AIDS). Pentamidine is an alternative drug to trimethoprim–sulfamethoxazole (see Chapter 59) and is available for injection or oral inhalation.

Mechanism

Exact mechanism of action has not been established; drug may interfere with nuclear metabolism and inhibit the synthesis of DNA, RNA, proteins, and phospholipids.

Uses

Alternative treatment of *Pneumocystis carinii* pneumonia (IV, IM)
Prevention of *Pneumocystis carinii* pneumonia in high-risk, HIV-infected patients
Treatment of trypanosomiasis and visceral leishmaniasis (investigational uses)

Dosage

Injection: 4 mg/kg once daily for 14 days; given by IV infusion or deep IM injection
Aerosol: 300 mg once every 4 weeks administered with a nebulizer

Fate

Well absorbed from IM injection sites but exists in the bloodstream only temporarily, because it is extensively bound to tissues; approximately one third of a dose is excreted unchanged by the kidneys within 6 hours; the remainder is very slowly eliminated over several weeks; drug does not enter the CNS in appreciable amounts. Plasma concentrations after aerosol administration are low.

Common Side Effects

Injection: Elevated serum creatinine and liver function tests, nausea, anorexia, fever, hypotension, rash, hypoglycemia, sterile abscess or pain at IM injection site
Aerosol: Metallic taste, shortness of breath, anorexia, fatigue, cough, dizziness, rash, pharyngitis, nausea, chills, vomiting, bronchospasm

Significant Adverse Reactions

Confusion, hallucinations, anemia, neuralgia, hyperkalemia, phlebitis, thrombocytopenia, acute renal failure, hypocalcemia, ventricular tachycardia, arrhythmias, Stevens-Johnson syndrome.

Too-rapid IV administration can result in headache, dizziness, tachycardia, vomiting, and possibly fainting.

CAUTION

The incidence of adverse reactions is significantly higher in patients with AIDS receiving pentamidine than in patients with other conditions.

Contraindications

No absolute contraindications. *Cautious use* in people with hypotension; hypoglycemia; hypocalcemia; leukopenia; thrombocytopenia; anemia; renal or hepatic disease; arrhythmias; and in pregnant women.

Nursing Management

Pretherapy Assessment

Assess and record baseline data necessary for detection of adverse effects of pentamidine: General: VS, body weight, skin color, temperature, and integrity; GI: biliary function; GU: renal function (urinalysis, BUN, creatinine); CVS: hematologic function, baseline electrocardiogram; CNS: neurologic function; Laboratory: glucose, calcium.

Review medical history and documents for existing or previous conditions that:

a. require cautious use of pentamidine: impaired renal or hepatic function; hypotension; hypoglycemia; hypocalcemia; leukopenia; thrombocytopenia; arrhythmias.
b. contraindicate use of pentamidine: allergy to pentamidine, history of anaphylactoid reaction to inhaled or parenteral pentamidine; if diagnosis of *P carinii* pneumonia has been confirmed, there are no absolute contraindications; **pregnancy (Category C)**; lactation (safety not established, avoid use in nursing mothers).

Nursing Interventions

Medication Administration

Inject into large muscle mass, rotate sites, and apply warm compresses to site when giving IM. Because injection is painful and may cause sterile abscesses, intermittent IV infusion is preferred route of administration.

Prepare patient for confinement to bed in supine position before IV infusion. Keep patient supine during infusion.

Closely monitor patient during administration; fatalities have been reported.

Routinely rotate IV sites and assess frequently for pain, redness, and swelling because phlebitis may occur.

Ensure that emergency equipment and drugs, including vasopressors, are available to treat hypotension during infusion.

Monitor blood pressure at least every 15 minutes during IV infusion, every 0.5 hour for 2 hours after infusion is terminated, and every 4 hours thereafter until stable because sudden, severe hypotension may develop.

Surveillance During Therapy

Monitor for toxicity and interactions.

Monitor temperature, and institute measures to control, as needed. Although fever is a symptom of the illness, it may rapidly rise as high as 40°C (104°F) shortly after drug infusion.

After infusion, when patient is not dizzy and blood pressure is stable, help patient out of bed and protect from injury until all potentially hazardous reactions have subsided.

Monitor results of BUN and serum creatinine determinations, measure and record intake and output, and assess for edema because acute renal failure may occur. If signs of impending dysfunction appear, dosage should be adjusted.

Check patient's pulse at least twice daily to detect arrhythmias because cardiac function may be affected.

Monitor results of liver function tests because hepatic dysfunction may occur.

Assess patient for signs of hypoglycemia. Blood glucose

can be monitored with fingerstick methods. If hypoglycemia occurs, increased food intake (five to six small meals per day) may control the problem.

Before initiating pentamidine prophylaxis, assess symptomatic patients to exclude the presence of *active Pneumocystis carinii* pneumonia. The dose of aerosolized pentamidine is insufficient to *treat* acute pneumocystis pneumonia.

Interpret results of diagnostic tests and contact practitioner as appropriate.

Patient Teaching

Instruct patient about possible adverse side effects of pentamidine: metallic taste in mouth; GI upset.

Implement other interventions for patient with AIDS (eg, protect from infection, provide emotional support, promote adequate nutrition, prevent transmission of HIV virus to others).

Instruct patients who experience bronchospasm or cough with aerosolized pentamidine to use an inhaled bronchodilator before each pentamidine dose.

Note that the safety and efficacy of the inhalant solution in children has not been established.

Instruct patient to notify practitioner if patient experiences: pain at injection site; confusion; hallucinations; unusual bleeding or bruising; weakness or fatigue.

• Spectinomycin

Trobicin

An antibiotic related to the aminoglycosides, spectinomycin is used IM for alternative treatment of gonorrhea in patients hypersensitive to penicillins, or for eradication of organisms resistant to penicillins.

Mechanism

Inhibits protein synthesis in the bacterial cell at the 30S ribosomal subunit; bacteriostatic at normal doses; active against most strains of *Neisseria gonorrhoeae;* not effective against *Treponema* (syphilis).

Uses

Treatment of acute gonorrheal urethritis, proctitis, and cervicitis due to susceptible strains of *Neisseria gonorrhoeae* (usually in patients sensitive to penicillins or tetracyclines or when organisms are resistant to these drugs).

Dosage

Adults and children weighing more than 100 lb (45 kg): usually 2 g (5 mL) IM in a single dose; in areas where antibiotic resistance is known to be present, 4 g (10 mL) divided into two equal parts and injected at different sites

Children weighing less than 100 lb (45 kg) (safety has *not* been established): 40 mg/kg IM

Fate

Absorption from IM injection site is rapid; serum levels peak in 1 to 2 hours and effective levels are still present at 8 hours; not significantly protein bound; excreted by the kidneys in a biologically active form.

Common Side Effects

Irritation and soreness at injection site.

Significant Adverse Reactions

Urticaria, fever, dizziness, nausea, chills, insomnia, and reduced urine output.

Multiple doses have elicited decreases in hemoglobin and hematocrit and creatinine clearance, and elevations in BUN, alkaline phosphatase, and alanine aminotransferase.

Contraindications

Treatment of pharyngeal infections due to *Neisseria gonorrhoeae. Cautious use* in people with a history of allergies, in infants and young children, and in pregnant or nursing women.

Nursing Management

Pretherapy Assessment

Assess and record baseline data necessary for detection of adverse effects of spectinomycin: General: VS, body weight, skin color, temperature, and integrity; GI: biliary function; GU: renal function (urinalysis, BUN, creatinine); CVS: hematologic function; CNS: neurologic function; Laboratory: culture of infected site.

Review medical history and documents for existing or previous conditions that:

a. require cautious use of spectinomycin: history of allergy, use in infants or small children.
b. contraindicate use of spectinomycin: allergy to spectinomycin; treatment of pharyngeal infections due to *Neisseria gonorrhoeae*; **pregnancy (Category B)**; lactation (safety not established, avoid use in nursing mothers).

Nursing Interventions

Medication Administration

Expect person known to have been exposed recently to gonorrhea to be treated the same as one proven to have gonorrhea by culture.

Inject IM deeply into upper outer quadrant of buttocks using a 20-gauge needle. Administer no more than 5 mL per injection.

Reconstitute powder for injection with accompanying diluent, and mix thoroughly. Use within 24 hours.

Surveillance During Therapy

Monitor for toxicity and interactions.

Monitor for signs of hypersensitivity, which may require discontinuation of drug.

Monitor CBC, urinalysis, and liver and kidney function test results obtained over the course of therapy.

Interpret results of diagnostic tests and contact practitioner as appropriate.

Patient Teaching

Instruct patient regarding the importance of completing the full course of therapy as prescribed, that is, not to discontinue the drug once signs and symptoms of the infection being treated subside.

Inform patient of the consequences of not taking or abruptly discontinuing the spectinomycin.

Instruct patient that the prescribed drug is to be taken for the condition for which it is prescribed, and not to be used to treat any other infections.
Explain the need for a serologic test for syphilis, which should be performed at the time of diagnosis and again after 3 months (the drug may mask or delay symptoms of incubating syphilis).
Instruct patient about possible adverse side effects of spectinomycin: nausea; rash; fever; chills; insomnia; reduced urine output.
Instruct patient on appropriate action to take if side effects occur: notify practitioner if infection worsens; or dark-colored urine, yellowing of the skin or eyes, skin rash, or itching occurs.

• Trimetrexate

Neutrexin

Trimetrexate is a synthetic folate antagonist indicated for the treatment of *Pneumocystis carinii* pneumonia in immunocompromised patients, such as those with AIDS.

Mechanism

Competitive inhibitor of dihydrofolate reductase, the enzyme necessary for activation of folic acid that is required for purine synthesis, and the subsequent synthesis of DNA, RNA, and proteins. A selective toxic effect occurs in *Pneumocystis* organisms if leucovorin (activated form of folic acid) is administered along with trimetrexate. Mammalian cells have a specific carrier-mediated process for uptake of leucovorin that provides a source of activated folic acid necessary for normal cellular biosynthetic activities. *Pneumocystis* organisms lack this carrier-mediated transport process and therefore are subjected to the cytotoxic effects of trimetrexate.

Uses

Alternative therapy for the treatment of moderate to severe *Pneumocystis carinii* pneumonia in immunocompromised patients who are intolerant or refractory to trimethoprim–sulfamethoxazole therapy.

NOTE: leucovorin must be administered concurrently.

Dosage

Slow IV infusion over 60 to 90 minutes of 45 mg/m^2 for 21 days. Leucovorin is administered concurrently, either IV (20 mg/m^2 every 6 hours) or orally (20 mg/m^2 4 times per day for 24 days).

Fate

Trimetrexate has a terminal half-life that ranges from 7 to 15 hours; metabolism involves oxidative *O*-demethylation followed by glucuronidation conjugation; excretion is primarily renal; plasma protein binding is approximately 95% and appears to decrease with increased dosage, which suggests saturable binding.

Common Side Effects

Nausea, vomiting, rash, pruritus, fatigue.

Significant Adverse Reactions

Hematologic toxicity that includes neutropenia, thrombocytopenia, and anemia; hepatotoxicity, nephrotoxicity, allergic reactions.

Contraindications

No specific contraindications other than the development of allergy. Safety during pregnancy, lactation, or in children has not been established. Trimetrexate is fetotoxic and teratogenic in rats and rabbits.

Interactions

Drugs that induce or inhibit P-450 enzymes may decrease or increase plasma concentrations of trimetrexate, respectively. This includes drugs such as cimetidine, and the imidazole antifungal agents (ketoconazole, itraconazole, miconazole).

Nursing Management

See Methotrexate (Chapter 74).

• Vancomycin

Lyphocin, Vancocin, Vancoled

Vancomycin is a bactericidal glycopeptide antibiotic active against many gram-positive organisms, such as streptococci, staphylococci (including penicillinase-producing ones), *Clostridium difficile*, *Corynebacterium* sp, and *Listeria* sp. In addition, it appears to be bacteriostatic against enterococci. The potential for serious toxicity, however, limits its systemic usefulness to treatment of life-threatening infections in patients allergic or unresponsive to less toxic antibacterial drugs. In many instances, it is the only drug effective in cases of methicillin-resistant *Staphylococcus aureus* infection, a life-threatening infection. A related drug, teicoplanin, which exhibits a similar spectrum of activity and a longer duration of action, is expected to become available shortly.

Vancomycin may also be administered orally for treatment of staphylococcal enterocolitis and antibiotic-induced pseudomembranous colitis (for which it is usually considered to be the drug of choice), because it is poorly absorbed from the GI tract.

Mechanism

Inhibits bacterial cell wall synthesis by binding to precursors of the cell wall, such as the D-alanyl-D-alanine portion of the precursor units; drug may also inhibit bacterial RNA synthesis and damage bacterial cytoplasmic membranes. There appears to be no cross-resistance between vancomycin and any other antibiotic.

Uses

Treatment of serious staphylococcal infections (eg, endocarditis, septicemia, pneumonia, osteomyelitis) in patients who cannot tolerate or who do not respond to penicillins, cephalosporins, or other, less toxic antibiotics
Treatment of staphylococcal enterocolitis (oral use only)
Treatment of antibiotic-induced pseudomembranous colitis caused by *Clostridium difficile*

Dosage

Oral, IV (Slow Infusion)

Adults: 500 mg every 6 hours *or* 1 g every 12 hours
Children: 44 mg/kg/day in divided doses (maximum 2 g/day)
Prevention of bacterial endocarditis in penicillin-allergic

patients undergoing dental procedures or upper respiratory tract surgery:

Adults: 1 g IV infused over 30 to 60 minutes 0.5 to 1 hour before surgery; then oral erythromycin 500 mg every 6 hours for 8 doses

Children: 20 mg/kg IV infused over 30 to 60 minutes as above; then 10 mg/kg oral erythromycin every 6 hours for 8 doses

Prevention of bacterial endocarditis in penicillin-allergic patients undergoing GI or genitourinary surgery:

Adults: 1 g IV infused over 60 minutes *plus* 1.5 mg/kg gentamicin IM or IV concurrently 1 hour before procedure

Children weighing less than 27 kg: 20 mg/kg IV slowly over 1 hour *and* 2 mg/kg gentamicin IM or IV concurrently 1 hour before procedure

Oral Only

Pseudomembranous colitis (adults): 500 mg to 2 g every 6 to 8 hours for 7 to 10 days

Fate

Poorly absorbed orally, although measurable plasma levels have occurred after oral use in treating colitis; IV administration yields rapid attainment of effective serum levels; half-life is 4 to 8 hours in adults and 2 to 3 hours in children; half-life increases in renal failure; widely distributed in the body but does not readily cross the blood–brain barrier; penetrates into pleural, pericardial, ascitic, and synovial fluid in the presence of inflammation; approximately 80% of injected drug is excreted by the kidneys.

Common Side Effects

Nausea with oral administration.

Significant Adverse Reactions

Parenteral administration: "red neck" syndrome (fever, chills, erythema of the neck and back, paresthesias—usually seen with too-rapid injection); macular rash, urticaria, eosinophilia, ototoxicity, (tinnitus, hearing loss); nephrotoxicity, anaphylactoid reactions, pain and thrombophlebitis with IV injection, superinfections, dyspnea, wheezing, pruritus, hypotension, phlebitis, elevated serum creatinine or BUN, and thrombocytopenia.

Contraindications

Concurrent use with other ototoxic or nephrotoxic drugs (see Interactions). *Cautious use* in patients with renal impairment, hearing disturbances, and in neonates, elderly people, and pregnant or nursing women.

Interactions

Increased ototoxicity and nephrotoxicity can result from concurrent use of vancomycin with aminoglycosides, polymyxin B, colistin, amphotericin B, cisplatin, bumetanide, furosemide, and ethacrynic acid.

The action of vancomycin may be antagonized by concurrent use of bacteriostatic antibiotics (eg, example, tetracyclines, erythromycins).

Antivertigo and antinausea drugs (eg, meclizine, dimenhydrinate, promethazine) may mask the ototoxic effects of vancomycin.

Nursing Management

Pretherapy Assessment

Assess and record baseline data necessary for detection of adverse effects of vancomycin: General: VS, body weight, skin color, temperature, and integrity; GI: biliary function; GU: renal function (urinalysis, BUN, creatinine); CVS: hematologic function; CNS: neurologic function (eighth cranial nerve function), auditory function; Laboratory: culture of infected site.

Review medical history and documents for existing or previous conditions that:

a. require cautious use of vancomycin: impaired renal function; hearing disturbances; use in neonates and the elderly.
b. contraindicate use of vancomycin: allergy to vancomycin; **pregnancy (Category C)**; lactation (safety not established).

Nursing Interventions

Medication Administration

Seek clarification if prescribed orally for systemic infection because drug is poorly absorbed from GI tract.

Dilute contents of one vial (500 mg) in 30 mL water to prepare oral solution, and administer by mouth or by nasogastric tube.

Dilute powder for injection with 10 mL sterile water for injection, then add to 100 to 200 mL infusion solution for intermittent IV infusion. Infuse over 20 to 30 minutes every 6 hours. Drug should be administered IV by intermittent infusion if possible.

Dilute 1 to 2 g powder in sufficient vehicle and administer by slow IV drip over 24 hours if continuous IV infusion is necessary,

Closely observe IV infusion site for signs of extravasation, which can cause severe irritation and necrosis.

Instruct patient to report any pain in extremity used for infusion, and closely observe extremity for signs of thrombophlebitis when administering IV. The risk of thrombophlebitis can be reduced by mixing drug with 200 mL or more of glucose or saline solution.

Surveillance During Therapy

Monitor for signs of hypersensitivity, which may require discontinuation of drug.

Monitor for signs of "red neck" syndrome: fever, chills, erythema of the neck and back, paresthesias.

Monitor CBC, urinalysis, and liver and kidney function test results obtained over the course of therapy.

Monitor results of hematologic studies, urinalyses, and liver and kidney function tests, which should be performed periodically on any patient receiving the drug.

Assess patient for signs of possible nephrotoxicity (oliguria, proteinuria, urinary casts), and notify drug prescriber immediately if these occur.

Ensure that serial tests of auditory function and vancomycin serum levels, which should be performed on any patient with borderline renal function and on elderly patients, are obtained as prescribed (peak therapeutic serum concentrations = 25–40 μg/mL, trough = 10–15 μg/mL).

Interpret results of diagnostic tests and contact practitioner as appropriate.

Monitor intake–output, observing for signs and symptoms of possible renal impairment and dehydration secondary to GI side effects (vomiting, diarrhea).

Monitor for possible drug–drug and drug–nutrient interactions: increased ototoxicity and nephrotoxicity with concurrent use of aminoglycosides, polymyxin B, amphotericin B, cisplatin, bumetanide, furosemide, and ethacrynic acid; action antagonized by concurrent use of bacteriostatic antibiotics (tetracyclines and erythromycins); masking of ototoxic effect by antivertigo–antinausea agents; increased neuromuscular blockade with competitive neuromuscular blockers.

Patient Teaching

Instruct patient regarding the importance of completing the full course of therapy as prescribed.

Instruct patient to report tinnitus or other auditory disturbances *immediately* because drug must be discontinued to prevent deafness, which may progress despite cessation of therapy.

Instruct patient about possible adverse side effects of vancomycin: nausea; changes in hearing; superinfections in the mouth, vagina.

Instruct patient on appropriate action to take if side effects occur:

Notify practitioner if early signs of hematologic or hepatic toxicity (sore throat, fever, mucosal ulceration, malaise, pallor, jaundice) occur.

Notify practitioner of any unusual bleeding. Rationale: hypoprothrombinemia and bleeding tendencies due to decreased synthesis of vitamin K by intestinal microflora may occur.

Notify practitioner if ringing in the ears, loss of hearing; difficulty voiding; rash; flushing occur.

Selected Bibliography

Armstrong D, Bernard E: Aerosol pentamidine. Ann Intern Med 109:852, 1988

Polk RE, et al: Vancomycin and the red-man syndrome: Pharmacodynamics of histamine release. J Infect Dis 157:502, 1988

Salamone FR, Cunha BA: Update on pentamidine for the treatment of *Pneumocystis carinii* pneumonia. Clin Pharm 7:501, 1988

Uttley AH, et al: Vancomycin-resistant enterococci. Lancet 1:57, 1988

Weinthal J, Frost JD, Briones G, Cairo MS: Successful *Pneumocystis carinii* pneumonia prophylaxis using aerosolized pentamidine in children with acute leukemia. J Clin Oncol 12:136, 1994

West BC, et al: Aplastic anemia associated with parenteral chloramphenicol. Rev Infect Dis 10:1048, 1988

Nursing Bibliography

A new Rx for bacterial vaginosis. Emergency Medicine 23(2):77, 1991

Oral therapy for strep carriers. Emergency Medicine 23(18):77, 1991

Rubin LG, Tucci V, Cerenado E, Eliopoulos G, Isenberg H: Vancomycin resistant *Enterococcus faecun* in hospitalized children. Infection Control and Hospital Epidemiology 13:700, 1992

Ulrich M: Leprosy in women: Characteristics and repercussions. Soc Sci Med 37:445, 1993

68
Antitubercular Agents

Aminosalicylic acid
Capreomycin
Cycloserine
Ethambutol
Ethionamide
Isoniazid
Pyrazinamide
Rifabutin
Rifampin
Streptomycin

Tuberculosis, an infection caused by *Mycobacterium tuberculosis*, is most commonly confined to the lungs and is characterized by severe inflammation, tissue necrosis, and frequently by the development of open cavities, all of which can impair pulmonary function. In some cases, the offending pathogen gains access to the blood or lymph, and the infection may spread to other body tissues as well. Transmission of the disease is usually by inhalation of cough-expelled droplets from infected people.

The incidence of tuberculosis is increasing, both in the United States and throughout the world. These increases are concentrated primarily in specific epidemiologic groups that are characterized as racial and ethnic minorities, foreign-born immigrants, people with human immunodeficiency virus (HIV) infection, homeless people living in shelters, and prison inmates. HIV infection is the greatest risk factor for tuberculosis, and tuberculosis is often the initial manifestation of HIV infection. Testing for HIV infection is recommended in all patients with tuberculosis.

Drug therapy for tuberculosis is very effective, provided strict patient compliance can be ensured, but it may be complex, difficult, and prolonged. Infections tend to be chronic, and the microorganisms can exhibit extended periods of inactivity, making complete eradication difficult. The pathogen rapidly develops resistance to single-drug antitubercular therapy and, perhaps even more serious, increasing numbers of bacterial strains are proving resistant to some multiple-drug regimens. To minimize the emergence of resistant strains, therefore, antitubercular agents are almost always administered as combinations of two, three, or four drugs. Moreover, combination therapy allows use of lower doses of each individual drug than would be required if each were used alone, thereby reducing the likelihood of adverse effects.

Antitubercular drugs vary markedly both in efficacy and toxicity, and may be divided into first-line and second-line drugs on the basis of these differences. The first-line drugs are almost always used to initiate treatment of a newly diagnosed infection, inasmuch as they are the most dependable and least toxic agents when used in low- to moderate-dose combination therapy. Second-line drugs, in contrast, are often less effective and usually more toxic than the first-line drugs, and hence are reserved for treatment of resistant infections. Classification of the available antitubercular drugs in this text is as follows:

First-line drugs
- Ethambutol
- Isoniazid (INH)
- Pyrazinamide
- Rifampin
- Streptomycin

Second-line drugs
- Aminosalicylic acid and salts
- Capreomycin
- Cycloserine
- Ethionamide

For the initial treatment of uncomplicated tuberculosis, the recommended drug regimen includes INH, rifampin, and pyrazinamide, with or without other drugs for a minimum of 6 months. Although the initial phase of therapy usually requires daily administration of the drugs, subsequent administration may be daily, twice weekly, or three times weekly. Patients in whom drug-resistant tuberculosis is suspected or likely should receive an initial regimen consisting of *four* drugs given daily. The four-drug regimen usually consists of INH, rifampin, pyrazinamide, and ethambutol or streptomycin given daily for 2 months, followed by daily INH and rifampin or three times weekly INH, rifampin, and pyrazinamide for the remainder of the treatment period. Treatment is continued for at least 6 to 9 months and for several months after bacterial cultures become negative. Patients with HIV infection or those with acquired immunodeficiency syndrome should also receive the four-drug regimen. In these cases, therapy is more prolonged and patients are monitored periodically for evidence of relapse after therapy is complete.

Although para-aminosalicylic acid (PAS) was formerly widely used with INH, it is poorly tolerated by many patients, and the GI distress caused by the large doses that are required often reduces patient compliance. PAS is still a valuable adjunctive drug, but, as indicated, it has been replaced in many INH drug regimens by ethambutol or rifampin. Streptomycin is likewise an effective antitubercular drug, but must be given only in combination with other drugs such as INH, PAS, ethambutol, and rifampin, because resistance develops rapidly. It is used principally for extensive pulmonary or disseminated tuberculosis. The second-line drugs, because of their toxicity, are indicated only where treatment with the first-line drugs has failed. In addition, pyrazinamide is most effective during the first few months of treatment and is often the first drug to be eliminated from the treatment regimen.

Because there are numerous differences among the clinically available antitubercular drugs, they are considered individually in the following sections.

• Para-aminosalicylate Sodium (PAS)

P.A.S. Sodium

(CAN) Nemasol

The sodium salt of PAS contains 73% aminosalicylic acid equivalent and 10.9% sodium. It is used *in combination with* INH, rifampin, or streptomycin to delay the emergence of bacterial resistance to these first-line antitubercular drugs. PAS should *never* be used as the sole therapeutic agent in treating tuberculosis.

Mechanism

PAS is bacteriostatic in action; it inhibits mycobacterial folic acid synthesis by competing with enzyme systems for incorporation of para-aminobenzoic acid (PABA).

Uses

Adjunctive treatment of tuberculosis in combination with INH, rifampin, or streptomycin to delay development of resistance.

Dosage

Adults: 14 to 16 g/day in two to three divided doses
Children: 275 to 420 mg/kg/day in three to four divided doses

Fate

Well absorbed orally; widely distributed, concentrating in pleural tissue; half-life is about 1 hour; rapidly excreted in the urine, 80% to 90% within 8 to 10 hours, as both intact drug and metabolites.

Common Side Effects

GI distress, nausea, anorexia, diarrhea.

Significant Adverse Reactions

GI: vomiting, abdominal pain, epigastric burning, ulceration, gastric hemorrhage
Hypersensitivity: fever, skin rash, malaise, joint pain, mononucleosis-like syndrome, jaundice, hepatitis, pancreatitis
Hematologic: leukopenia, agranulocytosis, thrombocytopenia, hemolytic anemia
Other: goiter, hypokalemia, acidosis, vasculitis, Löffler's syndrome (fever, cough, dyspnea), encephalopathy, crystalluria

Contraindications

Salicylate hypersensitivity. *Cautious use* in people with impaired renal or hepatic function, gastric ulcer, congestive heart failure and other situations requiring sodium restriction; goiter; or hematologic abnormalities.

Interactions

PAS plasma levels may be increased by probenecid, salicylates, or sulfinpyrazone.
PAS may decrease absorption of rifampin, folic acid, digoxin, and vitamin B_{12}.
PAS may increase INH plasma levels by reducing its rate of metabolism.
Urinary acidifiers (eg, ammonium chloride, ascorbic acid) increase the possibility of PAS crystalluria.
PAS may potentiate the action of oral anticoagulants.

Nursing Management

Pretherapy Assessment

Assess and record baseline data necessary for detection of adverse effects of PAS: General: vital signs (VS), body weight, skin color, temperature, and integrity; GI: biliary function; Genitourinary (GU): renal function (urinalysis, blood urea nitrogen [BUN], creatinine); Cardiovascular system (CVS): hematologic function; Central nervous system (CNS): neurologic function; thyroid function.
Review medical history and documents for existing or previous conditions that:
a. require cautious use of PAS: impaired renal or hepatic function; gastric ulcer; congestive heart failure; goiter; hematologic abnormalities.
b. contraindicate use of PAS: allergy to PAS, salicylate; **pregnancy (Category C)**.

Nursing Interventions

Medication Administration

Administer oral form of drug with meals to minimize GI upset.
Administer PAS on schedule to ensure stable steady-state concentrations for the duration of therapy.
Administer only in conjunction with other antitubercular agents.
Reduce the risk of stomatitis through frequent mouth care.
Initiate a meal schedule that provides small, frequent meals if GI upset occurs.
Provide ready access to bathroom and interventions directed at symptom relief if diarrhea occurs.
Discard dosage form if it has a purple-brown color because drug deteriorates in sunlight, water, or heat.

Surveillance During Therapy

Monitor for signs of hypersensitivity, which may require discontinuation of drug.
Monitor complete blood count (CBC), urinalysis, and liver and kidney function test results obtained over the course of therapy.
Interpret results of diagnostic tests and contact practitioner as appropriate.
Monitor intake–output, observing for signs and symptoms of possible renal impairment and dehydration secondary to GI side effects (vomiting, diarrhea).
Interpret results of the following urine tests cautiously because the drug may interfere with them: protein, urobilinogen, vanillylmandelic acid, and glucose determinations with copper sulfate reagents (Clinitest tablets).
Monitor for possible drug–drug and drug–nutrient interactions: see Interactions.

Patient Teaching

Instruct patient regarding the importance of completing the full course of therapy as prescribed.
Inform patient of the consequences of not taking or abruptly discontinuing the PAS.
Instruct patient that the prescribed drug is to be taken for

the condition for which it is prescribed, and not to be used to treat any other infections.

Instruct patient to take drug with food to minimize GI upset. Suggest use of sugar-free gum or candy to eliminate the sour or bitter aftertaste that sometimes ensues.

Instruct patient to take drug dissolved in water (the sodium salt of PAS is freely soluble in water) if the powder is used. Powder is available in preweighed packets and in bulk containers.

Instruct patient not to use tablets or solutions (made from powder) that have turned brown or purple because discoloration indicates deterioration of drug.

Teach patient how to recognize and report indications of hypersensitivity (eg, skin eruptions, fever, malaise, fatigue, pruritus, joint pain). If these appear, all drugs should be discontinued, if necessary, to prevent development of liver or kidney damage or pancreatitis. Therapy may be resumed with low doses once symptoms have abated, but patient should be observed closely.

Instruct patient to avoid excessive intake of cranberry or prune juice because they tend to acidify urine, which increases the danger of crystalluria.

Instruct patient about possible adverse side effects of PAS: loss of appetite, nausea, vomiting, diarrhea.

Instruct patient on appropriate action to take if side effects occur:

- Notify practitioner if early signs of hematologic or hepatic toxicity (sore throat, fever, mucosal ulceration, malaise, pallor, jaundice) occur.
- Notify practitioner of any unusual bleeding. Rationale: hypoprothrombinemia and bleeding tendencies due to decreased synthesis of vitamin K by intestinal microflora may occur.

• Capreomycin

Capastat

Capreomycin is a polypeptide antibiotic used in combination with other appropriate drugs as an alternative antitubercular agent when the first-line drugs are ineffective. Capreomycin is both ototoxic and nephrotoxic and must be administered cautiously.

Mechanism

Not established; bacteriostatic against human strains of *Mycobacterium tuberculosis*; exhibits a neuromuscular blocking action in large doses; no cross-resistance with other tuberculostatic drugs.

Use

Adjunctive therapy of pulmonary tuberculosis in patients intolerant of or resistant to first-line drug regimens (ie, INH, ethambutol, rifampin, streptomycin).

Dosage

IM only: 1 g/day for 60 to 120 days, followed by 1 g two to three times a week (maximum 20 mg/kg/day).

Fate

Not appreciably absorbed when administered orally; peak serum levels in 1 to 2 hours after IM injection; excreted essentially unchanged in the urine, 50% within 12 hours.

Common Side Effects

Elevated BUN and nonprotein nitrogen, subclinical hearing loss (5–10 dB), and eosinophilia (with daily injections).

Significant Adverse Reactions

Hematuria, proteinuria, abnormal urinary sediment, renal tubular necrosis, tinnitus, vertigo, anorexia, clinically apparent hearing loss, leukocytosis, leukopenia, abnormal liver function test results, pain and induration of IM injection site, urticaria, maculopapular skin rash, hypokalemia.

Contraindications

Concurrent administration with streptomycin or other ototoxic drugs (eg, aminoglycosides, polymyxin, colistin); severe renal impairment. *Cautious use* in patients with renal or hepatic dysfunction, auditory impairment, history of allergies; in children and during pregnancy.

Interactions

Capreomycin may enhance the muscle-relaxing action of neuromuscular blocking agents, polypeptide antibiotics, aminoglycosides, and general anesthetics.

The potential for nephrotoxicity is increased by combined use of capreomycin with aminoglycosides, cephalothin, high-ceiling diuretics, polymyxins, and vancomycin.

Ototoxic effects of capreomycin can be potentiated by aminoglycosides, ethacrynic acid, bumetanide, furosemide, and vancomycin.

Nursing Management

Pretherapy Assessment

Assess and record baseline data necessary for detection of adverse effects of capreomycin: General: VS, body weight, skin color, temperature, and integrity; GI: biliary function; GU: renal function (urinalysis, BUN, creatinine); CVS: hematologic function; CNS: neurologic function; thyroid function; vestibular function; Laboratory: CBC, serum potassium.

Review medical history and documents for existing or previous conditions that:

a. require cautious use of capreomycin: impaired renal or hepatic function; auditory impairment, history of allergies, use in children.
b. contraindicate use of capreomycin: allergy to capreomycin; use with streptomycin or other ototoxic agents (aminoglycosides, polymyxins, colistin); severe renal impairment; **pregnancy (Category C)**; lactation (little is known about secretion into breast milk, use caution).

Nursing Interventions

Medication Administration

Administer capreomycin on schedule to ensure stable steady-state concentrations for the duration of therapy.

Administer only in conjunction with other antitubercular agents.
Reduce the risk of stomatitis through frequent mouth care.
Inject IM deeply into large muscle, and observe for inflammation and bleeding.

Surveillance During Therapy

Monitor for signs of hypersensitivity, which may require discontinuation of drug.
Monitor intake–output and check urine samples and laboratory findings for indications of renal toxicity (eg, hematuria; urinalysis showing casts, red cells, white cells, or protein; BUN above 30 mg/dL). If these appear, drug should be discontinued to prevent serious kidney damage. Renal function tests should be performed regularly during therapy.
Monitor CBC, urinalysis, and liver and kidney function test results obtained over the course of therapy.
Interpret results of diagnostic tests and contact practitioner as appropriate.
Monitor for possible drug–drug and drug–nutrient interactions: increased nephrotoxicity and ototoxicity if used with other nephrotoxic or ototoxic agents; increased neuromuscular activity if used with nondepolarizing neuromuscular blockers.

Patient Teaching

Instruct patient regarding the importance of completing the full course of therapy as prescribed.
Inform patient of the consequences of not taking or abruptly discontinuing the capreomycin.
Instruct patient that the prescribed drug is to be taken for the condition for which it is prescribed, and not to be used to treat any other infections.
Explain implications of drug's ototoxicity. Patient should understand that any sign of hearing impairment or vertigo must be promptly reported to appropriate person because drug needs to be discontinued immediately to prevent development of serious ear disorders. Also, audiometric and vestibular function tests should be performed periodically during therapy.
Teach patient how to recognize and report symptoms of potassium deficiency (eg, paresthesias, muscle cramping, palpitations), and explain that serum potassium levels are usually checked frequently because hypokalemia may occur during prolonged therapy.
Instruct patient about possible adverse side effects of capreomycin: dizziness, vertigo, loss of hearing.
Instruct patient on appropriate action to take if side effects occur: notify practitioner if skin rash, loss of hearing, decreased urine output, or palpitations occur.

• Cycloserine

Seromycin

A broad-spectrum antibiotic, cycloserine is effective against a variety of gram-positive and gram-negative bacteria as well as *Mycobacterium tuberculosis*. A second-line drug in the treatment of tuberculosis, it can also be used for acute urinary tract infections unresponsive to commonly used drugs. Major untoward reactions are CNS toxicity (eg, convulsions, psychosis, depression) and allergic reactions.

Mechanism

Inhibits cell wall synthesis in susceptible bacteria by antagonizing D-alanine, an essential factor in bacterial cell wall synthesis; bactericidal at usual therapeutic doses.

Uses

Alternative treatment of active tuberculosis in conjunction with other tuberculostatic drugs when first-line therapy has failed
Alternative treatment of acute urinary tract infections, especially those due to *Enterobacter* and *Escherichia coli*, only where other antimicrobial agents are ineffective and the infecting organism has demonstrated sensitivity to cycloserine

Dosage

Oral: initially 250 mg twice a day for 2 weeks; maintenance dose is 500 to 1000 mg/day in divided doses as necessary; do not exceed 1 g/day.

Fate

Well absorbed orally; peak plasma levels attained in 3 to 4 hours; widely distributed, including the CNS; half-life is 10 hours; excreted primarily in the urine, both as active drug and metabolites.

Significant Adverse Reactions

Neurotoxicity (*dose-related*; symptoms include vertigo, paresthesias, irritability, headache, aggression, hyperreflexia, drowsiness, tremor, dysarthria, confusion, disorientation, loss of memory, convulsions, localized clonic seizures, psychoses, suicidal tendencies, coma).

Other adverse reactions are skin rash, allergic dermatitis, photosensitivity, elevated serum transaminase, vitamin B_{12} or folic acid deficiency, megaloblastic anemia.

Contraindications

Epilepsy, severe anxiety, psychoses, excessive alcohol consumption, depression, and severe renal insufficiency. *Cautious use* in patients with liver or kidney impairment, in young children, and in pregnant women.

Interactions

Cycloserine can potentiate the effects of monoamine oxidase (MAO) inhibitors and phenytoin.
Ethionamide, INH, and alcohol can enhance the neurotoxic effects of cycloserine.
Cycloserine can increase the excretion of the B-complex vitamins.

Nursing Management

Pretherapy Assessment

Assess and record baseline data necessary for detection of adverse effects of cycloserine: General: VS, body weight, skin color, temperature, and integrity; GI: biliary function; GU: renal function (urinalysis, BUN, creatinine); CVS: hematologic function, electrocardiogram; CNS: neurologic function; Laboratory: culture of infected site.

Review medical history and documents for existing or previous conditions that:

a. require cautious use of cycloserine: impaired renal or hepatic function; use in children.

b. contraindicate use of cycloserine: allergy to cycloserine; epilepsy; severe anxiety; psychosis; excessive alcohol consumption; depression; severe renal insufficiency; **pregnancy (Category C)**; lactation (safety not established, avoid use in nursing mothers).

Nursing Interventions

Medication Administration

Administer oral form of drug with meals, with a full glass of water.

Reduce the risk of stomatitis through frequent mouth care.

Be prepared to administer oxygen, artificial respiration, intravenous fluids, vasopressors, and anticonvulsants in case convulsions or other manifestations of CNS toxicity occur. Because CNS toxicity is related to serum drug levels, high dosage (greater than 500 mg/day) or inadequate renal clearance predisposes to neurotoxicity.

Initiate a meal schedule that provides small, frequent meals if GI upset occurs.

Protect patient from exposure to sunlight and ultraviolet light. Use sunscreen (not containing PABA) or protective clothing.

Surveillance During Therapy

Monitor results of hematologic, renal excretion, liver function, and serum drug level studies, which should be performed periodically during therapy. Serum drug level should be determined at least weekly if patient is receiving large doses or exhibits reduced renal function. Dosage should be adjusted if serum level exceeds 30 μg/mL or if renal impairment as indicated by creatinine clearance develops (see package instructions).

Monitor for signs of hypersensitivity (including photosensitivity), which may require discontinuation of drug.

Monitor CBC, urinalysis, and liver and kidney function test results obtained over the course of therapy.

Interpret results of diagnostic tests and contact practitioner as appropriate.

Monitor for possible drug–laboratory test interactions.

Monitor for possible drug–drug and drug–nutrient interactions: potentiation of effects of MAO inhibitors and phenytoin; ethionamide, INH, and alcohol potentiate neurotoxic effects of cycloserine; increase in excretion of B-complex vitamins.

Provide for patient safety needs to minimize environmental hazards and risk of injury if CNS side effects develop.

Patient Teaching

Instruct patient regarding the importance of completing the full course of therapy as prescribed.

Inform patient of the consequences of not taking or abruptly discontinuing the cycloserine.

Instruct patient that the prescribed drug is to be taken for the condition for which it is prescribed, and not to be used to treat any other infections.

Emphasize the importance of informing drug prescriber immediately if symptoms of allergic dermatitis or CNS toxicity occur (see Significant Adverse Reactions) because dosage should be reduced or drug discontinued to avoid more serious untoward reactions. Anticonvulsants, pyridoxine, or sedatives may be effective in controlling CNS toxicity.

Instruct patient about possible adverse side effects of cycloserine: drowsiness; tremor; disorientation; depression; personality change; numbness and tingling.

Instruct patient on appropriate action to take if side effects occur: notify practitioner if skin rash, headache, tremors, shaking, confusion, or dizziness occur.

• Ethambutol

Myambutol

(CAN) Etibi

A synthetic, orally administered tuberculostatic drug effective against actively dividing mycobacteria, ethambutol is a first-line drug for treatment of pulmonary tuberculosis. It is most often used in combination with INH, rifampin, or streptomycin, depending on the resistance of the organism, because it is somewhat less active alone than other first-line drugs. Ethambutol may have adverse effects on visual acuity, and monthly eye examinations are recommended during therapy.

Mechanism

Inhibits protein synthesis and impairs cellular metabolism, thus blocking multiplication of bacterial cells; does not exhibit cross-resistance with other agents; bacteriostatic in action.

Uses

Treatment of pulmonary tuberculosis, in combination with INH, rifampin, pyrazinamide, or streptomycin.

Dosage

Initial treatment: 15 mg/kg as a single oral dose every 24 hours with INH

Retreatment: (patients having previous antituberculosis treatment) 25 mg/kg as a single oral dose every 24 hours with at least one other antitubercular drug to which the organism is susceptible; decrease to 15 mg/kg after 60 days

Fate

Readily absorbed from GI tract; absorption unaffected by the presence of food; peak serum level occurs in 2 to 4 hours; no accumulation has been reported in patients with normal kidney function; approximately 50% excreted unchanged in the urine, 20% to 25% eliminated unchanged in the feces, and remainder excreted as metabolites in the urine.

Significant Adverse Reactions

CNS: decreased visual acuity due to optic neuritis (eg, altered color perception, blurred vision), fever, malaise,

headache, dizziness, confusion, disorientation, paresthesias, hallucinations
GI: abdominal pain, GI upset, vomiting, anorexia
Allergic–hypersensitivity: pruritus, dermatitis, joint pain, anaphylactic reactions
Other: elevated serum uric acid, acute gout, transient impairment of liver function, epidermal necrolysis, thrombocytopenia

Contraindications

Optic neuritis; children younger than 12 years of age. *Cautious use* in patients with hepatic or renal dysfunction, hyperuricemia, or history of acute gout; during pregnancy.

Interactions

Ethambutol may reduce the effectiveness of uricosuric drugs such as probenecid and sulfinpyrazone.
Aluminum-containing antacids may impair oral absorption of myambutol.

Nursing Management

Pretherapy Assessment

Assess and record baseline data necessary for detection of adverse effects of ethambutol: General: VS, body weight, skin color, temperature, and integrity; GI: biliary function; GU: renal function (urinalysis, BUN, creatinine); CVS: hematologic function; CNS: neurologic function, ophthalmologic examination.
Review medical history and documents for existing or previous conditions that:
a. require cautious use of ethambutol: impaired renal or hepatic function; hyperuricemia, history of acute gout.
b. contraindicate use of ethambutol: allergy to ethambutol; optic neuritis; use in children younger than 12 years of age; **pregnancy (Category B)**; lactation (safety not established, avoid use in nursing mothers).

Nursing Interventions

Medication Administration

Administer oral form of drug with meals, with a full glass of water.
Reduce the risk of stomatitis through frequent mouth care.
Must be used in combination with other antitubercular agents.
Provide small, frequent meals if GI upset occurs.
Ensure that visual function is tested before therapy is initiated. It should be retested periodically during treatment (monthly if drug is administered in high dosages).
Expect dosage to be reduced in patient with impaired renal function. Dosage should be based on desired serum level of drug (eg, 2–5 μg/mL).

Surveillance During Therapy

Interpret aminotransferase and serum uric acid findings cautiously because drug can increase levels.
Monitor results of renal excretion, liver function, CBC, and ophthalmologic examinations.
Monitor for signs of hypersensitivity (including photosensitivity), which may require discontinuation of drug.
Interpret results of diagnostic tests and contact practitioner as appropriate.
Monitor for possible drug–drug and drug–nutrient interactions: may reduce the effectiveness of uricosuric agents (probenecid, sulfinpyrazone); oral absorption impaired by aluminum-containing antacids.

Patient Teaching

Instruct patient regarding the importance of completing the full course of therapy as prescribed.
Inform patient of the consequences of not taking or abruptly discontinuing the ethambutol.
Instruct patient that the prescribed drug is to be taken for the condition for which it is prescribed, and not to be used to treat any other infections.
Instruct patient about possible adverse side effects of ethambutol: nausea; vomiting; epigastric distress; skin rashes or lesions; disorientation; confusion; drowsiness; dizziness.
Instruct patient on appropriate action to take if side effects occur: notify practitioner if skin rash or changes in vision (blurring, altered color perception) occur.

• Ethionamide

Trecator-SC

Mechanism

Not established; probably similar to that of INH; may inhibit peptide synthesis in mycobacterial cells.

Use

Alternative therapy of active tuberculosis in combination with other effective antitubercular drugs when treatment with first-line drugs (INH, ethambutol, pyrazinamide, rifampin, streptomycin) has failed

Dosage

Adults: 0.5 to 1 g/day in divided doses with at least one other antitubercular drug and pyridoxine (50 mg/day)—see Patient Teaching, below
Children: optimum dosage is not established; 4 to 5 mg/kg every 8 hours has been suggested

Fate

Well absorbed orally and distributed widely in the body, including the CNS; peak serum levels attained in 3 to 4 hours; excreted largely in the urine, almost entirely as metabolites.

Common Side Effects

GI upset (nausea, vomiting, cramping), salivation, metallic taste, stomatitis, diarrhea, anorexia, drowsiness, asthenia.

Significant Adverse Reactions

Neurotoxicity: blurred vision, diplopia, optic neuritis, peripheral neuritis, olfactory disturbances, dizziness, headache, restlessness, tremors, convulsions, psychosis
GI: hepatitis, jaundice
Other: orthostatic hypotension, impotence, gynecomastia,

acne, skin rash, alopecia, pellagra-like syndrome, thrombocytopenia

Contraindications

Severe hepatic dysfunction. *Cautious use* in patients with diabetes mellitus, liver or renal impairment, in children, and during pregnancy (fetal damage has been reported in experimental animals).

Interactions

Ethionamide can enhance the neurotoxicity of cycloserine and may intensify the adverse effects of other tuberculostatic agents.
Ethionamide may increase the neurotoxic effects of alcohol.
Ethionamide may potentiate the hypotensive effects (especially orthostatic) of antihypertensive drugs.
Ethionamide may interfere with the management of diabetes by hypoglycemic drugs.

Nursing Management

Pretherapy Assessment

Assess and record baseline data necessary for detection of adverse effects of ethionamide: General: VS, body weight, skin color, temperature, and integrity; GI: biliary function; GU: renal function (urinalysis, BUN, creatinine); CVS: hematologic function; CNS: neurologic function, ophthalmologic examination.
Review medical history and documents for existing or previous conditions that:
a. require cautious use of ethionamide: impaired renal or hepatic function; diabetes mellitus; use in children.
b. contraindicate use of ethionamide: allergy to ethionamide; severe hepatic dysfunction; **pregnancy (Category B)**; lactation (safety not established, avoid use in nursing mothers).

Nursing Interventions

Medication Administration

Administer oral form of drug with meals, with a full glass of water.
Reduce the risk of stomatitis through frequent mouth care.
Must be used in combination with other antitubercular agents.
Provide small, frequent meals if GI upset occurs.
Ensure that visual function is tested before therapy is initiated. It should be retested periodically during treatment (monthly if drug is administered in high dosages).

Surveillance During Therapy

Monitor results of renal excretion, liver function, CBC, and ophthalmologic examinations.
Ensure that serum aminotransferases (ALT, AST) are measured before therapy is initiated. They also should be determined at 2- to 4-week intervals throughout therapy.
Monitor for signs of hypersensitivity, which may require discontinuation of drug.
Interpret results of diagnostic tests and contact practitioner as appropriate.
Monitor for possible drug–drug and drug–nutrient interactions: may enhance the neurotoxicity of cycloserine; may intensify adverse effects of other tuberculostatic agents; may increase neurotoxic effects of alcohol; may potentiate the hypotensive effects of antihypertensives; may interfere with the effectiveness of hypoglycemic agents.

Patient Teaching

Instruct patient regarding the importance of completing the full course of therapy as prescribed.
Inform patient of the consequences of not taking or abruptly discontinuing the ethionamide.
Instruct patient that the prescribed drug is to be taken for the condition for which it is prescribed, and not to be used to treat any other infections.
Caution patient to avoid excessive use of alcohol to minimize danger of neurotoxicity.
Instruct patient with diabetes to monitor blood sugar carefully because management of diabetes mellitus may be more difficult. Dosage of hypoglycemic drugs should be adjusted on the basis of blood glucose determinations.
Explain that 50 mg per day of vitamin B_6 may be prescribed during therapy (when used with INH, ethionamide may contribute to INH-induced pyridoxine deficiency).
Instruct patient about possible adverse side effects of ethionamide: nausea; vomiting; epigastric distress; metallic taste; stomatitis; skin rashes or lesions; blurred vision; diplopia; optic neuritis; hepatitis; disorientation; confusion; drowsiness; dizziness.
Instruct patient on appropriate action to take if side effects occur: notify practitioner if skin rash, changes in vision (blurring, altered color perception) or yellowing of the skin or eyes occur.

• Isoniazid (INH)

Laniazid, Nydrazid
(CAN) Isotamine, PMS Isoniazid

A first-line drug of choice for most cases of active tuberculosis, INH is usually prescribed in combination with pyrazinamide and rifampin, with or without ethambutol, or all three, to delay the emergence of resistant strains. It is also indicated for prophylactic use in high-risk patients, such as household members of infected people or people with positive tuberculin skin test reactions. A major danger associated with INH is severe and sometimes fatal hepatitis. The risk of development of hepatitis increases with advancing age and alcohol consumption (see Significant Adverse Reactions).

Mechanism

Not completely established; drug is bactericidal; may interfere with biosynthesis of lipids, proteins, nucleic acid, and mycolic acid, the latter leads to bacterial cell wall destruction in susceptible organisms; resistance frequently develops rapidly when INH is used alone; can antagonize the activity of vitamin B_6.

Uses

Treatment of all forms of active tuberculosis due to susceptible organisms, usually in combination with other tuberculostatic drugs

Prophylaxis in high-risk patients such as household members or close associates of actively infected people or people evidencing positive tuberculin skin test reactions in the absence of positive bacteriologic findings; also used in people younger than 35 years (especially children younger than 7 years) with positive skin test reactions, patients with hematologic diseases (eg, leukemia, Hodgkin's disease) or diabetes, people undergoing immunosuppressive therapy or prolonged treatment with corticosteroids, and after a gastrectomy

Dosage

Active tuberculosis

Adults: 5 mg/kg/day in a single dose (maximum 300 mg/day)

Children: 10 to 20 mg/kg/day in a single dose (maximum 500 mg/day)

Prophylaxis

Adults: 300 mg/day in a single dose for 6 to 12 months

Children: 10 mg/kg/day in a single dose for 6 to 12 months

NOTE: Pyridoxine (vitamin B_6) is given concurrently with INH at a dosage of 15 to 50 mg a day (see Nursing Management).

Fate

Completely absorbed from the GI tract; absorption is reduced by food; peak blood levels in 1 to 2 hours, declining to 50% or less within 6 hours; widely distributed in the body, including cerebrospinal, pleural, and ascitic tissues; less than half is excreted unchanged in the urine—most of the remainder is acetylated or hydrolyzed by the liver and metabolites are removed by the kidneys; rate of acetylation is genetically determined and may be slow (in approximately 50% of blacks and whites) or rapid (rest of blacks and whites, Orientals, and Eskimos); rate of acetylation does *not* alter clinical efficacy of INH but may influence toxicity (ie, slow acetylators are more prone to elevated blood levels and increased toxic reactions, including peripheral neuropathies; rapid acetylators are more likely to develop hepatitis); liver disease can prolong clearance of INH.

Common Side Effects

Paresthesias, peripheral neuropathy (especially in malnourished, diabetic, or alcoholic people), and mild hepatic dysfunction (transient elevation of serum transaminase).

Significant Adverse Reactions

CNS: optic neuritis, toxic encephalopathy, memory impairment, toxic psychosis, convulsions

GI: nausea, vomiting, epigastric distress

Hepatic: bilirubinemia, bilirubinuria, jaundice, severe (occasionally fatal) hepatitis

Hematologic: hemolytic or aplastic anemia, agranulocytosis, eosinophilia, thrombocytopenia

Allergic–hypersensitivity: fever, skin rashes (morbilliform, maculopapular, purpuric, exfoliative), vasculitis, lymphadenopathy

Other: vitamin B_6 deficiency, hyperglycemia, metabolic acidosis, gynecomastia, pellagra, rheumatoid, or systemic lupus-like symptoms, irritation at IM injection site

Contraindications

Acute liver disease, previous adverse reaction with INH. *Cautious use* in patients with chronic liver disease, renal dysfunction, diabetes, convulsive disorders, psychoses, a history of allergic reactions; in alcoholics and in pregnant or nursing women.

Interactions

INH can increase serum levels of phenytoin by reducing its metabolism.

The efficacy of INH may be reduced when used with corticosteroids.

Alcohol increases the risk of INH-induced hepatitis.

INH can potentiate the pharmacologic and toxicologic effects of carbamazepine and benzodiazepine antianxiety agents.

Antacids reduce GI absorption of INH if they are given together.

Disulfiram and INH can impair coordination and elicit behavioral changes.

Concurrent use of INH and rifampin may increase the likelihood of hepatotoxicity, whereas combined use of INH and cycloserine can increase CNS toxicity.

INH may exhibit MAO-inhibitory activity and can potentiate sympathomimetic amines, leading to increased blood pressure.

INH has been reported to potentiate anesthetics, anticoagulants, anticonvulsants, hypoglycemics, antihypertensives, antiparkinsonian agents, anticholinergics, antidepressants, narcotics, and sedatives, although the clinical importance of these potential interactions has not been definitely established.

Nursing Management

Pretherapy Assessment

Assess and record baseline data necessary for detection of adverse effects of INH: General: VS, body weight, skin color, temperature, and integrity; GI: biliary function; GU: renal function (urinalysis, BUN, creatinine); CVS: hematologic function; CNS: neurologic function, ophthalmologic examination; Laboratory: blood glucose.

Review medical history and documents for existing or previous conditions that:

a. require cautious use of INH: impaired renal function; diabetes mellitus; chronic liver disease; convulsive disorders; psychoses; history of allergic reactions; alcoholism.

b. contraindicate use of INH: allergy to INH; INH-associated hepatic dysfunction; acute hepatic disease; **pregnancy (Category C)**; lactation (secreted in breast milk; observe infants for adverse effects).

Nursing Interventions

Medication Administration

Administer oral form of drug with a full glass of water, 1 or 2 hours after meals.

Reduce the risk of stomatitis through frequent mouth care.
Provide small, frequent meals if GI upset occurs.
Expect to administer IM only if oral route is unavailable or impractical. Inform patient that IM injection may be irritating or painful.
Expect supplemental vitamin B_6 (10–100 mg/day) to be prescribed to minimize neurotoxic effects, especially in malnourished or diabetic patient or slow acetylator of INH (see Fate). INH is available in fixed combinations with vitamin B_6 (100 mg INH/5 mg vitamin B_6; 100 mg/10 mg; and 300 mg/30 mg) as Teebaconin and Vitamin B_6 and P-I-N Forte.
Note that INH is available in fixed combinations with rifampin as Rifamate or Rimactane/INH Dual Pack.

Surveillance During Therapy

Monitor results of renal excretion, liver function, CBC, and ophthalmologic examinations.
Monitor carefully for indications of hepatic dysfunction (anorexia, malaise, nausea, vomiting, darkening of urine, paresthesias, jaundice). Drug should be discontinued immediately if these occur. Monthly liver function tests should be performed during therapy.
Ensure that serum aminotransferase is measured before therapy is initiated. It also should be determined at 2- to 4-week intervals throughout therapy.
Monitor for signs of hypersensitivity, which may require discontinuation of drug.
Interpret results of diagnostic tests and contact practitioner as appropriate.
Monitor for possible drug–drug and drug–nutrient interactions: see Interactions.

Patient Teaching

Instruct patient regarding the importance of completing the full course of therapy as prescribed.
Inform patient of the consequences of not taking or abruptly discontinuing the INH. Because adverse effects, especially hepatotoxicity and neurotoxicity, are more prevalent at higher doses, recommended dosages should not be exceeded. Conversely, consequences of skipping doses or discontinuing therapy without prescriber knowledge may also be serious because insufficient dosage permits resistant strains to emerge, and relapse rates are high if treatment is terminated prematurely.
Instruct patient that the prescribed drug is to be taken for the condition for which it is prescribed, and not to be used to treat any other infections.
Caution patient to reduce intake of alcohol to minimize risk of hepatitis and the danger of neurotoxicity.
Instruct patient to obtain periodic ophthalmic examinations during therapy and to notify drug prescriber if visual disturbances occur.
Instruct patient with diabetes to monitor blood sugar carefully. Dosage of hypoglycemic medication should be adjusted as needed to maintain control because INH can elevate blood sugar *or* potentiate the action of hypoglycemic drugs.
Instruct patient about possible adverse side effects of INH: nausea; vomiting; epigastric distress; skin rashes or lesions; blurred vision; diplopia; optic neuritis; hepatitis; disorientation; confusion; drowsiness; dizziness.
Instruct patient on appropriate action to take if side effects occur: notify practitioner if skin rash, changes in vision (blurring, altered color perception), yellowing of the skin or eyes, darkening of urine, numbness or tingling in hands or feet occur.

• Pyrazinamide

(CAN) PMS Pyrazinamide, Tebrazid

Pyrazinamide is a first-line tuberculostatic agent, commonly used in combination with other primary drugs (INH, ethambutol, rifampin, streptomycin). Principal adverse effects are hepatotoxicity (the incidence of which ranges from 2%–20% and depends on the dosage) and hyperuricemia.

Mechanism

Not established; primarily bacteriostatic, possibly interferes with protein synthesis; active only at slightly acidic pH.

Uses

Initial treatment of active tuberculosis, in combination with other first-line drugs in patients in whom resistance is anticipated.

Dosage

15 to 30 mg/kg once daily; not to exceed 2 g/day when given as a daily regimen; alternatively: 50 to 70 mg/kg twice weekly

Fate

Readily absorbed orally; peak serum levels in 2 hours; half-life is 9 to 10 hours; widely distributed in the body, partially metabolized by the liver and excreted in the urine primarily (70%) as metabolites with some unchanged drug.

Significant Adverse Reactions

Hepatic dysfunction (fever, anorexia, malaise, hepatomegaly, abdominal tenderness, splenomegaly, jaundice, yellow atrophy of the liver), GI distress, arthralgia, anemia, dysuria, urinary retention, hyperuricemia, acute gout, skin rash, urticaria, and photosensitivity.

Contraindications

Severe liver damage; in children. *Cautious use* in patients with a history of gout or hyperuricemia, diabetes mellitus, impaired renal function, peptic ulcer, acute intermittent porphyria; and in alcoholics.

Interactions

Pyrazinamide can interfere with the uricosuric action of probenecid and sulfinpyrazone.
Pyrazinamide may alter the dosage requirements for insulin or oral hypoglycemic drugs in patients with diabetes.

Nursing Management

Pretherapy Assessment

Assess and record baseline data necessary for detection of adverse effects of pyrazinamide: General: VS, body weight, skin color, temperature, and integrity; GI: biliary function; CVS: hematologic function; CNS: neurologic function, ophthalmologic examination; Laboratory: blood glucose, serum and urine uric acid.

Review medical history and documents for existing or previous conditions that:

a. require cautious use of pyrazinamide: impaired renal function; diabetes mellitus; peptic ulcer; history of gout; alcoholism.
b. contraindicate use of pyrazinamide: allergy to pyrazinamide; severe liver damage; **pregnancy (Category C)**; lactation (secreted in breast milk; observe infants for adverse effects).

Nursing Interventions

Medication Administration

Administer oral form of drug with a full glass of water, 1 or 2 hours after meals.

Reduce the risk of stomatitis through frequent mouth care.

Provide small, frequent meals if GI upset occurs.

Administer only in conjunction with other antitubercular agents.

Surveillance During Therapy

Monitor results of renal excretion, liver function, CBC, and ophthalmologic examinations.

Monitor carefully for indications of hepatic dysfunction (anorexia, malaise, nausea, vomiting, darkening of urine, paresthesias, jaundice). Drug should be discontinued immediately if these occur. Monthly liver function tests should be performed during therapy.

Ensure that serum aminotransferase is measured before therapy is initiated. It also should be determined at 2- to 4-week intervals throughout therapy.

Monitor serum uric acid; arrange for discontinuation of therapy if patient is hyperuricemic with acute gouty arthritis.

Monitor for signs of hypersensitivity (including photosensitivity), which may require discontinuation of drug.

Interpret results of diagnostic tests and contact practitioner as appropriate.

Monitor for possible drug–drug and drug–nutrient interactions: can interfere with uricosuric action of probenecid, sulfinpyrazone; alter dosage requirements for insulin and hypoglycemics in patients with diabetes.

Patient Teaching

Instruct patient regarding the importance of completing the full course of therapy as prescribed.

Inform patient of the consequences of not taking or abruptly discontinuing the pyrazinamide.

Instruct patient that the prescribed drug is to be taken for the condition for which it is prescribed, and not to be used to treat any other infections.

Instruct patient with diabetes to monitor blood sugar carefully. Dosage of hypoglycemic medication should be adjusted as needed to maintain control because pyrazinamide can elevate blood sugar *or* potentiate the action of hypoglycemic drugs.

Instruct patient about possible adverse side effects of pyrazinamide: loss of appetite; nausea; vomiting; skin rash; sensitivity to sunlight.

Instruct patient on appropriate action to take if side effects occur: notify practitioner if fever; malaise; loss of appetite; nausea; vomiting; darkened urine; yellowing of skin and eyes; severe pain in great toe, instep, ankle, heel, knee, or wrist occur.

• *Rifabutin*

Mycobutin

Rifabutin is an antimycobacterial agent similar to rifampin but with a specific indication—namely, prevention of disseminated *Mycobacterium avium* complex (MAC) disease in patients with advanced HIV infection. Rifabutin does *not* appear to be prophylactic against *Mycobacterium tuberculosis*, and patients with active tuberculosis should not be given rifabutin alone, because emergence of strains resistant to both rifampin and rifabutin has occurred. Patients requiring prophylaxis against both *M tuberculosis* and *M avium* complex, however, may be given INH and rifabutin concurrently. The usual dose of rifabutin is 300 mg orally, once daily, although it may be given in two divided doses if nausea and vomiting occur. Because neutropenia has been associated with rifabutin administration, periodic hematologic studies are necessary. Other common side effects include rash and GI distress. The drug colors most body fluids (saliva, perspiration, urine, tears) brown-orange, and soft contact lenses may become permanently stained.

• *Rifampin*

Rifadin, Rimactane

(CAN) Rofact

A derivative of the antibiotic rifamycin B, rifampin is a first-line bacteriostatic antitubercular drug. It is most often used in combination with INH and ethambutol, because resistance develops rapidly if it is given alone. The drug should be taken on an uninterrupted schedule, because intermittent therapy is associated with a higher incidence of adverse reactions, especially involving the liver and kidneys.

Mechanism

Inhibits DNA-dependent RNA polymerase activity in bacterial cells, thus interfering with nucleic acid synthesis; active against a number of gram-positive and gram-negative organisms; no apparent cross-resistance with other antitubercular drugs.

Uses

Treatment of pulmonary tuberculosis in conjunction with at least one other tuberculostatic drug (eg, INH, ethambutol)

Alternative chemoprophylaxis treatment in INH-resistant *Mycobacterium tuberculosis*

Treatment of asymptomatic carriers of *Neisseria meningitidis* to eliminate meningococci from the nasopharynx (*not* indicated for meningococcal infections)

Investigational uses include treatment of staphylococcal infections, Legionnaires' disease not responsive to erythromycin, gram-negative bacteremia in infancy, leprosy (with dapsone), and prophylaxis of *Haemophilus* meningitis

Dosage

Pulmonary tuberculosis

Adults: 600 mg/day in a single oral dose
Children older than 5 years: 10 to 20 mg/kg day in a single dose

Meningococcal carriers

Adults: 600 mg/day for 4 consecutive days
Children older than 5 years: 10 to 20 mg/kg/day for 4 consecutive days

Fate

Oral absorption is nearly complete; peak blood levels vary widely and occur between 1 and 4 hours; 70% to 80% protein bound; metabolized in the liver and excreted both in the feces (via bile) and to a lesser extent in the urine as both free drug and deacetylated metabolites; half-life varies from 1.5 to 5 hours but is progressively shortened during the initial weeks of therapy because microsomal enzyme induction accelerates the drug's metabolism.

Common Side Effects

Elevation of liver enzymes, rash, mild GI distress, flu-like syndrome at high doses (fever, chills, myalgia, and occasionally eosinophilia, thrombocytopenia, and hemolytic anemia).

Significant Adverse Reactions

GI: anorexia, vomiting, diarrhea, cramping, flatulence, sore mouth, pancreatitis, pseudomembranous colitis
CNS: headache, drowsiness, fatigue, dizziness, ataxia, confusion, visual disturbances, muscle weakness, generalized numbness, hearing disturbances
Allergic–hypersensitivity: pruritus, urticaria, rash, acneiform lesions, fever
Hepatic–renal: abnormal liver function test results (elevated BUN, serum bilirubin, serum transaminase, alkaline phosphatase), hepatitis, hemoglobinuria, hematuria, proteinuria, renal insufficiency, acute renal failure
Hematologic: transient leukopenia, thrombocytopenia, decreased hemoglobin, hemolytic anemia, eosinophilia
Other: conjunctivitis, elevated serum uric acid, menstrual irregularities, osteomalacia, myopathy

Contraindications

Not to be given on an *intermittent* dosage schedule (increased incidence of adverse reactions). *Cautious use* in patients with hepatic or renal disease or a history of alcoholism; in pregnant women and in children younger than 5 years of age.

Interactions

Rifampin induces microsomal enzymes and thus may decrease the effects of other drugs metabolized by these liver enzymes, for example, oral anticoagulants, estrogens, progestins, metoprolol, propranolol, quinidine, clofibrate, corticosteroids, oral hypoglycemics, and methadone.
PAS administered concurrently can impair GI absorption of rifampin and can reduce rifampin serum levels.
The action of rifampin can be potentiated by probenecid or INH, which compete for hepatic uptake.
Concomitant use of rifampin and alcohol may increase the incidence of hepatotoxicity.

Nursing Management

Pretherapy Assessment

Assess and record baseline data necessary for detection of adverse effects of rifampin: General: VS, body weight, skin color, temperature, and integrity; GI: biliary function; GU: renal function (urinalysis, BUN, creatinine); CNS: neurologic function (gait, muscle strength), ophthalmologic examination.
Review medical history and documents for existing or previous conditions that:
a. require cautious use of rifampin: impaired renal or hepatic function; history of alcoholism.
b. contraindicate use of rifampin: allergy to rifampin; severe liver damage (predisposes to fatal hepatotoxicity); **pregnancy (Category C)**; lactation (secreted in breast milk; discontinue nursing if drug is necessary).

Nursing Interventions

Medication Administration

Administer oral form of drug with a full glass of water, 1 or 2 hours after meals.
Reduce the risk of stomatitis through frequent mouth care.
Provide small, frequent meals if GI upset occurs.
Not to be administered on an intermittent dose schedule.

Surveillance During Therapy

Monitor results of renal excretion, liver function, CBC, and ophthalmologic examinations.
Monitor carefully for indications of hepatic dysfunction (anorexia, malaise, nausea, vomiting, darkening of urine, paresthesias, jaundice). Drug should be discontinued immediately if these occur. Monthly liver function tests should be performed during therapy.
Ensure that serum aminotransferase is measured before therapy is initiated. It also should be determined at 2- to 4-week intervals throughout therapy.
Monitor serum uric acid; arrange for discontinuation of therapy if patient is hyperuricemic with acute gouty arthritis.
Monitor for signs of hypersensitivity, which may require discontinuation of drug.
Interpret results of diagnostic tests and contact practitioner as appropriate.
Notify laboratory of drug use if serum folate and vitamin B_{12} determinations are required; alternative testing methods must be used because rifampin can interfere with standard assays for serum folate and vitamin B_{12}.
Monitor for possible drug–drug and drug–nutrient interactions: induces microsomal enzymes and may decrease effects of other drugs metabolized by these enzymes; when used with PAS, can impair rifampin absorption; action can be potentiated by probenecid or INH, which impair hepatic uptake; when used with alcohol, increases risk of hepatotoxicity.

Patient Teaching

Instruct patient regarding the importance of completing the full course of therapy as prescribed.

Inform patient of the consequences of not taking or abruptly discontinuing the rifampin.

Instruct patient that the prescribed drug is to be taken for the condition for which it is prescribed, and not to be used to treat any other infections.

Instruct patient to report development of flu-like symptoms (fever, chills, headache, muscle aches) because they may signal impending hepatorenal dysfunction, especially if drug has been used intermittently.

Teach patient how to recognize and immediately report appearance of jaundice-like symptoms (yellowing of skin or sclerae, pruritus, darkened urine, light-colored stools). Liver function must be evaluated periodically during therapy.

Inform patient to note occurrence of sore throat, unusual bleeding or bruising, or excessive weakness, indications of possible blood dyscrasias, and to inform prescriber immediately if they occur. Hematologic studies should be performed.

Inform patient that drug may impart a harmless red-orange color to urine, feces, saliva, sputum, sweat, and tears. Inform premenopausal woman that menstrual irregularities may occur.

Discuss use of alternative contraceptive methods with woman using oral contraceptive during rifampin therapy because effectiveness of oral contraceptives may be reduced.

Instruct patient about possible adverse side effects of rifampin: red-orange discoloration of body fluids, tears, sweat, saliva, urine, feces, sputum; contact lenses may be permanently stained; nausea; vomiting; epigastric distress; skin rashes or lesions; numbness; tingling; drowsiness; fatigue.

Instruct patient on appropriate action to take if side effects occur: notify practitioner if fever; malaise; loss of appetite; nausea; vomiting; darkened urine; yellowing of skin and eyes; muscle or bone pain; skin rash or itching occur.

• Streptomycin

An aminoglycoside antibiotic effective against *Mycobacterium tuberculosis*, streptomycin usually is considered a primary drug. It is most often used in combination with INH, rifampin, or ethambutol for control of more severe infections. Resistance develops rapidly, and hence combination therapy is necessary to maintain effectiveness. It is administered IM only; thus, patient compliance during prolonged therapy may be poor. The principal danger associated with use of streptomycin is ototoxicity, both vestibular and auditory, and patients receiving the drug must be observed carefully. Streptomycin has been reviewed in Chapter 64, and only the dosage regimen for use in tuberculosis is given here.

Dosage

Usual regimen is 1 g streptomycin IM with an appropriate dose of additional antitubercular drugs, such as INH, ethambutol, or rifampin; reduce streptomycin dosage to 1 g two or three times a week as symptoms improve.

Use smaller doses in the elderly or in patients with impaired renal function.

Nursing Management

Refer to Chapter 64.

Selected Bibliography

American Academy of Pediatrics: Chemotherapy for tuberculosis in infants and children. Pediatrics 89:161, 1992

Barnes PF, Barrows SA: Tuberculosis in the 1990s. Ann Intern Med 119:400, 1993

Bloom BR, Murray CJ: Tuberculosis: Commentary on a reemergent killer. Science 257:1055, 1992

Davidson PT, Le HQ: Drug treatment of tuberculosis—1992. Drugs 43:651, 1992

Elpern EH, Girzadas AM: Tuberculosis update: New challenges of an old disease. Med Surg Nursing 2(3):176, 1993

Gaston B: TB: Return of an old scourge. Journal of Emergency Medicine Service 19(1):70, 1994

Goble M, et al: Treatment of 171 patients with pulmonary tuberculosis resistant to isoniazid and rifampin. N Engl J Med 328:527, 1993

Lordi GM, Reichman LB: Treatment of tuberculosis. Am Fam Physician 44:219, 1992

Starke JR: Multidrug therapy for tuberculosis in children. Pediatr Infect Dis J 9:785, 1990

Nursing Bibliography

Allen M: Tuberculosis: The other epidemic. Journal of the Association of Nurses in AIDS Care 26:341, 1991

Barker P, Lewis D: Tuberculosis: The past helps to understand the present. Critical Care Nursing Quarterly 13(2):73, 1990

Boutotte J: Tuberculosis: The second time around . . . and how you can help to control it. Nursing '93 23(5):42, 1993

Busillo C: Multidrug resistant *Mycobacterium tuberculosis* in patients with human immunodeficiency virus infection. Chest 102:797, 1992

CDC draft guidelines for T.B. renew infection control debate. Hospital Infection Control 20(3):36, 1993

Franckhauser M: Tuberculosis in the 1990's. Nurse Practitioner Forum 4(1):30, 1993

Gray M: Medications for a growing concern: Tuberculosis. Orthopedic Nursing 12(2):75, 1993

Lancaster E: Tuberculosis comeback: Impact on long term care facilities. Journal of Gerontological Nursing 19(7):16, 1993

Morris J: Homeless individuals and drug-resistant tuberculosis in South Texas. Chest 102:802, 1992

Pokalo C: Tuberculosis: The return of a monster. Today's OR Nurse 14(10):31, 1992

T.B.—It can threaten your future. American Nurse 24(5):40, 1992

69
Antimalarial Agents

Chloroquine
Hydroxychloroquine
Mefloquine
Primaquine
Pyrimethamine
Sulfadoxine and Pyrimethamine
Quinacrine
Quinine

Malaria is a parasitic disease that is still prevalent in many areas of the world, especially Southeast Asia, Africa, and Central and South America. Four species of the protozoan *Plasmodium* can cause malaria in humans, and these are described briefly in the following:

Plasmodium falciparum: causes malignant tertian (MT) malaria, a severe, often fulminating infection that may progress to a fatal outcome if not treated quickly and vigorously; prompt therapy is usually highly successful, however, and relapses usually do not occur, but inadequate treatment can lead to periodic outbreaks owing to multiplication of parasites persisting in the blood

Plasmodium vivax: causes benign tertian (BT) malaria, a less severe disease than that produced by the *P falciparum* strain, having a low mortality but characterized by periodic relapses that may continue for years if untreated

Plasmodium malariae: causes quartan malaria; so named because the attacks of chills and high fever reoccur every 4 days rather than every 3 days as in the tertian form of the disease; outbreaks tend to appear in localized regions of the tropics; clinical signs may remain dormant for many years, and relapses do occur, but less frequently than with the *P vivax* organism

Plasmodium ovale: causes ovale tertian malaria, a rare form of relapsing malaria similar to but milder and more readily cured than the vivax infection

Malaria is usually transmitted to humans by the bite of the female *Anopheles* mosquito, which deposits the infective sporozoites, formed in the blood of the mosquito by the union of male and female gametocytes, into the human. The sporozoites localize in the liver, where they form primary tissue schizonts. These then grow and multiply into merozoites. This is the preerythrocytic or symptom-free stage of the infection. When mature, the merozoites are released from the liver and invade the erythrocytes (red blood cells) to begin the blood cycle phase of the infection. Young parasites in the red blood cell, termed *trophozoites*, grow and divide into mature schizonts, also known as *blood merozoites*. Periodically, the blood merozoites burst from the ruptured cells and invade a new group of erythrocytes, beginning the process anew. This periodic (every 3–4 days) rupturing of infected erythrocytes is responsible for the characteristic fever and chills that accompany acute attacks of malaria.

Another phase of the plasmodial life cycle, which occurs in infections caused by *P vivax*, *P ovale*, and possibly *P malariae*, is termed the exoerythrocytic cycle. After the release of most of the mature merozoites from the liver, some parasites in the merozoite stage of these three forms of *Plasmodium* remain in the liver and continue to multiply in liver cells for extended periods. Relapses developing months or even years after the initial infection can then occur as new merozoites are released from the liver cells to reinvade erythrocytes. Thus, malarial attacks can occur for several years unless these exoerythrocytic forms are eradicated during the primary treatment phase.

Finally, some of the merozoites that invade erythrocytes do not undergo the above-described process of *asexual* reproduction but instead differentiate into male and female gametocytes. On ingestion into a female mosquito (ie, when the mosquito draws blood from an infected human by a bite), sexual fertilization of the female gametocyte by the male gametocyte occurs in the gut of the mosquito, giving rise to new infective sporozoites.

Drug therapy of malaria may be directed toward prevention of infection, suppression of clinical symptoms, treatment of acute attacks, or prevention of relapses.

Prevention of infection: Drugs that kill the malarial organisms during their preerythrocytic (exoerythrocytic) stages are termed *causal prophylactics*; however, no drug is available that can *selectively* destroy sporozoites at therapeutic levels that are considered safe. Prophylaxis of malaria is best accomplished by mosquito control.

Suppression of clinical symptoms: Inhibition of the erythrocytic stage of the cycle can prevent development of clinical symptoms in an infected person. Several antimalarial drugs (ie, chloroquine, hydroxychloroquine, pyrimethamine, mefloquine) act in this manner, but acute attacks can occur when therapy is discontinued if exoerythrocytic forms of the organism are still present.

Treatment of acute attacks: Interruption of erythrocytic parasite multiplication can terminate the symptoms of an acute malarial attack, and drugs acting in this way are termed *schizonticides*. The 4-aminoquinolines usually are considered drugs of choice in this case, but they do not completely eliminate the parasite from the body; hence the possibility of relapse exists, especially with the *P vivax* strains.

Prevention of relapse: Drugs that eradicate the exoerythrocytic parasites (secondary tissue forms) can prevent relapse infections, and such treatment is sometimes referred to as a *radical cure*. The only available drug producing a radical cure in *P vivax* malaria is primaquine, which is usually given in combination with a drug (eg, chloroquine) that suppresses the erythrocyte cycle as well.

Combination suppressive therapy and radical cure (eg, with chloroquine and primaquine) is widely used in travelers to areas in which malaria is endemic. Therapy is begun before arrival and repeated at weekly intervals during and for at least 2 months after return from the malarial region to ensure that in the event infection occurs, clinical symptoms are suppressed and any secondary tissue forms are eradicated.

Prophylaxis may also be accomplished by use of the combination product sulfadoxine and pyrimethamine (Fansidar) beginning 1 to 2 days before exposure to an endemic area, continuing during the stay, and then for 4 to 6 weeks after departure.

An increasingly prevalent problem in treating malaria is the extent of acquired resistance that has developed to many antimalarial drugs. The most serious problem with resistance appears to be with *P falciparum*, because this species is responsible for most cases of malaria and most of the human mortality associated with the disease. Resistance of *P falciparum* to chloroquine, a mainstay in the treatment of malaria for many years, is increasing dramatically throughout the world, and there is increasing resistance to pyrimethamine–sulfadoxine, a combination considered to be the preferred alternative to chloroquine for prophylaxis of *P falciparum* malaria. When drug resistance is present or suspected, a relatively new drug, mefloquine, is used for both prophylaxis or treatment.

Owing to the many differences among them, the available antimalarial drugs are considered individually in the following sections.

• 4-Aminoquinolines

Chloroquine
Hydroxychloroquine

The 4-aminoquinolines are synthetic drugs that are particularly active against the erythrocytic forms of *P vivax* and *P malariae* and against most forms of *P falciparum*. Because they are ineffective against the exoerythrocytic forms, they do not prevent initial infection, nor do they prevent relapses in infected people. Their principal indications are as suppressive agents in *P vivax* or *P malariae* malaria and for terminating acute attacks of all types of malaria; these two drugs are reviewed together.

Mechanism

Not entirely known; appear to complex with DNA molecules of the parasite, thereby inhibiting RNA replication and subsequent nucleic acid synthesis; may also exert an amebicidal action and may exhibit antiinflammatory activity as well.

Uses

- Suppression and treatment of acute attacks of malaria due to *P vivax*, *P malariae*, *P ovale*, and susceptible strains of *P falciparum*
- Treatment of extraintestinal amebiasis (chloroquine, see Chapter 71)
- Treatment of systemic lupus erythematosus and rheumatoid arthritis (investigational use for hydroxychloroquine; Table 69-1)

Dosage

See Table 69-1.

Fate

Rapidly and completely absorbed orally; widely distributed in the body, attaining high concentrations in many tissues; approximately 50% protein bound; partially metabolized in the liver and slowly excreted by the kidneys; urinary elimination is enhanced by acidification of the urine; tissue levels are detectable for months and occasionally years, especially after termination of prolonged therapy.

Common Side Effects

Mild and transient headaches, GI distress, pruritus, visual disturbances (blurring, difficulty in focusing).

Significant Adverse Reactions

Usually seen with prolonged, high-dosage therapy:

- *CNS*: corneal edema or opacity, retinal changes, scotomata, optic atrophy, vertigo, tinnitus, impaired hearing, fatigue, psychic stimulation, convulsions, psychotic episodes
- *CV*: hypotension, ECG changes (T-wave inversion, widening of the QRS complex)
- *Dermatologic*: skin eruptions, pruritus, alopecia, dermatoses, skin and mucosal pigmentary changes
- *Hematologic*: blood dyscrasias
- *Other*: vomiting, diarrhea, stomach pain, anorexia, neuromyopathy, muscle weakness

Contraindications

Retinal damage, visual field changes, pregnancy, prolonged therapy in children, patients receiving bone marrow depressants or hemolytic drugs. *Cautious use* in patients with neurologic or hepatic disease, glucose-6-phosphate dehydrogenase (G-6-PD) deficiency, blood disorders, psoriasis, porphyria, severe GI disorders, or alcoholism; in infants or small children; and in pregnant or nursing women.

Interactions

- Liver toxicity may be increased by combined use of other known hepatotoxic drugs.
- Gold compounds, antiinflammatory drugs, and other agents known to cause drug sensitization and dermatitis may increase the dermatologic side effects of the 4-aminoquinolines.
- Excretion of the 4-aminoquinolines may be enhanced by urinary acidifiers (eg, ammonium chloride) and reduced by urinary alkalinizers (eg, sodium bicarbonate).
- The action of antipsoriatic drugs may be antagonized by the 4-aminoquinolines, and a severe psoriatic attack can be precipitated.
- Monoamine oxidase inhibitors can increase the toxicity of 4-aminoquinolines by impairing their hepatic inactivation.
- The GI absorption of 4-aminoquinolines may be decreased by concurrent administration of kaolin or magnesium trisilicate.

Nursing Management

See Table 69-1. In addition:

Pretherapy Assessment

Assess and record baseline data necessary for detection of adverse effects of 4-aminoquinolines: General: vital

Table 69-1. **4-Aminoquinolines**

Drug	*Usual Dosage Range*	*Nursing Considerations*
Chloroquine *Aralen* *(CAN) Novo-chloraquine*	**Treatment of acute attack** *Adults* Oral: 600 mg (base) initially followed by 300 mg (base) 6 h, 24 h, and 48 h later IM: 160–200 mg (base) initially; repeat in 6 h; (maximum 800 mg base/24 h) *Children* Oral: 10 mg/kg (base) initially, followed by 5 mg/kg (base) 6 h, 24 h, and 48 h later IM: 5 mg/kg (base) initially; repeat in 6 h (maximum 10 mg/kg base in a 24-h period) **Suppression (oral only)** *Adults* 300 mg (base) once weekly, beginning 2 wk before exposure; continue for 6–8 wk after leaving endemic area *Children* 5 mg/kg (base) weekly as for adults **Treatment of amebiasis** Oral: 600 mg (base) daily for 2 d, then 300 mg (base) daily for 2–3 wk IM: 160–200 mg (base) injected daily for 10–12 d	Indicated for treatment of acute attacks and suppressive therapy of all forms of malaria; also used with an amebicide for treatment of extraintestinal amebiasis (see Chapter 71); for radical cure of *P vivax* malaria, should be combined with primaquine; parenteral therapy should be terminated and oral therapy initiated as soon as possible; children and infants are very susceptible to adverse effects from parenteral chloroquine; do *not* exceed 5 mg/kg base for any single injection in young children; may be used for treating symptoms of rheumatoid arthritis (150 mg of base in a single daily dose), but hydroxychloroquine is preferred
Hydroxychloroquine Sulfate *Plaquenil*	**Treatment of acute attack** *Adults* 620 mg (base) initially, followed by 310 mg (base) 6 h, 24 h, and 48 h later *Children* 10 mg/kg (base) initially, followed by 5 mg/kg (base) 6 h, 24 h, and 48 h later **Suppression** *Adults and children* 5 mg/kg (base) once weekly beginning 2 wk before exposure (maximum 310 mg base per week); continue for 6–8 wk after leaving endemic area **Rheumatoid arthritis** Initially 400–600 mg/d in a single dose; reduce to 200–400 mg/d when optimum response is observed **Lupus erythematosus** Initially 400 mg once or twice a day; continue for weeks or months, but reduce to 200–400 mg/d when possible	Used for suppression and treatment of all forms of susceptible malaria and for treatment of rheumatoid arthritis and systemic lupus erythematosus; children's dose should never exceed adult dose; radical cure of *P vivax* and *P malariae* malaria requires concomitant therapy with primaquine; several weeks may be required to demonstrate an effect in rheumatoid arthritis; safe use in juvenile arthritis has not been established

signs (VS), body weight, skin color, temperature, and integrity; GI: biliary function; Genitourinary (GU): renal function (urinalysis, blood urea nitrogen [BUN], creatinine); CNS: neurologic function (gait, muscle strength), ophthalmologic examination; Cardiovascular system: ECG; Laboratory: G-6-PD.

Review medical history and documents for existing or previous conditions that:

a. require cautious use of 4-aminoquinolines: neurologic or hepatic dysfunction; G-6-PD deficiency; blood dyscrasias; psoriasis; porphyria; use in infants and small children.
b. contraindicate use of 4-aminoquinolines: allergy to 4-aminoquinolines; ophthalmic disorders; prolonged therapy in children; use with bone marrow suppressants or hemolytic agents; **pregnancy (Category C)**; lactation (secreted in breast milk; safety not established).

Nursing Interventions

Medication Administration

Administer oral form of drug with a full glass of water, 1 or 2 hours after meals.

Reduce the risk of stomatitis through frequent mouth care.

Provide small, frequent meals if GI upset occurs.

Double-check pediatric doses, children are very susceptible to overdosage.

Seek clarification if more than 5 mg/kg intramuscular (IM) is prescribed as a single dose for a child. Rationale: children are very susceptible to adverse reactions.

Provide ready access to bathroom facilities.

Surveillance During Therapy

Monitor results of blood counts, which should be obtained regularly during therapy.

Monitor results of renal excretion, liver function, complete blood count (CBC), and ophthalmologic examinations.
Monitor for signs of hypersensitivity, which may require discontinuation of drug.
Interpret results of diagnostic tests and contact practitioner as appropriate.
Monitor for possible drug–drug and drug–nutrient interactions; see Interactions.

Patient Teaching

Instruct patient regarding the importance of completing the full course of therapy as prescribed.
Inform patient of the consequences of not taking or abruptly discontinuing the 4-aminoquinolines.
Instruct patient that the prescribed drug is to be taken for the condition for which it is prescribed, and not to be used to treat any other infections.
Explain that weekly suppressive treatment is started at least 2 weeks before anticipated exposure and continued for at least 8 weeks after leaving endemic area. The drug should be taken on the same day each week.
Instruct patient to obtain baseline and periodic ophthalmologic examinations during and after prolonged therapy and to report promptly any visual disturbances, because retinal damage is frequently irreversible and may progress even after therapy has been terminated.
Warn patient to be alert for and to report development of muscular weakness or impaired reflexes, especially during prolonged therapy. Treatment should be discontinued if these develop.
Instruct patient to observe for appearance of dermatologic reactions (rash, pruritus, pigmentary changes) and to notify drug prescriber if any occur because dosage should be lowered or an alternative drug should be used.
Inform patient that drug may harmlessly discolor urine yellow-brown.
Inform patient that certain strains of *P falciparum* are resistant to 4-aminoquinolines and may require treatment with quinine or other appropriate antimalarial drugs.
Instruct patient about possible adverse side effects of 4-aminoquinolines: stomach pain, loss of appetite, nausea, vomiting, or diarrhea.
Instruct patient on appropriate action to take if side effects occur: notify practitioner if blurring of vision, loss of hearing, ringing in the ears, muscle weakness, or fever occur.

• Mefloquine

Lariam

Mefloquine is a structural analogue of quinine that is primarily indicated for the prophylaxis or treatment of malaria caused by strains of *P falciparum* that are resistant to chloroquine or pyrimethamine–sulfadoxine. In addition, mefloquine may be considered for use against chloroquine-susceptible strains of *P falciparum* and *P vivax*. The effectiveness of mefloquine against *P ovale* and *P malariae* has not been documented.

Mechanism

Not known; mefloquine is a potent schizonticidal drug that has very little effect on either gametocytes or the hepatic stages of *P vivax* infection.

Uses

Suppression and treatment of acute attacks of *P falciparum* and *P vivax* malaria, including chloroquine- and other multidrug-resistant strains of *P falciparum*.

Dosage

Treatment of acute infection: 1250 mg as a single dose, with at least 8 oz of water
Prophylaxis: 250 mg once weekly for 4 weeks, then 250 mg every other week; therapy should be started 1 week before travel, continued weekly during travel, and continued for 4 weeks after leaving infected areas.
Children: 1/4 to 1 tablet weekly as above, depending on body weight

Fate

Well absorbed orally; highly bound to plasma proteins (98%), concentrated in erythrocytes, and extensively distributed to the tissues, including the CNS; metabolized by the liver and excreted largely in the feces; half-life ranges from 15 to 33 days.

Common Side Effects

Nausea, vomiting, dizziness.

Significant Adverse Reactions

CNS: tinnitus, vertigo, visual disturbances, psychotic episodes, depression, convulsions
CV: bradycardia, possible ECG changes
Dermatologic: pruritus, rash, alopecia
Other: diarrhea, abdominal pain, loss of appetite, myalgia

Contraindications

Hypersensitivity to mefloquine or related drugs; see contraindications for quinine, which may also apply to mefloquine; *Cautious use* in patients with a history of epilepsy or psychiatric disorders; and in pregnancy.

Interactions

Risk of convulsions may be increased with chloroquine and other drugs that lower the seizure threshold.
Mefloquine may lower serum concentrations of valproic acid.
ECG disturbances and cardiac arrest may be caused by beta-adrenergic blockers, quinine, quinidine, and other cardiac depressants.

Nursing Management

Pretherapy Assessment

Assess and record baseline data necessary for detection of adverse effects of mefloquine: General: VS, body weight, skin color, temperature, and integrity; GI: biliary function; GU: renal function (urinalysis, BUN, creatinine); CNS: neurologic function, ophthalmologic examination; Laboratory: hematocrit (Hct), aminotransferase levels, cultures for sensitivity in acute treatment.

Review medical history and documents for existing or previous conditions that:
a. require cautious use of mefloquine: history of epilepsy or psychiatric disorders.
b. contraindicate use of mefloquine: allergy to mefloquine and related agents; **pregnancy (Category C)**; lactation (secreted in breast milk; safety not established).

Nursing Interventions

Medication Administration

Administer oral form of drug with a full glass of water, 1 or 2 hours after meals.
Provide small, frequent meals if GI upset occurs.
Provide ready access to bathroom facilities.
Arrange for treatment with primaquine in acute *P vivax* infection. Rationale: mefloquine does not eliminate exoerythrocytic parasites and relapse may occur.

Surveillance During Therapy

Monitor results of blood counts, which should be obtained regularly during therapy.
Monitor results of renal excretion, liver function, CBC, and ophthalmologic examinations.
Monitor for signs of hypersensitivity, which may require discontinuation of drug.
Interpret results of diagnostic tests and contact practitioner as appropriate.
Monitor for possible drug–drug and drug–nutrient interactions: increased risk of convulsions when used with chloroquines; increased risk of cardiac toxicity when used with quinine and quinidine (delay use of mefloquine at least 12 hours after last dose of quinine or quinidine); decreased serum concentrations and effectiveness of valproic acid.

Patient Teaching

Instruct patient regarding the importance of completing the full course of therapy as prescribed.
Inform patient of the consequences of not taking or abruptly discontinuing the mefloquine.
Instruct patient that the prescribed drug is to be taken for the condition for which it is prescribed, and not to be used to treat any other infections.
Explain that weekly suppressive treatment is started at least 1 week before anticipated exposure and continued for at least 4 weeks after leaving endemic area. The drug should be taken on the same day each week.
Instruct patient to obtain baseline and periodic ophthalmologic examinations during and after prolonged therapy and to report promptly any visual disturbances, because retinal damage is frequently irreversible and may progress even after therapy has been terminated.
Instruct patient about possible adverse side effects of mefloquine: dizziness; visual disturbances; headache; joint pain; nausea; vomiting; diarrhea.
Instruct patient on appropriate action to take if side effects occur: notify practitioner if anxiety, depression, restlessness, confusion, or palpitations occur.

• Primaquine phosphate

Primaquine

Primaquine phosphate is a synthetic 8-aminoquinoline derivative that eliminates the tissue or exoerythrocytic forms of the organism, thereby preventing relapse of *P vivax* malaria. Primaquine is not effective alone during an acute attack, but is administered in combination with chloroquine or hydroxychloroquine, which destroy the blood or erythrocytic forms.

Mechanism

Not completely established; appears to produce mitochondrial swelling in parasitic cells, thereby disrupting energy metabolism and impairing protein synthesis; prevents development of blood (erythrocytic) forms of *P vivax* malaria; also active against gametocytes of *P falciparum*.

Use

Prevention of relapse (radical cure) of *P vivax* malaria.

Dosage

Adults: 26.3 mg daily for 14 days
Children: 0.5 mg/kg/day for 14 days

Fate

Well absorbed orally; plasma levels are maximum within 2 to 3 hours but fall rapidly thereafter; relatively low levels are found in the lung, liver, heart, skeletal muscles, or brain; rapidly and completely metabolized and excreted largely in the urine; metabolism is impaired by quinacrine (see Interactions).

Common Side Effects

Epigastric distress.

Significant Adverse Reactions

Usually with large doses: nausea, vomiting, abdominal cramping, headache, impaired visual accommodation, pruritus, granulocytopenia, leukopenia, hemolytic anemia, and methemoglobinemia.

Contraindications

In patients receiving quinacrine (see Interactions), acutely ill patients; rheumatoid arthritis, lupus erythematosus, granulocytopenia, concurrent therapy with potentially hemolytic drugs or bone marrow depressants. *Cautious use* in pregnant women.

Interactions

Quinacrine can potentiate the toxicity of primaquine, presumably by impairing its metabolism.

Nursing Management

Pretherapy Assessment

Assess and record baseline data necessary for detection of adverse effects of primaquine: General: VS, body weight, skin color, temperature, and integrity; Laboratory: Hct, hemoglobin, G-6-PD in deficient patients.
Review medical history and documents for existing or previous conditions that:
a. require cautious use of primaquine: anemia.
b. contraindicate use of primaquine: allergy to prima-

quine and related agents; acutely ill, suffering from hematologic suppression; rheumatoid arthritis; lupus erythematosus; granulocytopenia; **pregnancy (Category C)**; lactation (secreted in breast milk; safety not established).

Nursing Interventions

Medication Administration

Administer oral form of drug with a full glass of water, 1 or 2 hours after meals.
Provide small, frequent meals if GI upset occurs.
Provide ready access to bathroom facilities.
Arrange for concurrent treatment with chloroquine.
Note that primaquine (45-mg base) is available in fixed combination with chloroquine (300-mg base) as Aralen Phosphate with Primaquine Phosphate for prophylaxis of malaria in areas in which the disease is endemic. Adult dosage is 1 tablet weekly during exposure and for 8 weeks after leaving endemic area.

Surveillance During Therapy

Monitor for signs of developing hemolytic anemia (darkened urine, fall in hemoglobin or erythrocyte count, chills, fever, precordial pain). Dark-skinned people are particularly susceptible to hemolytic anemia owing to a congenital deficiency of erythrocyte G-6-PD. Drug should be discontinued if hemolytic anemia occurs.
Monitor results of blood cell counts and hemoglobin determinations, which should be performed regularly during therapy. Recommended dosages should not be exceeded.
Monitor results of blood counts, which should be obtained regularly during therapy.
Monitor for signs of hypersensitivity, which may require discontinuation of drug.
Interpret results of diagnostic tests and contact practitioner as appropriate.
Monitor for possible drug–drug and drug–nutrient interactions: increased toxicity if taken with quinacrine; increased bone marrow suppression if taken with drugs that cause bone marrow suppression.

Patient Teaching

Instruct patient regarding the importance of completing the full course of therapy as prescribed.
Inform patient of the consequences of not taking or abruptly discontinuing the primaquine.
Explain to patient with parasitized red cells or one treated for acute attack of *P vivax* malaria that chloroquine should be taken concurrently with primaquine to destroy the erythrocytic parasites.
Instruct patient that the prescribed drug is to be taken for the condition for which it is prescribed, and not to be used to treat any other infections.
Instruct patient about possible adverse side effects of primaquine: stomach pain, loss of appetite, nausea, vomiting, abdominal cramps.
Instruct patient on appropriate action to take if side effects occur: notify practitioner if darkening of urine; severe abdominal cramps; GI distress; persistent nausea or vomiting occur.

• *Pyrimethamine*

Daraprim

A folic acid antagonist that interferes with development of fertilized gametes in the mosquito, pyrimethamine is used for prophylaxis of malaria due to susceptible strains. Its slow onset of action reduces its usefulness in treating acute attacks. Commonly given with a fast-acting schizonticide such as chloroquine to provide both transmission control and suppressive (*not* radical) cure.

Mechanism

Selectively inhibits the enzyme dihydrofolate reductase in protozoal cells, thereby blocking conversion of dihydrofolic acid to tetrahydrofolic acid, an essential step in protozoal cell metabolism; reduces sporogony (ie, reproduction of spores) in the mosquito but does not destroy gametocytes; plasmodial resistance can develop rapidly when pyrimethamine is used alone.

Uses

Prophylaxis of malaria due to susceptible strains of *Plasmodia* (usually in combination with a 4-aminoquinoline during acute attacks)
Treatment of toxoplasmosis, in combination with a sulfonamide

Dosage

Malaria:

Prophylaxis

Adults and children older than 10 years: 25 mg once a week
Younger children: 6.25 to 12.5 mg once a week
Drug is given for at least 6 to 10 weeks

Treatment of Acute Attacks

25 mg daily for 2 days, then 12.5 to 25 mg a week in combination with a rapid-acting schizonticide (chloroquine, quinine).

Toxoplasmosis:

Adults: 50 to 75 mg daily with 1 to 4 g/day of a sulfapyrimidine for 1 to 3 weeks; reduce dose by one-half and continue for another 4 to 5 weeks
Children: 1 mg/kg/day in 2 divided doses; after 2 to 4 days, reduce dose by one-half and continue for 1 month.

Fate

Well absorbed orally; plasma half-life is about 4 days, but effective levels are maintained for up to 2 weeks; excreted mainly in the urine, slowly over a period of several weeks.

Common Side Effects

Gastric upset, skin rash.

Significant Adverse Reactions

Usually with larger doses, as used for toxoplasmosis: anorexia, vomiting, atrophic glossitis, megaloblastic anemia, leukopenia, thrombocytopenia, pancytopenia, hemolytic anemia in patients with a G-6-PD deficiency, convulsions with overdosage.

Contraindications

No absolute contraindications. *Cautious use* in patients with convulsive disorders or G-6-PD deficiency, and in pregnant women.

Interactions

The action of pyrimethamine can be impaired by folic acid or para-aminobenzoic acid (PABA).

Pyrimethamine can increase quinine blood levels by competing for protein-binding sites.

Nursing Management

Pretherapy Assessment

Assess and record baseline data necessary for detection of adverse effects of pyrimethamine: General: VS, body weight, skin color, temperature, and integrity; Laboratory: Hct, hemoglobin, G-6-PD in deficient patients.

Review medical history and documents for existing or previous conditions that:

a. require cautious use of pyrimethamine: seizures, G-6-PD deficiency.

b. contraindicate use of pyrimethamine: allergy to pyrimethamine; **pregnancy (Category C)**; lactation (secreted in breast milk; safety not established).

Nursing Interventions

Medication Administration

Administer oral form of drug with a full glass of water, 1 or 2 hours after meals.

Provide small, frequent meals if GI upset occurs.

Provide ready access to bathroom facilities.

Arrange for decreased dosage or discontinuation if signs of folate deficiency develop.

Surveillance During Therapy

Monitor patient treated for toxoplasmosis very closely because the dose used is 10 to 20 times the dosage used for malaria, and it approaches the toxic level. Recommended dosage for malaria suppression should not be exceeded because incidence of untoward reactions is significantly higher at elevated dosage levels.

Monitor for signs of GI adverse effects: trophic glossitis, anorexia, stomach upset, vomiting.

Monitor results of blood cell counts and hemoglobin determinations, which should be performed regularly during therapy. Recommended dosages should not be exceeded.

Monitor results of blood counts, which should be obtained regularly during therapy.

Monitor for signs of hypersensitivity, which may require discontinuation of drug.

Interpret results of diagnostic tests and contact practitioner as appropriate.

Monitor for possible drug–drug and drug–nutrient interactions: action impaired by folic acid or para-aminobenzoic acid; can increase quinine blood concentrations by competing for protein binding.

Patient Teaching

Instruct patient regarding the importance of completing the full course of therapy as prescribed.

Inform patient of the consequences of not taking or abruptly discontinuing the pyrimethamine.

Instruct patient that the prescribed drug is to be taken for the condition for which it is prescribed, and not to be used to treat any other infections.

Caution patient immediately to report signs of possible developing blood dyscrasia (fever, sore throat, mucosal ulceration, bruising or bleeding).

Explain that weekly blood counts (including platelet counts) are required during high-dosage therapy because the drug should be discontinued if hematologic abnormalities occur. Folinic acid (leucovorin) may be given (3–9 mg IM daily for 3 days) to return depressed platelet or white blood cell count to normal.

Instruct patient about possible adverse side effects of pyrimethamine: stomach pain, loss of appetite, nausea, vomiting, abdominal cramps.

Instruct patient on appropriate action to take if side effects occur: notify practitioner if darkening of urine; severe abdominal cramps; GI distress; persistent nausea or vomiting occur.

• Sulfadoxine and Pyrimethamine

Fansidar

A fixed combination of sulfadoxine (500 mg) and pyrimethamine (25 mg) is available for prophylaxis of malaria and for treatment of susceptible strains of *Plasmodia* resistant to chloroquine.

Mechanism

The two drugs block sequential enzymatic steps involved in the biosynthesis of folinic acid, a necessary intermediate in the parasitic cellular synthesis of purines, pyrimidines, and certain amino acids. Thus, protein and nucleic acid production is impaired in the plasmodial organisms.

Uses

Treatment of *P falciparum* malaria in chloroquine-resistant cases

Prophylaxis of malaria in travelers to areas where chloroquine-resistant *P falciparum* is endemic

Dosage

Acute Attacks

Adults: 2 to 3 tablets (500 mg/25 mg) as a single dose, either alone or in sequence with quinine or primaquine

Children: 1/2 to 2 tablets according to age, as above

Prophylaxis

1/4 to 1 tablet once weekly or 1/2 to 2 tablets once every 2 weeks according to age; first dose is given 1 or 2 days before entering the endemic area; dosing is continued during the stay and for 4 to 6 weeks after return

Fate

Both drugs are well absorbed orally; peak serum concentrations are attained in 2 to 8 hours; elimination half-life is prolonged, averaging 7 days for sulfadoxine and 4.5 days for pyrimethamine.

Significant Adverse Reactions

See sulfonamides (Chapter 59) and pyrimethamine (this chapter).

NOTE: Although all adverse reactions reported for the sulfonamides and pyrimethamine are *theoretically* possible with Fansidar, not all have been documented thus far for this combination drug.

Rarely, toxic epidermal necrolysis, Stevens-Johnson syndrome, leukopenia, fulminant hepatic necrosis.

Contraindications

Megaloblastic anemia due to folate deficiency; sulfonamide hypersensitivity; pregnancy, and lactation; in infants younger than 2 months of age. *Cautious use* in patients with renal or hepatic impairment, folate deficiency, severe allergy, or bronchial asthma.

CAUTION

If signs of folic acid deficiency develop, discontinue drug and administer leucovorin in doses of 5 to 15 mg IM daily for at least 3 days to restore depressed platelet or white cell count.

Interactions

See sulfonamides (Chapter 59) and pyrimethamine (this chapter).

Nursing Management

Refer to Chapter 59.

Patient Teaching

Also see discussion of individual drugs.

- Help patient develop plan to maintain adequate fluid intake to prevent crystalluria or stone formation.
- Instruct patient to notify drug prescriber at first sign of fever, sore throat, abnormal bruising, pallor, jaundice, rash, pruritus, pharyngitis, or glossitis, possible indications of developing toxicity.
- Explain to patient receiving prophylactic treatment for 2 months or longer that drug will be discontinued if the count of any formed blood element is significantly reduced or if active bacterial or fungal infection develops, because leukopenia may occur.
- Encourage women with childbearing potential to practice contraception during therapy.

• Quinacrine

Atabrine

Although quinacrine is an effective antimalarial, its use in malaria largely has been supplanted by more active and less toxic drugs. It has been used for both treatment and suppression of malaria, inasmuch as it destroys both erythrocytic forms of *P vivax*, *P falciparum*, and quartan malaria as well as gametocytes of *P vivax* and quartan malaria. Quinacrine is ineffective, however, against *P falciparum* gametocytes and all sporozoites. The drug also may be used in the treatment of tapeworm infestations and giardiasis, and this application is considered in Chapter 70.

Mechanism

Not completely established; may interfere with nucleic acid synthesis by blocking DNA replication and interfering with transcription of RNA.

Uses

- Treatment and suppression of susceptible strains of *Plasmodia*
- Treatment of giardiasis and cestodiasis (tapeworm infestations; see Chapter 70)

Dosage

Treatment

Adults and children older than 8 years: 200 mg with 1 g sodium bicarbonate every 6 hours for 5 doses, then 100 mg 3 times a day for 6 days
Children (4–8 years): 200 mg 3 times a day the first day, then 100 mg every 12 hours for 6 days
Children (1–4 years): 100 mg 3 times a day the first day, then 100 mg once daily for 6 days

Suppression

Adults: 100 mg daily
Children: 50 mg daily

Fate

Readily absorbed from GI tract; maximum plasma levels occur in 1 to 3 hours; highly protein bound; widely distributed in the body and binds to many tissues; slowly excreted by the kidneys, and accumulation of drug in the body is gradual.

Common Side Effects

Nausea, abdominal cramping, diarrhea, headache, dizziness, and yellowing of the urine, skin, and nails.

Significant Adverse Reactions

GI: vomiting
Dermatologic: skin eruptions, contact dermatitis, exfoliative dermatitis
CNS: nervousness, vertigo, irritability, insomnia, emotional changes, nightmares, transient psychosis, convulsions (rare)
Hematologic: (rare) aplastic anemia, agranulocytosis, bone marrow depression
Other: hepatitis, corneal edema or deposits

Contraindications

Psoriasis, porphyria, and combined use with primaquine (see Interactions). *Cautious use* in patients with hepatic or renal disease, alcoholism, history of psychosis, G-6-PD deficiency, during pregnancy, and in small children and patients older than 60 years of age.

Interactions

- Quinacrine increases the toxicity of primaquine and may potentiate the effects of other hepatotoxic drugs.
- Quinacrine may produce a disulfiram-like reaction with alcohol (see Chapter 81).
- The anticoagulant effects of heparin, an acidic drug, may be antagonized by quinacrine, a basic drug.
- The adverse effects of quinacrine can be potentiated by

monoamine oxidase inhibitors, which reduce its hepatic metabolism.

Urinary alkalinizers can increase the effects of quinacrine by delaying its urinary excretion.

Nursing Management

Pretherapy Assessment

Assess and record baseline data necessary for detection of adverse effects of quinacrine: General: VS, body weight, skin color, temperature, and integrity; CNS: neurologic function, ophthalmologic examination; Laboratory: CBC, urinalysis, stool for ova and parasites.

Review medical history and documents for existing or previous conditions that:

a. require cautious use of quinacrine: psoriasis, porphyria, hepatic disease, alcoholism.
b. contraindicate use of quinacrine: allergy to quinacrine; concomitant use with primaquine; **pregnancy (Category C)**; lactation (secreted in breast milk; safety not established).

Nursing Interventions

Medication Administration

Administer oral form of drug with a full glass of water, 1 or 2 hours after meals.

Provide small, frequent meals if GI upset occurs.

Provide ready access to bathroom facilities.

Surveillance During Therapy

Monitor for signs of GI adverse effects: trophic glossitis, anorexia, stomach upset, vomiting.

Monitor results of blood cell counts and hemoglobin determinations, which should be performed regularly during therapy. Recommended dosages should not be exceeded.

Monitor results of blood counts, which should be obtained regularly during therapy.

Monitor for signs of hypersensitivity, which may require discontinuation of drug.

Interpret results of diagnostic tests and contact practitioner as appropriate.

Monitor for possible drug–drug and drug–nutrient interactions: see Interactions.

Patient Teaching

Instruct patient regarding the importance of completing the full course of therapy as prescribed.

Inform patient of the consequences of not taking or abruptly discontinuing the quinacrine.

Instruct patient that the prescribed drug is to be taken for the condition for which it is prescribed, and not to be used to treat any other infections.

Caution patient immediately to report signs of possible developing blood dyscrasia (fever, sore throat, mucosal ulceration, bruising or bleeding).

Instruct patient on appropriate action to take if side effects occur: notify practitioner if darkening of urine; severe abdominal cramps; GI distress; persistent nausea or vomiting occur.

• Quinine Sulfate *(Pregnancy Category X)*

Legatrin, Quinamm, and other manufacturers

(CAN) Novoquinine

A natural alkaloid from the bark of the cinchona tree, quinine is an effective antimalarial drug that has been largely replaced by more active and less toxic drugs. It is used in conjunction with pyrimethamine and sulfadiazine or tetracycline, however, for treatment of *Plasmodia* resistant to other antimalarials, especially chloroquine-resistant *P falciparum* strains. Owing to its skeletal muscle-relaxant effects, it also is used occasionally for relief of nocturnal leg cramps. It usually is available over the counter, although some preparations may be restricted to prescription-only status.

Mechanism

Not completely established; may inhibit protein synthesis in malarial organisms by complexing with parasite DNA and may interfere with cellular metabolism; suppresses oxygen uptake and carbohydrate metabolism of *Plasmodia*; actively schizonticidal for all forms of malaria and gametocidal for *P vivax* and *P malariae* strains; also possesses an analgesic, antipyretic, skeletal muscle-relaxant, oxytocic, and hypoprothrombinemic action; exerts muscle-relaxing action by increasing refractory period of muscle cells, decreasing excitability of the motor end plate, and altering distribution of calcium within the muscle fiber.

Uses

Adjunctive treatment of chloroquine-resistant *P falciparum* malaria, along with pyrimethamine and sulfadiazine or tetracycline and in combination with other antimalarials for radical cure of relapsing *P vivax* malaria

Prevention and relief of nocturnal leg cramps

Dosage

Malaria

Adults: 600 to 650 mg every 8 hours for 5 to 7 days
Children: 8 to 10 mg/kg every 8 hours for 5 to 7 days

Leg cramps

260 to 300 mg at bedtime

Fate

Rapidly absorbed orally; peak plasma levels occur in 1 to 3 hours; highly (70%–80%) protein bound; widely distributed in the body, except to the CNS; metabolized by the liver and excreted in the urine, largely as metabolites with some (10%) unchanged drug.

Common Side Effects

Cinchonism (tinnitus, headache, dizziness, GI upset, visual disturbances)—frequently seen at full therapeutic doses.

Significant Adverse Reactions

CNS: temporary deafness, fever, apprehension, restlessness, excitement, confusion, delirium, syncope, hypothermia, convulsions

Ophthalmic: photophobia, amblyopia, scotomata, di-

plopia, mydriasis, altered color perception, optic atrophy
GI: vomiting, stomach cramps, diarrhea
Allergic–hypersensitivity: rash, pruritus, flushing, urticaria, facial edema, asthma-like reaction
Hematologic: hypoprothrombinemia, hemolytic anemia, thrombocytopenia, agranulocytosis
Other: (usually observed with very large doses) hypotension, respiratory depression, muscle paralysis

Contraindications

Pregnancy, myasthenia gravis, G-6-PD deficiency, tinnitus, and optic neuritis. *Cautious use* in patients with cardiac arrhythmias (quinine has cardiovascular actions similar to quinidine), angina, renal impairment, or a history of allergic reactions; and in nursing mothers.

Interactions

Pyrimethamine may increase blood levels of quinine, possibly leading to toxic effects.
Quinine can enhance the effects of skeletal muscle relaxants and increase their respiratory depressant action.
Quinine may potentiate the effects of oral anticoagulants through its hypoprothrombinemic action.
The urinary excretion of quinine can be reduced by urinary alkalinizers (eg, sodium bicarbonate, acetazolamide).
Aluminum-containing antacids can delay or reduce the oral absorption of quinine.
Owing to its similarity to quinidine, quinine may increase plasma levels of digoxin and digitoxin if given concurrently, as has been documented for quinidine.

Nursing Management

Pretherapy Assessment

Assess and record baseline data necessary for detection of adverse effects of quinine: General: VS, body weight, skin color, temperature, and integrity; GI: biliary function; GU: renal function (urinalysis, BUN, creatinine); CVS: hematologic function, ECG; CNS: neurologic function, ophthalmologic examihation, audiologic examination; Laboratory: CBC, differential, prothrombin time, G-6-PD in appropriate patients.
Review medical history and documents for existing or previous conditions that:
a. require cautious use of quinine: impaired renal function; G-6-PD deficiency (risk of hemolytic anemia); cardiac arrhythmias; angina; history of allergic reactions.
b. contraindicate use of quinine: allergy to quinine, tinnitus, optic neuritis, myasthenia gravis, history of backwater fever; **pregnancy (Category X)**; lactation (appears in breast milk; use with caution; do not use in patients with G-6-PD deficiency).

Nursing Interventions

Medication Administration

Administer oral form of drug with meals, with a full glass of water to decrease GI upset.
Administer quinine on schedule to ensure stable steady-state concentrations for the duration of therapy.
Administer with pyrimethamine and sulfadiazine or tetracycline for malaria.
Reduce the risk of stomatitis through frequent mouth care.
Initiate a meal schedule that provides small, frequent meals if GI upset occurs.
Provide ready access to bathroom and interventions directed at symptom relief if diarrhea occurs.

Surveillance During Therapy

Monitor for presence of cinchonism (tinnitus, headache, nausea, vision disturbance, GI upset, nervousness, CVS effects).
Monitor for signs of hypersensitivity (rashes, pruritus, flushing, sweating, facial edema, asthmatic symptoms), which may require discontinuation of drug.
Monitor CBC, urinalysis, and liver and kidney function test results obtained over the course of therapy.
Interpret results of diagnostic tests and contact practitioner as appropriate.
Monitor intake–output, observing for signs and symptoms of possible renal impairment and dehydration secondary to GI side effects (vomiting, diarrhea).
Monitor for possible drug–laboratory test interactions: false-positive elevated 17-ketogenic steroid concentrations.
Monitor for possible drug–drug and drug–nutrient interactions; see Interactions.
Provide for patient safety needs to minimize environmental hazards and risk of injury if CNS side effects develop.

Patient Teaching

Instruct patient regarding the importance of completing the full course of therapy as prescribed; that is, not to discontinue the drug once signs and symptoms of the infection being treated subside.
Inform patient of the consequences of not taking or abruptly discontinuing the quinine.
Instruct patient that the prescribed drug is to be taken for the condition for which it is prescribed, and not to be used to treat any other infections.
Inform patient that this drug should not be taken during pregnancy.
Instruct patient about possible adverse side effects of quinine: dizziness, fainting, confusion, blurred vision, diarrhea, nausea, stomach cramps, vomiting, decreased hearing, ringing in the ears.
Teach patient how to recognize and report symptoms of cinchonism (tinnitus, dizziness, visual disturbances, headache, GI distress), and inform patient that dosage will be reduced or drug will be discontinued if symptoms occur. Effects usually disappear quickly when drug is stopped.
Instruct patient on appropriate action to take if side effects occur:
Notify practitioner if headache; marked changes in vision; unusual bleeding or bruising; severe ringing

in the ears; marked loss of hearing; fever or chills occur.

Notify practitioner of any unusual bleeding. Rationale: hypoprothrombinemia and bleeding tendencies due to decreased synthesis of vitamin K by intestinal microflora may occur.

Selected Bibliography

Clark IA, Rockett KA: Immunizing against toxic malarial antigens. Parasitology Today 10(1):6; 1994

Gilles HM: Malaria: An overview. J Infect 18:11, 1989

Keystone JS: Prevention of malaria. Drugs 39:337, 1990

Olliaro P: How *Plasmodium* secures nutrients: New targets for drugs? Parasitology Today 10(1):4, 1994

Schlesinger PH, et al: Antimalarial agents: Mechanism of action. Antimicrob Agents Chemother 32:793, 1988

WHO: Severe and complicated malaria. Trans R Soc Trop Med Hyg 84(Suppl 2):542, 1990

Nursing Bibliography

Rangel-Frausto M, Edmond M: Malaria: Protection of the international traveler. Infection Control and Hospital Epidemiology 14(3):154, 1993

70

Anthelmintics

Diethylcarbamazine
Mebendazole
Niclosamide
Oxamniquine
Piperazine
Praziquantel
Pyrantel
Quinacrine
Thiabendazole

Anthelmintics are drugs used to facilitate the expulsion from the body of parasitic worms or helminths. Helminthiasis or worm infection is the most common disease in the world today. Although endemic in many tropical countries, helminthiasis is by no means limited to these areas, but is found in increasing numbers in many temperate climates as well. Poor living conditions, inadequate sanitation, lack of careful hygiene, and malnutrition are major contributory factors to the high incidence of helminthiasis in underdeveloped countries.

Helminthic infections are caused by two principal types of worms, roundworms (nematodes) and flatworms (cestodes, trematodes). Table 70-1 lists the major species of each type of worm and the drugs that are most effective against each helminth. Most nematodal infections are confined to the intestinal tract and include parasites such as roundworms, pinworms, whipworms, hookworms, and threadworms. Tissue-invading nematodes such as filarial worms and pork roundworms (*Trichinella*), however, can enter body organs, including the heart, liver, lungs, skeletal muscle, and CNS, in which case eradication is often quite difficult and more serious sequelae can ensue.

Cestodal infestations can occur with several types of tapeworms, the most common being the beef tapeworm (*Taenia saginata*). These infections are usually localized in the GI tract, although larvae of the pork tapeworm (*Taenia solium*) can occasionally gain access to the systemic circulation, resulting in inflammatory and granulomatous reactions in other organs (eg, cysticercosis).

Tissue-invading trematodes or blood flukes are responsible for a chronic infection termed *schistosomiasis*, or bilharziasis, which is widespread throughout Africa and parts of South America. Complications may range from minor conditions such as rash, itching, or headache to severe damage to vital organs. Other trematodes include the lung, liver, and intestinal flukes.

Accurate diagnosis of the invading helminth is essential for the successful treatment of the infestation, because many anthelmintic drugs are highly specific for a particular infection. Diagnosis is usually accomplished by obtaining a stool specimen or removing worms from the outer anal area with cellophane tape. Once the type of worm involved has been determined, selection of an appropriate anthelmintic drug can be made. Although a large number of different kinds of chemicals have been used in the past for treating the different types of worm infestations, they have been replaced by fewer but more effective and less toxic agents. Most of these newer anthelmintic drugs are not appreciably absorbed after oral administration, and thus they attain high levels in the GI tract, while systemic toxicity is largely avoided. Another advantage of certain of the newer drugs (mebendazole, thiabendazole, praziquantel) is that they have a broad spectrum of action and thus are effective against several types of helminths. These drugs are particularly valuable in mixed infections or when the diagnosis is uncertain.

An important aspect of successful anthelmintic therapy is proper patient education with regard to personal hygiene. Because many worms are primarily transmitted by transfer of eggs (ova) by hands, food, or contaminated articles such as toilet paper, towels, clothes, or sheets, it is imperative that patients be instructed in the necessary procedures for minimizing spread of the infection. Important measures that should be stressed are careful washing of hands after each bowel movement; daily or more frequent changes of underwear, towels, and bedding; and avoidance of scratching of the perianal area. Nail biting should also be strongly discouraged. Diagnosis of pinworm infection in one family member makes it imperative that all other family members be tested as well, because this infection commonly affects an entire family.

The principal drugs used to treat nematodal and cestodal infections (see Table 70-1) are discussed in detail in this chapter. Other anthelmintic drugs, such as niridazole, bithionol, ivermectin, metrifonate, and suramin, are used principally for certain filarial or trematodal infections and are available only on request from the Parasitic Disease Drug Service of the Centers for Disease Control. These agents are reviewed briefly in Table 70-2. Still other drugs that are occasionally used in certain helminthic infections (eg, emetine, chloroquine, paromomycin) have additional therapeutic actions as well, and are reviewed elsewhere in this book.

• Diethylcarbamazine

Hetrazan

Mechanism

Appears to immobilize small worms (microfilaria), increasing their susceptibility to phagocytosis by fixed tissue macrophages; does not appear to alter phagocytosis in the bloodstream; considered the drug of choice for filarial infections.

NOTE: Available without charge *only* from the manufacturer.

Uses

Treatment of filarial worm infections (Bancroft's filariasis, loiasis, onchocerciasis)
Treatment of roundworm infections (ascariasis)
Treatment of tropical eosinophilia

Table 70-1. **Helminthiasis Classification and Treatment**

Class of Helminth	*Disorder*	*Suggested Drugs of Choice* — *Primary*	*Secondary**
Nematodes			
Roundworm			
Ascaris lumbricoides	Ascariasis	Mebendazole, pyrantel pamoate	Piperazine, thiabendazole, diethylcarbamazine
Hookworm			
Necator americanus *Ancylostoma duodenale*	Uncinariasis	Mebendazole	Pyrantel pamoate, thiabendazole
Whipworm			
Trichuris trichiura	Trichuriasis	Mebendazole	Thiabendazole
Threadworm			
Strongyloides stercoralis	Strongyloidiasis	Thiabendazole	Mebendazole
Cutaneous larva migrans			
Ancylostoma braziliense	Creeping eruption	Thiabendazole	
Capillary worm			
Capillaria philippinensis	Capillariasis	Mebendazole	Thiabendazole
Pinworm			
Enterobius vermicularis	Enterobiasis	Mebendazole, pyrantel pamoate	Thiabendazole, piperazine
Pork roundworm			
Trichinella spiralis	Trichiniasis, trichinosis	Corticosteroids	Thiabendazole, mebendazole
Filarial worms			
Wuchereria bancrofti	Filariasis	Diethylcarbamazine	
Brugia malayi	Filariasis	Diethylcarbamazine	
Loa loa	Loiasis	Diethylcarbamazine	
Onchocerca volvulus	Onchocerciasis	Ivermectin†	Diethylcarbamazine, suramin†
Guinea worm			
Dracunculus medinensis	Dracunculiasis	Niridazole,† metronidazole	Mebendazole, thiabendazole
Rat lungworm			
Angiostrongylus cantonensis	Angiostrongyliasis	Thiabendazole	Mebendazole
Cestodes			
Tapeworms			
Beef			
Taenia saginata	Taeniasis	Niclosamide	Praziquantel
Pork			
Taenia solium	Taeniasis	Niclosamide, praziquantel	Paromomycin, mebendazole
Fish			
Diphyllobothrium latum	Diphyllobothriasis	Niclosamide	Dichlorophen, praziquantel, paromomycin
Dwarf			
Hymenolepis nana	Hymenolepiasis	Niclosamide, praziquantel	Mebendazole, paromomycin
Trematodes			
Blood flukes			
Schistosoma haematobium	Schistosomiasis (bilharziasis)	Praziquantel, metrifonate†	Niridazole,† stibocaptate†
Schistosoma mansoni	Schistosomiasis	Praziquantel, oxamniquine	Niridazole,† stibocaptate†
Blood flukes			
Schistosoma japonicum	Schistosomiasis	Praziquantel, niridazole†	Niridazole†
Schistosoma mekongi	Schistosomiasis	Praziquantel	Niridazole†
Lung flukes			
Paragonimus westermani	Paragonimiasis	Praziquantel	Chloroquine, bithionol†
Liver flukes			
Opisthorchis viverrini	Opisthorchiasis	Praziquantel	Mebendazole
Fasciola hepatica	Fascioliasis	Praziquantel, bithionol†	Metronidazole, emetine
Clonorchis sinensis	Clonorchiasis	Praziquantel	Mebendazole
Intestinal fluke			
Fasciolopsis buski	Fasciolopsiasis	Niclosamide, praziquantel	Tetrachloroethylene, hexylresorcinol

* Secondary drugs are often *ineffective* and seldom used alone.
† Available only by request from the Parasitic Disease Drug Service, Centers for Disease Control, Atlanta, GA 30333.

Table 70-2. **Anthelmintic Drugs Available by Request to Centers for Disease Control***

Drug	*Principal Indications*	*Usual Dosage Range*	*Remarks*
Bithionol *Actamer, Bitin, Lorothidol*	Lung fluke (*Paragonimus*) and liver fluke (*Fasciola*) infections	30–50 mg/kg orally in 2 or 3 divided doses on alternate days for 10 to 15 d	Alternative drug for treating lung fluke infections; GI side effects are common; use with *caution* in children younger than 8 years of age
Ivermectin *Mectizan*	Onchocerciasis	3 mg for 15–25 kg; 6 mg for 26–44 kg; 9 mg for 45–64 kg; 15 mg for 65 kg or more, orally in a single dose	Primary drug for onchocerciasis and possibly for the treatment of strongyloidiasis and trichuriasis; adverse effects usually mild and of short duration
Metrifonate *Bilarcil*	Schistosomiasis	7.5–10 mg/kg as a single dose; repeat twice at 2-week intervals	One of the drugs of choice for *S haematobium* infections; *not* effective against *S mansoni* or *S japonicum*; well tolerated; minimal side effects
Niridazole *Ambilhar*	Schistosomiasis, guinea worm infections	25 mg/kg/d orally in 2 or 3 divided doses for 7 d	Primary drug for *S japonicum* infections and alternative drug for other schistosomal infections; high incidence of side effects (70%), especially GI and allergic; CNS toxicity can occur, especially at high doses; patients must be hospitalized; usually contraindicated in cardiac, liver, or renal disease, hypertension, epilepsy, psychiatric disorders, GI ulceration, or hemorrhage
Suramin *Antrypol, Bayer 205, Belganyl, Germanin, Moranyl, Naganol, Naphuride*	Onchocerciasis (filarial worm infection), African trypanosomiasis (sleeping sickness)	1 g by *slow* IV injection weekly for 4 to 7 weeks	Used to eradicate adult filariae of *Onchocerca volvulus* after treatment with diethylcarbamazine to eliminate microfilariae; also effective in early stages of African trypanosomiasis before CNS involvement; proteinuria can occur; avoid extravasation because severe pain can result

* Parasitic Disease Drug Service, Bureau of Epidemiology, Centers for Disease Control, Atlanta, GA 30333.

Dosage

Filarial worm infections

2 mg/kg orally three times a day for 3 to 4 weeks; this dosage can be given for 3 to 5 days to treat large numbers of patients known to harbor microfilariae, as a public health measure

Roundworm infections

Adults: 13 mg/kg/day in a single dose for 7 days
Children: 6 to 10 mg/kg 3 times a day for 7 to 10 days

Tropical eosinophilia

13 mg/kg/day for 4 to 7 days

Fate

Well absorbed orally; peak blood levels occur in 3 to 4 hours; widely distributed in the body; excreted primarily in the urine, both as metabolites and unchanged drug.

Common Side Effects

Headache, weakness, lassitude, malaise, nausea, joint pain, and leukocytosis; in patients with onchocerciasis, facial edema, pruritus of the eyes, and skin rash are common.

Significant Adverse Reactions

Vomiting, skin rash, lymphadenopathy, tachycardia, visual disturbances, GI upset, abdominal pain, anorexia, fever, and severe allergic reactions due to release of helminthic proteins.

Contraindications

No absolute contraindications. *Cautious use* in people with a history of allergic reactions and in debilitated or malnourished patients.

Nursing Management

Nursing Interventions

Medication Administration

Note that when diethylcarbamazine is used to treat onchocerciasis, it is given in combination with suramin to kill adult worms as well as the microfilaria.

Surveillance During Therapy

Monitor patient for development of allergic reactions, especially during treatment for onchocerciasis. Have antihistamines, corticosteroids, and epinephrine available.

Patient Teaching

Teach patient personal hygiene measures to help minimize the danger of reinfection.

• Mebendazole

Vermox

Mechanism

Blocks uptake and use of glucose by worms, thereby depleting endogenous glycogen, reducing energy supply below that necessary for survival; worms are cleared from the GI tract over several days.

Uses

Treatment of single or mixed whipworm, pinworm, roundworm, and hookworm infestations
Alternative therapy for trichinosis, onchocerciasis, taeniasis, and infestation with liver flukes

Dosage

Whipworm, hookworm, and roundworm

Adults and children: 100 mg twice a day for 3 consecutive days; if necessary, repeat in 2 weeks

Pinworm

Adults and children: 100 mg as single dose

Fate

Only 5% to 10% of an oral dose is absorbed; approximately 2% of an administered dose is excreted in the urine, both as unchanged drug and a metabolite; the remainder is excreted in the feces.

Significant Adverse Reactions

Usually with massive infections: abdominal pain, nausea, vomiting, and diarrhea due to expulsion of worms; fever; neutropenia (high doses).

Contraindications

No absolute contraindications. *Cautious use* in children younger than 2 years of age and in pregnant women.

Nursing Management

Pretherapy Assessment

Assess and record baseline data necessary for detection of adverse effects of mebendazole: General: vital signs (VS), body weight, skin color and temperature; GI: bowel sounds, output; Laboratory: culture for ova and parasites.

Review medical history and documents for existing or previous conditions that:

a. require cautious use of mebendazole: use in children younger than 2 years of age.
b. contraindicate use of mebendazole: allergy to mebendazole; **pregnancy (Category C)**; lactation (appears in breast milk; avoid use in nursing mothers).

Nursing Interventions

Medication Administration

Administer drug with meals (chewed, swallowed whole, or crushed and mixed with food) with a full glass of water to decrease GI upset.
Administer mebendazole on schedule to ensure stable steady-state concentrations for the duration of therapy.
Expect a second course of therapy to be initiated if patient is not cured 3 weeks after initial treatment.
Note that fasting or posttreatment purging is not required with mebendazole.
Initiate a meal schedule that provides small, frequent meals if GI upset occurs.
Provide ready access to bathroom and interventions directed at symptom relief if diarrhea occurs.
Arrange for disinfection and treatment of all environmental factors.

Surveillance During Therapy

Monitor for adverse effects, toxicity, and interactions.
Monitor for signs of hypersensitivity.

Patient Teaching

Inform patient that tablets may be chewed, swallowed whole, or crushed and mixed with food.
Instruct patient that the prescribed drug is to be taken for the condition for which it is prescribed, and not to be used to treat any other infections.
Inform patient that this drug should not be taken during pregnancy.
Instruct patient about possible adverse side effects of mebendazole: nausea, abdominal pain, diarrhea.
Instruct patient on appropriate action to take if side effects occur: notify practitioner if fever, return of symptoms, severe diarrhea occur.

• Niclosamide

Niclocide

Mechanism

Inhibits oxidative phosphorylation in the mitochondria of cestodal parasites and may also stimulate adenosine triphosphatase; the head (scolex) and proximal segments of the worm are killed on contact, and the parasite is released from its attachment on the intestinal wall; the partially digested worms are then expelled in the feces; drug does not appear to produce any hematologic, renal, or hepatic abnormalities.

Use

Treatment of cestodal (tapeworm) infections—see Table 70-1 (drug of choice).

Dosage

Tablets are thoroughly chewed and swallowed with a little water.

Taenia/Diphyllobothrium infections

Adults: 2 g in a single dose
Children: 1.0 to 1.5 g in a single dose, depending on weight

CAUTION

In the treatment of *pork* tapeworm infections, a purgative *must be given* within 1 to 2 hours after niclosamide, because the lethal action of the drug is against the adult worm but not the ova, which can be liberated into the lumen of the gut. Subsequently, they may be absorbed and may invade other tissues (muscles, liver, lung, brain), leading to a condition termed *cysticercosis*, which can produce muscle pain, weakness, nervousness, convulsions, and paralysis.

Hymenolepis nana (dwarf tapeworm) infections

Adults: 2 g as a single dose daily for 7 days
Children weighing 34 kg (75 lb) and more: 1.5 g the first day, then 1 g daily for 6 days
Children weighing less than 34 kg (75 lb): 1.0 g the first day, then 0.5 g daily for 6 days

Fate

Not absorbed from the GI tract, excreted in the feces.

Common Side Effects

Nausea, vomiting, anorexia, diarrhea.

Significant Adverse Reactions

GI: constipation, rectal irritation or bleeding
CNS: headache, drowsiness, dizziness
Dermatologic: skin rash
Other: fever, oral irritation, bad taste in mouth, sweating, palpitations, weakness, backache, irritability, alopecia

Contraindications

No absolute contraindications. *Cautious use* in pregnant or nursing women and in children younger than 2 years of age.

Nursing Management

Pretherapy Assessment

Assess and record baseline data necessary for detection of adverse effects of niclosamide: General: VS, body weight, skin color and temperature; GI: bowel sounds, output; Laboratory: culture for ova and parasites.
Review medical history and documents for existing or previous conditions that:
a. require cautious use of niclosamide: use in children younger than 2 years of age.
b. contraindicate use of niclosamide: allergy to niclosamide; **pregnancy (Category B)**; lactation (appears in breast milk; avoid use in nursing mothers).

Nursing Interventions

Medication Administration

Administer drug with meals (chewed, swallowed whole, or crushed and mixed with food) with a full glass of water to decrease GI upset.
Administer niclosamide on schedule to ensure stable steady-state concentrations for the duration of therapy.
Initiate a meal schedule that provides small, frequent meals if GI upset occurs.
Provide ready access to bathroom and interventions directed at symptom relief if diarrhea occurs.
Arrange for a mild laxative if drug-induced constipation is severe.
Arrange for disinfection and treatment of all environmental factors.

Surveillance During Therapy

If *Taenia* or *Diphyllobothrium* segments or ova are still present in the stool 7 days after treatment, expect treatment to be repeated. A negative stool for at least 3 months is the criterion for cure.
Monitor for adverse effects, toxicity, and interactions.
Monitor for signs of hypersensitivity.

Patient Teaching

Inform patient that tablets may be chewed, swallowed whole, or crushed and mixed with food.
Instruct patient regarding the importance of completing the full course of therapy as prescribed; that is, not to discontinue the drug once signs and symptoms of the infection being treated subside.
Inform patient of the consequences of not taking or abruptly discontinuing the niclosamide.
Instruct patient that the prescribed drug is to be taken for the condition for which it is prescribed, and not to be used to treat any other infections.
Advise patient to use a mild laxative, if needed, to relieve constipation.
With patient treated for *Hymenolepis* infection, emphasize the importance of continuing treatment for the entire 7 days, as recommended, to ensure complete destruction of both mature and larval stages of the worm.
Inform patient that this drug should not be taken during pregnancy.
Instruct patient about possible adverse side effects of niclosamide: nausea, abdominal pain, diarrhea, drowsiness, dizziness.
Instruct patient on appropriate action to take if side effects occur: notify practitioner if fever, rash, severe abdominal pain, marked weakness, or dizziness occur.

• Oxamniquine

Vansil

Mechanism

Not completely established; may cause a shift in worms from the mesentery to the liver, where they die; appears to be more toxic to male schistosomes than to females, but surviving female worms no longer lay eggs.

Use

Treatment of all stages (acute, subacute, chronic) of *Schistosoma mansoni* infections.

Dosage

Adults: 12 to 15 mg/kg as a single oral dose
Children weighing less than 30 kg: 20 mg/kg in two divided doses with a 2- to 8-hour interval between doses

Fate

Readily absorbed orally; peak serum concentration in 1 to 2 hours; plasma half-life is about 1 to 3 hours; extensively metabolized and excreted in the urine, largely as inactive metabolites.

Common Side Effects

Drowsiness, dizziness.

Significant Adverse Reactions

Headache, anorexia, abdominal pain, nausea, vomiting, urticaria, liver enzyme elevations, and, rarely, convulsions.

Contraindications

No absolute contraindications. *Cautious use* in patients with a history of convulsive disorders and in pregnant or nursing women.

Nursing Management

Pretherapy Assessment

Assess and record baseline data necessary for detection of adverse effects of oxamniquine: General: VS, body weight, skin color and temperature; GI: bowel sounds, output; Laboratory: culture for ova and parasites.

Review medical history and documents for existing or previous conditions that:

a. require cautious use of oxamniquine: history of convulsive disorders.

b. contraindicate use of oxamniquine: allergy to oxamniquine; **pregnancy (Category C)**; lactation (appears in breast milk; avoid use in nursing mothers).

Nursing Interventions

Medication Administration

Administer drug with meals with a full glass of water to decrease GI upset.

Administer oxamniquine on schedule to ensure stable steady-state concentrations for the duration of therapy.

Initiate a meal schedule that provides small, frequent meals if GI upset occurs.

Provide ready access to bathroom and interventions directed at symptom relief if diarrhea occurs.

Arrange for disinfection and treatment of all environmental factors.

Surveillance During Therapy

Monitor for adverse effects, toxicity, and interactions.

Monitor for signs of hypersensitivity.

Patient Teaching

Instruct patient that the prescribed drug is to be taken for the condition for which it is prescribed, and not to be used to treat any other infections.

Instruct patient about possible adverse side effects of oxamniquine: nausea, abdominal pain, diarrhea, drowsiness, dizziness.

Instruct patient on appropriate action to take if side effects occur: notify practitioner if fever, rash, severe abdominal pain, marked weakness, or dizziness occur.

Instruct patient to take drug with food to improve tolerance.

Urge patient to exercise caution in performing hazardous tasks because drug causes drowsiness and dizziness in about a third of patients.

Inform patient that drug may color urine a harmless orange-red.

• Piperazine

Mechanism

Produces flaccid paralysis in worms, possibly by blocking acetylcholine, resulting in expulsion of the helminths by normal peristaltic movement.

Uses

Alternative treatment of roundworm and pinworm infestations.

Dosage

Roundworm

Adults: 3.5 g once daily for 2 days

Children: 75 mg/kg/day as a single dose for 2 days; may repeat in 1 week in severe infections; if repeat therapy is impractical or for mass therapy as a public health measure, 150 mg/kg may be given in a single dose

Pinworm

Adults and children: 65 mg/kg/day for 7 consecutive days (maximum daily dose, 2.5 g)

Fate

Oral absorption is variable; a portion of the absorbed drug is metabolized and excreted in the urine; remainder is eliminated in the feces or urine as unchanged drug.

Significant Adverse Reactions

Usually with high doses:

GI: nausea, vomiting, diarrhea, abdominal cramping

CNS: headache, vertigo, muscular weakness, hyporeflexia, blurred vision, paresthesias, tremors, choreiform movements, convulsions, impaired memory, EEG abnormalities, worsening of epileptic seizures

Allergic–hypersensitivity: fever, urticaria, arthralgia, purpura, lacrimation, eczematous skin eruptions, rhinorrhea, bronchospasm, erythema multiforme

Contraindications

Renal or hepatic impairment, convulsive disorders. *Cautious use* in patients with anemia, severe malnutrition, or neurologic disorders, and in pregnant women.

Interaction

Piperazine may increase the severity of extrapyramidal reactions caused by antipsychotic drug administration.

Nursing Management

Pretherapy Assessment

Assess and record baseline data necessary for detection of adverse effects of piperazine: General: VS, body weight, skin color and temperature; GI: bowel sounds, output; Laboratory: culture for ova and parasites.

Review medical history and documents for existing or previous conditions that:
a. require cautious use of piperazine: history of convulsive disorders.
b. contraindicate use of piperazine: renal or hepatic impairment; convulsive disorders; allergy to piperazine; **pregnancy (Category C)**; lactation (appears in breast milk; avoid use in nursing mothers).

Nursing Interventions

Medication Administration

Administer drug on an empty stomach, 1 hour before or 2 hours after meals.
Administer piperazine on schedule to ensure stable steady-state concentrations for the duration of therapy.
Initiate a meal schedule that provides small, frequent meals if GI upset occurs.
Provide ready access to bathroom and interventions directed at symptom relief if diarrhea occurs.
Arrange for disinfection and treatment of all environmental factors.

Surveillance During Therapy

Monitor for adverse effects, toxicity, and interactions.
Monitor for signs of hypersensitivity.

Patient Teaching

Instruct patient regarding the importance of completing the full course of therapy as prescribed; that is, not to discontinue the drug once signs and symptoms of the infection being treated subside.
Instruct patient that the prescribed drug is to be taken for the condition for which it is prescribed, and not to be used to treat any other infections.
Instruct patient about possible adverse side effects of piperazine: nausea, abdominal pain, headache, muscle weakness, dizziness, paresthesias.
Instruct patient on appropriate action to take if side effects occur: notify practitioner if vomiting, diarrhea, labored breathing, rash, severe abdominal pain, marked weakness, confusion, or dizziness occur.

• Praziquantel

Biltricide

Praziquantel is an anthelmintic that exhibits a rather broad spectrum of activity and a low overall incidence of serious adverse effects. It is considered a first-line drug in schistosomal infections, and it is also active against other trematodes as well as cestodes (see Table 70-1). In addition, praziquantel may also be useful in the treatment of cysticercosis, a serious complication of cestodal infections in which the larvae of *Taenia* invade other organs of the body, leading to fatigue, muscle pain, weakness, nervousness, and possibly convulsions or general paralysis.

Mechanism

Increases cell membrane permeability of susceptible worms, altering intracellular calcium and leading to paralysis; also produces vacuolization and subsequent disintegration of the surface tegmentum of the parasite, leading to death of the schistosomal organism.

Uses

Treatment of schistosomal infections (ie, *Schistosoma haematobium, Schistosoma mansoni, Schistosoma japonicum*)—drug of choice
Treatment of lung, liver, and intestinal flukes—drug of choice
Alternative treatment of cestodal (tapeworm) infections

Dosage

Schistosomiasis: 20 mg/kg 3 times a day for 1 day, at intervals of 4 to 6 hours; may repeat in 2 to 3 months
Cestodal infections: 10 to 25 mg/kg as a single dose followed by a purgative in 2 hours; tissue stage: 50 mg/kg in 3 divided doses daily for 14 days

Fate

Rapidly and almost completely (80%) absorbed orally; peak serum levels occur within 1 to 3 hours; metabolized in the liver and excreted largely by the kidneys.

Common Side Effects

Headache, dizziness, anorexia.

Significant Adverse Reactions

Abdominal discomfort, elevated liver enzymes, fever, urticaria, pruritus, diarrhea, arthralgia, myalgia (more frequent in heavily infected patients and those receiving high doses).

Contraindications

Ocular cysticercosis (parasite destruction may cause irreparable lesions). *Cautious use* in pregnant or nursing women and in children younger than 4 years of age.

Nursing Management

Pretherapy Assessment

Assess and record baseline data necessary for detection of adverse effects of praziquantel: General: VS, body weight, skin color and temperature; GI: bowel sounds, output; Laboratory: liver function tests, culture for ova and parasites.
Review medical history and documents for existing or previous conditions that:
a. require cautious use of praziquantel: children younger than 4 years of age.
b. contraindicate use of praziquantel: allergy to praziquantel; **pregnancy (Category B)**; lactation (appears in breast milk; patient should not nurse on day of treatment or for 72 hours after treatment).

Nursing Interventions

Medication Administration

Administer drug with meals with a full glass of water to decrease GI upset.
Note that when schistosomiasis or another trematodal infection is associated with cysticercosis, the patient should be hospitalized.
Administer praziquantel on schedule to ensure stable steady-state concentrations for the duration of therapy.

Initiate a meal schedule that provides small, frequent meals if GI upset occurs.
Provide ready access to bathroom and interventions directed at symptom relief if diarrhea occurs.
Arrange for disinfection and treatment of all environmental factors.

Surveillance During Therapy

Monitor for adverse effects, toxicity, and interactions.
Monitor for signs of hypersensitivity.

Patient Teaching

Instruct patient regarding the importance of completing the full course of therapy as prescribed; that is, not to discontinue the drug once signs and symptoms of the infection being treated subside.
Inform patient of the consequences of not taking or abruptly discontinuing the praziquantel.
Instruct patient that the prescribed drug is to be taken for the condition for which it is prescribed, and not to be used to treat any other infections.
Instruct patient about possible adverse side effects of praziquantel: nausea, abdominal pain, dizziness, headache.
Instruct patient on appropriate action to take if side effects occur: notify practitioner if fever, rash, severe abdominal pain, marked weakness, or dizziness occur.

• Pyrantel

Antiminth, Reese's Pinworm

Mechanism

Paralyzes worms, probably by a depolarizing neuromuscular blocking action that may result from inhibition of cholinesterase enzyme; thus, worms are expelled by peristalsis.

Uses

Treatment of roundworm and pinworm infections.

Dosage

Adults and children: 11 mg/kg in a single dose (1 mL suspension/4.5 kg (10 lb) of body weight; maximum dose 1 g).

Fate

Poorly absorbed orally; plasma levels are maximum in 1 to 3 hours but are quite low; metabolized in the liver; greater than 50% of an oral dose is excreted unchanged in the feces and less than 7% in the urine as both unchanged drug and metabolites.

Common Side Effects

Anorexia, nausea, abdominal cramping.

Significant Adverse Reactions

GI: vomiting, diarrhea, tenesmus, elevated aspartate aminotransferase (transient)
CNS: headache, dizziness, drowsiness, insomnia
Allergic–hypersensitivity: rash, fever

Contraindications

No absolute contraindications. *Cautious use* in patients with liver dysfunction, in pregnant women, and in children younger than 2 years of age.

Nursing Management

Nursing Interventions

Patient Teaching

Inform patient that drug may be taken without regard to presence of food or time of day and that use of a laxative is not necessary.
Stress the importance of meticulous hygiene for complete eradication of the parasites because pinworm infection is readily transmitted from person to person.

• Quinacrine

Atabrine

Quinacrine may occasionally be used as an alternative drug in the management of tapeworm infections, but it has largely been replaced by other more effective, less toxic agents such as niclosamide, praziquantel, or mebendazole. It apparently acts by causing the head of the worm to detach from the intestinal wall; the worm is then expelled by use of a purgative. Because rather high doses of quinacrine are required to treat tapeworm infections, side effects are common. Nausea and vomiting are frequently produced by the drug, as well as dizziness, headache, abdominal cramping, and signs of CNS stimulation (eg, anxiety, restlessness, confusion, aggression, and psychotic behavior). Treatment with quinacrine is best carried out in the hospital.

Dosage depends on the type of parasite present and is usually administered in divided amounts. For treating beef, pork, or fish tapeworm, adults are given four doses of 200 mg each, 10 minutes apart, together with 600 mg of sodium bicarbonate with each dose. Children are given a total dose of 400 to 600 mg in three to four divided doses at 10-minute intervals, together with 300 mg sodium bicarbonate with each dose. A saline purge is administered 1 to 2 hours later to remove the worm from the intestinal tract. The expelled worm is stained yellow.

Quinacrine is also indicated for the treatment of giardiasis, an intestinal protozoal infection caused by the flagellated protozoan *Giardia lamblia*. This disease is the most common protozoal infection in developed countries and is transmitted by cysts in contaminated food or water. Travelers or campers are particularly at risk, as are people living in crowded, unhygienic conditions. Diagnosis of giardiasis is made by identification of cysts or active trophozoites in fecal specimens. Because most infected people are largely asymptomatic, the disease is difficult to recognize and treat.

Adult dosage for quinacrine in giardiasis is 100 mg three times a day for 5 to 7 days. Children are given 7 mg/kg/day in three divided doses after meals for 5 days. A repeat course may be given 2 weeks later, if necessary.

Quinacrine has also been used in the treatment of malaria, and this application is discussed in Chapter 69.

• Thiabendazole

Mintezol

Mechanism

Not established; broad-spectrum anthelmintic that also possesses antiinflammatory and analgesic activities; appears to enhance T-cell function; may interfere with enzyme systems in helminths; suppresses egg and larval production by *Trichinella spiralis* (pork roundworm) and reduces fever and eosinophilia; it is a first-line drug against threadworm infections and cutaneous larva migrans, but despite its broad spectrum of activity, it is not recommended as first choice in other nematodal infections.

Uses

Treatment of threadworm (*Strongyloides*) and rat lungworm (*Angiostrongylus*) infections—drug of choice
Treatment of cutaneous larva migrans (creeping eruption)—drug of choice
Alternative treatment of pinworm, whipworm, hookworm, roundworm, and guinea worm infections
Symptomatic treatment of invasive trichinosis

Dosage

Usual dosage schedule is 2 doses per day for 2 successive days.

Adults and children weighing less than 67.5 kg (150 lb): 10 mg/lb per dose
Adults and children weighing more than 67.5 kg (150 lb): 1.5 g per dose

Maximum daily dose is 3 g.

Fate

Well absorbed orally; peak plasma levels occur in 1 to 2 hours; metabolized in the liver and excreted largely (90%) within 24 hours in the urine.

Common Side Effects

Anorexia, nausea, vomiting, dizziness.

Significant Adverse Reactions

GI: diarrhea, epigastric distress, cramping, perianal rash
CNS: lethargy, drowsiness, giddiness, headache, tinnitus, irritability, blurred vision, numbness
Allergic–hypersensitivity: pruritus, fever, flushing, chills, angioedema, erythema multiforme, lymphadenopathy, anaphylaxis
Renal–hepatic: enuresis, malodor of the urine, crystalluria, hematuria, cholestasis, jaundice, parenchymal liver damage, elevated aspartate aminotransferase
Other: hypotension, bradycardia, hyperglycemia, leukopenia

Contraindications

No absolute contraindications. *Cautious use* in patients with impaired kidney or liver function, anemia, or malnutrition, and in pregnant or nursing women.

Nursing Management

Pretherapy Assessment

Assess and record baseline data necessary for detection of adverse effects of thiabendazole: General: VS, body weight, skin color and temperature; GI: bowel sounds, output; Laboratory: culture for ova and parasites.
Review medical history and documents for existing or previous conditions that:
a. require cautious use of thiabendazole: use in children younger than 2 years of age.
b. contraindicate use of thiabendazole: allergy to thiabendazole; **pregnancy (Category C)**; lactation (avoid use in nursing mothers).

Nursing Interventions

Medication Administration

Administer drug with meals (chewed or crushed and mixed with food) with a full glass of water to decrease GI upset.
Administer thiabendazole on schedule to ensure stable steady-state concentrations for the duration of therapy.
Initiate a meal schedule that provides small, frequent meals if GI upset occurs.
Provide ready access to bathroom and interventions directed at symptom relief if diarrhea occurs.
Arrange for a mild laxative if drug-induced constipation is severe.
Arrange for disinfection and treatment of all environmental factors.

Surveillance During Therapy

Monitor for adverse effects, toxicity, and interactions.
Monitor for signs of hypersensitivity.
Observe patient for development of hypersensitivity reactions (fever, chills, skin rash). If any appear, the drug should be discontinued. Fatalities have occurred from severe erythema multiforme (Stevens-Johnson syndrome).

Patient Teaching

Inform patient that tablets should be chewed or crushed and mixed with food; oral suspension also may be given.
Instruct patient regarding the importance of completing the full course of therapy as prescribed; that is, not to discontinue the drug once signs and symptoms of the infection being treated subside.
Inform patient of the consequences of not taking or abruptly discontinuing the niclosamide.
Instruct patient that the prescribed drug is to be taken for the condition for which it is prescribed, and not to be used to treat any other infections.
Advise patient to use a mild laxative, if needed, to relieve constipation.
Inform patient that this drug should not be taken during pregnancy.
Warn patient to avoid performing hazardous tasks during therapy because dizziness, drowsiness, and other CNS side effects may occur.

Selected Bibliography

Breckenridge EE: Clinical pharmacokinetics of anthelmintic drugs. Clin Pharmacokinet 15:67, 1988

Crompton DWT: Hookworm disease: Current status and new directions. Parasitology Today 5:1, 1989

Drugs for parasitic infections. Med Lett Drugs Therap 34:17, 1992

Nokes C, Bundy DAP: Does helminth infection affect mental processing and educational development? Parasitology Today 10:14, 1994

Ottesen EA, et al: A controlled trial of ivermectin and diethylcarbamazine in lymphatic filariasis. N Engl J Med 322:1113, 1990

Nursing Bibliography

Aggarwal S: Diagnosis and management of neurocysticercosis. Hospital Practice 28(4):106, 1993

Booth S: Factors influencing self diagnosis and treatment of perceived helminthic infection in a rural Guatemalan community. Soc Sci Med 37:531, 1993

71
Amebicides

Chloroquine
Emetine
Iodoquinol
Metronidazole
Paromomycin

The term *amebiasis* refers to infection with the organism *Entamoeba histolytica*, a protozoan that usually invades the lower intestinal tract but may be found in the liver, lungs, brain, and other organs as well. Amebiasis affects approximately 10% of the world's population, is endemic in many tropical regions, and is present in many people in the United States, especially those exposed to poor sanitary conditions.

The disease can be manifested in one of several ways:

Asymptomatic intestinal amebiasis: presence of the organism in the intestinal tract without evidence of clinical symptoms; treatment is indicated because these patients are at risk for development of GI pathology and can serve as carriers, spreading the infection to other, less resistant people

Symptomatic intestinal amebiasis: presence of overt clinical symptoms ranging from mild manifestations (such as diarrhea, cramping, and flatulence) to severe dysentery with accompanying bloody diarrhea, vomiting, fever, and dehydration. Intestinal mucosal scarring and ulceration can promote systemic absorption of the protozoa, leading to the third stage of the disease, extraintestinal amebiasis

Extraintestinal amebiasis: presence of organisms in other body organs, most commonly the liver and lungs; may result in liver necrosis, amebic hepatitis, lung abscesses, and empyema; organisms can also invade the heart, causing pericarditis, and the CNS, leading to brain abscesses

The drugs used in the treatment of amebiasis can be characterized on the basis of their predominant site of action. That is, some agents (eg, iodoquinol, carbarsone, diloxanide) are active only against organisms present in the lumen of the intestine, whereas others (eg, emetine, chloroquine) are effective against parasites found in the bowel wall and other tissues. Still other drugs (eg, metronidazole) are claimed to affect both intestinal and extraintestinal protozoa. To understand better the rationale for the use of a particular drug in the different stages of amebiasis, it is helpful to review briefly the two-stage life cycle of *Entamoeba histolytica*.

The organism is transmitted from person to person through ingestion of amebic cysts, a form in which the protozoa are extremely resistant to destruction outside the body. The cysts are likewise unaffected by gastric juice, and they pass intact to the small intestine, where some develop into motile trophozoites that can invade the intestinal mucosa, be absorbed systemically, and find their way to other organs in the body. The remaining cysts are excreted intact, and they can thus continue the reinfective cycle in another person.

Interruption of this cycle can be accomplished in several ways. Most drugs for treating amebiasis are amebicidal, directly killing or inhibiting the growth and maturation of the trophozoites, whereas some drugs exhibit a cystocidal action. Because most of the effective amebicides have the potential to elicit serious untoward reactions, their use should be undertaken only on a definitive diagnosis of *Entamoeba histolytica* as the causative agent, and patients must be closely observed during therapy for development of adverse reactions.

There is lack of general agreement as to the preferred drug regimens for treating the several forms of amebiasis. *Luminal* amebicides (iodoquinol, diloxanide) are used principally in the treatment of asymptomatic or mild intestinal forms of amebiasis. In addition, they are frequently given together with a systemic or mixed amebicide to eradicate an infection completely.

Systemic amebicides (dehydroemetine, chloroquine) are useful in invasive forms of amebiasis such as amebic dysentery or hepatic abscesses. They are infrequently used today, however, because the preferred drug in most cases of symptomatic intestinal or systemic amebiasis is metronidazole, a *mixed* amebicide effective against both intestinal and systemic forms of the disease.

Metronidazole, however, has been demonstrated to be carcinogenic in mice and rats, and some clinicians believe that it should be reserved for use in severe, acute intestinal amebiasis with hepatic abscesses. In treating symptomatic intestinal or systemic amebiasis, metronidazole is usually used together with the luminal drugs diloxanide or iodoquinol, because metronidazole is well absorbed and may fail to reach effective amebicidal levels in the large intestine. Emetine is also active against both intestinal and extraintestinal organisms, but is a potentially dangerous drug and must be administered parenterally in a hospital setting under close supervision.

Other drugs that may be effective in intestinal forms of amebiasis are the antibiotics tetracycline, erythromycin, and paromomycin. Of these, however, only paromomycin is sometimes used as an alternative drug in chronic intestinal amebiasis, usually in conjunction with one or more other luminal amebicides.

Dehydroemetine and diloxanide are not available for general use in the United States but may be obtained by request from the Parasitic Disease Drug Service of the Centers for Disease Control. They are briefly discussed in Table 71-1. Diloxanide alone is viewed by many as the drug of choice for eradication of microorganisms from asymptomatic carriers of the disease, and it is also considered as a primary drug for treatment of milder intestinal infections, sometimes combined with iodoquinol.

The amebicides are discussed individually in this chapter. Several drugs used in amebiasis (eg, paromomycin, chloroquine) are also effective in other disease states, and have been reviewed elsewhere. Only those aspects of their pharmacology

Table 71-1. **Amebicides Available by Request from the Centers for Disease Control***

Drug	Usual Dosage Range	Remarks
Dehydroemetine *Mebadin*	Adults and children: 1–1.5 mg/kg/d IM *or* SC for up to 5 d (maximum 100 mg/d)	Clinical indications are the same as for emetine, but the incidence and severity of cardiovascular complications may be somewhat less; usually given in combination with diloxanide and a tetracycline, followed by chloroquine if hepatic amebiasis is present; daily dose may be divided into 2 parts; use very *cautiously* in patients with cardiac disease or neuromuscular disorders
Diloxanide furoate *Furamide*	Adults: 500 mg 3 times a day for 10 d Children: 20 mg/kg/d in 3 divided doses for 10 d; repeat in several weeks if necessary	Relatively nontoxic intestinal amebicide regarded by many as the drug of choice for asymptomatic and mild symptomatic intestinal amebiasis; ineffective alone against extraintestinal parasites; may be combined with metronidazole in moderate to severe intestinal disease; mild GI distress and flatulence have been reported; GI absorption is appreciable, and much of an oral dose is excreted in the urine within 48 h, largely as metabolites

* Parasitic Disease Drug Service, Centers for Disease Control, Atlanta, Georgia 30333.

related to the treatment of amebic infections are considered here.

• Chloroquine

Aralen

(CAN) Novo-Chloroquine

Primarily used as an antimalarial drug, chloroquine is also effective in the treatment of amebic liver abscesses (often with emetine), because chloroquine localizes in the liver in a concentration several hundred times greater than in the plasma. The drug is largely ineffective against intestinal organisms because it is rapidly absorbed; therefore, it is always given either in combination with or after other drugs active against intestinal amebiasis. When used in hepatic amebiasis, chloroquine also may be combined with metronidazole or diloxanide or both to ensure that all protozoa are eradicated. Chloroquine is discussed fully in Chapter 69, and only information pertinent to its use in amebiasis is presented here.

Uses

Treatment of extraintestinal amebiasis, in combination with other amebicides active against intestinal forms.

Dosage

Oral: (phosphate salt) 1 g/day for 2 days, then 500 mg/day for at least 2 to 3 weeks
IM: (hydrochloride salt) 200 to 250 mg/day for 10 to 12 days; oral therapy should be substituted as soon as possible
Children: maximum single dose is 5 mg (base)/kg

Nursing Management

See Chapter 69.

• Emetine *(Pregnancy Category X)*

Emetine is a potent amebicide effective against both intestinal and extraintestinal tissue parasites. Its use is restricted to severe cases of amebic dysentery and amebic hepatitis or liver abscesses, inasmuch as the drug can cause serious untoward reactions related to cumulative toxicity as well as a wide range of milder adverse effects. The close structural analogue dehydroemetine is available as Mebadin from the Centers for Disease Control in Atlanta; it is equally effective and may be somewhat less toxic (see Table 71-1).

Mechanism

Exerts a direct lethal action on trophozoites, probably blocking protein synthesis by interfering with attachment of t-RNA to the ribosomes; much more effective against motile forms than against cysts; exhibits some anticholinergic and antiadrenergic action; may depress cardiac conduction and contraction; electrocardiographic (ECG) changes have occurred.

Uses

Symptomatic treatment of acute amebic dysentery or acute episodes of chronic amebic dysentery, in combination with other amebicides
Treatment of amebic hepatitis and amebic abscesses in other tissues, in combination with an amebicide effective against intestinal parasites
Alternative treatment of balantidiasis, fascioliasis, and paragonimiasis

Dosage

Deep SC injection is preferred; may be given IM.

Acute amebic dysentery
65 mg/day SC or IM for 3 days to 5 days, in a single or two divided doses

Amebic hepatitis or abscesses

65 mg/day SC or IM for 10 days
Children (younger than 8 years): maximum 10 mg/day
Children (older than 8 years): maximum 20 mg/day

CAUTION

Do not extend therapy beyond 10 days or exceed a total dose of 650 mg in adults, because cumulative toxicity can occur. Do not repeat a course of therapy until 6 to 8 weeks have elapsed.

Fate

Well absorbed from SC or IM injection sites; widely distributed in the body (eg, kidney, spleen, lungs), highest concentrations being found in the liver; excreted very slowly by the kidneys, some drug still present in the body 60 days after administration; danger of cumulative toxicity is appreciable.

Common Side Effects

Pain, tenderness, stiffness, and local muscle weakness at injection sites; nausea, diarrhea, abdominal pain, dizziness, fainting.

Significant Adverse Reactions

GI: vomiting
CV: hypotension, tachycardia, precordial pain, cardiac dilation, ECG abnormalities (T-wave inversion, QT prolongation), gallop rhythm, dyspnea, congestive heart failure, and arrhythmias
Neuromuscular: muscle stiffness and weakness, tremors
Dermatologic: urticarial, eczematous, or purpuric skin lesions

Contraindications

Organic heart or kidney disease; pregnancy; in children (except those with severe dysentery not controlled by other amebicides) and people receiving a course of emetine therapy within the previous 2 months; IV injection of the drug. *Cautious use* in people with liver disease, ECG abnormalities; in nursing mothers and in elderly or debilitated people.

Nursing Management

Pretherapy Assessment

Assess and record baseline data necessary for detection of adverse effects of emetine: General: vital signs (VS), body weight, skin color and temperature; CNS: orientation, reflexes, affect, bilateral grip strength; GI: bowel sounds; Laboratory: blood urea nitrogen, urinalysis, renal function tests.

Review medical history and documents for existing or previous conditions that:

a. require cautious use of emetine: liver disease, ECG abnormalities.
b. contraindicate use of emetine: allergy to any ingredient; organic heart or kidney disease; in children (except those with severe dysentery not controlled by other amebicides); a course of emetine therapy within the previous 2 months; IV injection of the drug; **pregnancy (Category X)**; lactation (excreted in breast milk, mothers should not nurse while taking these agents).

Nursing Interventions

Medication Administration

Confine patient to bed and observe very carefully during therapy and for several days thereafter.

Monitor pulse and blood pressure several times a day. Drug should be discontinued if tachycardia, marked drop in blood pressure, neuromuscular symptoms, muscle weakness, or severe GI symptoms occur.

Handle solution carefully and avoid contact with eyes and mucous membranes because solution is very irritating

Administer by deep IM or SC injection. Inadvertent IV injection can cause severe toxic effects.

Provide for frequent oral hygiene.

Surveillance During Therapy

Notify drug prescriber if fatigability or listlessness occurs, or if patient experiences muscle stiffness, pain, or tenderness, especially in the neck or upper extremities, because these are often early signs of more serious neuromuscular toxicity. Drug should be discontinued.

Monitor results of ECG, which should be obtained before initiating therapy, after the fifth dose, on completion of treatment, and again 1 week later. Although ECG changes are common and are not an absolute indication for discontinuing therapy, the patient must be carefully observed for additional complications (eg, dyspnea, arrhythmias).

Monitor intake–output, and note any change in renal function. Report immediately.

Observe number, consistency, and character of stools. Fecal examinations should be repeated for up to 3 months after therapy to ensure elimination of parasites.

Monitor ECG, blood pressure, and pulse frequently.

Carefully monitor laboratory studies and patient for indications of adverse reactions.

Interpret results of diagnostic tests and contact practitioner as appropriate.

Monitor for possible drug–drug and drug–nutrient interactions; see Interactions.

Patient Teaching

Instruct patient to avoid strenuous activity for several weeks after termination of therapy.

Inform patient that the following may occur as a result of therapy: diarrhea, weakness, fatigue.

Teach the patient that the effects of this drug may last for weeks and to inform the practitioner during this period if any of the following occur: muscle pain, headache, dizziness, fainting, palpitations, extreme weakness.

• Iodoquinol (diiodohydroxyquin)

Yodoxin

(CAN) Diodoquin

An iodinated hydroxyquinoline, iodoquinol is effective in intestinal amebiasis, especially in asymptomatic carriers. It is relatively nontoxic and inexpensive and has been used for mass treatment.

Mechanisms

Not established; exerts a direct amebicidal action against both motile and cystic forms of trophozoites; action is restricted to the intestinal tract owing to poor oral absorption.

Uses

Treatment of asymptomatic or mild to moderate acute or chronic intestinal amebiasis
Treatment of giardiasis (investigational use)

Dosage

Adults: 650 mg orally three times a day for 20 days
Children: 40 mg/kg/day in three divided doses for 20 days (maximum 2 g/day)

Fate

Poorly absorbed from the GI tract; eliminated largely in the feces.

Common Side Effects

Gastric distress (diarrhea, nausea, abdominal discomfort).

Significant Adverse Reactions

Rare at usual doses: vomiting, abdominal cramping, pruritus ani, urticaria, skin eruptions, headache, vertigo, fever, chills, thyroid enlargement. Optic neuritis, optic atrophy, and peripheral neuropathy have occurred with long-term therapy.

Contraindications

Hypersensitivity to iodides, hepatic damage. *Cautious use* in patients with thyroid disorders and in pregnant or lactating women.

Nursing Management

Pretherapy Assessment

Assess and record baseline data necessary for detection of adverse effects of iodoquinol: General: VS, body weight, skin color and temperature; CNS: orientation, reflexes, affect, bilateral grip strength; Laboratory: liver, thyroid function function tests, protein-bound serum iodine.
Review medical history and documents for existing or previous conditions that:
a. require cautious use of iodoquinol: thyroid disorders.
b. contraindicate use of iodoquinol: allergy to any ingredient; hypersensitivity to iodides; hepatic damage; **pregnancy (Category C)**; lactation (excreted in breast milk, mothers should not nurse while taking these agents).

Nursing Interventions

Medication Administration

Determine whether patient is allergic to iodide before administering initial dose.
Question prescription of iodoquinol for prophylaxis or treatment of nonspecific or "travelers' " diarrhea. It is *not* indicated for these conditions, although it has been used for them.
Interpret results of thyroid function tests cautiously because drug can interfere with some of them by increasing protein-bound serum iodine levels.
Administer after meals, providing small, frequent meals if GI upset occurs.

Surveillance During Therapy

Monitor for toxicity; blurring of vision (optic neuritis); fatigue, numbness (peripheral neuropathy).
Carefully monitor laboratory studies and patient for indications of adverse reactions.
Interpret results of diagnostic tests and contact practitioner as appropriate.
Monitor for possible drug–drug and drug–nutrient interactions; see Interactions.
Provide for patient safety needs if CNS or visual effects occur.

Patient Teaching

Instruct patient to be alert for development of ocular or neurologic disturbances, especially during prolonged high-dosage therapy, and to inform drug prescriber if they occur because the drug should be discontinued. Long-term therapy should be avoided.
Inform patient that periodic ophthalmologic examinations are advisable during therapy, especially in young children.
Teach patient how to recognize signs of hypersensitivity reactions (pruritus, urticaria, chills, fever). Instruct patient to notify drug prescriber if they occur.
Inform patient that the following may occur as a result of therapy: GI upset, diarrhea, weakness, fatigue.
Teach the patient that the effects of this drug may last for weeks and to inform the practitioner during this period if any of the following occur: severe GI upset; skin rash; blurring of vision; unusual fatigue; fever.

• Metronidazole

Flagyl, MetroGel, Metro I.V., Protostat

(CAN) Apo-Metronidazole, Neo-Tric, Novonidazol, PMS Metronidazole

Metronidazole exerts a direct amebicidal and trichomonacidal action against *Entamoeba histolytica* and *Trichomonas vaginalis*, respectively. It is considered the drug of choice for oral treatment of trichomoniasis in both women and men. In addition, it is used in treating acute intestinal amebiasis, both symptomatic and asymptomatic, as well as amebic liver abscess. The drug has been reported to be carcinogenic in mice and rats, and *unnecessary* use should be avoided; however, metronidazole remains a valuable drug for the therapy of both amebiasis and trichomoniasis.

In addition to its use as both an amebicide and trichomonacide, metronidazole is also available both orally and IV for the treatment of serious infections caused by susceptible anaerobic bacteria. Parenteral metronidazole has demonstrated clinical activity against the following organisms: anaerobic gram-negative bacilli, including *Bacteroides* and *Fusobacterium* sp; anaerobic gram-positive bacilli, including *Clostridium* sp; and anaerobic gram-positive cocci, including *Peptococcus* and *Peptostreptococcus* sp. Necessary surgical procedures should always be performed in conjunction with drug treatment, and in mixed aerobic–anaerobic infections, appropriate antibiotics should be included in the drug regimen. The principal hazard connected with parenteral metronidazole therapy is the possibility of convulsive seizures and development of peripheral neuropathy. The benefit–risk ratio must be critically evaluated in patients who show evidence of abnormal neurologic signs.

Finally, metronidazole is available as a topical gel for treatment of the inflammatory papules and erythema of rosacea, and also as a vaginal gel for treatment of bacterial vaginosis.

Mechanism

Not entirely established; appears to disrupt the structure of DNA in susceptible organisms, causing strand breakage and loss of helical structure; destroys most organisms within 24 to 48 hours.

Uses

Treatment of acute intestinal amebiasis (amebic dysentery) and amebic liver abscess

Treatment of symptomatic and asymptomatic trichomoniasis in both sexes (oral only)

Treatment of serious infections caused by susceptible anaerobic bacteria, especially *Bacteroides* sp (including strains resistant to clindamycin and chloramphenicol), *Clostridium* sp (including pseudomembranous colitis resulting from *Clostridium difficile* overgrowth), *Eubacterium, Peptococcus*, and *Peptostreptococcus* sp (IV)

Preoperative, intraoperative, or postoperative prophylaxis of infection in patients undergoing surgery classified as potentially contaminated, such as colorectal, abdominal, or gynecologic surgery

Treatment of rosacea (topical only)

Treatment of bacterial vaginosis (intravaginally only)

Investigational uses include 1) hepatic encephalopathy, 2) treatment of giardiasis or *Gardnerella vaginalis* infections, 3) Crohn's disease, and 4) as a radiosensitizer to render tumors more susceptible to radiation

Dosage

Amebiasis

Adults: 500 to 750 mg three times a day orally for 5 to 10 days

Children: 35 to 50 mg/kg/day orally in three divided doses for 10 days

Trichomoniasis

250 mg three times a day orally for 7 days *for men and women; alternatively*, 2 g in a single dose or two divided doses; allow 4 to 6 weeks between courses of therapy when a repeat treatment is necessary

Anaerobic infections

Initially 15 mg/kg infused over 1 hour; maintenance doses, 7.5 mg/kg infused over 1 hour every 6 hours for 7 to 10 days; maximum dose, 4 g/24-hour period; may change to oral therapy (7.5 mg/kg every 6 hours) as condition warrants

Prophylaxis of postoperative infection

15 mg/kg infused over 30 to 60 minutes and completed at least 1 hour before surgery, followed by 7.5 mg/kg infused over 30 to 60 minutes at 6 and 12 hours after the initial dose

Rosacea

Apply in a thin film twice daily; may require 3 to 6 weeks of therapy for significant response

Bacterial vaginosis

One full applicator applied intravaginally twice a day for 5 days

Fate

Well absorbed from GI tract; peak serum levels occur in 1 to 2 hours; widely distributed in the body and diffuses well into all tissues; slightly (20%) bound to plasma proteins; plasma half-life is approximately 8 hours; excreted largely in the urine, both as unchanged drug (20%) and 2-hydroxymethyl metabolite; both parent compound and metabolite have antibacterial activity.

Common Side Effects

Especially orally: nausea, metallic taste, anorexia, epigastric distress.

Significant Adverse Reactions

CAUTION

Prolonged oral administration of metronidazole in rodents has been associated with an increased incidence of neoplastic tumors, especially hepatic and mammary. Unnecessary use of the drug for extended periods in humans should be avoided.

Oral

GI: vomiting, diarrhea, abdominal cramping, furry tongue, glossitis, stomatitis, candidal overgrowth

CNS: dizziness, vertigo, incoordination, ataxia, paresthesia, numbness, confusion, depression, irritability, insomnia

Allergic–hypersensitivity: pruritus, flushing, urticaria, fever

Urinary: dysuria, cystitis, polyuria, incontinence, darkened urine

Other: leukopenia, nasal congestion, xerostomia, dyspareunia, decreased libido, proctitis, pyuria, flattened T wave, joint pain

IV

See Oral; in addition, convulsions, seizures, peripheral neuropathy, thrombophlebitis with IV infusion

Topical

Dryness and redness

Vaginal

Candidal overgrowth, abdominal pain and cramping

Contraindications

Blood dyscrasias, organic CNS disease, first trimester of pregnancy (unless absolutely necessary, eg, *severe*, life-threatening infections). *Cautious use* in patients with liver or kidney disease, persistent fungal infections; in alcoholics (see Interactions), and in pregnant or nursing women.

Interactions

Alcohol ingestion may elicit a disulfiram-like reaction (abdominal cramps, vomiting, severe headache, hypotension); see Chapter 81.

Metronidazole may potentiate the effects of oral anticoagulants.
The effectiveness of metronidazole may be reduced when used with phenobarbital or phenytoin, drugs that may increase its rate of metabolism.
Cimetidine may reduce the metabolism of metronidazole.

Nursing Management

Pretherapy Assessment

Assess and record baseline data necessary for detection of adverse effects of metronidazole: General: VS, body weight, skin color and temperature; CNS: orientation, reflexes, affect; GI: abdominal examination; liver palpation; Laboratory: liver function function tests, complete blood count, urinalysis.
Review medical history and documents for existing or previous conditions that:
a. require cautious use of metronidazole: liver or kidney disease, history of seizures, persistent fungal infections; in alcoholics.
b. contraindicate use of metronidazole: allergy to metronidazole; blood dyscrasias; organic CNS disease; candidiasis; **pregnancy (Category B)**; lactation (excreted in breast milk, mothers should not nurse while taking these agents).

Nursing Interventions

Medication Administration

Closely follow package instructions for preparing IV infusion solution. Order of mixing is important. Do *not* refrigerate neutralized solution because precipitate may form. Use within 24 hours.
Protect IV solution from light.
Administer oral doses with food.
Provide small, frequent meals if GI upset becomes a problem.
Ensure ready access to bathroom facilities if diarrhea occurs.

Surveillance During Therapy

Observe patient for symptoms of CNS toxicity (eg, mood changes, incoordination, ataxia). Drug should be discontinued if these occur.
Observe patient carefully for signs of peripheral neurologic dysfunction, especially with IV administration. Persistent peripheral neuropathy has occurred in some patients on prolonged therapy. Benefit–risk ratio of continued therapy must be critically evaluated.
Monitor results of total and differential leukocyte counts, which should be performed before and periodically during therapy because drug can elicit leukopenia.
Carefully monitor laboratory studies and patient for indications of adverse reactions.
Interpret results of diagnostic tests and contact practitioner as appropriate.
Monitor for possible drug–drug and drug–nutrient interactions; see Interactions.

Patient Teaching

Instruct patient to take oral drug with food to minimize GI upset.
Inform patient that drug may cause an unpleasant metallic taste.
Inform patient that drug may harmlessly darken urine.
Stress the importance of adhering to prescribed dosage (see CAUTION under Significant Adverse Reactions) and of completing the full course of therapy.
Inform patient that ingestion of alcohol in any form (eg, cough preparations, mouthwashes) can result in a disulfiram-like reaction (vomiting, diarrhea, flushing, hypotension, abdominal pain).
Teach patient how to recognize signs of secondary fungal (candidal) overgrowth, which may result from drug use. If glossitis, stomatitis, vaginitis, vaginal discharge, diarrhea, or furry tongue occur, appropriate antifungal medicine is required.
Caution women treated for trichomoniasis that concurrent treatment of the male sexual partner is usually necessary to prevent reinfection.

Paromomycin

Humatin

An aminoglycoside-like drug, paromomycin exhibits an antibacterial action resembling that of neomycin. In addition, it exerts an amebicidal action in the intestinal tract but is not appreciably absorbed orally, and is therefore ineffective in extraintestinal amebiasis.

Mechanism

Direct amebicidal action in vivo and in vitro; may also reduce the population of intestinal microbes essential for proliferation of protozoa.

Uses

Treatment of acute and chronic intestinal amebiasis, usually as an alternative drug to other more potent and specific amebicides
Adjunctive therapy in management of hepatic coma

Dosage

Amebiasis: 25 to 35 mg/kg/day in three divided doses for 5 to 10 days
Hepatic coma: 4 g/day in divided doses for 5 to 6 days

Fate

Not significantly absorbed orally; excreted largely in the feces; systemically absorbed drug is excreted very slowly by way of the kidneys.

Common Side Effects

Nausea, anorexia, GI upset, diarrhea.

Significant Adverse Reactions

Abdominal cramps, pruritus ani, headache, vertigo, skin rash, malabsorption state, and overgrowth of nonsusceptible organisms.

Contraindications

Intestinal obstruction, ulcerative bowel lesions. *Cautious use* in patients with preexisting hearing loss, vestibular damage, or renal dysfunction.

Nursing Management

See Chapter 64 for complete discussion of aminoglycosides; in addition:

Nursing Interventions

Medication Administration

Note that paromomycin is an aminoglycoside derivative. Although it has the potential to elicit serious untoward reactions (nephrotoxicity, ototoxicity) and to interact with a number of other drugs (see Chapter 64 for complete discussion of aminoglycosides), the incidence of such reactions is quite low because paromomycin is poorly absorbed.

Administer with meals, providing small, frequent meals if GI upset occurs.

Patient Teaching

Instruct patient to take drug with meals to minimize GI upset.

Inform patient that stools are usually examined weekly during and for at least 6 weeks after termination of therapy.

Teach patient how to recognize signs of secondary fungal (candidal) overgrowth, which may result from drug use. If glossitis, stomatitis, vaginitis, vaginal discharge, diarrhea, or furry tongue occur, appropriate antifungal medicine should be instituted.

Selected Bibliography

Dooley CP, O'Morain CAO: Recurrence of hepatic amebiasis after successful treatment with metronidazole. J Clin Gastroenterol 10:339, 1988

Holtan NR: Giardiasis: A crimp in the lifestyle of campers, travelers, and others. Postgrad Med 83:54, 1988

Panosian CB: Parasitic diarrhea. Infect Disease Clin North Amer 2:685, 1988

Plaisance KI, Quintilliani R, Nightingale CM: The pharmacokinetics of metronidazole and its metabolites in critically ill patients. J Antimicrob Chemother 21:195, 1988

Roberson DH, et al: Treatment failure in *Trichomonas vaginalis* infections in females: Concentrations of metronidazole in plasma and vaginal content during normal and high dosage. J Antimicrob Chemother 21:373, 1988

Nursing Bibliography

Peppercorn M, Shelly D, Sobel J: Metronidazole: Versatile antimicrobial. Patient Care 27:137, 1993

Pogson C: Acanthamoeba keratitis. Journal of Ophthalmic Nursing and Technology 12(3):114, 1993

Widmer A: Amebiasis. Infection Control and Hospital Epidemiology 12:735, 1991

72

Antifungal Agents

Drugs for treating systemic infections only

Flucytosine
Fluconazole
Itraconazole

Drugs for treating both systemic and topical infections

Amphotericin B
Ketoconazole
Miconazole
Nystatin

Drugs for treating topical infections only

Oral administration only

Griseofulvin

Cutaneous administration only

Ciclopirox
Econazole
Haloprogin
Iodochlorhydroxyquin
Naftifine
Oxiconazole
Sulconazole
Terbinafine
Tolnaftate
Triacetin
Undecylenic Acid

Vaginal administration only

Butoconazole
Tioconazole
Terconazole

Cutaneous and vaginal administration

Clotrimazole

Drugs for treating ophthalmic infections only

Natamycin

Fungal, or mycotic, infections are responsible for a number of pathologic conditions in humans that, with few exceptions, remain difficult to treat. Fungal diseases are conventionally categorized as either topical (cutaneous, superficial) or deep (systemic) infections. Although this classification is convenient, it should be recognized that organisms responsible for local infections of the skin, nails, vagina, or GI tract (such as *Candida*) can also invade deeper body organs, resulting in systemic involvement and serious complications. Because there are only a few effective systemic antifungal drugs, most of which are relatively toxic in the doses needed to eliminate deep mycotic infections, successful treatment of systemic fungal diseases is one of the most difficult tasks in chemotherapy.

Reflecting the classification of fungal diseases into topical or deep infections, antifungal drugs can be categorized in much the same way, although it should be noted that some drugs are used in treating *both* superficial and systemic infections.

The organisms responsible for the common fungal infections, together with the preferred drugs for treating each disease, are listed in Table 58-1, Chapter 58. Most systemic fungal infections respond best to amphotericin B. Flucytosine is indicated for serious candidal or cryptococcal infections and is synergistic with amphotericin B against these organisms. Fluconazole, itraconazole, ketoconazole,and miconazole are viewed as rather broad-spectrum antifungal agents, but some questions exist as to their clinical efficacy in many fungal diseases. In addition, relapses have frequently occurred with use of these agents. Oral nystatin is indicated for intestinal candidiasis and for local fungal infections of the mouth and throat. Topical or vaginal monilial infections caused by *Candida* species can be effectively controlled by several antifungal drugs, such as butoconazole, terconazole, clotrimazole, miconazole, and nystatin. Cutaneous dermatophytal infections (eg, tinea) of the skin, hair, or nails (including ringworm, athlete's foot, jock itch) can be controlled either by oral griseofulvin (severe ringworm) or one of the topically effective antifungal drugs such as ciclopirox, econazole, haloprogin, terbinafine, tolnaftate, triacetin, or undecylenic acid. Natamycin is an antifungal agent used locally in the eye for treatment of fungal conjunctivitis, blepharitis, and keratitis.

The systemic antifungal agents are reviewed individually in detail in this chapter. The topically effective drugs are then listed in Table 72-1, along with their indications, dosage ranges, and specific information relating to each drug.

Systemic Antifungal Agents

• Amphotericin B

Fungizone

An antibiotic produced by a strain of *Streptomyces*, amphotericin is a first-line drug for many severe progressive and potentially fatal systemic fungal infections, but because of its serious toxicity, it should not be used to treat trivial or clinically insignificant fungal diseases. It is also used topically to treat cutaneous or mucosal candidal (monilial) infections.

Mechanism

Fungistatic or fungicidal depending on organism and concentration of drug; binds to sterols (eg, ergosterol) in fungal cell membrane, thus increasing cell permeability and allowing leakage of cellular constituents; no effect on bacteria, viruses, or rickettsiae; potentiates the effects of flucytosine and other antibiotics by allowing penetration of these drugs into the fungal cell

Uses

Treatment of serious and potentially fatal systemic fungal infections, such as aspergillosis, blastomycosis, coccidioidomycosis, cryptococcosis, disseminated candidiasis (moniliasis), histoplasmosis, mucormycosis, and sporotrichosis (see Table 58-1)

Alternative treatment of American mucocutaneous leishmaniasis (intravenous [IV] only)

Treatment of cutaneous and mucocutaneous candidal (monilial) infections (topically only)

Malseed, RT; Goldstein, FJ; and Balkon, N: PHARMACOLOGY: DRUG THERAPY AND NURSING CONSIDERATIONS, Fourth Edition.

Dosage

IV infusion:

Initially 0.25 mg/kg/day infused over 6 hours; may increase gradually to 1 mg/kg/day or 1.5 mg/kg every other day as tolerance permits; total treatment time is usually several months, although some serious infections can require 9 to 12 months of therapy; maximum daily dose is 1.5 mg/kg; total dosage can range from 1.5 g for blastomycosis to 4 g for life-threatening infections such as rhinocerebral phycomycosis

Intrathecal/intraventricular:

0.1 mg initially, increased gradually up to 0.5 mg every 48 to 72 hours (investigational use only)

Topical:

Apply liberally to lesions two to four times a day for 1 to 4 weeks depending on response

Fate

Poorly absorbed from GI tract and not given orally; after IV infusion, drug is highly (90%–95%) bound to plasma proteins and has a plasma half-life of 24 hours; diffuses well into inflamed pleural and peritoneal cavities and joints but poorly into most other body tissues; slowly excreted by the kidneys (elimination half-life is 15 days), a small fraction in a biologically active form; drug can be detected in the urine for at least 7 weeks after termination of therapy

Common Side Effects

IV: fever, chills, nausea, vomiting, diarrhea, headache, dyspepsia, impaired renal function (hypokalemia, azotemia, renal tubular acidosis, nephrocalcinosis), anorexia, weight loss, malaise, muscle and joint pain, abdominal cramping, pain at injection site, phlebitis, normochromic–normocytic anemia

Significant Adverse Reactions

IV: maculopapular rash, pruritus, tinnitus, hearing loss, blurred vision, vertigo, flushing, peripheral neuropathy, blood pressure alterations, arrhythmias, cardiac arrest, blood dyscrasias, coagulation defects, anuria, oliguria, hemorrhagic gastroenteritis, convulsions, anaphylactic reaction, acute liver failure

Topical: drying of the skin, irritation, pruritus, erythema, burning, contact dermatitis, skin discoloration

Contraindications

No absolute contraindications if the situation being treated is potentially life-threatening. *Cautious use* in pregnant women and in patients with renal impairment, blood dyscrasias, neurologic disorders, or peptic ulcer.

Interactions

Hypokalemia induced by amphotericin B may be increased by diuretics or corticosteroids and poses a danger in patients receiving digitalis drugs.

Amphotericin B can enhance the effect of peripherally acting muscle relaxants, for example, curare, gallamine, succinylcholine.

Concomitant use of corticosteroids, antibiotics, or antineoplastics with amphotericin B can increase the incidence of superinfections and blood dyscrasias.

Aminoglycosides, cyclosporine, and other nephrotoxic or ototoxic drugs can have additive toxic effects with amphotericin B.

Flucytosine, minocycline, and rifampin can potentiate the antifungal activity of amphotericin B.

Nursing Management

Pretherapy Assessment

Assess and record baseline data necessary for detection of adverse effects of amphotericin B: General: vital signs (VS), body weight, skin color and temperature; central nervous system (CNS): orientation, reflexes, affect; GI: abdominal examination; liver palpation; Lab: liver function tests, complete blood count (CBC), urinalysis.

Review medical history and documents for existing or previous conditions that:

a. require cautious use of amphotericin B: renal impairment; blood dyscrasias; neurologic disorders; peptic ulcer.
b. contraindicate use of amphotericin B: allergy to amphotericin B; **pregnancy (Category B)**, lactation (safety not established).

Nursing Interventions

Medication Administration

Administer IV only to hospitalized patients with a confirmed diagnosis of progressive, potentially fatal fungal disease. Ensure that patient is closely supervised during administration.

Infuse IV slowly and observe infusion site for signs of inflammation. Extravasation may lead to thromboses and thrombophlebitis. Simultaneous infusion of heparin may decrease the incidence of thrombophlebitis.

Be prepared to administer aspirin, antihistamines, antiemetics, or small doses of corticosteroids to lessen the severity of adverse reactions (eg, fever, headache, vomiting).

Add 10 mL sterile water for injection to powder, shake, then dilute further (1:50) with 5% dextrose injection of pH above 4.2. Do *not* reconstitute with saline solution because precipitate may form. Powder contains no preservative or bacteriostatic agent.

Store vials in refrigerator, protect against exposure to light, and use IV solutions immediately after preparing.

Ensure that the mean pore diameter is greater than 1 μm to allow passage of the colloidal dispersion of the drug if an in-line membrane is used during IV infusion.

Surveillance During Therapy

Monitor results of the following laboratory studies, which should be performed at least weekly during therapy: liver function studies, blood urea nitrogen (BUN), serum creatinine and potassium, and hemogram. Drug should be discontinued if liver function is abnormal, if BUN exceeds 40 mg/dL, or if serum creatinine exceeds 3 mg/dL.

Monitor intake–output and observe for oliguria, hematuria, or cloudy urine. Notify drug prescriber of any change in renal function because nephrotoxicity develops after a few months in most patients. The azotemia that develops during therapy is usually reversible, but if total dose exceeds 4 g, *persistent* renal damage often ensues.

Assess patient's auditory and vestibular function frequently, and instruct patient to report any changes immediately because drug is ototoxic.

Monitor patient for symptoms of hypokalemia (muscle weakness or cramping, drowsiness, paresthesias). If they occur, potassium supplementation should be provided.

Interpret results of the following laboratory tests cautiously because amphotericin can interfere with them: serum aminotransferases (ALT, AST), BUN, serum creatinine, hematocrit, hemoglobin, and platelet count.

Carefully monitor laboratory studies and patient for indications of adverse reactions.

Interpret results of diagnostic tests and contact practitioner as appropriate.

Monitor for possible drug–drug and drug–nutrient interactions: Refer to **Interactions**.

Patient Teaching

Instruct patient to apply topical preparation liberally and to rub gently but well into lesions.

Inform patient that some skin drying and discoloration may occur with use of cream preparation, but generally not with the lotion or ointment. Lotion may stain nail lesions, however.

Inform patient that topical preparation can stain clothes or other fabrics, but that the stain can be removed easily by washing with soap and water or by using a standard cleaning fluid.

Teach patient how to recognize signs of hypersensitivity reaction to topical preparation (rash, pruritus, erythema) and report to prescriber.

• Fluconazole

Diflucan

Fluconazole is an orally active triazole derivative structurally related to ketoconazole and miconazole (chemically referred to as imidazoles). Replacement of the imidazole ring with the triazole ring results in increased antifungal activity and an expanded antifungal spectrum. Fluconazole is effective in the treatment of serious oropharyngeal/esophageal candidiasis and cryptococcal meningitis, one of the most common opportunistic infections in patients with acquired immunodeficiency syndrome (AIDS). Fluconazole is well tolerated and is associated with a significantly lower incidence of adverse effects compared with amphotericin B or ketoconazole. Although less effective than amphotericin B for the initial treatment of cryptococcal meningitis, fluconazole may be the drug of choice for suppressive therapy to prevent recurrence of infection.

Mechanism

Fluconazole is considered to be fungistatic in action; the drug inhibits fungal cytochrome P-450 enzymes required for the synthesis of ergosterol (the principle sterol in fungal cell membranes), resulting in increased membrane permeability, leakage of cellular contents and inhibition of cellular growth; fluconazole has little affinity for mammalian P-450 enzymes

Uses

Treatment of oropharyngeal and esophageal candidiasis, and serious systemic candidal infections (peritonitis, pneumonia, and urinary tract infections)

Treatment of meningitis caused by *Cryptococcus neoformans*

Dosage

Oral:

Oropharyngeal candidiasis: 200 mg on day 1, followed by 100 mg once daily for a minimum of 2 weeks

Esophageal candidiasis: 200 mg on day 1, followed by 100 mg once daily for a minimum of 3 weeks and for at least 2 weeks after resolution of symptoms

Systemic candidiasis: 400 mg on day 1, followed by 200 mg once daily for a minimum of 4 weeks and for at least 2 weeks after resolution of symptoms

Cryptococcal meningitis: 400 mg on day 1, followed by 200 mg once daily for at least 10 to 12 weeks after cerebrospinal fluid (CSF) cultures become negative

IV infusion: 200 mg/hour, given as a constant infusion for up to 14 days

Fate

Oral bioavailability is greater than 90% and is not affected by food; plasma half-life ranges from 20 to 50 hours; approximately 60% to 80% of fluconazole is excreted unchanged in the urine, dosage should be adjusted in patients with reduced renal function; CSF concentrations are usually 60% to 90% of plasma concentrations; plasma protein binding is only 11% to 12%.

Common Side Effects

Nausea, headache, skin rash

Significant Adverse reactions

GI: vomiting, diarrhea, abdominal pain

Dermatologic: diffuse rash, pruritus, exfoliative skin disorders

Hepatic: increased concentrations of liver enzymes and bilirubin

CNS: dizziness, delirium, coma, psychiatric disturbances, paresthesia of hands and feet

Other: anemia and reductions in other blood cells, fever, hypotension, arthralgia, myalgia, edema, oliguria

Contraindications

No specific contraindications. *Cautious use* in patients with preexisting liver dysfunction or skin conditions; patients with AIDS appear to experience greater incidences of adverse effects; safety during pregnancy has not been established.

Interactions

Concomitant use of fluconazole and oral anticoagulants may increase the prothrombin time; other drugs whose effects may be increased by fluconazole include cyclosporine and phenytoin.

Concomitant use of fluconazole and oral contraceptives may reduce oral contraceptive effectiveness.

Plasma concentrations of fluconazole may be increased by hydrochlorothiazide, and reduced by either cimetidine or rifampin.

Nursing Management

Pretherapy Assessment

Assess and record baseline data necessary for detection of adverse effects of fluconazole: General: VS, body weight, skin color and temperature; CNS: orientation, reflexes, affect; GI: abdominal exam, bowel sounds; Lab: renal function tests, CBC, culture of area involved.

Review medical history and documents for existing or previous conditions that:

a. require cautious use of fluconazole: renal impairment; preexisting liver dysfunction or skin conditions.

b. contraindicate use of fluconazole: allergy to fluconazole; **pregnancy (Category C)**, lactation (safety not established).

Nursing Interventions

Medication Administration

Arrange for culture of area before initiation of therapy.

Infuse IV only; drug is not intended for IM or SC use.

Do not add any supplemental medication to the fluconazole.

Provide small, frequent meals if GI upset occurs.

Assure ready access to bathroom facilities if diarrhea occurs.

Surveillance During Therapy

Monitor injection sites and veins for signs of phlebitits.

Monitor renal function tests weekly; discontinue drug at any sign of renal toxicity.

Carefully monitor laboratory studies and patient for indications of adverse reactions.

Interpret results of diagnostic tests and contact practitioner as appropriate.

Monitor for possible drug–drug and drug–nutrient interactions: Refer to **Interactions**.

Patient Teaching

Teach patient that the following are a result of drug therapy: nausea, vomiting, diarrhea, headache.

Instruct the patient to report any of the following to the practitioner if they occur: rash; changes in stool or urine color; difficulty breathing; increased tears or salivation.

• Flucytosine

Ancobon

(CAN) Ancotil

A synthetic pyrimidine, structurally related to the antineoplastic drug fluorouracil, flucytosine is an orally effective systemic antifungal drug that is considered a secondary agent in treating deep-seated mycotic infections caused by *Candida* and *Cryptococcus* species. It is much less toxic than amphotericin B but is less effective as well, and resistance frequently develops rapidly. Thus it is used mainly in combination with amphotericin B for treating cryptococcal infections such as meningitis.

Mechanism

Probably converted to 5-fluorouracil in fungal cells (but not normal mammalian cells); acts as a competitive inhibitor of nucleic acid synthesis; host cells apparently lack the enzyme that converts drug to active metabolite and are thus unaffected

Uses

Treatment of serious systemic candidal infections (endocarditis, septicemia, urinary) or cryptococcal infections (meningitis, septicemia, pulmonary or urinary)—frequently given in combination with amphotericin B, with which it has a synergistic effect against *Candida* and *Cryptococcus*

Investigational use in the treatment of chromomycosis

Dosage

50 to 150 mg/kg/day orally in divided doses every 6 hours

Fate

Well absorbed orally; peak plasma concentrations occur within 1 to 2 hours; minimally bound to plasma proteins; widely distributed in the body; drug levels in CSF reach 50% to 80% of those in the serum; not significantly metabolized but excreted largely unchanged (70–90%) in the urine; serum half-life is 3 to 6 hours.

Common Side Effects

Nausea, diarrhea, skin rash, vomiting

Significant Adverse Reactions

Anemia, leukopenia, thrombocytopenia, pancytopenia, hepatomegaly, enterocolitis, elevation of ALT, AST, BUN, and serum creatinine; less frequently, headache, vertigo, drowsiness, confusion, and hallucinations

Contraindications

No absolute contraindications. *Cautious use* in patients with impaired renal function, bone marrow depression, hematologic disorders; during pregnancy or lactation; and in persons receiving radiation therapy or cancer chemotherapy.

Interactions

Flucytosine can potentiate the antifungal effects and toxicity of amphotericin B

Concurrent use with other bone marrow–depressing drugs (eg, antineoplastics, pyrazolones) may increase the toxic effects of both drugs

Concurrent use with cytosine may inactivate the antifungal activity of flucytosine

Nursing Management

Pretherapy Assessment

Assess and record baseline data necessary for detection of adverse effects of flucytosine: General: VS, body weight, skin color and temperature; CNS: orientation, reflexes, affect; GI: bowel sounds; liver evaluation; GU: renal function; Lab: renal and liver function tests, CBC.

Review medical history and documents for existing or previous conditions that:

a. require cautious use of flucytosine: impaired renal function; bone marrow depression; hematologic disorders; radiation therapy or cancer chemotherapy.
b. contraindicate use of flucytosine: allergy to flucytosine; **pregnancy (Category C)**, lactation (safety not established).

Nursing Interventions

Medication Administration

Provide small frequent meals if GI upset occurs.
Assure ready access to bathroom facilities if diarrhea occurs.
Administer capsules a few at a time over a 15-minute period to minimize the incidence of nausea and vomiting.

Surveillance During Therapy

Ensure that the renal, hepatic, and hematologic status of patient has been determined before therapy is initiated. These parameters should also be assessed at frequent intervals during therapy. Liver enzyme levels should be ascertained frequently during therapy.
Monitor intake–output. Serum drug levels should be assayed frequently to ensure normal excretion.
Monitor results of culture and sensitivity tests, which should be performed periodically during therapy, because drug resistance may develop during prolonged therapy.
Carefully monitor laboratory studies and patient for indications of adverse reactions.
Interpret results of diagnostic tests and contact practitioner as appropriate.
Monitor for possible drug–drug and drug–nutrient interactions: Refer to **Interactions**.
Provide for patient safety needs and protect from injury or infection if bone marrow suppression occurs.

Patient Teaching

Teach patient that the following are a result of drug therapy: nausea, vomiting, diarrhea, sedation, dizziness, confusion.
Instruct the patient to report any of the following to the practitioner if they occur: rash, severe nausea, vomiting, diarrhea, fever, sore throat, unusual bleeding or bruising.

• Griseofulvin

Microsize—Fulvicin U/F, Grifulvin V, Grisactin
Ultramicrosize—Fulvicin P/G, Grisactin Ultra, Gris-Peg

(CAN) Grisovin-FP

An orally administered fungistatic antibiotic that is effective only against dermatophyte infections of the skin, hair, and nails, griseofulvin is available as either a microsize or ultramicrosize particle formulation. Ultramicrosize griseofulvin exhibits approximately 1.5 times the biologic activity of microsize griseofulvin largely because of improved GI absorption; thus a 330-mg dose of ultramicrosize yields antifungal activity comparable to a 500-mg dose of the microsize formulation. However, there is no evidence that the ultramicrosize formulation is clinically superior with regard to efficacy or safety.

Mechanism

Localizes in keratin precursor cells in skin, nails, and hair and disrupts the mitotic spindle, thus arresting cell division; new keratin that is subsequently formed strongly binds griseofulvin and becomes resistant to fungal invasion; no effect on bacteria, yeasts, or fungi other than dermatophytal organisms

Uses

Treatment of fungal infections of the skin, hair, or nails caused by the following dermatophytes: *Epidermophyton, Microsporum*, or *Trichophyton*

CAUTION

Not effective in systemic mycotic infections, candidiasis, tinea versicolor, or bacterial infections—should not be used in trivial infections that respond to topical agents alone

Dosage

Adults: 500 mg to 1 g microsize *or* 330 to 750 mg ultramicrosize daily in a single dose or divided doses
Children: 11 mg/kg microsize daily *or* 7 mg/kg ultramicrosize daily in a single dose *or* divided doses

Fate

Oral absorption is somewhat variable, the ultramicrosize preparation being absorbed more efficiently than the microsize formulation. Peak plasma levels occur in approximately 4 hours, and drug is detectable in the skin within 4 to 8 hours. Griseofulvin exhibits a greater affinity for diseased skin than normal skin. Its plasma half-life is approximately 24 hours; it is metabolized in the liver and slowly excreted in the urine, mainly as metabolites.

Common Side Effects

Skin rash, urticaria

Significant Adverse Reactions

GI: nausea, vomiting, diarrhea, epigastric distress, flatulence, stomatitis
Neurologic: paresthesias, fatigue, headache, dizziness, insomnia, confusion, peripheral neuritis, blurred vision, impaired motor skills, syncope
Hematologic: leukopenia, neutropenia, granulocytopenia
Allergic: angioedema, serum sickness, photosensitivity, erythema multiforme, lupuslike syndrome
Other: proteinuria, estrogenlike effects in children

Contraindications

Porphyria, severe liver disease, systemic lupus erythematosus, prophylaxis of *non*established fungal infections. *Cautious use* in patients with renal dysfunction, penicillin allergy; in alcoholics (refer to **Interactions**); and in pregnant women.

Interactions

Griseofulvin can reduce the activity of oral anticoagulants and oral contraceptives.
Activity of griseofulvin may be diminished by barbiturates, glutethimide, diphenhydramine, orphenadrine, and phenylbutazone through enzyme induction.

The effects of alcohol may be potentiated by griseofulvin, producing tachycardia and flushing.

Nursing Management

Pretherapy Assessment

Assess and record baseline data necessary for detection of adverse effects of griseofulvin: General: VS, body weight, skin color and temperature; CNS: orientation, reflexes, affect; GI: bowel sounds; liver evaluation; Lab: renal and liver function tests, CBC.

Review medical history and documents for existing or previous conditions that:

a. require cautious use of griseofulvin: renal dysfunction; penicillin allergy; in alcoholics (refer to **Interactions**).

b. contraindicate use of griseofulvin: allergy to griseofulvin, penicillins; porphyria; severe liver disease; systemic lupus erythematosus; prophylaxis of *non*-established fungal infections; **pregnancy (Category C)**, lactation (safety not established).

Nursing Interventions

Medication Administration

Provide small frequent meals if GI upset occurs.

Assure ready access to bathroom facilities if diarrhea occurs.

Protect patient from exposure to ultraviolet light.

Continue administration until infection is irradicated: tinea capitis (4–6 weeks), tinea corporis (2–4 weeks), tinea pedis (4–8 weeks), tinea unguium–fingernails (4 months), toenails (6 months).

Surveillance During Therapy

Monitor results of hematologic studies, which should be performed at least weekly during therapy. Renal and hepatic function should be monitored periodically during prolonged treatment. Griseofulvin has produced hepatocellular necrosis and liver tumors in mice, impaired spermatogenesis in rats, and embryotoxic and teratogenic effects in rats and dogs. Although these effects have not been demonstrated in humans, caution is required when using drug for extended periods, and it should not be used for minor or trivial fungal infections, nor for infections due to organisms other than susceptible dermatophytes.

Carefully monitor laboratory studies and patient for indications of adverse reactions.

Interpret results of diagnostic tests and contact practitioner as appropriate.

Monitor for possible drug–drug and drug–nutrient interactions: Refer to **Interactions**.

Provide for patient safety needs if CNS effects occur.

Patient Teaching

Suggest taking drug with meals to reduce GI irritation and to improve absorption (a high-fat diet increases absorption).

Stress the necessity of continuing treatment until infecting organism is completely eradicated, as indicated by clinical and laboratory examinations. Beneficial effects may not be noticeable for several weeks to months. Average duration of treatment is 4 to 6 weeks for scalp ringworm and at least 4 to 6 months for fingernail and toenail fungal infections.

Instruct patient to report the development of fever, sore throat, mucosal irritation, or extreme malaise because these might indicate a developing blood dyscrasia.

Warn patient that flushing and tachycardia can occur with ingestion of alcohol.

Advise patient to avoid exposure to intense sunlight because photosensitivity can occur.

Teach patient interventions that minimize incidence of reinfection, and instruct patient to keep infected areas dry because moisture enhances fungal growth.

Teach patient how to recognize and report overgrowth of nonsusceptible fungi (diarrhea, perianal itching, stomatitis, "black tongue").

If patient is allergic to penicillin, warn him or her to watch for early signs of a hypersensitivity reaction because cross-sensitivity to penicillins can occur.

Teach patient that the following are a result of drug therapy: nausea, vomiting, diarrhea, sedation, dizziness, confusion, sensitivity to light.

Instruct the patient to report any of the following to the practitioner if they occur: rash, severe nausea, vomiting, diarrhea, fever, sore throat, unusual bleeding or bruising.

• Itraconazole

Sporanox

Itraconazole is a triazole derivative structurally related to fluconazole that has a broad spectrum of antifungal activity. The drug is well tolerated and appears to be safer than either amphotericin B or ketoconazole; it should prove to be a useful replacement for ketoconazole in certain infections. Itraconazole appears promising for the treatment of aspergillosis, blastomycosis, histoplasmosis, sporotrichosis, and coccidioidomycosis; the role of itraconazole in therapy is still being evaluated.

Mechanism

Similar to fluconazole, inhibition of fungal cytochrome P-450 enzymes necessary for ergosterol synthesis and cell membrane integrity; triazoles bind more selectively to fungal P-450 than to the corresponding mammalian enzymes, and this may account for the reduced toxicity of these drugs

Uses

Treatment of blastomycosis and histoplasmosis in both immunocompromised and nonimmunocompromised patients

Investigational uses include treatment of superficial dermatophytoses and candidiasis; systemic mycoses involving candidiasis, cryptococcal infections, aspergillus, coccidioidomycosis, and paracoccidioidomycosis

Dosage

Adults: 200 to 400 mg orally, once daily taken with food; doses greater than 200 mg given in two divided doses; in severe infections loading doses of 200 mg 3 times a day for the first 3 days can be given.

Fate

Absorption is increased by food and administration with meals is recommended; drug is widely distributed, with many tissue levels higher than plasma levels; CSF levels, however, are negligible; plasma protein binding is approximately 95%; itraconazole is eliminated in both the urine and the bile after extensive metabolism, drug metabolism appears to be a saturable process with half-life increasing from approximately 20 hours to 30 hours after several weeks of treatment.

Common Side Effects

Nausea, headache, rash

Significant Adverse Reactions

Diarrhea, abdominal pain, edema, fever, pruritus, dizziness, psychiatric disturbances, hypertension, hepatic dysfunction, hypokalemia

Contraindications

Concurrent use with terfenadine; itraconazole may increase terfenadine plasma levels that potentially can cause life-threatening cardiac dysrhythmias. *Cautious use* in patients with hepatic disease.

Interactions

Plasma concentrations of cyclosporine, digoxin, sulfonylureas, terfenadine, astemizole, or warfarin may be increased by concurrent therapy with itraconazole.

Isoniazid, phenytoin, rifampin and H-2 antagonist drugs (eg, cimetidine, ranitidine; see Chapter 16) can reduce itraconazole plasma concentrations.

Nursing Management

Refer to **Fluconazole** and **Ketoconazole**. In addition:

Pretherapy Assessment

Pregnancy (Category C), lactation (excreted in breast milk; should not be used in nursing mothers).

Nursing Interventions

Medication Administration

Coadmininstration with terfenadine or astemizole in contraindicated.

Drug should be administered with meals.

Patient Teaching

Patient should be instructed to report any signs and symptoms of liver dysfunction (unusual fatigue, anorexia, nausea, jaundice, dark urine, pale stool)

Instruct patient to take this drug with food.

• Ketoconazole

Nizoral

Ketoconazole is structurally an imidazole that is used orally for treating a variety of oral and systemic fungal infections. It is less toxic than amphotericin B but somewhat less effective as well. Gastrointestinal complaints are common, and serious hepatotoxicity has been reported. A topical cream is also available (Table 72-1).

Mechanism

The action of the imidazoles is similar to that of the triazoles, inhibition of cytochrome P-450 enzymes that are necessary for the synthesis of ergosterol and cell membrane integrity; ketoconazole can also inhibit mammalian P-450 enzymes that are involved in the synthesis of male sex hormones and to a lesser extent adrenal steroidogenesis, which contributes to the increased toxicity of the imidazoles compared with the triazoles

Uses

Oral

Treatment of the following fungal infections: candidiasis, oral thrush, chronic mucocutaneous candidiasis, candiduria, histoplasmosis, blastomycosis, coccidioidomycosis, paracoccidioidomycosis, and chromomycosis

Treatment of severe, resistant, cutaneous dermatophytal infections not responding to topical therapy or oral griseofulvin

Investigational uses include treatment of onychomycosis (caused by *Trichophyton* or *Candida* species), pityriasis versicolor (tinea versicolor), recurrent vaginal candidiasis, and in advanced prostatic carcinoma and Cushing's syndrome to reduce androgen or adrenal steroidogenesis

Topical

Refer to **Table 72-1**. In addition:

Treatment of tinea corporis, tinea cruris, and tinea versicolor

Dosage

Oral

Adults: 200 mg once daily (400 mg once daily in very serious infections)

Children (older than 2 years): 3.3 to 6.6 mg/kg/day as a single daily dose

Minimum treatment is 1 to 2 weeks for candidiasis, 4 weeks for recalcitrant dermatophytal infections, and 6 months for other systemic mycotic infections.

Topical

Refer to **Table 72-1**.

Fate

Well absorbed orally; peak serum levels occur in 1 to 2 hours; tablet dissolution requires an acidic environment; highly (95%–99%) protein-bound; cerebrospinal fluid penetration is negligible; undergoes extensive hepatic metabolism; excreted largely (80%–90%) in the bile and feces (through enterohepatic circulation) with approximately 10% to 15% of drug excreted in the urine

Common Side Effects

Nausea, vomiting, GI upset, pruritus; in addition, elevated serum transaminase occurs in 5% to 10% of patients.

Significant Adverse Reactions

Abdominal pain, diarrhea, dizziness, lethargy, headache, fever, chills, photophobia, impotence, gynecomastia, thrombocytopenia, hepatic dysfunction, and oligospermia

Contraindications

Treatment of fungal meningitis. *Cautious use* in persons with liver dysfunction and in pregnant or nursing women.

Interactions

GI absorption of ketoconazole may be impaired by antacids, histamine-2 antagonists, anticholinergics, and other drugs that reduce stomach acidity.
Ketoconazole can enhance the anticoagulant effect of coumarins, elevate the plasma level of cyclosporine, and increase the bioavailability of corticosteroids while also reducing corticosteroid clearance.
Rifampin and isoniazid can reduce blood levels of ketoconazole if given concurrently.
Use of ketoconazole and phenytoin may alter the metabolism of one or both drugs.
Theophylline blood levels may be decreased by ketoconazole.

Nursing Management

Pretherapy Assessment

Assess and record baseline data necessary for detection of adverse effects of ketoconazole: General: VS, body weight, skin color and temperature; CNS: orientation, reflexes, affect; GI: bowel sounds; liver evaluation; genitourinary (GU): renal function; Lab: liver function tests, CBC.
Review medical history and documents for existing or previous conditions that:
a. require cautious use of ketoconazole: liver dysfunction.
b. contraindicate use of ketoconazole: allergy to ketoconazole; fungal meningitis; **pregnancy (Category C)**, lactation (safety not established).

Nursing Interventions

Medication Administration

Administer with food to decrease GI upset.
Provide small frequent meals if GI upset occurs.
Do not administer with antacids.
Assure ready access to bathroom facilities if diarrhea occurs.
Protect patient from exposure to ultraviolet light.
Continue administration until infection is irradicated: candidiasis (1–2 weeks), other systemic mycoses (6 months), tinea versicolor (2 weeks).
Discontinue topical application if sensitivity or chemical reaction occurs.

Surveillance During Therapy

Monitor results of liver function tests, which should be performed before therapy is initiated and at intervals of several weeks during treatment. *Transient* elevations in liver enzymes occur frequently and do not require discontinuation of therapy. Persistent elevations or presence of clinical signs of hepatic injury, however, require immediate termination of treatment because liver disorders, although rare, are potentially fatal.
Note that ketoconazole can decrease synthesis of cortisol and testosterone, especially with higher doses. The clinical significance of these effects remains to be determined.
Carefully monitor laboratory studies and patient for indications of adverse reactions.
Interpret results of diagnostic tests and contact practitioner as appropriate.
Monitor for possible drug–drug and drug–nutrient interactions: Refer to **Interactions**.
Provide for patient safety needs if CNS effects occur.

Patient Teaching

Instruct patient not to take any other drugs, including over-the-counter (OTC) preparations, unless prescribed. If drugs or substances that reduce gastric acidity are taken within 2 hours of ketoconazole, GI absorption may be impaired (refer to **Interactions**).
Emphasize the importance of continuing treatment until *all* clinical and laboratory tests indicate that the active fungal infection has abated. In general, candidiasis requires a minimum of 2 weeks of therapy, whereas systemic mycotic infections may require 6 months or more of therapy.
Teach patient that the following are a result of drug therapy: nausea, vomiting, diarrhea, sedation, dizziness, confusion, stinging, irritation (topical).
Instruct the patient to report any of the following to the practitioner if they occur: rash, severe nausea, vomiting, diarrhea, fever, sore throat, unusual bleeding or bruising.

• Miconazole

Monistat I.V.

A broad-spectrum antifungal agent, miconazole is used intravenously for treatment of severe systemic fungal infections as well as topically and vaginally for control of cutaneous and mucocutaneous candidal and dermatophytal infections. The discussion that follows focuses on the systemic use of miconazole; its topical application is considered in Table 72-1.

Mechanism

Similar to ketoconazole; alters the permeability of the fungal cell membrane by interfering with ergosterol synthesis resulting in loss of cell constituents and ultimately cellular death

Uses

Alternative treatment of coccidioidomycosis, paracoccidioidomycosis, cryptococcosis, petriellidiosis, and chronic mucocutaneous candidiasis
Topical treatment of cutaneous and mucocutaneous candidal and dermatophytal infections (see Table 72-1)

Dosage

Intravenous

Adults: 200 to 3,600 mg/day depending on disease and severity, divided over three infusions of 30 to 60 minutes each; dilute standard injection (10 mg/mL) in 200 mL fluid before infusing
Coccidioidomycosis: 1,800 to 3,600 mg/day
Cryptococcosis: 1,200 to 2,400 mg/day
Petriellidiosis: 600 to 3,000 mg/day

Candidiasis: 600 to 1,800 mg/day
Paracoccidioidomycosis: 200 to 1,200 mg/day
Children: 20 to 40 mg/kg/day in divided infusions; maximum is 15 mg/kg/infusion

CAUTION

Treatment is continued until clinical and laboratory tests no longer indicate the presence of an active fungal infection (usually a minimum of 3–4 weeks), because inadequate treatment can result in recurrence of the infection.

Intrathecal

20 mg undiluted solution every 3 days to 7 days as adjunct to IV infusion in fungal meningitis

Bladder instillation

200 mg diluted solution (10 mg/200 mL)

Fate

Highly bound to plasma protein; penetration into CSF is poor; rapidly metabolized in the liver and excreted both in the urine and feces, mainly as inactive metabolites; elimination half-life is 20 to 25 hours.

Common Side Effects

(IV use only) Phlebitis, pruritus, nausea, febrile reactions, rash, vomiting

Significant Adverse Reactions

(IV use only) Diarrhea, drowsiness, flushing, anorexia, hyponatremia, decreased hematocrit, thrombocytopenia, hyperlipemia (due to the castor oil vehicle), and arrhythmias (with too-rapid IV administration)

Contraindications

No absolute contraindications. *Cautious use* in persons with anemia, hyperlipemia; in pregnant women or nursing mothers; and in young children.

Interactions

The effects of oral anticoagulants may be enhanced by IV miconazole.
Miconazole and amphotericin B are mutually antagonistic and the antifungal activity of the combination is less than that of either drug used alone.
Miconazole may potentiate the action of the oral hypoglycemic drugs.
The metabolism of phenytoin may be reduced by concurrent use of miconazole.

Nursing Management

Refer to **Ketoconazole**. In addition:

Nursing Interventions

Medication Administration

Initiate administration only in hospitalized patients, and monitor patient closely during therapy. An initial dose of 200 mg should be given to assess patient's reaction.
Administer IV infusion slowly (over a 30–60-minute period) to minimize the danger of tachycardia and arrhythmias.
Dilute injection in 200 mL sodium chloride or 5% dextrose solution.
Observe infusion site for signs of phlebitis.
If nausea and vomiting become problematic, collaborate with drug prescriber to implement effective interventions (eg, slowing infusion rate, reducing dose, avoiding mealtime drug administration, administering prophylactic antiemetic medication).

Surveillance During Therapy

Monitor results of hemoglobin, hematocrit, electrolyte, and lipid determinations, which should be performed at the beginning of therapy and regularly thereafter.

• Nystatin, Oral

Mycostatin, Nilstat

(CAN) Nadostine

Nystatin is a fungicidal antibiotic obtained from a species of *Streptomyces*. It is used principally in the treatment of candidal infections of the skin, mucous membranes, and intestinal tract. After oral administration, it is poorly absorbed and thus is effective only against candidal infections of the oral cavity and intestinal tract. The drug is available as an oral tablet (which is swallowed whole) for the treatment of intestinal candidiasis and also as an oral suspension (which is retained in the mouth as long as possible before swallowing) for the treatment of candidiasis of the oral cavity. Those indications are discussed here, whereas the topical use of nystatin is considered in Table 72-1.

Mechanism

Binds to sterols in the membrane of fungal cells, altering its permeability; the resultant leakage of intracellular components leads to cellular death

Uses

Treatment of intestinal candidiasis (oral tablet)
Treatment of candidiasis of the oral cavity (oral suspension)
Treatment of cutaneous and mucocutaneous candidal infections (for topical and vaginal application, see Table 72-1)

Dosage

Intestinal Candidiasis

500,000 to 1 million U (1 or 2 tablets) three times a day; continue for at least 48 hours after clinical cure

Oral Candidiasis

Adults and children: 400,000 to 600,000 U (4–6 mL oral suspension) four times a day (one-half dose in each side of mouth—retain for as long as possible before swallowing); continue for at least 48 hours after symptoms have disappeared
NOTE: The oral retention of the drug may be improved by the use of nystatin "popsicles," which are formulated to contain 250,000 U. Alternatively, nystatin vaginal tablets may be given orally and dissolved in the mouth.
Infants: 200,000 U four times a day, as above

(*text continues on page 736*)

Table 72-1. **Topical/Vaginal Antifungal Agents**

Drug	Preparations	Usual Dosage Range	Nursing Considerations
Amphotericin B, topical *Fungizone*	Cream: 3% Ointment: 3% Lotion: 3%	Apply liberally 2–4 times a day; duration of therapy ranges from 1–2 wk for simple infections (eg, candidiasis) to several months for onychomycoses	Used for treating cutaneous and mucocutaneous candidal infections; similar to nystatin in activity; cream may have a drying effect and discolor the skin; lotion and ointment may stain nail lesions; redness, itching, and burning have occurred with all preparations; discoloration of clothing or fabrics is removable by washing in soap and water or cleaning fluid; also used parenterally; see separate discussion
Butoconazole *Femstat*	Vaginal cream: 2%	1 applicator full into vagina at bedtime for 3 days; may give for 6 days if necessary	Used for vulvovaginal candidiasis; a 3-day course of therapy is usually sufficient except in pregnant women, who should receive the drug for 6 days; avoid during the first trimester of pregnancy; vulvar and vaginal itching and burning can occur
Ciclopirox *Loprox*	Cream: 1% Lotion: 1%	Apply twice a day	Broad-spectrum antifungal used for tinea pedis, tinea cruris, tinea corporis, candidiasis, and tinea versicolor due to *Malassezia furfur*; penetrates hair, hair follicles, sebaceous glands, and dermis; do *not* use occlusive dressings; if no clinical improvement occurs within 4 wk, reevaluate therapy; very low incidence of irritation, sensitization, or phototoxicity; safety and efficacy in children younger than 10 yr of age have not been established
Clotrimazole *Femcare, Gyne-Lotrimin, Lotrimin, Mycelex* *(CAN) Canestan, Myclo*	Cream: 1% Solution: 1% Lotion: 1% Troches: 10 mg Vaginal tablets: 100 mg, 500 mg Vaginal cream: 1%	*Topical*: massage into infected area twice a day *Vaginal*: 1 100-mg tablet inserted at bedtime for 7 days *or* 1 applicator full of vaginal cream inserted at bedtime for 7–14 days; *alternatively*, 1 500-mg tablet used *once only* *Oral*: 1 troche dissolved in mouth 5 times a day for 14 days	Broad-spectrum antifungal used topically for dermatophytal infections, candidiasis, and tinea versicolor and vaginally for vulvovaginal candidiasis; vaginal tablet and cream are available over-the-counter; topical application may cause burning, stinging, peeling, itching, urticaria, and edema; clinical improvement usually occurs within 7 days; discontinue if severe irritation or hypersensitivity reactions occur; vaginal application has resulted in mild burning, rash, urinary frequency, and lower abdominal cramping; use of a sanitary pad will prevent staining of clothing; in case of treatment failure, presence of other pathogens (eg, *Trichomonas, Haemophilus vaginalis*) should be suspected; stress importance of taking full course of therapy; oral use results in prolonged salivary levels of drug; nausea, vomiting, and abnormal liver function test (eg, elevated AST) occur in approximately 15% of patients using troches
Econazole *Spectazole* *(CAN) Ecostatin*	Cream: 1%	Apply once or twice a day	Broad-spectrum antifungal with good activity against dermatophytes, yeasts, and some gram-positive bacteria; after topical application, inhibitory concentrations of drug have been found as deep as the middle region of the dermis; low incidence of burning, itching, and erythema; apply after cleansing affected area; treat candidal infections, tinea cruris, and tinea corporis for 2 wk and tinea pedis for 4 wk

(*continued*)

Table 72-1. **Topical/Vaginal Antifungal Agents (Continued)**

Drug	*Preparations*	*Usual Dosage Range*	*Nursing Considerations*
Haloprogin *Halotex*	Cream: 1% Solution: 1%	Apply liberally 2 times a day for 2–4 wk	Indicated for superficial fungal infections of the skin and for tinea versicolor; side effects include irritation, burning, vesicle formation, and pruritis—may worsen pre-existing lesions; avoid contact with eyes; if no improvement is noted within 4 wk, patient's condition should be reevaluated
Iodochlorhydroxyquin (Clioquinol) *Vioform*	Cream: 3% Ointment: 3%	Apply 2–3 times a day for a maximum of 1 wk	Antibacterial and antifungal agent used in treatment of cutaneous fungal infections and inflammatory skin conditions (eg, eczema); do *not* use in the presence of superficial viral conditions, tuberculosis, vaccinia, or varicella; infrequently elicits skin irritation but can stain skin, hair, or fabrics; may be absorbed systemically if used on widespread areas, and can interfere with thyroid function tests because drug contains iodine; available in combination with hydrocortisone (Vioform-HC) as prescription only, but can be sold over-the-counter when used alone
Ketoconazole *Nizoral*	Cream: 2%	Apply once or twice daily for at least 2 wk	Broad-spectrum antifungal used topically for treatment of tinea corporis and tinea cruris as well as tinea versicolor caused by *Malassezia furfur*; resistance has not been reported; pruritis, stinging, and dermal irritation have occurred; *cautious use* in pregnant women; also used orally—see separate discussion
Miconazole *Micatin, Monistat-Derm, Monistat-3, Monistat 7, Zeasorb-AF*	Cream: 2% Lotion: 2% Powder: 2% Spray: 2% Vaginal cream: 2% Vaginal suppositories: 100 mg, 200 mg	*Topical*: apply twice a day for 2–4 wk *Vaginal*: 1 applicator full or 1 suppository (100 mg) vaginally at bedtime for 7 days *or* 1 suppository (200 mg) once daily for 3 days	Indicated for cutaneous dermatophytal and candidal infections, tinea versicolor, and vulvovaginal candidiasis; vaginal cream and suppositories are available over-the-counter; rarely causes burning or irritation topically; avoid eyes; use lotion rather than cream between the toes or fingers to avoid maceration effects; clinical improvement should occur in 1–2 wk; diagnosis should be reevaluated after 4 wk if good response is not evident; pathogens other than *Candida* should be ruled out before using drug for vaginitis, because it is effective only against candidal vulvovaginitis; 100-mg suppository (Monistat 7) is given for 7 days and 200-mg suppository (Monistat-3) is used only for 3 days; advise patient to insert high into vagina, to use sanitary napkin to prevent staining, to complete full course of therapy, and to avoid sexual intercourse during treatment to prevent reinfection; burning, itching, and irritation can occur—notify physician; use *cautiously* during pregnancy, especially the first trimester; perform urine and blood glucose studies in patients who do not respond to treatment, because persistent candidal vulvovaginitis may be related to unrecognized diabetes mellitus; also used IV for severe systemic fungal infections; see separate discussion

(*continued*)

Table 72-1. **Topical/Vaginal Antifungal Agents (Continued)**

Drug	Preparations	Usual Dosage Range	Nursing Considerations
Naftifine *Naftin*	Cream: 1%	Apply twice a day for at least 2 wk	Broad-spectrum agent used for treating tinea corporis and tinea cruris; some systemic absorption occurs, and drug and metabolites can appear in the urine and feces; burning, stinging, erythema, itching, dryness of skin are noted with topical use; avoid contact with eyes, nose or mouth; do *not* use occlusive dressings
Nystatin *Mycostatin, Nilstat, Nystex, O-V Statin* *(CAN) Nyaderm*	Cream: 100,000 U/g Ointment: 100,000 U/g Powder: 100,000 U/g Vaginal tablets: 100,000 U Troches: 200,000 U	*Topical*: apply 2–3 times a day for at least 1 wk after clinical cure *Vaginal*: 1 tablet inserted vaginally daily for 14 days *Oral*: 1–2 troches dissolved in mouth 4–5 times a day for up to 14 days	Used in treating cutaneous and vaginal infections caused by *Candida* species; troches and oral suspension (see nystatin, oral) are used to treat oral candidiasis; no detectable blood levels are noted after topical application; irritation is rare, and drug does not stain skin or mucous membranes; avoid contact with eyes; powder may be dusted into shoes and socks as well as onto feet; symptomatic relief of cutaneous infections usually occurs within 72 h; vaginal application should be continued for entire 14 days, even though clinical symptoms disappear within a few days; lack of response suggests presence of other pathogens besides *Candida*; no adverse effects or complications have been reported when drug is used during pregnancy; also available in oral tablets for treatment of intestinal candidiasis—see separate discussion
Oxiconazole *Oxistat*	Cream: 1%	Apply once daily for 2–4 wk	Broad-spectrum topical antifungal used to treat tinea pedis, tinea cruris, and tinea corporis; low incidence of itching, burning, and erythema with topical use; avoid eyes; systemic absorption is low
Sulconazole *Exelderm*	Topical solution: 1%	Massage small amount of solution into affected area once or twice daily	Broad-spectrum antifungal used for treating tinea cruris, tinea corporis, and tinea versicolor; efficacy in tinea pedis (athlete's foot) has *not* been demonstrated; itching, burning, or stinging on application is rare; avoid contact with eyes; improvement usually occurs within 1 week; continue treatment for 3–4 wk
Terbinafine *Lamisil*	Cream: 1%	Apply twice daily to affected area for 1–4 wk	Used for tinea pedis, tinea cruris or tinea corporis due to *Epidermophyton floccosum, Trichophyton mentagrophytes*, or *T. rubrum*; also effective in treating cutaneous candidiasis and tinea versicolor; do not use longer than 4 wk; avoid occlusive dressings
Terconazole *Terazol 3, Terazol 7*	Vaginal cream: 0.4% Vaginal suppositories: 80 mg	1 applicatorful at bedtime daily for 7 days (Terazol 7) or 3 consecutive days (Terazol 3) 1 suppository once daily for 3 days	Effective in treating vulvovaginitis caused by *Candida* only; systemic absorption can be as high as 15%; *cautious use* in pregnant and nursing women; headache is very common (25%); therapeutic effect is not altered by menstruation
Tioconazole *Vagistat*	Vaginal ointment: 6.5%	1 applicatorful once only, prior to bedtime	Single-dose antifungal for vaginal candidiasis; burning and itching are most common side effects

(*continued*)

Table 72-1. **Topical/Vaginal Antifungal Agents (Continued)**

Drug	Preparations	Usual Dosage Range	Nursing Considerations
Tolnaftate *Aftate, Tinactin, and other manufacturers* *(CAN) Pitrex*	Cream: 1% Gel: 1% Solution: 1% Liquid aerosol: 1% Powder: 1% Powder aerosol: 1%	Apply small amount 2–3 times a day for 2–6 wk as necessary	Effective in treating cutaneous dermatophytal infections, eg, athlete's foot, jock itch, or ringworm; inactive systemically, virtually nontoxic, nonirritating, and nonsensitizing; serious or chronic fungal infections may require concomitant use of griseofulvin; powder is used only as adjunctive therapy; liquids or solutions are preferred in hairy areas; not effective against *Candida* therefore, if patient does not improve within several weeks, additional antifungal therapy is indicated; discontinue treatment if irritation occurs or condition worsens; available without prescription
Triacetin *Fungoid, Ony-Clear Nail*	Cream: 25% Ointment: 25% Tincture (Fungoid): with cetylpyridinium and chloroxylenol Aerosol spray (Ony-Clear)	Apply 2 to 3 times a day; continue for at least 1 wk after symptoms have subsided	Indicated for milder superficial fungal infections (eg, nail fungus, athlete's foot, ringworm, monilial impetigo); cleanse affected area with alcohol or soap and water before application; cover treated areas; avoid eyes; use *cautiously* in patients with impaired circulation; may stain certain fabrics; treatment of nail fungus may require several months
Undecylenic acid and salts *Caldesene, Cruex, Desenex, and other manufacturers*	Cream: 8%, 20% Ointment: 22% Powder: 10%, 15%, 19% Foam: 10% Soap	Apply as needed several times a day	Fungistatic and weak antibacterial activity; mainly used for athlete's foot, jock itch, or ringworm *exclusive* of nails and hairy areas; also employed for relief or prevention of diaper rash, prickly heat, groin irritation, and other minor skin irritations; do *not* use if skin is broken or severely abraded; area should be cleansed well before application; use with *caution* in patients with impaired circulation; powder is recommended only as adjunctive therapy—ointments, creams, and liquids are used as primary therapy in most body areas

Fate

No detectable systemic blood levels after oral administration; excreted largely unchanged in the stool

Significant Adverse Reactions

Nausea, vomiting, GI distress, and diarrhea with large oral doses

Nursing Management

Nursing Interventions

Patient Teaching

Urge patient to complete the entire prescribed course of therapy to minimize the danger of reinfection or relapse.

Instruct patient using the oral suspension to place one-half of the dose in each side of the mouth, retain there as long as possible (at least several minutes), then swallow.

Ophthalmic Antifungal Agent

• *Natamycin*

Natacyn

An antibiotic obtained from a species of *Streptomyces*, natamycin is fungicidal against a variety of organisms. It is not absorbed orally and is used only in the eye for treatment of localized fungal infections.

Mechanism

Binds to sterols in fungal cell membrane, altering the cell permeability, thus allowing escape of essential cell constituents; not effective against bacteria.

Uses

Treatment of fungal blepharitis, conjunctivitis, and keratitis caused by susceptible organisms (drug of choice for *Fusarium solani* keratitis).

Dosage

One drop in affected eye every 1 to 2 hours for 3 to 4 days, then reduce to one drop six to eight times a day for 14 to 21 days, depending on the severity of the infection

Fate

No appreciable systemic absorption after topical administration

Significant Adverse Reactions

Conjunctival hyperemia or chemosis, blurred vision, and photosensitivity

Nursing Management

Nursing Interventions

Patient Teaching

Explain proper dosing procedure and importance of completing entire course of therapy to prevent recurrence.
Inform patient that bottle must be shaken well before use and dropper should not be contaminated by touching eyes, fingers, or other surfaces.
Instruct patient to wait at least 5 minutes before using any other drops in eyes.
Instruct patient to notify drug prescriber if irritation occurs or condition appears to deteriorate.
Inform patient that condition should be reevaluated if clinical improvement is not evident within 7 to 10 days. Additional laboratory tests are usually required to determine if other organisms are present.

Topical/Vaginal Antifungal Agents

A number of drugs possessing antifungal activity are employed topically or intravaginally for the treatment of cutaneous infections, for example, ringworm, athlete's foot, "jock itch," or mucocutaneous infections, such as vulvovaginal moniliasis. They are listed alphabetically in Table 72-1 along with dosage and other relevant information. Griseofulvin, an orally administered drug discussed earlier in the chapter, is also employed for treating ringworm (*Tinea*) infections of the skin, hair, or nails. Ketoconazole may also be administered orally for treating recurrent, resistant vaginal candidal infections.

Selected Bibliography

Bodey GP: Topical and systemic antifungal agents. Med Clin North Am 72:637, 1988

Cleary JD, Taylor JW, Chapman SW: Itraconazole in antifungal therapy. Ann Pharmacother 26:502, 1992

Gallis HA, Drew RH, Pickard WW: Amphotericin B: Thirty years of clinical experience. Rev Infect Dis 12:308, 1990

Grant SM, Clisssold SP: Fluconazole: A review of its pharmacodynamic and pharmacokinetic properties, and therapeutic potential in superficial and systemic mycoses. Drugs 39:877, 1990

Itraconazole. Med Lett Drugs Ther 35:7, 1993

Lyman CA, Walsh TJ: Systemically administered antifungal agents. A review of their clinical pharmacology and therapeutic applications. Drugs 44:9, 1992

Martin E et al: Novel aspect of amphotericin B action: Accumulation in human monocytes potentiates killing of phagocytosed *Candida albicans*. Antimicrob Agents Chemother 38(1):13, 1994

Stratton CW: Antifungal agents: The old and the new. Infect Dis Newslett 9:41, 1990

Nursing Bibliography

Karp R, Meldahl R, McCabe R: Candida albicans: Purulent pericarditis treated successfully without surgical drainage. Chest 102(3):953, 1992

Lesher J, Levine N, Treadwell P: Antifungals in office dermatology. Patient Care March 15:59, 1994

White G: Management of fungal infections. Nursing Standards 6(9):38, 1991

73
Antiviral Agents

Acyclovir
Amantadine
Didanosine
Famciclovir
Foscarnet
Ganciclovir
Idoxuridine
Ribavirin
Rimantadine
Stavudine
Trifluridine
Vidarabine
Zalcitabine
Zidovudine

Viruses are responsible for a large number of diseases, and the number of available antiviral drugs continues to increase. However, one obstacle to effective antiviral treatment in many instances is the fact that virus particles replicate within host (ie, human) cells by means of the enzyme systems of the invaded cell. Thus, drugs interfering with intracellular viral replication frequently damage the host cell as well and are often quite toxic if given systemically. However, increased knowledge of viral function has suggested that certain processes are unique to the virus particle and thus may be amenable to selective modification without damage to the host cell. Further, host cells often display surface receptors for viral particles, providing another site for antiviral drug action.

Many viral diseases are of short duration and are often clinically asymptomatic until the infectious process within the host cells is well advanced, by which time the body's own defense mechanisms have already come into play. Thus, to be maximally effective, drugs that block viral replication should be administered *before* the onset of the disease. Such is the case with use of amantadine or rimantadine as prophylactic agents against influenza A virus. Conversely, some viral infections, such as herpesvirus, continue to manifest viral replication even after symptoms have appeared. In these diseases, inhibition of *further* viral replication may speed healing and thus serves as the basis for use of drugs such as acyclovir, famciclovir, idoxuridine, and vidarabine in herpetic infections.

Most viral diseases are best managed prophylactically, either by active (attenuated or killed virus vaccines) or in some cases passive (viral antibodies) immunization. Once the disease has appeared, however, immunization is of little value, and most common viral infections (such as colds or "flu") are usually best treated symptomatically. Specific antiviral drugs have a limited therapeutic application in these instances, largely for the reasons already outlined.

The most serious viral disease today is AIDS, the acquired immunodeficiency syndrome caused by the HIV (human immunodeficiency) virus. Although no cure for this dread disease has been attained, several anti-AIDS drugs have become available. Although far from ideal drugs in terms of side effects and cost, zidovudine, didanosine, stavudine, and zalcitabine have at least afforded a degree of palliation and appear to slow the progression of the disease.

• Acyclovir

Zovirax

Acyclovir is a nucleoside of guanine with in vitro antiviral activity against herpes simplex types 1 and 2, varicella-zoster, Epstein–Barr, and cytomegalovirus. Normal cellular thymidine kinase enzyme does not use acyclovir; hence, the drug *selectively* inhibits viral cell replication with minimal toxicity for normal uninfected cells and is thus well tolerated by most patients. Acyclovir is available for oral, topical, or intravenous (IV) administration. Oral acyclovir can reduce the frequency and severity of recurrences in up to 95% of patients. Topical application of the drug also can shorten healing time and reduce pain when applied to primary lesions but generally has no significant beneficial effect on *recurrent* genital lesions. Intravenous infusion is used in severe infections or in immunocompromised patients.

Mechanism

Converted by herpes simplex virus–coded thymidine kinase into acyclovir monophosphate, which is further transformed into the diphosphate and triphosphate, the latter representing the active form of the drug; acyclovir triphosphate interferes with herpes simplex virus DNA polymerase, thus blocking viral replication, and can also be incorporated into growing chains of DNA by viral DNA polymerase, thereby terminating further growth of the DNA chain.

Uses

Topical

Management of initial episodes of herpes genitalis and limited, non–life-threatening mucocutaneous herpes simplex infections in immunocompromised patients

Intravenous infusion

Treatment of initial and recurrent mucosal and cutaneous herpes simplex (HSV-1 and HSV-2) infections in immunocompromised patients

Treatment of *severe* initial episodes of herpes genitalis in patients who are *not* immunocompromised

Oral

Treatment of initial episodes of genital herpes (HSV-2)

Management of recurrent episodes of genital herpes

Treatment of acute herpes zoster (shingles) and chickenpox (varicella) infections (see also famciclovir)

Dosage

IV infusion:

Adults: 5 to 10 mg/kg over 1 hour, every 8 hours for 7 to 10 days

Malseed, RT; Goldstein, FJ; and Balkon, N: PHARMACOLOGY: DRUG THERAPY AND NURSING CONSIDERATIONS, Fourth Edition.

Children (younger than 12): 250 to 500 mg/m^2 over 1 hour every 8 hours for 7 to 10 days

Oral:

Genital herpes: Initially, 200 mg every 4 hours 5 times a day for 10 days, then 400 mg twice a day for up to 12 months

Shingles: 800 mg every 4 hours 5 times a day for 7 to 10 days

Chickenpox: 20 mg/kg 4 times a day for 5 days

Topical: Apply to lesions every 3 hours 6 times a day for 7 days

Fate

Oral acyclovir is slowly and incompletely absorbed, and absorption is unaffected by food; peak plasma levels occur in 1.5 to 2 hours; widely distributed into most body tissues; concentrations in cerebrospinal fluid are approximately one-half those in plasma; protein binding is low (10%–30%); plasma half-life is 2 to 3 hours in patients with normal kidney function; excreted primarily unchanged by the kidneys (60%–90%), with approximately 15% of dose excreted as a metabolite

Systemic absorption after topical application is minimal.

Common Side Effects

IV: inflammation at injection site after extravasation, elevated serum creatinine, rash, urticaria

Topical: burning or stinging at application site, pruritus

Oral: nausea, vomiting, diarrhea, headache

Significant Adverse Reactions

IV: sweating, hypotension, headache, nausea, hematuria, thrombocytosis, nervousness, and renal damage; *rarely*, encephalopathic changes (eg, lethargy, confusion, tremors, agitation, seizures, hallucinations, and coma)

Topical: rash, vulvitis

Oral: dizziness, vertigo, fatigue, insomnia, irritability, depression, skin rash, acne, accelerated hair loss, anorexia, arthralgia, fever, sore throat, palpitations, muscle cramping, lymphadenopathy, edema, menstrual abnormalities, and superficial thrombophlebitis

Contraindications

No absolute contraindications. *Cautious use* in patients with renal, hepatic, neurologic or electrolyte abnormalities; hypoxia; dehydration; and in pregnant or nursing women.

Interactions

Probenecid increases the half-life of acyclovir and reduces the rate of urinary elimination.

Zidovudine may increase the drowsiness and lethargy caused by acyclovir.

Nursing Management

Pretherapy Assessment

Assess and record baseline data necessary for detection of adverse effects of acyclovir: General: vital signs (VS), body weight, skin color and temperature; central nervous system (CNS): orientation, reflexes, affect; genitourinary (GU): output; Lab: blood urea nitrogen (BUN), creatinine clearance (C_{Cr}).

Review medical history and documents for existing or previous conditions that:

a. require cautious use of acyclovir: renal, hepatic, neurologic or electrolyte abnormalities; hypoxia; dehydration; seizures; congestive heart failure (CHF).
b. contraindicate use of acyclovir: allergy to acyclovir; **pregnancy (Category C)**, lactation (safety not established).

Nursing Interventions

Medication Administration

Assure ready access to bathroom facilities if diarrhea occurs.

Protect patient from exposure to ultraviolet light.

Administer IV infusion *slowly* because bolus injection can cause precipitation of acyclovir crystals in renal tubules. Adequate hydration should be ensured during infusion (urine flow should be sufficient to minimize danger of precipitation).

Observe infusion site for signs of phlebitis or inflammation.

Dissolve powder in 10 mL sterile water for injection, which yields a concentration of 50 mg/mL. Remove desired dose and add it to appropriate infusion solution. Infusion concentrations of 7 mg/mL or less are recommended because higher concentrations are more likely to cause inflammation and phlebitis on extravasation.

Use prepared solution (50 mg/mL) within 12 hours. Once diluted, each dose should be used within 24 hours.

Refer to enclosed package information for dosage modification based on creatinine clearance in patient with renal impairment.

Use a finger cot or rubber glove when applying ointment.

Surveillance During Therapy

Monitor results of complete blood counts with differentials, which should be performed before initiating therapy and at midtreatment each time the drug is used to detect development of blood dyscrasias.

Carefully monitor laboratory studies and patient for indications of adverse reactions.

Interpret results of diagnostic tests and contact practitioner as appropriate.

Monitor for possible drug–drug and drug–nutrient interactions: Refer to **Interactions**.

Provide for patient safety needs if CNS effects occur.

Patient Teaching

Caution patient to adhere to prescribed dosage, frequency of administration, and length of treatment.

Explain to patient, as supportively as possible, that there is no evidence that episodic treatment with any acyclovir drug forms (IV, oral, or topical) eliminates either contagiousness, which is present when the virus is shedding, or recurrence.

Explain to patient that ointment should be applied only cutaneously (it should not be used in the eyes).

Warn patient to use caution in driving or engaging in other hazardous activities until drug effects are known because transient dizziness may occur.

Teach patient how to recognize early signs of possible

blood dyscrasia (fever, sore throat, bleeding, or fatigue) and stress importance of reporting these to prescriber.

Urge patient to seek treatment for recurrence promptly. The sooner acyclovir therapy is initiated, the more effective it is.

Teach patient that the following are a result of drug therapy: nausea, vomiting, diarrhea, sedation, dizziness, confusion.

Instruct the patient to report any of the following to the practitioner if they occur: rash; difficulty urinating; increased severity or frequency of recurrences.

• Famciclovir

Famvir

Famciclovir is a new antiviral drug, related to acyclovir, that is indicated for the management of acute herpes zoster (shingles). It is available in 500-mg tablets, which are taken every 8 hours for 7 days. In addition to relieving the pain and speeding healing of the lesions, famciclovir may shorten the duration of postherpetic neuralgia, the pain that persists even after the lesions have healed. Refer to the discussion of acyclovir for additional information.

• Amantadine

Symmetrel

An orally effective drug that exhibits antiviral activity against influenza A viruses as well as an antiparkinsonian action, amantadine is used for the *prevention* of Asian (A) type viral infections in high-risk patients and as adjunctive therapy in Parkinson's disease and in drug-induced extrapyramidal reactions. In addition, the drug also may be effective in shortening the duration of viral symptoms (fever, chills) if taken early in the course of infection. The antiviral activity of amantadine appears to be specific for A virus strains, and there is no evidence that the drug is effective for either prophylaxis or treatment of other viral diseases. The antiparkinsonian actions of the drug are discussed in detail in Chapter 28, and only its antiviral activity is considered here.

Mechanism

Inhibits viral replication at an early stage, probably by preventing the uncoating of viral nucleic acid and blocking the release of nucleic acids into host cells; increases release of dopamine from nerve endings in the CNS (see Chapter 28)

Uses

Prevention and symptomatic management of Asian (A) influenza infections, especially in high-risk patients (eg, those with heart disease, pulmonary disease, or immunodeficiency states) or in cases in which contact with the virus is likely, for example, in hospital wards or infected households

Symptomatic treatment of Parkinson's disease or drug-induced extrapyramidal reactions, usually in combination with levodopa (see Chapter 28)

Dosage

Adults and children older than 12: 200 mg daily as a single dose or in two divided doses

Children 9 to 12 years: 100 mg twice a day

Children 1 to 9 years: 4.4 mg/kg to 8.8 mg/kg daily in two or three divided doses

Refer also to Chapter 28.

Fate

Readily absorbed orally; peak serum levels occur in 2 to 4 hours, but 48 hours is required for drug to reach maximal tissue concentrations; excreted largely unchanged in the urine, 50% of a dose within 20 to 24 hours.

Common Side Effects

Dizziness, lightheadedness, anxiety, irritability, confusion, mild depression, orthostatic hypotension, urinary hesitancy, and constipation

Significant Adverse Reactions

CV: congestive heart failure

Neurologic: fatigue, weakness, headache, nervousness, insomnia, tremors, convulsions, slurred speech, blurred vision, oculogyric crisis. Hallucinations and psychotic reactions have occurred, especially in older persons

GI: nausea, vomiting, anorexia, dry mouth

Others: leukopenia, neutropenia, livedo reticularis (skin mottling), skin rash, eczematoid dermatitis, peripheral edema

Contraindications

Pregnancy. *Cautious use* in patients with epilepsy or a history of convulsive disorders, congestive heart failure, peripheral edema, renal impairment, orthostatic hypotension, liver disease, history of skin rash or other allergic dermatoses; in psychotic patients; and in elderly or debilitated patients.

Interactions

Amantadine may exhibit additive atropine-like effects with anticholinergic drugs, tricyclic antidepressants, or antihistamines

Excessive CNS stimulation may occur with combined use of amantadine and other CNS stimulants (eg, amphetamines, methylphenidate)

Decreased urinary excretion of amantadine has occurred when hydrochlorothiazide plus triamterene was administered concurrently

Nursing Management

Refer to **Chapter 28**. In addition:

Nursing Interventions

Medication Administration

Note that amantadine does *not* suppress antibody response and therefore can be used in conjunction with influenza A virus vaccine until antibody response develops. It is administered for 2 to 3 weeks after the vaccine has been given. When given alone for prophylaxis, it should be continued for the duration of the epidemic, usually 6 to 8 weeks.

Patient Teaching

Refer also to **Chapter 28**.

Instruct patient to avoid taking drug too close to bedtime because insomnia may occur.
Warn patient not to engage in hazardous activities because dizziness, confusion, and blurred vision can occur, especially early in therapy.
Instruct patient to change position slowly to minimize the danger of orthostatic hypotension.
Inform patient that livedo reticularis (mottling of skin, usually of lower extremities) may occur but that it will subside when drug is discontinued or dosage is reduced.

• Foscarnet

Foscavir

Foscarnet is a pyrophosphate analogue of phosphonoacetic acid that has potent antiviral activity against herpes types 1 and 2, varicella-zoster, cytomegalovirus (CMV), and Epstein–Barr viruses. It has also been shown to inhibit HIV replication. Foscarnet is active against acyclovir- and ganciclovir-resistant herpesvirus, including CMV.

Mechanism

Foscarnet inhibits DNA polymerase and the reverse transcriptases of retroviruses by blocking the pyrophosphate binding site; this action prevents viral chain elongation.

Use

Treatment of CMV retinitis in patients with AIDS

Dosage

IV infusion: Initially, 60 mg/kg over 1 hour every 8 hours for 2 to 3 weeks
Maintenance: 90 to 120 mg/kg/day over 2 hours

Fate

Distributed throughout the body; cerebrospinal fluid (CSF) levels are variable; half-life ranges from 2 to 8 hours and is increased with renal impairment; foscarnet accumulates in bone and the slow release from bone may increase the terminal half-life after chronic therapy; 80% to 90% of the drug is excreted unchanged in the urine

Common Side Effects

Fever, nausea, anemia, abnormal renal function

Significant Adverse Reactions

CNS: dizziness, visual disturbances, paresthesia, neuralgia, seizures
Psychiatric: depression, anxiety, sleep disorders, psychotic episodes
GI: vomiting, diarrhea, abdominal pain, gastrointestinal ulceration, pancreatitis, abnormal liver function
Hematologic: anemia, pancytopenia, coagulation disorders
Respiratory: cough, dyspnea, inflammation of upper respiratory tract, bronchitis, pneumonia
Dermatologic: rash, acne, alopecia, pruritus, psoriasis
Urinary: abnormal renal function, increased serum creatinine, urinary tract infections
CV: hypertension, electrocardiogram (ECG) abnormalities, and arrhythmias
Other: electrolyte disturbances involving magnesium, phosphate, calcium, and potassium

Contraindications

No absolute contraindications. *Cautious use* in patients with preexisting renal impairment, cardiac disturbances, or history of seizures.

Interactions

Other nephrotoxic drugs, such as aminoglycosides, amphotericin B, cyclosporine, and pentamidine, may have additive effects with foscarnet.

Concurrent use of foscarnet and pentamidine may cause hypercalcemia, which also may occur with other drugs that elevate serum calcium.

Concurrent use of foscarnet with zidovudine, or other drugs that decrease blood cell proliferation, may increase the likelihood of developing anemia.

Nursing Management

Pretherapy Assessment

Assess and record baseline data necessary for detection of adverse effects of foscarnet: General: VS, body weight, skin color and temperature; CNS: orientation, reflexes, affect, ophthalmic examination; GU: output; Lab: BUN, C_{Cr}.
Review medical history and documents for existing or previous conditions that:
a. require cautious use of foscarnet: renal, hepatic, neurologic, or electrolyte abnormalities; seizures.
b. contraindicate use of foscarnet: allergy to foscarnet; **pregnancy (Category C)**, lactation (safety not established).

Nursing Interventions

Medication Administration

Drug is administered by controlled intravenous infusion, using either a central venous line or a peripheral vein.
Drug is chemically incompatible with 30% dextrose, amphotericin B, and solutions containing calcium.
Physical incompatibility reported with acyclovir, ganciclovir, trimetrexate, pentamidine, vancomycin, trimethoprim/sulfamethoxazole, diazepam, digoxin, phenytoin, leucovorin, and phenothiazines.
Assure ready access to bathroom facilities if diarrhea occur
Observe infusion site for signs of phlebitis or inflammation.

Surveillance During Therapy

Monitor results of complete blood counts with differentials, which should be performed before initiating therapy and at midtreatment each time the drug is used to detect development of blood dyscrasias.
Carefully monitor laboratory studies and patient for indications of adverse reactions.
Interpret results of diagnostic tests and contact practitioner as appropriate.
Monitor for possible drug–drug and drug–nutrient interactions: Refer to **Interactions**.
Provide for patient safety needs if CNS effects occur.

Patient Teaching

Explain to patient, as supportively as possible, that there is no evidence that treatment with foscarnet is curative for CMV retinitis and that they may continue to experience progression of retinitis.
Teach patient that the following are a result of drug therapy: fever, nausea, anemia, abnormal renal function.
Instruct the patient to report any of the following to the practitioner if they occur: rash; difficulty urinating; increased severity or frequency of recurrences.

• Ganciclovir

Cytovene

Ganciclovir is a synthetic nucleoside analog of 2-deoxyguanosine that is active against several types of viruses, including cytomegalovirus (CMV), herpes types 1 and 2, varicella-zoster, and Epstein-Barr. It is indicated *only* for treatment of CMV retinitis in immunocompromised patients, but it is being evaluated for use in other CMV infections.

Mechanism

Converted to the triphosphate by cellular kinases on entry into host cells; ganciclovir triphosphate inhibits viral DNA synthesis by competitive inhibition of viral DNA polymerases and by direct incorporation into viral DNA, resulting in termination of viral DNA elongation

Uses

Treatment of CMV retinitis in immunocompromised patients, including individuals with AIDS
Prophylaxis in transplant patients at risk for CMV disease
Investigational uses include treatment of other CMV infections such as pneumonitis or colitis and treatment of CMV infections in noncompromised patients

Dosage

IV infusion: Initially, 5 mg/kg over 1 hour every 12 hours for 14 to 21 days
Maintenance: 5 mg/kg over 1 hour once daily *or* 6 mg/kg once daily 5 days each week

Fate

After IV infusion, plasma half-life is 2 to 4 hours; the major route of elimination is glomerular filtration and renal excretion, with more than 90% of the dose appearing as unmetabolized drug in the urine

Common Side Effects

Granulocytopenia, thrombocytopenia

NOTE: The above two adverse effects occur in 20% to 40% of immunocompromised patients who receive ganciclovir. Granulocytopenia usually occurs within the first 2 weeks of therapy but may occur anytime. Withdrawal of ganciclovir usually results in recovery of cell counts within 3 to 7 days.

Significant Adverse Reactions

CNS: ataxia, confusion, bizarre dreams, dizziness, headache, somnolence, tremor, psychosis, coma
GI: nausea, diarrhea, anorexia, vomiting, abdominal pain
CV: hypertension, arrhythmia
Dermatologic: pruritus, urticaria, alopecia
Genitourinary: increased BUN and serum creatinine, hematuria
Other: fever, rash, anemia, chills, edema, malaise, dyspnea, decreased blood glucose, abnormal liver function values, anemia, pain and inflammation at injection site

Contraindications

No absolute contraindications. *Cautious use* in patients with preexisting cytopenias, reduced renal function, liver impairment, in elderly persons, in pregnant or nursing women, and in children.

Interactions

Other cytotoxic drugs, such as dapsone, flucytosine, vincristine, vinblastine, amphotericin B, adriamycin, and pentamidine may have additive effects with ganciclovir.
Probenecid may reduce the renal clearance of ganciclovir.
Concurrent use of ganciclovir and imipenem–cilastatin has resulted in generalized seizures.
Concurrent use of ganciclovir and zidovudine may result in severe granulocytopenia.
Concurrent use of other nephrotoxic drugs, such as aminoglycosides and cyclosporine may increase serum creatinine.

Nursing Management

Pretherapy Assessment

Assess and record baseline data necessary for detection of adverse effects of ganciclovir: General: VS, body weight, skin color and temperature; CNS: orientation, reflexes, affect, ophthalmic examination; GU: output; CVS: perfusion, edema; Lab: complete blood count (CBC), hematocrit (Hct), BUN, C_{Cr}, liver function tests.
Review medical history and documents for existing or previous conditions that:

a. require cautious use of ganciclovir: preexisting cytopenias; reduced renal function; liver impairment; use in elderly persons.
b. contraindicate use of ganciclovir: allergy to ganciclovir, acyclovir; **pregnancy (Category C)**, lactation (safety not established).

Nursing Interventions

Medication Administration

Assure ready access to bathroom facilities if diarrhea occurs.
Observe infusion site for signs of phlebitis or inflammation.
Do not exceed recommended dosage, because doses above 6 mg/kg or rates of infusion faster than 1 hour usually result in increased toxicity.
Do not administer ganciclovir IM or SC, because severe tissue irritation can occur because of the high pH (11) of the solution.
Ensure adequate hydration during administration of ganciclovir because drug is eliminated largely unchanged in the kidneys.

Use care to avoid extravasation during infusion, because drug solution is quite irritating; use veins with adequate blood flow to facilitate rapid dilution and distribution of drug.

Surveillance During Therapy

Perform neutrophil and platelet counts every 2 days during twice-daily dosing and weekly thereafter because of the frequency of granulocytopenia and thrombocytopenia. Severe neutropenia (500 cells/mm^3) or thrombocytopenia (25,000 platelets/mm^3) necessitates dose interruption until marrow recovery is evident.

Monitor serum creatinine or creatinine clearance every 2 weeks. Dosage is reduced accordingly if creatinine clearance decreases to below 80 mL/1.73 m^2/min.

Note than ganciclovir is carcinogenic and teratogenic, and causes impaired spermatogenesis in animals, although human studies are lacking. Use during pregnancy and in women of childbearing potential with caution.

Carefully monitor laboratory studies and patient for indications of adverse reactions.

Interpret results of diagnostic tests and contact practitioner as appropriate.

Monitor for possible drug–drug and drug–nutrient interactions: Refer to **Interactions**.

Provide for patient safety needs if CNS effects occur.

Patient Teaching

Caution patient to adhere to prescribed dosage, frequency of administration, and length of treatment.

Urge patients to have regular ophthalmologic examinations because retinitis is not cured by ganciclovir and condition ultimately deteriorates.

Impress patients with the necessity of using contraceptive measures during treatment, because drug may cause birth defects.

Teach patient that the following are a result of drug therapy: rash, fever, pain at the injection site, decreased blood count leading to susceptibility to infection.

Instruct the patient to report any of the following to the practitioner if they occur: bruising, bleeding, pain at injection site, fever, infection.

• *Idoxuridine*

Herplex, Stoxil

Idoxuridine (IDU) is a structural analogue of thymidine, an essential intermediate in DNA synthesis. Because it is rapidly inactivated by enzymes, IDU is used only locally in the eye for the treatment of herpes simplex keratitis, a viral disease that affects the cornea.

Mechanism

Incorporated into viral DNA, producing a faulty molecule incapable of reproduction, thus blocking herpes viral cell replication

Use

Treatment of herpes simplex (herpetic) keratitis

NOTE: Idoxuridine will control the infection but has no effect on accumulated scarring or progressive loss of vision.

Dosage

Ophthalmic solution: 1 drop every hour during the day and every 2 hours at night; reduce as improvement is noted

Ophthalmic ointment: Instill five times a day every 4 hours.

Fate

Short-acting and quickly inactivated by nucleotidases

Common Side Effects

Periorbital burning, irritation, lacrimation

Significant Adverse Reactions

Pain, inflammation, pruritus, and edema of eyes and eyelids; photophobia; local allergic reactions; corneal clouding, vascularization, or stippling; prolonged use can result in follicular conjunctivitis, blepharitis, conjunctival hyperemia, and corneal epithelial staining

Interactions

Concurrent use of a boric acid solution may increase the severity of local irritation.

Nursing Management

Nursing Interventions

Medication Administration

Note that improvement of keratitic lesions may be enhanced by concomitant use of topical corticosteroids. Steroid should be withdrawn several days before discontinuing idoxuridine. Corticosteroids should *not* be used without idoxuridine.

Patient Teaching

Teach patient how to administer eye drops or ointment (see Chapter 2).

Instruct patient to store ophthalmic solution in refrigerator, except for Herplex Liquifilm, which requires no refrigeration.

Stress the importance of continuing therapy for at least 5 to 7 days after healing is complete to prevent recurrence of infection, which is common with short courses of therapy.

Instruct patient to notify drug prescriber if improvement is not noted within 7 or 8 days, in epithelial infections, or if pain, itching, or swelling occurs, because drug should be discontinued.

• *Ribavirin*

Virazole

Ribavirin has demonstrated antiviral activity against respiratory syncytial virus (RSV), influenza A and B viruses, and herpes simplex virus. When administered as an aerosol, ribavirin retards replication of RSV in infants and reduces the severity and duration of the illness. Aerosol ribavirin has also been shown to be effective against influenza A and B, and oral ribavirin (an investigational dosage form) has been reported to be active in other viral diseases such as acute and chronic hepatitis, herpes genitalis, measles, and Lassa fever.

Mechanism

Not completely established; appears to interfere with guanidine monophosphate formation and subsequent nucleic acid synthesis in viral particles

Uses

Treatment of selected hospitalized infants and young children with severe lower respiratory tract infections caused by respiratory syncytial virus
Investigational uses include aerosol treatment of influenza A and B virus infection and oral therapy of hepatitis virus, measles, and Lassa fever

Dosage

Administer 12 to 18 hours a day for at least 3 but no more than 7 days.

Aerosol is delivered to an oxygen hood; alternatively, a face mask or oxygen tent may be used.

Fate

Administration by aerosolization results in significant systemic absorption; plasma half-life is 8 to 10 hours; ribavirin and its metabolites accumulate in red blood cells, with a half-life of approximately 40 days.

Significant Adverse Reactions

Rash, hypotension, conjunctivitis, reticulocytosis, worsening of respiratory status, bacterial pneumonia, pneumothorax, apnea, cardiac arrest (rare)

Contraindications

Pregnancy (drug is potentially teratogenic). *Cautious use* in persons with chronic obstructive lung disease, persons taking digitalis drugs (refer to **Interactions**) and in nursing mothers.

Interactions

Use of ribavirin can increase the likelihood of digitalis toxicity.

Nursing Management

Nursing Interventions

Medication Administration

Administer by aerosol only, use only a Viratek Small Particle Aerosol Generator (SPAG) Model SPAG-2 (operator's manual contains operating instructions), and avoid concomitant administration of other aerosol preparations.
Prepare aerosol solution with either sterile water for injection or sterile water for inhalation without preservatives or any other additive. Package insert contains preparation instructions.
Inspect solution before using. Discard if discolored or cloudy.

Surveillance During Therapy

Closely monitor patient's respiratory status. Assess rate and character of respirations, and auscultate lungs for abnormal breath sounds before initiation of therapy and frequently thereafter. Observe patient for signs of dyspnea; apnea; rapid, shallow respirations; intercostal and substernal retraction; nasal flaring; limited lung excursion; cyanosis; and evidence of pneumothorax.
Monitor cardiac rhythm continuously to detect cardiac arrhythmias.
Check blood pressure frequently to detect hypotension.
Monitor intake–output and assess fluid status frequently.
Monitor results of CBCs with differentials, which should be performed frequently during therapy, especially if treatment is prolonged, because drug may cause a precipitous drop in hemoglobin, hematocrit, and red blood cells.
Observe patient simultaneously receiving mechanical ventilation for signs of worsening pulmonary function. Obstruction may cause inadequate ventilation and gas exchange if ribavirin precipitates or fluid accumulates in tubing. Check equipment, including endotracheal tube, every 2 hours.

• Rimantadine

Flumadine

Rimantadine is a viral prophylactic agent, similar to amantadine, that is used for prophylaxis against various strains of influenza A virus. The recommended dose is 100 mg orally, twice a day, except in patients with severe renal or hepatic disease and in elderly patients, in whom the dose should be reduced to 100 mg once daily. Rimantadine is claimed to elicit fewer CNS side effects than amantadine. Concurrent administration of aspirin or acetaminophen may reduce peak serum concentrations of rimantadine. Refer to **amantadine** for Nursing Management and other additional information.

• Trifluridine

Viroptic

A halogenated pyrimidine, trifluridine exhibits in vivo antiviral activity against herpes simplex virus types 1 and 2 and vaccinia virus. The drug is also active in vitro against some strains of adenovirus. Its clinical application is currently restricted to ophthalmic infections caused by sensitive organisms, and the drug is often effective in patients unresponsive to idoxuridine and vidarabine.

Mechanism

Not established; interferes with DNA synthesis in cultured mammalian cells

Uses

Treatment of primary keratoconjunctivitis and recurrent epithelial keratitis due to herpes simplex viruses 1 and 2
Treatment of epithelial keratitis in patients intolerant of or unresponsive to idoxuridine or vidarabine
Treatment of ophthalmic infections caused by vaccinia virus or adenovirus (clinical efficacy not definitely established)
Prophylaxis of herpes simplex virus keratoconjunctivitis and epithelial keratitis (efficacy not definitely established)

Dosage

1 drop of ophthalmic solution every 2 hours while awake until corneal ulcer has healed, then 1 drop every 4 hours for 7 days

Fate

Intraocular penetration following topical application is good; systemic absorption is negligible; half-life is approximately 15 minutes

Common Side Effects

Mild, transient burning or stinging

Significant Adverse Reactions

Palpebral edema, superficial punctate keratopathy, epithelial keratopathy, stromal edema, irritation, hypersensitivity reactions, hyperemia, and increased intraocular pressure

Contraindications

No absolute contraindications. *Cautious use* in patients with glaucoma and in pregnancy or lactation.

Nursing Management

Nursing Interventions

Medication Administration

Administer only after diagnosis of herpetic keratitis has been established because drug is ineffective against bacterial, fungal, or chlamydial infections. Recommended dosage should not be exceeded. Alternative forms of therapy should be considered if clinical improvement does not occur within 7 days or if *complete* reepithelialization is not evident within 14 days. To avoid ocular toxicity, drug should not be used longer than 21 days under any circumstances.

Patient Teaching

Teach patient how to administer eye drops (see Chapter 2).
Inform patient that a transient stinging sensation may occur on instillation.
Instruct patient to store drug under refrigeration because elevated temperatures accelerate its degradation.

• Vidarabine

Vira-A

Vidarabine is a pyrimidine derivative that possesses antiviral activity against herpes simplex virus types 1 and 2. It may be used systemically in the treatment of herpes simplex virus encephalitis, or ophthalmically for keratoconjunctivitis and epithelial keratitis. Prompt diagnosis of herpes encephalitis, a frequent complication of cancer immunosuppressive therapy, and treatment by vidarabine can reduce mortality from 70% to approximately 25%. However, patients already in a comatose state at the time therapy is initiated do not appear to benefit from the drug. When applied locally in the eye, vidarabine is often effective in patients resistant to or intolerant of idoxuridine.

Mechanism

Converted into nucleotides, which can inhibit viral DNA synthesis, presumably by interfering with viral DNA polymerase; mammalian cell DNA synthesis is also inhibited, but to a lesser extent; metabolized to hypoxanthine arabinoside, which may act synergistically with the parent compound against DNA viruses

Uses

Treatment of herpes simplex virus encephalitis (IV only)
Treatment of herpes zoster (shingles) in immunocompromised patients
Treatment of superficial and recurrent epithelial keratitis and acute keratoconjunctivitis caused by herpes simplex virus types 1 and 2 (ophthalmic only)

Dosage

IV: 15 mg/kg/day infused over 12 to 24 hours for 10 days
Shingles: 10 mg/kg/day for 5 days
Ophthalmic: 1/2-inch ophthalmic ointment in lower conjunctival sac five times a day at 3-hour intervals until reepithelialization occurs; continue twice a day for another 7 days

Fate

IV infusion: rapidly deaminated to hypoxanthine arabinoside, the principal metabolite, which is quickly distributed in the body but possesses only 1/10 the in vitro antiviral activity of vidarabine; half-life of vidarabine is 1 hour, and hypoxanthine arabinoside is 3.5 hours; excreted primarily by the kidneys
Ophthalmic application: if cornea is normal, only trace amounts of drug or metabolite are detectable in the aqueous humor; systemic absorption following ocular administration is negligible

Common Side Effects

Temporary visual haze with ophthalmic application

Significant Adverse Reactions

IV: anorexia, nausea, vomiting, diarrhea; tremor, dizziness, ataxia, confusion, hallucinations, psychosis; decreased hemoglobin and hematocrit values, hematemesis, reduced white blood cell count and platelet count; weight loss, malaise; rash, pruritus, pain at injection site, and elevated total bilirubin and AST
Ophthalmic: irritation, ocular pain, photophobia, lacrimation, burning, superficial punctate keratitis, punctal occlusion, foreign body sensation, hypersensitivity reactions

Contraindications

No absolute contraindications. *Cautious use* of IV infusion during pregnancy and lactation, and in patients with impaired renal or liver function or in CNS infections other than herpes encephalitis.

Interactions

Concurrent use of allopurinol may interfere with vidarabine metabolism.

Nursing Management

Nursing Interventions

Medication Administration

Administer only after diagnosis of herpes simplex virus has been established because drug is ineffective against infections caused by other viral species or bacterial and fungal infections. Drug should not be used to treat trivial infections, and recommended dosage and duration of therapy should not be exceeded because vidarabine has exhibited mutagenic and carcinogenic potential in laboratory animals, although the significance of this for humans is not yet known.

Avoid rapid or bolus IV injections, and do not administer SC or IM because drug is poorly soluble and erratically absorbed.

Prepare infusion just before administration. To prepare, shake vial well, then withdraw and transfer desired dose (solution contains 200 mg/mL) into prewarmed (35–40°C) fluid (any IV solution is suitable *except* biologic or colloidal fluids such as protein solutions or blood products). Thoroughly agitate until completely clear, then run through an in-line filter (0.45 μm or smaller) to ensure that undissolved particles are removed. Do not refrigerate. Use within 48 hours.

Surveillance During Therapy

Monitor results of hematologic tests (eg, hemoglobin, hematocrit, white blood cells, platelets), which should be performed periodically during systemic therapy because vidarabine can alter them.

Patient Teaching

Teach patient how to administer ophthalmic ointment.

Inform patient using ophthalmic preparation that photophobia or a temporary clouding of vision may occur. Advise caution in operating machinery or performing other hazardous tasks.

Stress importance of adhering to prescribed ophthalmic dosage and frequency of administration. Drug prescriber should be notified if improvement is not observed within 7 days or if condition worsens during therapy. If complete reepithelialization has not occurred within 21 days, alternative treatment may be prescribed.

Drugs Used to Treat AIDS

• Zidovudine

Retrovir

Zidovudine, formerly known as azidothymidine (AZT), was the first available anti-AIDS drug. It appears to slow the replication of the human immunodeficiency virus (HIV), the causative agent of AIDS, thus allowing for some immunologic reconstruction in persons afflicted with the virus. To date, however, *no* cures have been reported in HIV-infected patients, and the drug must be viewed as merely palliative.

Mechanism

Thymidine analogue converted by thymidine kinase into the triphosphate derivative, which is the active form; inhibits viral RNA-dependent DNA polymerase (reverse transcriptase), which decreases viral DNA synthesis and viral replication; drug is also incorporated into DNA by viral reverse transcriptase, where it causes termination of viral DNA chain elongation. Treatment with zidovudine does *not* reduce the risk of transmission of the virus through sexual contact or blood contamination.

Uses

Management of patients with symptomatic HIV infection (ie, AIDS or AIDS-related complex—ARC) who have a history of cytologically confirmed *Pneumocystis carinii* pneumonia *or* an absolute CD4 (T_4 helper/inducer) lymphocyte count of less than 500/mm^2

Management of children older than 3 months of age who have HIV-related symptoms or who are asymptomatic but have abnormal laboratory values indicating HIV-related immunosuppression

Dosage

Oral:

Adults: 200 mg every 4 hours around the clock; after 1 month, dose may be reduced to 100 mg every 4 hours

Children (3 months to 12 years of age): 180 mg/m^2 every 6 hours, not to exceed 200 mg every 6 hours.

IV infusion:

Adults: 1 to 2 mg/kg over 1 hour every 4 hours around the clock

Fate

Oral absorption is rapid and peak plasma levels occur within 1 hour; plasma protein binding is 35% to 40%; drug is quickly metabolized in the liver; plasma half-life is approximately 1 hour; metabolites and some unchanged drug are eliminated in the urine

Common Side Effects

Headache, nausea, GI pain, skin rash, fever, myalgia, insomnia, asthenia

Significant Adverse Reactions

CAUTION

The most frequent adverse effects occurring with zidovudine are anemia and granulocytopenia. The frequency of occurrence is directly related to dosage and duration of therapy and inversely related to T_4 lymphocyte number, hemoglobin, and granulocyte count at the outset of therapy. Anemia usually occurs within 4 to 6 weeks of therapy and frequently requires blood transfusion. Myelosuppression is generally reversible but often recurs even with dosage reduction, which may necessitate repeated transfusions.

GI: anorexia, diarrhea, vomiting, dysphagia, flatulence, mouth ulcers, bleeding gums, edema of the tongue, rectal bleeding

CNS: dizziness, paresthesias, somnolence, anxiety, confusion, nervousness, syncope, depression

Respiratory: dyspnea, cough, nosebleed, sinusitis, pharyngitis, hoarseness, rhinitis

Urinary: dysuria, polyuria, urinary frequency

Dermatologic/hypersensitivity: pruritus, urticaria, acne

Other: vasodilation, arthralgia, muscle spasm, tremor, photophobia, hearing loss, amblyopia, chills, body odor, hyperalgesia, lymphadenopathy, altered taste

Contraindications

No absolute contraindications. *Cautious use* in the presence of liver or kidney disease, compromised bone marrow function, and in pregnant or nursing women.

Interactions

Use of drugs that are nephrotoxic or cytotoxic (eg, amphotericin B, flucytosine, dapsone, pentamidine, vincristine, vinblastine) may increase the risk of toxicity during zidovudine administration

Drugs that are likely to produce hematologic toxicity (chloramphenicol, carbamazepine, adriamycin, interferon) increase the likelihood of such effects with zidovudine

Drugs that can inhibit the metabolism (glucuronidation) of zidovudine (such as probenecid, indomethacin, aspirin, acetaminophen) by competitive antagonism may potentiate the toxic effects of the drug

Nursing Management

Pretherapy Assessment

Assess and record baseline data necessary for detection of adverse effects of zidovudine: General: VS, body weight, skin color and temperature; CNS: orientation, reflexes, affect; Lab: CBC, Hct, BUN, C_{Cr}, liver, kidney function tests.

Review medical history and documents for existing or previous conditions that:

a. require cautious use of zidovudine: liver or kidney disease; compromised bone marrow function.

b. contraindicate use of zidovudine: allergy to any component; **pregnancy (Category C)**, lactation (safety not established, do not administer to nursing mothers).

Nursing Interventions

Medication Administration

Assure ready access to bathroom facilities if diarrhea occurs.

Surveillance During Therapy

Monitor results of CBCs with differentials, which should be performed before initiation of therapy and at least every 2 weeks thereafter because hematologic toxicity is common (refer to **CAUTION** under Significant Adverse Reactions).

Assess patient for evidence of opportunistic infection. Zidovudine does not reduce patient's predisposition to infection. It may, in fact, increase it by suppressing bone marrow.

Carefully monitor laboratory studies and patient for indications of adverse reactions.

Interpret results of diagnostic tests and contact practitioner as appropriate.

Monitor for possible drug–drug and drug–nutrient interactions: See interactions.

Provide for patient safety needs if CNS effects occur.

Patient Teaching

Caution patient to adhere to prescribed dosage, frequency of administration, and length of treatment.

Ensure that patient understands dosage regimen: Drug is to be taken every 4 hours around the clock.

Warn patient not to take any other drugs, including over-the-counter (OTC) preparations, unless specifically ordered (refer to **Interactions**).

Explain the importance of maintaining close medical supervision. The patient should be evaluated at least weekly during early stages of therapy.

Supportively explain to patient that drug does not reduce risk of transmitting HIV.

Advise patient to notify drug prescriber if condition worsens or any unusual symptoms develop.

Teach patient that the following are a result of drug therapy: rash, fever, pain at the injection site, decreased blood count leading to susceptibility to infection.

Instruct the patient to report any of the following to the practitioner if they occur: bruising, bleeding, pain at injection site, fever, infection.

• Didanosine

Videx

Didanosine or dideoxyinosine (ddI) was the second drug approved for the treatment of AIDS and is indicated for treatment of advanced HIV infection in patients who cannot tolerate zidovudine or who are experiencing deterioration during zidovudine therapy. Like zidovudine, didanosine appears to slow replication of HIV and allow some recovery of immunologic function. The effect of didanosine on patient survival and its usefulness with other agents are still under evaluation.

Mechanism

Action similar to zidovudine; didanosine is a nucleoside analogue of deoxyadenosine that is activated by cellular enzymes to the active triphosphate form; activated form inhibits viral reverse transcriptase activity and interferes with viral DNA synthesis, viral replication, and DNA chain elongation

Uses

Treatment of adults and children older than 6 months of age with advanced HIV infection who cannot tolerate zidovudine or who are experiencing deterioration during zidovudine therapy

Dosage

Adults:
- (over 60 kg) 200 mg (tablets) or 250 mg (powder for solution) twice a day
- (under 60 kg) 125 mg (tablets) or 167 mg (powder for solution) twice a day

Children: (based on body surface area) 25 to 125 mg twice a day

Fate

Didanosine is rapidly degraded by gastric acid; consequently, all oral preparations contain buffering agents to increase the pH of the stomach; bioavailability ranges from 20% to 40% and is significantly decreased by food; distribution occurs throughout the body, with CSF levels approximately 20% of that in the plasma; drug metabolism of didanosine appears to follow the same pathway as that of endogenous purines; elimination is primarily renal but also involves the intestinal tract; half-life is between 1 and 2 hours; however, the intracellular half-life ranges between 12 and 24 hours; plasma protein binding is insignificant.

Common Side Effects

Nausea, headache, dizziness, rash, pruritus, insomnia, myalgia

Significant Adverse Reactions

Peripheral neuropathy: tingling, burning, numbness or pain in the distal extremities
Pancreatitis: abdominal pain, severe epigastric pain, vomiting

CAUTION

Pancreatitis is a serious toxicity that can be fatal. The levels of serum amylase, lipase, and triglycerides may increase before the development of pancreatitis, and patients receiving didanosine should be monitored for signs of pancreatitis.

Hematologic: granulocytopenia, anemia, leukopenia, thrombocytopenia
Other: diarrhea, asthenia, CNS depression, arthritis, dry mouth, alopecia, hyperuricemia (high doses), hepatitis, seizures

Contraindications

No specific contraindications. *Cautious use* in patients with a previous history of neuropathy, pancreatitis, liver dysfunction, renal impairment, and hyperuricemia; the buffered tablets and powders of didanosine contain a large amount of sodium and may be a concern for patients on sodium-restricted diets.

Interactions

The antacids (magnesium or aluminum) present in the didanosine preparations may reduce the absorption of fluoroquinolone or tetracycline antimicrobial drugs; thus these drugs should be administered 2 hours before or after didanosine.

Nursing Management

Refer to **Zidovudine**.

• Zalcitabine

Hivid

Zalcitabine is a pyrimidine analogue of cytidine that is also referred to as dideoxycytidine (ddC). Zalcitabine is currently indicated for the treatment of advanced HIV infection *in combination with zidovudine*.

Mechanism

Zalcitabine is activated to its triphosphate form by cellular enzymes. Like zidovudine and didanosine, the activated triphosphate inhibits the reverse transcriptase of HIV to interfere with both viral DNA synthesis and replication; triphosphate form is incorporated into the viral DNA chain, where it also functions as a chain terminator; as with the other drugs used in AIDS, zalcitabine appears to allow some recovery of immunologic function.

Uses

Treatment of advanced HIV infection in combination with zidovudine

Dosage

0.75 mg (orally) together with 200 mg zidovudine every 8 hours

Fate

Zalcitabine is well absorbed after oral administration, bioavailability is usually greater than 80% but is reduced in the presence of food; distribution is not as extensive as with didanosine; CSF levels are relatively low and variable; drug metabolism appears to be minimal with elimination primarily by way of the urinary tract; half-life ranges from 1 to 3 hours.

Common Side Effects

Fever, rash, aphthous stomatitis

Significant Adverse Reactions

Peripheral neuropathy: tingling, numbness, and a burning sensation in the distal extremities that may progress to severe pain

CAUTION

Neuropathy is potentially *irreversible* when drug is continued while symptoms progress.

Pancreatitis: may occur alone with zalcitabine or in combination with zidovudine, usually accompanied by an increase in serum amylase
Other: gastrointestinal disturbances, headache, dizziness, myalgia

Contraindications

No specific contraindications. *Cautious use* in patients with renal or hepatic impairment and in patients with known risk factors for pancreatitis.

Interactions

The risk of peripheral neuropathy is increased by concurrent use of drugs such as chloramphenicol, cisplatin, dapsone, didanosine, disulfiram, hydralazine, phenytoin, nitrofurantoin, isoniazid, vincristine, and others.
The risk of pancreatitis is increased by use of pentamidine or didanosine.

Nursing Management

Pretherapy Assessment

Assess and record baseline data necessary for detection of adverse effects of zalcitabine: General: VS, body weight, skin color and temperature; CNS: orientation, reflexes, affect, peripheral sensation; Lab: CBC, Hct, BUN, C_{Cr}, liver and kidney function tests, serum amylase, triglycerides.
Review medical history and documents for existing or previous conditions that:
a. require cautious use of zalcitabine: liver or kidney disease; compromised bone marrow function.
b. contraindicate use of zalcitabine: allergy to any component; **pregnancy (Category C)**, lactation (safety not established, do not administer to nursing mothers).

Nursing Interventions

Medication Administration

Assure ready access to bathroom facilities if diarrhea occurs.

Surveillance During Therapy

Monitor results of CBCs with differentials, which should be performed before initiation of therapy and at least every 2 weeks thereafter because hematologic toxicity is common (refer to **CAUTION** under Significant Adverse Reactions).
Assess patient for evidence of opportunistic infection.
Carefully monitor laboratory studies and patient for indications of adverse reactions.
Interpret results of diagnostic tests and contact practitioner as appropriate.
Monitor for possible drug–drug and drug–nutrient interactions: Refer to **Interactions**.
Provide for patient safety needs if CNS effects occur.

Patient Teaching

Caution patient to report early signs of peripheral neuropathy (numbness, tingling, burning, "shooting" pain); drug must be discontinued if symptoms progress.
Caution patient to adhere to prescribed dosage, frequency of administration, and length of treatment.
Warn patient not to take any other drugs, including OTC preparations, unless specifically ordered (refer to **Interactions**).
Explain the importance of maintaining close medical supervision. The patient should be evaluated at least weekly during early stages of therapy.
Supportively explain to patient that drug does not reduce risk of transmitting HIV.
Advise patient to notify drug prescriber if condition worsens or any unusual symptoms develop.

Zidovudine, didanosine, and zalcitabine are the forerunners for what is hoped to be a spate of new drugs that will provide improved quality and length of life to AIDS victims and perhaps ultimately a cure for this dread disease. Other antiviral and immunomodulating drugs (see Chapter 78) are currently undergoing clinical trials for the treatment of AIDS, ARC, and AIDS-associated diseases, such as pneumocystis pneumonia and Kaposi's sarcoma.

• Stavudine

Zerit

Stavudine is a new antiviral drug that is indicated for the treatment of adults with advanced HIV infection and who are either intolerant of existing therapies or who have experienced severe immunologic compromise while being treated with the older drugs (eg, zidovudine, didanosine). The drug is administered orally in a dosage of 40 mg twice a day. It may be taken without regard to meals.

Selected Bibliography

Brooke GL: HIV disease: A review for the family physician. Part 1: Evaluation and conventional therapy. Hosp Pract 42:971, 1990
Brooke GL: HIV disease: A review for the family physician. Part II: Secondary infection, malignancy and experimental therapy. Hosp Pract 42:1299, 1990
Douglas RG: Prophylaxis and treatment of influenza. N Engl J Med 322:443, 1990
Drugs for viral infections. Med Lett Drugs Ther 34:31, 1992
Fischl MA: Combination antiretroviral therapy for HIV infection. Hosp Pract 29(1):43, 1994
Hirsch MS: Chemotherapy of human immunodeficiency virus infections. J Infect Dis 161:845, 1990
Richman DD: Antiviral therapy of HIV infection. Annu Rev Med 42:69, 1991
Richman DD: HIV drug resistance. Ann Rev Pharmacol Toxicol 33:149, 1993
Shelton MJ, O'Donnell AM, Morse GD: Didanosine. Ann Pharmacother 26:660, 1992
Smith MS, Koerber KL, Pagano JS: Long-term persistence of zidovudine resistance mutations in plasma isolates of human immunodeficiency virus Type 1 of dideoxyinosine-treated patients removed from zidovudine therapy. J Infect Dis 169(1):184, 1994
White DA, Gold JW: Medical management of AIDS patients. Med Clin North Am 76:1, 1992

Nursing Bibliography

Anostasi J, Rivera J: Understanding prophylactic treatment for HIV infections. Am J Nurs 94(2):36, 1994
Nettina S, Kauffman F: Sexually transmitted genital lesions: Diagnosis and management. Nurse Prac 15(1):20, 1990

74
Antineoplastic Agents

Alkylating Agents
- Busulfan
- Carboplatin
- Carmustine
- Chlorambucil
- Cisplatin
- Cyclophosphamide
- Dacarbazine
- Ifosfamide
- Lomustine
- Mechlorethamine
- Melphalan
- Pipobroman
- Streptozocin
- Thiethylenethiophosphoramide
- Uracil mustard

Antimetabolites
- Cytarabine
- Floxuridine
- Fludarabine
- Fluorouracil
- Mercaptopurine
- Methotrexate
- Thioguanine

Natural Products
- Asparaginase
- Bleomycin
- Dactinomycin
- Daunorubicin
- Doxorubicin
- Etoposide
- Idarubicin
- Mitomycin
- Mitoxantrone
- Paclitaxel
- Pentostatin
- Pegaspargase
- Plicamycin
- Teniposide
- Vinblastine
- Vincristine

Hormonal, Antihormonal, and Gonadotropin-Releasing Hormone Analogues

Hormonal
- Androgens
- Estrogens
- Progestins
- Prednisone

Antihormonal
- Aminoglutethimide
- Flutamide
- Mitotane
- Tamoxifen

Gonadotropin-Releasing Hormone Analogues
- Goserelin
- Leuprolide

Miscellaneous Antineoplastic Agents
- Aldesleukin
- Altretamine
- BCG
- Cladribine
- Hydroxyurea
- Interferon
- Levamisole
- Procarbazine

Cancer, a disease that occurs in all human and animal populations, affects tissues composed of dividing cells. The exact cause of most cancers is still unknown, but infections as well as environmental factors (chemicals, fiber particles, radiation) and genetic factors are all capable of inducing a normal cell to become neoplastic—that is, to multiply abnormally.

Cancer may be characterized by the following:

Cells grow excessively because normal growth-controlling mechanisms are impaired.
Cells and tissues are undifferentiated.
Cells exhibit invasiveness and have the ability to metastasize (ie, establish themselves at sites distant from their original location).
Cells have acquired heredity (ie, properties of the original cancerous cells).
Cells demonstrate increased synthesis of macromolecules from nucleosides and amino acids.

Treatment of cancer many involve surgery, radiation, immunotherapy, or chemotherapy. Previously, chemotherapy with antineoplastic drugs was used mainly to supplement surgery or radiation therapy in an attempt to eradicate any remaining metastatic tumor cell foci. Today, however, chemotherapy is an accepted and vital part of most cancer regimens. Some neoplastic diseases are, in fact, treated primarily with chemotherapy. In many patients undergoing cancer chemotherapy, a significantly prolonged survival time and, in some cases, complete remission have been achieved (Table 74-1).

The antineoplastic agents may be classified in a variety of ways. The broadest classification and the one used for this discussion is based on mechanism of action and source of the drug. Thus, the antineoplastic drugs include the following:

Alkylating agents
Antimetabolites
Natural products
Hormones, antihormones and gonadotropin-releasing hormone analogues
Miscellaneous agents

Antineoplastic agents also may be classified on the basis of their differential effects on normal and malignant cell metabolism. To understand this classification, it is important to review the phases of cell division:

G_1—*post*mitotic phase; a number of enzymes are synthesized during this phase
S—period of DNA synthesis for chromosomes
G_2—*pre*mitotic phase; specialized protein and RNA synthesis and formation of mitotic spindle
M—mitosis
G_0—temporarily nondividing cells, cell differentiation, or cell death

Some antineoplastic agents inhibit cells during a specific phase of the mitotic cycle and are referred to as *cell-cycle specific* (CCS). The therapeutic response to CCS agents is usually schedule dependent; that is, therapeutic blood levels must be maintained for a sufficient period to allow large numbers of cells to enter the S phase so that the greatest possible number of cells will be killed. Other antineoplastic agents are cytotoxic during any phase of the cell cycle and are referred to as *cell-cycle nonspecific* (CCNS). Cell-cycle nonspecific agents are dose dependent and are usually more effective if given in large intermittent doses. Cell-cycle specific and cell-cycle nonspecific agents are listed in Table 74-2.

To understand the complex pharmacology of the antineoplastic agents more fully, it is necessary to review the general principles of cancer chemotherapy.

Table 74-1. **Neoplastic Diseases Showing a Good Response to Chemotherapy**

Disease	***Antineoplastic Agents****
Acute lymphocytic leukemia (pediatric)	*Induction*: vincristine + prednisone ± asparaginase or doxorubicin *Maintenance*: methotrexate + 6-mercaptopurine
Acute myelogenous leukemia (adult)	Doxorubicin or daunorubicin + cytarabine *or* mitoxantrone + cytarabine ± daunorubicin
Breast cancer	Estrogens, progestins, and tamoxifen Cyclophosphamide + methotrexate + fluorouracil ± prednisone *or* cyclophosphamide + doxorubicin ± fluorouracil
Burkitt's lymphoma	Cyclophosphamide *or* cyclophosphamide + methotrexate + vincristine
Choriocarcinoma	Methotrexate ± dactinomycin
Diffuse histiocytic lymphoma	CHOP (cyclophosphamide, doxorubicin, vincristine, prednisone) *or* BACOP (bleomycin, doxorubicin, cyclophosphamide, vincristine, prednisone) *or* COMA (cyclophosphamide, vincristine, methotrexate, cytarabine) *or* COPP (cyclophosphamide, vincristine, procarbazine, prednisone) *or* MACOP-B (methotrexate, bleomycin, doxorubicin, cyclophosphamide, vincristine, prednisone) *or* ProMACE-MOPP (prednisone, methotrexate, doxorubicin, cyclophosphamide, etoposide–mechlorethamine, vincristine, procarbazine, prednisone) *or* COP-BLAM (cyclophosphamide, vincristine, prednisone, bleomycin, doxorubicin, procarbazine)
Ewing's sarcoma	Cyclophosphamide + doxorubicin + vincristine
Hairy cell leukemia	Interferon
Hodgkin's disease	MOPP (mechlorethamine, vincristine, procarbazine, prednisone) *or* ABVD (doxorubicin, bleomycin, vinblastine, dacarbazine) *or* CVPP (chlorambucil, vinblastine, procarbazine, prednisone) ± carmustine
Lung cancer (small cell)	CAV (cyclophosphamide, doxorubicin, vincristine) *or* etoposide + cisplatin *or* CEP (cyclophosphamide, etoposide, cisplatin)
Retinoblastoma	Cyclophosphamide
Rhabdomyosarcoma	VAC (vincristine, dactinomycin, cyclophosphamide) ± doxorubicin
Testicular cancer	Vinblastine + bleomycin + cisplatin *or* cisplatin + etoposide + bleomycin
Wilms' tumor	Dactinomycin + vincristine ± doxorubicin ± cyclophosphamide

* (±) indicates a possibly beneficial addition.

The goal of cancer therapy is to destroy or remove all neoplastic cells with minimal effect on normal host cells.

The maximum chance for cure exists when the tumor cell burden is at a minimum and tumors have a high growth fraction (ie, a high proportion of tumor cells are actively dividing).

A given dose of antineoplastic agent kills a constant *percentage* of cells, not a constant *number*.

Cell-cycle specific agents are more effective than cell-cycle nonspecific agents in tumors with a large, bulky mass.

Before a change to another agent, treatment with an antineoplastic agent should continue until either the desired response is obtained or toxicity occurs.

Toxicity is often the limiting factor in the usefulness of an antineoplastic agent, and the risk of toxicity is increased if the patient has received prior chemotherapy or radiation treatment. Because the disease is so often fatal, however, the risk of serious toxicity is relatively acceptable in most instances.

Malignant cells may exhibit resistance to some antineoplastic agents, thus limiting their usefulness. Resistance may be natural or acquired, that is, either the tumor is resistant from the start of therapy (natural), or resistance occurs after therapy has begun and results from drug-induced adaptation or mutation of malignant cells (acquired).

Drug scheduling is important. High-dose intermittent therapy is usually more effective, less toxic, and less immunosuppressive than low-dose, continuous therapy. Toxicity may be reduced and cell resistance delayed by administering combinations of drugs in cycles or sequence (see discussion of combination chemotherapy at the end of the chapter).

Factors such as the age, sex, and physical condition

Table 74-2. **Cell-Cycle–Specific and Cell-Cycle–Nonspecific Agents**

Cell-Cycle–Specific	***Cell-Cycle–Nonspecific***
Antimetabolites	*Alkylating agents*
Cytarabine	Busulfan
Fludarabine	Carboplatin
Mercaptopurine	Carmustine
Methotrexate	Chlorambucil
Thioguanine	Cisplatin
	Cyclophosphamide
	Dacarbazine
	Ifosfamide
	Lomustine
	Mechlorethamine
	Melphalan
	Pipobroman
	Streptozocin
	Triethylenethiophosphoramide
Natural products	*Natural products*
Bleomycin	Dactinomycin
Etoposide	Daunorubicin
Placitaxel	Doxorubicin
Teniposide	Idarubicin
Vinblastine	Mitoxantrone
Vincristine	*Antimetabolites*
Miscellaneous	Floxuridine
Hydroxyurea	Fluorouracil
	Miscellaneous
	Cladribine
	Procarbazine

of the patient, prior treatment, and altered renal or hepatic function can influence the outcome of chemotherapy.

When dosage of antineoplastic agents is based on weight, children tolerate relatively larger doses of drugs than do older patients. Dosage may be more accurately calculated in adults and children using body surface area; mg/kg doses may be conveniently converted to mg/m^2 doses by multiplying by 40.

Although a variety of drugs are employed in cancer chemotherapy, a number of nursing considerations are common to all antineoplastic drugs; these are outlined below. Specific interventions and considerations pertaining to individual drugs are given with the respective discussions of each group.

General Nursing Management—Antineoplastic Drugs

Nursing Interventions

Medication Administration

Avoid skin or eye contact and inhalation of vapors or powders when handling cytotoxic drugs. Protective gloves should be worn, particularly when working with solutions, because many of these drugs are potent vesicants and all are potential carcinogens. Guidelines for handling cytotoxic drugs have been published by several national agencies.

Assess administration site frequently for earliest signs of extravasation if cytotoxic drugs are given IV. Certain agents cause thrombophlebitis and severe tissue necrosis; among these are carmustine, dacarbazine, dactinomycin, daunorubicin, doxorubicin, etoposide, mechlorethamine, mithramycin, mitomycin, streptozocin, vinblastine, and vincristine. The following guidelines are recommended to reduce the risk of extravasation and to treat it:

To reduce the risk of extravasation:

- Choose a vein that travels a straight course long enough to accept the length of the needle. Veins of the dorsum of the hand, ventral surface of the forearm, or antecubital fossa are preferred.
- Avoid bruised, sclerosed, or inflamed veins and veins that travel through hematomas or ecchymotic areas.
- Avoid using an arm where axillary node dissection has been performed or an arm affected by the superior vena cava syndrome.
- Alternate sites of drug administration.
- Use 21-, 23- or 25-gauge butterfly needle, when possible, because it can be secured easily and causes minimal irritation. The small needle is easy to position, and the presence of blood return can be noted in the tubing.
- Allow for visualization of the injection site, the proximal portion of the butterfly tubing, and the surrounding area, including most of the arm, when securing a butterfly catheter or tubing.
- Always check needle position and flow by administering 5 to 10 mL normal saline before injecting cytotoxic agent.
- Administer drug by slow, steady IV push or by IV infusion through injection port of tubing.
- Flush tubing and vein with 5 to 10 mL normal saline after administration of drug.
- Instruct patient to immediately report any discomfort or other unusual sensation.
- Stop injection immediately and administer drug through another site if there is any doubt about patency of vein (eg, redness, swelling).

To treat extravasation:

- Stop infusion. Leave needle in place.
- Aspirate as much of drug as possible.
- Administer specific antidote, if available.
- Administer 100 to 200 mg hydrocortisone *or* 4 mg dexamethasone through the *same* needle.
- Inject 1% to 2% lidocaine into area to reduce pain (optional).
- Apply ice packs for 24 to 36 hours.
- Apply warm, moist compresses after the first 24 to 36 hours. Check site frequently.
- Elevate injection site above the level of the heart.
- Tissue necrosis may be treated by surgically excising the ulcer and covering the wound with a xenograft (usually pigskin) for 48 to 72 hours. The xenograft is then replaced by a split-thickness skin graft, and the extremity is immobilized for 5 to 7 days.

Obtain patient's *lean* body weight. Medication dosages should be calculated on this basis, particularly if patient is obese or has edema or ascites. Dosages should, however, be adjusted, wherever possible, to account for clinical response and development of adverse reactions.

Implement nursing interventions to prevent or minimize bleeding if platelet count is low. Avoid giving injections.

Collaborate with dietitian, practitioner, patient, and family to plan measures to help maintain or attain optimal nutritional status. In addition to the usual reasons for concern with nutritional status, therapy is most successful when the patient is well nourished.

Implement nursing interventions to prevent or minimize nausea and vomiting. Highly emetogenic drugs include cisplatin, dacarbazine, dactinomycin, mechlorethamine, and streptozocin. With these drugs, as well as many others, it is often necessary to give an effective dose of an appropriate antiemetic drug 30 to 60 minutes before the antineoplastic agent is administered. Bland food or antacids given before administration of an oral agent may reduce nausea and vomiting caused by local irritation, but the presence of food in the stomach may impair absorption of some agents.

Inform practitioner if patient vomits after receiving an oral antineoplastic agent. If the medication was not absorbed, a dosage adjustment may be required.

Be prepared to assist with one of the following procedures to minimize hair loss if medication is given by IV push and if widely metastatic tumors (ie, leukemia) are *not* being treated: 1) apply scalp tourniquet before drug administration and retain for at least 5 minutes afterwards; 2) apply ice compress to scalp 15 minutes before and for 30 minutes after drug administration.

Be prepared to administer antihistamines, steroids, epinephrine, and oxygen to treat hypersensitivity reaction.

Surveillance During Therapy

Monitor results of blood, liver, and renal studies, which should be performed before initiation of therapy and periodically during therapy, to assess the effectiveness and toxicity of therapy. The frequency at which studies are done varies with the agent or agents used and the patient's clinical status.

Frequently assess patient for signs of developing myelosuppression (unusual bleeding or bruising, fever, sore throat, mucosal ulceration, weakness).

Check patient's temperature frequently, especially if the granulocyte count is very low, because susceptibility to infection is increased by these drugs. If potential for rectal irritation exists, avoid taking the temperature rectally, because thermometer may irritate rectal mucosa.

Inspect patient's mouth frequently, particularly for evidence of stomatitis or infection.

Place patient in protective isolation and monitor carefully for signs of infection if bone marrow depression becomes severe.

Assess patient's hepatic status frequently for signs of developing dysfunction (jaundice, yellowing of eyes, hepatomegaly, anorexia, right hypochondriac tenderness, clay-colored stools, dark urine).

Assess patient's pulmonary status frequently for signs of possible pulmonary fibrosis (fever, cough, shortness of breath).

Be alert for indications of CNS toxicity (dizziness, headache, convulsions, confusion, fatigue, slurred speech, paresthesias).

Assess patient frequently for loss of taste and for tingling in face, fingers, or toes, symptoms of possible peripheral neuropathy.

Monitor patient for indications of hyperuricemia (swelling of feet or lower legs, joint pain, stomach pain), which can lead to uric acid nephropathy.

Observe patient for rash or dermatitis, which may signal drug hypersensitivity.

Provide appropriate emotional support. Involve other health team members, patient, and patient's significant others in nursing care plans to ensure consistency and continuity of care.

Ensure that patient has opportunities to privately discuss self-concept, body image, and sexuality. Many anticancer drugs cause both subjective and objective changes that elicit widespread alterations in feelings about self.

Monitor intake and output, and collaborate with patient to develop plan to maintain fluid intake at 2 to 3 L/day to ensure that urine output is adequate for drug excretion, to prevent dehydration related to excessive vomiting, and to minimize risks of hyperuricemia and uric acid nephropathy.

Use appropriate interventions for mouth care. Anorexia, nausea and vomiting, xerostomia, increased risk of dental caries, bleeding tendencies, heightened susceptibility to infection, and numerous other potential problems need to be considered. Soft-bristled toothbrushes, special mouth rinses, avoidance of certain foods (tart, spicy, hot, rough-textured), and use, when prescribed, of antifungal agents formulated for intraoral use to treat fungal overgrowth of the mouth all may be helpful, depending on the patient's condition.

Patient Teaching

Instruct patient to notify prescriber if a dose of medication is missed. The next dose should not be doubled; instead, the regular dosing schedule should be resumed.

Explain that drug effects may not become manifest for several weeks.

Stress the importance of adhering to prescribed regimen and avoiding all nonprescribed drugs, including over-the-counter (OTC) medications.

Discuss the importance of observing for development of side effects and informing appropriate care provider if they occur.

Reassure patient that dosage adjustment can often reduce incidence and severity of untoward reactions.

Inform patient that alopecia may occur, but that it is transient. Encourage use of wigs, scarves, and hats until normal regrowth occurs, usually 4 to 8 weeks after therapy ends. Transient regrowth may occur during therapy, but hair is often of a different texture, and color will be lost as therapy continues.

Counsel male or female patient regarding the possibility of birth defects or sterility, which can occur after therapy is terminated as well as during therapy.

Alkylating Agents

The alkylating agents were developed during the 1940s as a result of research on chemical warfare agents, notably the mustard gases. Of these compounds, the nitrogen mustards were found to have a marked cytotoxic action on lymphoid tissue, and clinical research was then initiated that led to development of chemically related derivatives.

The alkylating agents used in chemotherapy may be divided into six different chemical groups as follows:

Nitrogen mustards: chlorambucil, cyclophosphamide, ifosfamide, mechlorethamine, melphalan, uracil mustard
Ethylenimines: thiotepa
Alkyl sulfonates: busulfan
Triazenes: dacarbazine
Nitrosoureas: carmustine, lomustine, streptozocin
Miscellaneous alkylator-like agents: carboplatin, cisplatin, pipobroman

The alkylating agents are discussed as a group, and then individual drugs are listed in Table 74-3.

Mechanism

Alkylating agents are polyfunctional compounds that produce highly reactive carbonium ions that form covalent linkages with nucleophilic centers such as amino, carboxyl, hydroxyl, imidazole, phosphate, and sulfhydryl groups. The most important site of alkylation is the number 7 nitrogen in the purine base guanine. This may cause cross-linking of DNA strands and miscoding of the genetic message, resulting in abnormal base pairing. Destruction of the guanine ring and DNA chain breakage ensues, inhibiting DNA replication, transcription of RNA, and normal nucleic acid function. Cross-linking of DNA strands thus appears to be the major cytotoxic effect of the alkylating agents.

Uses

Refer to Table 74-3

Dosage

Refer to Table 74-3

Fate

The oral agents busulfan, chlorambucil, cyclophosphamide, lomustine, melphalan, pipobroman, and uracil mustard generally exhibit rapid absorption, but melphalan and uracil mustard may be incompletely absorbed. All alkylating agents are widely distributed throughout the body and exhibit some protein binding. Carmustine and lomustine are rapidly transported across the blood–brain barrier. Most agents are metabolized in the liver to inactivate metabolites; however, cyclophosphamide and ifosfamide must be metabolized to become active. All alkylating agents are eliminated by way of the kidney as both inactive metabolites and unchanged drug.

Common Side Effects

Myelosuppression (leukopenia, thrombocytopenia, anemia), nausea, vomiting, and anorexia

Cisplatin: nephrotoxicity and hyperuricemia
Cyclophosphamide: gonadal suppression
Streptozocin: nephrotoxicity

Significant Adverse Reactions

(Not all reactions observed with all drugs)

GI: diarrhea, abdominal cramping, stomatitis, glossitis, colitis
Renal: hyperuricemia, uric acid nephropathy, hemorrhagic cystitis (especially ifosfamide)
Hypersensitivity: dermatitis, maculopapular skin eruption, urticaria, fever, alopecia, pruritus, facial edema, anaphylacticlike reaction, erythema multiforme
Neurologic: headache, confusion, tinnitus, weakness, ataxia, peripheral neuropathies, dizziness, paralysis, depression, hyperactivity, convulsions
Respiratory: pulmonary fibrosis, dyspnea, wheezing
CV: tachycardia, hypotension, flushing, sweating
Other: hepatic dysfunction, jaundice, hepatitis, gynecomastia, impotence, myxedema, myalgia, metallic taste, melanoderma, hyperpigmentation, pain at IV injection site or along vein

CAUTION

All alkylating agents have been shown to be teratogenic and/or carcinogenic (owing to a direct cellular action or immunosuppression) and to cause testicular and ovarian suppression.

Contraindications

Leukopenia, thrombocytopenia or anemia caused by previous chemotherapy or radiation therapy, hepatotoxicity, renal toxicity, and known hypersensitivity

Interactions

The toxicity of *chlorambucil* and *cyclophosphamide* may be increased when used concurrently with barbiturates, chloral hydrate, or phenytoin, because of induction of liver microsomal enzymes.
Cisplatin used concurrently with aminoglycosides may increase nephrotoxicity and ototoxicity.
Allopurinol and chloramphenicol may increase the toxicity of *cyclophosphamide*.
Corticosteroids may decrease the activity of *cyclophosphamide* by inhibiting microsomal enzymes.
Cyclophosphamide and *thiotepa* may decrease serum pseudocholinesterase and thereby enhance the effect of succinylcholine.
Cyclophosphamide used concurrently with daunorubicin or doxorubicin may increase cardiotoxicity.
Dacarbazine may potentiate the activity of allopurinol by inhibiting xanthine oxidase.
The metabolism of *dacarbazine* may be enhanced by phenobarbital and phenytoin because of induction of liver microsomal enzymes.
Most *alkylating agents* may antagonize the effects of antigout medications by increasing serum uric acid levels; dosage adjustments of the antigout medications may be necessary.
Alkylating agents cause immunosuppression, which may result in a generalized vaccinia after immunization with smallpox vaccine.
Corticosteroids used concurrently with *streptozocin* may increase the hyperglycemic effect of *streptozocin*.

(text continues on page 760)

Table 74-3. Alkylating Agents

<table>
<tr><th>Drug</th><th>Usual Dosage Range</th><th>Uses</th><th>Nursing Considerations</th></tr>
<tr><td>Busulfan
Myleran</td><td>Adults
Initially: 4–12 mg/day
Maintenance: 2 mg once or twice a week to 1–4 mg/day
Children
Induction: 0.06–0.12 mg/kg/day or 1.8–4.6 mg/m^2/day</td><td>Chronic myelogenous leukemia (DOC)
Polycythemia vera</td><td>May increase uric acid levels in blood and urine; pulmonary fibrosis usually occurs with long-term therapy—onset after 8 mo–10 yr (average, 4 yr); treatment is usually unsatisfactory and death usually occurs within 6 mo of diagnosis; can induce severe bone marrow hypoplasia</td></tr>
<tr><td>Camustine (BCNU)
BiCNU</td><td>75–100 mg/m^2 by IV infusion over 1–2 h for 2 consecutive days or 200 mg/m^2 in a single dose no more frequently than every 6–8 wk
A suggested guide for subsequent dosage adjustment is the following:
<table>
<tr><th colspan="2">Nadir after Prior Dose</th><th>% of Prior Dose to be Given</th></tr>
<tr><th>Leukocytes</th><th>Platelets</th><th></th></tr>
<tr><td>Above 4000</td><td>Above 100,000</td><td>100%</td></tr>
<tr><td>3000–3999</td><td>75,000–99,999</td><td>100%</td></tr>
<tr><td>2000–2999</td><td>25,000–74,999</td><td>70%</td></tr>
<tr><td>Below 2000</td><td>Below 25,000</td><td>50%</td></tr>
</table></td><td>Brain tumors (DOC)
Multiple myeloma (in combination with prednisone)
Hodgkin's disease (in combination with other approved drugs in patients who experience relapse while on primary therapy or fail to respond to the primary therapy)
Non-Hodgkin's lymphomas (in combination with other drugs; see above)
May also be useful in Burkitt's tumor, Ewing's sarcoma, malignant melanoma (in combination with vincristine), in hepatic carcinoma when given by intraarterial injection, and in mycosis fungoides</td><td>Unopened vials of dry powder must be stored under refrigeration—oily film on bottom of the vial is sign of decomposition, and vial should be discarded; preparation of solution: dissolve contents of vial with 3 mL absolute alcohol diluent and then add 27 mL sterile water for injection—resulting solution contains 3.3 mg/mL; further dilution in 500 mL 0.5% dextrose or 0.9% sodium chloride results in a solution stable for 48 h when refrigerated and protected from light; contact with skin may cause transient hyperpigmentation; may increase bilirubin, alkaline phosphatase, AST, and BUN levels; a 0.1–0.4% solution in 95% alcohol applied topically 1–2 times/day for 2 wk has been used to treat mycosis fungoides; pulmonary fibrosis and pneumonitis occur, primarily with high cumulative dose (1200–1400 mg/m^2) or long-term therapy (5 mo), but also may occur with short-term, low-dose therapy</td></tr>
<tr><td>Carboplatin
Paraplatin</td><td>360 mg/m^2 by infusion over 15 min–1 h; repeat every 4 wk
A suggested guide for subsequent dosage adjustment is the following:
<table>
<tr><th colspan="2">Nadir after Prior Dose</th><th>% of Prior Dose to be Given</th></tr>
<tr><th>Neutrophils</th><th>Platelets</th><th></th></tr>
<tr><td>Above 2000</td><td>Above 100,000</td><td>125%</td></tr>
<tr><td>500–2000</td><td>50,000–100,000</td><td>100%</td></tr>
<tr><td>Below 500</td><td>Below 50,000</td><td>75%</td></tr>
</table>
<table>
<tr><th colspan="2">Renal Impairment</th></tr>
<tr><th>Creatinine Clearance</th><th>Dose</th></tr>
<tr><td>41–59 mL/min</td><td>250 mg/m2</td></tr>
<tr><td>16–40 mL/min</td><td>200 mg/m2</td></tr>
</table></td><td>Palliative treatment of ovarian carcinoma
May also be useful in small cell and non-small cell lung carcinoma and head and neck tumors</td><td>To prepare solution, dissolve contents of vials in sterile water for injection, 5% dextrose, or 0.9% sodium chloride; solutions are stable for 8 h at room temperature; do not use needles, IV sets, or other equipment containing aluminum, as drug may form a precipitate with loss of potency; drug may be used in patients previously treated with cisplatin; no pre- or posttreatment hydration or forced diuresis is required; reduce dosage in patients with impaired kidney function</td></tr>
<tr><td>Chlorambucil
Leukeran</td><td>Adults
Initially: 0.1–0.2 mg/kg/day for 3–6 wk (4–12 mg/day for the average patient)
Maintenance: 2–6 mg/day, not to exceed 0.1 mg/kg/day; may be as low as 0.03 mg/kg/day
Macroglobulinemia: 2–10 mg/day or 8 mg/m^2/day for 10 days; repeat every 6–8 wk</td><td>Chronic lymphocytic leukemia (DOC)
Malignant lymphomas
Hodgkin's disease
Choriocarcinoma
Ovarian carcinoma
Breast carcinoma
Macroglobulinemia
Nephrotic syndrome
Uveitis (intractable, idiopathic)</td><td>Give dose 1 h before breakfast or 2 h after evening meal; may increase serum and urine uric acid levels; can severely depress bone marrow function; teratogenic in humans; sterility has occurred in both sexes</td></tr>
</table>

(continued)

Table 74-3. **Alkylating Agents (Continued)**

Drug	Usual Dosage Range	Uses	Nursing Considerations
	Nephrotic syndrome: 0.1–0.2 mg/kg/day for 8–12 wk Uveitis: 0.1 mg/kg/day *Children* 0.1–0.2 mg/kg/day *or* 4.5 mg/m²/day		
Cisplatin *Platinol, Platinol-AQ*	*As a single agent* 100 mg/m² IV once every 4 wk *Testicular tumors* 20 mg/m² IV for 5 days every 3 wk for 3 courses *in combination with* Bleomycin: 30 U IV on day 2 of each week for 12 doses and Vinblastine: 0.15 mg/kg–0.2 mg/kg IV on days 1 and 2 of each week every 3 wk for 4 courses Maintenance for patients who respond: vinblastine 0.2 mg/kg IV every 4 wk for 2 yr *Ovarian tumors* 50 mg/m² IV once every 3 wk on day 1 *in combination with* Doxorubicin: 50 mg/m² IV once every 3 wk on day 1 A repeat dose should not be given until serum creatinine is below 1.5 mg/dL or BUN is below 25 mg/dL, platelets are over 100,000/mm³, and WBCs are over 4000/mm³ *Advanced bladder carcinoma* 50 mg to 70 mg/m² IV once every 3–4 wk; patients receiving prior radiation or chemotherapy should start at 50 mg/m² IV once every 4 wk *Non-small cell lung carcinoma* 75 mg–120 mg/m² IV once every 3–6 wk *Neuroblastoma and osteosarcoma in children* 90 mg/m² IV once every 3 wk *or* 30 mg/m² IV once weekly Renal Impairment Creatinine Clearance — Dosage 10–50 mL/min — 75% usual dose < 10 mL/min — 50% usual dose	Metastatic testicular tumors (DOC) Metastatic ovarian tumors (DOC) Lymphoma Squamous cell carcinoma of head and neck Advanced bladder carcinoma (DOC) Cervical cancer (DOC) Prostatic carcinoma Non-small cell lung carcinoma Neuroblastoma Osteosarcoma	Preparation of solution: dissolve contents of vial in 10 mL sterile water for injection; solution is stable for 20 h at room temperature—do *not* refrigerate; hydrate patient with 1–2 L fluid infused over 8–12 h before treatment; dilute drug in 1–2 L 5% dextrose in 0.3% or 0.45% saline containing 37.5 g mannitol, and infuse over 6–8 h; maintain urinary output of 100 mL/h for 24 h after therapy to reduce danger of nephrotoxicity; do *not* use needles, IV sets, or equipment containing aluminum to administer cisplatin—a black precipitate of platinum will form; may increase BUN, serum creatinine, AST, and serum uric acid levels; may decrease creatinine clearance and serum calcium, magnesium, and potassium levels; high-frequency hearing loss may occur in one or both ears, more commonly in children
Cyclophosphamide *Cytoxan, Neosar*	*Oral* Adult: 1–5 mg/kg/day Children: induction: 2–8 mg/kg *or* 60–250 mg/m² for 6 or more days Maintenance: 2–5 mg/kg or 50–150 mg/m² twice a week *IV* Adult: induction—40–50 mg/kg in divided doses over 2–5 days. Maintenance: 10–15 mg/kg every 7–10 days *or* 3–5 mg/kg twice a week *or* 1.5–3 mg/kg daily	Hodgkin's disease Non-Hodgkin's lymphomas (DOC) Follicular lymphomas Lymphocytic lymphosarcoma Reticulum cell sarcoma Lymphoblastic lymphosarcoma Burkitt's lymphoma (DOC) Multiple myeloma (DOC) Leukemias: Chronic lymphocytic leukemia Chronic granulocytic leukemia Acute myelogenous and monocytic leukemia	To prepare solution: Reconstitute with sterile water for injection or bacteriostatic water for injection (paraben preserved only); use 5 mL for the 100-mg vial, 10 mL for the 200-mg vial, 25 mL for the 500-mg vial, 50 mL for the 1-g vial, and 100 mL for the 2-g vial; lyophilized powder dissolves much more quickly than regular powder; solution is stable for 24 h at room temperature or 6 days refrigerated; may be given IM, IV push, intra-

(*continued*)

Table 74-3. **Alkylating Agents (Continued)**

Drug	*Usual Dosage Range*	*Uses*	*Nursing Considerations*
	Children: induction—2–8 mg/kg *or* 60–250 mg/m² in divided doses for 6 or more days; Maintenance: 10–15 mg/kg every 7–10 days *or* 30 mg/kg every 3–4 wk Reduce induction dose by 1/3–1/2 in patients with bone marrow depression Hepatic impairment: bilirubin 3.1–5.0 mg/dL or SGOT > 180, reduce dose by 25%; bilirubin > 5.0 mg/dL omit dose Renal impairment: GFR < 10 mL/min, decrease dose by 50% Immunosuppressant nephrotic syndrome: 2–2.5 mg/kg/day Rheumatoid arthritis: 1.5–3 mg/kg/day	Acute lymphoblastic leukemia Mycosis fungoides Neuroblastoma (DOC) Adenocarcinoma of ovary (DOC) Retinoblastoma (DOC) Carcinoma of breast or lung (DOC) Ewing's sarcoma (DOC) Other uses: Prevent transplant rejection Rheumatoid arthritis Nephrotic syndrome Systemic lupus erythematosus	peritoneally, intrapleurally, or by IV infusion in 5% dextrose, 5% dextrose in 0.9% saline; may suppress positive reactions to skin tests; may increase uric acid levels of urine and serum; may produce false-positive Pap test; secondary malignancies have been observed, most frequently of the urinary bladder; may cause syndrome of inappropriate antidiuretic hormone secretion (SIADH); manifested as tiredness, weakness, confusion, agitation; an oral solution may be prepared by dissolving the powder for injection in aromatic elixir to a concentration of 1–5 mg/mL—refrigerate and use within 14 days; tablets contain tartrazine
Dacarbazine *DTIC-Dome*	IV: 2–4.5 mg/kg/day for 10 days, repeated every 28 days *or* 250 mg/m²/day for 5 days, repeated every 21 days	Metastatic malignant melanoma (DOC) Hodgkin's disease Investigational uses include: Soft tissue sarcomas Neuroblastoma	To prepare solution: Add 9.9 mL sterile water for injection to 100 mg vial *or* 19.7 mL sterile water for injection to 200-mg vial, giving a concentration of 10 mg/mL; solution, colorless or clear yellow in color, is stable 8 h at room temperature or 72 h refrigerated, and protected from light—a change in color to pink indicates decomposition; may be given by IV push over 1 min *or* by IV infusion over 30 min, diluted in 250 mL 5% dextrose in water or 0.9% sodium chloride; severe pain along injected vein can occur—dilute drug, infuse slowly, and avoid extravasation; may increase alkaline phosphatase, BUN, AST, ALT
Ifosfamide *Ifex*	IV: 1.2 g/m²/day for 5 days; repeat every 21 days *or* when leukocytes are more than 4,000 and platelets are more than 100,000	Germ cell testicular cancer *Other uses*: Lung, breast, ovarian, pancreatic, and gastric cancer; acute leukemias (except AML) and malignant lymphoma	To prepare solution: Use 20 mL sterile water for injection *or* bacteriostatic water for injection; solutions are stable for 1 wk at room temperature or up to 3 wk when refrigerated; solutions may be further diluted in 5% dextrose, 0.9% saline, lactated Ringer's solution, or sterile water for injection and are stable up to 6 wk when refrigerated; to prevent bladder toxicity (gross hematuria, hemorrhagic cystitis), patient should be hydrated with 2 L oral or IV fluid daily; incidence of hemorrhagic cystitis may be reduced by IV administration of mesna (Mesnex) in a dosage equal to 20% of the ifosfamide dose, given with ifosfamide and again at 4 and 8 h after ifosfamide
Lomustine (CCNU) *CeeNU*	*Oral* Adults and children: 100–130 mg/	Brain tumors (DOC) Hodgkin's disease	May cause transient elevation of liver function tests; available as a

(*continued*)

Table 74-3. **Alkylating Agents (Continued)**

Drug	Usual Dosage Range	Uses	Nursing Considerations
	m^2 as a single dose, repeated every 6 wk A suggested guide for subsequent dosage adjustment is the following: Nadir after Prior Dose — Leukocytes / Platelets / % of Prior Dose to be Given: Above 4000 / Above 100,000 / 100% 3000–3999 / 75,000–99,999 / 75%–100% 2000–2999 / 25,000–74,999 / 50%–75% Below 2000 / Below 25,000 / 0–50%	Investigational uses include: Lung and breast carcinoma Malignant melanoma Multiple myeloma Gastrointestinal carcinoma Renal cell carcinoma	dose pack containing two 10-mg capsules, two 40-mg capsules, and two 100-mg capsules
Mechlorethamine (Nitrogen Mustard, HN_2) *Mustargen*	IV: 0.4 mg/kg as a single dose *or* in divided doses of 0.1–0.2 mg/kg/day; repeat every 3–6 wk Intracavitary: 0.4 mg/kg diluted in 50–100 mL 0.9% saline; 0.2 mg/kg may be used intrapericardially Ointment and solution: apply once daily (up to 4 times/day in severe cases) to entire skin surface for 6–12 mo until response has occurred, then every 2–7 days for up to 3 yr	Hodgkin's disease (DOC) Lymphosarcoma Chronic myelocytic and lymphocytic leukemia Bronchogenic carcinoma Polycythemia vera Mycosis fungoides (DOC) Intracavitary injection to control malignant effusions	Do *not* use drug if vial contains water droplets before reconstitution. To prepare solution: Reconstitute with 10 mL sterile water for injection or 0.9% sodium chloride injection; use immediately; discard unused portion after neutralizing with aqueous solution containing equal parts of 5% sodium bicarbonate and 5% sodium thiosulfate; any equipment used for administration (gloves, tubing, glassware) should be neutralized for 45 min in this solution; avoid inhalation of powder or vapors; avoid contact with skin or mucous membranes—if contact occurs, wash 15 min with water, followed by 2% sodium thiosulfate solution; administer IV dose by injection into tubing of running IV; change position of patient every 5–10 min for 1 h after intracavitary injection. A topical solution may be prepared by dissolving 10 mg in 20–60 mL water or sodium chloride and made fresh daily; an ointment may be prepared (0.01%–0.04%) by dissolving drug in absolute alcohol and mixing into an anhydrous ointment base; use protective gloves to apply topical preparations; use minimal application to perineum, axillary, inguinal, inframammary areas, and inside bends of elbows and backs of knees
Melphalan (L-PAM, Phenylalanine Mustard, L-Sarcolysin) *Alkeran*	0.15 mg/kg/day for 7 days followed by a rest period of 2–6 wk, then 0.05 mg/kg/day maintenance *or* 0.1–0.15 mg/kg/day for 2–3 wk *or* 0.25 mg/kg/day for 4 days followed by a rest period of 2–4 wk, then 2–4 mg/day maintenance *or* 0.2 mg/kg/day for 5 days followed by a rest period of 4–5 wk (for ovarian carcinoma) *or* 7 mg/m^2/day for 5 days every 5–6 wk	Multiple myeloma (DOC) Malignant melanoma Breast, lung, and ovarian carcinoma Testicular seminoma Reticulum cell and osteogenic sarcoma Polycythemia vera Amyloidosis	May increase uric acid levels in blood and urine; acute, nonlymphatic leukemia has developed in some patients with multiple myeloma treated with melphalan; benefit/risk ratio must be determined on an individual basis

(*continued*)

Table 74-3. **Alkylating Agents (Continued)**

Drug	*Usual Dosage Range*	*Uses*	*Nursing Considerations*
Pipobroman *Vercyte*	Polycythemia vera: 1 mg/kg/day for 30 days, then increase to 1.5–3 mg/kg/day if no response. Maintenance—0.1–0.2 mg/kg/day when hematocrit has been reduced to 50%–55% Chronic myelocytic leukemia: 1.5–2.5 mg/kg/day until leukocyte count approaches 10,000, then maintenance dose of 7–175 mg/day as required	Polycythemia vera Chronic myelocytic leukemia (resistant to other therapy)	May increase uric acid levels in blood and urine; may increase serum potassium. *Not* recommended for children younger than 15 yr
Streptozocin *Zanosar*	IV: 500 mg/m²/day for 5 consecutive days every 4–6 wk *or* 1 g/m² once a week for 2 wk; thereafter, dosage may be increased to a maximum of 1.5 g/m² weekly for 2–4 wk; may be given by rapid IV injection, short infusion (10–15 min), long infusion (6 h), or continuous 5-day infusion Renal impairment: 50%–75% of usual dose based on creatinine clearance	Metastatic islet cell carcinoma of the pancreas (DOC) Advanced Hodgkin's disease Investigational use: Malignant carcinoid tumors, palliative treatment of metastatic colorectal cancer	Dry powder must be stored under refrigeration and protected from light; preparation of solution; reconstitute with 9.5 mL 5% dextrose in water or 0.9% sodium chloride; solution is stable for 12 h at room temperature; solution is preservative-free and should *not* be used for more than one dose; a change in color from pale gold to brown indicates decomposition; adequate patient hydration may reduce renal toxicity; hypophosphatemia may be first sign of renal toxicity
Triethylenethiophosphoramide *Thiotepa*	IV: 0.3–0.4 mg/kg at 1–2 wk intervals, *or* 0.5 mg/kg every 1–4 wk, *or* 0.2 mg/kg/day for 5 days repeated every 2–4 wk; may be given by IV push Local, intratumor: 0.6–0.8 mg/kg; maintenance dose, 0.07–0.8 mg/kg every 1–4 wk Intracavitary: 0.6–0.8 mg/kg diluted in 10–20 mL 0.9% saline Bladder instillation: 30–60 mg at weekly intervals diluted in 30–60 mL sterile water for injection; patient should retain for 2 h with frequent repositioning; repeat once weekly for 4 wk; volume may be reduced to 30 mL if discomfort occurs Intrathecal (investigational): 1–10 mg/m² 1 or 2 times/wk (1 mg/mL)	Superficial papillary carcinoma of the urinary bladder (DOC) Adenocarcinoma of the breast and ovary Intracavitary injection to control malignant effusions Lymphomas Investigational uses: Malignant meningeal neoplasms	Dry powder must be stored under refrigeration. To prepare solution: Reconstitute with 1.5 mL sterile water for injection; solution should be clear to slightly opaque—if *grossly* opaque, discard; solution is stable 5 days under refrigeration; compatible with procaine 2% and epinephrine HCl 1:1,000 for local injection; dehydrate patients 8–12 h before bladder instillation; may increase uric acid levels in blood and urine; has been used IM, although not approved by the FDA
Uracil Mustard	Initially 1–2 mg/day until improvement or bone marrow depression occurs; then 1 mg/day for 3 out of 4 wk maintenance *or* Initially 3–5 mg/day for 7 days not to exceed 0.5 mg/kg during this period, then 1 mg/day for 3 out of 4 wk maintenance	Chronic lymphocytic leukemia Non-Hodgkin's lymphomas Chronic myelocytic leukemia Polycythemia vera (early stage) Mycosis fungoides	May increase uric acid levels in blood and urine; total dosage of 1 mg/kg greatly increases the risk of irreversible bone marrow depression; capsules contain tartrazine

DOC, drug of choice

Streptozocin should not be used concurrently with nephrotoxic medications such as aminoglycoside antibiotics, cephalothin, cisplatin, or polymyxins.
Phenytoin may protect pancreatic beta cells from the cytotoxic effects of *streptozocin*, thus reducing its therapeutic effect in patients with islet cell tumors.
Myelosuppression caused by *carmustine* may be enhanced by cimetidine.
Carmustine and *cyclophosphamide* may decrease the effects of digoxin by decreasing its GI absorption.
Carmustine and *cisplatin* may decrease the effects of phenytoin.
Cisplatin used concurrently with loop diuretics (bumetanide, ethacrynic acid, furosemide) may increase the ototoxicity of both drugs.
Cyclophosphamide may increase the effects of succinylcholine, resulting in periods of prolonged respiratory depression.
Carboplatin may potentiate the renal effects of other nephrotoxic drugs.

NOTE: Ifosfamide is a new antineoplastic agent with no reported drug interactions at this time. Because of its structural similarity to cyclophosphamide, however, drug interactions similar to those seen with cyclophosphamide may occur when using ifosfamide.

Nursing Management

Refer to general discussion of nursing considerations for all antineoplastic drugs. In addition:

Nursing Interventions

Medication Administration

Monitor patient for tachycardia, hypotension, or shortness of breath, when administering carboplatin, cisplatin, or mechlorethamine, because anaphylactoid reactions, which necessitate supportive measures, can occur.
Check patient receiving cyclophosphamide or ifosfamide for hematuria or dysuria. Withhold drug and notify practitioner at first sign of hemorrhagic cystitis.
Closely monitor patient receiving first dose of streptozocin for signs of hypoglycemia caused by sudden release of insulin. Have IV dextrose available.

Surveillance During Therapy

Assess auditory function frequently if patient is receiving cisplatin or mechlorethamine. Tinnitus or impaired hearing may signal ototoxicity. Periodic audiometric testing is recommended.
Work with patient in planning to maintain adequate hydration to reduce risk of hemorrhagic cystitis if cyclophosphamide or ifosfamide is prescribed. Give drug early in morning to prevent accumulation in bladder during night.

Antimetabolites

The *antimetabolites* are structural analogues of normally occurring metabolites that interfere with the synthesis of nucleic acids by competing with purines or pyrimidines in metabolic pathways. The antimetabolites themselves also may be incorporated into nucleic acids, resulting in a cell product that fails to function. Antimetabolites act during the S phase of the cell cycle (see Introduction). They can be divided into three groups: folic acid antagonists (methotrexate), purine antagonists (mercaptopurine, thioguanine), and pyrimidine antagonists (floxuridine, fluorouracil, cytarabine, fludarabine). They are considered here as a group, then listed individually in Table 74-4.

Mechanism

Folic acid antagonists bind to the enzyme dihydrofolate reductase, thereby preventing reduction of folic acid to tetrahydrofolic acid. This limits the availability of one-carbon fragments necessary for purine and thymidine synthesis, thereby blocking DNA synthesis and cell replication.

Purine antagonists are analogues of the natural purines hypoxanthine, guanine, and adenine. These agents must be metabolized to active nucleotides that then can interfere with the synthesis of natural purines, thus preventing normal nucleic acid synthesis.

The *pyrimidine antagonists* floxuridine and fluorouracil compete for the enzyme thymylate synthetase, preventing synthesis of thymidine, an essential substrate of DNA, and thereby blocking DNA synthesis. Cytarabine and fludarabine are metabolized by deoxycytidine kinase to the nucleotide triphosphates (ARA–CTP and 2-fluro-ara-ATP, respectively), which are inhibitors of DNA polymerase, an enzyme necessary for the conversion of RNA into DNA.

Uses

Refer to Table 74-4

Dosage

Refer to Table 74-4

Fate

The oral agents mercaptopurine and methotrexate are well absorbed from the GI tract, whereas thioguanine is poorly absorbed. Cytarabine, fludarabine, and methotrexate are widely distributed and cross the blood–brain barrier. Mercaptopurine and methotrexate are moderately protein bound. All agents are largely metabolized in the liver (except methotrexate) and are excreted by the kidneys as inactive metabolites and unchanged drug. Floxuridine and fluorouracil are also partially eliminated by the lungs as carbon dioxide.

Common Side Effects

Myelosuppression (leukopenia, thrombocytopenia, anemia); nausea, vomiting, diarrhea, stomatitis, glossitis, hepatotoxicity (thioguanine and methotrexate), gastritis (fluorouracil and methotrexate); hyperuricemia, renal toxicity; interstitial pneumonitis; CNS disturbances (methotrexate and fludarabine)

Significant Adverse Reactions

(Not all reactions observed with all drugs)

Dermatologic: skin rash, freckling, dermatitis, hyperpigmentation, alopecia
CNS: ataxia, vertigo, anorexia
Ocular: blurred vision, photophobia, lacrimation
Renal/hepatic: hyperuricemia, uric acid nephropathy, hepatic dysfunction, cholestasis

Table 74-4. **Antimetabolites**

Drug	Usual Dosage Range	Uses	Nursing Considerations
Cytarabine (Cytosine Arabinoside, ARA-C) *Cytosar-U*	*Induction—IV infusion*: 100–200 mg/m²/day *or* 3 mg/kg/day as a continuous IV infusion over 24 h (or in divided doses by rapid IV injection) for 5–10 days and repeated approximately every 2 wk *Maintenance—IM, SC*: 1–1.5 mg/kg once or twice a week at 1–4 wk intervals *or* 70–200 mg/m²/day by rapid IV injection in divided doses or continuous IV infusion for 2–5 days repeated every 30 days *Investigational use for refractory acute myelogenous leukemia*: 2–3 g/m² IV infusion over 1–2 h every 12 h for 4–12 doses Combination therapy: *See* Table 74-8 *Stop therapy* if leukocyte count falls below 1,000 or platelet count below 50,000; resume usually after 5–7 drug-free days and when above levels are reached *Intrathecal injection (investigational)*: 5–75 mg/m² *or* 30–100 mg every 3–7 days or once daily for 4–5 days	Acute myelogenous leukemia (DOC) Also useful for: Acute lymphocytic leukemia Chronic myelogenous leukemia Meningeal leukemia Non-Hodgkin's lymphomas	To prepare solution: Reconstitute vials with bacteriostatic water for injection (0.9% benzyl alcohol) 5 mL/100-mg vial; 10 mL/500-mg vial; 10 mL/1-g vial, 20 mL/2-g vial; use 5–10 mL Elliott's B solution, lactated Ringer's solution, or patient's own cerebrospinal fluid to reconstitute for intrathecal injection; solution may be stored at room temperature for 48 h; discard any hazy or cloudy solution; infusion solutions may be prepared in 0.9% sodium chloride or dextrose 5%; solutions are stable at room temperature for 7 days; reconstitute with smaller volumes (1–2 mL) for SC injection; may increase AST levels and uric acid levels in blood and urine; usual pediatric dose is equivalent to the adult dose; less nausea, vomiting, diarrhea if given IV infusion rather than IV injection, but danger of hematologic toxicity is increased
Floxuridine *FUDR*	Intra-arterial infusion *only*; 0.1–0.6 mg/kg/day by continuous infusion; 0.4–0.6 mg/kg/day for hepatic artery infusion; continue therapy until toxicity occurs, usually 14–21 days, with 2-wk rest between courses	Palliative management of GI adenocarcinoma metastatic to liver, pancreas, or biliary tract Head and neck tumors Also, bladder, breast, cervical, ovarian and prostatic carcinoma	Reconstitute with 5 mL sterile water for injection; solution stable for 14 days under refrigeration; further dilution in 0.9% sodium chloride *or* 5% dextrose is necessary for infusion; dilution is stable for 24 h; may increase serum alkaline phosphatase, LDH, AST, ALT, and bilirubin levels
Fludarabine *Fludara*	*IV infusion*: 25 mg/m² over 30 min daily for 5 days every 28 days	Chronic lymphocytic leukemia Other uses: Non-Hodgkin's lymphoma Macroglobulinemic lymphoma Prolymphocytic leukemia Mycosis fungoides Hairy-cell leukemia Hodgkin's disease	Reconstitute with sterile water for injection; if solution contacts skin, wash thoroughly with soap and water; severe bone marrow depression can occur; large doses are frequently associated with severe neurologic effects, including blindness
Fluorouracil (5-Fluorouracil, 5-FU) *Adrucil*	*Initially*: 12 mg/kg IV injection over 1–2 min once daily for 4 days; maximum daily dose 800 mg; if no toxicity, give 6 mg/kg on days 6, 8, 10, and 12 (For *poor-risk patients*, reduce dose 50%) *Maintenance*: repeat above schedule every 30 days after last day of previous treatment *or* 10–15 mg/kg IV once a week, not to exceed 1 g/wk; dosage based on actual body weight unless patient is obese or has fluid retention *Oral*: 15–20 mg/kg/day for 5–8 days; dilute in water or bicarbonate buffer solution rather than juice	Palliative management of carcinoma of colon, rectum, stomach, and pancreas (DOC) Treatment of breast, ovarian, cervical, and liver carcinomas	Solution may discolor slightly during storage but may still be used safely; crystal precipitate may be redissolved by heating to 60°C—allow to cool to body temperature before using; infusions may be prepared using 0.9% sodium chloride *or* 5% dextrose; solutions are stable for 24 h; incompatible with cytarabine and methotrexate; may increase 5-hydroxyindole acetic acid (5-HIAA) in urine; may decrease plasma albumin; FDA has *not* approved the drug for oral use; oral doses are associated with a very brief clinical response

(continued)

Table 74-4. **Antimetabolites (Continued)**

Drug	Usual Dosage Range	Uses	Nursing Considerations
Mercaptopurine (6-Mercaptopurine, 6-MP) *Purinethol*	*Adults* Initially 2.5 mg/kg *or* 80–100 mg/m² daily in single or divided doses; if no response and no toxicity after 4 wk increase to 5 mg/kg/day *Maintenance*: 1.5–2.5 mg/kg *or* 50–100 mg/m² daily *Children* 2.5 or 75 mg/m² daily (Calculate all doses to nearest 25 mg) *Inflammatory bowel disease* 1.5 mg/kg/day; gradually increase to 2.5 mg/kg/day as necessary	Acute lymphocytic (DOC) and myelogenous leukemia Chronic myelogenous leukemia Other uses: Non-Hodgkin's lymphoma Polycythemia vera Inflammatory bowel disease Psoriatic arthritis	Decrease dose of mercaptopurine to 1/3–1/4 usual dose if given concurrently with allopurinol; may increase uric acid levels in blood and urine; rarely used as a single agent for maintenance of remissions in acute leukemia; may falsely increase serum glucose and uric acid levels when the SMA (sequential multiple analyzer) is used
Methotrexate (MTX) *Folex, Folex-PFS, Methotrexate-LPF, Rheumatrex DosePak*	*Choriocarcinoma*: 15–30 mg/day orally or IM for 5 days; repeat for 3–5 courses with 1–2-wk rest between courses *Leukemia*: induction—3.3 mg/m² IM, IV or orally daily for 4–6 wk combined with prednisone 60 mg/m² daily; maintenance—30 mg/m² orally or IM twice a week *or* 2.5 mg/kg IV every 14 days Children: 20–30 mg/m² orally or IM once a week *Meningeal leukemia*: 10–15 mg/m² intrathecally every 2–5 days; maximum, 15 mg; maximum pediatric dose, 12 mg *Burkitt's lymphoma* Stage I and II: 10–25 mg orally daily for 4–8 days then rest 1 wk Stage III: Up to 1 g/m²/day combined with cyclophosphamide and vincristine *Mycosis fungoides* Oral: 2.5–10 mg/day for weeks or months as needed IM: 50 mg once a week *or* 25 mg twice a week *Psoriasis* Oral: Three schedules may be used: 10–25 mg once a week to a maximum of 50 mg/wk *or* 2.5 mg every 12 h for 3 doses or every 8 h for 4 doses once a week, to a maximum of 30 mg/wk *or* 2.5 mg/day for 5 days, skip 2 days, and repeat; maximum 6.25 mg/day (this schedule may cause increased liver toxicity) IM, IV: 10–25 mg once a week to a maximum of 50 mg/wk *High-dose methotrexate* IV infusion: 100 mg/m²–15 g/m² over 4–24 h every 1–3 wk; follow with calcium leucovorin rescue (see below) *Calcium leucovorin "rescue"* Oral, IV, IM: 10–15 mg/m² every 6 h starting 1–24 h after methotrexate and continue for 24–72 h; (dosage and schedule vary according to protocol and methotrexate dose)	Trophoblastic tumors such as gestational choriocarcinoma, chorioadenoma destruens, or hydatidiform mole (DOC) Acute lymphocytic leukemia (DOC), prophylaxis of meningeal leukemia (DOC), breast, lung, and epidermoid cancers of head and neck, Burkitt's lymphoma (DOC), lymphosarcoma, mycosis fungoides, severe psoriasis, rheumatoid arthritis, osteosarcoma	Monitor urinary chorionic gonadotropin to determine effectiveness of therapy in choriocarcinoma; level should return to less than 50 IU/24 h after 3–4 courses of therapy; use preservative-free solution in treating meningeal leukemia; reconstitute with Elliott's B solution, 0.9% sodium chloride, lactated Ringer's solution, or patient's own cerebrospinal fluid; powders may be reconstituted with sterile water for injection, 0.9% sodium chloride injection, of 5% dextrose in water; solution is stable for 7 days at room temperature but should be used within 24 h because it is not preserved; for high-dose methotrexate therapy use preservative-free solution and dilute in 0.9% sodium chloride or 5% dextrose in water; patient should be well hydrated and urine alkalinized with sodium bicarbonate (3 g every 3 h for 12 h before therapy) to prevent renal toxicity; may increase uric acid levels in blood and urine; CNS toxicity is commonly associated with intrathecal injection; methotrexate is excreted in breast milk; calcium leucovorin is used to "rescue" from high methotrexate doses (see Usual Dosage Range)—dose of calcium leucovorin should be equal to or higher than dose of methotrexate

(continued)

Table 74-4. **Antimetabolites (Continued)**

Drug	Usual Dosage Range	Uses	Nursing Considerations
	Rheumatoid arthritis: 2.5 mg orally every 12 h for 3 doses, *or* 7.5 mg orally as a single dose once a week; may increase to a maximum of 20 mg/wk Alternatively, 7.5–15 mg IM once a week		
Thioguanine *TG, 6-Thioguanine*	*Induction* Adults and children: 2 mg/kg/day, *or* 75–200 mg/m²/day in 1–2 divided doses; may increase to 3 mg/kg/day *Maintenance* Adults and children: 2–3 mg/kg/day *or* 75–400 mg/m²/day Calculate all doses to nearest 20 mg	Acute lymphocytic and myelogenous leukemia (DOC) Chronic myelogenous leukemia	May increase uric acid levels of blood and urine

CV: myocardial ischemia, angina
Hypersensitivity: fever, anaphylaxis, arthralgia
Other: gastrointestinal (GI) ulceration, osteoporosis, pneumonia, thrombophlebitis, cellulitis, Guillain–Barré syndrome

CAUTION

Antimetabolite agents have been shown to be carcinogenic in animal studies and thus may present an oncogenic risk in humans. The antimetabolites are potential mutagens and teratogens and also cause ovarian and testicular suppression.

Contraindications

Leukopenia, thrombocytopenia or anemia caused by previous chemotherapy or radiation therapy; hepatotoxicity; and renal toxicity

In addition, do not use mercaptopurine or thioguanine in a patient who has demonstrated prior resistance to either of the two agents because there is usually complete cross-resistance.

Interactions

Cytarabine and *methotrexate* used concurrently can have either a synergistic or antagonistic effect.

Fluorouracil is incompatible with cytarabine, diazepam, doxorubicin, and methotrexate; complete flushing of IV line between injections is recommended.

The absorption of *fluorouracil* when given orally is decreased by the presence of food.

Concomitant administration of *mercaptopurine* and allopurinol increases both the antineoplastic and toxic effects of mercaptopurine; reduce the dose of mercaptopurine to one-third to one-fourth the usual dose.

Alcohol may enhance the possibility of *methotrexate*-induced hepatotoxicity.

Chloramphenicol, phenylbutazone, phenytoin, para-aminobenzoic acid, salicylates, sulfonamides, and tetracyclines can displace *methotrexate* from binding sites and cause increased toxicity.

Probenecid, salicylates, and nonsteroidal anti-inflammatory agents can block the tubular secretion of *methotrexate* and thus increase its toxicity.

Pyrimethamine used concurrently with *methotrexate* can cause increased toxicity because of similar folic acid antagonist actions.

Concurrent use of high-dose methotrexate and procarbazine may increase the nephrotoxicity of methotrexate.

Methotrexate may enhance the hypoprothrombinemic effect of oral anticoagulants such as warfarin.

Concurrent use of *methotrexate* and asparaginase may block the antineoplastic action of methotrexate by inhibiting cell synthesis; administer asparaginase 9 to 10 days before or within 24 hours after administering methotrexate; the toxic effect of methotrexate also may be reduced.

Vitamin preparations containing folic acid may decrease the effect of *methotrexate*.

Most *antimetabolite agents* may antagonize the effects of antigout medications by increasing serum uric acid levels; dosage adjustments of the antigout medications may be necessary.

Antimetabolite agents cause immunosuppression, which may result in a generalized vaccinia after immunization with smallpox vaccine.

Concurrent use of *fluorouracil* and allopurinol may reduce the hematologic toxicity of fluorouracil.

Mercaptopurine may increase or decrease the anticoagulant effect of warfarin.

Cytarabine and *methotrexate* may decrease the effects of digoxin by impairing its GI absorption; however, absorption from digoxin capsules (Lanoxicaps) may *not* be decreased.

The toxicity of *fluorouracil* and *methotrexate* may be increased when used concurrently with thiazide diuretics.

Mercaptopurine may reverse the effects of nondepolarizing muscle relaxants, such as pancuronium and atracurium.

Mercaptopurine and *methotrexate* may decrease the effects of phenytoin.

The toxic effects of *methotrexate* may be enhanced when used concurrently with etretinate to treat psoriasis.

Nursing Management

Refer to general discussion of nursing considerations for all antineoplastic drugs. In addition:

Nursing Interventions

Medication Administration

Monitor patient for tachycardia, hypotension, and shortness of breath when administering cytarabine or methotrexate, because anaphylactoid reactions, which require supportive measures, can occur.

Do *not* confuse the notations 5-FU, 6-MP, or 6-thioguanine, when administering fluorouracil, mercaptopurine, or thioguanine, which is how these drugs are often written, with the numbers of vials or tablets to be administered. In these instances, these numbers are part of the drug names.

Use an IV infusion pump to administer floxuridine, which is given intraarterially.

Natural Products

The natural products commercially available for use as chemotherapeutic agents include an enzyme, antibiotics, and plant derivatives. Asparaginase, an enzyme isolated from *Escherichia coli*, and pegaspargase, a modified version of asparaginase, are used to treat acute lymphocytic leukemia. Bleomycin, dactinomycin, daunorubicin, doxorubicin, mithramycin, mitomycin, and pentostatin are antineoplastic antibiotics produced from fermentation processes of several different strains of the *Streptomyces* fungus and are used to treat a wide range of malignant diseases. Idarubicin is a synthetic analogue of daunorubicin, and mitoxantrone is a synthetic anthracenedione that is structurally related to the anthracyclines such as daunorubicin and doxorubicin. Vinblastine and vincristine are plant alkaloids isolated from periwinkle (*Vinca rosea*); both agents have a broad spectrum of antitumor activity. Etoposide and teniposide are semisynthetic podophyllotoxins derived from the root of the May apple or mandrake plant (*Podophyllum*) and are used to treat a variety of cancers (Table 74-5). Paclitaxel is a natural product derived from the bark of the Pacific yew tree and used in treating metastatic ovarian cancer as well as a variety of other cancers.

Mechanism

Asparaginase/pegaspargase: Because they lack the enzyme asparagine synthetase, some tumor cells are unable to synthesize asparagine, an amino acid necessary for the synthesis of DNA and essential cellular proteins. Such cells must rely on an exogenous source of asparagine from the bloodstream. The administration of asparaginase or pegaspargase hydrolyzes serum asparagine to aspartic acid, which the tumor cells cannot use. Normal cells are able to synthesize asparagine and are therefore much less affected by the agent.

Antibiotics: The antibiotics work by inhibiting synthesis of DNA or RNA. Bleomycin causes rupture of DNA strands, thereby inhibiting DNA synthesis. Dactinomycin and plicamycin anchor to DNA and inhibit DNA-dependent RNA synthesis. Daunorubicin, doxorubicin, and idarubicin bind to adjoining nucleotide pairs of DNA and inhibit DNA and DNA-dependent RNA synthesis; idarubicin also interacts with the enzyme topoisomerase II. Mitoxantrone inhibits DNA synthesis and possesses cytocidal action on both proliferating and nonproliferating cells. Mitomycin acts like an alkylating agent causing cross-linking between DNA strands, thus inhibiting duplication. Pentostatin inhibits the enzyme adenosine deaminase, especially in malignant T cells, which interferes with DNA synthesis.

Plant derivatives: Vinblastine and vincristine inhibit mitosis during metaphase by binding to or crystallizing microtubular proteins, thus preventing their proper polymerization. At high concentrations, these agents also inhibit DNA-dependent synthesis. Etoposide inhibits mitosis at high concentrations (>10 μg/mL) by causing lysis of cells entering mitosis, and at low concentrations (0.3–10 μg/mL) by inhibiting cells from entering prophase; the net effect is inhibition of DNA synthesis; teniposide has a similar action. Paclitaxel also interferes with normal microtubular function, resulting in inhibition of DNA synthesis

Uses

Refer to Table 74-5

Dosage

Refer to Table 74-5

Fate

All of the natural products are administered parenterally and for the most part are widely distributed to most body tissues and organs, primarily the liver, kidneys, heart, and lungs. Asparaginase is not extensively distributed, and its metabolic fate is not well known. Plicamycin is the only natural product that crosses the blood–brain barrier. The agents are metabolized in the liver to some degree and are excreted in the urine or feces (through the bile) as inactive metabolites or unchanged drug.

Common Side Effects

Myelosuppression (leukopenia, thrombocytopenia, anemia; less commonly, agranulocytosis and pancytopenia), nausea, vomiting, alopecia, and anorexia

Daunorubicin, doxorubicin, and *idarubicin*: congestive heart failure

Asparaginase: hypersensitivity reactions, pancreatitis, hepatotoxicity, hypofibrinogenemia

Bleomycin: pneumonitis, hyperpigmentation, erythema, cutaneous edema and tenderness, hyperthermia

Dactinomycin: GI ulceration

Dactinomycin and doxorubicin: stomatitis, esophagitis

Plicamycin: hemorrhagic diathesis

Pentostatin: fever, rash

Vincristine: neurotoxicity, hyperuricemia, paralytic ileus, constipation

Paclitaxel: peripheral neuropathy, hypersensitivity reactions

(*text continues on page 769*)

Table 74-5. **Natural Products**

Drug	*Usual Dosage Range*	*Uses*	*Nursing Considerations*
Asparaginase *Elspar*	**Children** *Regimen 1* Asparaginase: 1,000 IU/kg/day IV for 10 days starting day 22 Vincristine: 2 mg/m² IV once a week on days 1, 8, 15; maximum single dose is 2 mg Prednisone: 40 mg/m²/day in 3 divided doses for 15 days, then 20 mg/m² for 2 days, 10 mg/m² for 2 days, 5 mg/m² for 2 days, and 2.5/m² for 2 days *Regimen 2* Asparaginase: 6,000 IU/m² IM every 3 days for 9 doses starting day 4 Vincristine: 1.5 mg/m² IV for 4 doses on days 1, 8, 15, 22 Prednisone: 40 mg/m²/day in 3 divided doses for 28 days, then taper over 14 days Sole induction agent: 200 IU/kg IV daily for 28 days **Adults** Induction: 10,000 IU/m² every 1–2 wk Intra-arterial: 20,000 IU/day for 7–10 days	Acute lymphocytic leukemia in children *Other uses* Acute myelocytic leukemia, chronic lymphocytic leukemia, Hodgkin's disease, lymphosarcoma, reticulum cell sarcoma, melanosarcoma, hypoglycemia due to islet cell tumors	Adult usage is primarily investigational; may be administered via the hepatic artery for insulin-secreting pancreatic islet cell tumors; store intact vial under refrigeration; for IV use, reconstitute with 5 mL 0.9% sodium chloride for injection and inject over at least 30 min into running IV of 0.9% sodium chloride *or* 5% dextrose; for IM use reconstitute with 2 mL 0.9% sodium chloride; do *not* inject more than 2 mL into one site; avoid vigorous shaking during reconstitution; solution is stable for 8 h at room temperature—discard solution if cloudy; *not* recommended as the sole induction agent unless combined chemotherapy is inappropriate because of toxicity or other factors; intradermal skin test is recommended before initiation of therapy and when more than 7 days have elapsed between doses (up to 35% of patients exhibit hypersensitivity reactions); give 0.1 mL (2 IU) test solution and observe for at least 1 h for erythema or wheal; to prepare skin test solution reconstitute vial with 5 mL 0.9% sodium chloride; withdraw 0.1 mL (200 IU) and inject into 9.9 mL 0.9% sodium chloride for injection giving test solution of 20 IU/mL; desensitization should be used on any positive reactors; inject 1 IU IV and double the dose every 10 min, provided there is no reaction, until total accumulated dose is equal to the dose for that day; may increase AST, ALT, alkaline phosphatase, bilirubin values; may increase blood ammonia, glucose, and uric acid levels; may increase urinary uric acid levels and decrease serum albumin and calcium; gelatinous fiberlike particles may develop in IV infusion on standing; solution may be administered through a 5-μm filter to remove particles without loss of potency; do not administer thru a 0.2-μm filter, loss of potency may result; (see also Pegaspargase)
Bleomycin *Blenoxane*	*Squamous cell carcinoma, lymphosarcoma, reticulum cell sarcoma, testicular carcinoma*: 0.25–0.5 U/kg (10–20 U/m²) IV, IM, or SC once or twice a week to a total of 300–400 U IV infusion: 0.25 U/kg/day *or* 15 U/m²/day over 24 h for 4–5 days *Hodgkin's disease*: as above until 50% response occurs, then 1U daily *or* 5 U weekly IV or IM Intra-arterial infusion for squamous cell carcinoma of head, neck, or cervix: 30–60 U/day over 1–24 h *Malignant effusion* Intrapleural: 15–120 U in 100 mL 0.9% sodium chloride allowed to dwell for 24 h	Squamous cell carcinoma of head and neck (DOC), mouth, tongue, nasopharynx, oropharynx, sinus, palate, lip, buccal mucosa, gingiva, epiglottis, skin, larynx, penis, cervix, vulva Lymphomas Hodgkin's disease Reticulum cell sarcoma Lymphosarcoma Testicular carcinomas (DOC) Embryonal cell carcinoma Choriocarcinoma	For IM or SC use, reconstitute with 1–5 mL sterile water for injection, 0.9% sodium chloride, 5% dextrose, or bacteriostatic water for injection; for IV use, reconstitute with 5 mL 0.9% sodium chloride or 5% dextrose and administer slowly over 10 min; solution is stable 14 days at room temperature and 28 days refrigerated; give test dose of 2 U for first 2 doses in lymphoma patients because of possibility of anaphylactoid reaction; pneumonitis occasionally progressing to pulmonary fibrosis occurs in 10%–40% of patients at total doses of 200–400 U; if bleomycin has been used to treat malignant effusions, ½ of the administered dose should be counted toward this total; be alert for symptoms such as dry

(*continued*)

Table 74-5. **Natural Products (Continued)**

Drug	***Usual Dosage Range***	***Uses***	***Nursing Considerations***
	Intraperitoneal: 60–120 U in 100 mL 0.9% sodium chloride allowed to dwell for 24 h *Warts*: 0.2–0.8 U intralesionally every 2–4 wk to a maximum of 2 U (prepare solution of 15 U/15 mL of 0.9% sodium chloride) Reduce dose in patients with impaired renal function Serum Creatinine — Dose 1.5–2.5 — 1/2 normal dose 2.5–4.0 — 1/4 normal dose 4.0–6.0 — 1/5 normal dose 6.0–10.0 — 1/10–1/20 normal dose	Teratocarcinoma (DOC) Malignant effusions Verruca vulgaris (warts)	cough, dyspnea, and fine rales; fatal in 1% of patients; cutaneous allergic reactions are also common; fever and chills occur in 25% of patients 3–6 h after administration and last 4–12 h; becomes less frequent with continued use
Dactinomycin *Actinomycin D, Cosmegen*	*Adults*: 0.01–0.015 mg/kg/day IV for 5 days every 4–6 wk, *or* 0.5 mg/m^2 (maximum, 2 mg) IV once a week for 3 wk *Children*: 0.01–0.015 mg/kg/day IV for 5 days or a total dose of 2.5 mg/m^2 IV in divided doses over 7 days; may repeat every 4–6 wk *Isolation perfusion* Upper extremity: 0.035 mg/kg Lower extremity: 0.05 mg/kg Dosage should be based on body surface area in obese or edematous patients	Wilms' tumor (DOC) Rhabdomyosarcoma Carcinoma of testis and uterus Ewing's sarcoma Osteosarcoma Choriocarcinoma *Investigational uses*: Kaposi's sarcoma, malignant melanoma, Paget's disease, management of acute organ rejection in kidney and heart transplants	Reconstitute with 1.1 mL sterile water for injection (preservative-free); administer directly into tubing of running IV of 0.9% sodium chloride or 5% dextrose; may dilute and infuse over 10–15 min; AVOID EXTRAVASATION; NEVER administer IM or SC; solution is *theoretically* stable at room temperature for long periods but should be discarded within 24 h to prevent bacterial contamination; may increase uric acid levels of blood and urine; hyperpigmentation occurs if skin has been previously irradiated; nausea and vomiting are common during first few hours and may persist for up to 24 h
Daunorubicin *Cerubidine*	**Adults** *Single agent* 30–60 mg/m^2/day IV on days 1–3 every 3–4 wk *or* 0.8–1 mg/kg/day IV for 3–6 days repeated every 3–4 wk *Combination* Daunorubicin: 45 mg/m^2/day IV on days 1–3 of first course and days 1 and 2 of subsequent courses Cytarabine: 100 mg/m^2/day IV infusion daily for 7 days for the first course and daily for 5 days for subsequent courses Total cumulative dose of daunorubicin should not exceed 550 mg/m^2 in adults, 300 mg/m^2 in children older than 2 yr or 10 mg/kg in children younger than 2 yr **Children** (see also below) *Combination* Daunorubicin: 25–45 mg/m^2 IV once a week for 4–6 wk Vincristine: 1.5 mg/m^2 IV once a week for 4–6 wk Prednisone: 40 mg/m^2 daily orally *Note*: For children younger than 2 yr or less than 0.5 m^2 body surface, dosage is based on body weight Reduce dose in patients with impaired hepatic or renal function Serum Bilirubin — Serum Creatinine — Dose 1.2 mg to 3 mg/dL — — 3/4 normal dose Above 3 mg/dL — Above 3 mg/dL — 1/2 normal dose	Acute myelogenous leukemia (DOC) Acute lymphocytic leukemia *Other uses* Neuroblastoma Ewing's sarcoma Wilms' tumor Non-Hodgkin's lymphoma Chronic myelogenous leukemia	Reconstitute with 4 mL sterile water for injection; solution is stable for 24 h at room temperature and 48 h under refrigeration; protect from exposure to sunlight; a change from red to blue-purple indicates deterioration; administer into the tubing of a rapidly flowing IV of 0.9% sodium chloride or 5% dextrose; AVOID EXTRAVASATION; NEVER administer IM or SC; may increase uric acid levels of blood and urine

(*continued*)

Table 74-5. **Natural Products (Continued)**

Drug	*Usual Dosage Range*	*Uses*	*Nursing Considerations*
Doxorubicin *Adriamycin-RDF, Adriamycin-PFS, Rubex*	*Adults*: 60–75 mg/m²/day IV repeated every 21 days *or* 25–30 mg/m²/day IV for 3 days repeated every 4 wk Alternatively, 20 mg/m² IV once weekly causes less cardiotoxicity Bladder instillation: 30 mg/30 mL of 0.9% sodium chloride instilled and retained for 30 min; repeat monthly *Children*: 30 mg/m²/day IV for 3 days repeated every 4 wk Total cumulative dose should not exceed 550 mg/m² Reduce dose in patients with impaired hepatic function Serum Bilirubin / BSP Retention / Dose 1.2–3 mg/dL / 9%–15% / 1/2 normal dose Above 3 mg/dL / Above 15% / 1/4 normal dose	Acute lymphocytic and myelogenous leukemia Wilms' tumor Neuroblastoma (DOC) Soft tissue and bone sarcomas (DOC) Thyroid carcinoma Hodgkin's disease Non-Hodgkin's lymphomas (DOC) Breast and ovarian carcinoma Bronchogenic carcinoma (DOC) Bladder carcinoma (DOC) Endometrial carcinoma Gastric carcinoma Retinoblastoma Pancreatic carcinoma Prostatic carcinoma Testicular carcinoma	Reconstitute powder with 0.9% sodium chloride injection according to package directions; solution is stable for 24 h at room temperature and 48 h under refrigeration; protect from exposure to sunlight; administer into the tubing of a rapidly flowing IV of 0.9% sodium chloride or 5% dextrose; local erythematous streaking along the vein or facial flushing may indicate too rapid administration; AVOID EXTRAVASATION; NEVER administer IM or SC; may increase uric acid levels of blood and urine; cardiotoxic effects can occur at cumulative doses above 550 mg/m² in most patients but may be seen at lower doses in patients who have received previous mediastinal irradiation or cyclophosphamide, dactinomycin or mitomycin therapy; in latter instances, dose should not exceed 400–450 mg/m²
Etoposide (VP-16-213) *VePesid*	*Testicular carcinoma* IV: 50–100 mg/m²/day for 5 days repeated every 3–4 wk In combination with other agents: 100 mg/m²/day on days 1, 3, and 5 repeated every 3–4 wk *Small cell lung carcinoma*: 35 mg/m²/day IV for 4 days to 50 mg/m²/day for 5 days; repeat every 3–4 wk; alternatively, 2 times IV dose orally rounded to the nearest 50 mg *Kaposi's sarcoma in AIDS patients* (investigational use): 150 mg/m²/day for 3 days; repeat every 4 wk	Refractory testicular tumors Small cell lung carcinoma *Investigational uses* Acute myelogenous leukemia Hodgkin's disease Non-Hodgkin's lymphomas Kaposi's sarcoma	Do *not* give by rapid IV push; severe hypotension may result. IV infusion prepared in 5% dextrose or 0.9% sodium chloride injection may be given over 30–60 min; infusion concentrations of 0.2 mg/mL are stable for 96 h at room temperature, and concentrations of 0.4 mg/mL are stable for 48 h in both glass and plastic containers; capsules must be stored under refrigeration; oral form is *not* indicated for testicular tumors; dosage reductions may be indicated in patients with impaired hepatic and renal function, although precise criteria for dosage adjustment have not been established
Idarubicin *Idamycin*	Induction: 12 mg/m² daily for 3 days by *slow IV infusion* in combination with Ara-C Maintenance: 100 mg/m² daily by continuous IV infusion for 7 days	In combination with other approved drugs for the treatment of acute myelogenous leukemia	Administer slowly into a free-flowing IV infusion; severe necrosis can occur upon extravasation; do *not* give IM or SC; caution in patients with preexisting heart disease—drug can precipitate congestive heart failure; *severe* myelosuppression has occurred
Mitomycin *Mutamycin*	IV: 10–20 mg/m² as a single dose repeated every 6–8 wk *or* 2 mg/m²/day IV for 5 days, skip 2 days, and repeat 2 mg/m²/day for 5 days; cycle may be repeated every 6–8 wk A suggested guide for subsequent dosage adjustment is the following: Nadir after Prior Dose — Leukocytes / Platelets / % of Prior Dose to be Given Above 4000 / Above 100,000 / 100% 3000–3999 / 75,000–99,999 / 100% 2000–2999 / 25,000–74,999 / 70% Below 2000 / Below 25,000 / 50% Doses greater than 20 mg/m² are no more effective than lower doses, but toxicity increases *Bladder instillation*: 20–40 mg of a solution of 1 mg/mL in water retained for 2–3 h; repeat weekly for 8 wk	Adenocarcinoma of stomach, pancreas, colon, rectum, and breast Squamous cell carcinoma of head, neck, lungs, and cervix (DOC) Malignant melanoma Chronic myelogenous leukemia Bladder carcinoma	Reconstitute with sterile water for injection: according to package directions; solution is stable 7 days at room temperature and 14 days if refrigerated; protect from light; may be diluted for IV infusion (5% dextrose, stable for 3 h at room temperature; 0.9% sodium chloride, stable 12 h; sodium lactate, stable 24 h); AVOID EXTRAVASATION; NEVER administer IM or SC; may increase BUN and serum creatinine levels; vomiting is usually transient (3–4 h), but nausea may persist up to 72 h; if disease shows no response after 2 courses of therapy, discontinue because likelihood of response is minimal

(*continued*)

Table 74-5. **Natural Products (Continued)**

Drug	*Usual Dosage Range*	*Uses*	*Nursing Considerations*
Mitoxantrone *Novantrone*	Initially, 12 mg/m²/day on days 1–3 as an IV infusion with 100 mg/m² cytosine arabinoside for 7 days as a continuous 24-h infusion; a second course of therapy may be given if response is incomplete as follows: 12 mg/m²/day of mitoxantrone on days 1 and 2 and 100 mg/m² of cytosine arabinoside on days 1–5	Acute nonlymphocytic leukemia Breast carcinoma Lymphoma Hepatic carcinoma	Solution must be diluted before IU administration with 0.9% sodium chloride or 5% dextrose injection; extravasation reactions are rare; avoid contact with skin (rinse immediately if contact occurs); do not mix in same syringe with heparin, because precipitate may form; spills may be cleaned using an aqueous solution of 5.5 parts calcium hypochlorite in 13 parts of water for each 1 part of mitoxantrone; may increase serum uric acid levels; urine may be blue-green for 24 h after administration and sclerae may be blue; cardiac toxicity may be less than that observed with daunorubicin or doxorubicin
Paclitaxel *Taxol*	*Metastatic carcinoma of the ovary*: 135 mg/m² IV infusion over 24 h every 3 weeks	Metastatic carcinoma of the ovary *Other uses*: Advanced head and neck cancer Small cell lung cancer Adenocarcinoma of upper GI tract Advanced prostate cancer Metastatic breast cancer Leukemias	Do not administer if neutrophil count is less than 1,500 cells/mm³; frequent blood counts must be performed; severe hypersensitivity reactions have occurred—patients should be pretreated with corticosteroids, H_2 antagonists, and diphenhydramine; alopecia is common; bone marrow suppression occurs frequently, is dose dependent, and is the limiting factor in therapy
Pentostatin (DCF) *Nipent*	IV: 4 mg/m² every other week. Hydration with dextrose (5%) in saline is required *before* and *after* pentostatin is given	Alpha-interferon—refractory hairy cell leukemia	Withhold drug treatment in patients with severe rash, active infection, creatinine clearance less than 60 mL/min, or evidence of CNS toxicity; caution in patients with reduced renal function; fever, nausea, fatigue, and rash are common
Pegaspargase *Oncaspar*	IM or IV: 2,500 IU/m² every 14 days	Acute lymphoblastic leukemia (in patients who have become hypersensitive to asparaginase)	Limit volume at IM site to 2 mL; use multiple sites if a larger volume is required; when used IV, give over 1–2 h; usually used in a combination regimen
Plicamycin *Mithracin (formerly mithramycin)*	*Testicular carcinoma*: 0.025–0.03 mg/kg/day IV infusion for 8 days to 10 days *or* 0.025–0.05 mg/kg/day IV on alternate days for 3–8 doses; repeat every 4 wk *Hypercalcemia and hypercalciuria*: 0.015–0.025 mg/kg/day for 3–4 days; may repeat at 1-wk intervals *or* 0.025 mg/kg IV over 4–6 h as a single dose; if no response in 48 h, a second dose may be given; subsequent doses are given every 3–7 days, depending on serum calcium level *Paget's disease*: 0.015 mg/kg/day IV for 10 days; reduce dose (by 25%–50%) in patients with impaired hepatic and renal function	Testicular carcinoma Hypercalcemia and hypercalciuria (not responsive to conventional treatment) associated with advanced neoplasms (see Chap. 41) *Investigational use*: Paget's disease	Store intact vial under refrigeration; alternate-day dosing may reduce toxicity; delayed toxicity may occur up to 72 h after medication has been discontinued after daily administration but *not* alternate-day administration; reconstitute with 4.9 mL sterile water for injection; stable 24 h at room temperature and 48 h refrigerated; dilute in 5% dextrose or 0.9% sodium chloride, and infuse over 4–6 h; AVOID EXTRAVASATION; may increase AST, ALT, LDH, BUN, serum creatinine levels; may decrease serum calcium, phosphorus, and potassium levels; be alert for epistaxis or hematemesis, early signs of possible hemorrhagic diathesis—inform physician immediately; dosages greater than 0.03 mg/kg/day or a duration of therapy longer than 10 days increases the potential of hemorrhagic diathesis
Teniposide (VM-26) *Vumon*	IV: 165 mg/m² in combination with cytarabine 300 mg/m² twice weekly for 8–9 doses	Alternate treatment of acute lymphocytic leukemia	Dilute with 5% dextrose injection or 0.9% sodium chloride; avoid extravasation; administer over 30–60 min or longer; hypotension can occur on too-rapid administration; reduce initial dosage in patients with Down's syndrome

(*continued*)

Table 74-5. **Natural Products** **(Continued)**

Drug	*Usual Dosage Range*	*Uses*	*Nursing Considerations*
Vinblastine *Alkaban-AQ, Velsar, Velban*	*Adults*: initially, 0.1 mg/kg *or* 3.7 mg/m² once every 7 days; increase in increments of 0.05 mg/kg *or* 1.8–1.9 mg/m² until tumor size decreases, leukocyte count falls to 3,000, or a maximum dose of 0.5 mg/kg or 18.5 mg/m² is reached (usual range is 0.15–0.2 mg/kg or 5.5–7.4 mg/m²); *maintenance* dose is 1 increment smaller than final initial dose repeated every 7–14 days *or* 10 mg once or twice a month *Children*: initially, 2.5 mg/m² once every 7 days; increase in increments of 1.25 mg/m² until leukocyte count falls to 3,000, tumor size decreases, or maximum dose of 7.5 mg/m² is reached; maintenance dose is 1 increment smaller than final initial dose repeated every 7–14 days Subsequent maintenance doses should not be given to adults *or* children until leukocyte count exceeds 4,000 Reduce dose by 50% in patients with a direct serum bilirubin greater than 3 mg/dL	*Frequently responsive* Hodgkin's disease Lymphosarcoma Renal carcinoma Reticulum cell sarcoma Neuroblastoma Advanced mycosis fungoides Histiocytosis X (Letterer-Siwe disease) Testicular carcinoma (DOC) Kaposi's sarcoma *Less responsive* Choriocarcinoma Breast carcinoma Chronic myelogenous leukemia *Investigational uses* Idiopathic thrombocytopenic purpura Auto-immune hemolytic anemia	Store unopened vial under refrigeration; reconstitute with 10 mL 0.9% sodium chloride; solution is stable 30 days under refrigeration; administer by IV push or through tubing of a running IV (0.9% sodium chloride or 5% dextrose) over 1 min; AVOID EXTRAVASATION; rinse syringe and needle with venous blood before withdrawing; if extravasation occurs, damage may be minimized by local injection of hyaluronidase and by following guidelines for treatment of extravasation outlined in general nursing considerations at the beginning of the chapter; may increase uric acid levels of blood and urine; Raynaud's phenomenon is seen with combined use of vinblastine and bleomycin for testicular carcinoma; response may not be seen in some patients until 4–12 wk of therapy have been completed
Vincristine *Oncovin, Vincasar PFS*	*Adults*: 0.01–0.03 mg/kg *or* 0.4 mg/m² to 1.4 mg/m² IV every 7 days as a single dose *Children* ≥ 10 kg: 1.5–2 mg/m² IV every 7 days as a single dose *Children < 10 kg*: 0.05 mg/kg IV once weekly Reduce dosage by 50% in patients with a direct serum bilirubin greater than 3 mg/dL Small daily doses are not recommended because severe toxicity can occur with no increased benefits	Acute lymphocytic leukemia (DOC) Hodgkin's disease (DOC) Lymphosarcoma Rhabdomyosarcoma (DOC) Neuroblastoma (DOC) Wilms' tumor (DOC) Carcinoma of lung and breast Cervical carcinoma Burkitt's lymphoma *Investigational uses* Ewing's sarcoma Multiple myeloma Idiopathic thrombocytopenic purpura Kaposi's sarcoma	Store unopened vial under refrigeration; protect from light; administer by IV push or through tubing of running IV (0.9% sodium chloride or 5% dextrose) over 1 min; for IV use *only*—intrathecal administration may be fatal; AVOID EXTRAVASATION (see vinblastine); neurotoxicity (numbness, weakness, myalgia, jaw pain, loss of deep tendon reflexes, motor difficulties, visual disturbances) can occur as soon as 2 mo after start of therapy and is usually progressive as long as treatment is continued; paralytic ileus can occur, more commonly in young children; syndrome of inappropriate antidiuretic hormone secretion has been noted, resulting in hyponatremia

Significant Adverse Reactions

(Not all reactions observed with all drugs)

GI: diarrhea, cheilitis, pharyngitis, esophagitis, hemorrhagic colitis, rectal bleeding

Hypersensitivity: skin rash, fever, chills, urticaria, angioedema, pruritus, anaphylactic reaction

Neurologic: agitation, drowsiness, headache, hypothermia, lethargy, malaise, irritability, confusion, syncope, paresthesias, peripheral neuritis, convulsions, motor incoordination

Ocular: blurred vision, conjunctivitis, lacrimation

Dermatologic: acne, hyperpigmentation, hyperkeratosis, thickening of nail beds, photosensitivity

Renal/hepatic: cystitis, polyuria, dysuria, uric acid nephropathy, electrolyte abnormalities, hepatotoxicity

Other: hyperglycemia, ototoxicity, Raynaud's phenomenon, pain at tumor or injection site, phlebitis, tissue necrosis on extravasation, pulmonary fibrosis

CAUTION

Natural products have been shown to be carcinogenic in animal studies and may present oncogenic risk. These agents are also potential mutagens and teratogens and can cause ovarian and testicular suppression.

Contraindications

Leukopenia, thrombocytopenia, or anemia caused by previous chemotherapy or radiation therapy; hepatotoxicity; renal toxicity; and known hypersensitivity

The use of *daunorubicin, doxorubicin*, and *idarubicin* in

patients with preexisting cardiac disease may increase the risk of cardiotoxicity (toxicity may occur at cumulative doses higher than 550 mg/m^2). Daunorubicin and doxorubicin are contraindicated in patients who have received previous treatment with complete cumulative doses of one of the agents. *Asparaginase* should not be used in patients with a history of pancreatitis.

Interactions

Most *natural products* may antagonize the effects of antigout medications by increasing serum uric acid levels; dosage adjustment of the antigout medications may be necessary.

Concurrent use of *asparaginase* and methotrexate may block the antineoplastic action of methotrexate by inhibiting cell synthesis; administer asparaginase 9 to 10 days before or within 24 hours after administering methotrexate; the toxic effect of methotrexate also may be reduced by this regimen.

The concurrent administration of *asparaginase, vincristine*, and prednisone may enhance the hyperglycemic effect, neurotoxicity, and myelosuppression of asparaginase; toxicity does not appear to be enhanced when asparaginase is administered *after* vincristine and prednisone.

Because *asparaginase* causes hyperglycemia, dosage adjustment of hypoglycemic medications may be necessary during asparaginase therapy.

Raynaud's phenomenon has occurred in patients with testicular carcinoma being treated with a combination of *bleomycin* and *vinblastine*; whether the cause is the disease, the chemotherapeutic agents, or a combination of these factors is not known.

Dactinomycin may decrease the effect of vitamin K, requiring an increase in the dose of vitamin K and close observation of the patient.

Daunorubicin is incompatible with heparin sodium and dexamethasone phosphate when mixed together.

Concurrent use of *cyclophosphamide, dactinomycin, idarubicin*, or *mitomycin* with *doxorubicin* may result in increased cardiotoxicity; the total dose of doxorubicin should not exceed 400 mg/m^2.

Doxorubicin is incompatible in solution with aminophylline, cephalothin, dexamethasone, fluorouracil, hydrocortisone, and sodium heparin.

Concurrent use of *cyclophosphamide* with *daunorubicin* may increase cardiac toxicity; the total dose of daunorubicin should not exceed 450 mg/m^2.

Administration of *doxorubicin* to a patient who has received *daunorubicin*, or vice versa, increases the risk of cardiotoxicity; neither agent should be used in a patient who has previously received complete cumulative doses of the other agent.

Concurrent use of *vincristine* with *doxorubicin* and prednisone can increase myelosuppression; avoid this combination.

Patients receiving *natural product antineoplastic agents* may develop a viral disease after immunization with a live virus vaccine for that disease.

Asparaginase may interfere with the interpretation of thyroid function tests by causing a rapid decrease of serum thyroxine-binding globulin within 2 days of administration of the drug; concentrations return to pretreatment levels within 4 weeks after the last dose of asparaginase.

Concurrent use of *dactinomycin* and radiation therapy may potentiate the effects of both and increase the toxicities of both; lower doses of both are suggested.

Concurrent use of *doxorubicin* with streptozocin may prolong the half-life of doxorubicin; therefore a reduction in dosage of doxorubicin is recommended.

The elimination of *etoposide* may be impaired in patients who have been previously treated with cisplatin.

Plicamycin can cause hypoprothrombinemia and inhibit platelet aggregation and therefore increase the risk of hemorrhage in patients receiving warfarin, heparin, thrombolytic agents, aspirin, dextran, dipyridamole, or valproic acid.

Concurrent use of *vincristine* with other neurotoxic drugs and spinal cord radiation therapy may produce increased neurotoxicity.

Bleomycin, doxorubicin, and *vincristine* may decrease the GI absorption of digoxin.

The concurrent administration of *bleomycin, vinblastine*, or *vincristine* with phenytoin may decrease the plasma levels of phenytoin.

Barbiturates can enhance the plasma clearance of *doxorubicin*.

Concomitant use of *etoposide or teniposide* and warfarin may increase the effects of warfarin.

Administration of *vinblastine* or *vincristine* may cause pulmonary distress in patients who are receiving or have received *mitomycin*.

Myelosuppression was more profound when *paclitaxel* was given after *cisplatin* than when given before.

Ketoconazole may inhibit the metabolism of *paclitaxel*.

Concurrent use of *pentostatin* and *fludarubine* may increase the risk of pulmonary toxicity.

Pentostatin enhances the effects of *vidarabine*; combined use may result in an increase in adverse effects of both drugs.

Nursing Management

Refer to general discussion of nursing considerations for all antineoplastic drugs. In addition:

Nursing Interventions

Medication Administration

Inject no more than 2 mL *asparaginase* intramuscularly (IM) at one site.

Inject *daunorubicin* and *doxorubicin* slowly. Facial flushing and erythematous streaking along the vein indicate that injection is too rapid.

Ensure that chest radiograph, electrocardiogram (ECG), and echocardiogram are obtained before, and every month during, therapy with *daunorubicin* or *doxorubicin*.

Ensure that pulmonary function studies have been completed before *bleomycin* therapy is initiated. Chest radiographs should be repeated every 2 weeks. Carbon dioxide diffusion capacity should be monitored monthly. Therapy should be discontinued if capacity falls below 30% to 35% of pretreatment value.

Surveillance During Therapy

In patients treated with *asparaginase*:

Observe for laryngeal constriction, hypotension, diaphoresis, facial edema, respiratory distress, fever, aches, chills, and loss of consciousness because hypersensitivity or acute anaphylactic reactions frequently occur. Because incidence increases with repeated doses, intradermal skin test should be repeated when more than 1 week passes between administrations.

Assess frequently for severe stomach pain with nausea and vomiting, possible indications of pancreatitis. Monitor results of serum amylase determinations, which should be performed often.

Observe for polyuria and polydipsia, potential signs of hyperglycemia. Monitor serum glucose determinations and check urine for glucose.

Monitor respiratory status of patient receiving *bleomycin* or *mitomycin*. Cough or shortness of breath may indicate pulmonary toxicity.

Assess frequently for wheezing, hypotension, and mental confusion, if patient is receiving *bleomycin*, during first 12 to 24 hours after administration of first two doses, because incidence of idiosyncratic anaphylactoid reaction is 1%. Risk of reaction may be reduced by giving diphenhydramine before administering bleomycin.

Assess cardiac status frequently if patient is receiving *daunorubicin* or *doxorubicin*. Dyspnea, tachycardia, hepatomegaly, and swelling of feet and lower legs may indicate cardiotoxicity.

If patient is receiving *plicamycin*, check laboratory findings for platelet count, bleeding time, and prothrombin time, which should be tested frequently during therapy, and monitor patient for episodes of epistaxis or hematemesis, signs of impending hemorrhagic syndrome.

Monitor patient for tetany or muscle cramps during therapy with *plicamycin*, possible indications of hypocalcemia. Monitor results of serum calcium, phosphorus, and potassium determinations, which should be obtained before, and at regular intervals during, therapy.

Assess neurologic status often if patient is receiving *vincristine* or *vinblastine*. Signs and symptoms of neurotoxicity (peripheral neuropathy) include loss of deep tendon reflexes, numbness, weakness, myalgias, motor difficulties, and visual disturbances.

Implement nursing interventions to prevent constipation and monitor bowel function during therapy with *vincristine*, because severe constipation may occur. Bulk-forming laxatives or stool softeners are often prescribed.

Be alert for development of anaphylactic-like reactions (eg, chills, fever, tachycardia, bronchospasm, dyspnea, hypotension) when *etoposide* is administered. Incidence is 1% to 2%.

Patient Teaching

Refer to general discussion of Patient Teaching for all antineoplastic drugs. In addition:

Inform patient receiving *daunorubicin* or *doxorubicin* that urine will be red for 24 to 48 hours after drug administration.

Explain to patient receiving mitomycin that purple bands in the nail beds may appear with repeated doses.

Hormonal, Antihormonal, and Gonadotropin-Releasing Hormone Analogue Agents

Hormonal agents have been used to successfully treat a variety of different types of neoplasms. Tumors that are sensitive to hormones may respond to the administration of natural or synthetic hormonal agents that delay tumor growth. Hormonal agents are not curative, however, because most lack a cytotoxic action. Still, they may provide the patient with prolonged palliation without major toxicities.

The principal hormones used as antineoplastic drugs are the sex hormones (androgens, estrogens, progestins) and the corticosteroids. Androgens, derivatives of testosterone, are used for the palliative treatment of advanced or disseminated breast cancer in *post*menopausal women when hormonal therapy is indicated. The androgens discussed in this section include the 17-alkylated compounds (dromostanolone, fluoxymesterone, testolactone) and testosterone propionate.

Estrogens are used for the palliative treatment of *post*menopausal breast cancer, advanced prostatic cancer, and male breast cancer in selected patients. The estrogens reviewed in this section include the estradiol compounds, whose steroidal structures closely resemble the natural hormone; estramustine, a phosphorylated combination of estradiol and mechlorethamine; and several nonsteroidal agents possessing estrogenic activity, such as chlorotrianisene and diethylstilbestrol (DES).

Progestins are steroidal compounds related to the natural hormone progesterone. Progestins have been used in the palliative treatment of carcinoma of the breast, endometrium, and renal cells. The progestational agents discussed in this section include hydroxyprogesterone caproate, medroxyprogesterone acetate, and megestrol acetate.

Corticosteroids are synthetic steroidal agents derived from the natural adrenal hormone cortisol (hydrocortisone). Corticosteroids, primarily prednisone, are used frequently in combination chemotherapy regimens for the treatment of acute and chronic lymphocytic leukemia, Hodgkin's and non-Hodgkin's lymphomas, multiple myeloma, and some breast cancers.

In addition to the hormonal drugs, six other agents are considered in this section. *Aminoglutethimide* is an antiadrenal agent used in the palliative treatment of *post*menopausal breast carcinoma and prostatic carcinoma. *Flutamide* is a nonsteroidal antiandrogen agent used in combination with leuprolide (see below) for the treatment of metastatic prostatic carcinoma. *Mitotane*, a derivative of the insecticide DDT, is used in the palliative treatment of inoperable adrenal cortical carcinoma. *Tamoxifen*, a nonsteroidal antiestrogen, is used for the palliative treatment of advanced breast cancer in premenopausal *and* postmenopausal women with estrogen receptor (ER)-positive tumors. *Leuprolide* and *goserelin* are gonadotropin-releasing hormone analogues used in the palliative treatment of advanced prostatic cancer when orchiectomy or estrogen therapy is either not indicated or is unacceptable to the patient.

The general discussion of these agents presented below is followed by a listing of individual agents in Table 74-6, where specific characteristics of each drug are given.

Mechanism

Hormonal agents

Androgens: The exact mechanism of the antitumor effect of androgens is unknown. In most cases, hormone receptors must be present in the tumor cell cytosol. Androgens bind to the receptor site, are transported into the cell nucleus, and block normal cell growth by inhibiting the transport of the natural growth hormone into the cell. In addition, androgens may inhibit estrogen synthesis, thus causing androgen-induced estrogen depletion.

Estrogens: The mechanism is thought to be essentially the same as proposed for androgens; the estrogens bind to the cell cytosol receptor, and this complex then translocates to the cell nucleus and blocks normal growth of the cell. Estrogens can also cause regression of some tumors by suppressing normal pituitary function. In men with prostatic cancer, estrogens decrease the amount of luteinizing hormone (LH) (ie, interstitial cell–stimulating hormone) secreted by the pituitary, which in turn decreases the amount of androgen secreted by the testes. The antitumor effect of estramustine may be attributable to estradiol, the alkylating activity of mechlorethamine, a direct effect of estramustine, or to a combination of these effects.

Progestins: The progestins may have a direct local effect on hormonally sensitive endometrial cells and also may decrease the amount of LH secreted by the pituitary gland. The antineoplastic effect of progestins on carcinoma of the breast is unclear.

Corticosteroids: The corticosteroids produce their antitumor effects by binding to corticosteroid receptors present in high numbers on lymphoid tumors. This binding appears to inhibit both cellular glucose transport and phosphorylation, thereby decreasing the amount of energy available for mitosis and protein synthesis, and ultimately resulting in cell lysis.

Antihormonal Agents

Aminoglutethimide: This agent blocks the conversion of cholesterol to pregnenolone by inhibiting the desmolase complex enzyme system in adrenal mitochondria, thus blocking the biosynthesis of all steroid hormones. Additionally, aminoglutethimide blocks the conversion of androgens to estrogens in peripheral tissues by blocking the aromatase enzyme. The net result is a medical adrenalectomy caused by the complete suppression of the adrenal cortex by aminoglutethimide.

Flutamide: This nonsteroidal antiandrogen exerts its antiandrogenic effect by competing with testosterone and its metabolites for the androgen binding sites on the receptor proteins in the cytoplasm of the prostate cells. Flutamide or a metabolite also interferes with the retention of the androgen-receptor complex in the nucleus, thus inhibiting prostatic-stimulated DNA synthesis.

Mitotane: This adrenal cytotoxic agent causes adrenal inhibition, apparently without cellular destruction. It exerts its principal action on the mitochondria of the adrenal cortex, although the exact biochemical mechanism of action is unknown. Mitotane modifies the peripheral metabolism of steroids and directly suppresses the adrenal cortex. Mitotane also alters the extra-adrenal metabolism of cortisol, even though plasma levels of corticosteroids do not fall. The drug apparently causes increased formation of 6β-hydroxycortisol.

Tamoxifen: Tamoxifen is a nonsteroidal estrogen antagonist that binds to estrogen receptor sites in the cytosol of the cell. This complex is translocated to the nucleus of the cell, where it acts as a false messenger and ultimately inhibits DNA synthesis. Tamoxifen is unlikely to cause a response in patients who have had a negative estrogen-receptor (ER) assay.

Leuprolide and goserelin: are gonadotropin-releasing hormone (GnRH) analogues, that have the same action as the naturally occurring hormone. Long-term administration inhibits gonadotropin secretion and suppresses ovarian and testicular steroidogenesis. These drugs reduce the number of pituitary GnRH or testicular LH receptors, causing pituitary or testicular desensitization, respectively. They may also inhibit the enzymes necessary for steroidogenesis.

In men, leuprolide and goserelin decrease serum levels of LH, follicle-stimulating hormone (FSH), testosterone, and dihydrotestosterone, with serum testosterone levels reaching castration levels after 2 to 4 weeks of continuous therapy. In women, there are decreased serum levels of LH, FSH, progesterone, and estrogen; the drugs suppress ovarian estrogen and androgen production by inhibiting pituitary gonadotropin release; serum estrogen levels in premenopausal women may be reduced to postmenopausal levels after 2 to 4 weeks of therapy

Uses

Refer to Table 74-6

Dosage

Refer to Table 74-6

Fate

The fate of the androgen, estrogen, progestin, and corticosteroid agents are reviewed in Chapters 45, 46, and 48. *Aminoglutethimide* is well absorbed from the GI tract, exhibits low protein binding, is metabolized in the liver, and is approximately 50% renally excreted. *Flutamide* is rapidly and completely absorbed orally, highly protein bound, rapidly and extensively metabolized in the liver, and excreted mainly in the urine. The antihormonal agent *mitotane* is approximately 40% absorbed from the GI tract and is excreted by the kidneys (10%–25%) as a water-soluble metabolite, in the bile (a small amount), and largely unchanged in the feces (60%). Mitotane is stored primarily in fatty tissues throughout the body, and blood levels are detectable up to 10 weeks after the medication has been discontinued. *Tamoxifen* is well absorbed orally, metabolized in the liver, and excreted primarily in the feces. *Leuprolide* is rapidly absorbed after subcutaneous administration. Its distribution, metabolism,

(*text continues on page 776*)

Table 74-6. **Hormonal, Antihormonal, and Gonadotropin-Releasing Hormones**

Drug	*Usual Dosage Range*	*Uses*	*Nursing Considerations*
ANDROGENS			
Fluoxymesterone *Android-F, Halotestin, Ora-Testryl*	10–40 mg/day in divided doses (0.05–1 mg/kg/day)	Advanced breast carcinoma	Indicated for women with inoperable cancer who are 1–5 yr *post*menopausal; continue treatment 8–12 wk to determine efficacy; if disease progresses during first 6–8 wk of IV therapy, consider alternate therapy; fewer androgenic side effects than testosterone; higher incidence of biliary stasis and jaundice than other androgens. Halotestin tablets contain tartrazine
Testolactone *Teslac*	Oral: 250 mg 4 times/day	Advanced breast carcinoma in women only	*See* Fluoxymesterone; may be used in *pre*menopausal women whose ovarian function has been terminated; devoid of androgenic activity at normal dosages
Methyltestosterone *Android, Oreton Methyl, Testred, Virilon*	Oral: 50–200 mg/day Buccal: 25–100 mg/day	Advanced breast carcinoma	*See* Fluoxymesterone; also, androgenic side effects are more common; painful, erythematous local reactions can occur at injection site; hypercalcemia may result if patient is immobilized or if bony metastases are present; crystals may develop at low temperatures but warming and shaking will redissolve them; moisture from wet needle or syringe may cloud solution but potency is not affected
Testosterone Cypionate *Andro-Cyp, Andronate, Depo-Testosterone, Depotest, Duratest, and others*	IM: 200–300 mg every 2–4 wk		
Testosterone Enanthate *Delatestryl, Everone, Testrin PA, and others*	IM: 200–400 mg every 2–4 wk		
Testosterone Propionate *Testex*	IM: 50–100 mg 3 times/wk		
ESTROGENS			
Chlorotrianisene *Tace*	Oral: 12–25 mg/day	Advanced prostatic carcinoma (DOC)	Also used for symptomatic treatment of menopausal symptoms and relief of postpartum breast engorgement (72-mg capsules; see Chap. 46)
Diethylstilbestrol *DES*	*Breast cancer* Oral: 1–5 mg 3 times/day *Prostatic cancer* Oral: 1–3 mg/day initially, then decrease to 1 mg/day	Advanced breast and prostatic carcinoma (DOC)	Dosage may be increased in advanced prostatic carcinoma, but incidence of thromboembolic complications increases with doses above 1 mg/day
Diethylstilbestrol Diphosphate *Stilphostrol*	Oral: 50–200 mg 3 times/day IV: 500 mg on day 1, 1,000 mg on days 2–5, then 250–500 mg 1–2 times/wk Maintenance: 250–500 mg IV once or twice a week	Advanced prostatic carcinoma (DOC)	Mix drug in 300 mL 5% dextrose or normal saline solution; administer slowly for 10–15 min at 20–30 drops/min then increase rate to run entire infusion in over 1 h
Estradiol *Estrace*	*Breast cancer* 10 mg 3 times/day *Prostatic cancer* 1–2 mg 3 times/day	Advanced breast and prostatic carcinoma	Continue breast cancer treatment for a minimum of 3 mo to determine efficacy

(continued)

Table 74-6. Hormonal, Antihormonal, and Gonadotropin-Releasing Hormones (Continued)

Drug	Usual Dosage Range	Uses	Nursing Considerations
Estradiol Cypionate *Depo-Estradiol, Depogen, Estro-Cyp, and others*	IM: initially 1–5 mg/wk Maintenance: 2–5 mg every 3–4 wk	Advanced prostatic carcinoma (DOC)	
Estradiol Valerate *Delestrogen, Gynogen LA, and others*	IM: 30 mg or more every 1–2 wk	Advanced prostatic carcinoma (DOC)	
Estramustine Phosphate Sodium *EMCYT*	14 mg/kg/day in 3–4 divided doses; maintenance therapy 10 mg/kg to 16 mg/kg/day in divided doses	Advanced prostatic carcinoma	Store in refrigerator and protect from light; continue treatment 1–3 mo to determine efficacy; may increase serum bilirubin, LDH, and AST concentrations
Estrogens, conjugated *Premarin*	*Breast cancer* 10 mg 3 times a day *Prostatic cancer* 1.25–2.5 mg 3 times/day	Advanced breast and prostatic carcinoma (DOC)	Continue breast cancer treatment 8–12 wk to determine efficacy; determine effectiveness in prostatic cancer by monitoring serum phosphate levels, which should decrease
Estrogens, esterified *Estratab, Menest*			
Estrone *Theelin*	IM: 2–4 mg 2–3 times/wk	Advanced prostatic carcinoma (DOC)	Continue treatment for 3 mo to determine efficacy
Ethinyl Estradiol *Estinyl*	*Breast cancer* 1 mg 3 times/day *Prostatic cancer* 0.15–2 mg/day	Advanced breast and prostatic carcinoma (DOC)	
Polyestradiol Phosphate *Estradurin*	IM: 40 mg every 2–4 wk; may increase to 80 mg	Advanced prostatic carcinoma (DOC)	Continue treatment for 3 mo to determine efficacy; reconstitute with sterile diluent provided; do *not* agitate violently; store at room temperature away from light for 10 days and discard at first sign of cloudiness or precipitate
PROGESTINS			
Hydroxyprogesterone caproate *Duralutin, Gesterol LA, Hylutin, Hyprogest*	IM: 1–7 g/wk	Advanced endometrial carcinoma (stage III or IV) (DOC)	Stop therapy when relapse occurs or after 12 wk with no objective response
Medroxyprogesterone Acetate *Amen, Curretab, Cycrin, Provera, Depo-Provera*	Oral, IM: 400–1000 mg/wk Maintenance: 400 mg/mo *or* adjusted to patient's needs	Endometrial and renal carcinoma (DOC)	Recommended *only* as adjunctive and palliative therapy in advanced inoperable cases; usually well tolerated even in large doses; gluteal abscesses have occurred
Megestrol Acetate *Megace*	*Breast cancer* 40 mg 4 times/day *Endometrial cancer* 40–320 mg/day in 4 divided doses	Breast and endometrial carcinoma (DOC) *Investigational use*: anorexia due to AIDS	Continue treatment at least 2 mo to determine efficacy; relatively nontoxic in doses up to 800 mg/day
CORTICOSTEROIDS			
Prednisone *Deltasone, Liquid Pred, Orasone and others*	*Acute and chronic lymphocytic leukemia* 40–60 mg/m²/day *Hodgkin's disease and non-Hodgkin's lymphomas* 40–100 mg/m²/day *Multiple myeloma* 75 mg/m²/day *Breast cancer* 40 mg/m²/day	Acute and chronic lymphocytic leukemia (DOC) Hodgkin's disease (DOC) Non-Hodgkin's lymphomas (DOC) Multiple myeloma (DOC) Some breast cancers	Never used alone but always as a part of combination chemotherapy regimens; side effects are minimized by alternate-day or intermittent therapy; concentrate solution is 30% alcohol and dye free

(*continued*)

Table 74-6. **Hormonal, Antihormonal, and Gonadotropin-Releasing Hormones (Continued)**

Drug	*Usual Dosage Range*	*Uses*	*Nursing Considerations*
ANTIHORMONAL AGENTS			
Aminoglutethimide *Cytadren*	*Antiadrenal*: 250 mg 2–3 times/day for 2 wk; maintenance—250 mg 4 times day to a maximum of 2 g/day *Breast and prostatic cancer* 250 mg 2–3 times/day for 2 wk; maintenance—250 mg 4 times/day in combination with hydrocortisone, 40 mg/day in 3 divided doses	Cushing's syndrome associated with adrenal carcinoma Investigational uses: Postmenopausal metastatic breast cancer and prostatic carcinoma	Serum acid phosphatase levels should decrease in patients with prostatic cancer if aminoglutethimide is producing a positive clinical response; replacement glucocorticoid therapy is usually required in patients with breast and prostatic cancer; replacement mineralocorticoid (fludrocortisone) may be necessary in 25%–50% of patients with Cushing's syndrome to prevent reduction of aldosterone, which could lead to hyponatremia and orthostatic hypotension; monitor thyroid function during prolonged therapy
Flutamide *Eulexin*	Oral: 250 mg 3 times/day at 8-h intervals	Metastatic prostatic carcinoma	Used in combination with gonadotropin-releasing hormone analogue agents (leuprolide); to provide maximal benefit, therapy must be started simultaneously with both drugs; monitor liver function in patients on long-term therapy; side effects include hot flashes, loss of libido, impotence, nausea, gynecomastia
Mitotane *Lysodren*	**Adults** Initially 8–10 g/day in 3 or 4 divided doses; adjust dosage to maximum tolerated dose (usually 2–16 g/day); maximum dose, 18–19 g/day *Cushing's syndrome*: Initially, 3–6 g/day in 3–4 divided doses; maintenance range is 500 mg twice a week to 2 g/day **Children** 0.1–0.5 mg/kg/day in divided doses *or* 1–2 g/day in divided doses; may be gradually increased to 5–7 g/day	Functional and nonfunctional adrenal cortical carcinoma (DOC) *Investigational use*: Cushing's syndrome	Continue therapy 3 mo to determine efficacy; may decrease protein-bound iodine and urinary 17-hydroxycorticosteroid levels; adrenocortical insufficiency can occur; replacement therapy may be necessary; periodic neurologic assessments are recommended for patients on therapy longer than 2 yr
Tamoxifen *Nolvadex*	10–20 mg twice a day	Advanced breast carcinoma (DOC)	May increase serum calcium levels; transient "flaring" of disease may occur during initial therapy—usually subsides rapidly; ocular toxicity is associated with long-term, high-dose therapy; can induce ovulation
GONADOTROPIN-RELEASING HORMONE ANALOGUE AGENTS			
Goserelin *Zoladex*	SC: 3.6-mg dose every 28 days	Advanced prostatic carcinoma	Synthetic gonadotropin-releasing hormone; chronic use leads to decreased testosterone levels; also useful in management of endometriosis
Leuprolide *Leupron*	*SC*: 1 mg/day Depot: 7.5 mg IM every 28–33 days	Advanced prostatic carcinoma (DOC) *Investigational uses* Pre- and postmenopausal breast cancer, polycystic ovarian disease, endometriosis, anovulation, amenorrhea	Patients may experience an increase in testosterone levels and worsening of signs and symptoms early in treatment: refrigerate before dispensing but may be stored at room temperature while in use; serum testosterone and prostatic acid phosphatase (PAP) levels should be assessed periodically to monitor therapeutic response; depot may be stored at room temperature

DOC, drug of choice

and excretion have not been conclusively determined. *Goserelin* is slowly absorbed during the first 8 days after injection, with more rapid and continuous absorption occurring during the remainder of the 28 day cycle

Common Side Effects

See Chapters 45, 46, and 48 for common side effects of corticosteroids, estrogens and progestins, and androgens, respectively.

Mitotane: anorexia, nausea, vomiting, diarrhea, skin rash, skin darkening; CNS toxicity (drowsiness, dizziness, depression)
Tamoxifen: nausea, vomiting, hot flashes
Aminoglutethimide: anorexia, nausea, vomiting; measles-like rash, itching (starting 10–15 days after initiation of therapy and lasting for 5–7 days), skin darkening; drowsiness, dizziness, lethargy, uncontrolled eye movements, headache, depression
Flutamide: hot flashes, loss of libido, gynecomastia, impotence; diarrhea, nausea, vomiting
Leuprolide and *goserelin*: hot flashes, gynecomastia, impotence; rash, itching; dizziness, headache, blurred vision, paresthesias; GI distress

Significant Adverse Reactions

See Chapters 45, 46, and 48 for significant adverse reactions of corticosteroids, estrogens and progestins, and androgens, respectively.

Mitotane: visual disturbances, hypersensitivity reactions (dyspnea, wheezing), generalized aching, hyperpyrexia, muscle twitching, hematuria, proteinuria, hemorrhagic cystitis
Tamoxifen: leukopenia, thrombocytopenia, hypercalcemia, increased bone pain, vaginal bleeding, menstrual irregularities, lactation, alopecia, photosensitivity, dizziness, headache, depression, anorexia, retinopathy, corneal changes, decreased visual acuity
Aminoglutethimide: myelosuppression (rare), hypotension, hypothyroidism (rare), hypersensitivity reactions (fever, skin rash, cholestatic jaundice, increased AST (rare)
Flutamide: elevated liver enzymes, hepatitis, edema, hypertension, myelosuppression (rare)
Leuprolide and *goserelin*: congestive heart failure, thrombophlebitis, peripheral edema, myalgia, increased bone or tumor pain, myocardial infarction (rare), pulmonary complications (rare)

Contraindications

(Especially as they apply to the use of these agents as antineoplastic drugs)

Androgens are contraindicated in carcinoma of the male breast, known or suspected prostatic cancer, and in *pre*menopausal women.
Estrogens are contraindicated in men or women with known or suspected cancer of the breast, except in appropriately selected patients being treated for metastatic disease.
Estrogen usage is contraindicated in known or suspected estrogen-dependent neoplasia.
Estrogen and *progestin* usage is contraindicated in active thrombophlebitis or thromboembolic disorders and in markedly impaired liver function.
The progestins *hydroxyprogesterone* and *medroxyprogesterone* are contraindicated in known or suspected breast carcinoma, known or suspected genital malignancy, and undiagnosed vaginal bleeding.
Aminoglutethimide is contraindicated in patients allergic to glutethimide (Doriden).
(See Chapters 45, 46, and 48 for additional information on contraindications of hormonal agents.)

Interactions

The androgens, particularly *fluoxymesterone* and *methyltestosterone*, may increase sensitivity to anticoagulants; the dosage of the anticoagulant may have to be decreased.
Androgens may enhance the effect of hypoglycemic agents.
Estrogens may reduce the effect of oral anticoagulants by increasing certain clotting factors in the blood.
The anticonvulsants carbamazepine, phenobarbital, phenytoin, and primidone may reduce the effect of *estrogens* because of increased estrogen metabolism caused by the induction of liver enzymes.
Concurrent use of rifampin and *estrogens* may result in decreased estrogenic activity due to enzyme induction.
Large doses of *estrogens* may enhance the side effects of tricyclic antidepressants and diminish their antidepressant effect.
Corticosteroids, when used concurrently with amphotericin B, may cause increased potassium depletion leading to hypokalemia.
Corticosteroids may increase *or* decrease the response to oral anticoagulants.
Corticosteroids cause hyperglycemia and thus may increase requirements for insulin or oral hypoglycemic agents.
Ephedrine, phenobarbital, phenytoin, and rifampin enhance the metabolism of *corticosteroids* through enzyme induction, thus decreasing corticosteroid activity.
Patients taking potassium-depleting diuretics and *corticosteroids* concomitantly may develop hypokalemia.
Corticosteroids may decrease blood salicylate levels by increasing the glomerular filtration rate and by decreasing renal tubular reabsorption of water.
Mitotane alters *corticosteroid* metabolism, and higher doses of corticosteroids may be needed to treat adrenal insufficiency.
Mitotane and CNS depressants used concurrently may cause additive CNS depression.
Milk, milk products, and calcium-rich foods or drugs should not be taken with *estramustine phosphate sodium* since an insoluble, nonabsorbable calcium salt may be formed.
Concurrent administration of spironolactone and *mitotane* may antagonize the effects of mitotane.
Concurrent administration of *aminoglutethimide* and theophylline or digitoxin may decrease the effects of the latter two drugs.

Aminoglutethimide may reduce the anticoagulant effect of warfarin, whereas *tamoxifen* may increase warfarin's action.

The effects of dexamethasone and medroxyprogesterone may be decreased by *aminoglutethimide*, even for several days after discontinuation of aminoglutethimide.

Nursing Management

Refer to individual Nursing Considerations for androgens, estrogens, progestins, and corticosteroids. In addition:

Nursing Interventions

Surveillance During Therapy

Monitor patient with metastatic breast cancer being treated with an *androgen, estrogen, progestin*, or *tamoxifen* for signs of hypercalcemia (polyuria, polydipsia, weakness, constipation, mental sluggishness, or disorientation). Check results of serum calcium determinations, which should be obtained periodically.

Consider the possibility of intermittent porphyria if patient experiences moderate to severe abdominal pain during therapy with an *androgen, estrogen*, or *progestin*.

Frequently assess neurologic status of patient receiving *testolactone*. Numbness or tingling of fingers, toes, or face may indicate peripheral neuropathy.

Be prepared to discontinue drug and administer steroids if patient receiving *aminoglutethimide* or *mitotane* experiences unusual stress, shock, or severe trauma, because normal adrenal response is suppressed.

Provide opportunity (ie, time, privacy) for patient to discuss feelings about potential or actual changes in body image and sexuality.

Implement interventions to increase patient mobility to reduce susceptibility to hypercalcemia, as needed.

Monitor patient receiving aminoglutethimide for signs of hypotension related to reduced aldosterone production.

Patient Teaching

Refer to Patient Teaching for androgens, estrogens, progestins, or corticosteroids. In addition:

Warn patient receiving mitotane or aminoglutethimide to exercise caution in performing hazardous tasks because drowsiness, dizziness, or weakness may occur, especially during early therapy.

Teach patient receiving aminoglutethimide precautions to prevent postural hypotension.

Review patient information package insert with patient before therapy with an *estrogen, leuprolide*, or a *progestin* is initiated to ensure that patient understands information.

Warn patient treated with *leuprolide* or *tamoxifen* that a transient flare of disease, with increased symptoms and bone pain, often occurs. Hot flashes may also occur with leuprolide.

Recommend use of contraceptive measures if patient is receiving an *estrogen, progestin, tamoxifen*, or *mitotane*.

Inform male patient receiving an estrogen that the gynecomastia that can occur may be prevented by pretreatment low-dose breast irradiation.

Explain that *leuprolide* therapy may impair fertility and decrease libido.

Miscellaneous Antineoplastic Agents

The agents discussed in this section are classified as miscellaneous agents because their mechanism(s) of action or source does not correspond with the other classes of antineoplastic agents.

Mechanism

Aldesleukin: Aldesleukin is a human recombinant interleukin protein that stimulates cellular immunity by enhancing lymphocyte mitogenesis, lymphocyte cytotoxicity, induction of killer cell activity, and the production of *gamma*-interferon.

Altretamine: The exact mechanism of action is unknown; drug structurally resembles one of the alkylating agents; however, it does not appear to demonstrate alkylating effects.

BCG: BCG is a freeze-dried suspension of *Mycobacterium bovis* that produces an inflammatory reaction in the urinary bladder that appears to reduce cancerous lesions.

Cladribine: Cladribine is a purine nucleoside analogue that accumulates within certain malignant lymphocytes and monocytes after phosphorylation to produce a cytotoxic effect.

Hydroxyurea: The exact mechanism of action is not completely established. Hydroxyurea causes an immediate inhibition of DNA synthesis without interfering with the synthesis of RNA or protein. It is a cell-cycle–specific agent for the S phase of cell division.

Interferon: The interferons are synthetic protein chains consisting of 165 amino acids produced by recombinant DNA technology using genetically engineered *Escherichia coli*. The exact mechanism of action of the interferons is unknown; however, it is known that interferons have antiviral, antiproliferative, and immunomodulatory activities, and any or all of these activities are important to the antitumor action of the interferons.

The interferons bind to specific membrane receptors on the surface of the cell and initiate a complex sequence of intracellular events that includes the induction of several enzymes (synthetases, protein kinases, and endonucleases). This process, in part, is responsible for the cellular responses to interferon: inhibition of virus replication in virus-infected cells, suppression of cell proliferation, and enhancement of the phagocytic activity of macrophages and augmentation of the specific cytotoxicity of lymphocytes for target cells.

Levamisole: Levamisole is a immunomodulator used in combination with fluorouracil in the treatment of Dukes' stage C colon cancer. The drug appears to restore depressed immune function, especially of T cells.

Procarbazine: The exact mechanism of action is not completely established. Procarbazine may inhibit DNA, RNA, and protein synthesis; however, no cross-resistance with other alkylating agents has been demonstrated. It is cell-cycle specific for the S phase of cell division.

Uses

Refer to Table 74-7

Dosage

Refer to Table 74-7

Fate

Aldesleukin is rapidly distributed to extravascular and extracellular spaces after IV administration. It is rapidly metabolized by the kidney with little or no bioactive protein excreted in the urine.

Altretamine is readily absorbed from the GI tract, but undergoes rapid and extensive metabolism in the liver followed by excretion by the kidneys and intestinal tract.

Cladribine is administered by IV infusion. Its half-life is approximately 5 hours, and 41% to 45% of the drug excreted unchanged in the urine along with metabolites.

Hydroxyurea is readily absorbed from the GI tract and readily crosses the blood–brain barrier. It is metabolized in the liver and excreted by the kidneys as urea and hydroxyurea and by the lungs as carbon dioxide.

Interferon is readily absorbed from IM or SC injection sites and is distributed principally to the blood and kidneys. It is metabolized in the kidneys, and the products of renal catabolism are almost completely reabsorbed with negligible renal excretion.

Levamisole is rapidly absorbed from the GI tract and extensively metabolized by the liver with the metabolites excreted mainly by the kidneys.

Procarbazine is rapidly and completely absorbed from the GI tract and readily crosses the blood–brain barrier. It is metabolized by the liver to active metabolites and excreted by the kidneys and lungs.

Common Side Effects

Aldesleukin: fever, chills, rigors, pruritus, and GI disturbances
Altretamine: nausea, vomiting, mild sensory neuropathy, anemia
BCG: fever, malaise, chills, dysuria and other bladder disturbances
Cladribine: nausea, rash, headache, fatigue, neutropenia, injection site reactions
Hydroxyurea: myelosuppression (leukopenia), drowsiness
Interferon: leukopenia and thrombocytopenia (occur frequently but are generally mild); flulike syndrome—anorexia, nausea, vomiting, diarrhea; altered taste sensation, dizziness, tiredness
Levamisole: nausea, diarrhea, dermatitis, altered taste sensation
Procarbazine: myelosuppression (leukopenia, thrombocytopenia, anemia); nausea, vomiting, diarrhea; fever, chills, sweating, myalgia, arthralgia

Significant Adverse Reactions

Aldesleukin: hypotension, tachycardia, cardiac arrhythmias, pulmonary edema and congestion, jaundice, myelosuppression, elevated laboratory test abnormalities (bilirubin, blood urea nitrogen [BUN], serum creatinine, liver enzymes), CNS disturbances, oliguria and anuria, arthralgia, infection
Altretamine: moderate to severe sensory neuropathy, myelosuppression, increased serum creatinine
BCG: leukopenia, abdominal pain, myalgia, arthralgia, infection, hepatitis
Cladribine: myelosuppression, abdominal pain, edema, tachycardia, myalgia, arthralgia, breathing difficulties
Hydroxyurea: GI disturbances, stomatitis, neurotoxicity (headache, dizziness, disorientation, hallucinations, convulsion), hyperuricemia, dysuria, uric acid nephropathy, maculopapular rash, facial edema, alopecia
Interferon: cardiotoxicity (edema, hypotension, angina, arrhythmias, tachycardia, congestive heart failure, myocardial infarction [high doses]); neurotoxicity (paresthesias, numbness, depression, nervousness, sleep disturbances, seizures, hallucinations); hyperuricemia; proteinuria; elevated serum creatinine and BUN; alopecia with long-term therapy
Levamisole: leukopenia, arthralgia, dizziness, paresthesias, CNS depression, infection
Procarbazine: neurotoxicity (paresthesias, decreased tendon reflexes, peripheral neuropathies, depression, insomnia, nightmares, tremors, ataxia, convulsions); dermatologic toxicity (pruritus, dermatitis, alopecia, photosensitivity, hyperpigmentation); ophthalmic toxicity (diplopia, nystagmus, photophobia, papilledema, retinal hemorrhage); pneumonitis, hepatotoxicity, dysuria, orthostatic hypotension, tachycardia, hypertensive crisis, impaired hearing

Contraindications

Hydroxyurea and *procarbazine* therapy should not be initiated in any patient with marked bone marrow depression. Patients hypersensitive to any alfa-interferon also may be intolerant of *recombinant interferon alfa-2a*, *alfa-2b* or *alfa-n3*. Also patients hypersensitive to mouse immunoglobulin may also be hypersensitive to *interferon alfa-2a, recombinant*. Retreatment with *aldesleukin* is contraindicated in patients who previously experienced cardiac arrhythymias or chest pain. *BCG* should not be given to patients on immunosuppressive or corticosteroid therapy, or those with depressed immune systems.

Interactions

Aldesleukin may increase the hypotensive effects of antihypertensive drugs and increase the toxic effects of other drugs that cause renal, cardiac, liver, and myelotoxic effects.
Altretamine duration of action and toxicity may be increased by cimetidine, which inhibits microsomal drug metabolism; monoamine oxidase (MAO) inhibitors and concurrent use of altretamine may cause severe orthostatic hypotension.
Hydroxyurea may antagonize the effects of antigout medications by increasing serum uric acid; dosage adjustment of the antigout medications may be necessary.
Levamisole may produce a disulfiramlike reaction with alcohol; concurrent use of levamisole and fluorouracil has caused increased phenytoin plasma levels.
Procarbazine and ethanol ingestion may cause a dis-

Table 74-7. **Miscellaneous Antineoplastic Agents**

Drug	Usual Dosage Range	Uses	Nursing Considerations
Aldesleukin *Interleukin-2, IL-2, Proleukin*	*Metastatic renal cell carcinoma* 600,000 IU/kg by IV infusion every 8 h for 14 doses; repeat in 9 days	Adult metastatic renal cell carcinoma *Investigational uses* Kaposi's sarcoma Metastatic melanoma Colorectal cancer Non-Hodgkin's lymphoma	Do not use in patients with impaired cardiac or pulmonary function; may result in hypotension and reduced organ perfusion; neutrophil function may be impaired, with increased risk of infection
Altretamine *Hexalen*	*Ovarian cancer* Oral: 260 mg/m^2/day for 14 or 21 days in a 28-day cycle, daily dose given as 4 divided doses after meals and bedtime	Persistent or recurrent ovarian cancer	Synthetic cytotoxic drug used as a single agent in palliative therapy of recurrent ovarian cancer; neurotoxicity can occur—perform regular neurologic examinations; monitor peripheral blood counts
BCG, Intravesical *TheraCys*	*Carcinoma of urinary bladder* 3 vials (50 mg/vial) intravesically once weekly for 6 weeks followed by 1 treatment at 3, 6, 12, 18, and 24 months after initial treatment	Primary and relapsed carcinoma of the urinary bladder	Promotes a local inflammatory reaction in urinary bladder, which may reduce superficial cancerous lesions; do not use in patients with impaired immune function or urinary tract infections
Cladribine (CdA) *Leustatin*	Hairy cell leukemia 0.09 mg/kg in 500 mL 0.9% sodium chloride injection infused IV continuously for 24 h, repeat for 7 days	Hairy cell leukemia *Investigational uses* Cutaneous T cell lymphoma Chronic lymphocytic leukemia Non-Hodgkin's lymphoma Acute myeloid leukemia Autoimmune hemolytic anemia Mycosis fungoides	High doses are associated with neurologic toxicity, often irreversible; bone marrow suppression can occur, but is usually reversible; acute nephrotoxicity has occurred especially at high doses and in conjunction with whole body irradiation
Hydroxurea *Hydrea*	*Solid tumors* Intermittent therapy: 80 mg/kg as a single dose every third day Continuous therapy: 20–30 mg/kg daily as a single dose *Carcinoma of head and neck* 80 mg/kg as a single dose every third day; used concomitantly with radiation *Myelocytic leukemia* 20–30 mg/kg daily as a single dose *Malignant melanoma* 60–80 mg/kg as a single dose every third day either alone or in combination with radiation *or* 20–30 mg/kg daily as a single dose	Acute and chronic myelocytic leukemia Malignant melanoma Ovarian carcinoma Squamous cell carcinoma of head and neck (excluding the lip) *Investigational uses* Advanced prostatic carcinoma Lung carcinoma Psoriasis Hypereosinophilia syndrome	Discontinue therapy if leukocytes are less than 2,500 and platelets are less than 100,000; drowsiness occurs with large doses; hydroxyurea should be started at least 7 days before radiation therapy and continued during and after radiation therapy; contents of capsules may be emptied into a glass of water and taken immediately if patient is unable to swallow capsules (some inert material may not dissolve and may float on the surface); may increase serum uric acid, BUN, and creatinine levels; dysuria may occur but is usually temporary; intermittent therapy causes less toxicity; continue therapy 6 wk to determine efficacy
Interferon Alfa-2a, Recombinant *Roferon-A*	*Hairy cell leukemia* IM, SC Induction: 3 million IU/day for 16–24 wk Maintenance: 3 million IU 3 times/wk; reduce dose by 50% if severe adverse effects occur *Kaposi's sarcoma* Induction: 36 million IU daily IM or SC for 10–12 wk Maintenance: 3 million IU 3 times/wk; reduce dose by 50% if severe adverse effects occur Some dosage regimens for investigational uses:	Hairy cell leukemia and Kaposi's sarcoma (in patients 18 yr and older) *Investigational uses* Renal carcinoma Bladder carcinoma (instillation) Non-Hodgkin's lymphomas Malignant melanoma Mycosis fungoides Condylomata accuminata (genital warts) (by intralesional injection) Chronic myelogenous leukemia Multiple myeloma Cervical and ovarian cancer Osteosarcoma Cutaneous T cell lymphoma	Interferon alfa-2a and 2b are *not* interchangeable; store solution in refrigerator; do *not* shake or freeze; patients should be well hydrated during initiation of therapy to prevent hypotension due to fluid depletion; patients should be treated for 6 mo to determine efficacy of therapy; maintenance therapy may be continued for up to 20 mo; neutralizing antibodies to alfa-2a have been detected in 27% of patients but *no* clinical significance has been determined; patients with platelet counts less than 50,000/mm^3 should receive SC injection

(*continued*)

Table 74-7. **Miscellaneous Antineoplastic Agents (Continued)**

Drug	Usual Dosage Range	Uses	Nursing Considerations
	Chronic myelogenous leukemia IM: 5 million IU/m²/day *Non-Hodgkin's lymphomas* IM: 50 million IU/m² 3 times/wk; reduce a dose as needed if side effects occur *Renal cell carcinoma* IM: 20 million IU/m²/day *or* 5 times a week *or* 3 times/wk *Malignant melanoma* IM: 12–50 million IU/m² 3 times/wk *Mycosis fungoides* IM: 50 million IU/m² 3 times/wk *Multiple myeloma* IM: 2–100 million IU/m²/day	Chronic non-A, non-B hepatitis Cytomegaloviruses Cutaneous warts Herpes keratoconjunctivitis Herpes simplex Papillomaviruses Rhinoviruses *Vaccinia* virus *Varicella zoster* Viral hepatitis B	*not* IM injection; premedicate patient with acetominophen to minimize flulike syndrome and administer at night to minimize persistent fatigue; lyophilized powder is stable for 30 days when refrigerated after reconstitution
Interferon Alfa-2b, Recombinant *Intron-A*	*Hairy cell leukemia*: 2 million IU/m² IM *or* SC 3 times/wk; may require 6 mo or longer therapy; reduce dose by 50% if severe adverse effects occur *Condylomata accuminata*: 1 million IU/lesion 3 times/wk for 3 wk (maximum response usually occurs within 4–8 wk—if response is inadequate after 12 wk, a second course may be initiated *Kaposi's sarcoma*: 30 million IU/m² IM or SC 3 times/wk; reduce dose by 50% if severe adverse effects occur	Hairy cell leukemia and Kaposi's sarcoma (in patients 18 years of age or older) Condylomata accuminata *Investigational uses* See Interferon alfa-2A	See interferon alfa-2A, recombinant Use only the 10-million IU vial reconstituted with 1 mL or diluent for intralesional injection; use of other strengths results in a hypertonic solution; after reconstitution with bacteriostatic water for injection the clear, colorless to light yellow solution is stable for 30 days when refrigerated; prothrombin time (PT) and partial thromboplastin time (PTT) may be increased

Preparation of Solution

Vial Strength	Amount of Diluent	Final Concentration
3 million IU	1 mL	3 million IU/mL
5 million IU	1 mL	5 million IU/mL
10 million IU	2 mL	5 million IU/mL
25 million IU	5 mL	5 million IU/mL
50 million IU	1 mL	50 million IU/mL

Drug	Usual Dosage Range	Uses	Nursing Considerations
Interferon Alfa-n3 *Alferon N*	*Condylomata Accuminata* 250,000 IU/lesion 2 times/wk for 8 weeks	Condylomata accuminata *Investigational uses* See Interferon alfa-2A	See interferon alfa-2A; manufactured using human leukocytes; cautious use in patients with cardiovascular or pulmonary disease, diabetes, coagulation disorders and severe myelosuppression, may impair fertility
Levamisole *Ergamisole*	Oral: 50 mg every 8 h for 3 days following surgery Maintenance: 50 mg every 8 h every 2 weeks	In combination with fluorouracil in Duke's stage C colon cancer	Immunomodulator used to increase survival time and reduce recurrence after resection for colon cancer (Duke's stage C); may cause agranulocytosis—monitor for early signs (flulike symptoms, bruising) and perform frequent blood counts
Procarbazine *Matulane*	**Adults** *Initially* 2–4 mg/kg/day (to the nearest 50 mg) in single or divided doses the first week; then 4–6 mg/kg/day until leukocytes fall below 4000, platelets below 100,000 or a maximum clinical response is obtained	Hodgkin's disease (DOC) Non-Hodgkin's lymphomas (DOC) *Investigational uses* Lung carcinoma Malignant melanoma Brain tumors Multiple myeloma Polycythemia vera Mycosis fungoides	Tolerance to GI side effects usually develops within several days; fever, chills, and sweating are most common during early stages of therapy; use in children is limited; undue toxicity such as tremors, coma, and convulsions have occurred; dosage must be individually adjusted

(*continued*)

Table 74-7. **Miscellaneous Antineoplastic Agents (Continued)**

Drug	Usual Dosage Range	Uses	Nursing Considerations
	Following recovery from hematologic toxicity: 1–2 mg/kg/day; maintenance—1–2 mg/kg/day **Children** *Initially* 50 mg/m² daily for 1 wk; then 100 mg/m² daily (to the nearest 50 mg) until hematologic toxicity occurs or maximum response occurs, then 50 mg/m² daily after recovery; maintenance—50 mg/m² daily		

ulfiramlike reaction and have an additive CNS-depressant effect.

Concurrent use of *procarbazine* with tricyclic antidepressants, MAO inhibitors, or phenothiazines, may cause a severe hypertensive crisis.

Thiazide diuretics administered concurrently with *procarbazine* may cause enhanced hypotension.

CNS depressants such as narcotic analgesics and barbiturates used concurrently with *procarbazine* may cause enhanced CNS depression and hypotension in some patients but may cause excitation, rigidity, sweating, hyperpyrexia, and hypertension in others.

Procarbazine may enhance the effects of insulin and oral hypoglycemic medications; dosage adjustment of hypoglycemic agents may be necessary.

Guanethidine, levodopa, methyldopa, or reserpine used concurrently with *procarbazine* may result in hypertension and excitation.

Sympathomimetics such as amphetamines, epinephrine, ephedrine, isoproterenol, methylphenidate, and phenylpropanolamine used concurrently with *procarbazine* may cause hyperpyrexia and a severe hypertensive crisis.

Ingestion of foods with a high tyramine content (see Nursing Alerts) may cause a severe hypertensive crisis in a patient on *procarbazine* therapy.

Concurrent use of any of the miscellaneous agents with live virus vaccines may potentiate the replication of the vaccine virus, increase the side effects and adverse reactions of the vaccine virus, or decrease the patient's antibody response to the vaccine because the patient's normal defense mechanisms are suppressed.

Concurrent use of *procarbazine* with dextromethorphan (a cough suppressant found in many nonprescription cough preparations) may cause excitation and hyperpyrexia.

Interferon may increase the effects of theophylline and aminophylline by decreasing their clearance.

The gastrointestinal absorption of digoxin may be impaired by concurrent administration of *procarbazine*.

Concurrent administration of *procarbazine* and high-dose methotrexate may increase the nephrotoxicity of methotrexate.

Nursing Management

Refer to general discussion of Nursing Management for all antineoplastic agents. In addition:

Nursing Interventions

Medication Administration

The following points pertain to a patient receiving *procarbazine*:

- Before initiating therapy, be sure that the patient has not taken another MAO inhibitor within the previous 14 days or tricyclic antidepressants within the previous 10 days.
- Check ingredients of all medications before administering. Sympathomimetic agents, which can precipitate potentially lethal hypertensive crises, are present in many prescription and OTC preparations, such as cough, cold, asthma, hay fever, and allergy formulations, appetite depressants, and antiemetics.
- Institute preventive measures and monitoring procedures appropriate for MAO inhibitors (refer to **MAO Inhibitors**).

The following points pertain to a patient receiving *interferon*:

- Ensure that baseline laboratory determinations of complete blood count, peripheral and bone marrow hairy cells, and liver and renal function are obtained before initiating administration. Monitor results of tests obtained during therapy, usually every month, to assess response to drug.
- Monitor intake and output, and work with patient to develop plan to maximize fluid intake. Patient should be well hydrated, especially during initial stages of therapy, to prevent hypotension from fluid depletion.
- Monitor blood pressure and vital signs because cardiotoxicity may occur, particularly if patient has a history of heart disease or cancer is in advanced stage.
- Carefully evaluate for evidence of neuropsychiatric

(*text continues on page 793*)

Table 74-8. **Combination Chemotherapeutic Regimens**

Acronym	*Drug*	*Dosage*	*Indications*
ABVD	A—doxorubicin B—bleomycin V—vinblastine D—dacarbazine	25 mg/m² IV days 1 and 14 10 U/m² IV days 1 and 14 6 mg/m² IV days 1 and 14 375 mg/m² IV days 1 and 14 Repeat every 28 days for 6–8 cycles	Hodgkin's disease
AC-BCG	A—doxorubicin C—cyclophosphamide BCG—bacille Calmette Guérin	40 mg/m² IV days 1 and 14 200 mg/m² IV days 3–6 1 vial by scarification on days 8 and 15 Repeat every 3–4 wk	Ovarian carcinoma
A Ce (AC)	A—doxorubicin Ce—cyclophosphamide	40 mg/m² IV day 1 200 mg/m² PO days 3–6 Repeat every 21–28 days	Breast carcinoma
ACE	A—doxorubicin C—cyclophosphamide E—etoposide	45 mg/m² IV day 1 1 g/m² IV day 1 50 mg/m²/day IV days 1–5 Repeat every 21 days	Small cell lung carcinoma
ACMF	A—doxorubicin C—cyclophosphamide M—methotrexate F—fluorouracil	40 mg/m² IV day 1 1 g/m² IV day 1 30 mg to 40 mg/m² IV days 21, 28, and 35 400 mg to 600 mg/m² IV days 21, 28, and 35 Repeat every 42 days	Breast carcinoma
A-COPP	A—doxorubicin C—cyclophosphamide O—vincristine P—procarbazine P—prednisone	60 mg/m² IV day 1 300 mg/m² IV days 14 and 20 1.5 mg/m² IV days 14 and 20 (maximum, 2 mg) 100 mg/m² PO days 14–28 40 mg/m² PO days 1–27 (first and fourth cycles) days 14–27 (second, third, fifth, and sixth cycles) Repeat every 42 days for 6 cycles	Hodgkin's disease
ACV	A—doxorubicin C—cyclophosphamide V—vincristine	75 mg/m² IV days 1 and 43 40 mg/kg IV day 21 0.04 mg/kg IV day 22	Ewing's sarcoma
AD	A—doxorubicin D—dacarbazine	60 mg/m² IV day 1 (adequate marrow) 45 mg/m² IV day 1 (inadequate marrow) 250 mg/m² IV days 1–5 (adequate marrow) 200 mg/m² IV days 1–5 (inadequate marrow)	Soft tissue and bony sarcomas
ADIC	A—doxorubicin DIC—dacarbazine	50 mg/m² IV day 1 250 mg/m² IV days 1–5 Repeat every 3–4 wk	Advanced sarcomas
Ad-OAP (AOAP)	Ad—doxorubicin O—vincristine A—cytarabine P—prednisone	40 mg/m² IV day 1 2 mg IV day 1 70 mg/m² continuous infusion days 1–7 *or* 100 mg/m² continuous infusion days 5–9 100 mg/day on days 1–5 Repeat after 2 wk	Acute myelocytic leukemia
Adria + BCNU	Adria—doxorubicin BCNU—carmustine	30 mg/m² IV day 1 30 mg/m² IV day 1 Repeat every 21–28 days	Multiple myeloma
AMV	A—doxorubicin M—mitomycin V—vinblastine	30 mg/m² IV every 4 wk 10 mg/m² IV every 8 wk 6 mg/m² IV every 4 wk	Breast carcinoma
AP	A—doxorubicin P—cisplatin	50 mg/m² IV every 21 days 50 mg/m² IV every 21 days	Ovarian carcinoma
Ara-C + ADR	Ara-C—cytarabine ADR—doxorubicin	100 mg/m² continuous IV infusion for 7–10 days 30 mg/m² IV days 1–3	Acute myelocytic leukemia
Ara-C + DNR + PRED + MP	Ara-C—cytarabine DNR—daunorubicin PRED—prednisone MP—mercaptopurine	80 mg/m² IV days 1–3 25 mg/m² IV day 1 40 mg/m² PO daily 100 mg/m² PO daily Repeat weekly until remission, then monthly for maintenance	Acute myelocytic leukemia (in children)
Ara-C + 6-TG	Ara-C—cytarabine 6-TG—thioguanine	100 mg/m² IV every 12 h for 10 days 100 mg/m² PO every 12 h for 10 days Repeat every 30 days until remission, then repeat monthly for 5 days for maintenance	Acute myelocytic leukemia

(continued)

Table 74-8. **Combination Chemotherapeutic Regimens (Continued)**

Acronym	*Drug*	*Dosage*	*Indications*
AV	A—doxorubicin V—vincristine	60–75 mg/m^2 day 1 1.4 mg/m^2 days 1 and 8 Repeat every 3 wk	Breast carcinoma
BACON	B—bleomycin A—doxorubicin C—lomustine O—vincristine N—mechlorethamine	30 U IV (6 h after vincristine) 40 mg/m^2 IV day 1; repeat every 4 wk 65 mg/m^2 PO day 1; repeat every 4–8 wk 0.75–1 mg IV day 2; repeat every week for 6 wk 8 mg/m^2 IV day 1 (30 min after lomustine); repeat every 4 wk	Squamous cell carcinoma of lung
BACOP	B—bleomycin A—doxorubicin C—cyclophosphamide O—vincristine P—prednisone	5 U/m^2 IV days 15 and 22 25 mg/m^2 IV days 1 and 8 650 mg/m^2 IV days 1 and 8 1.4 mg/m^2 IV days 1 and 8 60 mg/m^2 PO days 15–28 Repeat every 28 days for 6 cycles	Non-Hodgkin's lymphomas
BCAP	B—carmustine C—cyclophosphamide A—doxorubicin P—prednisone	50 mg/m^2 IV day 1 200 mg/m^2 IV day 1 20 mg/m^2 IV day 2 60 mg/m^2 PO days 1–5 Repeat every 4 wk	Multiple myeloma
B-CAVe	B—bleomycin C—lomustine A—doxorubicin Ve—vinblastine	5 U/m^2 IV days 1, 28, 35 100 mg/m^2 PO day 1 60 mg/m^2 IV day 1 5 mg/m^2 IV day 1 Repeat every 6 weeks for 9 cycles	Hodgkin's disease
BCMF	B—bleomycin C—cyclophosphamide M—methotrexate F—fluorouracil	7.5 U/m^2 continuous infusion days 1–3 300 mg/m^2 IV day 5 30 mg/m^2 IV day 5 300 mg/m^2 IV day 5 Repeat every 3 wk	Squamous cell carcinoma of head and neck
BCNU + 5-FU	BCNU—carmustine 5-FU—fluorouracil	40 mg/m^2 IV days 1–5 10 mg/kg IV days 1–5 Repeat every 6 wk	Gastric carcinoma
BCOP	B—carmustine C—cyclophosphamide O—vincristine P—prednisone	100 mg/m^2 IV day 1 600 mg/m^2 IV day 1 1 mg/m^2 IV days 1 and 14 40 mg/m^2 PO days 1–7 Repeat every 28 days	Non-Hodgkin's lymphomas
BCVPP	B—carmustine C—cyclophosphamide V—vinblastine P—procarbazine P—prednisone	100 mg/m^2 IV day 1 600 mg/m^2 IV day 1 5 mg/m^2 IV day 1 100 mg/m^2 PO days 1–10 60 mg/m^2 PO days 1–10 Repeat every 28 days for 6 cycles	Hodgkin's disease
B-DOPA	B—bleomycin D—dacarbazine O—vincristine P—prednisone A—doxorubicin	4 U mg/m^2 IV days 2 and 5 150 mg/m^2 IV days 1–5 1.5 mg/m^2 PO days 1 and 5 40 mg/m^2 PO days 1–6 60 mg/m^2 IV day 1 Repeat every 21 days	Hodgkin's disease
BEP	B—bleomycin E—etoposide P—cisplatin	30 U IV weekly 100 mg/m^2/day IV days 1–5 20 mg/m^2/day IV days 1–5 Repeat every 3 wk for 4 cycles Reduce dose of etoposide by 20% if patient received prior radiotherapy	Testicular carcinoma
BHD	B—carmustine H—hydroxyurea D—dacarbazine	100 mg or 150 mg/m^2 IV day 1; repeat every 6 wk 1480 mg/m^2/day PO days 1–5; repeat every 3 wk 100 mg or 150 mg/m^2/day IV days 1–5; repeat every 3 wk	Malignant melanoma
BLEO-MTX	BLEO—bleomycin MTX—methotrexate	15 U IV every 4 days–14 days 15 mg/m^2 IV every 4–14 days	Head and neck carcinoma

(continued)

Table 74-8. **Combination Chemotherapeutic Regimens (Continued)**

Acronym	*Drug*	*Dosage*	*Indications*
B-MOPP	B—bleomycin	2 U/m^2 IV days 1 and 8	Hodgkin's disease
	M—mechlorethamine	6 mg/m^2 IV days 1 and 8	
	O—vincristine	1.4 mg/m^2 IV days 1 and 8	
	P—procarbazine	100 mg/m^2 PO days 1–4	
	P—prednisone	50 mg/m^2 PO days 1–14 cycles 1 and 4 only	
		Repeat every 28 days	
BM	B—bleomycin	5 U/day IV days 1–7	Carcinoma of cervix
	M—mitomycin	10 mg IV day 8	
		Repeat every 2 wk	
BOPP	B—carmustine	80 mg/m^2 IV day 1	Hodgkin's disease
	O—vincristine	1.4 mg/m^2 IV days 1 and 8	
	P—procarbazine	50 mg PO day 1; 100 mg PO day 2; 100 mg/m^2/day PO days 3–14	
	P—prednisone	40 mg/m^2 PO days 1–14	
		Repeat every 28 days for 6 cycles	
BVD	B—carmustine	65 mg/m^2 IV days 1–3	Malignant melanoma
	V—vincristine	1–1.5 mg IV weekly	
	D—dacarbazine	250 mg/m^2 IV days 1–3	
		Repeat every 6 wk	
CAF	C—cyclophosphamide	100 mg/m^2 PO days 1–14	Breast carcinoma
	A—doxorubicin	30 mg/m^2 IV days 1 and 8	
	F—fluorouracil	500 mg/m^2 IV days 1 and 8	
		Repeat every 4 wk until total dose of 450 mg/m^2 doxorubicin is administered; then discontinue doxorubicin and replace with methotrexate 40 mg/m^2 IV and increase fluorouracil to 600 mg/m^2 IV	
CAM	C—cyclophosphamide	600 mg/m^2 IV day 1	Prostatic carcinoma (advanced)
	A—doxorubicin	40 mg/m^2 IV day 1	
	M—methotrexate	15 mg/m^2 PO days 9, 13, 16, 20	
		Repeat every 21 days	
CAMP	C—cyclophosphamide	300 mg/m^2 IV days 1 and 8	Lung carcinoma (non–oat cell)
	A—doxorubicin	20 mg/m^2 IV days 1 and 8	
	M—methotrexate	15 mg/m^2 IV days 1 and 8	
	P—procarbazine	100 mg/m^2 PO days 1–10	
		Repeat every 28 days	
CAP	C—cyclophosphamide	400 mg/m^2 IV day 1	Adenocarcinoma of lung
	A—doxorubicin	40 mg/m^2 IV day 1	
	P—cisplatin	60 mg/m^2 IV day 1	
		Repeat every 4 wk for 10 cycles	
CAP	C—cyclophosphamide	650 mg/m^2 IV day 1	Bladder carcinoma
	A—doxorubicin	50 mg/m^2 IV day 1	
	P—cisplatin	100 mg/m^2 IV day 1 or 2	
		Repeat every 3–4 wk	
CAV	C—cyclophosphamide	500 mg/m^2 IV day 1	Non–small cell lung carcinoma
	A—doxorubicin	50 mg/m^2 IV day 1	
	V—vincristine	1.4 mg/m^2 IV day 1 (not to exceed 2 mg)	
	or	Repeat every 28 days	
	C—cyclophosphamide	750 mg/m^2 IV day 1	Small-cell lung carcinoma
	A—doxorubicin	50 mg/m^2 IV day 1	
	V—vincristine	2 mg IV day 1	
		Repeat every 21 days	
CAVe	C—lomustine	100 mg/m^2 PO day 1	Hodgkin's disease
	A—doxorubicin	60 mg/m^2 IV day 1	
	Ve—vinblastine	5 mg/m^2 IV day 1	
		Repeat every 6 wk for 9 cycles	
CCV	C—cyclophosphamide	700 mg/m^2 IV days 1 and 22	Oat-cell carcinoma of lung
	C—lomustine	70 mg/m^2 PO day 1	
	V—vincristine	2 mg IV days 1 and 22	
		Repeat every 6 wk	
CCV-AV	C—lomustine	100 mg/m^2 PO day 1	Oat-cell carcinoma of lung
	C—cyclophosphamide	1 g/m^2 IV days 1 and 22	
	V—vincristine	2 mg IV days 1, 22, 42, 63	
	AV—doxorubicin	75 mg/m^2 IV days 42 and 63	
		Repeat every 12 wk	

(continued)

Table 74-8. **Combination Chemotherapeutic Regimens (Continued)**

Acronym	Drug	Dosage	Indications
CD	C—cisplatin D—doxorubicin *or* C—cytarabine D—daunorubicin	50–60 mg/m² IV day 1 50–60 mg/m² IV day 1 Repeat every 21–28 days 100 mg/m² IV infusion over 24 h daily for 7 days 45 mg/m² IV days 1–3	Prostatic carcinoma (advanced) Acute myelocytic leukemia
CDC	C—carboplatin D—doxorubicin C—cyclophosphamide	300 mg/m² IV day 1 40 mg/m² IV day 1 500 mg/m² IV day 1 Repeat every 28 days	Ovarian carcinoma
CDV	C—cyclophosphamide D—dacarbazine V—vincristine	750 mg/m² IV day 1 250 mg/m² IV days 1–5 1–5 mg/m² IV day 1 Repeat every 22 days	Neuroblastoma
CEV	C—cyclophosphamide E—etoposide V—vincristine	1000 mg/m² IV day 1 50 mg/m² IV day 1, then 100 mg/m²/day PO on days 2–5 1.4 mg/m² IV day 1 Repeat every 3 wk	Small-cell lung carcinoma
CFB	C—cisplatin F—fluorouracil B—bleomycin	100 mg/m²/day continuous IV infusion day 1 1,000 mg/m²/day continuous IV infusion days 1–4 30 U/m² continuous IV infusion day 1, then 7.5 U/day continuous IV infusion days 2–4	Head and neck carcinoma
CFD	C—cyclophosphamide F—fluorouracil D—doxorubicin	500 mg/m² IV day 1 500 mg/m² IV day 1 50 mg/m² IV day 1 Repeat every 21 days	Prostatic carcinoma (advanced)
CHL + PRED	CHL—chlorambucil PRED—prednisone	0.4 mg/kg PO 1 day every other week, increase by 0.1 mg/kg every 2 wk until toxicity or control 100 mg PO days 1 and 2 every other week	Chronic lymphocytic leukemia
CHOP	C—cyclophosphamide H—doxorubicin O—vincristine P—prednisone	750 mg/m² IV day 1 50 mg/m² IV day 1 1.4 mg/m² IV day 1 (maximum 2 mg) 60 mg/day PO days 1–5 Repeat every 21–28 days for 6 cycles	Non-Hodgkin's lymphoma
CHOP-BCG	CHOP—(as above) *plus* BCG—bacille Calmette Guérin	 1 vial by scarification days 7 and 14	Non-Hodgkin's lymphoma
CHOP-Bleo	C—cyclophosphamide H—doxorubicin O—vincristine P—prednisone Bleo—bleomycin	750 mg/m² IV day 1 50 mg/m² IV day 1 1.4 mg/m² IV day 1 (maximum, 2 mg) 100 mg/m²/day days 1–5 4 U IV days 1 and 8 or 15 U IV days 1 and 5 Repeat every 21–28 days	Non-Hodgkin's lymphoma
CHOR	C—cyclophosphamide H—doxorubicin O—vincristine R—radiation	750 mg/m² IV days 1 and 22 50 mg/m² IV days 1 and 22 1 mg IV days 1, 8, 15, 22 3000 rad total dose in daily fractions over 2 wk starting day 36	Lung carcinoma
CISCA	CIS—cisplatin C—cyclophosphamide A—doxorubicin	100 mg/m² IV infusion over 2 h day 2 650 mg/m² IV day 1 Increase to 1,000 mg/m² when doxorubicin is discontinued 50 mg/m² IV day 1; discontinue at 450 mg/m² total dose; repeat every 21 days	Urinary carcinoma
$CISCA_{II}VB_{IV}$	CIS—cisplatin C—cyclophosphamide A—doxorubicin V—vinblastine B—bleomycin	100–120 mg/m² IV day 3 500 mg/m² IV days 1 and 2 40–45 mg/m² IV days 1 and 2 *alternating with* 3 mg/m²/day IV as a continuous infusion for 5 days 30 U/day IV as a continuous infusion for 5 days	Testicular carcinoma
CMC-High dose	C—cyclophosphamide M—methotrexate C—lomustine	1,000 mg/m² IV days 1 and 29 15 mg/m² IV twice wk for 6 wk 100 mg/m² PO day 1	Lung carcinoma

(continued)

Table 74-8. **Combination Chemotherapeutic Regimens (Continued)**

Acronym	*Drug*	*Dosage*	*Indications*
CMC-V	C—cyclophosphamide M—methotrexate C—lomustine V—vincristine	700 mg/m^2 IV day 1 20 mg/m^2 PO days 18 and 21 70 mg/m^2 PO day 1; repeat every 28 days 2 mg IV days 1, 8, 15, 22; then 1.3 mg/m^2 IV every 4 wk	Small-cell carcinoma of the lung
CMF	C—cyclophosphamide M—methotrexate F—fluorouracil	100 mg/m^2 PO days 1–14 40–60 mg/m^2 IV days 1 and 8 600 mg/m^2 IV days 1 and 8 Repeat every 28 days; above age 60, reduce methotrexate dose to 30 mg/m^2 and fluorouracil dose to 400 mg/m^2	Breast carcinoma
CMFP	C—cyclophosphamide M—methotrexate F—fluorouracil P—prednisone	100 mg/m^2 PO days 1–14 60 mg/m^2 IV days 1 and 8 700 mg/m^2 IV days 1 and 8 40 mg/m^2 PO days 1–14 Repeat every 28 days	Breast carcinoma
CMFT	C—cyclophosphamide M—methotrexate F—fluorouracil T—tamoxifen	100 mg/m^2/day PO days 1–14 40 mg/m^2 IV days 1 and 8 400 mg/m^2/day IV days 1 and 8 10 mg PO 2 times/day ongoing Repeat every 4 wk	Breast carcinoma
CMFVP (Cooper's regimen)	C—cyclophosphamide M—methotrexate F—fluorouracil V—vincristine P—prednisone	2 mg/kg PO daily 0.75 mg/kg IV weekly for 8 wk; then every other week 12 mg/kg IV weekly for 8 wk, then every other week 0.035 mg/kg IV weekly (maximum, 2 mg) 0.75 mg/kg PO days 1–10 then taper	Breast carcinoma
COMA or COMLA	C—cyclophosphamide O—vincristine M—methotrexate L—leucovorin A—cytarabine	1.5 g/m^2 IV 1.4 mg/m^2 IV days 1, 8, 15 120 mg/m^2 PO Give leucovorin 25 mg PO every 6 h 4 doses starting 6 h after methotrexate 300 mg/m^2 IV bolus 16 h after methotrexate Repeat every 7–14 days for 8 cycles through days 22–71	Non-Hodgkin's lymphoma
COAP	C—cyclophosphamide O—vincristine A—cytarabine P—prednisone	100 mg/m^2 IV days 1–5 1 mg IV days 1, 8, 15, 22 200 mg/m^2 IV days 1–5 or 100 mg/m^2 IV days 1–10 100 mg/day PO days 1–5 Repeat after 2-wk interval	Acute myelocytic leukemia
COP	C—cyclophosphamide O—vincristine P—prednisone	1,000 mg/m^2 IV day 1 1.4 mg/m^2 IV day 1 (maximum, 2 mg) 60 mg/m^2 PO days 1–5 Repeat every 21 days for 6 cycles	Non-Hodgkin's lymphoma
COP-BLAM	C—cyclophosphamide O—vincristine P—prednisone BL—bleomycin A—doxorubicin M—procarbazine	400 mg/m^2 day 1 1 mg/m^2 IV day 1 40 mg/m^2 PO days 1–10 15 U IV day 14 40 mg/m^2 IV day 1 100 mg/m^2 PO days 1–10 Repeat every 21 days	Histiocytic lymphoma
COPP or C-MOPP	C—cyclophosphamide O—vincristine P—procarbazine P—prednisone	650 mg/m^2 IV days 1 and 8 1.4 mg/m^2 IV days 1 and 8 (maximum, 2 mg) 100 mg/m^2 PO days 1–14 40 mg/m^2 PO days 1–14 Repeat every 28 days for 6 cycles	Non-Hodgkin's lymphoma
CP	C—carmustine P—prednisone	150 mg/m^2 IV day 4 60 mg/m^2 PO days 1–4 Repeat every 42 days	Multiple myeloma
Hi-CP	C—cyclophosphamide P—prednisone	1,000 mg/m^2 IV day 1 60 mg/m^2 days 1–4 Repeat every 42 days	Multiple myeloma
CT	C—cytarabine T—thioguanine	1–3 mg/kg IV daily for 8–32 days 2–2.5 mg/kg PO daily for 8–32 days Thioguanine usually given in morning and cytarabine 8–10 h later	Acute myelocytic leukemia

(*continued*)

Table 74-8. **Combination Chemotherapeutic Regimens (Continued)**

Acronym	*Drug*	*Dosage*	*Indications*
CV	C—cyclophosphamide V—vincristine	10 mg/kg IV every other week 0.05 mg/kg IV on the alternate weeks Continue treatment 12 wk or longer	Neuroblastoma
CVB	C—cisplatin V—vinblastine B—bleomycin	20 mg/m² IV days 1–5; repeat every 3 wk for 3 cycles 0.2 mg/kg IV days 1 and 2; repeat every 3 wk for 12 wk; then 0.3 mg/kg IV every 4 wk for 2 yr 30 U IV weekly for 12 wk	Testicular carcinoma
CVB	C—lomustine V—vinblastine B—bleomycin	100 mg/m² PO day 1 6 mg/m² IV days 1 and 8 15 U/m² IV days 1 and 8 Repeat every 28 days	Hodgkin's disease
CVI	C—carboplatin V—etoposide I—ifosfamide	300 mg/m² IV day 1 60–100 mg/m² IV day 1 1.5 g/m² IV days 1, 3, and 5 Repeat cycle every 28 days	Non-small cell lung carcinoma
CVP	C—cyclophosphamide V—vincristine P—prednisone	400 mg/m² PO days 2–6 1.4 mg/m² IV day 1 (maximum, 2 mg) 40 mg/m² PO days 1–14 Repeat every 28 days for 6 cycles	Non-Hodgkin's lymphoma
CVPP	C—cyclophosphamide V—vinblastine P—procarbazine P—prednisone	300 mg/m² IV days 1 and 8 10 mg/m² IV days 1, 8, 15 100 mg/m² PO days 1–15 40 mg/m² PO days 1–15 (cycles 1 and 4 only) Repeat every 28 days	Hodgkin's disease
CVPP/CCNU	C—cyclophosphamide V—vinblastine P—procarbazine P—prednisone CCNU—lomustine	600 mg/m² IV day 1 6 mg/m² IV day 1 100 mg/m² PO days 1–14 40 mg/m² days 1–14 75 mg/m² day 1 (alternate cycles) Repeat every 28 days	Hodgkin's disease
CY-VA-DIC	CY—cyclophosphamide V—vincristine A—doxorubicin DIC—dacarbazine	500 mg/m² IV day 1 1.4 mg/m² IV days 1 and 5 (maximum, 2 mg) 50 mg/m² IV day 1 250 mg/m² IV days 1–5 Repeat every 21 days	Soft tissue sarcomas
DA	D—daunorubicin A—cytarabine	45 mg/m² IV days 1–3 100 mg/m² IV days 1–10 Repeat as needed	Acute myelocytic leukemia
DAT	D—daunorubicin A—cytarabine (Ara-C) T—thioguanine	60 mg/m² IV days 5–7 100 mg/m² IV over 30 min twice a day for 7 days 100 mg/m² PO every 12 h for 7 days Repeat every 30 days with 5 days' therapy of cytarabine and thioguanine alternating with a single dose of daunorubicin	Acute myelocytic leukemia
DC	D—doxorubicin C—cisplatin	60 mg/m² IV day 1 at 6 A.M. 60 mg/m² IV day 1 at 6 P.M.	Ovarian carcinoma
DMC	D—doxorubicin M—methotrexate C—citrovorum factor (calcium leucovorin)	2.5 mg/kg/day IV days 1–3 200–750 mg/kg/24 h IV infusion day 14 9 mg PO every 6 h for 12 doses starting 12 h after methotrexate infusion Repeat every 28 days	Osteogenic sarcoma
DOAP	D—daunorubicin O—vincristine A—cytarabine P—prednisone	60 mg/m² IV day 1 1 mg IV days 1, 8, 15, 22 200 mg/m² IV days 1–5 or 100 mg/m² IV days 1–10 100 mg/day PO days 1–5 Repeat after 2-wk interval	Acute myelocytic leukemia
FAC	F—fluorouracil A—doxorubicin C—cyclophosphamide	500 mg/m² IV days 1 and 8 50 mg/m² IV day 1 500 mg/m² IV day 1 Repeat every 3 wk	Breast carcinoma
FAM	F—fluorouracil A—doxorubicin M—mitomycin	600 mg/m² IV days 1, 2, 28, 36 30 mg/m² IV days 1 and 28 10 mg/m² IV day 1 Repeat every 8 wk	Lung or gastric carcinoma

(*continued*)

Table 74-8. **Combination Chemotherapeutic Regimens (Continued)**

Acronym	Drug	Dosage	Indications
	or		Pancreatic carcinoma
	F—fluorouracil	600 mg/m² IV wk 1, 2, 5, 6, 9	
	A—doxorubicin	30 mg/m² IV wk 1, 5, 9	
	M—mitomycin	10 mg/m² IV wk 1 and 9	
FAP	F—fluorouracil	500 mg/m² IV day 1	Bladder carcinoma
	A—doxorubicin	50 mg/m² IV day 1	
	P—cisplatin	100 mg/m² IV day 1; reduce to 50–75 mg/m² after 3 doses	
		Repeat every 4 wk	
FCP	F—fluorouracil	8 mg/kg/day IV for 5 days	Breast carcinoma
	C—cyclophosphamide	4 mg/kg/day for 5 days	
	P—prednisone	30 mg/day PO tapered to 10 mg/day	
	(±) vincristine	1.4 mg/m² IV days 1 and 5	
FIVB (FDVB)	F—fluorouracil	10 mg/kg IV days 1–5	Colorectal carcinoma
	I—dacarbazine	3 mg/kg IV days 1 and 2	
	V—vincristine	0.025 mg/kg IV day 1	
	B—carmustine	1.5 mg/kg IV day 1	
		Repeat every 4–6 wk	
FL	F—flutamide	250 mg PO 3 times/day	Prostatic carcinoma
	L—leuprolide	1 mg SC daily or 7.5 mg depot injection IM every 28 days	
FOMi	F—fluorouracil	300 mg/m² IV days 1–4	Lung carcinoma (non–small cell)
	O—vincristine	2 mg IV day 1	
	Mi—mitomycin	10 mg/m² IV day 1	
		Repeat every 3 wk for 3 cycles then every 6 wk	
HOP	H—doxorubicin	80 mg/m² IV day 1	Non-Hodgkin's lymphoma
	O—vincristine	1.4 mg/m² IV day 1 (maximum, 2 mg)	
	P—prednisone	100 mg/m² PO days 1–5	
		Repeat every 3 wk	
ID	I—ifosfamide	5 g/m² IV over 24 h day 1 along with mesna 1 g/m² IV bolus before ifosfamide, then 4 g/m² IV continuous over 32 h	Soft tissue sarcoma
	D—doxorubicin	40 mg/m² IV day 1	
		Repeat cycle every 21 days	
IMF	I—ifosfamide	1.5 g/m² IV days 1 and 8 along with mesna IV at 20% of ifosfamide dose given before ifosfamide and again at 4 h and 8 h after ifosfamide	Breast carcinoma
	M—methotrexate	40 mg/m² IV days 1 and 8	
	F—fluorouracil	600 mg/m² IV days 1 and 8	
		Repeat cycle every 28 days	
M-2 Protocol	vincristine	0.03 mg/kg IV day 1 (maximum, 2 mg)	Multiple myeloma
	carmustine	0.5 mg/kg IV day 1	
	cyclophosphamide	10 mg/kg IV day 1	
	melphalan	0.25 mg/kg PO days 1–14	
	prednisone	1 mg/kg PO days 1–7, then taper to day 21	
		Repeat every 35 days	
MA	M—mitomycin	10 mg/m² IV day 1	Breast carcinoma or Adenocarcinoma of lung
	A—doxorubicin	50 mg/m² IV days 1 and 22	
		Repeat every 6 wk	
MAC	M—methotrexate	15 mg IM days 1–5	Choriocarcinoma
	A—dactinomycin	8–10 μg/kg IV days 1–5	
	C—chlorambucil	8–10 mg PO days 1–5	
		Repeat every 10–14 days	
MACC	M—methotrexate	40 mg/m² IV day 1	Lung carcinoma (non–oat cell)
	A—doxorubicin	40 mg/m² IV day 1	
	C—cyclophosphamide	400 mg/m² IV day 1	
	C—lomustine	30 mg/m² PO day 1	
		Repeat every 21 days	
MACM	M—mitomycin	8 mg/m² IV day 1	Squamous cell carcinoma of lung
	A—doxorubicin	60 mg/m² IV day 1	
	C—lomustine	60 mg/m² PO day 1	
	M—methotrexate	40 mg/m² IV day 1	
		Repeat every 4 wk	

(*continued*)

Table 74-8. **Combination Chemotherapeutic Regimens (Continued)**

Acronym	***Drug***	***Dosage***	***Indications***
MACOP-B	M—methotrexate	400 mg/m² IV wk 2, 6, 10 given as 100 mg/m² IV bolus and 300 mg/m² IV infusion over 4 h followed in 24 h by leucovorin calcium 15 mg PO every 6 h for 6 doses	Non-Hodgkin's lymphoma
	A—doxorubicin	50 mg/m² IV weeks 1, 3, 5, 7, 9, 11	
	C—cyclophosphamide	350 mg/m² IV weeks 1, 3, 5, 7, 9, 11	
	O—vincristine	1.4 mg/m² IV wks 2, 4, 6, 8, 10, 12	
	P—prednisone	75 mg/day PO daily; dose tapered over the last 15 days	
	B—bleomycin *plus*	10 U/m² IV weeks 4, 8, 12	
	Co-trimoxazole	Two tablets twice a day throughout 12-week course of therapy	
MAID	M—mesna	240 mg/m² at 0, 4, and 8 h by IV bolus days 1–3	Advanced sarcomas
	A—doxorubicin	20 mg/m²/day continuous IV infusion days 1–3	
	I—ifosfamide	2500 mg/m²/day continuous IV infusion days 1–3	
	D—dacarbazine	300 mg/m²/day continuous IV infusion days 1–3	
MAP	M—melphalan	6 mg/m² PO days 1–4	Multiple myeloma
	A—doxorubicin	25 mg/m² IV day 1	
	P—prednisone	60 mg/m² PO days 1–4 Repeat every 4 wk	
M-BACOD	M—methotrexate	3 g/m² IV day 14 followed by leucovorin calcium 10 mg/m² IV in 24 h and 10 mg/m² PO every 6 h for 72 h	Non-Hodgkin's lymphoma
	B—bleomycin	4 U/m² IV day 1	
	A—doxorubicin	45 mg/m² IV day 1	
	C—cyclophosphamide	600 mg/m² IV day 1	
	O—vincristine	1 mg/m² IV day 1	
	D—dexamethasone	6 mg/m² PO days 1–5 Repeat every 21 days	
MBD	M—methotrexate	40 mg/m² IM days 1 and 15	Head and neck carcinoma
	B—bleomycin	10 U IM weekly	
	D—cisplatin (*cis*-diamminedichloroplatinum)	50 mg/m² IV day 4 Repeat every 21 days	
MC	M—mitoxantrone	12 mg/m²/day IV days 1 and 2	Acute myelocytic leukemia
	C—cytarabine	100 mg/m²/day IV days 1–5 by continuous infusion Repeat cycle in 4 wk	
MCBP	M—melphalan	4 mg/m² PO days 1–4	Multiple myeloma
	C—cyclophosphamide	300 mg/m² IV day 1	
	B—carmustine	30 mg/m² IV day 1	
	P—prednisone	60 mg/m² PO days 1–4 Repeat every 4 wk	
MCC	M—methotrexate	10 mg/m² PO twice a week	Non–small cell lung carcinoma
	C—cyclophosphamide	500 mg/m² IV every 21 days	
	C—lomustine (CCNU)	50 mg/m² PO every 42 days	
MCP	M—melphalan	6 mg/m² PO days 1–4	Multiple myeloma
	C—cyclophosphamide	500 mg/m² PO day 1	
	P—prednisone	60 mg/m² PO days 1–4 Repeat every 4 wk	
MF	M—mitomycin	15–20 mg/m² IV day 1; repeat every 8 wk; reduce dose 50% after second dose	Colorectal carcinoma
	F—fluorouracil	1 g/m² continuous IV infusion over 24 h days 1–4 Repeat every 4 wk	
M-F	M—methotrexate	125–250 mg/m² IV	Head and neck carcinoma
	F—fluorouracil	600 mg/m² IV 1 h later	
	Leucovorin rescue	10 mg/m² IV or PO at 24 h then 10 mg/m² PO every 6 h for 5 doses Repeat every 7 days	
MOB	M—mitomycin	20 mg/m² IV day 1	Squamous cell carcinoma of cervix
	O—vincristine	0.5 mg/m² IV twice a week for 12 wk	
	B—bleomycin	6 U/m² IM or IV 6 h after vincristine twice a week for 12 wk Repeat every 6 wk	

(continued)

Table 74-8. **Combination Chemotherapeutic Regimens (Continued)**

Acronym	*Drug*	*Dosage*	*Indications*
MOPP	M—mechlorethamine O—vincristine P—procarbazine P—prednisone	6 mg/m² IV days 1 and 8 1.4 mg/m² IV days 1 and 8 (maximum, 2 mg) 100 mg/m² PO days 1–14 40 mg/m² PO days 1–14 Repeat every 28 days for 6 to 8 cycles	Hodgkin's disease
MOPP-LO BLEO	M—mechlorethamine O—vincristine P—procarbazine P—prednisone BLEO—bleomycin	6 mg/m² IV days 1 and 8 1.5 mg/m² IV days 1 and 8 (maximum, 2 mg) 100 mg/m² PO days 2–7, 9–12 40 mg/m² PO days 2–7, 9–12 2 U/m² IV days 1 and 8 Repeat every 28 days for 6 cycles	Hodgkin's disease
MP	M—melphalan P—prednisone	0.25 mg/kg PO days 1–4 2 mg/kg PO days 1–4 Repeat every 6 wk	Multiple myeloma
MPL + PRED (MP)	MPL—melphalan PRED—prednisone	8 mg/m² PO days 1–14 75 mg/m² PO days 1–7 Repeat every 28 days for 6 cycles	Multiple myeloma
MTX + MP	MTX—methotrexate MP—mercaptopurine	20 mg/m² IV weekly 50 mg/m²/day PO Continue until relapse or remission for 3 yr	Acute lymphocytic leukemia
MTX + MP + CTX	MTX—methotrexate MP—mercaptopurine CTX—cyclophosphamide	20 mg/m² IV weekly 50 mg/m²/day PO 200 mg/m² IV weekly Continue until relapse or remission for 3 yr	Acute lymphocytic leukemia
MV	M—mitomycin V—vinblastine	20 mg/m² IV day 1 0.15 mg/kg IV days 1 and 22 Repeat every 6–8 wk	Breast carcinoma
M-VAC	M—methotrexate V—vinblastine A—doxorubicin C—cisplatin	30 mg/m² IV days 1, 15, 22 3 mg/m² IV days 2, 15, 22 30 mg/m² IV day 2 70 mg/m² IV day 2 Repeat every 28–35 days	Genitourinary carcinoma
MVPP	M—mechlorethamine V—vinblastine P—procarbazine P—prednisone	6 mg/m² IV days 1–8 6 mg/m² IV days 1 and 8 100 mg/m² PO days 1–14 40 mg/day PO days 1–14 Rest 28 days and repeat for 6 or more cycles	Hodgkin's disease
MVVPP	M—mechlorethamine V—vincristine V—vinblastine P—procarbazine P—prednisone	0.4 mg/kg IV day 1 1.4 mg/m² IV days 1, 8, 15 6 mg/m² IV days 22, 29, 36 100 mg/m² PO days 22–43 40 mg/m² PO days 1–22 (taper over 14 days) Repeat every 57 days	Hodgkin's disease
OAP	O—vincristine A—cytarabine P—prednisone	1 mg IV days 1, 8, 15, 22 200 mg/m² IV days 1–5 or 100 mg/m² IV days 1–10 100 mg PO days 1–5 Repeat after 2-wk interval	Acute myelocytic leukemia
PA	P—cisplatin A—doxorubicin	50–60 mg/m² IV 50–60 mg/m² IV Repeat every 3–4 wk	Adenocarcinoma of prostate
PAC-5	P—cisplatin A—doxorubicin C—cyclophosphamide	20 mg/m² IV days 1–5 (total dose, 300 mg/m²) 50 mg/m² IV day 1 (total dose, 450 mg/m²) 750 mg/m² IV day 1 (increase dose 20% after stopping cisplatin and doxorubicin) Repeat every 3 wk	Ovarian carcinoma
PCV	P—procarbazine C—lomustine V—vincristine	60 mg/m² PO days 8–21 110 mg/m² PO day 1 1.4 mg/m² IV days 8 and 29 Repeat every 6–8 wk	Primary malignant brain tumors
PEB	P—cisplatin E—etoposide B—bleomcyin	20 mg/m² IV days 1–5 100 mg/m² IV days 1–5 30 U/day IV on day 2, then weekly for 12 consecutive wk	Testicular carcinoma

(*continued*)

Table 74-8. **Combination Chemotherapeutic Regimens (Continued)**

Acronym	*Drug*	*Dosage*	*Indications*
POCC	P—procarbazine	100 mg/m² PO days 1–14	Lung carcinoma
	O—vincristine	2 mg IV days 1 and 8	
	C—cyclophosphamide	600 mg/m² IV days 1 and 8	
	C—lomustine	60 mg/m² PO day 1	
		Repeat every 28 days	
POMP (low dose)	P—prednisone	150 mg/day PO days 1–5	Acute myelocytic leukemia
	O—vincristine	2 mg/day IV day 1	
	M—methotrexate	5 mg/m²/day IV days 1–5	
	P—mercaptopurine	500 mg/m² IV days 1–5	
		Repeat every 2–3 wk as tolerated	
Pro-MACE-MOPP	Pro—prednisone	60 mg/m² PO days 1–14	Non-Hodgkin's lymphomas
	M—methotrexate	1500 mg/m² IV day 14 followed in 24 h by *leucovorin calcium* 50 mg/m² PO every 6 h for 5 doses	
	A—doxorubicin	25 mg/m² IV days 1 and 8	
	C—cyclophosphamide	650 mg/m² IV days 1 and 8	
	E—etoposide	120 mg/m² IV days 1 and 8	
		Repeat every 28 days	
	MOPP	Standard MOPP therapy after remission and repeated every 28 days	
PVB	P—cisplatin	20 mg/m²/day IV days 1–5 every 3 wk for 4 doses	Testicular carcinoma
	V—vinblastine	0.2–0.4 mg/kg IV day 1 every 3 wk for 4 doses	
	B—bleomycin	30 U IV day 2 and then weekly for 12 consecutive wk	
SCAB	S—streptozocin	500 mg/m² IV days 1 and 15	Hodgkin's disease
	C—lomustine	100 mg/m² PO day 1	
	A—doxorubicin	45 mg/m² IV day 1	
	B—bleomycin	15 U/m²mg/m²s 1 and 8	
		Repeat every 28 days	
SMF (or FMS)	S—streptozocin	1000 mg/m² IV days 1, 8, 29, 35	Pancreatic carcinoma
	M—mitomycin	10 mg/m² IV day 1	
	F—fluorouracil	600 mg/m² IV days 1, 8, 29, 35	
		Repeat every 8 wk	
T-2 protocol	*Cycle No. 1*		Ewing's sarcoma
	Month 1		
	dactinomycin	0.45 mg/m² IV days 1–5	
	doxorubicin	20 mg/m² IV days 20–22	
	radiation	Days 1–21, then rest 2 wk	
	Month 2		
	doxorubicin	20 mg/m² IV days 8–10	
	vincristine	1.5–2 mg/m² IV day 24 (maximum, 2 mg)	
	cyclophosphamide	1200 mg/m² IV day 24	
	radiation	Days 8–28	
	Month 3		
	vincristine	1.5–2 mg/m² IV days 3, 9, 15 (maximum, 2 mg)	
	cyclophosphamide	1200 mg/m² IV day 1	
	Cycle No. 2		
	Repeat Cycle No. 1 without radiation		
	Cycle No. 3		
	Month 1		
	dactinomycin	0.45 mg/m² IV days 1–5	
	doxorubicin	20 mg/m² IV days 20–22	
	Month 2		
	vincristine	1.5–2 mg/m² IV days 8, 15, 22, 28 (maximum, 2 mg)	
	cyclophosphamide	1200 mg/m² IV days 8 and 22	
	Month 3		
	No drugs given for 28 days		
	Cycle No. 4		
	Repeat Cycle No. 3		

(continued)

Table 74-8. **Combination Chemotherapeutic Regimens (Continued)**

Acronym	*Drug*	*Dosage*	*Indications*
TODD	T—thioguanine O—vincristine D—pyrimethamine D—dexamethasone	2 mg/kg PO days 1–5 2 mg/m² IV day 1 1.5 mg/kg PO days 1–5 2 mg/m² PO 3 times/day on days 1–5 Repeat every 11 days with 6-day rest period	Acute lymphocytic leukemia
TRAMPCO(L)	T—thioguanine	100 mg/m² PO days 1–3 Increase to 4–5 days after first course	Acute leukemia
	R—daunorubicin	40 mg/m² IV day 1	
	A—cytarabine	100 mg/m² IV days 1–3 Increase to 4–5 days after first course	
	M—methotrexate	7.5 mg/m² IV or IM days 1–3 Increase to 4–5 days after first course	
	P—prednisolone	200 mg PO days 1–3 Increase to 4–5 days after first course	
	C—cyclophosphamide	100 mg/m² IV days 1–3 Increase to 4–5 days after first course	
	O—vincristine	2 mg IV day 1	
	L—L-asparaginase	8000 U/m² IV days 1–28 in first 2 courses Repeat every 2–4 wk with wider spacing in patients with good response	
TRAP	T—thioguanine R—daunorubicin (rubidomycin) A—cytarabine P—prednisone	100 mg/m²/day PO days 1–5 40 mg/m²/day IV day 1 100 mg/m²/day IV or IM days 1–5 30 mg/m²/day PO days 1–5	Acute myelocytic leukemia
VAC	V—vincristine A—dactinomycin C—cyclophosphamide	1.5 mg/m² IV every week for 10–12 wk 0.5 mg/day IV days 1–5; repeat every 4 wk 5–7 mg/kg/day IV days 1–5; repeat every 4 wk	Ovarian carcinoma
VAC	V—vincristine A—doxorubicin C—cyclophosphamide	1 mg IV day 1 50 mg/m² IV day 1 750 mg/m² IV day 1	Lung carcinoma
VAC Pulse	V—vincristine A—dactinomycin	2 mg/m² IV weekly for wk 1–12 (maximum, 2 mg) 0.015 mg/kg IV days 1–5 of wk 1 and 13, then every 3 mo for 5 or 6 courses (maximum, 0.5 mg/day)	Sarcoma
	C—cyclophosphamide	10 mg/kg IV or PO for 7 days Repeat every 6 wk for 2 yr	
VAC Standard	V—vincristine A—dactinomycin	2 mg/m² IV weekly for wk 1–12 (maximum, 2 mg) 0.015 mg/kg IV days 1–5; repeat every 3 mo for 5 or 6 courses (maximum, 0.5 mg a day)	Sarcoma
	C—cyclophosphamide	2.5 mg/kg PO daily for 2 yr	
VAD	V—vincristine A—doxorubicin D—dexamethasone	0.4 mg/day IV continuous infusion days 1–4 9 mg/m²/day continuous IV infusion days 1–4 40 mg PO daily, days 1–4	Multiple myeloma
VAP	V—vincristine A—doxorubicin P—prednisone	2 mg/m² IV weekly for 6 wk 25 mg/m² IV weekly for 6 wk 60 mg/m² PO days 1–28	Acute lymphocytic leukemia
VBAP	V—vincristine B—carmustine A—doxorubicin P—prednisone	1 mg IV day 1 30 mg/m² IV day 2 30 mg/m² IV day 2 60 mg/m² PO days 2–5 Repeat every 3 wk	Multiple myeloma
VBD	V—vinblastine B—bleomycin D—cisplatin	6 mg/m² IV days 1 and 2 15 U/m² IV days 1–5 by 24-h infusion 50 mg/m² IV day 5 Repeat every 28 days	Melanoma
VBP	V—vinblastine	0.2 mg/kg IV days 1 and 2; repeat every 3 wk for 5 courses	Testicular carcinoma
	B—bleomycin	30 U/week IV 6 h after vinblastine on the second day of each week for 12 wk until total dose of 360 U	
	P—cisplatin	20 mg/m² IV days 1–5, 6 h after vinblastine Repeat every 3 wk for 3 courses	
VC	V—etoposide C—carboplatin	100–200 mg/m² IV days 1–3 50–125 mg/m² IV days 1–3 Repeat cycle every 28 days	Small cell lung carcinoma

(continued)

Table 74-8. **Combination Chemotherapeutic Regimens (Continued)**

Acronym	Drug	Dosage	Indications
VCAP	V—vincristine C—cyclophosphamide A—doxorubicin P—prednisone	1 mg IV day 1 100 mg/m² PO days 1–4 25 mg/m² IV day 2 60 mg/m² PO days 1–4 Repeat every 4 wk	Multiple myeloma
VCR-MTX-CF or VMC	VCR—vincristine MTX—methotrexate CF—citrovorum factor (calcium leucovorin)	2 mg/m² IV for one dose (maximum, 2 mg) 3,000–7,500 mg/m² IV 6-h infusion starting 30 min after vincristine 15 mg IV every 3 h for 8 doses, then 15 mg PO every 3 h for 8 doses	Osteogenic sarcoma
VM	V—vinblastine M—mitomycin	5 mg/m² IV 6 mg/m² IV Repeat every 2 wk	Adenocarcinoma of lung
VMCP	V—vincristine M—melphalan C—cyclophosphamide P—prednisone	1 mg IV day 1 5 mg/m² PO days 1–4 100 mg/m² PO days 1–4 60 mg/m² PO days 1–4 Repeat every 3 wk	Multiple myeloma
VP	V—vincristine P—prednisone	2 mg/m² IV every week for 4–6 wk (maximum, 2 mg) 60 mg/m² PO daily for 4 wk, then taper wks 5–7	Acute lymphocytic leukemia
VP-L-Asparaginase (VPAsp)	V—vincristine P—prednisone Asp—L-asparaginase	2 mg/m² IV every week for 4–6 wk (maximum, 2 mg) 60 mg/m² PO daily for 4–6 wk, then taper 10,000 U/m² IV days 1–14	Acute lymphocytic leukemia
VP plus Daunorubicin	V—vincristine P—prednisone daunorubicin	1.5 mg/m² IV weekly for 4–6 wk 40 mg/m² PO daily for 4–6 wk 25 mg/m² IV weekly for 4–6 wk	Acute lymphocytic leukemia

changes such as depression, sleep disturbances, or hallucinations, because neurotoxicity may occur.

When possible, administer *alfa-2a interferon* in the morning to maximize accuracy of assessment for toxicity. A consistent time of administration is also important.

When possible, administer *alfa-2b interferon* at night to minimize impact of side effects.

Surveillance During Therapy

Carefully monitor intake and output during therapy with hydroxyurea, as well as results of BUN and serum creatinine determinations, because renal function may be temporarily impaired. If patient with renal impairment receives hydroxyurea, auditory and visual hallucinations or increased hematologic toxicity may develop.

If patient is receiving interferon, provide for patient safety needs to prevent falls because of gait alterations that can be caused by neurotoxicity.

Patient Teaching

Refer to general discussion of Patient Teaching for all antineoplastic agents. In addition:

The following points pertain to a patient receiving *procarbazine*:

Teach precautions appropriate for MAO inhibitors (refer to discussion of MAO Inhibitors).

Warn patient to exercise caution while performing potentially hazardous tasks because drowsiness, dizziness, or blurred vision may occur.

Warn fertile woman to use effective contraceptive measures.

Inform patient that flulike symptoms may occur during initiation of *procarbazine* therapy and usually occur 2 to 6 hours after a dose of *interferon*. Reassure patient that symptoms tend to abate with continued therapy. Premedication with acetaminophen may help control this response to interferon.

Inform patient that postirradiation erythema may be exacerbated if patient receiving *hydroxyurea* has had previous radiation therapy.

Combination Chemotherapy

Combination chemotherapy is currently in widespread use in the treatment of many neoplastic diseases to produce higher response rates and longer periods of remission than can be obtained with single-agent therapy. Combinations of agents are also used to delay the emergence of resistance in the tumor cells and to obtain a synergistic therapeutic effect with minimal toxicity.

The general principles used for the selection of agents to be used for a combination chemotherapeutic regimen are as follows:

I. Each agent used in the regimen must be *clinically active* in the specific disease.
II. To obtain synergism, each agent must have a *different*

mechanism of action. Agents are used to block different sites in biochemical pathways or to inhibit critical cell functions. Three different types of blockade have been described:

A. *Sequential blockade*: the inhibition of two different steps of the same biochemical pathway
B. *Concurrent blockade*: the blockade of parallel metabolic pathways leading to a common end product
C. *Complementary inhibition*: inhibition at different sites in the synthesis of large polymeric molecules

III. The agents used must have *different toxicities* or *different timing* of a similar toxicity. This reduces cumulative toxicity to a single-organ system and allows for individual agents to be used in full clinical doses.

IV. Agents are *scheduled* with respect to tumor cell kinetics to potentiate the effect of each agent in the regimen. Both cell-cycle–specific and cell-cycle–nonspecific agents are used in regimens to simultaneously kill both dividing and nondividing cell fractions in the tumor. Careful intermittent scheduling has also proved to be less immunosuppressive and less toxic than continuous daily therapy.

V. Each agent should be administered at the maximum dose tolerated by the patient, and such dose should be close to or beyond the *minimum effective dosage* of each agent as a single agent.

Table 74-8 lists a number of currently used combination chemotherapeutic regimens according to their commonly known acronyms. Individual drug components of the combination are given along with the recommended dosage and indications.

Selected Bibliography

Bar MH et al: Metastatic melanoma treated with combined bolus and continuous infusion of interleukin-2 and lymphokine-activated killer cells. J Clin Oncol 8:1138, 1990

Black DJ, Livingston RB: Antineoplastic drugs in 1990: Parts I and II. Drugs 39:489(I);652(II), 1990

Buroker TR et al: Randomized comparison of two schedules of fluorouracil and leucovorin in the treatment of advanced colorectal cancer. J Clin Oncol 12(1):14, 1994

Hoskins PJ, Swenerton KD: Oral etoposide is active against platinum-resistant epithelial ovarian cancer. J Clin Oncol 12(1):60, 1994

Moertel CG et al: Levamisole and fluorouracil for adjuvant therapy of resected colon carcinoma. N Engl J Med 322:352, 1990

Moore MJ: Clinical pharmacokinetics of cyclophosphamide. Clin Pharmacokinet 20(3):194, 1991

Piro LD et al: Lasting remission in hairy-cell leukemia induced by a single infusion of 2-chlorodeoxyadenosine. N Engl J Med 322:1117, 1990

Nursing Bibliography

Grajny A, Christie D, Tichy A, Talashek M: Chemotherapy: How safe for the caregiver. Home Health Care Nurse 11(5):51, 1993

Miaskowski C: Chemotherapy update. Nurs Clin North Am 26(2):331, 1991

Nichols G: Update on the biologic agents in home care of the cancer client. Home Health Care Nurse 11(5):30, 1991

Pate R: The role of chemotherapy treatment in the treatment of lung cancer. Nurs Clin North Am 27(3):653, 1992

Rogers B: Taxol: A promising new drug of the 90's. Oncology Nursing Forum 20(10):1483, 1993

IX

Nutrients, Fluids, and Electrolytes

75
Vitamins

Water-Soluble Vitamins	**Fat-Soluble Vitamins**
Vitamin B_1	Vitamin A
Vitamin B_2	Vitamin D
Vitamin B_3	Vitamin E
Vitamin B_5	Vitamin K
Vitamin B_6	
Vitamin B_{12}	
Vitamin C	

Vitamins are organic substances required by the body for synthesis of essential cofactors that catalyze metabolic reactions. The body does not have the capacity to provide enough of all the essential vitamins; hence, dietary sources are necessary. The average diet in developed countries is usually more than adequate in supplying most required vitamins, and there is seldom need for additional vitamins in most otherwise healthy persons. There are, however, certain situations in which vitamin supplementation can be justified. Vitamin deficiency states can result from inadequate nutritional intake, impaired absorption; increased requirements, malnutrition (eg, from starvation, anorexia, extreme diets, food faddism), pathologic conditions (gastrointestinal [GI] disorders, hyperthyroidism, intestinal surgery, carcinomas), alcoholism, prolonged stress, dialysis, and a variety of other conditions. Provided that a definite vitamin deficiency can be demonstrated on the basis of clinical symptoms, *selective* replacement of those vitamins that are lacking is indicated. Use of multivitamin formulations for replacement therapy, however, is usually unnecessary and can become a significant expense as well. A much more reasonable approach is to supply the deficient vitamin or vitamins in the amounts required to eliminate the symptoms of the vitamin deficiency state. For example, thiamine is indicated for beriberi, niacin for pellagra, ascorbic acid for scurvy, and cyanocobalamin for pernicious anemia. It is important, however, to regard vitamins as *drugs;* as such, they should be used only where there is valid indication. Injudicious or excessive intake of vitamins is at best wasteful and may result in development of untoward reactions. Moreover, continued self-medication with vitamin preparations may delay recognition or mask the symptoms of a more serious underlying disease. Vitamin supplementation should be undertaken only after consultation with a healthcare professional, and the type and amount of individual vitamins prescribed should be based on a clinical assessment of the patient's diet, health status, and presenting symptoms.

The Food and Nutrition Board of the National Academy of Sciences periodically provides guidelines for recommended intake of individual nutrients, including vitamins. The recommended dietary allowances (RDAs) are *not* requirements but are suggested daily intakes of vitamins and other nutrients that, based on current scientific data, are believed to be adequate for the nutritional needs of most healthy persons under normal environmental conditions. Recommended dietary allowances vary with sex and age, and additional allowances are made for special circumstances, such as during pregnancy and lactation. As noted, RDA values apply to *healthy* persons and are not intended to cover nutritional requirements in disease or other abnormal situations. They are subject to periodic revision, and values do change as population subgroups with unique nutritional requirements emerge.

The U.S. Food and Drug Administration (FDA) regulates the labeling of vitamin and mineral products sold as foods or drugs and has designated an "official" U.S. RDA for each substance, which serves as the legal standard for nutritional labeling of those products controlled by the Administration. In general, U.S. RDAs represent the highest male or female RDA for each nutrient. Previously, these U.S. RDAs were labeled "minimum daily requirements" (MDRs), but this term has become obsolete. The current RDAs for the various vitamins are listed in Table 75-1.

Vitamins and Minerals as Therapy

During the last decade or so, more and more health practitioners have been using vitamins and minerals to treat various disorders, even though there is lack of widespread approval. Some vitamin-based therapies have become standard, but many are still controversial and require verification. Many practitioners of "natural" medicines use various nutritional supplements for a wide variety of disorders ranging from depression to menstrual cramps. Some recent epidemiologic studies have shown the value of supraphysiologic doses of some of the vitamins for certain medical conditions. It is not uncommon today to see people using megadoses (greatly exceeding U.S. RDA) of vitamins and minerals for all kinds of illnesses. Recent examples include large doses (up to several grams) of vitamin C for the treatment of the common cold and vitamins A and E for treating various skin disorders. Despite occasional claims that such therapy is effective, many physicians and scientists maintain that this practice is financially wasteful and potentially hazardous to health. It is well known that excessively high doses of vitamins A, B_6, D, as well as some minerals like selenium, can cause potentially dangerous pharmacologic effects. Unfortunately, there simply is little information on the long-term effects of megadoses of normally innocuous vitamins.

For those vitamins used as "therapy," it is important to note that there are some well-established medical practices for their use. For example, vitamin A derivatives have been used for severe acne, cyanocobalamin (vitamin B_{12}) is an effective treatment for pernicious anemia, and niacin (vitamin B_3) can lower cholesterol and triglyceride levels in patients who have coronary artery disease.

Other potential therapeutic applications for the B vitamins include: 1) thiamine (B_1) for the treatment of depression, air and sea sickness, hangovers, neuralgia, and shingles; 2) riboflavin

Table 75-1. Vitamins: Recommended Dietary Allowances, Sources, and Symptoms of Deficiency States

Vitamin	Major Dietary Sources	Recommended Dietary Allowances (RDAs)*			Principal Symptoms of Deficiency States
		Infants	Children	Adults	
I. Water-Soluble					
B Complex					
Thiamine (B_1)	Liver; whole grain, enriched bread and cereals; pork	0.3–0.4 mg	0.7–1.0 mg	1.0–1.5 mg	Anorexia, constipation, beriberi (cardiac complications, peripheral neuritis)
Riboflavin (B_2)	Organ meats, milk, eggs, green vegetables, enriched bread and flour	0.4–0.5 mg	0.8–1.2 mg	1.2–1.8 mg	Stomatitis, glossitis, ocular itching or burning, photophobia, facial dermatitis, cheilosis, corneal vascularization
Nicotinic acid (Niacin, B_3)	Liver, fish, poultry, red meat, enriched bread and cereals	5–6 mg	9–14 mg	14–20 mg	Pellagra (nervousness, insomnia, dermatitis, diarrhea, confusion, delusions)
Pantothenic acid (B_5)	Organ meats, egg yolks, beef, peanuts, whole grains, cauliflower	†	†	†	Weakness, fatigue, mood changes, dizziness, "burning-foot" syndrome
Pyridoxine (B_6)	Red meat, liver, yeast, whole grains, soybeans, green vegetables	0.3–0.6 mg	1.0–1.4 mg	1.4–2.0 mg	Anemia, CNS lesions, epileptic convulsions in children
Cyanocobalamin (B_{12})	Red meat, milk, egg yolk, oysters, clams	0.3–0.5 μg	0.7–1.4 μg	2 μg	Pernicious anemia, glossitis, paresthesias, muscle incoordination, confusion
Vitamin C (Ascorbic acid)	Citrus fruits, tomatoes, green vegetables, potatoes, strawberries, green peppers	35 mg	45 mg	50–60 mg	Scurvy (petechiae, bleeding gums, bruising, impaired wound healing, loosened teeth)
II. Fat-Soluble					
Vitamin A	Fish liver oils, eggs, milk, butter, green and yellow vegetables, tomatoes, squash	2,000–2,100 IU	2,500–3,500 IU	4,000–5,000 IU	Night blindness, xerophthalmia, keratinization of epithelial tissues, increased susceptibility to infection, retarded growth and development
Vitamin D	Fish liver oils, egg yolk, milk, butter, margarine, salmon, sardines	300–400 IU	400 IU	200–400 IU	Rickets, osteomalacia
Vitamin E	Wheat germ, vegetable oils, green leafy vegetables, nuts, cereals, eggs, dairy products, meats	4–6 IU	9–10 IU	12–15 IU	Not established in humans; *possibly* hemolytic anemia, muscular lesions and necrosis, creatinuria
Vitamin K	Green leafy vegetables, liver, cheese, egg yolks, tomatoes, meats, cereals	5–10 μg	15–30 μg	40–80 μg	Hypoprothrombinemia, hemorrhage

* Average daily intake over time.

† RDA is not established

(B_2) for treating certain drug-induced psychoses, and for treating alcoholics; 3) niacin (B_3) for lowering elevated triglyceride and cholesterol levels as well as in the management of anxiety, depression, schizophrenia, autism, arthritis, diabetes, and hypoglycemia; 4) pantothenic acid (B_5) for relieving the symptoms of allergy, helping to overcome constipation, treating peptic ulcers, and treating a variety of skin problems like eczema; 5) pyridoxine (B_6) for symptoms of premenstrual syndrome (PMS), such as tension, acne, migraine, and fluid retention, as well as depression associated with birth control pills, and for the relief of symptoms of diabetes, carpal tunnel syndrome, heart disease, asthma, arthritis, skin disorders, bladder cancer, mental illness, calcium oxalate kidney stones, rare types of anemia, and side effects of certain antituberculosis drugs; 6) cyanocobalamin (B_{12}) for management of depression, fatigue, anxiety, insomnia, neuralgias, asthma, and seborrheic dermatitis.

In addition, biotin has been used for treating infants with eczema, and in diabetic patients and kidney dialysis patients. Folic acid may be helpful in treating canker sores, cervical dysplasias, heart disease, gout, psoriasis, and most recently in preventing certain birth defects. Ascorbic acid (vitamin C), a relatively nontoxic vitamin, is currently widely touted as an antioxidant for prevention of various cancers, cardiovascular diseases, and viral and bacterial infections and for protecting the body against harmful effects of smoking, radiation therapy, and pollution. It also may help to improve immune function. Vitamin A, also reputed to be an antioxidant, is used to treat acute infections, acne, peptic ulcers, to stem excess menstrual bleeding, and to promote wound healing. Beta-carotene, a water-soluble precursor to vitamin A, is also a good antioxidant that is widely promoted for preventing cardiovascular disease, certain types of cancer, and for modifying aging effects. Vitamin D has been promoted in menopause to help increase absorption of dietary calcium as well as being used in conjunction with calcium for leg cramps, night sweats, and hot flashes. Vitamin E is also an antioxidant and may help prevent cardiovascular disease and cancers, improve circulation, prevent blood clots, slow aging, help in fibrocystic breast disease, possibly prevent miscarriages, relieve premenstrual tension, and help prevent cataracts. Vitamin K combined with vitamin C has been used to relieve nausea and vomiting during pregnancy, and may be useful in managing recurrent nose bleeds and heavy menstrual bleeding. It is evident that vitamins have been promoted for a vast array of human ills, and their use continues to expand as new reports of their potential effectiveness appear regularly.

It should be noted that the principal candidates for vitamin supplements are pregnant women, who usually do need larger amounts of iron and other nutrients; the elderly, who may eat less and tend to absorb nutrients less efficiently; heavy drinkers, who need thiamine and folic acid; cigarette smokers, who generally have low levels of vitamin C; strict vegetarians, who may need vitamin B_{12}; dieters, who may miss certain needed vitamins; the chronically ill, whose medications may inhibit nutrient absorption; and patients recovering from surgery or infection, who need nutrients to help overcome the stress of illness.

One final note related to vitamin and mineral supplements is the recent surge of interest in so-called "medical" foods, "designer" foods, or "nutraceuticals." Like the use of vitamins and minerals in amounts above the norm, certain foods are now promoted in higher quantities in the diet for purported specific healthful and medical benefits. Some do contain vitamins, but many have other natural nutrients or unique food-derived compounds that may have potential physiological and pharmacological benefit. Tables 75-2 and 75-3 provide examples of "designer foods" and foods with medical properties that may be useful in treating certain medical disorders. Most of these are preventative and supportive in nature and in no way should replace standard medications, particularly for acute medical conditions.

Vitamins are commonly classified as either water-soluble (B complex, C) or fat soluble (A, D, E, and K). They are reviewed in that order in this chapter.

Water-Soluble Vitamins

Certain vitamins are readily soluble in water and are found together in many of the same foods. They are therefore usually grouped together as the water-soluble vitamins. They include the B complex group and ascorbic acid (vitamin C). These substances are readily excreted in the urine and thus are potentially much less toxic after large doses than are the fat-soluble vitamins, which are metabolized slowly and can be stored in significant amounts in the body.

B Complex Vitamins

The vitamin B complex group is composed of a number of compounds that differ in structure and biologic activity but are obtained from many of the same sources, most notably liver and yeast. Two B complex vitamins, cyanocobalamin (vitamin B_{12}) and folic acid (vitamin B_9) have been reviewed in Chapter 36,

Table 75-2. **"Designer Foods"**

Phytochemicals	*Botanical Source*	*Purported Properties*
Allicin, ajoene	Garlic	Stimulates biochemical pathways involving glutathione, which detoxifies foreign materials; intercepts activated carcinogens before they attach to DNA; inhibits prostaglandin E-2, which is linked to tumor promotion. Has antimicrobial properties
Flavonoids, phenolics, carotenoids, saponins and triterpenoids	Citrus fruits	Enhance body's detoxification system. Have antioxidant effects. Regulate enzymes produced by cancer cells. Phenolics stimulate synthesis of glutathione, the body's "detoxifier." Carotenoids quench damaging oxygen free radicals. Saponins and triterpenoids may block cells' receptors for estrogen, which may protect against breast cancer. Inhibits prostaglandin E-2, which is linked to tumor promotion
Alpha-linoleic acid, phenolic lignans	Flaxseed	These fatty acids diminish cholesterol formation, lignans have antiestrogenic activity, which may lower breast cancer risk. Inhibits prostaglandin E-2, which is linked to tumor promotion
Glycyrrhizic acid, other related triterpenoids, phenolics	Licorice	Antibiotic properties; phenolics inhibit key enzymes overproduced by cancer cells. Inhibits prostaglandin E-2, which is linked to tumor promotion
Isoflavones	Soybeans	Isoflavones inhibit activity of tyrosine kinases, which are overproduced when normal cells are transformed into cancer cells
Indoles, betacarbolenes	Cabbage-family members	Favor estrogen deactivation and excretion, which minimizes tumor activation pathway
Phenolic acids	Umbelliferous vegetables, eg, parsley, celery	Possible antiulcer properties

Table 75-3. **Foods with Reported Medical Properties**

Food	*Constituents*	*Purported Medical Properties*
Apple	Pectin, caffeic acid	Lowers cholesterol, blood pressure. Juice antimicrobial, antidiarrheal properties. Possible protectant against cancer
Banana and plantain	Fiber in unripe plantain, pectin	Prevents and heals ulcers, helps lower blood cholesterol. Stimulates proliferation of cells in stomach lining and release of protective mucous
Broccoli	Indoles, glucosinolates, dithiolthiones, carotenoids	Lowers risk of cancer
Cabbage	Chlorophyll, dithiolthiones, flavonoids, indoles, isothiocyanates, phenolic, caffeic and ferulic acid, vitamins E and C, "growth factor," mucinlike substances	Lowers risk of colonic cancer, juice helps prevent and heal ulcers, stimulates immune system, kills microbes, is classed as desmutagen (cancer antagonist)
Chili pepper	Capsaicin, vitamin C	Increases mucous secretion in lung, acts as expectorant, alleviates chronic bronchitis and emphysema, decongestant, diminishes clot formation (fibrinolytic), topically effective analgesic used in "cluster" headaches, induces secretion of endorphin
Spices, eg, cumin, cinnamon, ginger, mustard	Various active principles	Reduced cholesterol levels in animals
Fenugreek	Various active principles, fiber	Helps control sugar levels in diabetics

because they are primarily indicated in the treatment of pernicious anemia; cyanocobalamin is discussed here only as a nutritional supplement. The remaining B complex vitamins are examined individually in this chapter.

• Vitamin B_1 (Thiamine)

Biamine, Thiamilate

(CAN) Betaxin, Bewon

Thiamine, or vitamin B_1, is an organic molecule that combines with adenosine triphosphate (ATP) to form thiamine pyrophosphate, a coenzyme essential for carbohydrate metabolism. Thiamine requirements are closely linked to caloric intake, and clinical manifestations of thiamine deficiency can range from mild (anorexia, weakness, paresthesias, hypothermia, hypotension) to moderate (polyneuritis, sensory and motor defects, cardiovascular disease) to severe (Wernicke's encephalopathy, Korsakoff's psychosis). Beriberi, a thiamine deficiency characterized by GI disturbances, peripheral neurologic complications ("dry beriberi"), and cardiovascular disease ("wet beriberi"), is frequently observed in far eastern countries, where the diet consists largely of polished rice, which is very low in thiamine. In contrast, in the United States, alcoholism is the most common cause of thiamine deficiency.

Mechanism

Interacts with ATP to form thiamine pyrophosphate, a coenzyme that functions in the decarboxylation of alpha-keto and pyruvic acids and in the utilization of pentose by the hexose–monophosphate shunt.

Uses

Prevention and treatment of thiamine deficiency states (Table 75-1)

Dosage

Oral: 5 to 30 mg/day

IM (Beriberi): 10 mg to 20 mg three times a day for 2 weeks, supplemented with a daily oral multivitamin containing 5 to 10 mg thiamine

IV (Beriberi with myocardial failure; Wernicke–Korsakoff syndrome): up to 30 mg three times a day

CAUTION

When thiamine is to be administered IV, perform an intradermal sensitivity test before injection, because deaths have resulted from thiamine hypersensitivity after IV use.

Fate

Oral absorption is limited to 8 to 15 mg/day. As intake exceeds the minimal requirement (1–2 mg), tissue stores become saturated, and the excess appears in the urine, either as unchanged thiamine or as a pyrimidine metabolite.

Significant Adverse Reactions

(Usually with large doses) Feeling of warmth, pruritus, urticaria, sweating, nausea, restlessness, weakness, cyanosis, dyspnea, tightness of the throat, angioedema, pulmonary edema, and GI hemorrhage

Interactions

Thiamine is unstable in alkaline solutions, for example, with carbonates or citrates.

Nursing Management

Pretherapy Assessment

Assess and record baseline data necessary for detection of adverse effects of thiamine: General: vital signs (VS), body weight, skin color and temperature; GI: biliary function; genitourinary (GU): renal function; Lab: urinalysis, blood urea nitrogen (BUN), creatinine; cardiovascular system (CVS): hematologic function.

Review medical history and documents for existing or previous conditions that:

a. require cautious use of thiamine: gallbladder disease; diabetes mellitus, gout

b. contraindicate use of thiamine: allergy to thiamine; peptic ulcer; **pregnancy (Category—undetermined)**

Nursing Interventions

Medication Administration

Be prepared to administer thiamine to thiamine-deficient patient before a glucose load is delivered to avert the sudden worsening of symptoms of Wernicke's encephalopathy (eg, ataxia, diplopia, tremor, agitation) that may occur after IV glucose administration.

Expect appropriate supplementary therapy to be instituted because multiple vitamin and nutrient deficiencies usually accompany thiamine deficiency.

Do *not* use thiamine in combination with alkaline solutions (eg, citrates, carbonates, bicarbonates, barbiturates) because it is unstable in alkaline or neutral solutions.

Note that clinically significant thiamine depletion can occur within 3 weeks in the total absence of dietary thiamine.

Administer thiamine in divided doses with food to improve absorption.

Expect to administer thiamine to patients receiving total parenteral nutrition (TPN) as requirements increase as carbohydrate utilization increases.

Surveillance During Therapy

Monitor patient for allergic reactions to parenteral thiamine, which may range from itching and rash to anaphylactic cardiovascular collapse.

Monitor patient for significant adverse effects of high-dose thiamine therapy, including pruritus, urticaria, sweating, nausea, restlessness, weakness, cyanosis, dyspnea, tightness of the throat, angioedema, pulmonary edema, and GI hemorrhage.

Interpret results of diagnostic tests and contact practitioner as appropriate.

Patient Teaching

Instruct patient that the dosage form should be kept in a cool, dark place to ensure thiamine stability.

Instruct the patient to take thiamine with food.

Instruct patient to check dosage form expiration dates: potency diminishes rapidly after 3 months.

• Vitamin B_2 (Riboflavin)

Riboflavin, or vitamin B_2, derives its name from the presence of the sugar ribose as a component of the molecule and from the fact that the remainder of the structure is a yellow-pigmented compound termed a *flavin*. Riboflavin functions as a coenzyme that plays an essential role in the metabolism of a variety of cellular respiratory proteins.

Mechanism

Converted to one of two riboflavin-containing biologically active coenzymes, flavin mononucleotide (FMN) and flavin adenine dinucleotide (FAD), which play a vital metabolic role in the action of tissue respiratory flavoproteins

Uses

Prevention and treatment of riboflavin deficiency (ariboflavinosis)—see Table 75-1

Dosage

Oral: 5 to 25 mg/day

Fate

Well absorbed orally; widely distributed in the body but very little is stored; in small amounts, approximately 10% is excreted in the urine; larger doses are eliminated in increasing proportion in the urine; drug is present in the feces but probably represents vitamin synthesized by intestinal microorganisms.

Interactions

Riboflavin may inhibit the activity of tetracyclines when mixed together in solution.

Nursing Management

Pretherapy Assessment

Assess and record baseline data necessary for detection of adverse effects of riboflavin: General: VS, body weight, skin color and temperature; GI: biliary function; GU: renal function; Lab: urinalysis, BUN, creatinine; CVS: hematologic function.

Review medical history and documents for existing or previous conditions that:

a. require cautious use of riboflavin: none

b. contraindicate use of riboflavin: allergy to riboflavin; **pregnancy (Category—undetermined)**

Nursing Interventions

Medication Administration

Expect appropriate supplementary therapy to be instituted because multiple vitamin and nutrient deficiencies usually accompany riboflavin deficiency.

Administer riboflavin in divided doses with food to improve absorption.

Surveillance During Therapy

Interpret results of diagnostic tests and contact practitioner as appropriate.

Patient Teaching

Instruct patient that the dosage form should be kept in a cool, dark place to ensure thiamine stability.

Instruct the patient to take riboflavin with food.

Reassure patient that symptoms of riboflavin deficiency (sore throat, stomatitis, glossitis, corneal vascularization, cheilosis, seborrheic dermatitis, blepharospasm, photophobia) usually disappear shortly after beginning replacement therapy.

Inform patient that riboflavin will impart a harmless yellowish color to urine. The color may, however, interfere with urinary catecholamine determinations.

Instruct patient to check dosage form expiration dates: potency diminishes rapidly after 3 months.

• *Vitamin B_3 (Nicotinic Acid, Niacin)*

Nia-Bid, Niacor, Niacels, Nico-400, Nicobid, Nicolar, Nicotinex, Slo-Niacin

(CAN) Novoniacin, Tri-B3

Nicotinic acid or niacin (vitamin B_3) is a B complex vitamin that serves as a constituent of two important coenzymes, NAD (coenzyme I) and NADP (coenzyme II). These coenzymes function in several oxidation–reduction reactions required for cellular and tissue respiration. Niacin is an essential dietary constituent, the lack of which results in pellagra, a condition that primarily affects the skin, GI tract, and CNS, and is often characterized by the three "Ds," that is, dermatitis, diarrhea, and dementia. In addition to its value in treating pellagra and other nicotinic acid deficiency states, niacin is also employed in large doses as adjunctive therapy in several forms of hyperlipidemia and hypercholesterolemia. These latter indications are reviewed in Chapter 35. Finally, its vasodilatory action has led to its use as a circulatory aid in peripheral vascular diseases, but there is no conclusive evidence that the drug has a clinically beneficial effect in patients with circulatory impairment.

Large doses of nicotinic acid have been employed in treating schizophrenia as part of what has been termed *orthomolecular psychiatry*. There is no convincing evidence that such treatment is effective, and use of high doses of nicotinic acid may be associated with significant toxicity, including liver damage, arrhythmias, peptic ulceration, sensory neuropathy, hyperglycemia, dermatoses, and GI distress.

Mechanism

Niacin functions as a component of NAD and NADP, coenzymes vital to cellular metabolism. Large doses exert a hypolipemic effect, presumably by reducing triglyceride synthesis and blocking the release of very low-density lipoproteins (VLDLs) from the liver; it may also increase cholesterol oxidation and inhibit mobilization of free fatty acids; niacin exerts a direct, although relatively weak, relaxing effect on peripheral vascular smooth muscle.

Uses

Prevention and treatment of pellagra and other niacin deficiency states

Adjunctive therapy of hypercholesterolemia and hyperbetalipoproteinemia (Types IIb, III, IV, and V); see Chapter 35

Symptomatic treatment of peripheral vascular disorders (conclusive evidence of beneficial effect is lacking)

Dosage

Oral:

Niacin deficiency: 10 to 100 mg/day

Pellagra: up to 500 mg/day, depending on severity of symptoms

Hyperlipidemias: 1 to 2 g three times a day (maximum, 6 g/day)

IV (preferred), IM or SC (for vitamin deficiencies only)

Dosage and duration of therapy dependent on patient response

Fate

Readily absorbed orally and widely distributed; peak serum concentrations occur in 45 minutes; approximately one-third of a normal oral dose is excreted unchanged in the urine; with very large doses, the principal urinary excretory product is the unchanged drug.

Common Side Effects

Cutaneous flushing and sensation of warmth, especially in the face or neck area; GI distress

Significant Adverse Reactions

(Especially with large doses) Headache, tingling, skin rash, pruritus, increased sebaceous gland activity, dryness of the skin, jaundice, allergic reactions, keratosis nigricans, activation of peptic ulcer, abdominal pain, vomiting, diarrhea, hypotension (orthostatic), dizziness, hyperuricemia, toxic amblyopia, and decreased glucose tolerance

Contraindications

Active peptic ulcer, severe hepatic dysfunction, severe hypotension, hemorrhaging or arterial bleeding. *Cautious use* in patients with glaucoma, jaundice, liver disease, peptic ulcer, gallbladder disease, diabetes, gout, or angina; in children, and in pregnant or nursing women.

Interactions

Niacin may have additive blood pressure-lowering effects with antihypertensive drugs.

Niacin can reduce the effectiveness of oral hypoglycemic agents by elevating blood glucose levels.

Niacin may reduce the uricosuric action of sulfinpyrazone or probenecid.

Nursing Management

Pretherapy Assessment

Assess and record baseline data necessary for detection of adverse effects of niacin: General: VS, body weight, skin color and temperature; GI: biliary function; Lab: liver function, serum uric acid, glucose tolerance.

Review medical history and documents for existing or previous conditions that:

a. require cautious use of niacin: glaucoma, jaundice, liver disease, peptic ulcer, gallbladder disease, diabetes, gout, or angina
b. contraindicate use of niacin: allergy to nicotinic acid, or nicotinamide; allergy to aspirin (formulations containing tartrazine); active peptic ulcer, severe hepatic dysfunction, severe hypotension, hemorrhaging or arterial bleeding; **pregnancy (Category A)** for RDA dosage, **pregnancy (Category C)** for parenteral usage

Nursing Interventions

Medication Administration

Expect therapy to begin with small doses to minimize untoward reactions. Dosage should be increased gradually to optimal level. Initial therapeutic response usually occurs within 24 to 48 hours.

Administer parenteral therapy, which is indicated only for severe niacin deficiency (not for hyperlipidemia), by slow IV injection, if possible.

Administer oral drug with food to minimize GI upset.

Arrange for one aspirin 30 min before dose of niacin to minimize flushing in patients to whom it is distressing.

Surveillance During Therapy

Monitor patient for changes in liver function during long-term therapy.
Monitor patient for signs of orthostatic hypotension.
Interpret results of diagnostic tests and contact practitioner as appropriate.

Patient Teaching

Instruct patient that the dosage form should be kept in a cool, dark place to ensure drug stability.
Instruct patient to take drug during meals to minimize GI upset and to swallow with cold water. Hot beverages should be avoided because they may intensify vasodilation.
Inform patient that tingling, itching, headache, or a sensation of warmth, especially in the area of the head, neck, and ears, can occur shortly after administration, but that these effects usually subside with continued therapy. For vitamin replacement therapy, niacinamide may be used instead of niacin if flushing is severe or bothersome (see nicotinamide).
Warn patient not to engage in hazardous activities because dizziness or weakness can occur, especially during early therapy.
Advise patient to avoid prolonged exposure to bright sunlight.
Instruct patient to check dosage form expiration dates: potency diminishes rapidly after 3 months.

• Nicotinamide

Niacinamide

An amide of nicotinic acid, nicotinamide provides a source of niacin that can be used by the body but is devoid of hypolipidemic and vasodilatory effects. Thus, it is indicated only for treatment of niacin deficiency states, in which it is preferred by many patients, who find the flushing and paresthesias resulting from niacin itself unpleasant. Nicotinamide is available for oral or parenteral administration, and dosage is highly individual and based on symptoms and response. The usual dosage range is 50 mg 3 to 10 times a day. Other than a reduced incidence of circulatory side effects, the pharmacology of nicotinamide is essentially similar to that of nicotinic acid.

• Vitamin B_5 (Calcium Pantothenate)

Pantothenic acid is often referred to as vitamin B_5. Because pantothenic acid is found abundantly in the normal diet, deficiency states are quite rare. Although it is a necessary nutrient, the daily requirement is not known and no RDAs are available. Pantothenic acid in the form of its calcium salt is commonly found in multivitamin preparations, but its presence is probably unnecessary. It is incorporated into coenzyme A, which functions as a cofactor for a variety of essential metabolic activities such as oxidative metabolism of carbohydrates, gluconeogenesis, synthesis and degradation of fatty acids, and synthesis of sterols and steroid hormones. Recommended dosage is 5 to 10 mg/day, although up to 10 g/day has been employed. Because no spontaneously occurring pantothenic acid deficiency state has been reported in humans, it use as an exogenous supplement is probably unnecessary.

• Vitamin B_6 (Pyridoxine)

Beesix, Nestrex

Naturally occurring substances that exhibit vitamin B_6 activity include pyridoxine in plants and pyridoxal and pyridoxamine in animals. All three compounds possess similar biologic activity and thus should be regarded as different forms of vitamin B_6, although pyridoxine is the most commonly used term. Pyridoxine functions as a coenzyme at different stages in the metabolism of carbohydrates, fats, and proteins. The need for pyridoxine increases with the amount of protein in the diet.

Mechanism

All three forms of vitamin B_6 are converted in vivo to pyridoxal phosphate or pyridoxamine phosphate, the physiologically active forms that serve as coenzymes for a number of essential metabolic reactions. Such reactions include decarboxylation, transamination, and transulfuration of amino acids, conversion of tryptophan to serotonin or niacin, and glycogenolysis.

Uses

Treatment of pyridoxine deficiency, as seen, for example, with inadequate dietary intake, inborn errors of metabolism (eg, pyridoxine-dependent convulsions, pyridoxine-responsive anemia) or drug-induced depletion (eg, from isoniazid, alcohol, oral contraceptives)
Investigational uses include control of nausea and vomiting in pregnancy or that resulting from radiation, reversal of the neurologic symptoms of hydrazine poisoning, symptomatic treatment of the premenstrual syndrome, and treatment of oxalate kidney stones

Dosage

Dietary deficiency: 10 to 20 mg/day orally for 3 weeks, followed by an oral multivitamin containing 2 to 5 mg pyridoxine (see Nursing Considerations)
Pyridoxine dependency syndrome: up to 600 mg/day initially, reduced to 25 to 50 mg/day for life
Isoniazid-induced deficiency: 50 to 200 mg daily
Isoniazid overdosage (10 g or more): give an equal amount of pyridoxine (4 g IV injection, followed by 1 g IM every 30 min)

Fate

Well absorbed orally; converted to pyridoxal phosphate; and pyridoxamine phosphate; half-life is 15 to 20 days; metabolized in the liver to 4-pyridoxic acid, which is excreted in the urine

Significant Adverse Reactions

(Usually only with large doses) Paresthesias, somnolence, flushing, reduced serum folic acid levels, and pain at injection site

Contraindications

No absolute contraindications. *Cautious use* in nursing mothers (may inhibit lactation).

Interactions

Pyridoxine can reduce the effectiveness of levodopa by accelerating its peripheral metabolism.
Pyridoxine requirement may be increased in patients taking isoniazid, cycloserine, oral contraceptives, hydralazine, or penicillamine.

Concomitant administration of pyridoxine may decrease serum levels of phenobarbital and phenytoin.

Nursing Management

Pretherapy Assessment

Assess and record baseline data necessary for detection of adverse effects of **pyridoxine**: General: VS, body weight, skin color and temperature; CNS: orientation.

Review medical history and documents for existing or previous conditions that:

a. require cautious use of pyridoxine: use in nursing mothers (may inhibit lactation).

b. contraindicate use of pyridoxine: none.

Nursing Interventions

Medication Administration

Advocate pyridoxine supplementation for alcoholic patient to prevent neurologic complications because a substantial number of alcoholics have a significant deficiency. Pyridoxine deficiency is also common in patients taking isoniazid, and it may occur with use of oral contraceptives and certain other drugs (refer to Interactions).

Expect symptoms to be controlled with a multivitamin preparation once pyridoxine levels are restored because selective pyridoxine dietary deficiency is rare.

Surveillance During Therapy

Monitor patient for changes in neurologic function during long-term therapy.

Interpret results of diagnostic tests and contact practitioner as appropriate.

Patient Teaching

Instruct patient that the dosage form should be kept in a cool, dark place to ensure drug stability.

Instruct patient to take drug during meals to minimize GI upset.

Instruct patient to check dosage form expiration dates: potency diminishes rapidly after 3 months.

• Vitamin B_{12} (Cyanocobalamin)

Cyanocobalamin, or vitamin B_{12}, is essential for normal growth and development, cell reproduction, hematopoiesis, and nucleoprotein and myelin synthesis. Insufficient GI absorption of cyanocobalamin, due primarily to decreased availability of intrinsic factor, leads to pernicious anemia and is treated with large oral or parenteral doses (see Chapter 36). Oral preparations containing less than 500 μg cyanocobalamin are *not* indicated for pernicious anemia but are employed solely as a nutritional supplement, especially in persons on strict vegetarian diets. The recommended dosage range is 25 to 250 μg/day, although it should be remembered that the RDA for cyanocobalamin is only 3 μg in adults.

• Vitamin C (Ascorbic Acid)

Various Manufacturers

Vitamin C, or ascorbic acid, is an essential dietary substance that plays a major role in many metabolic reactions as well as the formation and maintenance of collagen and intracellular ground substance. The name *ascorbic acid* is a condensation of the term *antiscorbutic vitamin*. It is derived from the compound's ability to prevent scurvy, the principal ascorbic acid deficiency state. In normal therapeutic doses, ascorbic acid elicits few demonstrable pharmacologic effects except in the scorbutic person (ie, the patient with symptoms of scurvy). This disease is occasionally observed in elderly or debilitated persons, drug addicts, alcoholics, and others with poor diets. It is characterized by degenerative changes in connective tissue, bones, and capillaries. The symptoms of ascorbic acid deficiency (swollen and bleeding gums, petechiae, easy bruising, delayed wound healing, loosened teeth, joint pain, and bloody stools) are usually readily relieved by 200 to 400 mg ascorbic acid daily for several days; they can be prevented from recurring by small (50–100 mg) daily supplemental doses of the vitamin. Although very large amounts (megadoses) of ascorbic acid have been advocated for a wide variety of disease states (refer to opening of chapter), ranging from prophylaxis of the common cold to treatment of carcinomas, *conclusive evidence* for the vitamin's effectiveness in megadose quantities for any of the proposed indications is lacking. In addition to ascorbic acid itself, a sodium salt and a calcium salt are also available.

Mechanism

Participates in a number of essential biologic functions, for example, formation of collagen and intracellular ground substance, cellular respiration, microsomal drug metabolism, steroid synthesis, tyrosine metabolism, and conversion of folic acid to folinic acid; important for the maintenance of tooth and bone matrix and capillary integrity, and may aid wound healing; reduces pH of the urine

Uses

Prevention and treatment of scurvy and other ascorbic acid deficiency states

Adjunctive therapy in extensive or deep burns, delayed wound healing, chronic or severe illnesses, and a variety of other disease states and stressful situations (effectiveness has not been conclusively demonstrated)

Acidification of the urine, usually in conjunction with a urinary anti-infective (eg, methenamine)

Dosage

Oral:

Treatment of deficiency states: 300 to 1,000 mg/day as needed

Prophylaxis: 75 to 150 mg/day

Wound healing: 300 to 500 mg/day for 7 to 10 days; much larger amounts have been used

Burns: 1 g to 2 g/day

IM, SC, IV:

Up to 2 g/day may be given as needed for severe deficiency states; maintenance dose is 100 to 250 mg once or twice a day

Fate

Readily absorbed orally or parenterally and widely distributed; partly metabolized and excreted in the urine both as metabolites and unchanged drug; renal threshold is 1.5 mg/dL plasma, and the amount excreted markedly increases with large doses

Significant Adverse Reactions

(Usually with large doses) Diarrhea, precipitation of oxalate or urate renal stones, soreness at IM or SC injection sites, and dizziness or faintness with too rapid IV injection

Contraindications

Use of sodium ascorbate injection in patients on sodium-restricted diets. *Cautious use* in patients with glucose-6-phosphate dehydrogenase deficiency, hyperuricemia, or renal impairment, and in pregnant women.

Interactions

Large doses of ascorbic acid lower urinary pH and thus may reduce excretion of acidic drugs (eg, salicylates, barbiturates) and increase excretion of basic drugs (eg, quinidine, atropine, amphetamines, tricyclic antidepressants, phenothiazines).

Ascorbic acid increases serum levels of estrogen, and may result in increased adverse effects if given concurrently.

Large doses of ascorbic acid may shorten the prothrombin time in patients receiving oral anticoagulants.

Ascorbic acid can interfere with the effectiveness of disulfiram when it is used in the alcoholic patient (see Chapter 81).

Ascorbic acid in large doses may enhance the absorption of oral iron.

Mineral oil can retard absorption of ascorbic acid.

Ascorbic acid is chemically incompatible with penicillin G potassium and should not be mixed in the same syringe.

Smoking may slightly reduce ascorbic acid serum levels; conversely, ascorbic acid can enhance excretion of nicotine, perhaps resulting in an increased desire to smoke.

Nursing Management

Pretherapy Assessment

Assess and record baseline data necessary for detection of adverse effects of ascorbic acid: General: VS, body weight, skin color and temperature; GU: output, pH.

Review medical history and documents for existing or previous conditions that:

a. require cautious use of ascorbic acid: glucose-6-phosphate dehydrogenase deficiency, hyperuricemia, or renal impairment, and in pregnant women.
b. contraindicate use of ascorbic acid: use in patients on sodium-restricted diets.

Nursing Interventions

Medication Administration

Inject IV slowly to avoid dizziness and possible fainting.

Surveillance During Therapy

Interpret results of diagnostic tests and contact practitioner as appropriate.

Interpret results of urine glucose, serum uric acid, and urinary steroid determinations cautiously because large doses may result in false readings.

Patient Teaching

Instruct patient that the dosage form should be kept in a cool, dark place to ensure drug stability.

Instruct patient to take drug during meals to minimize GI upset.

Instruct patient to check dosage form expiration dates: potency diminishes rapidly after 3 months.

Fat-Soluble Vitamins

Unlike the B complex and C vitamins, vitamins A, D, E, and K are poorly soluble in water but dissolve readily in fats. This property is responsible for certain characteristics that distinguish the fat-soluble vitamins from their water-soluble counterparts. Whereas the B and C vitamins are readily absorbed orally, the fat-soluble vitamins require the presence of sufficient amounts of bile salts in the GI tract for adequate absorption. However, their absorption may be impaired by the presence of mineral oil or other fatty vehicles that can sequester the vitamins in the lumen of the intestine. Compared with the water-soluble vitamins, vitamins A, D, E, and K are stored in much larger amounts in body tissues such as adipose tissue, liver, and muscles. From these storage depots, small amounts are released over extended periods to meet nutritional needs; hence symptoms of a fat-soluble vitamin deficiency usually develop only after long periods of inadequate intake, that is, not until body stores are depleted. Loss of fat-soluble vitamins in the urine is minimal, and excretion proceeds at a slow rate. This relatively inefficient excretion of most fat-soluble vitamins can result in accumulation to toxic levels if *excessive* quantities of the vitamins are ingested to supplement the diet, and such a practice should be discouraged.

Characteristics of the fat-soluble vitamins are listed in Table 75-1, along with their recommended dietary allowances. The four vitamins making up the fat-soluble group are reviewed below. In addition, two vitamin A analogues, (tretinoin, isotretinoin) used in treatment of severe acne and other types of skin conditions, and a third analogue (etretinate) useful in recalcitrant psoriasis are reviewed in Chapter 79.

• Vitamin A

Aquasol A, Del-Vi-A

The term *vitamin A* is commonly used to refer to a group of several biologically active compounds. Vitamin A_1 (retinol) is the principal naturally occurring substance and is formed from precursors termed *carotenes*, the most important of which is beta-carotene (provitamin A). The average adult receives about one-half the daily dietary intake of vitamin A as preformed retinol and the remainder as carotene precursors. Vitamin A_2 (3-dehydroretinol) occurs mixed with retinol in many dietary sources. Most currently used preparations are synthetic retinol esters, which have largely replaced the natural vitamin A products previously extracted from fish liver oils, inasmuch as they are generally better absorbed and provide more consistent blood levels of the vitamin.

The potency of vitamin A preparations is expressed as international units (IU), one IU being equal to 0.3 μg retinol. Activity is expressed as retinol equivalents (RE), 1 RE having the activity of 1 μg retinol (3.33 IU) or 6 μg beta-carotene (10 IU). Vitamin A is required for growth of bones and teeth, integrity of epithelial tissue, normal functioning of the retina (especially visual adaptation to darkness), reproduction, and embryonic development. In addition, vitamin A deficiency can lower resistance to infection and reduce adrenal cortical steroid production. Deficiencies are rarely observed when reasonable dietary practices are followed, and liver stores of vitamin A are usually sufficient to satisfy requirements of the vitamin for up to 2 years.

Mechanism

Complex and incompletely understood; among the actions ascribed to vitamin A are increased synthesis of RNA, proteins, steroids, mucopolysaccharides, and cholesterol; prevents growth retardation and preserves the integrity of epithelial cells; also necessary for formation of rhodopsin, a photosensitive pigment important for vision in dim light; may enhance healing of wounds

Uses

Treatment of vitamin A deficiency states (eg, biliary or pancreatic disease, colitis, hepatic cirrhosis, celiac disease, regional enteritis)
Prophylaxis of vitamin A deficiency during periods of increased requirements, for example, infancy, pregnancy, lactation, severe illness

Dosage

Adults:
- Oral: 100,000 to 500,000 IU/day for 3 days, then 50,000 IU/day for 2 weeks, then 10,000 to 20,000 IU/day for 2 months
- IM: 100,000 IU/day for 3 days, then 50,000 IU/day for 2 weeks

Children:
- Oral: 10,000 to 15,000 IU/day as a dietary supplement
- IM (1–8 yr): 17,500 to 35,000 IU/day for 10 days

Infants
- IM: 7,500 to 15,000 IU/day for 10 days

Fate

Gastrointestinal absorption of vitamin A preparations is good in the presence of bile acids, pancreatic lipase, and dietary fat; aqueous dispersions of the synthetic vitamin are more rapidly absorbed than oil solutions; peak plasma concentrations occur in approximately 3 to 4 hours; most of a dose is stored in the liver, with smaller amounts stored in many other body tissues; vitamin E increases tissue storage of vitamin A; plasma levels increase substantially when hepatic storage sites are saturated; slowly released from liver; serum concentrations can be maintained for months by hepatic stores; transported in the plasma as retinol bound to retinol-binding protein; excretion probably occurs primarily in the bile as a glucuronide, with small amounts appearing in the urine.

Significant Adverse Reactions

(Due to overdosage: hypervitaminosis A syndrome)
CNS: fatigue, irritability, malaise, lethargy, night sweats, vertigo, headache, increased intracranial pressure (may be manifested as papilledema)
Dermatologic: drying and fissuring of skin and lips, alopecia, gingivitis, pruritus, desquamation, increased pigmentation, tender swellings on the extremities
Musculoskeletal: retarded growth, arthralgia, premature closure of the epiphyses, bone pain
GI: abdominal pain, vomiting, anorexia
Other: liver and spleen enlargement, jaundice, leukopenia, hypomenorrhea, polydipsia, polyuria, hypercalcemia

Contraindications

Oral administration in patients with malabsorption syndrome, hypervitaminosis A; administration by the IV route. *Cautious use* in the presence of impaired renal or hepatic function and in pregnant women.

Interactions

Mineral oil, cholestyramine resin, and colestipol may impair absorption of vitamin A.
Increased plasma vitamin A levels have occurred in women taking oral contraceptives.

Nursing Management

Pretherapy Assessment

Assess and record baseline data necessary for detection of adverse effects of vitamin A: General: VS, body weight, skin color and temperature; GU: output, pH; Lab: liver function, urinalysis, CBC.
Review medical history and documents for existing or previous conditions that:
a. require cautious use of vitamin A: impaired renal or hepatic function and in pregnant women.
b. contraindicate use of vitamin A: oral administration in patients with malabsorption syndrome, hypervitaminosis A; administration by the IV route.

Nursing Interventions

Medication Administration

Administer IM *only* when oral administration is not feasible, such as, for example, when vomiting, unconsciousness, steatorrhea, or other malabsorption states are present.
Question administration of large doses over prolonged periods because tissue accumulation can occur. Blood levels do not necessarily reflect total body concentration because liver storage is usually extensive.
Note that preparations containing up to 25,000 IU are available without prescription. Stronger preparations require a prescription.

Surveillance During Therapy

Interpret results of diagnostic tests and contact practitioner as appropriate.
Monitor patient for signs of hypervitaminosis A syndrome; including CNS, dermatologic, musculoskeletal, GI, and hepatosplenic symptoms.

Patient Teaching

Instruct patient that the dosage form should be kept in a cool, dark place to ensure drug stability.
Warn fertile woman that use of vitamin A in excess of the RDA (ie, 6,000 IU) during pregnancy can cause fetal abnormalities.
Instruct patient to avoid using mineral oil while taking vitamin A (refer to Interactions).
Instruct patient to discontinue drug and notify prescriber

if signs of hypervitaminosis A appear (refer to Significant Adverse Reactions). Symptoms subside quickly, but some, such as tender swellings in the extremities, may remain for months.

Vitamin D Preparations

Calcifediol
Calcitriol
Cholecalciferol
Dihydrotachysterol
Ergocalciferol

The term *vitamin D* is commonly applied to two related fat-soluble substances, ergocalciferol (D_2) and cholecalciferol (D_3), which are formed from the provitamins ergosterol and 7-dehydrocholesterol, respectively, by ultraviolet (UV) irradiation. The principal source of endogenous vitamin D in humans is the synthesis of D_3 from 7-dehydrocholesterol on exposure to the UV rays of the sun. Vitamin D_3 is then converted by hepatic microsomal enzymes to calcifediol (25-hydroxycholecalciferol), the principal transport form of vitamin D_3. Calcifediol possesses minor intrinsic vitamin D activity and is further metabolized in the kidney to calcitriol (1,25 dihydroxycholecalciferol), the most active form of vitamin D_3. Ergocalciferol and cholecalciferol, as well as calcifediol and calcitriol, are available for clinical use, as is dihydrotachysterol, a vitamin D analogue that is converted by the liver to 25-hydroxydihydrotachysterol, which elevates serum calcium levels.

Vitamin D_2 is the form usually found in commercial vitamin preparations and in fortified milk, bread, and cereals. Because in humans there is no difference in activity between vitamin D_2 and D_3, *vitamin D* is used as the collective term for all substances, natural and synthetic, having similar activity.

Dosage of the vitamin is measured in international units (IU), one IU of vitamin D activity being equal to 0.025 μg cholecalciferol.

After a general discussion of vitamin D, the individual vitamin D preparations are listed in Table 75-4.

Mechanism

Enhances the active absorption of calcium and phosphorus from the small intestine, facilitates their resorption from bone, and promotes their reabsorption by the renal tubules; plasma levels of calcium and phosphorus are therefore maintained at levels adequate for neuromuscular activity, mineralization of bone, and other calcium-dependent functions

Uses

Prevention or treatment of vitamin D deficiency (cholecalciferol)
Treatment of refractory (vitamin D–resistant) rickets (ergocalciferol)
Treatment of familial hypophosphatemia and hypoparathyroidism (ergocalciferol, dihydrotachysterol)

Table 75-4. **Vitamin D Preparations**

Drug	Usual Dosage Range	Nursing Considerations
Calcifediol *Calderol*	Initially, 300–350 μg/wk, on a daily or alternate-day schedule; may increase at 4-wk intervals as needed Usual maintenance range, 50–100 μg/day	Hydroxylated metabolite of cholecalciferol; used for management of metabolic bone disease or for hypocalcemia in patients on chronic renal dialysis; principal serum transport form of vitamin D_3; converted in the kidneys to calcitriol; increases serum calcium and decreases alkaline phosphatase and parathyroid hormone levels
Calcitriol *Calcijex, Rocaltrol*	Initially, 0.25 μg/day; increase by 0.25-μg/day increments at 4–8 wk intervals; hemodialysis patients generally require doses of 0.5–1 μg/day *Hypoparathyroidism*: 0.5–2.0 μg daily	Most active metabolite of vitamin D; potent hypercalcemic agent primarily used for treating hypocalcemia in patients undergoing renal dialysis; avoid magnesium-containing antacids because hypermagnesemia may occur, and do not give other vitamin D supplements during therapy; advise patients to note occurrence of weakness, vomiting, or muscle or bone pain, as these may indicate hypercalcemia
Cholecalciferol *Delta-D*	400–1,000 IU daily	Used as a dietary supplement in vitamin D deficiency states; precursor of calcifediol and calcitriol; available over-the-counter
Dihydrotachysterol *DHT, Hytakerol*	Initially, 0.8–2.4 mg daily for several days Maintenance doses are 0.2–1 mg daily as needed to maintain normal serum calcium levels	Potent vitamin D preparation that is more effective than ergocalciferol in mobilizing calcium from bone but shorter acting; primarily used in treating tetany and symptoms of hypoparathyroidism; maximal hypercalcemic effects require 1–2 wk to develop; safety margin with drug is rather small; be alert for symptoms of hypercalcemia
Ergocalciferol *Calciferol, Drisdol*	*Vitamin D–resistant rickets*: 50,000–500,000 IU daily, depending on severity of disease *Hypoparathyroidism*: 50,000–200,000 IU daily *plus* 500 mg elemental calcium 6 times daily *Hypophosphatemia*: 10,000–80,000 IU daily plus 1–2 g/day of elemental phosphorus	Usually administered orally, but IM administration is necessary in patients with GI, liver, or biliary disease associated with malabsorption of vitamin D; range between therapeutic and toxic doses is small; serum calcium concentration is maintained between 9 mg and 10 mg/dL; use with *caution* in patients with impaired kidney function or kidney stones

Treatment of metabolic bone disease or hypocalcemia in patients on chronic renal dialysis (calcifediol, calcitriol)

Treatment of acute, chronic, or latent forms of postoperative tetany or idiopathic tetany

Dosage

Refer to Table 75-4

Fate

Well absorbed from the intestine, D_3 more completely and more rapidly than D_2; bile is essential for absorption; stored primarily in the liver, with small amounts in skin, bones, and CNS; in the plasma, vitamin D is bound to albumin and alpha globulins; plasma half-life of the various derivatives varies from 24 hours (ergocalciferol) up to 20 days (calcifediol); primary route of excretion is the bile; very small amounts are found in the urine.

Significant Adverse Reactions

(Usually from overdosage: hypervitaminosis D syndrome)

Renal: polyuria, nocturia, elevated BUN, hypercalciuria, azotemia, nephrocalcinosis, proteinuria, urinary casts, renal insufficiency

GI: anorexia, nausea, vomiting, constipation or diarrhea, metallic taste, dry mouth

Other: acidosis, anemia, weakness, headache, irritability, photophobia, conjunctivitis, pancreatitis, hypertension, arrhythmias, vascular and soft-tissue calcification, muscle stiffness and pain, bone demineralization, mental retardation in children, dwarfism, hyperthermia, elevated serum transaminases (ALT and AST)

Contraindications

Hypercalcemia, malabsorption syndrome, hypervitaminosis D, and renal osteodystrophy with hyperphosphatemia. *Cautious use* in patients with a history of renal stones and in pregnant or nursing women and young children.

Interactions

Mineral oil and cholestyramine resin can impair vitamin D absorption.

Phenytoin, primidone, and barbiturates may reduce the effectiveness of vitamin D by increasing its metabolic inactivation.

Thiazide diuretics may potentiate vitamin D–induced hypercalcemia in hypoparathyroid patients.

Vitamin D may increase the likelihood of cardiac arrhythmias with digitalis drugs.

Magnesium-containing antacids used together with vitamin D may result in development of hypermagnesemia.

Nursing Management

Pretherapy Assessment

Assess and record baseline data necessary for detection of adverse effects of vitamin D: General: VS, body weight, skin color and temperature; GU: output, pH; CNS: orientation, taste; Lab: serum calcium, phosphorus, magnesium, alkaline phosphatase, liver function, urinalysis, CBC.

Review medical history and documents for existing or previous conditions that:

a. require cautious use of vitamin D: history of renal stones and in pregnant or nursing women and young children.
b. contraindicate use of vitamin D: allergy to vitamin D, tartrazine, or aspirin; hypercalcemia, malabsorption syndrome, hypervitaminosis D, and renal osteodystrophy with hyperphosphatemia; **pregnancy (Category C)**, lactation: secreted in breast milk.

Nursing Interventions

Medication Administration

Ensure that patient's diet is critically evaluated before vitamin D supplementation is initiated. Supplementation is usually unnecessary for patient who eats fortified foods and is exposed to normal amounts of sunlight.

Be prepared to administer ergocalciferol IM in patient with gastrointestinal, biliary, or liver disease associated with vitamin D malabsorption.

Collaborate with drug prescriber and dietician regarding calcium intake during treatment. Drug is often given with supplemental calcium salts or high-calcium foods because proper amount of additional calcium enhances therapeutic response.

Surveillance During Therapy

Interpret results of diagnostic tests and contact practitioner as appropriate.

Monitor patient for signs of hypervitaminosis D syndrome; including CNS, dermatologic, musculoskeletal, GI, and hepatosplenic symptoms.

Closely monitor results of serum calcium level determinations (normal range, 9–11 mg/dL), which should be obtained biweekly during early therapy, and assess patient for evidence of hypercalcemia or hypervitaminosis D (refer to Significant Adverse Reactions), because the range between therapeutic and toxic doses of vitamin D is very small. If hypercalcemia occurs, drug should be discontinued and supportive measures instituted (eg, high fluid intake, restriction of dietary calcium, laxatives).

Be prepared to administer intravenous diuretics, corticosteroids (150 mg/day cortisone or equivalent), and sodium citrate (2.5% IV infusion) if overdosage is severe.

Monitor results of serum phosphorus, magnesium, and alkaline phosphatase and 24-hour urinary calcium and phosphorus determinations, which should be obtained periodically during treatment.

Institute appropriate interventions to enhance patient's compliance with drug regimen, dietary recommendations, and calcium supplementation (when indicated) to minimize danger of untoward reactions

Patient Teaching

Instruct patient that the dosage form should be kept in a cool, dark place to ensure drug stability.

Instruct patient to discontinue drug and notify prescriber if signs of hypervitaminosis D appear (refer to Significant Adverse Reactions). Symptoms subside quickly, but some, such as tender swellings in the extremities, may remain for months.

Warn pregnant women not to exceed RDA (400 IU/day) because high doses have been associated with fetal abnormalities in animal studies.

Warn patient of the hazards of excessive or indiscriminate use of vitamin D, and explain that dosage levels are individually adjusted as the deficiency abates.

Inform patient that improvement may develop slowly (7–10 days) and that effects may persist for up to 30 days after therapy is terminated.

• Vitamin E

Aquasol E and other manufacturers

The term *vitamin E* is commonly used generically to describe eight naturally occurring tocopherols possessing vitamin E activity. Alpha-tocopherol constitutes approximately 90% of the tocopherols found in animal tissues, is the most biologically active of the eight, and is available both naturally, in vegetable oils and other foods, and synthetically. Because the potencies of the different forms of vitamin E vary somewhat, dosage is standardized in international units (IUs) according to activity.

Although RDAs have been published for vitamin E, deficiencies of vitamin E in humans are rare, inasmuch as adequate amounts are supplied in the ordinary diet. Low levels have occasionally been noted in severely malnourished infants and in patients with prolonged fat malabsorption or acanthocytosis.

Mechanism

Incompletely understood; action appears to be caused by its antioxidant properties; prevents oxidation of essential cellular constituents and formation of toxic oxidation products; may serve as a cofactor in enzyme reactions, play a role in hematopoiesis and hemoglobin formation, protect red blood cells from hemolysis, interfere with platelet aggregation, and enhance utilization of vitamin A

Uses

Prevention or treatment of vitamin E deficiency states

Investigational uses include reduction of the toxic effects of oxygen therapy on lung parenchyma (bronchopulmonary dysplasia) and the retina (retrolental fibroplasia), prevention of hemolytic anemia in infants, and temporary relief of minor skin disorders.

Other purported uses for vitamin E include prevention of cardiovascular disease, cancer, aging, premenstrual syndrome, nocturnal leg cramps, and to improve athletic performance, although conclusive evidence for these actions is lacking.

Dosage

Oral (deficiency states): 50 to 1,000 IU/day have been employed, depending on severity (RDA is approximately 15 IU)

Fate

Readily absorbed from GI tract if fat absorption is adequate; widely distributed in the body and stored in tissues for extended periods, providing a continual source of the vitamin; placental transfer is poor; largely excreted in the feces by way of the bile, smaller amounts appearing as metabolites in the urine

Significant Adverse Reactions

Minimal, even at very large doses; occasionally GI distress, muscle weakness

A *hypervitaminosis E syndrome* has been described, characterized by fatigue, headache, nausea, weakness, diarrhea, flatulence, blurred vision, and dermatitis.

Interactions

Vitamin E may enhance the action of oral anticoagulants by reducing levels of vitamin K–dependent clotting factors.

Vitamin E can reduce the efficacy of oral iron preparations.

• Vitamin K

Phytonadione (K_1)
Menadiol sodium diphosphate (K_4)

The term *vitamin K* refers to two structurally similar compounds that possess the ability to promote hepatic synthesis of certain blood clotting factors. The primary source of vitamin K in humans is through absorption of phytonadione (vitamin K_1) synthesized in the gut by intestinal bacteria. In addition, vitamin K is found in many foods (Table 75-1), although in most cases these represent a minor source of usable vitamin. Vitamin K_1 (phytonadione) is the only naturally occurring vitamin K used clinically; however, this lipid-soluble derivative is also prepared synthetically. The other synthetic vitamin K compound employed therapeutically is menadiol sodium diphosphate (vitamin K_4), a water-soluble analogue that is approximately one-half as potent as menadione (K_3), to which it is converted in vivo. Phytonadione is the preferred drug for treating hypoprothrombinemia, because it is the most potent of the derivatives and exhibits the fastest onset and longest duration of action. However, adequate absorption of phytonadione occurs only in the presence of bile salts, whereas K_4 can be adequately absorbed without bile salts.

The available vitamin K derivatives are discussed as a group, then listed individually in Table 75-5. Phytonadione has been reviewed previously in Chapter 37 as an antidote to overdosage with oral anticoagulants and is considered only briefly here.

Mechanism

Promote hepatic synthesis of blood clotting factors II, VII, IX, and X, probably by functioning as an essential cofactor for microsomal enzyme systems that activate the precursors of these clotting factors

Uses

Treatment of vitamin K deficiency caused by antibacterial therapy

Treatment of hypoprothrombinemia secondary to impaired absorption or synthesis of vitamin K, for example, obstructive jaundice, biliary fistulas, ulcerative colitis, sprue, celiac disease, regional enteritis, intestinal resection, cystic fibrosis, salicylate therapy

Treatment of oral anticoagulant–induced prothrombin deficiency (phytonadione *only*)

Prophylaxis and treatment of hemorrhagic disease of the newborn (phytonadione *only*)

Table 75-5. **Vitamin K Preparations**

Drug	Usual Dosage Range	Nursing Considerations
K_1 (Phytonadione) *AquaMEPHYTON, Konakion, Mephyton*	*Hypoprothrombinemia and anticoagulant-induced prothrombin deficiency* 2.5–25 mg initially; repeat in 6–8 h after parenteral injection *or* 12–48 h after oral administration until prothrombin time is in desired range *Hemorrhagic disease of newborn* Prophylaxis: 0.5–2 mg IM *or* (less desirable) 1–5 mg to the mother 12–24 h before delivery Treatment: 1–2 mg SC *or* IM daily	Fat-soluble derivative that is the preferred antidote to oral anticoagulant overdose; only vitamin K preparation indicated for hemorrhagic disease of the newborn; requires bile salts for oral absorption; injection is available as an aqueous colloidal solution (AquaMEPHYTON) for IV, SC, or IM use and as an aqueous dispersion (Konakion) for IM use only; do *not* exceed 1 mg/min when injecting IV; use smaller doses as antidote for short-acting anticoagulants and larger doses for longer-acting anticoagulants; protect solutions from light
K_4 (Menadiol sodium diphosphate) *Synkayvite*	*Oral* 5–10 mg/day *Parenteral (SC, IM, IV)* Adults: 5–15 mg 1–2 times a day Children: 5–10 mg 1–2 times a day	Water-soluble derivative of vitamin K that is converted to menadione in vivo; approximately one-half as potent as menadione; well absorbed orally and does not require presence of bile salts; used principally for hypoprothrombinemia caused by obstructive jaundice, biliary fistulas, or administration of salicylates or antibiotics; single dose usually restores prothrombin time within 8–24 h; may induce hemolysis of erythrocytes in glucose-6-phosphate dehydrogenase–deficient patients; do not infuse together with other drugs; may be given with any IV fluid

Dosage

Refer to Table 75-5

Fate

Phytonadione is absorbed from the GI tract by way of the lymph and only in the presence of bile salts. Menadiol is absorbed directly into the bloodstream even in the absence of bile. Bleeding is controlled within 6 to 12 hours after oral administration and within 3 to 6 hours after parenteral injection. It is initially concentrated in the liver, but levels decline very rapidly. There is little accumulation in other tissues, and the drug is rapidly metabolized. It is excreted both in the bile and urine.

Common Side Effects

Flushing sensation with IV injection

Significant Adverse Reactions

Oral: GI upset, nausea, vomiting, headache

Parenteral: dizziness, tachycardia, weak pulse, chills, fever, sweating, hypotension, dyspnea, cyanosis, hypersensitivity reactions, anaphylaxis, pain and swelling at injection site, and erythematous skin reactions; in newborns, hyperbilirubinemia, kernicterus, and hemolytic anemia have occurred, especially with menadiol

Contraindications

Menadiol is contraindicated in infants and in women during the last few weeks of pregnancy and during labor (refer to Significant Adverse Reactions). *Cautious use* in patients with liver disease.

Interactions

Vitamin K antagonizes the anticoagulant action of coumarins and indanediones, but not heparin.

Mineral oil or cholestyramine may impair GI absorption of K_1 but *not* K_4.

Antibiotics may reduce endogenous vitamin K activity by decreasing its synthesis by intestinal flora. Increased bleeding can result.

Nursing Management

Refer to Phytonadione in Chapter 37, and to Table 75-5 for specific information on each derivative. In addition:

Pretherapy Assessment

Assess and record baseline data necessary for detection of adverse effects of vitamin K: General: VS, body weight, skin color and temperature; Lab: liver function, PT, CBC.

Review medical history and documents for existing or previous conditions that:

a. require cautious use of vitamin K: liver disease.
b. contraindicate use of vitamin K: allergy to any component of the preparation; use in infants and in women during the last few weeks of pregnancy and during labor.

Nursing Interventions

Medication Administration

Seek clarification before administering repeated large doses if initial response is poor because excessive dosage can further depress hepatic function.

Note that phytonadione is the only vitamin K analogue indicated for treating hemorrhagic disease of the newborn, especially in premature infants, because increased bilirubinemia, severe hemolytic anemia, and kernicterus, possibly resulting in brain damage or death, can occur with use.

Administer by SC or deep IM injection; use extreme caution if giving by the IV route.

Surveillance During Therapy

Interpret results of diagnostic tests and contact practitioner as appropriate.

Selected Bibliography

Alexander LJ: Ocular vitamin therapy. A review and assessment. Optometry Clin 2(4):1, 1992

Block G: Vitamin C and cancer prevention: the epidemiologic evidence. Am J Clin Nutr 53:270S, 1991

Block G, Abrams B: Vitamin and mineral status of women of childbearing potential. Ann NY Acad Sci 678:244, 1993

Chavance M, Herbeth B, Lemoine A, Zhu BP: Does multivitamin supplementation prevent infections in healthy elderly subjects? A controlled trial. Int J Vitamin Nutr Res 63(1):11, 1993

Der Marderosian AH: Foods and "Health Foods" as drugs. Acta Horticulturae 332:81, 1993

Dorgan JF, Schatzkin A: Antioxidant micronutrients in cancer prevention. Hematol Oncol Clin North Am 5(1):43, 1991

Linderborn KM: Independently living seniors and vitamin therapy: What nurses should know. J Gerontol Nurs 19(8):10, 1993

Meydani SN: Vitamin/mineral supplementation, the aging immune response, and risk of infection. Nutr Rev 51(4):106, 1993

Rumore MM: Vitamin A as an immunomodulating agent. Clin Pharm 12(7):506, 1993

Russell RM, Suter PM: Vitamin requirements of elderly people: An update. Am J Clin Nutr 58(1):4, 1993

Nursing Bibliography

E: The evidence grows stronger. University of California at Berkeley Wellness Letter, 9(5):2, 1993

Loken S, et al: Factors that influence therapeutic anticoagulation control. Nurse Prac Forum, 3(2):95, 1992

Rowell M: Eradication of vitamin A deficiency with five cents and a vegetable garden. J Ophthal Nur Technol 12(5):284, 1993

Vitamin D3 plus calcium to prevent fractures. Nurses Drug Alert 17(2):10, 1993

Vitamins with a vengeance. Emerg Med 24(4):274, 1992

Yen P: Casting some light on the sunshine vitamin. Geriatr Nurse 13(5):284, 1992

76

Nutrients, Minerals, Fluids, and Electrolytes

Oral Nutritional Supplements
- Potassium
- Fluoride
- Minerals and electrolytes
- Miscellaneous nutritional factors

Parenteral Nutritional Supplements
- Protein (amino acid) products
- Carbohydrate products
- Lipid products
- Parenteral electrolytes

The fluid composition of the body is normally kept reasonably constant despite the many stresses placed on it. Significant alterations in the volume and composition of the internal fluid environment can, however, result from disease, trauma, or drug therapy, as well as from a number of other external factors. Disturbances in fluid and electrolyte balance may involve changes in pH, volume, osmolarity, or concentrations of individual ions, and can seriously impair the normal metabolic activity of body organs. Thus, the chemical constituents of the body (ie, electrolytes, minerals, amino acids, fluids, proteins, lipids) are often administered either individually or in combination to correct acute or chronic deficiency states, and such a procedure is termed *nutritional replacement therapy*.

This chapter considers those nutrients, fluids, and electrolytes, both orally and parenterally administered, that are commonly used to supply the nutritional needs of patients suffering from a deficiency of one or more of these substances. The oral nutritional supplements are reviewed first, followed by a discussion of parenteral nutrients. Not all of the substances used as nutritional supplements are considered here, inasmuch as several have been mentioned in other chapters dealing with drugs affecting specific organs with which a particular mineral or electrolyte is intimately associated. Thus, calcium is discussed with parathyroid hormone and calcitonin in Chapter 43, iron is reviewed along with other drugs used to treat anemia in Chapter 36, and iodine and iodide salts are considered in Chapter 42 with the thyroid hormones. In addition, the vitamins are discussed in Chapter 75.

Oral Nutritional Supplements

Bioflavonoids
Calcium caseinate
l-Carnitine
Choline
Citrate
Corn oil
Fluoride
Glucose polymers
Inositol
Lactase
Lecithin
l-Lysine
Magnesium
Manganese
Medium-chain triglycerides
Methionine
Omega-3 polyunsaturated fatty acids
Oral electrolyte mixture
Para-aminobenzoic acid
Phosphorus
Potassium
Protein hydrolysates
Safflower oil
Sodium bicarbonate
Sodium chloride
l-Tryptophan
Threonine
Zinc

The substances used orally for correcting nutritional deficiency states include minerals, electrolytes, amino acids, proteins, and lipids, as well as a few other miscellaneous drugs. Perhaps the most widely used oral electrolytes are potassium and fluoride, and these preparations are considered individually in detail below. The remaining oral nutritional supplements are listed in Table 76-1.

• *Potassium*

Several manufacturers

Potassium is the principal intracellular cation and is essential for many vital physiologic processes, including nerve impulse transmission; skeletal, cardiac, and smooth muscle contraction; and maintenance of intracellular tonicity and renal function. Potassium depletion occurs most frequently as a result of diuretic therapy but may also be attributable to hyperaldosteronism, severe diarrhea, or diabetic ketoacidosis. It is usually accompanied by chloride loss as well and therefore frequently is associated with metabolic alkalosis. Symptoms of potassium depletion include muscle weakness, cramping, fatigue, disturbances in cardiac rhythm, and inability to concentrate urine. The salts of potassium available for oral use are the chloride, gluconate, acetate, citrate, and bicarbonate. When hypokalemia is associated with alkalosis, the chloride salt should be used. When acidosis is present, one of the other salts is indicated. When oral replacement therapy is not feasible (as with severe vomiting, prolonged diuresis, marked diabetic acidosis), parenteral (IV infusion) therapy is indicated (Table 76-2).

The usual adult dietary intake of potassium ranges from 40 to 120 mEq/day. Despite this variability in intake, renal regulatory mechanisms normally maintain plasma potassium levels within the narrow physiologic range of 3.5 to 5 mEq/L.

Table 76-1. **Oral Nutritional Supplements**

Drug	*Usual Dosage Range*	*Nursing Considerations*
MINERALS AND ELECTROLYTES		
Citrate *Bicitra, Polycitra, Oracit*	*Adults*: 15–30 mL diluted in water 4 times/day *Children*: 5–10 mL in water 4 times/day	Solutions of sodium citrate, potassium citrate, and citric acid used as systemic and urinary alkalinizers for treating chronic metabolic acidosis; also used in patients with uric acid nephropathy in conjunction with uricosuric drugs; do not use in persons with renal impairment, hyperkalemia, acute dehydration or myocardial damage
Magnesium *Almora, Magonate, Mag-Tab SR, Mag-Ox, Magtrate, Slow-Mag, Uro-Mag*	27–100 mg 2–4 times a day	RDAs are 200 mg (children 4–6 yr), 300–400 mg (adults); excessive amounts may produce diarrhea; necessary for a number of enzyme systems and for nerve conduction and muscle contraction; deficiency is rare in well-nourished persons
Manganese	20–50 mg/day	Need in human nutrition is not established; functions as a cofactor in many enzyme systems; localized primarily in mitochondria
Oral Electrolyte Mixture *Infalyte Oral, Pedialyte, Resol, Rehydralyte*	Dosage and volume of solution is based on child's age and degree of dehydration and weight loss	Used to replace water and electrolytes when food and fluid intake is sharply reduced (eg, postoperatively, starvation) or when fluid loss is excessive (eg, diarrhea, severe vomiting); severe continual diarrhea requires parenteral replacement therapy; use only in recommended volumes to prevent electrolyte overload; reduce intake when other electrolytes are reinstituted; do not use in the presence of intestinal obstruction, intractable vomiting, adynamic ileus, perforated bowel, or impaired renal function; *avoid* mixing with other electrolyte-containing liquids (milk, fruit juice)
Phosphorus *K-Phos Neutral, Neutra-Phos, Neutra-Phos-K, Uro-KP-Neutral*	1–2 tablets 4 times a day *or* Contents of 1 capsule mixed with 75 mL water 4 times a day *or* 75 mL reconstituted solution 4 times a day	Used as dietary supplement where diet is deficient, needs are increased, or GI absorption is impaired; RDAs are 800 mg (adults and children 1–10 yr) and 1,200 mg (children 11–18 yr and pregnant or lactating women); phosphate can lower urinary calcium levels; a laxative effect is common early in therapy; *contraindicated* in hyperkalemia and Addison's disease
Sodium Chloride *Slo-Salt*	0.5–1 g 3–6 times a day for prevention of dehydration and heat cramps	Used to replace excessive loss of sodium and chloride (eg, resulting from perspiration or extreme diuresis) and to counteract excessive salt restriction; use *cautiously* in patients with congestive heart failure, renal disease, circulatory insufficiency, or electrolyte disturbances (See also Table 76-2)
Sodium Bicarbonate	325 mg to 2 g up to 4 times a day (maximum, 16 g/day)	Used as a gastric, systemic, or urinary alkalinizer; *cautious use* in patients with congestive heart failure or renal impairment; 1 g provides 11.9 mmoi sodium and bicarbonate; also used parenterally (see Table 76-2)
Zinc Sulfate *Orazinc, Verazinc, Zinc-220, Zincate (CAN) Anuzinc, PMS Egozinc* **Zinc Gluconate**	25–50 mg elemental zinc a day	Important mineral for normal growth and repair of body tissues; symptoms of zinc deficiency include anorexia, loss of taste and olfactory sensation, mood changes, and growth retardation; used investigationally to treat delayed wound healing, acne, and rheumatoid arthritis, to improve the immune response in the elderly, and to delay onset of dementia in patients genetically at risk; RDAs are 10 mg (children 1–10 yr), 15 mg (adults), 20–25 mg (pregnant or lactating women); excessive doses may produce severe vomiting, dehydration and restlessness; GI upset can occur and can be minimized by taking drug with food or milk; zinc can impair oral absorption of tetracyclines
MISCELLANEOUS NUTRITIONAL FACTORS		
Bioflavonoids *Various manufacturers*	100–500 mg/day	Derived from green citrus fruits; previously used to reduce capillary fragility and referred to as vitamin P ("permeability"); *no evidence* that they are effective and no established need in human nutrition
Calcium Caseinate *Casec*	Variable according to patient's requirements	Used as an infant formula modifier or as a diet supplement; available in combination with sucrose as Gevral Protein

(*continued*)

Table 76-1. **Oral Nutritional Supplements (Continued)**

Drug	*Usual Dosage Range*	*Nursing Considerations*
l-Carnitine *Carnitor, VitaCarn*	Adults: 1–3 g a day Children: 50–100 mg/kg/day	Naturally occurring amino acid derivative synthesized from methionine and lysine; acts to facilitate fatty acid metabolism and subsequent energy production; used in patients with primary carnitine deficiency, which can result in elevated triglycerides and free fatty acids and impaired ketogenesis, and, in children, reduced growth and development; GI distress is common; drug may also produce an unpleasant body odor; has been used experimentally to improve athletic performance and treat toxicity due to valproic acid (see Chapter 27)
Choline	650 mg–2 g/day	A component of lecithin that has a lipotropic action and is essential for the formation of acetylcholine; average diet provides sufficient choline for body needs; has been used to treat fatty liver and cirrhosis, and to relieve symptoms of CNS disorders such as Huntington's disease and tardive dyskinesias; can cause GI disturbances and depression and imparts an unpleasant odor to the breath; used as free choline as well as bitartrate, chloride, and dihydrogen citrate salts
Corn Oil *Lipomul*	Adults: 45 mL 2–4 times a day Children: 30 mL 1–4 times a day	Used to increase caloric intake in malnourished or debilitated patients; use *cautiously* in persons with diabetes and gallbladder dysfunction; each dose contains 270 cal and 30 g fat
Glucose Polymers *Moducal, Polycose, Sumacal*	Add to foods or beverages and give in small, frequent feedings	Derived from cornstarch; supplies calories in patients unable to meet caloric needs with usual food intake or in patients on protein-, electrolyte-, and fat-restricted diets; *not* intended as the sole nutritional source; may be used for extended periods with diets containing all other essential nutrients
Inositol *(CAN) Linodil*	1–3 g/day in divided doses	An isomer of glucose possessing lipotropic activity in animals; physiologic role in humans is obscure and there is *no evidence* that it is clinically effective, although it has been used to treat liver disorders and disordered fat metabolism; dietary sources include mainly vegetables
Lactase *Dairy Ease, Lact-Aid, Lactrase*	5–15 drops per quart of milk, 1–3 chewable tablets with a meal, *or* 1–2 capsules either added to a quart of milk or taken along with milk or dairy products	Enzyme preparation used to facilitate digestion of milk lactose in patients with lactose intolerance
Lecithin *Phos Chol*	1–2 capsules/day	A source of choline, inositol, phosphorus, and linoleic and linolenic acids employed as a dietary supplement (see choline, above)
l-Lysine *Enisyl*	312–1500 mg/day	An essential amino acid used as a dietary supplement to increase utilization of vegetable proteins; also available in combination with other amino acids, vitamins, and minerals in a variety of combination products
Medium Chain Triglycerides *MCT*	15 mL 3–4 times a day	A dietary supplement for persons who cannot efficiently digest and absorb conventional long-chain fatty acids; medium-chain triglycerides are more rapidly hydrolyzed than conventional food fat and are not dependent on bile salts for emulsification; may be mixed with juices, poured on salads or other foods, incorporated into sauces, or used in cooking and baking; use with *caution* in persons with hepatic cirrhosis; one dose weighs approximately 14 g and contains 115 cal
Methionine	500 mg daily	Used as a dietary supplement; RDA has not been established
Omega-3 Polyunsaturated Fatty Acids *Several manufacturers*	1–2 capsules 3 times a day with meals	Used as dietary supplements to *possibly* reduce cholesterol and triglyceride concentrations, prolong bleeding times, and decrease platelet aggregation; no conclusive evidence that drug decreases risk of coronary artery disease; diarrhea is common at high doses; *cautious use* in patients receiving other drugs that reduce platelet aggregation; unlabeled uses include treatment of rheumatoid arthritis and psoriasis

(*continued*)

Table 76-1. **Oral Nutritional Supplements (Continued)**

Drug	Usual Dosage Range	Nursing Considerations
Para-aminobenzoic Acid (PABA) *Potaba* *(CAN) Pabanol, RV Paba Stick*	Adults: 12 g/day in 4–6 divided doses Children: 1 g/10 lb daily in divided doses	A substance found naturally associated with the B complex vitamins and essential for the functioning of a number of important biologic processes; considered "possibly effective" for scleroderma, dermatomyositis, morphea, pemphigus, and Peyronie's disease; dissolve tablets in liquid to minimize GI upset; drug should be taken with food; adverse reactions include anorexia, nausea, fever, and rash; use *cautiously* in patients with kidney impairment; do *not* give concurrently with sulfonamides, because PABA interferes with their antibacterial action; has no known human nutritional value; acts as a sunscreen when applied topically
Protein Hydrolysates *A/G Pro, PDP Liquid Protein, Propac*	Dosage depends on product formulation	Preparations of amino acids and peptides obtained by hydrolysis of larger proteins; used as dietary supplement to correct or prevent protein deficiency; optimum daily intake of dietary protein is 1 g/kg
Safflower Oil *Microlipid*	1–2 tbsp several times a day as necessary or administered by tube feeding	A caloric and fatty-acid supplement used in malnourished patients and other persons with fatty-acid deficiencies; contains 4,500 cal and 500 g fat per liter
Threonine	500 mg daily	Used as a dietary supplement; take on an empty stomach

Mechanism

Essential ion for maintenance of excitability of nerves and muscles, as well as acid–base balance

Uses

Prevention and treatment of hypokalemia, for example, resulting from diuretic therapy, prolonged vomiting or diarrhea, diabetes, hepatic cirrhosis, inadequate dietary intake, malabsorption, hyperaldosteronism, or nephropathy

Dosage

NOTE: The dosage of potassium (K^+) is given in milliequivalents (mEq) of the ion. Clinically available salts of potassium (with the potassium content) are as follows:

Potassium acetate 10.2 mEq K^+/g
Potassium bicarbonate 10 mEq K^+/g
Potassium chloride 13.4 mEq K^+/g
Potassium citrate 9.8 mEq K^+/g
Potassium gluconate 4.3 mEq K^+/g

Prevention of hypokalemia: 16 to 24 mEq/day
Treatment of deficiency states: 40 to 100 mEq/day

Fate

Oral potassium is well absorbed; renal excretion occurs primarily by secretion in the distal portion of the nephron; most of the filtered load of potassium is reabsorbed in the proximal tubule; fecal excretion is minimal and does not play a significant role in potassium hemostasis

Common Side Effects

Nausea, abdominal discomfort, vomiting, diarrhea

Significant Adverse Reactions

GI bleeding and perforation, hyperkalemia (paresthesias, flaccid paralysis, confusion, weakness, hypotension, respiratory distress, arrhythmias, cardiac depression, heart block)

Contraindications

Severe renal impairment with oliguria, anuria, or azotemia; Addison's disease; acute dehydration; heat cramps; hyperkalemia in patients receiving potassium-sparing diuretics; in addition, solid dosage forms of potassium are contraindicated in patients in whom there is delayed passage of contents through the GI tract. *Cautious use* in patients with systemic acidosis, acute dehydration, chronic renal dysfunction, cardiac disease, adrenal insufficiency, or peptic ulcer.

Interactions

Combinations of potassium salts with potassium-sparing diuretics or angiotensin-converting enzyme (ACE)-inhibitors can result in hyperkalemia.

Increased serum potassium decreases both toxicity and effectiveness of digitalis drugs.

Concurrent use of salt substitutes with potassium supplements can lead to hyperkalemia.

Concomitant administration of anticholinergics and oral potassium products may increase the likelihood of GI erosion because of slowed GI motility and delayed gastric emptying.

Nursing Management

Pretherapy Assessment

Assess and record baseline data necessary for detection of adverse effects of potassium: General: vital signs

(*text continues on page 818*)

Table 76-2. **Parenteral Electrolytes**

Drug	*Usual Dosage Range*	*Nursing Considerations*
Ammonium Chloride	Dependent on patient's status; not to exceed 1%–2% ammonium chloride or an administration rate faster than 5 mL/min	Indicated for treatment of metabolic alkalosis or hypochloremic states severe enough to cause signs of impending tetany (severe or protracted vomiting, gastric suction); generally given with 20–40 mEq potassium/L to correct accompanying hypokalemia; *contraindicated* in severe hepatic impairment because danger of ammonia retention is present, and in patients with primary respiratory alkalosis and high CO_2; *cautious use* in renal dysfunction, cardiac edema, or pulmonary insufficiency; administer by *slow* IV infusion and observe for signs of ammonia toxicity (sweating, irregular breathing, bradycardia, vomiting, twitching, arrhythmias); do *not* give SC, intraperitoneally, or rectally; solution should be diluted with normal saline; may increase excretion rate of basic drugs (eg, amphetamines, quinidine)
Calcium Chloride	**Slow IV injection only** *Hypocalcemia*: 500 mg–1 g at 1–3 day intervals *Magnesium intoxication*: 500 mg at once; repeat as necessary *Cardiac resuscitation*: 200–800 mg into the ventricular cavity *or* 500 mg–1 g IV	Indicated for treatment of hypocalcemia requiring a prompt elevation in serum calcium levels (eg, neonatal tetany, parathyroid deficiency, alkalosis); also used to prevent hypocalcemia during exchange transfusions, as adjunctive therapy in treating serious insect bites, for managing lead colic and magnesium intoxication, and for cardiac resuscitation (calcium chloride only) when epinephrine therapy is ineffective; calcium chloride is highly irritating and severe necrosis and sloughing can occur; other calcium salts are preferred where possible; IM administration of calcium salts (except chloride and gluconate—IV only) should be done only where IV administration is impractical or technically too difficult; do *not* mix calcium salts with sulfates, phosphates, carbonates, or tartrates in solution, because precipitation can occur; IV solutions should be warmed to body temperature and given slowly (0.5–2 mL/min); side effects are infrequent at recommended doses; use with caution in digitalized patients and in patients with arrhythmias; calcium may antagonize the effects of verapamil
Calcium Gluceptate	*Hypocalcemia* IM: 2–5 mL IV: 5–20 mL *Exchange transfusions in newborn* 0.5 mL after each 100 mL of blood is exchanged	
Calcium Gluconate	*Hypocalcemia* Adults: 15–30 mL of 10% solution as needed by IV infusion Children: 2–15 mL in divided doses *Magnesium intoxication*: Adults: 10–20 mL IV *Exchange transfusions*: Adults: 3 mL IV with each 100 mL citrated blood Neonates: 1 mL IV as above	
Magnesium Sulfate	*Mild magnesium deficiency* 1 g (2 mL 50% solution) IM every 6 h for 4 doses *Severe magnesium deficiency* IM: 2 mEq/kg within 4 h IV: 5 mg (40 mEq)/1,000 mL infused over 3 h *Total parenteral nutrition* Adults: 8–24 mEq/day Infants: 2–10 mEq/day	Indicated for replacement therapy in magnesium-deficiency states, especially when accompanied by signs of tetany, and for treating hypomagnesemia resulting from hyperalimentation; may also be employed in certain acute convulsive states (eg, toxemia, eclampsia, preeclampsia, epilepsy [1–4 g 10%–20% solution IV]), although other more effective and less toxic drugs are available (see Chap. 27); use with *extreme caution* in patients with renal impairment and observe closely for signs of overdosage (hypotension, respiratory depression, absence of patellar reflex); have respiratory assistance available; urine output should be maintained at a minimum of 100 mL/4 h; do *not* exceed 1.5 mL/min when infusing the 10% concentration (or equivalent volume of higher concentrations); dilute 50% solution to a concentration of 20% or less before infusing; however, the full-strength solution may be injected IM in adults; effects of CNS depressants can be potentiated by magnesium
Phosphate *Potassium Phosphate, Sodium Phosphate*	*Total parenteral nutrition* Adults: 10–15 mM phosphorus (310–465 mg elemental phosphorus) per liter of TPN solution Infants: 1.5–2 mM/kg/day	Primarily used to prevent or correct hypophosphatemia in patients undergoing hyperalimentation; *contraindicated* in diseases with high phosphate or low calcium levels; used IV only, diluted in a larger volume of fluid and slowly infused; monitor serum phosphorus, calcium, and sodium or potassium levels depending on which phosphate salt is used; be alert for symptoms of hypocalcemic tetany; use *cautiously* in patients with renal impairment, cardiac disease, arrhythmias, or adrenal insufficiency; symptoms of overdosage include weakness, confusion, paresthesias, hypotension, arrhythmias, flaccid paralysis, and ECG abnormalities

(*continued*)

Table 76-2. Parenteral Electrolytes (Continued)

Drug	Usual Dosage Range	Nursing Considerations
Potassium *Potassium acetate, Potassium chloride*	Dependent on patient's status and governed by serum potassium level and ECG pattern; if serum potassium is less than 2 mEq/L, maximum infusion rate is 40 mEq/h to a total of 400 mEq/day; if serum potassium is greater than 2.5 mEq/L, maximum infusion rate is 10 mEq/h to a maximum of 200 mEq/day	Indicated for the prevention or treatment of moderate to severe potassium deficiency states and as adjunctive therapy in the management of cardiac arrhythmias, especially those due to digitalis overdosage; *contraindicated* in patients with anuria, oliguria, azotemia, adrenocortical insufficiency, acute dehydration, hyperkalemia, and severe hemolytic reactions; dilute injections with large volumes of parenteral solutions and administer *slowly* IV; direct injection of undiluted solution may be *fatal*; use *cautiously* in patients with cardiac disease, especially those taking digitalis drugs; monitor serum potassium levels, ECG, and urine flow frequently during therapy; be aware that toxic effects of potassium on the heart may be increased if serum sodium or calcium levels decrease or serum pH is reduced; most frequent adverse reactions are nausea, vomiting, diarrhea, and abdominal pain; avoid extravasation as irritation is often severe and tissue necrosis can occur
Sodium Acetate, Sodium Bicarbonate, Sodium Lactate *Neut*	*Metabolic acidosis* Initially 2–5 mEq/kg by IV infusion over 4–8 h; adjust dose as necessary depending on clinical response *Cardiac arrest* Adults: initially 1 mEq/kg, followed by 0.5 mEq/kg every 10 min of arrest; use 7.5% *or* 8.4% solution Children under 2 yr: initially 1–2 mEq/kg over 1–2 min, followed by 1 mEq/kg every 10 min of arrest; use 4.2% solution	Indicated for acute treatment of metabolic acidosis, such as resulting from cardiac arrest, shock, or other circulatory insufficiency states, severe dehydration, or diabetic or lactic acidosis; also used to alkalinize the urine for treating certain drug intoxications and adjunctively in severe diarrhea to replace loss of bicarbonate; sodium lactate and sodium acetate are metabolized to bicarbonate, although conversion of lactate to bicarbonate is impaired in patients with hepatic disease; *contraindicated* in hypochloremia, metabolic or respiratory alkalosis, and hypocalcemia; use *cautiously* in patients with congestive heart failure, kidney impairment, edema, hypertension, or arrhythmias; do *not* exceed 8 mg/kg/day in small children, and infuse *slowly* because rapid injection or use of hypertonic solutions has resulted in decreased CSF pressure and intracranial hemorrhage; closely monitor pH and blood gases and electrolytes; avoid overdosage and subsequent production of alkalosis by giving repeated small doses; observe for signs of developing alkalosis (hyperirritability, restlessness, tetany) and discontinue drug; sodium bicarbonate is incompatible in solution with a wide variety of other drugs; administer alone to avoid undesirable interaction
Sodium Chloride intravenous infusion, Sodium Chloride diluents, Sodium Chloride injection (concentrated)	(Dependent on patient's status and preparation being used) Average adult dose: 1 L of 0.9% solution daily by IV infusion (see Nursing Considerations)	Used IV in various concentrations as a source of fluid and electrolytes; the 0.45% solution (hypotonic) is used when fluid loss exceeds electrolyte depletion; the 0.9% solution (isotonic) is most commonly used as replacement for fluid and sodium loss and as a diluent for many other drugs and nutrients; the 3% and 5% solutions (hypertonic) are indicated for hyponatremia and hypochloremia, extreme dilution of body fluids due to excessive water intake, and treatment of severe salt depletion; use with caution in patients with congestive heart failure, severe renal impairment, and edema with sodium retention; the 3% and 5% solutions should *not* be used when plasma sodium and chloride are elevated, normal, or even slightly decreased; monitor intake–output ratio and serum electrolytes; also use *cautiously* in patients with decompensated cardiovascular or nephrotic diseases and in patients receiving corticosteroids; infuse higher-strength solutions very slowly to avoid pulmonary edema
Tromethamine *Tham*	*Acidosis associated with cardiac arrest* 2–6 g (62–185 mL) injected into ventricular cavity *or* 3.6–10.8 g (111–333 mL) injected into a large peripheral vein; additional amounts as needed *Acidosis during cardiac bypass surgery* 9.0 mL/kg (2.7 mEq/kg) to a maximum of 1,000 mL in unusually severe cases *Correct acidity of ACD priming blood* 0.5–2.5 g (15–77 mL) added to each 500 mL blood (usually 2 g is adequate)	A highly alkaline, sodium-free organic amine that acts as a proton acceptor, combining with hydrogen ions to prevent or correct systemic acidosis associated with, for example, cardiac arrest or cardiac bypass surgery; also added to ACD priming blood to elevate pH; may function as an osmotic diuretic and increase urine flow and excretion of fixed acids, carbon dioxide, and electrolytes; *contraindicated* in anuria or uremia; should be administered slowly IV to avoid overdosage and alkalosis; may also be given by injection into ventricular cavity during cardiac arrest and by addition to pump oxygenator ACD blood or other priming fluid; treatment should not continue longer than a 24-h period; determine blood values (pH, P_{CO_2}, P_{O_2}, glucose), electrolytes, and urinary output before treatment and frequently during drug administration to assess progress of treatment; adjust dose so that blood pH does not increase above normal (7.35–7.45); drug may depress respiration; have respiratory assistance available; avoid extravasation, because severe inflammation, vascular spasm, and tissue necrosis can result; transient hypoglycemia may occur, especially in infants; use *cautiously* in children, in patients with impaired renal function, and in pregnant women

(VS), body weight, skin color and temperature; cardiovascular system (CVS): baseline electrocardiogram (ECG); Lab: serum potassium, serum electrolytes, bicarbonate.

Review medical history and documents for existing or previous conditions that:

a. require cautious use of potassium: systemic acidosis, acute dehydration, chronic renal dysfunction, cardiac disease, adrenal insufficiency, or peptic ulcer.
b. contraindicate use of potassium: severe renal impairment with oliguria, anuria, or azotemia; Addison's disease; acute dehydration; heat cramps; hyperkalemia in patients receiving potassium-sparing diuretics; in addition, solid dosage forms of potassium are contraindicated in patients in whom there is delayed passage of contents through the GI tract.

Nursing Interventions

Medication Administration

Administer oral drug after meals or with food and a full glass of water to decrease GI upset.

Provide small frequent meals if GI upset is severe.

Do *not* administer potassium chloride by intravenous (IV) push or in concentrated amounts by any route.

Administer only liquid dosage forms, never solid forms (ie, tablets, capsules, powders) to patient with reduced GI passage because gastric and intestinal ulceration can occur.

Surveillance During Therapy

Observe patient for development of severe vomiting, GI bleeding (ie, black stools), weakness, and abdominal pain or distention. Drug should be discontinued immediately if these occur.

Closely monitor results of acid–base balance, serum electrolyte, and ECG determinations during treatment to avoid potassium intoxication, which can result in arrhythmias and cardiac depression.

Monitor intake–output ratio and immediately report any significant change in renal function. Potassium intoxication with oral administration is rare in persons with normal kidney function.

Assist with evaluation of drug effects. *Serum* potassium concentrations are not always an accurate indication of total *intracellular* potassium levels. Treatment of potassium depletion, therefore, requires careful assessment of clinical status as well as laboratory evaluations.

Interpret results of diagnostic tests and contact practitioner as appropriate.

Patient Teaching

Instruct patient to swallow coated tablets whole because chewing them will increase likelihood of GI irritation. They should be taken with a full glass of water, preferably after meals or with food.

Instruct patient to avoid use of salt substitutes, many of which contain potassium, and excessive use of laxatives, which can alter electrolyte balance.

Instruct patient to dissolve powders or effervescent tablets in 4 to 8 oz cold water, juice, or other beverage, and to sip slowly.

• *Fluoride*

Luride, Pediaflor, Phos-Flur, and other manufacturers

(CAN) Fluoron, Karidium

The fluoride ion, used either orally or topically, is employed as an aid in the prevention of dental caries. It is most commonly administered to young children in combination with vitamins and minerals in the form of drops or chewable tablets. Fluoride can also be used as a mouthwash or oral gel by persons susceptible to dental caries. Sodium fluoride has also been employed in large doses in the management of osteoporosis. Although some studies have suggested a beneficial effect for fluoride in reducing the incidence of fractures, other studies have shown the opposite effects, that is, an increased likelihood of fractures. The use of sodium fluoride in the treatment of osteoporosis remains controversial.

Mechanism

Incorporated into external layers of dental enamel, making it more resistant to erosion by acid; may also facilitate osteoblastic activity of bone

Uses

Aid in prevention of dental caries where community water supplies are low in fluoride

Reduce dental decay caused by dryness of the mouth resulting from radiation therapy.

Treatment of osteoporosis; doses up to 60 mg/day, in combination with calcium, vitamin D, or estrogen (investigational use only)

Dosage

(Prevention of dental caries)

Oral: 0.25 to 1 mg/day, depending on age

Topical: 5 to 10 mL once a day as a mouth rinse after brushing; rinse for 1 minute, then expectorate

Fate

Rapidly absorbed orally, largely from the stomach; widely distributed and quickly deposited in teeth and bone; quickly excreted by the kidneys.

Significant Adverse Reactions

Eczema, atopic dermatitis, urticaria, nausea, GI distress, headache, weakness, staining of the teeth (topical only)

Prolonged overdosage can lead to mottling of the tooth enamel.

Acute ingestion of large doses of fluoride may cause excessive salivation, GI disturbances, irritability, tetany, hyperreflexia, seizures, and cardiac failure.

Contraindications

Supplemental fluoride should not be provided when the fluoride content of drinking water contains 0.7 ppm or more of fluoride. Persons on low-sodium or sodium-free diets should avoid fluoride as well. *Cautious use* in pregnant or nursing mothers and in persons with tartrazine sensitivity.

Nursing Management

Pretherapy Assessment

Assess and record baseline data necessary for detection of adverse effects of fluoride: General: VS, body weight, skin color and temperature; CVS: baseline ECG; Lab: serum potassium, serum electrolytes, bicarbonate.

Review medical history and documents for existing or previous conditions that:

a. require cautious use of fluoride: use in pregnancy or nursing mothers.

b. contraindicate use of fluoride: use in individuals on low-sodium or sodium-free diets; supplemental fluoride should not be provided when the fluoride content of drinking water contains 0.7 ppm or more of fluoride.

Nursing Interventions

Medication Administration

Oral drug should not be administered in the presence of dairy products, which will impair absorption.

Provide small frequent meals if GI upset is severe.

Surveillance During Therapy

Note that acute fluoride overdosage can result in excessive salivation and GI disturbances. Emesis, which invariably occurs with ingestion of large amounts, serves as a protective mechanism.

Interpret results of diagnostic tests and contact practitioner as appropriate.

Patient Teaching

Advise patient to use plastic container to dilute rinse or drops.

Instruct patient to take tablets or drops after meals but to avoid milk or dairy products with sodium fluoride tablets because GI absorption is reduced.

Encourage patient using rinse to apply immediately after brushing teeth and just before retiring at night. Instruct patient not to swallow while using rinse and to avoid eating or drinking for at least 30 minutes after use.

Instruct patient to notify drug prescriber if teeth become stained or mottled after repeated use.

Parenteral Nutritional Supplements

Parenteral nutritional supplementation is provided for a number of reasons, ranging from correction of simple acute dehydration to prolonged treatment of serious nutritional deficiencies resulting from such conditions as severe GI disorders, prolonged kidney failure, and extensive burns.

Substances provided in parenteral nutritional supplements include electrolytes, carbohydrates, fats, proteins, and vitamins. Administration of nutritional solutions through peripheral veins (ie, peripheral parenteral nutrition) is generally adequate if caloric requirements are minimal and can be partially satisfied with oral supplements and if nutritional therapy will only be required for 1 to 2 weeks. Conversely, in severely depleted patients or in patients who require prolonged supplemental nutrition, total parenteral nutrition (TPN) administered by a central venous catheter is usually indicated. This latter procedure, frequently termed *hyperalimentation*, is used to maintain an anabolic state when conventional oral or tube feeding is inappropriate and when peripheral IV therapy cannot meet the nutritional demands of the patient. Total parenteral nutrition is indicated after a major bowel resection, in the presence of obstructive or severe inflammatory conditions of the bowel, and in patients with prolonged paralytic ileus (such as after abdominal trauma or surgery). It is also employed to manage hypermetabolic states caused by severe trauma such as extensive burns, infections, or multiple injuries; to treat malabsorption states, such as, for example, those resulting from hepatic or pancreatic insufficiency, and as adjunctive therapy for patients receiving chemotherapy or radiation therapy or suffering from anorexia nervosa. In general, persons requiring 1,000 calories or more to maintain nutritional status are candidates for TPN.

Solutions used in TPN contain a protein source (amino acids) together with varying amounts of dextrose, vitamins, electrolytes, and trace minerals. In addition, other agents that may be added to TPN solutions include heparin, insulin, and cimetidine or another H_2 antagonist to prevent stress ulcers. Because of their high osmolarity, these solutions must be administered through a *large* vein having sufficient blood flow to provide adequate dilution so as to minimize the danger of phlebitis. For this reason, the solution is given into the superior vena cava through the subclavian vein, and the procedure is carried out by surgically implanting a catheter into the appropriate vessel. Although the technical details of the hyperalimentation procedure are not reviewed here, this form of nutritional therapy is a potentially hazardous one that requires personnel trained and experienced in the technique as well as in the care of patients undergoing the procedure.

The substances used for parenteral nutrition are considered individually; however, as previously indicated, several different kinds of nutrients are usually administered together, depending on the clinical status and nutritional requirements of the patient.

Protein (Amino Acid) Products

The protein products employed as parenteral nutrients include protein hydrolysates and mixtures of crystalline amino acids, with or without added electrolytes. Most products are used for central venous hyperalimentation, but some of the amino acid preparations can be employed as dilute solutions for peripheral parenteral feeding. These products provide a concentrated form of usable amino acids for protein synthesis as well as varying amounts of electrolytes, but they require addition of sufficient dextrose to provide for full caloric energy requirements when used for long-term hyperalimentation.

• Crystalline Amino-Acid Infusion

Aminosyn, FreAmine III, Novamine, ProcalAmine, Travasol, TrophAmine

Crystalline amino acids are hypertonic solutions of essential and nonessential *l*-amino acids or low-molecular-weight peptides with varying proportions of electrolytes that provide a substrate for protein synthesis and exert a protein-sparing effect. Preparations differ in degree of osmolarity, amino-acid ratios, and content of nitrogen. In addition to the general amino acid formulations listed, specialized formulations are available for use in patients with renal failure, hepatic failure/encephalopathy, or acute metabolic stress. These latter products are considered after the review of the general formulations.

Mechanism

Provide replacement of deficient amino acids and electrolytes; possess a nitrogen-sparing effect when used with a nonprotein caloric source; promote a positive nitrogen balance and increase protein synthesis

Uses

Prevention of nitrogen loss or treatment of negative nitrogen balance

Adjuncts in providing adequate nutrition, as a component product of total parenteral nutrition (ie, hyperalimentation) in full strength or peripheral parenteral nutrition in diluted form

Dosage

Dosage is flexible and depends on daily protein requirements, patient's clinical response, and metabolic activity; see individual package instructions; average adult dose is 2 L/day to provide 1 to 2 g protein/kg.

CAUTION

Solutions contain between 2.75% and 15% amino-acid concentration (both essential and nonessential) together with electrolytes, providing between 0.46 and 2.3 g/100 mL of nitrogen; some solutions also contain 5% to 25% dextrose.

Common Side Effects

Nausea, flushing, sensation of warmth (especially with rapid infusion)

Significant Adverse Reactions

Vomiting, chills, headache, abdominal pain, dizziness, allergic reactions, phlebitis, venous thrombosis, skin rash, papular eruptions; metabolic disturbances include acidosis, alkalosis, hypocalcemia, hypophosphatemia, hyperglycemia, glycosuria, hypovitaminosis, and other electrolyte imbalances

Contraindications

Anuria, oliguria, severe liver or kidney impairment, metabolic disorders involving impaired nitrogen utilization, decreased circulating blood volume, inborn errors of amino acid metabolism, hepatic coma or encephalopathy, and hyperammonemia. *Cautious use* in patients with cardiac insufficiency.

Interactions

Antianabolic drugs and tetracyclines may reduce the protein-sparing effects of amino acids.

Addition of calcium to the infusion may precipitate the phosphate ion.

Nursing Management

Pretherapy Assessment

Assess and record baseline data necessary for detection of adverse effects of parenteral amino acids: General: VS, body weight, skin color and temperature; CVS: baseline ECG; Lab: serum potassium, serum electrolytes, bicarbonate.

Review medical history and documents for existing or previous conditions that:

a. require cautious use of parenteral amino acids: cardiac insufficiency.
b. contraindicate use of parenteral amino acids: anuria, oliguria, severe liver or kidney impairment, metabolic disorders involving impaired nitrogen utilization, decreased circulating blood volume, inborn errors of amino acid metabolism, hepatic coma or encephalopathy, and hyperammonemia; **pregnancy (Category—unknown)**.

Nursing Interventions

Medication Administration

Dosage is flexible and dependent on daily protein requirements.

Solutions contain between 2.75% and 15% amino acid concentration (both essential and nonessential) together with electrolytes, providing between 0.46 and 2.3 g/100 mL of nitrogen; some solutions also contain 5% to 25% dextrose.

Use aseptic technique in mixing solutions and in the insertion and maintenance of central venous catheters because risk of sepsis is considerable. Use solution promptly after mixing and discard unused portion. Do not mix antibiotics with protein–carbohydrate hyperalimentation solutions.

Infuse slowly to minimize adverse effects, particularly hyperglycemia and glycosuria, which can, however, be controlled with insulin if necessary.

Do *not* premix amino acid infusions with fat emulsions. Instead, infuse simultaneously through a Y connector located near infusion site.

Do *not* administer simultaneously with blood through same infusion site because pseudoagglutination can occur.

Do *not* administer strongly hypertonic solutions (eg, stronger than 12.5% dextrose) by *peripheral* venous infusion. They should be given only through an indwelling central venous catheter whose tip is located in the superior vena cava.

Replace all IV administration sets every 24 to 48 hours.

Note that supplementary vitamins, minerals, electrolytes, heparin, or insulin may be administered cautiously through the indwelling catheter, but administration of any *other* medication or withdrawal or transfusion of blood by this route is *not* recommended.

Note that most amino acid infusions are indicated for hyperalimentation, *except for* Aminosyn 3.5%, FreAmine III 3% w/electrolytes, ProcalAmine, and Travasol 3.5% w/electrolytes.

Surveillance During Therapy

Monitor results of blood sugar determinations in diabetics and in patients with impaired glucose tolerance, which should be performed frequently, and test urine for sugar often because insulin dosage may need to be adjusted.
Ensure that sufficient dextrose (in the form of concentrated dextrose solutions) is administered to meet full caloric energy requirements when amino acid infusions are used for prolonged hyperalimentation,.
Monitor results of serum electrolyte determinations. Appropriate supplemental electrolyte solutions should be provided as necessary.
Be alert for signs of fatty acid deficiency (flaking skin, loss of hair), and assess results of plasma lipid level determinations. Intravenous fat emulsions will correct a deficiency.
Interpret results of diagnostic tests and contact practitioner as appropriate.

• Amino Acid Formulation for Renal Failure

Aminosyn-RF, Aminess, NephrAmine, RenAmin

Amino acid formulation for renal failure is indicated to provide nutritional support for uremic patients when oral nutrition is impractical and dialysis is not feasible. The products are used in conjunction with dextrose, electrolytes, and vitamins and are administered by central venous injection. Amino acid formulation for renal failure supplies only essential amino acids, thus allowing urea nitrogen to be recycled to glutamate, which serves as a precursor for synthesis of nonessential amino acids. Therefore, use of these products in uremic patients promotes utilization of retained urea and amelioration of azotemic symptoms. For urea reutilization to occur, however, it is essential to provide adequate calories and to restrict intake of nonessential nitrogen.

• Amino Acid Formulation for High Metabolic Stress

Aminosyn-HBC, Branch Amin, FreAmine HBC

Amino acid formulation for high metabolic stress is a mixture of essential and nonessential amino acids with high concentrations of the branched-chain amino acids isoleucine, leucine, and valine. Metabolic stress is often characterized by increased urinary excretion of nitrogen and by hyperglycemia, with decreased plasma levels of branched-chain amino acids. As a result, glucose utilization and fat mobilization are impaired. By supplying branched-chain amino acids, this formulation provides the substrates needed to meet the energy requirements of muscle and brain tissue.

• Amino Acid Formulation for Hepatic Failure or Hepatic Encephalopathy

HepatAmine

This formulation is very similar to that used for high metabolic stress, being a mixture of essential and nonessential amino acids with high concentrations of branched-chain amino acids. It is used for treating hepatic encephalopathy in patients intolerant of general-purpose amino acid injections. Replenishment of stores of branched-chain amino acids can reverse the abnormal plasma amino acid pattern seen in hepatic encephalopathy, with resultant improvement in mental status and EEG pattern. Nitrogen balance is also significantly improved.

Carbohydrate Products

Parenteral carbohydrate solutions are indicated primarily as a source of calories and fluid in patients with nutritional deficiencies who are unable to obtain the necessary nutrients orally. The available preparations include dextrose in water, alcohol in dextrose infusion, and a large number of products containing dextrose together with various electrolytes.

• Dextrose in Water Injection

D-2.5-W, D-5-W, D-10-W, D-20-W, D-25-W, D-30-W, D-38.5-W, D-40-W, D-50-W, D-60-W, D-70-W

Dextrose in water injection is available as solutions of varying concentrations of dextrose (D-glucose) in water for injection. Caloric content ranges from 85 cal/L (2.5%) to 2,380 cal/L (70%). The 5% solution is isotonic and along with the 2.5% and 10% solutions may be given by IV infusion into peripheral veins to provide calories when nonelectrolytic fluid is required. The 20% solution provides adequate calories in a minimal volume of water. The more concentrated solutions provide even greater caloric content with less fluid volume and may be irritating if given by peripheral infusion; they are usually administered by central venous catheters as a component of total parenteral nutrition (TPN). Dextrose is also available in several electrolyte solutions in various concentrations for IV infusion in patients having both a carbohydrate and an electrolyte deficit. Principal electrolytes used in fixed combination with dextrose are sodium, chloride, potassium, calcium, magnesium, phosphate, lactate, and acetate.

Mechanism

Provides a source of calories and fluid volume where nutritional or fluid deficiencies (or both) exist; dextrose is oxidized to CO_2 and water and provides 3.4 cal/g D-glucose; promotes glycogen deposition and reduces protein and nitrogen loss.

Uses

To provide nonelectrolytic fluid and caloric replacement (usually 5% or 10% solution)
Component of TPN, in conjunction with other solutions of proteins, electrolytes, fats, vitamins (usually 40%, 50%, 60%, or 70% solution)
Treatment of insulin hypoglycemia to restore blood glucose levels (50% solution)
Treatment of acute symptomatic hypoglycemia in the neonate or older infant to restore depressed blood glucose levels (25% solution)

Dosage

Dependent on patient's status and nutritional state

Fate

Approximately 95% is retained if infusion rate is 800 mg/kg/hr; essentially 100% retention occurs at 400 to 500 mg/kg/hr.

Significant Adverse Reactions

Thrombophlebitis (with prolonged infusion), irritation, tissue necrosis, infection at injection site, hypervolemia, mental confusion, hyperglycemia, glycosuria (especially with concentrated solutions or too-rapid administration), overhydration, congestion, and pulmonary edema

Contraindications

Diabetic coma; use of concentrated solutions in patients with intracranial hemorrhage or delirium tremens. *Cautious use* in patients with renal insufficiency, cardiac decompensation, hypervolemia, carbohydrate intolerance, or urinary tract obstruction.

Interactions

Dextrose infusions may alter insulin or oral hypoglycemic drug requirements and may cause vitamin B complex deficiency

Hyperglycemia and glycosuria may be intensified by diuretics that decrease glucose tolerance

Nursing Management

Pretherapy Assessment

Assess and record baseline data necessary for detection of adverse effects of dextrose in water injection: General: VS, body weight, skin color and temperature; CVS: baseline ECG; Lab: serum potassium, serum electrolytes, bicarbonate, glucose.

Review medical history and documents for existing or previous conditions that:

a. require cautious use of dextrose in water injection: renal insufficiency, cardiac decompensation, hypervolemia, carbohydrate intolerance, or urinary tract obstruction.

b. contraindicate use of dextrose in water injection: diabetic coma; use of concentrated solutions in patients with intracranial hemorrhage or delirium tremens.

Nursing Interventions

Medication Administration

Administer concentrated (hypertonic) solutions (25% or stronger) *slowly* by central venous catheter. They are very irritating and may cause thrombosis if given into a peripheral vein.

Be prepared to add appropriate electrolytes to infusion according to patient's electrolyte status.

Use only clear solutions. Discard unused portions.

Discontinue hypertonic dextrose infusion gradually. If infusion is terminated abruptly, 5% dextrose should be administered to avoid rebound hypoglycemia.

Surveillance During Therapy

Monitor results of blood sugar determinations in diabetics and in patients with impaired glucose tolerance, which should be performed frequently, and test urine for sugar often because insulin dosage may need to be adjusted.

Monitor results of serum electrolyte determinations. Appropriate supplemental electrolyte solutions should be provided as necessary.

Observe patient for signs of hyperglycemia or hyperosmolarity (confusion, unconsciousness). If they occur, infusion should be reduced or terminated.

Closely monitor blood and urine glucose determinations during prolonged infusions, especially with concentrated solutions. The maximum rate that dextrose can be infused without inducing glycosuria is 0.5 g/kg/hour.

Assess patient frequently for evidence of fluid overload, which could lead to congestive heart failure and pulmonary edema.

Interpret results of diagnostic tests and contact practitioner as appropriate.

• Alcohol in Dextrose Infusion

Alcohol in dextrose infusions are solutions of 5% dextrose in water containing 5% or 10% ethyl alcohol that provide a source of carbohydrate calories. They are not as commonly used as plain dextrose in water infusions because of the adverse effects of alcohol in many patients.

Mechanism

Supply a source of carbohydrate calories; may result in liver glycogen depletion and exert a protein-sparing action; alcohol can prevent premature labor, presumably by inhibiting release of oxytocin from the posterior pituitary

Uses

Aid in increasing caloric intake and replenishing fluids in nutritional deficiencies

Prevention of premature labor (IV infusion of 10% solution)—investigational use only

Dosage

1 to 2 liters 5% solution in a 24-hour period by *slow* IV infusion

Children: 40 mL/kg/24 hours

Fate

Alcohol is metabolized at a rate of 10 to 20 mL/hour (200–400 mL 5% solution).

Significant Adverse Reactions

(Usually with too-rapid infusion): Vertigo, flushing, sedation, confusion, alcoholic odor on breath, and pain and irritation at infusion site

Contraindications

Epilepsy, alcohol addiction, diabetic coma, urinary tract infections, severe kidney or liver impairment, shock. *Cautious use* in patients with diabetes or liver or renal impairment; in the presence of shock; during postpartum hemorrhage; after cranial surgery; and in pregnant or nursing women.

Interactions

Alcohol may shorten the duration of effect of phenytoin, warfarin, and tolbutamide.

Alcohol can potentiate the postural hypotensive effects of antihypertensive drugs, vasodilators, and diuretics.

Additive CNS depressive effects can occur between alcohol and other CNS depressants, such as barbiturates, benzodiazepines, meprobamate, glutethimide, narcotics, and phenothiazines.

An acute alcohol intolerance syndrome (eg, flushing, sweating, tachycardia, nausea) has occurred with concurrent administration of disulfiram, metronidazole, cefamandole, cefoperazone, and sulfonylurea hypoglycemic drugs.

Increased GI bleeding can occur with combined use of salicylates or other anti-inflammatory drugs.

Nursing Management

Pretherapy Assessment

Assess and record baseline data necessary for detection of adverse effects of alcohol in dextrose infusion: General: VS, body weight, skin color and temperature; Lab: serum potassium, serum electrolytes, bicarbonate, glucose.

Review medical history and documents for existing or previous conditions that:

a. require cautious use of alcohol in dextrose infusion: diabetes or liver or renal impairment; in the presence of shock; during postpartum hemorrhage; after cranial surgery; and in pregnant or nursing women.

b. contraindicate use of alcohol in dextrose infusion: epilepsy, alcohol addiction, diabetic coma, urinary tract infections, severe kidney or liver impairment, shock.

Nursing Interventions

Medication Administration

Use the largest available peripheral vein and a small-bore needle to minimize irritation. Infuse at a slow rate, and observe for signs of alcohol intoxication (slurred speech, drowsiness, flushing, dizziness).

Note that 10% solutions of ethyl alcohol can be used by IV infusion to delay labor, presumably by decreasing release of oxytocin from the pituitary. Commercially available alcohol and dextrose infusions are not approved by the Food and Drug Administration (FDA) for this particular indication.

Avoid extravasation during IV administration. Do not inject subcutaneously (SC).

Surveillance During Therapy

Monitor results of blood sugar determinations in diabetics and in patients with impaired glucose tolerance, which should be performed frequently, and test urine for sugar often because insulin dosage may need to be adjusted.

Monitor results of serum electrolyte determinations. Appropriate supplemental electrolyte solutions should be provided as necessary.

Observe patient for signs of hyperglycemia or hyperosmolarity (confusion, unconsciousness).

Interpret results of diagnostic tests and contact practitioner as appropriate.

Lipid Products

Fat emulsions designed for IV infusion are prepared from either soybean or safflower oil and contain a mixture of neutral triglycerides, which are largely polyunsaturated fatty acids. In addition, these products also contain 1.2% egg yolk phospholipids as an emulsifier and glycerin to adjust tonicity. Caloric content of the 10% IV fat emulsion is 1.1 cal/mL and that of the 20% emulsion is 2.0 cal/mL. These IV emulsions are isotonic and may be given by either peripheral or central venous routes.

• Intravenous Fat Emulsion

Intralipid 10%, 20%; Liposyn II 10%, 20%; Liposyn III 10%, 20%

Mechanism

Provide a source of calories and essential fatty acids in parenteral nutrition regimens.

Uses

Supplemental source of calories and fatty acids for patients requiring total parenteral nutrition (TPN) for extended periods whose caloric requirements cannot be met by glucose

Treatment of fatty acid deficiency states

Dosage

NOTE: Fat emulsion should constitute no more than 60% of the total caloric intake of the patient.

Total Parenteral Nutrition

Adults:

10%: initially 1 mL/minute for 15 to 30 minutes; infusion rate may be increased to 2 mL/minute; infuse only 500 mL first day, then gradually increase dose; maximum daily dose is 2.5 g/kg.

20%: initially 0.5 mL/minute for 15 to 30 minutes; infuse only 250 mL first day; maximum daily dose is 3 g/kg.

Children (refer to Significant Adverse Reactions):

10%: initially 0.1 mL/minute for 10 to 15 minutes

20%: initially 0.5 mL/minute for 10 to 15 minutes; gradually increase rate of each to 1 g/kg/4 hour; do not exceed 3 g/kg/day

Fatty Acid Deficiency

Supply 8% to 10% of the caloric intake by IV fat emulsion

Fate

Metabolized and used as a source of energy; cleared from the plasma in a manner similar to clearance of chylomicrons.

Significant Adverse Reactions

CAUTION

Infusion of IV fat emulsion in premature infants has resulted in some fatalities, presumably because of fat accumulation in the lungs. Follow dosage guidelines strictly; infusion rate should be as slow as possible, not to exceed 1 g/kg in 4 hours. Carefully monitor the infant's ability to clear the fat from the circulation between infusions, for

example, measurement of triglyceride or free fatty acid levels. Lipemia *must* clear between daily infusions.

Dyspnea, cyanosis, allergic reactions, nausea, vomiting, flushing, headache, fever, sweating, insomnia, dizziness, chest or back pain, hyperlipemia, hypercoagulability, thrombophlebitis, irritation at injection site, transient increase in liver enzymes; with prolonged administration, hepatomegaly, jaundice, leukopenia, thrombocytopenia, splenomegaly, seizures, and shock

Contraindications

Disturbed fat metabolism, acute pancreatitis; in premature infants with bilirubin levels above 5 mg/dL; in patients with severe egg allergies. *Cautious use* in patients with liver damage, pulmonary disease, anemia, or coagulation disorders, or where there is danger of fat embolism.

Nursing Management

Pretherapy Assessment

Assess and record baseline data necessary for detection of adverse effects of IV fat emulsion infusion: General: VS, body weight, skin color and temperature; Lab: liver profile, serum potassium, serum electrolytes, bicarbonate, glucose, complete blood count (CBC).

Review medical history and documents for existing or previous conditions that:

a. require cautious use of IV fat emulsion infusion: liver damage, pulmonary disease, anemia, or coagulation disorders, or where there is danger of fat embolism.

b. contraindicate use of IV fat emulsion infusion: disturbed fat metabolism, acute pancreatitis; in premature infants with bilirubin levels above 5 mg/dL; in patients with severe egg allergies.

Nursing Interventions

Medication Administration

Use only freshly opened solutions. Store preparations at 25°C or below, but do *not* freeze.

Carefully avoid disturbing the emulsion when mixing with electrolyte nutrient solutions or other additive solutions, and do not use filters. Observe emulsion for any separation; do not use if it appears disturbed.

When administering together with carbohydrate or protein/amino acid infusion solutions, infuse into separate peripheral site or through Y connector located near infusion site. To prevent backflow, ensure that lipid infusion line is higher than dextrose/amino-acid infusion line.

Expect also to administer products containing carbohydrates and amino acids because no more than 60% of patient's total caloric intake should come from IV fat emulsion.

Surveillance During Therapy

Monitor results of serum electrolyte determinations. Appropriate supplemental electrolyte solutions should be provided as necessary.

Assess patient's liver status frequently during extended administration. Drug should be discontinued if liver dysfunction is noted.

Monitor results of the following laboratory studies, which should be performed often: hemogram, blood coagulation, plasma, lipids, platelet count, and liver function tests. In neonates, platelet counts should be obtained daily. Infusion should be discontinued if significant abnormality occurs in any of these.

Note that use of this product may cause deposition of a brown pigment in the reticuloendothelial system ("intravenous fat pigment"). The cause and significance are unknown.

Electrolytes

Ammonium
Bicarbonate
Calcium
Chloride
Magnesium
Phosphate
Potassium
Sodium
Tromethamine

Parenteral electrolytes are sometimes supplied individually to correct a specific known deficiency (eg, hyponatremia, hypokalemia) but more commonly are used as combination electrolyte solutions for adjunctive treatment of nutritional disorders, dehydration, severe burns, trauma, and other emergency situations. Combined electrolyte solutions are also employed as part of the total parenteral nutrition (hyperalimentation) regimen. Serum electrolyte levels must be monitored closely during treatment, and the composition of the infusion solution as well as the rate of administration should be adjusted to provide as nearly optimal blood levels of each electrolyte as possible.

The parenteral electrolytes are listed in Table 76-2, along with their recommended dosage and nursing implications. Although the discussion afforded these preparations here is rather brief, anyone using these products routinely should become thoroughly familiar with their pharmacology and toxicology, because serious untoward reactions have occurred with improper selection or administration of parenteral electrolytes.

Selected Bibliography

Compher C, Mullen JL, Barker CF: Nutritional support in renal failure. Surg Clin North Am 71(3):597, 1991

Dudrick PS, Souba WW: Amino acids in surgical nutrition. Principles and practice. Surg Clin North Am 71(3):459, 1991

Edes TE: Nutritional support of critically ill patients. Guidelines for optimal management. Postgrad Med 89(5):193, 1991

Goepp JG, Katz SA: Oral rehydration therapy. Am Fam Physician 47(4): 843, 1993

Imm A, Carlson RW: Fluid resuscitation in circulatory shock. Crit Care Clin 9(2):313, 1993

Kaminski MV Jr, Blumeyer TJ: Metabolic and nutritional support of the intensive care patient. Crit Care Clin 9(2):363, 1993

Kelly KG: Advances in perioperative nutritional support. Med Clin North Am 77(2):465, 1993

Meguid MM, Muscaritolli M: Current uses of total parenteral nutrition. Am Fam Physician 47(2):383, 1993

Nagata MJ: Hypersensitivity reactions associated with parenteral nutrition: Case report and review of the literature. Ann Pharmacother 27(2):174, 1993

Sax HC, Souba WW: Enteral and parenteral feedings. Guidelines and recommendations. Med Clin North Am 77(4):863, 1993

Skaer TL: Total parenteral nutrition: clinical considerations. Clin Ther 15(2):272, 1993

Nursing Bibliography

Graves L: Disorders of calcium, phosphorus, and magnesium. Critical Care Nursing Quarterly 13(3):3, 1990

Innerarity S: Hyperkalemic emergencies. Critical Care Nursing Quarterly 14(4):32, 1992

Isley W: Serum sodium concentration abnormalities. Critical Care Nursing Quarterly 13(3):82, 1990

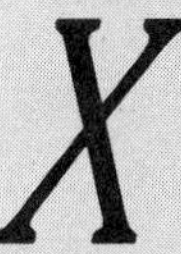

Drugs Affecting the Immune System

77 Serums and Vaccines

The ability of circulating antibodies to render a person resistant to a particular disease is known as *immunity*. Immunity may be natural or acquired. Persons born with resistance to a certain disease state are said to have *natural* immunity; however, this is a relatively rare occurrence. Most types of immunity are *acquired*, that is, attained during the person's lifetime, either by production of antibodies in response to an invasion by foreign microorganisms (*active* acquired immunity) or by utilization of antibodies obtained from an animal or another human immunized against a particular disease (*passive* acquired immunity). Active immunity, therefore, is acquired through contact with the antigen itself, which stimulates the body to produce its own specific antibodies to combat it. If the antibodies develop in response to exposure to an actual disease state, whether clinical symptoms are present or not, the active immunity is said to be *naturally acquired*. Conversely, if the antibodies form in response to inoculation into the body of killed or attenuated microorganisms or their toxic by-products, the active immunity is referred to as *artificially acquired*.

Agents for Active Immunity

Agents used for active immunity contain specific antigens that induce the formation of antibodies when injected into the body. These antigenic substances are of two types, toxoids and vaccines. *Toxoids* are toxins derived from microorganisms that have been modified (ie, detoxified), usually with formaldehyde, so that they are no longer toxic but are still antigenic, and thus are capable of stimulating antibody production. *Vaccines* are suspensions of whole microorganisms, either killed or chemically attenuated to reduce their virulence, which are capable of inducing the formation of antibodies without causing an outbreak of the disease. Active immunity with toxoids or vaccines requires several days or even weeks to develop, because sufficient antibody levels need to be attained. In some cases, more than one dose may be required. Thus, toxoids and vaccines are of limited value in treating *active* infections. Once acquired, however, active immunity can usually be made to last a lifetime, especially if reinforced by periodic "booster" doses at appropriate intervals.

A recommended schedule for the active immunization of infants and children is presented in Table 77-1. Because immunization schedules can change as newer vaccines are introduced (eg, varicella or chickenpox vaccine), the most recent recommendations of the American Academy of Pediatrics should be followed.

Toxoids

- Diphtheria toxoid
- Diphtheria and Tetanus toxoids
- Diphtheria and Tetanus toxoids and Pertussis vaccine (DTP)
- Diphtheria and Tetanus toxoids and Whole Cell Pertussis and *Haemophilus influenzae* Type B conjugate vaccines (DTP-HIB)
- Tetanus toxoid

Toxoids are generally prepared by treating exotoxins with formaldehyde, which renders them nontoxic but still antigenic. Stimulation of antibody production by toxoids can be increased by precipitating the toxoid with alum or adsorbing it onto colloids such as aluminum hydroxide. The precipitated or adsorbed products are absorbed and excreted more slowly, and they persist in tissues longer than do plain toxoids, resulting in higher antibody production. The principal disadvantage of these precipitated or adsorbed toxoids is that their use is frequently associated with pain, swelling, and tenderness at the injection site, especially in older children and adults. These reactions are sometimes quite severe. The most commonly employed toxoids are diphtheria and tetanus, which are usually given in combination with pertussis vaccine (as DTP) for routine immunization in preschool children. A newer preparation (Tetramune) also incorporates *Haemophilus influenzae*, Type B vaccine, but is not intended to replace the standard DTP in most children. Table 77-2 lists the currently available toxoids and combination products.

Vaccines

Bacterial:
- BCG
- Cholera
- *Haemophilus B* conjugate
- Meningococcal polysaccharide
- Mixed respiratory
- Plague
- Pneumococcal
- Staphage lysate
- Typhoid

Viral:
- Hepatitis B, recombinant
- Influenza
- Japanese encephalitis
- Measles

Table 77-1. **Recommended Schedule for Active Immunization of Normal Infants and Children**

Recommended Age	Immunization(s)	Comments
2 mo	DTP*, OPV†	Can be initiated as early as 2 weeks of age in areas of high endemicity or during epidemics
4 mo	DTP, OPV	2-month interval desired for OPV to avoid interference from previous dose
6 mo	DTP (OPV)	OPV is optional (may be given in areas with increased risk of poliovirus exposure)
15 mo	Measles, mumps, rubella (MMR)‡	MMR preferred to individual vaccines; tuberculin testing may be done
18 mo	DTP§‖ OPV‖	
24 mo	HIB-Conjugate vaccine#	
4–6 y**	DTP, OPV	At or before school entry
14–16 y	Td††	Repeat every 10 years throughout life

* DTP—Diphtheria and tetanus toxoids with pertussis vaccine
† OPV—Oral, poliovirus vaccine contains attenuated poliovirus types 1, 2, and 3
‡ MMR—Live measles, mumps, and rubella viruses in a combined vaccine
§ Should be given 6 to 12 months after the third dose
‖ May be given simultaneously with MMR at 15 months of age
\# *Haemophilus* b conjugate vaccine (may be given at 18 months in children at increased risk)
** Up to the seventh birthday
†† Td—Adult tetanus toxoid (full dose) and diphtheria toxoid (reduced dose) in combination
For all products used, consult manufacturer's package insert for instructions for storage, handling, and administration. Biologics prepared by different manufacturers may vary, and those of the same manufacturer may change from time to time. Therefore, the physician should be aware of the contents of the package insert.
(Report of the Committee on Infectious Diseases, American Academy of Pediatrics, 20th ed, p 9. Copyright American Academy of Pediatrics, 1986)

Measles and rubella
Measles, mumps, and rubella
Mumps
Poliovirus
Rubella
Rubella and mumps
Yellow fever

Vaccines are suspensions of killed or attenuated microorganisms of bacteria or viruses that are capable of stimulating antibody production but that are in themselves nonpathogenic. The live, attenuated vaccines are claimed to provide longer-lasting immunity in most cases than the killed or inactivated vaccines, although both types are quite effective in increasing antibody levels. Caution must be observed, however, in using a vaccine grown and cultivated in living tissues, for example, chick embryo, because allergic reactions can occur in patients hypersensitive to the specific animal proteins. However, influenza virus vaccine, although grown in embryonated eggs, is highly purified and is much less likely to elicit hypersensitivity reactions than are other vaccines. Conversely, live viral vaccines prepared by growing viruses in human cell culture (eg, rubella) are much less antigenic than animal-derived products.

Viral replication after administration of live attenuated virus vaccines may be enhanced in persons with immunodeficiency diseases or suppressed immune response, for example, persons with leukemia or other malignancies, acquired immunodeficiency virus (HIV), or persons receiving corticosteroids or cancer chemotherapeutic agents. Such patients should not be given live, attenuated virus vaccines.

In the case of certain viral vaccines, a subclinical disease state may be induced by the vaccine itself, accompanied by fever, myalgia, and other manifestations of the particular viral disease (eg, rash, urticaria, parotitis). These symptoms are generally mild and transient and usually require nothing more than symptomatic management with medications such as antipyretics or analgesics. Vaccines do not afford immediate protection, because several days or occasionally weeks are required to produce sufficient serum antibody levels. A second and occasionally a third injection at 4- to 8-week intervals are frequently given with certain vaccines to ensure adequate antibody levels. Active or imminent infections, therefore, require administration of one of the immune serums or antitoxins.

The bacterial and viral vaccines are listed in Table 77-3, along with dosage guidelines and pertinent remarks.

In addition to the commercially available vaccines listed in Table 77-3, other vaccines are available from the Centers for Disease Control in Atlanta for nonemergency use in persons at high risk for exposure in the laboratory. These products include botulinum toxoid (pentavalent) and smallpox vaccine.

Agents for Passive Immunity

Substances used to confer passive immunity are termed *immune serums* and consist of preformed antibodies derived from either human or animal sources. Human immune serums contain globulins possessing antibodies against a number of bacterial and viral diseases and are derived from human serum or

Table 77-2. **Toxoids**

Preparations	*Administration*	*Nursing Considerations*
Diphtheria Toxoid, Adsorbed, Pediatric	2 injections (0.5 mL) IM 6–8 wk apart, then a third dose 1 yr later *Booster*: 5–10-year intervals	Used in infants and children under 6 yr; do *not* administer subcutaneously; avoid giving during active infections or in patients receiving corticosteroids, because antibody response is diminished; *cautious use* in children with neurologic or convulsive disorders
Diphtheria and Tetanus Toxoids, Combined, Pediatric	*Infants 6 wk through 11 mo*: 3 injections (0.5 mL) IM at least 4 wk apart; a fourth injection is given after 6–12 mo *Booster*: 0.5 mL at 4–6 yr	Used only in children 6 yr or younger; indicated only where the triple antigen (DTP) is contraindicated; do *not* administer during acute infection or in patients receiving immunosuppressant drugs; note that pediatric preparation is 3–8 times as potent as adult preparation with respect to diphtheria toxoid; side effects include localized pain, swelling, and tenderness; drowsiness, fretfulness, and anorexia
Diphtheria and Tetanus Toxoids, Combined, Adult	2 injections (2 U diphtheria/0.5 mL) IM 4–6 wk apart, then a third dose 6–12 mo later *Booster*: 10-yr intervals	Reduced amount of diphtheria toxoid provides adequate immunization in adults with minimal risk of hypersensitivity reactions; tetanus toxoid content is identical in pediatric and adult preparations; *cautious use* during pregnancy and in debilitated individuals
Diphtheria and Tetanus Toxoids and Whole-Cell Pertussis Vaccine, Adsorbed (DTwP) *Tri-Immunol*	3 injections (0.5 mL) IM at 4–8-wk intervals, beginning at 2 mo, then a fourth dose 1 yr thereafter *Booster*: at 4–6 yr of age	Most commonly used preparation for routine immunization of young children; *not* recommended in adults or children over 7; may be used for all five doses (see under administration) *or* acellular DTP (see below); can be used for fourth and fifth doses. Diphtheria and tetanus toxoids are the preferred immunizing agent in adults and older children; use with *extreme caution* in children with history of CNS disease or convulsions because pertussis has caused neurologic side effects in a small percentage of children; *defer* administration during an acute febrile illness, shock, alterations in consciousness, extremely agitated behavior, or if patient is receiving immunosuppressive therapy; slight fever, malaise, and injection site pain frequently occur after injection
Diphtheria and Tetanus Toxoids and Acellular Pertussis Vaccine (DTaP) *Acel-Imune, Tripedia*	0.5 mL at 18 mo of age (at least 6 mo after third DTwP dose) *Booster*: at 4–6 yr of age	Use is restricted to *fourth and fifth doses* of a primary immunizing series; not recommended for adults or children younger than 15 mo of age or older than 7 yr of age; may elicit fewer side effects than DTwP; see above
Diphtheria and Tetanus Toxoids and Whole-Cell Pertussis and Haemophilus Influenzae Type B Conjugate Vaccines (DTwP-HIB) *Tetramune*	3 injections (0.5 mL) at 2-mo intervals, beginning at 2 mo of age, then a fourth dose at 15 mo of age *Booster*: at 4–6 yr of age with DTP or DTaP	Used for immunization of children 2 mo to 5 yr of age against diphtheria, tetanus, pertussis and *Haemophilus b* diseases. Children 15–18 mo of age may be given DTaP *plus* a *Haemophilus b* conjugate vaccine as separate injections
Tetanus Toxoid, Fluid or Adsorbed	Fluid: 0.5 mL at 3–8-wk intervals for 3 doses, then a fourth dose 6–12 mo later Adsorbed: 0.5 mL at 4–8-wk intervals for 2 doses, then a third dose 1 yr later *Booster*: Every 10 yr for each	Adsorbed toxoid gives higher antibody levels and longer protection than fluid toxoid and is the preferred agent; adsorbed preparation is given IM only, but fluid preparation can be administered IM or SC; do *not* use in patients with acute respiratory infection, active tetanus infection, or convulsive disorders, or in persons receiving immunosuppressive therapy; local irritation and erythema are *common*, especially in adults

plasma. Conversely, immune serums obtained by actively immunizing an animal against a specific disease, then removing and purifying the serum, which contains antibodies against that disease, are generally termed *antitoxins* or *antivenins*. Although both types of immune serums are effective in protecting against certain diseases, the human immune serums are much less likely to elicit hypersensitivity reactions, inasmuch as they do not contain foreign (ie, animal-derived) proteins.

Antitoxins/Antivenins

Black widow spider antivenin
Crotalidae antivenin
Diphtheria antitoxin
North American coral snake antivenin
Tetanus antitoxin

(text continues on page 835)

Table 77-3. **Vaccines**

Vaccine	*Administration*	*Nursing Considerations*
BACTERIAL		
BCG Vaccine *TICE BCG*	Percutaneous: 0.2–0.3 mL dropped onto skin, followed by application of a multiple-puncture disk; repeat in 2–3 mo. if patient remains tuberculin negative	Live, attenuated vaccine used in tuberculin-negative children exposed to persons with active tuberculosis; *contraindicated* in tuberculin-positive patients, burn patients, and persons receiving chronic corticosteroid therapy; do not inject IV, SC or intradermally; low incidence of untoward reactions but can produce skin ulceration and abscesses; *unused portion* and equipment should be disposed of as biohazardous material
Cholera Vaccine	*Adults*: 0.5 mL SC or IM followed in 1–4 wk by a second 0.5-mL dose *Children*: 0.2–0.3 mL SC or IM (or 0.2 mL intradermally); repeat in 1–4 wk *Booster*: 0.2–0.5 mL (depending on age) given *every 6 mo* as long as protection is desired	Used to protect travelers to or residents of countries where cholera is endemic or epidemic; *not* indicated for treatment of acute cholera infection; vaccine does *not* prevent development of a carrier state; immunity is short-lived (3–6 mo); therefore repeated dosages are necessary to confer long-lasting protection; injections *often* cause local pain, erythema, swelling, and a febrile reaction
Haemophilus b Conjugate Vaccine *HibTITER, Pedvax HIB, ProHIBiT*	Vaccination schedule differs depending on product used and child's age	Used for immunization of children 2–5 yr against disease caused by *H. influenzae* b; younger children (under 1 yr) may not be adequately protected; acute febrile reaction, erythema, and induration of injection site can occur; do *not* give during acute febrile illness or active infection; same product should be used throughout the vaccination series
Meningococcal Polysaccharide Vaccine *Menomune-A/C/Y/W-135*	0.5 mL SC as a single injection	Stimulates antibody production against *Neisseria meningitidis* groups A, C, Y, and W-135; used in persons 2 yr of age and older at risk in epidemic or endemic areas (eg, travelers, medical and laboratory personnel, household or institutional contacts); do *not* give intradermally or IV; local tenderness is common; other adverse reactions include chills, fever, malaise; *contraindicated* in presence of active infections, and in pregnant women
Mixed Respiratory Vaccine (MRV)	Initially, 0.05 mL SC; increase by 0.05–0.1 mL at 4–7 day intervals until a maximum of 1 mL is given; maintenance dosage 0.5 mL every 1–2 wk	Suspension of several strains of bacteria commonly found in respiratory infections; used to prevent bacterial hypersensitization in respiratory infections that can lead to asthma, urticaria, rhinitis; effectiveness has *not* been conclusively demonstrated; repeat doses should *not* be given until all local reactions from previous dose have disappeared; children's dose is the same as adults; local hypersensitivity reactions are common and are not a cause for alarm unless accompanied by fever or myalgia
Plague Vaccine	*Adults*: 1.0 mL IM, followed in 1–3 mo by 0.2 mL IM; third injection of 0.2 mL IM after 3–6 mo is recommended *Booster*: 0.1–0.2 mL at 6-mo intervals during active exposure *Children (under 10 yr)*: Reduce dose proportionately depending on age	Suspension of inactivated *Yersinia pestis* organisms grown in artificial media; repeated injections increase the likelihood of adverse reactions, especially local allergic effects; *common* initial side effects are malaise, headache, fever, local erythema, and mild lymphadenopathy; vaccine is recommended for those persons who must be in known plague areas and for persons working with the organism in laboratories or exposed to the organism in the environment
Pneumococcal Vaccine, Polyvalent *Pneumovax 23, Pnu-Imune 23*	0.5 mL SC *or* IM; revaccination at not less than 5-yr intervals	Used for protection against pneumococcal pneumonia and bacteremia resulting from any of the 23 most prevalent capsular types of *pneumococci*, accounting for some 90% of all cases; indicated in persons over 2 yr of age with increased risk of morbidity or mortality (eg, chronic debilitating disease or metabolic disorders, persons over 65, patients in chronic care facilities); also used to prevent pneumococcal otitis media in children under 2 yr who are at high risk, although not a recognized indication by the CDC. Protection is conferred for extended periods, and too frequent revaccination results in increasingly severe local reactions; do *not* inject IV or intradermally; local soreness and induration are very common within 2 days but quickly disappear; fever and myalgia are often noted within 24 h; *not* recommended in children under 2 yr

(*continued*)

Table 77-3. **Vaccines (Continued)**

Vaccine	*Administration*	*Nursing Considerations*
Staphage Lysate *SPL—Serologic Types I and III*	*Acute infections*: 0.05–0.2 mL, followed by increases of 0.1–0.2 mL at 1–2-day intervals to a maximum dose of 0.5 mL *Chronic or subacute infections*: 0.05–0.1 mL followed by increases of 0.1–0.2 mL at 2–4-day intervals to a maximum of 0.2–0.5 mL depending on severity of disease *Children* receive one-half the adult dose	Sterile staphylococcal vaccine used to treat staphylococcal infections or polymicrobial infections with a staphylococcal component; effectiveness has *not* been conclusively demonstrated; a skin test (0.025–0.05 mL intracutaneously) should be performed prior to initial use; may be administered by several routes (SC, intranasal, oral, topical, or irrigation) depending on site and severity of infection; malaise, fever, and chills can occur and local redness, itching, and swelling at injection site are common initially; following SC injection, the remaining solution in the 1-mL ampule may be given orally, topically, or intranasally to reinforce the SC dose
Typhoid Vaccine *Vivotif Berna Vaccine*	*Oral* 1 capsule on alternate days (1, 3, 5, 7) for 4 doses Booster: repeat dosage schedule every 5 years *Injection* *Adults*: Two 0.5-mL doses SC at 4-wk intervals *Booster*: 0.5 mL SC *or* 0.1 mL intradermally every 3 yr *Children under 10 yr*: Two 0.25-mL doses, SC, at least 4 wk apart *Booster*: 0.25 mL SC *or* 0.1 mL intradermally every 3 yr	Used for immunization against typhoid fever in persons exposed to a known typhoid carrier or travelling to areas where the disease is endemic; injection commonly causes local erythema, tenderness, and induration as well as malaise, headache, fever, and myalgia; do *not* administer during other active infections; oral capsules contain lyophilized bacteria made resistant to stomach acid; capsules should be taken one hour before meals and swallowed whole
VIRAL		
Hepatitis B Vaccine, Recombinant *Engerix-B, Recombivax HB*	*Adults*: 1.0 mL initially, IM, 1.0 mL at 1 mo, and 1.0 mL at 6 mo *Children under 10 yr*: 0.25 mL to 0.5 mL initially; repeat at 1 mo and 6 mo. *Booster (if necessary)*: at 5 yr to maintain immunity *Infants born to hepatitis B surface antigen-positive mothers* (see Nursing Considerations): 0.5 mL hepatitis B immune globulin at birth followed by 0.5 mL pediatric injection within 7 days, then again at 1 and 6 mo	Vaccine is a genetically engineered product made by programming common yeast cells to produce large quantities of the antigen portion of the virus contained in its outer coat; affords a high degree of protection (93%–99%) against hepatitis B virus, a significant health risk for health care professionals, drug abusers, homosexuals, patients undergoing hemodialysis or renal transplantation, cancer patients, and patients receiving multiple blood transfusions; protection lasts for 5 yr; hepatitis B infections have also been linked to hepatocellular carcinoma; effectiveness of vaccine in preventing hepatitis B when given *after* exposure to virus is not conclusively established, but vaccine has been given with hepatitis B immune globulin with no deleterious effects. Infants born to mothers who are hepatitis B surface antigen (HBsAg) positive are at high risk of becoming carriers of hepatitis B virus and of developing chronic infection sequelae; they should be treated beginning at birth according to the schedule given under Administration
Influenza Virus Vaccines *Flu-Imune, Fluogen, Flu-Shield, Fluzone*	*Over 8 yr*: 0.5 mL IM in a single dose *3–8 yr*: 2 doses of 0.5 mL IM at least 4 wk apart *Under 3 yr*: 2 doses of 0.25 mL IM at least 4 wk apart	Composition of vaccine changes yearly depending on prevalent virus strains; recommended in persons at high risk for adverse reactions from lower respiratory infections, such as those with heart disease, chronic pulmonary disease, renal dysfunction, diabetes, or debilitation; use with caution in hypersensitive persons, because vaccine is egg-grown, although it is highly purified; *defer* immunization in patients with acute respiratory disease or other active infection and in pregnant women during first trimester; not effective against *all* influenza viruses; available as "whole-virus," "split-virus," or purified surface antigen preparations—due to fewer febrile reactions, use only split-virus or purified surface antigen in children; antigenic response to vaccine may be lower than expected in immunocompromised patients
Japanese Encephalitis Vaccine *(JE-VAX)*	*Adults and children over 3 yr*: 1 mL SC on days 0, 7, and 30 *Children 1–3 yr*: 0.5 mL SC on days 0, 7, and 30	Used for active immunization against Japanese encephalitis (JE) virus, a mosquito-borne infection that is the leading cause of viral encephalitis in Asia; recommended for persons who will be spending at least 1 month in epidemic or endemic areas during the transmission season; approximately 20% of vaccine recipients experience mild to moderate local side effects (eg, erythema, rash, hives, swelling, etc); travel should not be undertaken for at least 10 days after vaccination due to possibility of delayed adverse reactions

(*continued*)

Table 77-3. **Vaccines (Continued)**

Vaccine	*Administration*	*Nursing Considerations*
Measles Vaccine—Rubeola *Attenuvax*	Administer reconstituted vaccine SC *Booster*: not necessary	Live, attenuated strain of measles virus grown in chick embryo tissue culture; most often given together with mumps and rubella vaccines as a single preparation (see MMR below); produces a mild measles infection (eg, fever, rash), which induces immunity in 97% of susceptible individuals; recommended in children 15 mo or older; revaccination is *not* required if child was over 12 mo when initially vaccinated; *contraindicated* in pregnancy; use *cautiously* in children with a history of febrile convulsions or cerebral injury; discard if not used within 8 h
Measles and Rubella Vaccine *M-R-Vax II*	Administer reconstituted vaccine SC *Booster*: not necessary	Indicated for simultaneous immunization against measles and rubella (German measles) in children over 15 mo; see measles vaccine and rubella vaccine for additional information; most frequently given together with mumps vaccine as a single preparation (see below).
Measles, Mumps, and Rubella Vaccine *M-M-R II*	Administer reconstituted vaccine SC Revaccination recommended upon entering school	Preferred preparation in children over 15 mo for immunization against measles, mumps, and rubella: highly effective (95%–98% of children develop effective antibody levels to all three viruses) and generally well tolerated; widely used preparation; immunity persists for at least 8 yr to 10 yr; thus revaccination is not required; see Nursing Considerations for measles, mumps, and rubella vaccines, individually
Mumps Vaccine *Mumpsvax*	Administer reconstituted vaccine SC *Booster*: not necessary	Used for immunization of children over 15 mo and adults; immunity is produced in 97% of children and 93% of adults with a single dose and persists for at least 10 yr; do *not* use in pregnant women; allergic reactions can occur (vaccine is derived from chick embryo); be prepared with epinephrine
Poliovirus Vaccine, Inactivated—IPV *IPOL*	2 doses (0.5 mL each) given SC at 2 and 4 mo of age followed by a third dose 6–12 mo after the second dose *Booster*: 4–6 yr of age	Indicated for polio immunization in persons with compromised immune systems; oral polio vaccine (Sabin) is vaccine of choice in other persons; dosage schedule is often integrated with that of DTP immunization and begun at 6–12 wk of age; see Table 77-1; vaccine should be clear red; do *not* use if cloudy, discolored, or precipitated; *defer* injections during periods of other active infections; hypersensitivity reactions can occur; have epinephrine injection available
Poliovirus Vaccine, Live Oral Trivalent—TOPV, Sabin *Orimune*	3 doses (0.5 mL each) given orally at 6–12 wk of age, 8 wk later, and 8 mo after the second dose *Booster*: 4–6 yr of age	Vaccine of choice for primary immunization against poliovirus; advantages over Salk vaccine are ease of administration, longer-lasting immunity, protection against infection by wild polioviruses, and lack of need for periodic booster doses; see Table 77-1; do *not* administer if persistent vomiting or diarrhea is present; store in a freezer, thaw before use, refrigerate vial after opening, and use contents within 7 days
Rubella Vaccine *Meruvax II*	Administer total volume of reconstituted vaccine SC	Live, attenuated rubella virus strains used to immunize against rubella in children from 15 mo to puberty; antibody levels persist for at least 6 yr; useful in adolescents and adults to prevent outbreaks in high risk situations; do *not* administer to pregnant women and use *cautiously* in women of childbearing age because congenital abnormalities can occur; usually given combined with measles and mumps vaccines (see MMR); side effects are usually transient (rash, urticaria, sore throat, malaise, fever, headache, lymphadenopathy); arthralgia is fairly common in women (12%–20%)
Rubella and Mumps Vaccine *Biavax II*	Administer total volume of reconstituted vaccine SC	Combination vaccine yielding effective antibody levels in 97% to 100% of susceptible children; may be given as early as 1 yr of age; not as frequently used as measles, mumps, and rubella vaccine (MMR); see Nursing Considerations for rubella and mumps vaccines, individually
Yellow Fever Vaccine *YF-Vax*	0.5 mL SC	Indicated for immunization of persons traveling to countries requiring vaccination against yellow fever; immunity develops within 7 days and can last for up to 10 yr; administer at least 1 mo apart from other live viruses; fever and malaise occur in about 10% of patients; keep frozen until reconstituted and then use within 1 h; do *not* use if vaccine has been exposed to temperatures above 5°C

Antitoxins and antivenins are prepared by repeatedly inoculating an animal, usually a horse, with a toxoid (eg, diphtheria, tetanus) or a venom (eg, from a snake or a black widow spider), then bleeding the animal and concentrating the antibody-containing fraction of the plasma. The partially purified antibodies or antitoxins can then be administered to humans to neutralize toxins produced by invading microorganisms or introduced by a bite.

It is imperative that a skin or conjunctival hypersensitivity test be performed before administering any of these preparations to determine if the patient exhibits an allergic reaction to the foreign serum. Package literature describing the appropriate hypersensitivity testing procedure should always be consulted before using one of these products. Even a negative sensitivity test result, however, does not completely rule out the possibility of an allergic reaction, and epinephrine injection should always be available when an antitoxin or antivenin is administered. Adverse reactions to antitoxins and antivenins range from local pain and erythema at the injection site to serum sickness and anaphylaxis, the incidence of the more serious allergic reactions being approximately 5% to 10%.

Information pertaining to the commercially available antitoxins and antivenins is presented in Table 77-4. In addition, botulism equine antitoxin and diphtheria equine antitoxin are available on request from the Centers for Disease Control in Atlanta.

Human Immune Serums

Cytomegalovirus immune globulin
Hepatitis B immune globulin
Immune globulin, human
Lymphocyte immune globulin

(*text continues on page 838*)

Table 77-4. **Antitoxins/Antivenins**

Antitoxin/Antivenin	*Administration*	*Nursing Considerations*
ANTIVENINS		
Black Widow Spider Species Antivenin *Antivenin Latrodectus mactans*	2.5 mL reconstituted antivenin IM *or* 2.5 mL in 10–50 mL saline by IV infusion	Used to treat persons bitten by black widow spider; prompt administration yields most effective results; give by IV infusion in severe cases or if patient is in shock; use of muscle relaxants appears to be most important during early reaction phase; test for sensitivity to horse serum prior to administration
Crotalidae Antivenin, Polyvalent	Dosage depends on severity of bite Mild: 2–4 vials IV Moderate: 5–9 vials IV Severe: 10–20 vials IV (Children and small adults may require larger doses; see Nursing Considerations) *NOTE*: may be given IM but is less effective than IV	Preparation of serum globulins containing protective antibodies against a number of crotalids, including pit vipers, rattlesnakes, cottonmouths, copper heads, bushmasters (see package instructions); administer as soon as possible after bite and immobilize patient to minimize spread of venom; do *not* administer at or around the site of the bite; children have less resistance and require proportionately larger doses than adults; subsequent injections depend on clinical response; IV use is mandatory if shock is present; administer within 4 h of bite if possible; test for sensitivity to horse serum before administration
North American Coral Snake Antivenin *Antivenin Micrurus fulvius*	3–5 vials (30–50 mL) slowly injected directly into IV infusion tubing or added to reservoir bottle of IV drip	Concentrated solution of serum globulins obtained from horses immunized against eastern coral snake venom; bitten area should be completely immobilized; first several milliliters of antivenin should be administered over a 5-min period and patient carefully observed for evidence of allergic reaction; 10 vials or more have been required in some persons with severe or multiple bites
ANTITOXINS		
Diphtheria Antitoxin	*Adults and children*: 20,000–120,000 U IM *or* IV depending on severity and duration of infection *Prophylaxis*: 10,000 U IM if sensitivity test is negative	Concentrated solution of purified globulins obtained from the serum of horses immunized against diphtheria toxin; delay in beginning therapy increases dosage requirements and reduces beneficial effects; continue treatment until all symptoms are controlled; appropriate antimicrobial agents should be used concurrently; nonimmunized patients exposed to diphtheria should receive a low dose (see Administration) to produce a temporary passive immunity; sensitivity testing is necessary before administration
Tetanus Antitoxin	*Treatment*: 50,000–100,000 U IV or IM *Prophylaxis*: 1500–5000 U IM or SC depending on body weight	Concentrated solution of serum globulins from horses immunized against tetanus toxin; indicated *only* when tetanus immune globulin (see Table 77-5) is not available; protection lasts about 2 wk with a single prophylactic dose; tetanus toxoid, adsorbed, is usually given with the antitoxin to initiate active immunization; most children are routinely immunized against tetanus and the need for the antitoxin seldom occurs

Table 77-5. **Human Immune Serums**

Immune Serum	*Administration*	*Nursing Considerations*
Cytomegalovirus Immune Globulin Intravenous, Human (CMV-IGIV)	150 mg/kg IV infusion within 72 hr of transplant; 100 mg/kg at 2, 4, 6 and 8 weeks posttransplant; 50 mg/kg at 12 and 16 weeks posttransplant	Used to reduce the probability of primary CMV disease in patients who receive a kidney transplant from a donor who is seropositive for CMV; administer through an IV line using a constant infusion pump; do not dilute CMV-IGIV more than 1:2 with any other IV solution; begin infusion at a rate of 15 mg/kg/h and increase at 30-min intervals to a maximum of 60 mg/kg/h; side effects may include flushing, chills, fever, cramping, nausea, vomiting, and wheezing
Hepatitis B Immune (HBIG) Globulin *H-BIG, Hep-B-Gammagee, HyperHep*	0.06 mL/kg IM as soon after exposure as possible; repeat in 1 mo *Prevention of carrier state*: 0.5 mL IM no later than 24 h after birth; repeat in 3 mo *Prophylaxis of infants born to HB_sAg-positive mothers*: 0.5 mL IM at birth	Solution of immunoglobulins containing a high titer of antibodies to hepatitis B surface antigen (HB_sAg); indicated for prophylaxis following accidental oral, parenteral, or direct mucous membrane exposure to antigen-containing materials such as blood or serum; also for prophylaxis of infants born to HB_sAg-positive mothers who are at risk of being infected or becoming chronic carriers; may be given at the same time or up to 1 mo preceding hepatitis B vaccine without altering the resultant immune response; solution should be stored at 2°C–8°C but *not* frozen
Immune Globulin—Intramuscular (ISG) *Gamma Globulin, Gamastan, Gammar*	*IM injection only* Hepatitis A: 0.02 mL/kg Immunoglobulin deficiency: 1.3 mL/kg initially, then 0.66 mL/kg every 3–4 wk Measles: 0.25 mL/kg Rubella: 0.55 mL/kg (pregnant women *only*) Varicella: 0.6–1.2 mL/kg	Solution of globulins obtained from pooled human serum, containing antibodies to a number of organisms; used to decrease the severity of certain diseases (hepatitis, measles, varicella) in persons exposed to an active infection; also indicated as replacement therapy for immunoglobulin deficiency states and as adjunctive treatment to antibiotics in severe bacterial infections or burns; may be of benefit in pregnant women exposed to rubella virus to lessen possibility of fetal damage, but routine use in early pregnancy cannot be justified; injections can be very painful
Immune Globulin, Intravenous (IGIV) *Gamimune N, Gammagard, Gammar-IV, Sandoglobulin, Venoglobulin 1*	*IV infusion only* 100–300 mg/kg once a month by IV infusion (0.01–0.04 mL/kg/min for 30 min) *Idiopathic thrombocytopenic purpura*: 400 mg/kg for 5 consecutive days	Provides *immediate* antibody levels; half-life is about 3 wk; preferred to immune globulin, IM, in patients requiring rapid increases in IgG antibodies, in patients with a small muscle mass, and in patients with bleeding tendencies; maltose is added to stabilize the protein, reducing the incidence of adverse effects; may cause a precipitous drop in blood pressure, especially at rapid infusion rates; monitor vital signs carefully during infusion; have epinephrine available for allergic reactions
Lymphocyte Immune Globulin—Anti-thymocyte Globulin (LIG, ATG) *Atgam*	*Allograft rejection* *IV infusion only* Adults: 10–30 mg/kg/day Children: 5–25 mg/kg/day (Given daily for 14 days, then every other day for a total of 21 doses in 28 days) *Aplastic anemia* 10–20 mg/kg daily for 8–14 days	A lymphocyte-selective immunosuppressant that reduces the number of circulating, thymus-dependent lymphocytes; used by *experienced personnel only* for management of allograft rejection in renal transplant patients and as an adjunct to other immunosuppressive therapy (eg, azathioprine, corticosteroids) to delay onset of first rejection; also used in severe aplastic anemia in patients unsuited for bone marrow transplantation; *discontinue* if anaphylaxis or *severe* thrombocytopenia or leukopenia occurs; frequently encountered adverse reactions are fever, chills, rash, pruritus, urticaria, leukopenia, and thrombocytopenia; drug must be diluted in saline before infusion; use within 12 h; do *not* dilute with dextrose solutions or highly acidic solutions because precipitation can occur; a dose should *not* be infused over less than 4 h; have resuscitative materials available (eg, epinephrine, antihistamines, steroids, etc.)
Tetanus Immune Globulin *Hyper-Tet*	*Treatment*: 3000–6000 U IM *Prophylaxis*: 250 U IM (children—4 U/kg)	Indicated for passive tetanus prophylaxis in persons not actively immunized or whose immunization status is uncertain; not generally necessary if person has had at least 2 doses of tetanus toxoid; produces effective levels of circulating antibodies for much longer periods than tetanus antitoxin; does not interfere with immune response to tetanus toxoid given at the same time; thorough cleansing of wounds and removal of all foreign particles is important to prevent infection; do *not* give IV

(*continued*)

Table 77-5. Human Immune Serums (Continued)

Immune Serum	*Administration*	*Nursing Considerations*
Rh_o(D) Immune Globulin *Gamulin Rh, HypRho-D, Rhesonativ, RhoGAM (CAN) Win Rho*	Inject contents of 1 vial IM for every 15 mL fetal packed red cell volume within 72 h following delivery, miscarriage, abortion, or transfusion (See package instructions for mixing and injecting directions) *Antepartum prophylaxis* 1 vial IM at 26 and 28 weeks gestation and again within 72 hr of Rh-incompatible delivery	Used to prevent sensitization in a subsequent pregnancy to the Rh_o(D) factor in an Rh-negative mother who has given birth to an Rh-positive infant by an Rh-positive father; also may be employed to prevent Rh_o(D) sensitization in Rh-negative patients accidentally transfused with Rh-positive blood; consult product information for blood typing and drug administration procedures; do *not* give IV; also available in microdose form (MICRhoGAM, Mini-Gamulin Rh, HypRho-D Mini-Dose) to prevent maternal Rh-immunization following miscarriage or abortion up to 12 weeks gestation
Varicella-Zoster Immune Globulin (human)—VZIG	*IM only*: 125 U/10 kg body weight to a maximum of 625 U; do *not* give fractional units	Globulin fraction of adult human plasma (primarily immunoglobulin G) with high titer of varicella-zoster antibodies; used for passive immunization of *immunodeficient* children following exposure to varicella; most effective if given within 96 h after exposure; *not* indicated prophylactically; do *not* administer IV; no more than 2.5 mL should be injected at a single IM site (1.25 mL maximum if patient weighs less than 10 kg); VZIG must be requested from regional distribution centers of American Red Cross Blood Services

Table 77-6. Rabies Prophylaxis Products

Immune Serum	*Administration*	*Nursing Considerations*
Antirabies Serum, Equine	40 U/kg (1000 U/55 lb) IM in a single dose Usually given together with HDVC, although *not* at the same site nor in the same syringe	Used in conjunction with HDVC (see below) to promote passive immunity to rabies when rabies immune globulin is unavailable; delays propagation of virus, thus allowing time for rabies vaccine to induce sufficient antibodies; give as soon as possible after exposure; sensitivity testing (intradermal or conjunctival) should be done before administration; up to 50% of the dose should be infiltrated into the tissue around the wound; adverse reactions include local pain, erythema, urticaria, and serum sickness
Rabies Immune Globulin, Human *Hyperab, Imogam*	20 U/kg (9 U/lb); 1/2 the dose IM and 1/2 the dose to infiltrate the wound	Used to provide rabies antibodies immediately; given in conjunction with HDCV vaccine; reduced risk of serum sickness compared to equine vaccine; should be given as soon as possible following exposure, but regardless of interval, immune globulin is still recommended; do *not* give repeated doses once vaccine has been administered; muscle soreness and low grade fever can occur
Rabies Vaccine, Human Diploid Cell Cultures (HDCV) Intramuscular *Imovax* ***Intradermal*** *Imovax I.D.*	*IM* Preexposure: 3 injections, IM, of 1.0 mL each on days 0, 7, and 28 Boosters: every 6 mo–2 yr as needed to maintain immunity in high-risk individuals Postexposure: 5 injections, IM, of 1.0 mL each on days 0, 3, 7, 14, and 28 with a dose of rabies immune globulin on day 0; a sixth dose is given 90 days after the first dose *Intradermal* Preexposure *only*; 3 injections (0.1 mL) on days 0, 7, and either 21 or 28	Preferred rabies prophylaxis product; IM injection may be used either pre- or postexposure; intradermal injection is *only* for prophylaxis preexposure; postexposure antibody response is virtually 100% with recommended 5 doses; preexposure vaccination is indicated for persons in contact with rabid animals or patients or those handling rabies virus or contaminated articles; postexposure treatment should also include rabies immune globulin; adverse reactions to vaccine are infrequent; local swelling and erythema have occurred; corticosteroids and other immunosuppressive agents can interfere with development of active immunity to vaccine—do *not* administer together

Tetanus immune globulin
$Rh_o(D)$ immune globulin
Varicella zoster immune globulin

Immune globulins containing antibodies against certain diseases can be obtained from human serum, and these products are generally preferred over animal-derived globulins because of their lower incidence of hypersensitivity reactions. Human immune globulins may be obtained from pooled plasma of human donors, in which case the preparation contains antibodies against a number of diseases (eg, hepatitis, rubella, varicella) or from the blood of persons recently recovered from or hyperimmunized against a *particular* disease, in which case the globulins contain high antibody titers against that particular disease. Protection against a particular disease occurs soon after administration but is of short duration, generally persisting for only 1 to 3 months.

Skin testing for hypersensitivity is meaningless with human immune serums, because intradermal injections frequently give rise to a local inflammatory response that can be misinterpreted as an allergic reaction. True hypersensitivity reactions to human immune globulins are extremely rare.

The human immune serums are listed in Table 77-5, along with dosages and other pertinent information. In addition, vaccinia immune globulin, human, is available on request from the Centers for Disease Control in Atlanta.

Rabies Prophylaxis Products

Antirabies serum, equine
Rabies immune globulin
Rabies vaccine, human diploid cell culture

Rabies is an acute viral disease of animals that can be transmitted to other animals and humans by the bite of an infected animal. Although many animals are susceptible to rabies, it occurs most commonly in dogs, cats, raccoons, skunks, coyotes, and wolves. The virus has a high affinity for the nervous system and is inevitably fatal unless appropriate immunologic therapy is instituted quickly.

Products used for rabies prophylaxis include the following:

- *Human diploid cell vaccine* (HDCV): suspension of Wistar rabies virus strain grown in human diploid cell cultures
- *Rabies immune globulin* (RIG): human immune globulin obtained from plasma of hyperimmunized donors
- *Antirabies serum, equine origin* (ARS): concentrated serum obtained from hyperimmunized horses

Postexposure treatment is best accomplished by a combination of active and passive immunization, that is, vaccine and immune globulin. For passive immunization, rabies immune globulin is the drug of choice; the equine antirabies serum should be used only when the immune globulin is unavailable. For active immunization, HDCV is used.

The rabies prophylaxis products are briefly reviewed in Table 77-6. It is important, however, that anyone using any of the products become thoroughly familiar with the indications, precautions, and general handling procedures of each particular preparation by consulting the product literature.

Selected Bibliography

ASHP therapeutic guidelines for intravenous immune globulin. ASHP Commission on Therapeutics. Clin Pharm 11:117, 1992

Bixler GS, Pillai S: The cellular basis of the immune response to conjugate vaccines. Contrib Microbiol Immunol 10:18, 1989

Gronski P, Selier FR, Schwick HG: Discovery of antitoxins and development of antibody preparations for clinical uses from 1890–1990. Molec Immunol 28:1321, 1991

Isaacs D, Menser M: Measles, mumps, rubella and varicella. Lancet 335:1384, 1990

Levine MM: Modern vaccines: Enteric infections. Lancet 335:958, 1990

Messner RL, Mufson MA: Pneumococcal vaccine: A focus for nursing. Adv Clin Care 5:11, 1990

Stiehm ER: Recent progress in the use of intravenous immunoglobulin. Curr Prob Pediatr 22:335, 1992

Update of adult immunization. Recommendations of the Immunization Practices Advisory Committee. Morbidity Mortality Weekly Report 40:1, 1991

Walker PD: Bacterial vaccines: Old and new, veterinary and medical. Vaccine 10:977, 1992

Werner SB: Sources of supply of selected immunobiologics, 1990. West J Med 153:503, 1990

Nursing Bibliography

Kefalas M: American children and immunizations: Part program initiatives. J Pediatr Nurs 8(6):403, 1993

Tittle K: Immunizations: Supporting the community's efforts. J Pediatr Nurs 8(2):132, 1993

78
Immunomodulators

Colony-Stimulating Factors
- Filgrastim
- Sargramostim

Immunosuppressants
- Azathioprine
- Cyclosporine
- Muromonab-CD3
- FK 506

Immune Serums
- Lymphocyte Immune Globulin

Interferons
- Interferon Beta-1b
- Interferon Gamma-1b

Overview of Immunology

The concept of *immunity* encompasses all the mechanisms used by the body to resist and defend itself against potentially harmful environmental factors, foreign substances, and abnormal cells.

Natural (Innate) Immunity

Natural or innate immunity includes all nonspecific, inherited mechanisms that collectively provide the first line of defense against a wide array of threatening factors. The principal components of natural immunity include physical, chemical, and cellular mechanisms.

Physical (Mechanical) Mechanisms

These serve as barriers to invasion of the body by extrinsic factors, and include the skin and mucous membranes.

Chemical Mechanisms

A wide array of chemical molecules participate in nonspecific defense. Some of these chemicals enhance the protective effects of the mechanical barriers (eg, the acidity of the sebum, gastric juice, and vaginal secretions), and retard microbial growth on the skin and mucous membranes. Other chemicals (eg, histamine, kinins, prostaglandins, and leukotrienes) act as mediators of inflammation.

The *interferons* and the *complement proteins* function in both nonspecific (natural) and specific (acquired) immune mechanisms, as is discussed later in this chapter.

Cellular Mechanisms

A variety of cells participate in nonspecific immunity through phagocytosis, cytolysis, and involvement in the inflammatory response. This "army" of cells includes neutrophils, monocytes, basophils, eosinophils, mast cells, natural killer cells, and macrophages.

Acquired (Adaptive) Immunity

Acquired or adaptive immune mechanisms exhibit two important characteristics that distinguish them from natural or innate mechanisms: *specificity* and *memory*.

There are two distinct but functionally interactive forms of specific adaptive immunity:

1. *Cellular (cell-mediated) immunity*: Cellular immunity uses activated T lymphocytes and their secretory products, collectively termed *lymphokines*, to eliminate virally infected cells and neoplastic (cancer) cells and provide immunity against most viral, parasitic, and fungal infections, and against a few bacteria. This form of immunity is also involved in delayed hypersensitivity reactions and organ transplant rejection.
2. *Humoral (antibody-mediated) immunity*: Humoral immunity provides protection against most bacteria and a few viruses through the production of highly specific gamma-globulin proteins termed *immunoglobulins* or *antibodies*.

Adaptive immune mechanisms are designed to destroy or eliminate specific molecules called *antigens* (*or immunogens*). Typically, such molecules are large (high molecular weight), chemically complex, and foreign to the body. Specific portions of the molecules that may activate an adaptive immune response are termed antigenic determinants or *epitopes*.

The cells central to the specific immune response are the *lymphocytes*. There are two major types of lymphocytes, B lymphocytes and T lymphocytes, both of which develop from multipotent stem cells in the bone marrow. The B lymphocytes (B cells) complete their maturation in the bone marrow. The immature T lymphocytes, however, migrate from the bone marrow to the thymus gland, where they acquire important surface proteins that serve as receptors and special markers. After becoming immunocompetent, the mature B and T cells are seeded in secondary lymphoid tissues, such as the spleen, lymph nodes, and tonsils.

Major Histocompatibility Complex Antigens

Genetically determined factors play a key role in the specific immune response. The major histocompatibility complex (MHC) antigens, also known as human leukocyte-associated (HLA) antigens, are glycoproteins (unique in each individual) encoded by a cluster of genes (MHC genes) located on the short arm of chromosome 6. There are two major classes of MHC (or HLA) antigens. *Class I MHC* antigens (which include HLA-A, HLA-B, and HLA-C antigens) are found on the surfaces of all nucleated cells. *Class II MHC* antigens (which include all HLA-D antigens) are found on B lymphocytes, macrophages, and other antigen-presenting cells (APCs).

T-Cell Maturation

During their maturation in the thymus gland, T lymphocytes acquire *T-cell receptors* (TCRs), which can recognize a specific antigen–MHC glycoprotein combination. T cells also acquire coreceptor molecules (either CD4 or CD8), which allow the T cells to bind to different classes of MHC molecules.

T cells that acquire CD4 coreceptors bind only to class II MHC glycoproteins, and functionally, such cells are *helper T cells* or *inducer T cells* (also termed T4 cells). The T4 cells appear to be the principal targets of the human immunodeficiency virus, which causes acquired immunodeficiency syndrome (AIDS).

T cells that acquire CD8 coreceptor molecules bind only to class I MHC glycoproteins. Functionally, such CD8 or T8 cells may be *cytotoxic T cells* or *suppressor T cells*.

T cells can respond to foreign antigens only when those antigens are associated with "self" antigens (ie, class I or class II MHC glycoproteins) on a cell surface. This requires the participation of APCs, described in the following section.

Antigen-Presenting Cells

APCs include B lymphocytes, macrophages, dendritic cells of the spleen and lymph nodes, and Langerhans' cells of the skin. APCs ingest exogenous antigens (free viruses, bacteria), extract specific peptide fragments of the antigen, and combine them with class I or II MHC glycoproteins. The entire antigen–MHC glycoprotein complex is subsequently displayed on the surface of the APC for eventual recognition by specific T cells bearing the appropriate TCR.

Activated macrophages secrete monokines, notably interleukin-1, which activates B-cell and T4-cell clones specific to the exogenous antigen, stimulates production of Interleukin-2 (IL-2) by activated T4 cells, and exerts a variety of systemic effects.

T Lymphocytes (Cellular Immunity)

There are several recognized functional subsets of T lymphocytes. The current classification is likely to change as more is learned about the complex activities and interactions of T cells.

Helper–Inducer T Cells (T4 Cells). Helper–inducer cells are endowed with CD4 coreceptor molecules, which allow them to interact with class II MHC glycoproteins. T4 cells facilitate or amplify responses by B cells through direct contact with B cells, as well as chemically, through the production of lymphokines such as IL-2.

T4 cells also stimulate proliferation of activated T8 cells through the actions of IL-2.

Cytotoxic T Cells. T cells that carry CD8 coreceptor molecules are activated when their complementary TCRs bind to specific peptide–MHC I glycoprotein complexes on the surfaces of infected or abnormal cells. When simultaneously exposed to IL-2, T8 cells proliferate and differentiate into *cytotoxic T cells*, which attack and destroy the target cells. Activated cytotoxic T cells secrete *perforins*, which create pores in the membranes of target cells and ultimately cause cytolysis. Cytotoxic T cells may also secrete *lymphotoxin*, which activates enzymes that cause DNA fragmentation in the target cell, resulting in eventual cell death.

Suppressor T Cells. Suppressor cells develop very slowly from activated T8 cells under the influence of IL-2 secreted by helper T cells. Suppressor cells inhibit both cytotoxic and helper T-cell activities, and they dampen B-cell responses to antigens. The ratio of helper T cells to suppressor T cells in the body is normally 2:1. This ratio is markedly reduced in AIDS; however, much remains to be learned about the modulating mechanisms of suppressor cells.

Memory T Cells. Even after the activation of suppressor cells, some helper T cells and cytotoxic T cells remain to function as memory cells that can be recruited to initiate immune responses to subsequent encounters with the same antigen.

Cytokines

Cytokines are relatively small protein molecules (produced by a variety of cells) that affect blood cell development and influence many immune-related responses.

Cytokines produced by macrophages and monocytes may also be called *monokines*, whereas those secreted by lymphocytes are termed *lymphokines*. By convention, once the amino acid sequence of a cytokine has been determined, its name becomes a sequentially numbered *interleukin*. Unfortunately, much confusion in nomenclature still exists because some cytokines, such as the interferons, have already become so established by name that the "interleukin rule" has not been applied universally. An overview of representative cytokines and their principal actions is presented in Table 78-1.

B Lymphocytes (Humoral Immunity)

The cell membranes of B lymphocytes are endowed with antibody molecules that serve as receptors for a specific antigen. When that antigen binds to the antibody receptor, the B cell becomes activated, proliferating and differentiating into *plasma cells* and *memory B cells*. Plasma cells are modified (enlarged) B lymphocytes possessing a highly developed endoplasmic reticulum, and are engaged in the production of antibodies specific to the antigen that led to their production. Memory B cells may be rapidly mobilized to become functional antibody-secreting plasma cells if the same antigen is encountered again at a later time.

Activated helper T (T4) cells greatly facilitate humoral immunity by binding to the antigen–MHC II complex on the surface of a B cell already bound to an antigen. T4 cells also secrete lymphokines (IL-2, IL-4, IL-6, and gamma-interferon), which chemically stimulate B-cell proliferation and differentiation.

Immunoglobulins (Antibodies)

Humoral immunity is mediated by modified gamma-globulin proteins called *immunoglobulins* or *antibodies*. Each immunoglobulin molecule is composed of four polypeptide chains (two long *heavy* chains and two shorter *light* chains) linked by disulfide bonds. There are five structural classes of immunoglobulins, named according to the type of heavy chain:

Table 78-1. **Cytokines and Their Principal Actions**

Cytokine	*Principal Actions*
Interferon-alpha	Antiviral; antiproliferative; induces class I MHC complex; increases production of cytotoxic T cells
Interferon-beta	See interferon-alpha
Interferon-gamma	Antiviral; activates macrophages; increases NK cell activity; induces expression of Class I and II MHC antigens; facilitates production of T-cell suppressor factor
Interleukin-1 (IL-1)	Activates T cells and differentiation of B cells; mediates inflammatory reactions; induces fever; stimulates production of lymphokines; facilitates differentiation of bone marrow stem cells to develop receptors for IL-2
Interleukin-2 (IL-2)	Enhances growth and differentiation of cytotoxic, helper, and suppressor T cells, and NK cells; increases NK cell activity; induces lymphokine production by T cells
Interleukin-3 (IL-3)	Enhances growth and differentiation of hematopoietic precursors; facilitates growth of mast cells
Interleukin-4 (IL-4)	Growth factor for antigen-primed B cell and T cells; increases cytotoxicity of killer T cells and macrophages; enhances Class II MHC antigen expression on B cells
Interleukin-5 (IL-5)	Stimulates B-cell activation and eosinophil proliferation; increases production of IgA and IgM antibodies by activated B cells; induces formation of IL-2 receptors on B cells
Interleukin-6 (IL-6)	Enhances differentiation of activated B cells and secretion of immunoglobulins; facilitates differentiation of killer T cells; induces acute-phase proteins
Interleukin-7 (IL-7)	Stimulates proliferation of pre-B, CD4-CD8-T cells
Tumor necrosis factor-alpha (TNF-alpha)	Mediates inflammation and septic shock; exhibits antitumor and antiparasitic action; stimulates production of lymphokines; activates macrophages and neutrophils; induces hemorrhagic necrosis of some tumors
Tumor necrosis factor-beta (TNF-beta)	Similar action to TNF-alpha; renders some tumors more susceptible to NK-mediated lysis
Granulocyte colony-stimulating factor	Stimulates growth and activation of neutrophil colonies
Macrophage colony-stimulating factor	Stimulates growth and activation of macrophage colonies
Granulocyte–macrophage colony-stimulating factor	Stimulates growth of neutrophil, eosinophil, and macrophage colonies; activates mature granulocytes and macrophages

MHC, major histocompatibility complex; NK, natural killer; CSF, colony-stimulating factor.

1. **IgM** immunoglobulins are the first antibodies produced in response to an antigen (the "primary response"). IgM molecules may also serve as antigen receptors on the surfaces of B lymphocytes.
2. **IgG** is the major circulating antibody, being the principal immunoglobulin secreted during the "secondary response." IgG is the only antibody capable of crossing the placenta.
3. **IgA** immunoglobulins are found in external secretions such as saliva, tears, and colostrum.
4. **IgE** immunoglobulins bind to the cell membranes of basophils and mast cells. When antigens bind to the IgE antibodies, the basophils and mast cells degranulate and release bioactive molecules (eg, histamine, kinins, prostaglandins) that mediate immediate (ie, type I) hypersensitivity reactions such as asthma and hay fever.
5. **IgD** immunoglobulins are present on cell membranes of circulating B lymphocytes, where they function as antigen receptors.

Antibodies protect the body from potentially harmful antigens by binding to antigens and rendering them inactive or by facilitating their removal by nonspecific immune mechanisms (eg, phagocytosis). Principal antigen–antibody interactions may be manifested in the following ways:

1. *Neutralization* (effective for inactivating bacterial toxins)
2. *Agglutination* (clumping of cells linked through lattices of antigen–antibody complexes)
3. *Precipitation* (causing otherwise soluble antigens to form insoluble clumps or precipitates)
4. *Opsonization* (enhancement of phagocytosis by coating cells with antibodies)
5. *Lysis* (induction of cell lysis by activation of complement proteins or by activation of natural killer cells).

Complement consists of a group of circulating proteins that are activated in a cascading sequence of reactions, triggered by antigen–antibody complexes (the *classical pathway*) or by exposure to certain microbial polysaccharide molecules (the *alternate pathway*). The activated complement system promotes chemotaxis, opsonization, inflammation, phagocytosis, and cell lysis.

The complexity of immune responses makes them vulnerable to altered functional states, be they hypofunctional (eg, immunodeficiency disorders), misdirected (eg, autoimmune diseases) or hyperfunctional (eg, allergic hypersensitivity states).

The three principal indications for immunomodulator therapy are prevention of organ transplantation rejection, treatment of autoimmune disease, and correction of primary immunodeficiency disorders. The various immunomodulating drugs are discussed in the following sections.

Colony-Stimulating Factors

Colony-stimulating factors, also known as cellular growth factors, are glycoproteins produced by recombinant DNA technology. They are used to stimulate the production of certain white blood cells (granulocytes, macrophages) by hematopoietic tissue within bone marrow. Colony-stimulating factors are used to accelerate the recovery of bone marrow cellular production after chemotherapy and/or radiation therapy, or when bone marrow transplantation engraftment has been delayed. There are two colony-stimulating factors available.

• Filgrastim

Neupogen

Filgrastim is a human granulocyte colony-stimulating factor produced by recombinant DNA technology in *Escherichia coli* bacteria. It regulates the production of neutrophils in bone marrow with minimal effects on other hematopoietic cell types.

Mechanism

Binds to specific cell surface receptors and stimulates neutrophil proliferation, enhanced phagocytic activity, antibody-dependent killing, and increased cell surface antigen activity.

Uses

Decrease incidence of infection in patients with nonmyeloid malignancies receiving anticancer drugs associated with a significant incidence of neutropenia and fever.

Dosage

5 μg/kg/day, administered SC or IV as a single daily dose. May be increased in increments of 5 μg/kg for each cycle according to severity of absolute neutrophil count.

Fate

Half-lives average 3 to 4 hours; single parenteral doses or daily IV doses over a 14-day period resulted in comparable half-lives.

Common Side Effects

Medullary bone pain; reversible elevations in uric acid, lactate dehydrogenase, and alkaline phosphatase; nausea, vomiting, skeletal pain, diarrhea.

Significant Adverse Reactions

Alopecia, fever, anorexia, dyspnea, headache, cough, skin rash, chest pain, weakness, sore throat, stomatitis, constipation.

Contraindications

No absolute contraindications. *Cautious use* in patients receiving cytotoxic chemotherapy, antiplatelet therapy, and in pregnant or lactating women.

Nursing Management

Pretherapy Assessment

Assess and record baseline data necessary for detection of adverse effects of filgrastim: General: vital signs (VS), body weight, skin color, temperature, and integrity; Cardiovascular system (CVS): electrocardiogram (ECG); Gastrointestinal (GI): output; Central nervous system (CNS): bilateral grip strength; Laboratory: hematologic profile, hematocrit, platelet count.

Review medical history and documents for existing or previous conditions that:

a. require cautious use of filgrastim: cytotoxic chemotherapy, radiation therapy, antiplatelet therapy, pregnancy and lactation.
b. contraindicate use of filgrastim: allergy to *E coli*-derived products, filgrastim, or any component of the product; **pregnancy (Category C)**.

Nursing Interventions

Medication Administration

Recommended starting dose is 5 μg/kg/day.

Administer once daily by bolus injection, by short IV infusion or continuous infusion.

Do not administer within 24 hours of cytotoxic chemotherapy.

Do not dilute dosage form with saline because precipitation of protein will occur.

Drug should be discontinued when absolute neutrophil count exceeds 10,000/mm^3.

Surveillance During Therapy

Monitor for toxicity and interactions.

Monitor for signs of hypersensitivity, which may require discontinuation of drug.

Monitor diagnostic test results obtained over the course of therapy.

Interpret results of diagnostic tests and contact practitioner as appropriate.

Patient Teaching

Instruct patient about expected actions and possible adverse effects of prescribed drug.

• Sargramostim

Leukine, Prokine

Sargramostim is a recombinant human granulocyte–macrophage colony-stimulating factor of 127 amino acids that stimulates proliferation of hematopoietic cells. It also activates mature granulocytes and macrophages.

Mechanism

Stimulates production and maturation of both granulocytes and macrophages from hematopoietic progenitor cells; accelerates bone marrow reproduction after radiation therapy and chemotherapy.

Uses

Accelerates myeloid recovery in patients with non-Hodgkin's lymphoma, acute lymphoblastic leukemia, and Hodgkin's disease undergoing bone marrow transplantation

Treatment of patients who have undergone bone marrow transplantation in which engraftment is delayed or has failed.

Investigational uses include correction of neutropenia in aplastic anemia treatment, decreased leukopenia secondary to myelosuppressive chemotherapy, increased white cell counts in patients with AIDS receiving zidovudine, and decreased transplantation-associated organ system damage in liver and kidney transplants

Dosage

250 μg/m²/day for 14 to 21 days as a 2-hour IV infusion. If engraftment has not occurred after 7 days, therapy may be repeated. A third course of 500 μg/m²/day for 14 days may be tried after another 7 days of therapy if necessary.

Common Side Effects

Fever, malaise, nausea, diarrhea, anorexia, GI upset, edema, alopecia, rash, dyspnea.

Significant Adverse Reactions

Headache, arthralgia, myalgia, bone pain, chills, stomatitis, liver abnormalities, bleeding, blood dyscrasias, sepsis, altered kidney function.

Contraindications

No absolute contraindications. *Cautious use* in patients with respiratory complications, fluid retention, renal or hepatic disorders, and in pregnant or nursing mothers.

Interactions

Concurrent use of corticosteroids or lithium may potentiate the myeloproliferative effects of sargramostim.

Nursing Management

Pretherapy Assessment

Assess and record baseline data necessary for detection of adverse effects of sargramostim: General: VS, body weight, skin color, temperature, and integrity; CVS: ECG; GI: output; CNS: bilateral grip strength; Laboratory: hematologic profile, hematocrit, platelet count, blood urea nitrogen (BUN), creatinine, hepatic profile, electrolytes.

Review medical history and documents for existing or previous conditions that:

a. require cautious use of sargramostim: cytotoxic chemotherapy, radiation therapy, antiplatelet therapy, pregnancy and lactation.

b. contraindicate use of sargramostim: allergy to sargramostim or any component of the product; excessive myeloid blasts in bone marrow or blood (>10%); **pregnancy (Category C)**.

Nursing Interventions

Medication Administration

Recommended starting dose is 250 μg/m²/day for 21 days.

Administer once daily as a 2-hour IV infusion.

Do not administer within 24 hours of cytotoxic chemotherapy or within 12 hours of radiation therapy.

Dilute dosage form with Sterile Water for Injection (USP).

Drug should be discontinued if blast cells appear or disease progression occurs.

Surveillance During Therapy

Monitor for toxicity and interactions.

Monitor for signs of hypersensitivity, which may require discontinuation of drug.

Monitor diagnostic test results obtained over the course of therapy.

Interpret results of diagnostic tests and contact practitioner as appropriate.

Patient Teaching

Instruct patient about expected actions and possible adverse effects of prescribed drug.

Immunosuppressants

Drugs that suppress the immune response are extremely valuable agents in preventing rejection of transplanted tissues and in treating diseases believed to result from overactivity of the body's immune system. The clinically available immunosuppressant drugs are reviewed in this section.

• Azathioprine

Imuran

Azathioprine is an immunosuppressive agent used to prevent rejection in renal transplantations. It is a potent bone marrow depressant, and frequent blood counts are necessary during therapy. Azathioprine has been used experimentally in treating other disorders believed to be the result of altered immunologic function, such as severe rheumatoid arthritis, systemic lupus erythematosus, and idiopathic thrombocytopenic purpura.

Mechanism

Not completely established; converted to 6-mercaptopurine, which appears to interfere with nucleic acid and protein synthesis and coenzyme function (see **mercaptopurine**, Chapter 74); may also alter cellular metabolism.

Uses

Adjunct for prevention of rejection in renal homotransplantation

Treatment of severe, active rheumatoid arthritis in patients not responsive to conventional therapy (ie, aspirin, nonsteroidal antiinflammatory drugs, corticosteroids, gold)

Treatment of chronic ulcerative colitis, generalized myasthenia gravis, Crohn's disease (*investigational use only*)

Dosage

Prevention of rejection: initially 3 to 5 mg/kg/day IV beginning at the time of transplant; switch to oral therapy as soon as feasible; usual maintenance range is 1 to 3 mg/kg/day

Rheumatoid arthritis: initially 1 mg/kg as a single dose or two divided doses; increase stepwise in 0.5 mg/kg/day increments at 4- to 6-week intervals if response is not satisfactory and no serious toxicity is noted; maximum dose is 2.5 mg/kg/day

Fate

Largely converted to 6-mercaptopurine after administration; most is metabolized in the liver and excreted by the kidneys; partially (30%) bound to plasma proteins.

Common Side Effects

Leukopenia, infections (fever, chills, sore throat, cold sores), nausea, vomiting.

Significant Adverse Reactions

Anemia, thrombocytopenia, bleeding, jaundice, diarrhea, alopecia, oral mucosal lesions, pancreatitis, arthralgia, steatorrhea, severe secondary infections, toxic hepatitis, and biliary stasis.

CAUTION

Azathioprine is carcinogenic in animals and may increase the risk of neoplasia, especially in transplant recipients. The benefit–risk ratio must be carefully assessed when using azathioprine; acute myelogenous leukemia and solid tumors have occurred in patients with rheumatoid arthritis receiving the drug.

Contraindications

Treatment of rheumatoid arthritis in pregnant women or in patients previously treated with alkylating agents. *Cautious use* in patients with liver or kidney dysfunction, during a clinically active infection, in pregnant or nursing women, and in women of childbearing potential.

Interactions

Allopurinol inhibits azathioprine and mercaptopurine metabolism, and can increase the toxic effects of these drugs.

Azathioprine may reverse the neuromuscular blocking activity of nondepolarizing muscle relaxants (eg, pancuronium).

Nursing Management

Pretherapy Assessment

Assess and record baseline data necessary for detection of adverse effects of azathioprine: General: VS, body weight, skin color, temperature, and integrity; CVS: ECG; GI: output; CNS: bilateral grip strength; Laboratory: renal and hepatic function tests, complete blood count (CBC).

Review medical history and documents for existing or previous conditions that:

a. require cautious use of azathioprine: liver or kidney dysfunction, a clinically active infection, women of childbearing potential.
b. contraindicate use of azathioprine: allergy to azathioprine; previous treatment with alkylating agents; **pregnancy (Category D)**.

Nursing Interventions

Medication Administration

Administer by the IV route if oral administration is not possible.

Administer in divided doses or with food if GI upset occurs.

Ensure ready access to bathroom facilities if diarrhea occurs.

Expect dosage to be reduced to one third to one fourth normal dose if azathioprine is given concurrently with allopurinol (see Interactions).

Surveillance During Therapy

Monitor results of complete blood counts and liver and kidney function tests, which should be performed at least weekly during initial therapy and every 2 to 3 weeks during prolonged treatment. Rapid fall in leukocyte count or persistently low level mandates a dosage reduction or drug withdrawal.

Assess patient carefully for indications of thrombocytopenia (abnormal bleeding or bruising, mucosal ulceration). Notify practitioner if any occur.

Observe for indications of hepatic dysfunction (pruritus, darkened urine, light-colored stools, yellowing of skin or sclerae), and alert drug prescriber if they occur.

Monitor intake–output ratio and renal clearance of drug to prevent accumulation toxicity.

Monitor for signs of hypersensitivity, which may require discontinuation of drug.

Monitor diagnostic test results obtained over the course of therapy.

Interpret results of diagnostic tests and contact practitioner as appropriate.

Patient Teaching

Instruct patient about expected actions and possible adverse effects of prescribed drug.

Teach patient interventions to reduce risk of infections; ensure that patient understands their importance. If infection develops, it should be treated immediately with appropriate drugs. In addition, the dosage of azathioprine may need to be reduced.

• Cyclosporine

Sandimmune

Cyclosporine (cyclosporin A) is an immunosuppressant that may be used to prolong and assist survival of allogeneic transplants involving the heart, kidneys, liver, and possibly also the bone marrow, pancreas, and lungs.

Mechanism

Not completely established; appears specifically and reversibly to inhibit T lymphocytes, including the T helper cell and T suppressor cell; lymphokine production is also impaired, and release of interleukin-2 or T-cell growth factor may be reduced.

Uses

Prevention of organ rejection in kidney, liver, or heart transplants, in conjunction with adrenal corticosteroids

Treatment of chronic rejection in patients previously treated with other immunosuppressive drugs

Dosage

Oral: initially 15 mg/kg/day, 4 to 12 hours before transplantation; continue for 1 to 2 weeks postoperatively, then taper by 5%/week to a maintenance level of 5 to 10 mg/kg/day

IV: initially 5 to 6 mg/kg/day 4 to 12 hours before transplantation, as a slow (2–6 hour) infusion of dilute solution (50 mg/20 to 100 mL of sodium chloride injection or 5% dextrose injection)

Fate

Oral absorption is erratic and incomplete; peak serum levels are attained in 3 to 4 hours; distributes to erythrocytes, granulocytes, leukocytes, and plasma, where it is approximately 90% protein bound; extensively metabolized and excreted primarily in the bile, with only about 60% of the dose eliminated in the urine.

Common Side Effects

Renal dysfunction, tremor, hirsutism, hypertension, gum hyperplasia, secondary infections.

Significant Adverse Reactions

CNS: headache, confusion, convulsions, flushing, paresthesias

GI: diarrhea, vomiting, abdominal pain, gastritis, peptic ulcer, anorexia, hepatotoxicity

Dermatologic: acne, brittle nails

Other: anxiety, depression, muscle weakness, joint pain, chest pain, visual disturbances, gynecomastia, difficulty in swallowing, upper GI bleeding, pancreatitis, mouth sores, constipation, night sweats, leukopenia, lymphoma, anemia, thrombocytopenia

Contraindications

No absolute contraindications. *Cautious use* in hypertensive patients (blood pressure elevations are common); in patients with renal or liver dysfunction, seizure disorders; and in pregnant or nursing women; although safety and efficacy have not been established in children, cyclosporine has been used in patients as young as 6 months with no apparent deleterious effects.

Interactions

Cyclosporine can enhance the nephrotoxicity of aminoglycosides, erythromycin, ketoconazole, calcium channel blockers, loop diuretics, and other drugs that can damage the kidney.

Ketoconazole and amphotericin B can elevate the plasma levels of cyclosporine.

Concomitant use of cyclosporine with other immunosuppressive drugs can result in increased susceptibility to infection and possible development of lymphoma.

Concurrent use of phenytoin, phenobarbital, carbamazepine, rifampin, or trimethoprim–sulfamethoxazole may reduce plasma levels of cyclosporine.

Nursing Management

Pretherapy Assessment

Assess and record baseline data necessary for detection of adverse effects of cyclosporine: General: VS, body weight, skin color, temperature, and integrity; CVS: peripheral perfusion; GI: output, gum evaluation; Laboratory: renal and hepatic function tests, CBC.

Review medical history and documents for existing or previous conditions that:

a. require cautious use of cyclosporine: liver or kidney dysfunction, hypertension, seizure disorders, women of childbearing potential.
b. contraindicate use of cyclosporine: allergy to cyclosporine or polyoxyethylated castor oil; **pregnancy (Category C)**.

Nursing Interventions

Medication Administration

Mix oral solution with milk or orange juice in a glass container (not styrofoam), preferably at room temperature, to mask the unpleasant taste. Stir well, and have patient drink *immediately*. Rinse mixing container with milk or juice, and have patient drink the second glass to ensure that all drug has been taken.

Use parenteral administration only if patient is unable to take oral solution.

Ensure ready access to bathroom facilities if diarrhea occurs.

Protect IV solution from light.

Ensure that adequate laboratory and supportive resources are readily available and that the patient is managed only by healthcare personnel skilled in administering and monitoring the drug.

Be prepared to treat severe allergic reactions with IV administration. Because the drug is highly insoluble, the IV form is prepared in a cremophor vehicle that is allergenic, and its use can result in anaphylactic reactions. Consequently, the patient should be transferred from IV to oral administration as soon as possible after surgery.

Seek clarification if any other immunosuppressant drugs (except adrenal steroids) are prescribed because serious toxicity can result (see Interactions).

Surveillance During Therapy

Observe for indications of hepatic dysfunction (pruritus, darkened urine, light-colored stools, yellowing of skin or sclerae), and alert drug prescriber if they occur.

Monitor intake–output ratio and renal clearance of drug to prevent accumulation toxicity.

Assess patient for occurrence of fever, sore throat, abnormal bruising, or unusual tiredness, possible early indications of a developing blood dyscrasia. Notify prescriber immediately if these occur.

Assess renal and hepatic status regularly, and monitor results of BUN and serum creatinine, bilirubin, and liver enzyme determinations, which should be performed frequently. Although serum creatinine and BUN are commonly elevated during therapy, they usually respond to dosage reduction. If persistent elevations do not respond to a dosage alteration, it may be necessary to substitute another immunosuppressant.

Monitor for signs of hypersensitivity, which may require discontinuation of drug.

Monitor results of cyclosporine blood level determinations, which should be obtained frequently with oral use, because oral absorption is erratic. Dosage should be adjusted as necessary to minimize toxicity due to excessive plasma levels.

Monitor diagnostic test results obtained over the course of therapy.

Interpret results of diagnostic tests and contact practitioner as appropriate.

Patient Teaching

Instruct patient about expected actions and possible adverse effects of prescribed drug.

Discuss potential risks of teratogenicity should pregnancy occur during therapy.

• Muromonab-CD3

Orthoclone OKT3

Mechanism

A monoclonal antibody to the T3 (CD3) antigen of human T cells; blocks T-cell function (which plays a major role in acute renal rejection) by reacting with and blocking the action of a molecule (CD3) in the membrane of human T cells that is essential for signal transduction; a rapid decrease in number of circulating T cells is observed within minutes after administration; reacts with most peripheral T cells in blood and body tissues.

Uses

Treatment of acute allograft rejection in renal transplant patients

Treatment of steroid-resistant acute allograft rejection in cardiac and hepatic transplant patients

Dosage

5 mg/day by IV bolus injection for 10 to 14 days, beginning once the renal rejection has been confirmed. Methylprednisolone (1 mg/kg, IV) is given before the first dose of muromonab-CD3 and hydrocortisone (100 mg, IV) is given 30 minutes after the first dose to minimize adverse reactions. Acetaminophen and antihistamines are also used to reduce early reactions.

Fate

Mean serum levels of drug will rise over the first 3 days, then level off during the remaining 7 to 10 days; antibodies to muromonab-CD3 have occurred and usually appear after approximately 21 days.

Common Side Effects

"First dose effects," such as fever, chills, wheezing, dyspnea, chest pain, nausea, diarrhea, vomiting, tremor.

Significant Adverse Reactions

Pulmonary edema, herpes infections, serum sickness, anaphylaxis.

Contraindications

Fluid overload. *Cautious use* in patients with fever and in pregnant women. A second course of therapy should be undertaken with caution, because drug-induced antibody formation in most patients may limit its effectiveness on repeat administration. Antibodies normally develop within several weeks of the start of therapy.

Nursing Management

Pretherapy Assessment

Assess and record baseline data necessary for detection of adverse effects of muromonab: General: VS, body weight, skin color, temperature, and integrity; CVS: peripheral perfusion; Laboratory: chest radiograph, renal and hepatic function tests, CBC.

Review medical history and documents for existing or previous conditions that:

a. require cautious use of muromonab: fever; previous administration of muromonab.
b. contraindicate use of muromonab: allergy to muromonab or any murine product; uncompensated heart failure or fluid overload; history of seizures or predisposed to seizures; **pregnancy (Category C)**; lactation.

Nursing Interventions

Medication Administration

Do not shake ampule, and draw solution into syringe through a low protein-binding filter, when preparing injection.

Administer drug only by IV bolus. It should *not* be given by IV infusion or in conjunction with other drug solutions.

Arrange for chest radiograph within 24 hours of initiation of treatment.

Ensure ready access to bathroom facilities if diarrhea occurs.

Arrange for use of acetaminophen if patient is febrile before treatment or in response to first dose.

Administer drug only in an area equipped to institute cardiac resuscitation.

Be prepared to administer IV methylprednisolone before the first dose and IV hydrocortisone 30 minutes after the first dose to minimize first-dose reaction (see Dosage).

Surveillance During Therapy

Closely monitor patient response for 48 hours after first dose to detect symptoms of first-dose reaction (see Common Side Effects), which usually occurs within the first hour after the first dose and lasts several hours. Vital signs should be checked every 15 minutes for the first hour, every half hour for the next hour, then every 2 hours.

Vital signs may be required every 4 hours for the duration of therapy. Temperature should be taken before treatment and several hours afterward to detect infection.

Monitor breath sounds to detect fluid. The patient with fluid overload is particularly susceptible to acute pulmonary edema, which may be fatal.

Implement appropriate measures for infection control. Because the drug destroys T cells, the patient is highly vulnerable to infection, particularly by viruses and opportunistic organisms.

Monitor for toxicity and interactions.

Assess patient for occurrence of fever, sore throat, abnormal bruising, or unusual tiredness, possible early indications of a developing blood dyscrasia. Notify prescriber immediately if these occur.

Monitor for signs of hypersensitivity, which may require discontinuation of drug.

Monitor diagnostic test results obtained over the course of therapy.

Interpret results of diagnostic tests and contact practitioner as appropriate.

Patient Teaching

Instruct patient about expected actions and possible adverse effects of prescribed drug.

Inform patient that a first-dose reaction involving fever, chills, difficulty breathing, and chest congestion may occur.

• FK 506

FK 506 is still an investigational immunosuppressant with properties similar to those of cyclosporine but approximately 100 times more potent in prolonging graft survival. The drug appears selectively to inhibit the transcription of certain lymphokine genes in T cells, and is undergoing trials in liver, kidney, and pancreatic transplantation. It is a well tolerated drug, the principal adverse effects reported thus far being nausea and vomiting. FK 506 does not display the nephrotoxic potential of cyclosporine and can be used as an alternative to cyclosporine when renal immunosuppression is required.

Immune Serums

• Lymphocyte Immune Globulin—Anti-Thymocyte Globulin

Atgam

Lymphocyte immune globulin (antithymocyte globulin—ATG) is a lymphocyte-selective immunosuppressant that decreases the number of circulating thymus-dependent lymphocytes. The antilymphocytic antibody binds to the surface of T cells, resulting in their destruction with the aid of serum complement. Thus, delayed hypersensitivity and cellular immunity are impaired while humoral antibody production is largely unaffected. ATG is used to prevent allograft rejection in renal transplant patients and also to treat severe aplastic anemia in patients who are unsuited for bone marrow transplantation. Investigational uses for ATG include other organ transplants, and treatment of multiple sclerosis, myasthenia gravis, and scleroderma. Lymphocyte immune globulin is listed in Table 77-5 (Chapter 77).

Interferons

Interferons are a family of naturally occurring proteins that exert antiviral and immunomodulatory effects. The three major classes of interferons have been identified as alfa, beta, and gamma, and they possess distinct biologic activity. Interferon-alfa products are reviewed in detail in Chapter 74, because they are principally used in certain neoplastic diseases. The other two types of interferons are discussed in this section.

• Interferon Beta-1b

Betaseron

Mechanism

Interferon beta-1b exhibits antiviral and immunoregulatory actions. The drug interacts with specific cell receptors on human cells, resulting in gene expression, which is believed to mediate the biologic effects.

Uses

Reduce frequency of exacerbations of multiple sclerosis in ambulatory patients

Investigational uses include treatment of AIDS and AIDS-related Kaposi's sarcoma, metastatic renal cell carcinoma, malignant melanoma, T-cell lymphoma, and acute non-A, non-B hepatitis

Dosage

0.25 mg SC every other day. Evidence of efficacy beyond 2 years is unknown.

Fate

Peak serum concentrations occur within 1 to 8 hours; elimination half-life is variable, ranging from 0.5 to 4 hours.

Common Side Effects

Headache, fever, flu-like symptoms, abdominal pain, diarrhea, GI upset, myalgia, sinusitis, decreased lymphocyte count, malaise.

Significant Adverse Reactions

NOTE: A large number of adverse reactions have been reported with use of interferon beta-1b. Among the more important are:

CNS: mental state alterations (confusion, emotional lability, depression, suicidal thoughts); may be related in part to the underlying condition

Genitourinary: menstrual disorders, breast pain, cystitis, urinary urgency

CV: hypertension, palpitations, tachycardia

Other: migraine headache, lymphadenopathy, myasthenia-like reaction, vomiting, hypoglycemia, conjunctivitis

Contraindications

Hypersensitivity to albumin. *Cautious use* in patients with depression or suicidal ideation, neutrophil count below $750/mm^3$, elevated serum transaminase or bilirubin, and in pregnant or nursing mothers.

Nursing Management

Pretherapy Assessment

Assess and record baseline data necessary for detection of adverse effects of interferon therapy: General: VS, body weight, skin color and temperature; CVS: peripheral perfusion, edema, ECG; GI: liver evaluation; Laboratory: renal and hepatic function tests, CBC.

Review medical history and documents for existing or previous conditions that:

a. require cautious use of interferon: depression or suicidal ideation, neutrophil count below 750/mm^3, elevated serum transaminase or bilirubin; and in nursing mothers.
b. contraindicate use of interferon: allergy to interferon, *E coli*-derived products or any component of the product; **pregnancy (Category C)**.

Nursing Interventions

Medication Administration

Dosage form should be kept refrigerated, neither frozen nor shaken; not stable after 12 hours at room temperature.

Drug should be administered SC in the right or left deltoid or the anterior thigh.

Provide small, frequent meals if GI upset occurs.

Surveillance During Therapy

Monitor for toxicity and interactions.

Assess patient for occurrence of fever, sore throat, abnormal bruising, or unusual tiredness, possible early indications of a developing blood dyscrasia. Notify prescriber immediately if these occur.

Monitor for signs of hypersensitivity, which may require discontinuation of drug.

Monitor diagnostic test results obtained over the course of therapy.

Interpret results of diagnostic tests and contact practitioner as appropriate.

Patient Teaching

Instruct patient about expected actions and possible adverse effects of prescribed drug.

• Interferon Gamma-1b

Actimmune

Mechanism

Possesses potent phagocyte-activating effects; stimulates generation of toxic oxygen metabolites, which are lethal to several microorganisms; enhances oxidative metabolism of tissue macrophages and natural killer cell activity; suppresses IgE levels and inhibits production of collagen; functions as part of a lymphokine-regulatory network.

Uses

Reducing frequency and severity of infections associated with chronic granulomatous disease.

Dosage

Body surface area > 0.5 m^2: 50 μg/m^2 SC, 3 times a week

Body surface area < 0.5 m^2: 1.5 μg/kg/dose SC, 3 times a week

Fate

Slowly absorbed after SC injection; mean elimination half-life is 6 hours; peak plasma concentrations attained within 6 to 7 hours; no accumulation of drug with repeated SC injections as directed.

Common Side Effects

Fever, headache, rash, chills, pain and redness at injection site, fatigue, diarrhea.

Significant Adverse Reactions

GI: vomiting, abdominal pain, anorexia

CNS: confusion, gait disturbances, parkinsonian symptoms, seizures

CV: tachycardia, hypotension, syncope, heart block

Other: pancreatitis, hepatic insufficiency, deep vein thrombosis, pulmonary embolism, bronchospasm, pneumonitis, hyperglycemia

Contraindications

No absolute contraindications. *Cautious use* in patients with seizure disorders, cardiac disease, asthma, and in pregnant or nursing mothers.

Interactions

Interferon gamma-1b may potentiate the myelosuppressive effects of other drugs having a similar action.

Interferon gamma-1b may decrease the hepatic metabolism of other drugs by reducing cytochrome-P450 concentrations in the liver.

Nursing Management

See Nursing Management under Interferon beta-1b.

A number of other drugs possessing immunomodulating properties have been discussed elsewhere in the text under different indications. Principal among these drugs are the interferons and interleukins being used in treating various cancers as well as chronic hepatitis, genital or venereal warts, and other viral infections (herpes, cytomegaloviruses, rhinoviruses, vaccinia, varicella). These antineoplastic drugs are reviewed in Chapter 74.

Corticosteroids have routinely been used either alone or as adjunctive agents in treating a variety of autoimmune disorders as well as neoplastic diseases. Although they exhibit immunosuppressive properties, they are principally used to control the inflammatory reactions that frequently accompany transplantation procedures or autoimmune diseases. Corticosteroids are considered in detail in Chapter 45.

Selected Bibliography

Ferrara JL, Deeg HJ: Graft-versus-host disease. N Engl J Med 324:667, 1991

Johnson HM, Bazer FW, Szente BE, Jarpe MA: How interferons fight disease. Sci Am 270(5):68, 1994

Life, death and the immune system (issue). Sci Am 269(9), 1993

Metcalf D: Control of granulocytes and macrophages: Molecular, cellular and clinical aspects. Science 254:529, 1991

Pellegrini S, Schindler C: Early events in signalling by interferons. Trends Biol Sci 18:338, 1993

Rose NR, Mackay IR: The Autoimmune Diseases. New York, Academic Press, 1992

Sinha AA, Lopez MT, McDevitt O: Autoimmune diseases: The failure of self tolerance. Science 248:1380, 1990

von Boehmer H, Kisielow P: How the immune system learns about self. Sci Am 265:74, 1991

Nursing Bibliography

Farivar J, Kriett J: Transplantation: A review of immunosuppressive agents. Critical Care Nursing Quarterly 15(4):13, 1993

Jarpe M: Nursing care of patients receiving long term infusion of neuromuscular blocking agents. Critical Care Nurse 12(7):58, 1992

Ross A: Nursing interventions for persons receiving immunosuppressive therapies for demyelinating pathology. Nursing Clinics of North America 28(4):829, 1993

Roth S: Nursing care of the patient undergoing combined kidney-pancreas transplantation. Critical Care Nursing Quarterly 14(3):30, 1991

White-Williams C: Immunosuppressive therapy following cardiac transplantation. Critical Care Nursing Quarterly 16(2):1, 1993

XI

Miscellaneous Agents

79

Dermatologic Drugs

Drugs are applied to the skin and mucous membranes for a variety of reasons and in a number of different dosage forms. A general classification of these drugs is presented in Table 79-1, and the drugs are discussed in this chapter in the order they appear in the table, except where they have been reviewed in another chapter, in which case appropriate reference is made.

Acne Aids

Topical preparations useful in treating acne vulgaris include tretinoin and isotretinoin, both forms of vitamin A, as well as benzoyl peroxide, sulfur preparations, tetracycline, erythromycin, clindamycin, and various keratolytics and astringents.

• Tretinoin

Retin-A

(CAN) Stie VAA, Vitamin A Acid

Tretinoin (retinoic acid) is available for topical application in the treatment of acne vulgaris. Its effectiveness approaches that of steroid–antibiotic combinations and usually surpasses that of most other available topical acne preparations. Its use is frequently associated with erythema and desquamation, however, and some patients do not tolerate the drug. Tretinoin is available as a gel, cream, or liquid.

In addition to its usefulness in treating acne, topical tretinoin has been advocated as a "wrinkle remover" for photoaged skin. Although much publicity has surrounded this potential application, a definitive statement regarding its suitability for treating wrinkled skin must await the results of additional clinical trials. Of particular concern is the frequent occurrence of a local dermatitis after application, often requiring the use of topical steroids.

Mechanism

Promotes epidermal cell turnover and facilitates desquamation; suppresses keratin synthesis and prevents formation of comedones.

Uses

- Treatment of acne vulgaris, especially grades I, II, and III; not effective against acne conglobata (ie, deep cystic nodules and extensive pustules)
- Treatment of several forms of skin cancer (investigational use)
- Treatment of premature skin aging and wrinkling (investigational use)

Dosage

Apply once a day for at least 4 to 6 weeks, at bedtime, and cover entire area lightly; reduce frequency of application as lesions respond.

Common Side Effects

Stinging, feeling of warmth, dryness, peeling, erythema.

Significant Adverse Reactions

Edema, blistering, pigmentary changes, photosensitivity, and contact dermatitis (rare).

Contraindications

No absolute contraindications. *Cautious use* in people with eczema and in pregnant or nursing women.

Interactions

- Increased skin peeling can occur if tretinoin is used with sulfur, resorcinol, benzoyl peroxide, or salicylic acid.
- Excessive skin drying can result from concomitant use of tretinoin and products containing high concentrations of alcohol, astringents, or lime.

Nursing Management

Pretherapy Assessment

- Assess and record baseline data necessary for detection of adverse effects of tretinoin: General: vital signs (VS), body weight, skin color, temperature, and integrity.
- Review medical history and documents for existing or previous conditions that:
  a. require cautious use of a tretinoin: eczema; and in nursing women.
  b. contraindicate use of a drug: allergy to tretinoin or components in the product; **pregnancy (Category B)**.

Nursing Interventions

Medication Administration

- Wash hands thoroughly immediately after applying tretinoin.
- Apply once a day, covering entire affected area.

Table 79-1. **Drugs Used for Dermatologic Disorders**

Drug Type	***Examples***
Acne aids	Benzoyl peroxide, tretinoin
Antibacterials	Bacitracin, neomycin, tetracycline
Antifungals	Clotrimazole, econazole, nystatin
Antihistamines	Diphenhydramine, pyrilamine
Antipsoriatics	Anthralin, coal tar
Antiseptics	Chlorhexidine, hexachlorophene
Antivirals	Acyclovir, idoxuridine
Corticosteroids	Betamethasone, fluocinolone
Enzymes	Collagenase, sutilains
Keratolytics	Cantharidin, podophyllum resin
Local anesthetics	Benzocaine, lidocaine
Pigmenting–depigmenting agents	Methoxsalen, hydroquinolone
Scabicides–pediculicides	Lindane, permethrin
Sunscreens	PABA, oxybenzone

PABA, paraaminobenzoic acid.

Do not apply to broken or sunburned skin.
Arrange to discontinue medication if skin becomes severely irritated.

Surveillance During Therapy

Monitor for signs of hypersensitivity, which may require discontinuation of drug.
Monitor diagnostic test results obtained over the course of therapy.
Interpret results of diagnostic tests and contact practitioner as appropriate.
Monitor for possible drug–laboratory test interactions.
Monitor for possible drug–drug and drug–nutrient interactions.

Patient Teaching

Instruct patient about expected actions and possible adverse effects of prescribed drug.
Caution patient to minimize exposure to sunlight or sunlamps because photosensitivity reactions can occur. Experimental animal studies have indicated a tumorigenic potential for tretinoin on exposure to ultraviolet (UV) light, although the significance of this effect in humans is not clear.
Warn patient to keep drug away from eyes, mouth, and other mucous membranes because irritation can occur.
Inform patient that slight stinging and feelings of warmth frequently occur, and dryness and peeling of skin are to be expected.
Inform patient that condition may *temporarily* worsen early in therapy owing to drug action on deeper, previously invisible lesions.
Instruct patient to notify drug prescriber if significant erythema or irritation occurs because the frequency of application may need to be reduced or the medication may need to be temporarily discontinued.

• ***Isotretinoin*** *(Pregnancy Category X)*

Accutane

Isotretinoin is an isomer of retinoic acid, a metabolite of retinol. It is used orally for treatment of *severe* acne and other cutaneous disorders of keratinization, such as ichthyosis, pityriasis, and other hyperkeratotic skin conditions. Because of its potential for eliciting serious untoward reactions, isotretinoin should be used with utmost caution and only under close supervision.

Mechanism

Not completely established; reduces sebum secretion and inhibits sebaceous gland differentiation; keratinization is also inhibited; elevates plasma triglycerides and cholesterol.

Uses

Treatment of severe, recalcitrant cystic acne in patients unresponsive to conventional therapy, including antibiotics (eg, tetracyclines)
Treatment of disorders of excessive keratinization (eg, ichthyosis, pityriasis, hyperkeratosis plantaris, rubra pilaris)
Treatment of cutaneous T-cell lymphoma (mycosis fungoides)

Dosage

Usually, 1 to 2 mg/kg/day in two divided doses for 15 to 20 weeks; a second course of therapy may be initiated after a 2-month drug-free interval. Doses of 0.05 to 0.5 mg/kg/day have been effective in some patients, but relapses are more common.

Fate

Oral bioavailability of the capsule dosage form is approximately 25%; peak plasma levels occur in about 3 hours; the drug is almost completely protein bound; elimination half-life averages

10 hours (range, 7–35 hours); excreted in the urine and feces in approximately equal amounts.

Common Side Effects

Cheilitis, eye irritation, conjunctivitis; dry skin, skin fragility, pruritus; nosebleed, dryness of the nose and mouth; nausea, vomiting, abdominal pain; lethargy; white cells in urine; triglyceride elevation, elevated sedimentation rate.

Significant Adverse Reactions

CAUTION

Isotretinoin should not be used in women who are pregnant or who intend to become pregnant, because numerous fetal abnormalities and spontaneous abortions have occurred. An effective means of contraception must be used during therapy and for at least 1 month before *and* after therapy.

Dermatologic: facial skin desquamation, nail brittleness, rash, alopecia, photosensitivity, skin infections, erythema nodosum, pigmentary changes, urticaria
GI: anorexia, regional ileitis, mild GI bleeding, inflammatory bowel disease, weight loss
CNS: insomnia, fatigue, paresthesias, headache, dizziness, visual disturbances, papilledema, corneal opacities
Musculoskeletal: arthralgia, joint and muscle pain and stiffness
Urinary: proteinuria, hematuria
Other: bruising, edema, respiratory infections, abnormal menses, herpes simplex infections, increased serum aminotransferases, alkaline phosphatase, and fasting serum glucose, elevated platelet counts, hyperuricemia, elevated cholesterol, decreased high-density lipoproteins

Contraindications

Pregnancy (drug causes fetal abnormalities), patients sensitive to parabens (preservatives in the formulation). *Cautious use* in obese, diabetic, or alcoholic patients, because triglyceride levels may be excessively high.

Interactions

Vitamin A supplements together with isotretinoin may result in increased toxicity.
Tetracyclines and isotretinoin can lead to pseudotumor cerebri or papilledema.
Concomitant ingestion of alcohol may further increase serum triglyceride levels.

Nursing Management

Pretherapy Assessment

Assess and record baseline data necessary for detection of adverse effects of isotretinoin: General: VS, body weight, skin color, temperature, and integrity; CNS: orientation, reflexes, ophthalmic examination; GI: mucous membranes, bowel sounds; Laboratory: serum triglycerides, high-density lipoproteins, sedimentation rate, complete blood count with differential, urinalysis, pregnancy test.

Review medical history and documents for existing or previous conditions that:
a. require cautious use of an isotretinoin: obesity, diabetes, or alcoholism, because triglyceride levels may be excessively high.
b. contraindicate use of isotretinoin: allergy to isotretinoin or components (parabens)in the product; **pregnancy (Category X)**.

Nursing Interventions

Medication Administration

Ensure that patient is not pregnant before administering.
Do not administer a second course of therapy within 8 weeks of prior course of isotretinoin therapy.
Administer with meals; do not crush capsules.
Do not administer vitamin supplements that contain vitamin A.
Discontinue use if signs of papilledema occur.
Discontinue use if visual disturbances, abdominal pain, rectal bleeding, or severe diarrhea occur.
Protect patient from exposure to the sun; arrange for use of sunscreen, protective clothing.
Provide for ready access to bathroom facilities if diarrhea occurs.
Provide small, frequent meals if GI distress occurs.

Surveillance During Therapy

Monitor triglycerides during therapy. Monitor results of serum lipid determinations, which should be performed before initiation of therapy and at weekly or biweekly intervals during therapy. Increased triglyceride and cholesterol levels and decreased high-density lipoprotein levels occur in up to 25% of patients, but they revert to pretreatment levels when therapy is terminated.
Monitor for signs of hypersensitivity, which may require discontinuation of drug.
Do not allow blood donation from a patient on isotretinoin because of ability to transfer teratogenic potential.
Monitor diagnostic test results obtained over the course of therapy.
Interpret results of diagnostic tests and contact practitioner as appropriate.
Monitor for possible drug–laboratory test interactions.
Monitor for possible drug–drug and drug–nutrient interactions.

Patient Teaching

With fertile woman, see CAUTION under Significant Adverse Reactions, and also see applicable portions of Patient Teaching for etretinate, later in this chapter; in addition:

Instruct patient about expected actions and possible adverse effects of prescribed drug.
Explain that periodic ophthalmic examinations should be performed during treatment and that any changes in visual function should be reported to drug prescriber.
Inform patient that acne may temporarily worsen during initial stages of therapy.
Discuss the importance of reducing caloric intake, dietary

fat, and alcohol consumption to minimize elevations in serum triglyceride levels.

Inform patient that musculoskeletal disorders may occur (incidence is 15%–20%), but that symptoms are usually mild, seldom require discontinuation of therapy, and disappear on cessation of drug.

Inform patient that if a second course of therapy is required, it will probably not begin until at least 8 weeks after termination of the first course. Clinical improvement may, however, continue during drug-free periods.

Caution patient to minimize exposure to sunlight or sunlamps because photosensitivity reactions can occur. Experimental animal studies have indicated a tumorigenic potential for tretinoin on exposure to UV light, although the significance of this effect in humans is not clear.

• Benzoyl Peroxide

Benzac, Desquam-X, Fostex, Oxy-10, and other manufacturers

Benzoyl peroxide is used as a liquid, soap, lotion, cream, or gel for treating mild to moderate forms of acne. Its effectiveness appears to be the result of its antibacterial activity against *Propionibacterium acnes*, the predominant organism found in sebaceous follicles and comedones. It is usually applied once or twice a day after cleaning the skin. Drying, scaling, and erythema can occur and if these reactions become severe, the dose should be reduced or the drug temporarily discontinued. Most dosage forms are available in 5% and 10% strengths.

• Sulfur Preparations

Liquimat, Xerac, and other manufacturers

Sulfur is used as a lotion, gel, cream, or soap in strengths of 2% to 5% as an aid in treating mild acne and oily skin conditions. A thin film is applied one to three times a day after cleaning the skin. Reddening and scaling of the skin occur frequently, and if severe, the drug should be discontinued.

• Topical Antibiotic Preparations

Several antibiotics (tetracycline, erythromycin, clindamycin) are available in alcoholic solutions or creams for topical application to acne lesions. These applications are discussed in Chapters 62, 63, and 67, respectively.

Antibacterials

Topically applied antibacterial drugs are used to prevent infection in minor skin wounds or abrasions and to treat superficial infections of the skin and mucous membranes due to susceptible organisms. Antibacterial drugs used most commonly for topical infections include bacitracin, neomycin, polymyxin B, and gentamicin. These agents may be applied alone or in combination with corticosteroids (eg, as Mycolog II, Cortisporin, Neo-Synalar, Lotrisone). These latter combinations are often used in treating diaper rash and eczema. In addition, mupirocin is a topical antibacterial drug indicated for treatment of impetigo due to *Staphylococcus aureus* or beta-hemolytic streptococci, and metronidazole (MetroGel) is an antiprotozoal–antibacterial agent used for treating inflammatory pustules and papules characteristic of rosacea. The various antibacterial drugs used topically are reviewed in detail in the appropriate chapters in the Antiinfective section of the text.

Antifungals

Superficial fungal infections (eg, candidiasis, tinea) usually respond well to topically applied antifungal drugs. Many different antifungal drugs are used topically in treating dermatophyte and yeast infections of the skin, nail beds, vagina, and other mucous membranes. The topical antifungal products are listed in Table 72-1. In addition, oral administration of griseofulvin or ketoconazole has been used in treating superficial fungal infections not responding to topically applied drugs; these indications are also discussed in Chapter 72.

Antihistamines

Topical antihistamines, in the form of creams or lotions, are sometimes used to relieve itching due to minor skin irritations. These drugs possess some local anesthetic activity but may cause localized irritation and sensitization, especially with prolonged use. Most topical antihistamine preparations contain either diphenhydramine or pyrilamine, often combined with an astringent, local anesthetic, or antipruritic (eg, camphor). These preparations should not be applied to raw, blistered, or oozing areas. A complete discussion of antihistamines is presented in Chapter 16.

Antipsoriatics

A variety of drugs has been used in the treatment of psoriasis, including topical use of corticosteroids, salicylic acid, coal tar, and anthralin, as well as systemic administration of corticosteroids, methotrexate, or etretinate, the latter agents being reserved for severe, recalcitrant forms of the disease. Topical and systemic corticosteroids are discussed in Chapter 45, salicylic acid is reviewed in Chapter 21, and methotrexate is considered in Chapter 74. The remaining antipsoriatic drugs are discussed in the following sections.

• Anthralin

Anthra-Derm, Drithocreme, Lasan

Anthralin is a mild irritant that reduces the proliferation of epidermal cells in psoriatic lesions by inhibiting the synthesis of nucleic protein. The drug is used as an ointment or cream (0.1%–1%) and applied as a thin layer once or twice a day. Treatment is continued until scales are removed or lesions are flattened. The drug should not be applied to the face, and application discontinued if inflammation or an allergic reaction develops.

Anthralin causes erythema and irritation of unaffected skin. Gloves should be worn when applying the drug and care must be taken to avoid unaffected skin. The drug will stain fabric and may cause temporary discoloration or white or gray hair if contact is made.

• Coal Tar Preparations

Shampoo: Denorex, DHS Tar, Ionil-T Plus, Neutrogena-T/Gel, Polytar, Tegrin
Bath Oils: Balnetar, Cutar, Polytar Bath, Zetar
Gel: Aquatar, Estar, P and S Plus, PsoriGel
Lotion/cream: Fototar, Oxipor VHC, Tegrin
Soap: Packer's Pine Tar, Polytar

Coal tar–containing products possess antipruritic, antieczematous, and keratoplastic activity and are used adjunctively in a variety of dermatologic disorders, including psoriasis, seborrheic and atopic dermatitis, and other chronic skin disorders. Available preparations include shampoos, bath emulsions, gels, creams, lotions, and soaps. These coal tar preparations should not be used when acute inflammation is present and should not be applied near the eyes or the genitorectal area. Frequency of use depends on the condition being treated, and can range from once daily to once weekly.

• Etretinate *(Pregnancy Category X)*

Tegison

Etretinate is related to vitamin A and is used in certain severe forms of psoriasis that have not responded to other modes of treatment. The drug is potentially toxic and is associated with a risk of fetal abnormalities. Patients using the drug must be closely supervised.

Mechanism

Decreases erythema and thickness of psoriatic lesions and promotes normalization of epidermal differentiation; may also decrease inflammation of the epidermis and dermis; can produce a wide range of adverse effects, and its use is restricted to patients unresponsive to or intolerant of conventional modes of antipsoriatic therapy.

Uses

Treatment of *severe, recalcitrant* psoriasis in patients unresponsive to systemic corticosteroids, methotrexate, psoralens plus UV light, or topical tar plus UV light.

Dosage

Initially: 0.75 to 1.0 mg/kg/day orally in divided doses
Maintenance dose: 0.5 to 0.75 mg/kg/day after 8 to 16 weeks of therapy

Fate

Oral absorption is good and may be increased by a high-lipid diet; drug undergoes significant first-pass hepatic metabolism and is more than 99% protein bound; has an extremely long half-life, and elimination is very slow. Prolonged dosing has been associated with the maintenance of detectable serum levels up to 3 years after therapy was discontinued. Excretion is by way of both the urine and bile.

Common Side Effects

Dry nose, sore mouth, chapped lips, thirst, nosebleed, dry skin, hair loss, itching, bone or joint pain, bruising, fatigue, muscle cramping, headache, fever, eye irritation, visual disturbances, nausea, anorexia.

Also, increased serum triglycerides, serum aminotransferases, alkaline phosphatase, and cholesterol can occur, as well as changes in serum potassium, calcium, and phosphorus.

Significant Adverse Reactions

CAUTION

Etretinate must not be used by women who are pregnant during therapy, and contraception should be practiced for some time after discontinuation of therapy (at least 2 years, owing to the drug's extremely slow elimination). Fetal abnormalities have been reported (also see Isotretinoin).

CNS: dizziness, lethargy, pain, anxiety, depression, emotional lability, flu-like symptoms, abnormal thinking, pseudotumor cerebri (benign intracranial hypertension)
Sensory: earache, otitis externa, lacrimation, hearing changes, photophobia, decreased night vision, scotoma
GI: constipation, diarrhea, weight loss, oral ulcers, altered taste, tooth cavities
CV: chest pain, postural hypotension, phlebitis, syncope, arrhythmias
Dermatologic: bullous eruption, urticaria, pyogenic granuloma, onycholysis, hirsutism, impaired wound healing, herpes simplex infections, skin odor, fissures, skin atrophy, gingival bleeding, decreased mucus secretion, rhinorrhea
Musculoskeletal: myalgia, gout, hyperostosis (see under Contraindications), hyperkinesia
Other: coughing, dysphonia, pharyngitis, proteinuria, glycosuria, urinary casts, hemoglobinuria, kidney stones, abnormal menses, atrophic vaginitis dysuria, polyuria or urinary retention, hepatotoxicity (see under Contraindications)

Contraindications

Use in women who are pregnant or who may become pregnant during or for up to 2 years after therapy. *Cautious use* in patients with liver dysfunction, hypertension, visual disturbances, and elevated serum lipids.

Interactions

The oral absorption of etretinate may be increased by the presence of milk.

Nursing Management

Pretherapy Assessment

Assess and record baseline data necessary for detection of adverse effects of etretinate: General: VS, body weight, skin color, temperature, and integrity; CNS: orientation, reflexes, ophthalmic examination; GI: mucous membranes, bowel sounds; Laboratory: hepatic function tests, electrolytes, cholesterol, serum triglycerides, high-density lipoproteins, sedimentation rate, complete blood count with differential, urinalysis, pregnancy test.

Review medical history and documents for existing or previous conditions that:
a. require cautious use of an etretinate: liver dysfunc-

tion, hypertension, visual disturbances, and elevated serum lipids.

b. contraindicate use of etretinate: allergy to etretinate or retinoids; **pregnancy (Category X)**.

Nursing Interventions

Medication Administration

Ensure that patient is not pregnant before administering.
Administer with meals; do not crush capsules.
Do not administer vitamin supplements that contain vitamin A.
Discontinue use if signs of papilledema occur.
Discontinue use if visual disturbances, abdominal pain, rectal bleeding, or severe diarrhea occur.
Protect patient from exposure to the sun; arrange for use of sunscreen, protective clothing.
Provide for ready access to bathroom facilities if diarrhea occurs.
Provide small, frequent meals if GI distress occurs.

Surveillance During Therapy

Monitor triglycerides during therapy. Monitor results of serum lipid determinations, which should be performed before initiation of therapy and at weekly or biweekly intervals during therapy. Increased triglyceride and cholesterol levels and decreased high-density lipoprotein levels occur in up to 25% of patients, but they revert to pretreatment levels when therapy is terminated.
Monitor for signs of hypersensitivity, which may require discontinuation of drug.
Do not allow blood donation from a patient on isotretinoin because of ability to transfer teratogenic potential.
Monitor diagnostic test results obtained over the course of therapy.
Interpret results of diagnostic tests and contact practitioner as appropriate.
Monitor for possible drug–laboratory test interactions.
Monitor for possible drug–drug and drug–nutrient interactions.

Patient Teaching

With fertile woman, see CAUTION under Significant Adverse Reactions, and also see applicable portions of Patient Teaching for isotretinoin; in addition:

With fertile woman (and sexual partner, as appropriate):

Ensure that patient is fully aware of drug's teratogenic potential (see CAUTION under Significant Adverse Reactions).
Verify that patient clearly understands the importance of effective contraception.
Explain that contraception needs to be used at least 1 month before the start of treatment, during treatment, and for as long as 2 years after cessation of treatment. As appropriate, help patient determine preferred form of contraception or refer her and her partner to available resources.
Explain that a pregnancy test will be performed several weeks before therapy is initiated and that the drug will be started shortly after the onset of the next normal menstrual period.

With any patient:

Discuss the need to control dietary fat intake because drug may cause elevation of serum lipids. Refer patient to dietitian for additional counseling as needed.
Instruct patient to avoid vitamin A supplements because of possible additive toxicity.
Inform patient that psoriasis may temporarily worsen during early treatment.
Instruct patient to notify drug prescriber immediately if pain or limitation of motion is experienced in ankles, pelvis, or knees. Periodic radiographs may be recommended to detect early hyperostosis (abnormal growth of bone tissue). Evidence of emerging calcification of tendons or ligaments requires drug discontinuation.
Teach patient how to recognize possible early indications of hepatitis (yellow skin and sclerae, light-colored stools, dark urine, flu-like symptoms) and stress importance of notifying prescriber. If hepatitis is diagnosed, drug will be discontinued.
Instruct patient to notify drug prescriber of any visual difficulties, which call for an ophthalmologic examination and, usually, drug discontinuation.
Teach patient how to recognize possible early symptoms of pseudotumor cerebri (headache, nausea, vomiting, blurred vision) and to report them. If papilledema is present, drug will be discontinued and patient will be referred for neurologic evaluation.
Warn patient who wears contact lenses that dry eyes may cause lens discomfort. Eye lubricants such as artificial tears may help.
Caution patient to avoid excessive exposure to sun because photophobia and photosensitivity may occur. Use of sunglasses and sunscreen is recommended.
Teach patient interventions to relieve xerostomia. Frequent dental care is recommended to monitor for development of caries. Drug may be discontinued if periodontal disease or candidal infection occurs.
Caution patient not to donate blood until several years after therapy has terminated to prevent transmission of teratogen to a pregnant woman.
Instruct patient about expected actions and possible adverse effects of prescribed drug.

Antiseptics

Several different types of compounds are useful as topical antiseptics or germicides for preoperative cleaning of the skin or for treatment of minor skin wounds or abrasions.

• *Benzalkonium Chloride*

Benza, Zephiran

Benzalkonium chloride is a cationic, surface-active agent that is either bactericidal or bacteriostatic, depending on concentration, toward a variety of bacteria as well as some viruses, fungi, and protozoa. The drug is available as a solution or tincture spray (1:750) or as a concentrate (17%). The aqueous solutions are used for antisepsis of the skin, mucous membranes, and wounds; for preoperative preparation of the skin; for preservation of ophthalmic solutions; for irrigation of the eye, body cavities, bladder and urethra; and for vaginal douching. The tincture spray is useful for preoperative skin preparation and for treatment of abrasions and minor superficial wounds.

The drug is rapid acting and has a relatively long duration of action, although it is inactivated by soaps or anionic detergents. Solutions can be irritating and the drug should not be used in occlusive dressings, casts, and anal or vaginal packs. Concentrations stronger than 1:5000 should not be applied to mucous membranes.

• *Chlorhexidine*

Exidine, Hibiclens, Hibistat, Peridex

Chlorhexidine is an effective antimicrobial agent against a wide range of microorganisms, including *Pseudomonas aeruginosa*. It may be used twice daily as an oral rinse (Peridex) for treatment of gingivitis, as a sudsing cleanser (4%) or drug-impregnated sponge (4%) for surgical scrub or skin wound cleaning, and as a topical germicidal rinse (0.5%). The drug should be kept out of the eyes and ears; deafness can occur if the drug reaches the middle ear through a perforation. Chlorhexidine 4% skin cleanser has also been used in treating acne vulgaris with some success.

• *Hexachlorophene*

phisoHex, Septisol Foam

Hexachlorophene is bacteriostatic against many gram-positive organisms and may be used as a liquid (3%) or a foam (0.23%) as a surgical scrub or skin cleanser. It is not intended for use on open cuts, burns, wounds, or mucous membranes or as an occlusive dressing, wet pack, or lotion. Rapid absorption can occur if hexachlorophene is applied to areas of lesioned skin, and toxic blood levels can ensue. Infants are particularly likely to absorb hexachlorophene in significant amounts and systemic toxicity may be manifested as CNS stimulation. The drug is *not* intended for routinely bathing infants. Occasional adverse reactions include dermatitis, photosensitivity, and peeling and dryness of the skin.

• *Povidone-Iodine*

Betadine, Iodex, Operand, Polydine

Povidone-iodine is a water-soluble complex of iodine with povidone containing 9% to 12% available iodine. The complex provides the germicidal action of iodine without undue irritation to skin and mucous membranes. The product is available in a variety of dosage forms and may be used as a surgical scrub, skin cleanser, perineal disinfectant, vaginal gel, mouthwash/gargle, or whirlpool concentrate.

• *Thimerosal*

Aeroaid, Mersol

Thimerosal is an organomercurial containing approximately 50% mercury. It possesses prolonged bacteriostatic and fungistatic activity against many common pathogens. Available preparations include a tincture, solution, and aerosol, all containing a concentration of 1:1000. Thimerosal may be used for treating contaminated wounds, for antisepsis of intact skin, for preoperative and postoperative use, and for local application to the eye, nose, throat, vagina, and urinary tract. Thimerosal should not be used with strong acids, salts of heavy metals, potassium permanganate, or iodine, because it is incompatible with these substances.

• *Triclosan*

Septi-Soft, Septisol

Triclosan is a bacteriostatic disinfectant used as a skin cleanser, shampoo, or hand wash. It may also be used as a hand or towel bath. It is active against a wide range of organisms.

Antiviral Drugs

Antiviral drugs used topically include idoxuridine, trifluridine, and vidarabine, which may be instilled into the eye for local viral infections, and acyclovir, which is used as an ointment for the management of initial episodes of herpes genitalis or other mucocutaneous herpes simplex viral infections. These agents are reviewed in Chapter 73.

Corticosteroids

A number of different corticosteroids are available for topical application for the treatment of inflammatory dermatoses. The relative potency of the various agents depends on several factors, including the concentration of drug applied, the type of vehicle used, and whether an occlusive dressing was applied. The topical corticosteroids are considered in Chapter 45 and a relative potency ranking of the available topical corticosteroid preparations in found in Table 45-2. Dermatologic disorders that usually respond well to topical corticosteroids include atopic, contact, eczematous, irritant and seborrheic dermatitis, as well as pruritus ani, lichen simplex, and mild psoriasis of the face and genitalia. Conditions that respond less well include discoid lupus erythematosus, sarcoidosis, pemphigus, vitiligo, acne cysts, keloids, hypertrophic lichen planus, and alopecia areata. Local side effects of corticosteroid administration include erythema, "wrinkled" skin, steroid acne, pustules and papules on the facial area, and hypertrichosis.

Enzymes

Several different enzymes are used topically for debriding surface ulcers, surgical or other types of wounds, and second- or third-degree burns. Their effectiveness varies with the condition of the wound or ulcer. To enhance their efficacy, the lesion or wound should be cleansed of as much debris as possible and any dry, dense eschar removed if possible before application of the enzyme. The various topical enzyme preparations are presented in Table 81-2, Chapter 81, along with the other types of available enzyme preparations.

Keratolytics

Keratolytics are desquamating agents that cause degeneration and sloughing of epidermal cells. They are used for various indications, such as removal of epithelial growths (eg, warts), excessive keratin in hyperkeratotic skin disorders, and psoriatic lesions.

• *Salicylic Acid*

Compound W, DuoFilm, Freezone, Keralyt, Occlusal, Trans-Ver-Sal

Salicylic acid, used as a gel, cream, liquid, ointment, transdermal patch, or plaster has long been used as a keratolytic in concentrations of between 2% and 6%. Concentrations of up to 20% in collodion are effective for the removal of common and plantar warts, and up to 50% concentrations in plasters can be used to remove corns and warts. Other uses for salicylic acid preparations include acne, seborrheic dermatitis, calluses, dandruff, and psoriasis. The various topical preparations of salicylic acid are listed in Table 21-1, Chapter 21, together with the other salicylates.

• *Cantharidin*

Cantherone, Verr-Canth

Cantharidin is an irritant substance, also known as *Spanish fly* or dried blister beetles. Its acantholytic action results from changes in epidermal cell membranes, leading to blister formation. This effect is confined to epidermal cells, and thus there is no scarring from topical application. The principal use for cantharidin is removal of benign epithelial growths, such as warts or molluscum contagiosum. The drug should not be applied to the anogenital area because it is a strong irritant. Application to the skin usually results in tingling, itching, or burning within several hours. Cantharidin can produce blisters on normal skin or mucous membranes and should be wiped immediately with acetone, alcohol, or tape remover if the drug is spilled on skin. Use of a mild antibacterial agent is recommended until tissue reepithelialization occurs.

• *Masoprocol*

Actinex

Masoprocol possesses antiproliferative activity against keratinocytes and is used as a 10% cream for the treatment of actinic (solar) keratoses. The drug is gently massaged into the areas twice a day for 28 days where actinic keratoses are present. Occlusive dressing should *not* be used. Transient burning sensations can occur immediately after application. Allergic contact dermatitis has been reported in up to 10% of patients receiving masoprocol application; the drug should be discontinued if sensitivity develops. The drug can stain clothing. Common side effects include erythema, flaking, itching, dryness, and localized edema.

• *Podofilox*

Condylox

Podofilox is a topical antimitotic drug used in the treatment of external genital warts (condylomata acuminatum). Correct diagnosis of the condition is important with use of podofilox, because it should *not* be used to treat squamous cell carcinoma, which often presents with a similar appearance. The topical solution is applied twice daily for 3 days, then withheld for 4 consecutive days; this cycle may be repeated up to four times until there is no visible wart tissue. Common side effects include burning, itching, pain, and inflammation at the application site. The minimum amount of solution necessary to cover the lesion should be applied with a cotton-tipped applicator. The efficacy of treatment for longer than 4 weeks has not been established.

• *Podophyllum Resin*

Pod-Ben 25, Podocon-25, Podofin

Podophyllum resin is a mixture of several substances that are cytotoxic to embryonic and tumor cells. It produces degeneration of epithelial cells and mitotic arrest. The principal applications for podophyllum resin are the treatment of condylomata acuminatum (genital warts) and other papillomas, verrucae, and multiple superficial keratoses. It is a powerful caustic and severe irritant, and is to be applied only by a physician. The drug should not be used in patients with diabetes or other conditions associated with compromised circulation; it should also be avoided on bleeding warts, moles, birthmarks, and any other unusual warts. Contact with the eyes or other healthy tissue should be avoided. Neuropathy has occurred after use of large amounts on widespread lesions. The minimum amount of contact time necessary to produce the desired results (commonly 1–4 hours) minimizes the danger of severe untoward reactions.

• *Urea*

Aquacare, Carmol 10, Ureacin

Urea (or carbamide) possesses a softening or moisturizing effect on the stratum corneum and can facilitate the solubilization of keratin. It is used as a cream or lotion (10%–40%) to promote hydration and remove excess keratin in dry skin or hyperkeratotic conditions. In addition, the 40% cream may be used to remove dystrophic nails without local anesthesia or surgery. Urea is normally applied two to four times a day and rubbed in completely. Concentrations greater than 10% may be associated with a stinging sensation on application.

Local Anesthetics

Topically applied local anesthetics are used for a variety of skin and mucous membrane disorders as well as for preparation for minor surgical procedures. The various local anesthetic preparations are discussed in Chapter 18.

Pigmenting–Depigmenting Agents

Normal skin pigmentation is the result of the presence of melanocytes in the basal layer of the epidermis. These cells have the ability to form the pigment melanin by oxidation of tyrosine. Subsequent activation of melanin occurs by exposure to radiant energy in the form of UV light.

Pigmenting Agents

• Psoralens

Methoxsalen
Trioxsalen

Two psoralen compounds, methoxsalen and trioxsalen, have the ability to increase the deposition of the pigment melanin in the skin in response to UV radiation. They may be used either orally or topically to facilitate repigmentation in patients with vitiligo, a disorder characterized by patchy areas of nonpigmented skin. The oral dosage form of these two drugs can also be used to increase tolerance to sunlight in people with fair complexions who suffer severe reactions on exposure. Finally, much interest is centered on the possible beneficial effects of these drugs in treating severe psoriasis, when followed by controlled exposure to long-wavelength UV light (320–400 nm). Such treatment, known as PUVA therapy, shows promise of being a very effective, albeit potentially toxic, form of therapy.

In vitiligo, repigmentation varies in time of onset, degree of completeness, and duration. Although some effect may be evident within several weeks after beginning therapy, significant repigmentation may take 6 to 12 months. The psoralens are effective in enhancing pigmentation only when followed by exposure of affected skin areas to UV light, either artificial or natural (sunlight).

The two drugs are reviewed together in the following, and listed individually in Table 79-2.

Mechanism

Not established; may increase the number of functional melanocytes and activate resting or dormant cells; also initiate a local inflammatory response; can increase synthesis of melanosomes and activity of tyrosinase, an enzyme involved in conversion of tyrosine to dihydroxyphenylalanine, a precursor of melanin; activity is dependent on the presence of functional melanocytes and activation of the psoralen agent by UV radiation, either artificial or sunlight.

Uses

Repigmentation of idiopathic vitiligo
Aid to increasing tolerance to sunlight (trioxsalen only)
Treatment of severe, recalcitrant, disabling psoriasis not responsive to other forms of therapy—given *only* in conjunction with controlled doses of long-wave UV radiation
Palliative treatment of cutaneous T-cell lymphoma, with long-wave UV radiation of white blood cells, in patients who have not responded to other forms of treatment (methoxsalen, oral)

Dosage

See Table 79-2.

Fate

Oral absorption is 95% complete; food appears to increase serum concentrations; after oral ingestion, skin sensitivity to UV radiation is maximal in 2 hours and disappears within 8 hours; psoralens are metabolized in the liver and excreted primarily (90%) in the urine; topical application produces a rapid sensitivity.

Common Side Effects

Nausea, pruritus, erythema.

Significant Adverse Reactions

CAUTION

Use of psoralens together with UV radiation must be undertaken only by healthcare personnel experienced in photochemical treatment of psoriasis and vitiligo. Severe adverse reactions can occur (burns, ocular damage, skin aging, skin cancer) and patients must be informed of the risks inherent in such treatment.

Topical: skin irritation, erythema, blistering
Oral: GI upset, nervousness, insomnia, depression, edema, dizziness, headache, hypopigmentation, ve-

Table 79-2. **Psoralens**

Drug	Usual Dosage Range	Nursing Considerations
Methoxsalen *Oxsoralen, Oxsoralen-Ultra, 8-MOP* *(CAN) Ultra MOP*	Topical: apply once weekly to small, well defined lesions, then expose area to UV light for 1 min; subsequent exposure times should be increased with caution Oral: 1 to 6 capsules/day in a single dose, followed in 2 h by a 15 min exposure to UV light; gradually increase exposure time to 30–40 min	Pigmentation may begin within several weeks, but significant repigmentation may require treatment for 6–9 mo; do *not* increase dosage of oral preparation; perform liver function tests periodically during therapy and stop drug if liver impairment occurs; Oxsoralen-Ultra capsules produce earlier onset time of photosensitization than regular oxsoralen capsules, even though dose is identical—do not use interchangeably; topical preparation is used only on small, well defined vitiliginous lesions that can be protected from excessive exposure; use of bandages or sunscreens or both may be necessary
Trioxsalen *Trisoralen*	*Vitiligo*: 10 mg/d, followed in 2–4 h by UV exposure ranging from 15–30 min *Sunlight tolerance*: 10 mg/d, 2 h before exposure to sun, for a maximum of 14 d	More active than methoxsalen, yet its median lethal dose is 6 times higher; do *not* increase dosage and lengthen exposure times only in gradual increments; discontinue drug if repigmentation is not evident within 3–4 mo

UV, ultraviolet.

siculation, nonspecific rash, urticaria, folliculitis, leg cramps, hypotension, severe burns from UV light, cataracts from UV exposure

Contraindications

Melanoma, invasive squamous cell carcinoma, aphakia, albinism, porphyria, acute lupus erythematosus, leukoderma of infectious origin; in children younger than 12 years of age (trioxsalen only); and concurrent use of a photosensitizing drug. *Cautious use* in patients with impaired liver function and in pregnant or nursing women.

Interactions

An increased danger of severe burns exists if psoralens are used together with known photosensitizing agents, such as anthralin, coal tar derivatives, griseofulvin, nalidixic acid, phenothiazines, sulfonamides, tetracyclines, and thiazide diuretics.

Nursing Management

Pretherapy Assessment

Assess and record baseline data necessary for detection of adverse effects of psoralens: General: VS, body weight, skin color, temperature, and integrity.

Review medical history and documents for existing or previous conditions that:

a. require cautious use of psoralens: impaired liver function; breast-feeding.

b. contraindicate use of psoralens: allergy to psoralens, melanoma, invasive squamous cell carcinoma, aphakia, albinism, porphyria, acute lupus erythematosus, leukoderma of infectious origin; in children younger than 12 years of age (trioxsalen only); and concurrent use of a photosensitizing drug; **pregnancy (Category C)**.

Nursing Interventions

Medication Administration

Protect hands of person applying agent to prevent photosensitization.

Apply to a well defined area of vitiligo; initial exposure should be conservative.

Surveillance During Therapy

Observe patient for signs of irritation or blistering, particularly during first few days of therapy when sensitivity to light is greatest. Prescribed dosage and exposure should not be exceeded, and patient should be under *constant* supervision during therapy because overdosage or overexposure can result in severe blistering and burning.

Monitor for signs of hypersensitivity, which may require discontinuation of drug.

Monitor diagnostic test results obtained over the course of therapy.

Interpret results of diagnostic tests and contact practitioner as appropriate.

Monitor for possible drug–laboratory test interactions.

Monitor for possible drug–drug and drug–nutrient interactions.

Patient Teaching

Instruct patient about expected actions and possible adverse effects of prescribed drug.

Ensure that patient is aware of risks inherent in treatment (see CAUTION under Significant Adverse Reactions).

Instruct patient to take oral preparation with food or milk to minimize GI distress, or to divide oral dose into two portions taken one half hour apart. Topical preparations should *not* be used at home; they should be applied and monitored only by trained personnel under strictly controlled light conditions.

Caution patient to protect lips and eyes during UV exposure periods.

Instruct patient receiving topical preparation to keep treated area protected from sunlight, except for desired exposure periods, because severe burns can occur if treated area is exposed to additional UV light.

Inform patient that a complete blood count, an antinuclear antibody test, liver and kidney function tests, and an ophthalmologic examination are recommended before therapy and at 6- to 12-month intervals during prolonged therapy.

Depigmenting Agents

Two agents are available for reducing hyperpigmentation of skin, but they differ in that one of the drugs, hydroquinone, usually produces a temporary lightening of skin areas, whereas the other drug, monobenzone, produces irreversible depigmentation.

• *Hydroquinone*

Eldopaque, Esoterica Regular, Porcelana, and other manufacturers

(CAN) Eldoquin, Solaquin

Hydroquinone is capable of interfering with the formation of melanin by inhibiting the enzymatic oxidation of tyrosine. Skin color begins to lighten usually after 3 to 4 weeks, but a good response may require up to 6 months. The drug may be applied twice a day as a cream (2%, 4%), lotion (2%), solution (3%), or gel (4%), often in combination with a sunscreening agent to minimize repigmentation on exposure to sunlight. Hydroquinone should be applied only to limited areas of the face, neck, hands, or arms; the drug is *not* to be used on irritated, denuded, or damaged skin. Because the effect of the drug is temporary, treated skin areas return to their original color when the drug is discontinued. Principal uses for hydroquinone are for reversible bleaching of hyperpigmented skin areas, such as freckles, chloasma, melasma, or senile lentigines.

• *Monobenzone*

(CAN) Benoquin

Monobenzone is used as a 20% cream for permanent depigmentation in patients with extensive vitiligo. It is *not* to be used on freckles, melasma, pigmented nevi, or hyperpigmentation resulting from photosensitization, inflammation, or other causes. It is a *potent* depigmenting agent. Depigmentation occurs within 1 to 4 months after initiation of therapy. Safety for use in pregnant women, nursing mothers, and children younger than 12 years of age has not been established. The cream is applied two to three times a day. If irritation, burning, or dermatitis occur on application, the drug should be discontinued.

Scabicides–Pediculicides

• *Crotamiton*

Eurax

Crotamiton is a scabicide with antipruritic properties. It is effective as a 10% cream or lotion for the eradication of scabies (*Sarcoptes scabiei*) and for treatment of pruritic skin conditions.

In treating scabies, two applications are made 24 hours apart, and a cleansing bath is taken 48 hours after the final application. The drug should not be applied to inflamed or denuded skin or to the eyes or mouth.

• *Lindane*

G-Well, Kwell, Scabene

Lindane is an effective scabicide and pediculicide that is used in treating head lice, crab lice, and scabies. The drug may be applied as a 1% cream, lotion, or shampoo. The cream or lotion is applied in sufficient quantity to cover the affected area, rubbed in, left in place for 8 to 12 hours, and then thoroughly washed off. Reapplication is necessary only if living lice are detected 7 days later. The shampoo is thoroughly worked through dry hair and allowed to remain for 5 minutes; it is then rinsed out and the hair dried. A fine-tooth comb may be used to remove any remaining nit shells.

Significant percutaneous absorption can result in CNS stimulation; oils may increase absorption and use of oil-based hair dressings or lotions should be avoided. The drug should not be applied to the face, nor to open wounds or abrasions, and unnecessary skin contact should be avoided. When used properly, the risk of adverse effects is extremely small.

• *Permethrin*

Elimite,Nix

Permethrin as active against lice, mites, ticks, and fleas, because it acts on the nerve cell membranes of the parasites to cause paralysis. The drug is available as a 5% cream that is massaged into the skin and left on for 8 to 14 hours before washing, and as a 1% cream rinse, which is applied to the hair and scalp, left on for 10 minutes, and washed out. A single treatment with either preparation is usually sufficient to remove the infestation. Itching and transient burning or stinging are the most frequently encountered side effects.

• *Pyrethrins*

Pyrethrins are available in combination with piperonyl butoxide or petroleum distillates in a number of over-the-counter pediculicides, such as A-200, RID, R and C Shampoo, and Tisit. The combinations exert a synergistic action against head lice, body lice, and pubic lice and can be applied either as a liquid, gel, or shampoo. The products are irritating to the eyes and mucous membranes, and should be discontinued if severe irritation occurs.

Sunscreens

Preparations useful as sunscreens provide either a chemical or physical barrier to sunlight. *Chemical* sunscreens absorb UV radiation in the medium wavelength range of 290 to 320 nm (UV-B range), which is the spectrum of UV light most responsible for burning. Long-wavelength (320–400 nm) UV light (UV-A range) can cause tanning but is a major risk factor for serious skin damage, and can deeply penetrate the dermis. *Physical* sunscreens reflect or scatter light in the spectrum of 290 to 700 nm and prevent its skin penetration.

Available sunscreens in each category include:

Chemical

1. Benzophenones (oxybenzone, dioxybenzone)
2. Paraaminobenzoic acid and esters (PABA, octyldimethyl PABA, glyceryl PABA)
3. Cinnamates (cinoxate, octylmethoxy cinnamate)
4. Salicylates (octylsalicylate, homosalate, ethylhexyl salicylate)
5. Miscellaneous (methyl anthranilate, digalloyl trioleate)

Physical

1. Titanium dioxide
2. Red petrolatum
3. Zinc oxide

Titanium dioxide and zinc oxide have a UV spectrum of 290 to 700 nm, protecting against both UV-A and UV-B light. Benzophenones protect within the range of 250 to 400 nm, whereas most other sunscreen products protect primarily within the UV-B range (280–320 nm).

Effectiveness of a sunscreen product usually is given by its sun protection factor (SPF), which indicates the relative resistance to sunburning afforded by the product. For example, an SPF of 6 means that the product affords six times the sun exposure protection as use of no sunscreen. Most people should use a sunscreen product with an SPF of at least 6 to 10, and people who tend to burn easily should use a 15 SPF product.

Sunscreens should be applied to all exposed areas and reapplied periodically to maintain an even film; some products are "water resistant" and do not wash off as rapidly.

Contact dermatitis can develop with some sunscreen products, particularly PABA or its esters, benzophenones, and cinnamates. Contact with the eyes should be avoided and use of the product discontinued if rash or other signs of hypersensitivity appear.

Selected Bibliography

Allen JG, Bloxham DP: The pharmacology and pharmacokinetics of the retinoids. Pharmacol Ther 40:1, 1989

Bigby M, Stern RS: Adverse reactions to isotretinoin. J Am Acad Dermatol 18:543, 1988

Lever L, Marks R: Current views on the aetiology, pathogenesis and treatment of acne vulgaris. Drugs 39:681, 1990

Maibach H (ed): Dermatotoxicology, 4th ed. Hemisphere Press, 1991

Maibach H, Surber C (eds): Topical Corticosteroids. Basel, Karger, 1992

Pathak MA, Fitzpatrick TB: The evolution of photochemotherapy with psoralens and UVA (PUVA): 200BC to 1992 AD. J Photochem Photobiol 14:3, 1992

Stolk LM, Siddiqui AH: Biopharmaceutics, pharmacokinetics and pharmacology of psoralens. Gen Pharmacol 19:649, 1988

80 Diagnostic Agents

In Vitro Diagnostic Aids
Intradermal Diagnostic Aids
In Vivo Diagnostic Aids
Radiographic Diagnostic Aids

Effective treatment of many disease states depends on a critical assessment of the underlying pathology. To accomplish this, a number of diagnostic agents are available that assist the clinician in evaluating the clinical status of the patient as well as the functional capacity of many body organs. In most instances, proper use of diagnostic agents requires specially trained personnel and a thorough knowledge of the agent being employed. The extensive array of available diagnostic drugs precludes an in-depth discussion of each agent in a general pharmacology text of this type. Thus, this chapter presents a brief review of the principles of diagnostic drug usage, followed by tabular listings of the categories of diagnostic agents. It is imperative, however, that healthcare personnel using these drugs thoroughly familiarize themselves with the pharmacology and toxicology of the particular diagnostic agent being employed.

For purposes of discussion, the various diagnostic agents can be grouped into one of the four following categories:

- *In vitro diagnostic aids*: agents usually employed at home or in the physician's office to monitor blood or urine levels of substances such as glucose, proteins, or ketones as well as pH; also included in this category are the pregnancy screening tests, as well as tests for the presence of occult blood in the urine or feces
- *Intradermal diagnostic biologicals*: agents used in skin tests for sensitivity to certain diseases, notably tuberculosis, coccidioidomycosis, and histoplasmosis.
- *In vivo diagnostic aids*: agents usually employed to evaluate the functional status of body organs such as the liver, kidney, heart, pancreas, stomach, adrenal cortex, or pituitary; used in a hospital setting and require skilled personnel for administration and interpretation
- *Radiographic diagnostic agents*: opaque contrast substances, usually barium or iodine compounds, that are impenetrable by x-rays; used to visualize internal structures such as the GI tract, kidneys, gallbladder, and bronchial tree

In Vitro Diagnostic Aids

A large number of preparations are used for rapid screening of the urine, feces, or blood for the presence of certain substances. These in vitro diagnostic aids commonly employ either 1) a reagent or tablet that is mixed in a test tube or on a slide with the sample to be analyzed or 2) a reagent-impregnated strip or tape that is dipped into the sample. Most are available without prescription, and complete instructions for performing the test and analyzing the results are provided with the package. A few of these aids, however, such as tests for diagnosing mononucleosis, sickle cell anemia, certain viruses, or the presence of beta-hemolytic streptococci, are prescription-only items and require that the user be familiar with the product to interpret the results accurately.

Another in vitro diagnostic aid is a pregnancy test that may be employed either in the home or in a care provider's office. They generally employ a reagent to be added to a urine sample. Although home test kits are certainly valuable as a preliminary screening method, confirmation of pregnancy should always be obtained professionally by use of one of the more established pregnancy-screening procedures performed in the physician's office, which measure the presence of chorionic gonadotropin in the urine.

The in vitro diagnostic aids are listed alphabetically by trade name in Table 80-1, together with their specific diagnostic use.

Intradermal Diagnostic Biologicals

The ability of selected biologic products to elicit a local allergic reaction after intradermal injection is used to assess sensitivity to, but not necessarily the active presence of, certain diseases. The most commonly employed skin test is the tuberculin test, although sensitivity to mumps, histoplasmosis, coccidioidomycosis, *Trichophyton*, and *Candida* also can be determined by intradermal testing. Interpretation of the tests is based on the appearance of a local hypersensitivity reaction at the site of intradermal injection, usually consisting of induration (tissue hardening) and, in some cases, erythema, in those patients previously exposed to the infecting organism.

Information relating to the available intradermal diagnostic drugs is presented in Table 80-2. Further information describing proper methods of administration and interpretation is provided with the individual drugs and should be consulted before performing the test.

In Vivo Diagnostic Aids

The diagnostic agents used to assess the functional capacity of internal body organs are termed in vivo diagnostic aids and are administered either orally or parenterally. These compounds frequently are designed to be concentrated in or excreted by the organ to be evaluated. Because they are administered systemically, a potential for untoward reactions does exist, and although these are generally mild and transient, patients should be observed carefully during, and for some time after, the testing procedure for development of more serious adverse reactions.

Several compounds that may be used for diagnostic pur-

(text continues on page 870)

Table 80-1. **In Vitro Diagnostic Agents**

Trade Name	*Diagnostic Uses*
Abbott HTLV I EIA	Antibodies to human T-lymphotropic Virus Type I
Abbott HIVAG-1	Immunoassay for HIV-1 antigens
Abbott HIVAB HIV-1 EIA	Immunoassay for antibodies to HIV-1
Abbott TestPack-Strep A	Immunoassay for group A streptococci from throat
Abbott TestPack Plus hCG-Urine	Pregnancy
Accusens T	Taste dysfunction
Acetest	Serum-urinary ketones
Advance	Pregnancy
Albustix	Urinary proteins
Answer	Pregnancy
Answer Ovulation	Ovulation time
Azostix	Blood urea nitrogen
Bactigen Meningitis Panel	*H. influenzae* (Type B), *N. meningitidis* (serogroups A/B/C/Y/W135), and *S. pneumoniae* in CSF, serum, urine, and blood
Bactigen Salmonella-Shigella	*Salmonella* and *Shigella* in cultures
Bili-Labstix	Urinary glucose, proteins, pH, blood, ketones, bilirubin
Biocult-GC	Gonorrhea
CAST	Human immunoglobulin E in serum
Chemstrip bG	Blood glucose
Chemstrip 2 GP	Urinary glucose, protein
Chemstrip-K	Urinary ketones
Chemstrip LN	Urinary leukocytes, nitrite
Chemstrip uG	Urinary glucose
Chemstrip uGK	Urinary glucose, ketones
Chemstrip 4 OB	Urinary glucose, protein, blood leukocytes
Chemstrip 6	Urinary glucose, proteins, pH, blood, ketones, leukocytes
Chemstrip 7	As above, plus bilirubin
Chemstrip 8	As above, plus urobilinogen
Chemstrip 9	As above, plus nitrite
Chemstrip 10 with SG	As above, plus specific gravity
Chlamydiazyme	Immunoassay for *C. trachomatis*
Clearblue	Pregnancy
Clearplan Easy	Ovulation time
Clinistix	Urinary glucose
Clinitest	Urinary glucose
ColoCare	Fecal occult blood
Color Ovulation Test	Ovulation time
Combistix	Urinary glucose, protein, pH
CS-T ColoScreen	Fecal occult blood
Culturette 10 Minute Group A Strep ID	Group A streptococcal antigen
Daisy 2	Pregnancy
Dextrostix	Blood glucose
Diascan-S	Blood glucose
Diastix	Urinary glucose
Early Detector	Fecal occult blood
Entero-Test	Upper GI bleeding, duodenal parasites, pH disorders
e.p.t. Stick Test	Pregnancy
EZ-Detect	Fecal occult blood
Facts Plus	Pregnancy
First Response	Pregnancy
First Response Ovulation Test	Ovulation time
Fortel Ovulation	Pregnancy
Gastroccult	Blood in gastric contents
Gastro-Test	Stomach pH
Glucostix	Blood glucose
Gonodecten	Gonorrhea
Gonozyme	Gonorrhea
Hema-Chek	Fecal occult blood
Hema-Combistix	Urinary glucose, protein, pH, blood
Hemastix	Urinary blood
Hematest	Fecal occult blood
HemeSelect	Fecal occult blood
Hemoccult	Fecal occult blood
Ictotest	Urinary bilirubin

(*continued*)

Table 80-1. **In Vitro Diagnostic Agents (Continued)**

Trade Name	*Diagnostic Uses*
Isocult Culture Tests	Various culture tests for *Candida, Neisseria gonorrheae, Pseudomonas aeruginosa, S. aureus*, group A beta-hemolytic streptococci, *Trichomonas vaginalis*, or general bacteriuria
Keto-Diastix	Urinary glucose, ketones
Ketostix	Urinary or blood ketones
Labstix	Urinary glucose, protein, pH, blood, ketones
Lung Check	Precancerous cells in sputum
Microstix-3	Urinary nitrite, bacteria
MicroTrak Chlamydia	*C. trachomatis* in tissue culture
MicroTrak HSV 1/HSV 2	Herpes simplex in tissue culture
MicroTrak *Neisseria Gonorrheae* Culture Test	*N gonorrheae* in culture
Mono-Diff Test	Mononucleosis
Mono-Lisa	Mononucleosis
Monospot	Mononucleosis
Monosticon Dri Dot	Mononucleosis
Mono-Sure	Mononucleosis
Mono-Test	Mononucleosis
Multistix	Urinary glucose, protein, pH, blood, ketones, bilirubin, urobilinogen
Multistix SG	As above, plus specific gravity
Multistix 7	Urinary glucose, protein, pH, blood, ketones, nitrite, leukocytes
Multistix 8 SG	As above, plus specific gravity
Multistix 9 SG	As above, plus bilirubin
Multistix 10 SG	As above, plus urobilinogen
Nimbus	Monoclonal antibody immunoassay
Nitrazine Paper	Urinary pH
N-Multistix	Urinary glucose, protein, pH, blood, ketones, bilirubin, urobilinogen, nitrite
N-Multistix SG	As above, plus specific gravity
Ovu QUICK Self-Test	Ovulation time
Ovu KIT Self-Test	Ovulation time
Phenistix	Phenylketonuria
Pregnosis	Pregnancy
Pregnospia	Pregnancy
Pregnosticon Dri-Dot	Pregnancy
RAMP Urine hCG Assay	Pregnancy
Rapid Test Strep	Group A streptococci
Recombigen HIV-1 LA Test	Human antibody to HIV-1
Respiracult Strep	Group A beta-hemolytic streptococci
Respiralex	Group A beta-hemolytic streptococci
Rotalex	Rotavirus in feces
Rubacell II	Rubella virus in serum or plasma
Rubazyme	Rubella virus in serum
Sickledex Test	Hemoglobin S (sickle cells)
Streptonase B	Streptococcal infection
Strepto-Sec	Beta-hemolytic streptococci, groups A, B, C, and G
Tes-Tape	Urinary glucose
TPM-Test	Serum *Toxoplasma gondii* antibodies
Tracer bG	Blood glucose
UCG-Slide Test	Pregnancy
Uricult	Urinary bacteriuria-uropathogens
Uristix	Urinary glucose, protein
Uristix 4	Urinary glucose, protein, nitrite, leukocytes
Virogen Herpes Test	Herpes virus antigens in culture
Virogen HSV Antibody Test	Herpes virus antibody in serum
Virogen Rotatest	Rotavirus in feces
Virogen Rubella Microlatex Test	Rubella virus antibody in serum
Virogen Rubella Slide Test	Rubella virus antibody in serum
Visidex II	Blood glucose

These products are available for use in the physician's office or at home. Other in vitro diagnostic tests are used primarily in commercial laboratories.

Table 80-2. Intradermal Diagnostic Biologicals

Diagnostic Agent	*Uses*	*Nursing Considerations*
Coccidioidin *BioCox, Spherulin*	Diagnosis of coccidioidomycosis Differentiation of coccidioidomycosis from other diseases with similar clinical findings, eg, histoplasmosis, sarcoidosis	Diluted with sodium chloride injection; 0.1 mL of 1:10,000 is injected intradermally; if negative, repeat with 1:1000 and finally 1:100; positive reaction is appearance of area of induration measuring 5 mm or greater; erythema without induration is considered negative; reaction is readable at 24 h and maximal at 36 h and is indicative that contact with the fungus has occurred in the past although patient does not necessarily have an active infection; false positive skin reactions do *not* occur
Histoplasmin *Histoplasmin, Diluted; Histolyn-CYL*	Diagnosis of histoplasmosis Differentiation of histoplasmosis from other mycotic or bacterial infections, eg, coccidioidomycosis, sarcoidosis	A sterile filtrate from cultures of *Histoplasma capsulatum*; 0.1 mL is injected intradermally into flexor surface of the forearm and reaction is read in 48–72 h; induration of 5 mm or greater is considered positive and may indicate a previous mild, subacute, or chronic infection with *Histoplasma capsulatum* or immunologically related organisms; little value in diagnosing acute, fulminating infections because a negative reaction usually occurs; large doses can produce severe erythema; usually given in conjunction with tuberculin test (see below)
Oidiomycin and Trichophyton Extracts	Detection of delayed hypersensitivity to *Trichophyton* or *Candida albicans*	Intradermal injection of antigens reacts with sensitized lymphocytes causing release of inflammatory mediators; efficacy of product in assessing delayed hypersensitivity is unproven
Mumps Skin Test Antigen *MSTA*	Determination of sensitivity to mumps virus	Suspension of killed mumps virus used to determine skin sensitivity to mumps; no longer considered effective at identifying immunity to mumps virus; following injection of 0.1 mL intradermally on inner surface of forearm, reaction is read in 24–36 h; erythema of 1.5 cm or more indicates sensitivity to virus and probable immunity; negative reaction suggests probable susceptibility; do *not* use in persons sensitive to chicken, eggs, or feathers because preparation is cultivated in chicken embryo
Skin Test Antigens, Multiple *Multitest CMI*	Detection of nonresponsiveness to antigens by means of delayed hypersensitivity skin testing	Applicator has eight test heads preloaded with delayed hypersensitivity skin test antigens to tetanus toxoid, diphtheria toxoid, *Streptococcus*, old tuberculin, *Candida, Trichophyton*, and *Proteus*; reactivity may be reduced in patients receiving drugs that suppress immunity or in patients with acute viral infections; test results are read at 24 h and 48 h; positive reaction is induration of 2 mm or greater at antigen site provided there is *no* induration at control site; do *not* apply on infected or inflamed skin; if periodic testing is done, rotate sites of application
Tuberculin Purified Protein Derivative—Tuberculin PPD *Aplisol, Sclavo-PPD Solution, Tubersol*	Aid in diagnosis of tuberculosis	Aqueous solution of a purified protein fraction from filtrates of cultured human strains of *Mycobacterium tuberculosis*; use only *fresh* tuberculin preparations for testing; injected intradermally (5 U) on the flexor or dorsal surface of the forearm; reaction is read in 48–72 h; induration of 10 mm or more is a positive reaction, whereas induration of 5 mm or less is negative; erythema is not of diagnostic significance but may indicate incorrect administration; retesting is indicated if induration measures 5–9 mm; positive reaction does not indicate an active infection but suggests further evaluation is necessary; positive reaction may also indicate previous BCG vaccination; preferred over old tuberculin (OT) test owing to greater purity; highly sensitive persons may experience vesiculation, ulceration, and necrosis, and persons suspected of being highly sensitive should receive an initial dose of only 1 U
Tuberculin PPD, Multiple Puncture Device *Aplitest, Sclavo Test-PPD, Tine Test PPD*	See tuberculin PPD	A single-use device consisting of four stainless steel tines coated with tuberculin PPD, standardized to give reactions equivalent to 5 U of intradermal tuberculin PPD
Old Tuberculin, Multiple Puncture Devices *Mono-Vacc Test, Tuberculin Old Tine Test*	See tuberculin PPD	Single-use, multiple puncture device standardized to give reactions equivalent to 5 U of standard solution of old tuberculin administered intradermally; test is read 48–96 h after administration; positive reaction is vesiculation or induration of 1 mm or greater, but further diagnostic tests are necessary to establish presence of infection; infrequently used preparation

Table 80-3. **In Vivo Diagnostic Aids**

Diagnostic Agent	*Uses*	*Nursing Considerations*
Aminohippurate Sodium *PAH*	Assessment of renal blood flow and tubular secretory mechanisms	Occasionally used to study certain aspects of kidney function; used by IV injection; not metabolized and excreted solely by the kidney; low plasma concentrations (1–2 mg/dL) are used to measure renal blood flow; higher concentrations (40–60 mg/dL) are employed to determine maximal tubular secretory capacity; may elicit nausea, feelings of warmth, and urge to defecate
L-Arginine *R-Gene 10*	Determination of pituitary human growth hormone reserve; diagnosis of panhypopituitarism, pituitary dwarfism, pituitary trauma, and other hypopituitary conditions	Stimulates pituitary to release growth hormone; dosage is 300 mL in adults and 5 mL/kg in children; rate of false positive reactions is 32% and false negative is 27%; do *not* use in patients with strong allergic tendencies; excessive infusion rates can result in irritation, nausea, vomiting, and flushing; have antihistamine available in case of allergic reactions; do *not* use if solution is not clean or if bottle lacks a vacuum; refer to package literature for interpretation of results
Bentiromide *Chymex*	Screening test for pancreatic exocrine insufficiency	A peptide containing 170 mg para-aminobenzoic acid (PABA) per 500 mg dose; following oral administration, bentiromide is hydrolyzed by pancreatic chymotrypsin, liberating PABA, which is excreted in the urine; if exocrine pancreatic function is normal, over 50% of the PABA contained in bentiromide appears in the urine within 6 h; patients should fast at least 8 h before receiving a test dose; diarrhea, headache, nausea, flatulence, and weakness can occur; instruct patient to urinate immediately before receiving bentiromide; falsely elevated readings can occur if the patient is taking other drugs metabolized to arylamines, such as acetaminophen, chloramphenicol, lidocaine, procaine, procainamide, sulfonamides, or thiazide diuretics
Benzylpenicilloylpolylysine *Pre-Pen*	Skin test for penicillin hypersensitivity in patients who have previously received penicillin and demonstrated a clinical hypersensitivity reaction	May be applied either by scratching forearm (preferred method) or by intradermal injection on upper outer arm surface; positive reaction consists of whealing, erythema, and itching; occurs usually within 10 min and is associated with an incidence of allergic reactions to systemic benzylpenicillin or penicillin G of greater than 20%; a negative skin test response predicts a less than 5% incidence of allergic complications; of doubtful value in assessing sensitivity to semisynthetic penicillins or cephalosporins; may produce an intense local inflammatory response and occasionally systemic allergic reactions
Cosyntropin *Cortrosyn* *(CAN) Synacthen Depot*	Diagnosis of adrenal cortical insufficiency	Synthetic subunit of human ACTH used IM or by IV infusion to differentiate primary (adrenal) from secondary (pituitary) adrenocortical insufficiency; in primary Addison's disease, 24-h urinary 17-hydroxycorticosteroid levels fail to rise following IV infusion and plasma cortisol levels do not increase significantly within 30 min following IM injection; secondary pituitary failure is characterized by a *slow increase* in urinary steroids following IV infusion; produces fewer allergic reactions than ACTH injection
Gonadorelin *Factrel*	Evaluation of hypothalamic–pituitary–gonadotropic function Evaluation of residual gonadotropic function following hypophysectomy Investigational uses include induction of ovulation and treatment of precocious puberty	Synthetic luteinizing hormone–releasing hormone (LHRH) structurally identical to natural LHRH possessing a gonadotropin-releasing effect on the anterior pituitary; used SC or IV; in females, test should be performed in early follicular phase of the menstrual cycle; do *not* give concurrently with gonadal hormones, glucocorticoids or spironolactone, because pituitary secretion of gonadotropins can be affected; SC injection can result in localized pain, swelling and itching; use during pregnancy only when clearly needed; refer to package prescribing information for testing method
Histamine Phosphate	Assessment of gastric acid secretory capacity Presumptive diagnosis of pheochromocytoma	Basal acid secretion is measured, then 0.01–0.04 mg histamine base/kg is injected SC and gastric contents are collected in four 15-min specimens and analyzed for volume, pH, and acidity; an antihistamine should be administered IM before histamine; many side effects noted and severe allergic reactions (eg, asthma) can occur; largely replaced by other, safer diagnostic measures (eg, pentagastrin) Once used for diagnosis of pheochromocytoma but rarely employed today with the availability of more accurate and less dangerous procedures
Hysteroscopy Fluid *Hyskon*	Aid in distending the uterine cavity and visualizing its surfaces	Introduced into uterine cavity via cannula under low pressure until uterus is sufficiently distended to permit adequate visualization; volume usually required is 50–100 mL; allergic reactions, including anaphylaxis, can result if drug is absorbed systemically; *do not* exceed 150 mmHg infusion pressure

(*continued*)

Table 80-3. **In Vivo Diagnostic Aids (Continued)**

Diagnostic Agent	*Uses*	*Nursing Considerations*
Indocyanine Green *Cardio-Green*	Determination of cardiac output, hepatic function, and liver blood flow Aid in ophthalmic angiography	A water-soluble dye that is injected IV, is quickly bound to plasma proteins, and is taken up almost exclusively by hepatic parenchymal cells; dilution of dye in blood samples obtained from different sites at various times following administration is an indication of blood flow in a particular area; adverse effects are minimal
Inulin	Measurement of glomerular filtration rate	Polymer of fructose given by IV infusion; drug is rapidly filtered by the kidneys and neither secreted nor reabsorbed; following a loading dose, samples of urine are collected at regular intervals and concentration of inulin in each sample is determined colorimetrically; normal adult inulin clearance is 100–160 mL/min
Mannitol	Measurement of glomerular filtration rate	An osmotic diuretic (see Chap. 39) that is also used to measure glomerular filtration rate (GFR); 100 mL of a 20% solution is diluted with 180 mg normal saline and infused at a rate of 20 mL/min; urine is collected by a catheter for a specific time period and a blood sample is drawn at the beginning and end of the collection period; mannitol concentrations (mg/mL) are determined for each sample and the GFR is calculated as mL of plasma that must be filtered to yield the amount of mannitol excreted per minute in the urine
Methacholine *Provocholine*	Assessment of bronchial airway hyperactivity	Cholinergic agent that is administered by inhalation in solutions of increasing concentration; pulmonary function (forced expiratory volume—FEV) is measured after each dose; requires trained personnel and emergency equipment, and medications must be readily available; may cause headache, throat irritation, lightheadedness, and itching
Metyrapone *Metopirone*	Diagnosis of hypothalamus–pituitary function	Used to test whether pituitary secretion of ACTH is adequate; ability of adrenals to respond to ACTH should be demonstrated by ACTH or cosyntropin test before giving metyrapone; following a 2-day rest period, 15 mg/kg is administered orally every 4 h for 6 doses, then urinary 17-hydroxycorticosteroids (17-OHCS) are collected for 24 h; normal pituitary function is indicated by a 2–4-fold increase in 17-OHCS over control levels obtained before drug administration; excessive excretion of 17-OHCS suggests Cushing's syndrome (adrenal hyperplasia), while subnormal excretion indicates hypopituitarism
Pentagastrin *Peptavlon*	Evaluation of gastric and secretory capacity	Action resembles that of natural gastrin, following SC injection of 6 μg/kg, acid secretion begins within 10 min, peaks in 20–30 min, and lasts 60–90 min; elicits fewer and less intense side effects than either histamine or betazole and is the preferred drug for measuring gastric acid secretion
Protirelin *Relefact TRH, Thypinone*	Adjunct in the evaluation of thyroid function Adjunct for adjustment of thyroid hormone dosage in hypothyroid patients	Synthetic peptide similar in action to thyrotropin-releasing hormone (TRH); following IV injection (adults—500 μg; children—7 μg/kg), protirelin causes release of thyroid-stimulating hormone (TSH) from anterior pituitary; TSH blood levels are determined before injection and again 30 min after injection; thyroid function is characterized by comparing baseline TSH serum levels to those obtained following drug injection; if test is repeated, allow an interval of 7 days; discontinue thyroid drugs at least 7 days before performing test; most common side effects are nausea, urinary urgency, flushing, lightheadedness, headache, dry mouth, and abdominal discomfort; patient should be supine during testing to minimize changes in blood pressure
Secretin *Secretin-Kabi*	Diagnosis of pancreatic exocrine disease or gastrinoma (Zollinger–Ellison syndrome) Aid in obtaining pancreatic cells for pathologic study	Hormone obtained from porcine duodenal mucosa that increases volume and bicarbonate content of pancreatic secretions; powder is dissolved in 10 mL sodium chloride injection and administered by slow IV injection (5 min) at a dose of 1 U–2 U/kg; samples are collected with a gastric tube and analyzed for volume, enzyme and bicarbonate content, occult blood, biliary pigment; *cautious use* in acute pancreatitis; frequently given with sincalide (see below)
Sermorelin *Geref*	Test for growth hormone secreting ability of the pituitary	Synthetic polypeptide equivalent to growth-hormone–releasing hormone; administered IV after an overnight fast; venous blood is sampled 15, 30, 45, and 60 min after injection; does *not* test for hypothalamic dysfunction as a cause of reduced GH secretion

(*continued*)

Table 80-3. **In Vivo Diagnostic Aids (Continued)**

Diagnostic Agent	*Uses*	*Nursing Considerations*
Sincalide *Kinevac*	To stimulate pancreatic or gallbladder secretions	Synthetic subunit of cholecystokinin that produces gallbladder contraction following IV injection; also enhances pancreatic secretions when given in combination with secretin; to contract gallbladder, 0.02 μg/kg is given by rapid (30–60 sec) IV injection, which may be repeated in 15 min at 0.04 μg/kg; for secretin–sincalide test of pancreatic function, 0.02 μg/kg is infused over a 30 min period beginning 30 min after the secretion infusion
Teriparatide *Parathar*	Differentiation of hypoparathyroidism from pseudohypoparathyroidism	Synthetic polypeptide hormone consisting of the 1–34 fragment of human parathyroid hormone; hypercalcemia may develop; systemic allergic reactions have occurred; does *not* discriminate between hypoparathyroidism and normal
Thyrotropin *Thytropar*	Differential diagnosis of thyroid failure and decreased thyroid reserve	Purified, lyophilized thyroid-stimulating hormone obtained from bovine anterior pituitary; increases iodine uptake by gland and formation and release of thyroid hormones; thyroid hyperplasia can occur; administered IM or SC (10 IU for 1–3 days), followed by radioiodine study 24 h after last dose; no response is indicative of thyroid failure; nausea, vomiting, headache, urticaria, tachycardia, and hypotension can occur, anaphylactic reactions have been reported; use *cautiously* in presence of coronary artery disease or heart disease
Tolbutamide Sodium *Orinase Diagnostic*	Diagnosis of pancreatic islet cell adenoma or diabetics	Patients with pancreatic cell insulinomas show a *sharp, intense* drop in blood glucose following IV injection of 1 g tolbutamide sodium; hypoglycemia may persist for several hours and may require treatment if symptoms are too intense; diabetic patients show a *gradual* decrease in blood glucose, whereas normal persons evidence a prompt reduction (15–20 min) associated with an elevation in serum insulin
D-Xylose *Xylo-Pfan*	Test for intestinal malabsorption states	Nonmetabolizable sugar given orally (25 g) to assess absorptive capacity of GI tract; normal values are 5–8 g in urine within 5 h and 40 mg/100 mL blood within 2 h

poses have been discussed in other chapters (eg, edrophonium for myasthenia gravis in Chapter 12; phentolamine for pheochromocytoma in Chapter 15; radioiodide 131 for thyroid function in Chapter 42) and are not considered here. Table 80-3 lists the important in vivo diagnostic drugs, together with their preparations, uses, and pertinent remarks. It should be recognized that the consideration given to the agents in this chapter is brief and is not intended to provide comprehensive information regarding their safe and effective use. Experienced personnel and proper facilities are necessary to derive maximum benefit from use of these diagnostic agents and to deal with any untoward reaction that may occur.

Radiographic Diagnostic Agents

With the exception of barium sulfate-containing products, the substances used for radiographic diagnostic procedures are principally iodine-containing compounds. These agents are opaque chemicals that are employed as contrast media to enhance visualization of internal structures by x-ray examination. Localization of a substance to the particular area to be visualized is accomplished either through direct instillation into an organ (eg, uterus, colon, bronchioles, spinal column) or by incorporation of the radiopaque drug into an organic compound whose properties determine its distribution in the body (eg, excretion by way of the bile or urine or plasma protein binding).

(*text continues on page 874*)

Table 80-4. **Barium-Containing Diagnostic Agents**

Suspension	
Baro-Cat	1.5%
Enecat	5%
Entrobar	50%
Epi-C	150%
Flo-Coat	100%
HD 85	85%
Liquid Barosperse	60%
Liquipake	100%
Prepcat	1.5%
Tomocat	5%
Powder for Suspension	
Baricon	98%
Barosperse	95%
HD 200 Plus	98%
Tonopaque	95%
Paste	
Anatrast	100%

Note: Additional barium-containing diagnostic agents available in Canada include Colobar DC, Colobar-400, Epi-C, Epistat 57, Epistat-61, Esobar, Esopho-Cat, E-Z-Cat, E-Z-HD, E-Z-Jug, E-Z-Paque, Gel-Unix, Liqui-Jug, Polibar, Readi-Cat, Recto-Barium, Ultra-R, Unibar-60.

Table 80-5. Iodinated Radiographic Diagnostic Agents

Trade Name	Dosage Form	Iodine Content	Composition	Diagnostic Uses
Amipaque	Injection	48.25%	13.5%, 18.75% metrizamide	Myelography Computed tomography (CT) of intracranial subarachnoid spaces Peripheral arteriography Pediatric angiocardiography
Angio-Conray	Injection	48%	80% iothalamate	Angiocardiography Aortography
Angiovist 282	Injection	28%	60% diatrizoate meglumine	Angiography Arthrography Cholangiography Discography Excretory urography Peripheral arteriography Pyelography Splenoportography Venography
Angiovist 292	Injection	29.2%	52% diatrizoate meglumine and 8% diatrizoate sodium	See Angiovist 282
Angiovist 370	Injection	37%	66% diatrizoate meglumine and 10% diatrizoate sodium	See Angiovist 282
Bilivist	Capsules	61.4%	500 mg ipodate sodium	Cholangiography Cholecystography
Bilopaque	Capsules	57.4%	750 mg tyropanoate sodium	Cholecystography
Cholebrine	Tablets	62%	750 mg iocetamic acid	Cholecystography
Cholografin	Injection	5.1%	10.3% iodipamide meglumine	Cholecystography Cholangiography
Cholografin	Injection	26%	52% iodipamide meglumine	Cholecystography Cholangiography
Conray	Injection	28.2%	60% iothalamate meglumine	Cerebral angiography Drip infusion pyelography Peripheral arteriography Urography Venography
Conray-30	Injection	14.1%	30% iothalamate meglumine	Infusion Urography
Conray-43	Injection	20.2%	43% iothalamate meglumine	Lower extremity venography
Conray-325	Injection	32.5%	54.3% iothalamate sodium	Excretory urography
Conray-400	Injection	40%	66.8% iothalamate sodium	Angiocardiography Aortography Excretory urography IV pyelography Renal arteriography
Cysto-Conray	Instillation solution	20.2%	43% iothalamate meglumine	Cystography Cystourethrography Retrograde pyelography
Cysto-Conray II	Instillation solution	8.1%	17.2% iothalamate meglumine	Cystography Cystourethrography Retrograde pyelography
Cystografin	Instillation solution	14.1%	30% diatrizoate meglumine	Cystourethrography Retrograde pyelography
Cystografin-Dilute	Instillation solution	8.5%	18% diatrizoate meglumine	Retrograde cystourethrography
Diatrizoate-60	Injection	29.2%	52% diatrizoate meglumine and 8% diatrizoate sodium	See Angiovist 282, above Computed tomography (CT)
Diatrizoate meglumine 76%	Injection	35.8%	76% diatrizoate meglumine	Aortography Excretory urography Pediatric angiocardiography Peripheral arteriography
Ethiodol	Injection	37%	Ethiodized oil	Hysterosalpingography Lymphography

(continued)

Table 80-5. Iodinated Radiographic Diagnostic Agents (Continued)

Trade Name	Dosage Form	Iodine Content	Composition	Diagnostic Uses
Gastrografin	Oral/rectal solution	37%	66% diatrizoate meglumine and 10% diatrizoate sodium	GI radiography
Hexabrix	Injection	32%	39.3% ioxaglate meglumine and 19.6% ioxaglate sodium	Cerebral angiography Coronary arteriography Peripheral arteriography Visceral arteriography Digital angiography Peripheral venography Excretory urography Computed tomography (CT)
Hypaque 20%	Instillation solution	12%	20% diatrizoate sodium	Retrograde pyelography
Hypaque 25%	Injection	15%	25% diatrizoate sodium	Drip-infusion pyelography (excretory urography)
Hypaque 50%	Injection	30%	50% diatrizoate sodium	Angiography (cerebral and peripheral) Aortography Cholangiography Hysterosalpingography Intraosseous venography Splenoportography
Hypaque-M 75%	Injection	38.5%	50% diatrizoate meglumine and 25% diatrizoate sodium	Abdominal aortography Angiocardiography Arteriography (coronary, peripheral, and renal) Urography
Hypaque-M 90%	Injection	46.2%	60% diatrizoate meglumine and 30% diatrizoate sodium	Abdominal aortography Angiocardiography Arteriography (coronary and peripheral) Hysterosalpingography Urography
Hypaque-Cysto	Instillation solution	14.1%	30% diatrizoate meglumine	Retrograde cystourethrography
Hypaque Meglumine 30%	Injection	14.1%	30% diatrizoate meglumine	Infusion urography Computed tomography (CT)
Hypaque Meglumine 60%	Injection	28.2%	60% diatrizoate meglumine	Arthrography Cerebral angiography Cholangiography Discography Excretory urography Peripheral arteriography and venography Splenoportography
Hypaque Sodium	Liquid	24.9%	2.4 g diatrizoate sodium/mL	GI radiography
Hypaque Sodium	Powder for oral solution	59.8%		GI radiography
Hypaque-76	Injection	37%	66% diatrizoate meglumine and 10% diatrizoate sodium	See Angiovist 282, above
Isovue 300	Injection	30%	61% iopamidol	Angiography Arteriography IV contrast enhancement
Isovue 370	Injection	37%	75.5% iopamidol	See Isovue 300, above
Isovue-M 200	Injection	20%	40.8% iopamidol	Contrast enhancement Intrathecal neuroradiology Ventriculography
Isovue-M 300	Injection	30%	61.2% iopamidol	See Isovue-M 200, above
MD-60	Injection	29.2%	52% diatrizoate meglumine and 8% diatrizoate sodium	See Angiovist 282, above
MD-76	Injection	37%	66% diatrizoate meglumine and 10% diatrizoate sodium	See Angiovist 282, above
MD-Gastroview	Oral/rectal solution	37%	66% diatrizoate meglumine and 10% diatrizoate sodium	See Angiovist 282, above

(*continued*)

Table 80-5. **Iodinated Radiographic Diagnostic Agents (Continued)**

Trade Name	*Dosage Form*	*Iodine Content*	*Composition*	*Diagnostic Uses*
Optiray 160	Injection	16%	34% Ioversol	Angiography
Optiray 240	Injection	24%	51% Ioversol	Angiography Venography
Optiray 320	Injection	32%	68% Ioversol	Angiography Arteriography Aortography Computed tomography (CT) Urography
Omnipaque	Injection		Iohexol equivalent to 18%, 24%, 30%, or 35% iodine	Intrathecal or intravascular radiography
Oragrafin Calcium	Granules for oral suspension	61.7%	3 g ipodate calcium/8-g packet	Cholangiography Cholecystography
Oragrafin Sodium	Capsules	61.4%	500 mg ipodate sodium	Cholecystography
Renografin-60	Injection	29%	52% diatrizoate meglumine and 8% diatrizoate sodium	Arthrography Cerebral angiography Cholangiography Computed tomography (CT) Discography Excretory urography Peripheral arteriography Pyelography Splenoportography Venography
Renografin-76	Injection	37%	66% diatrizoate meglumine and 10% diatrizoate sodium	See Renografin-60, above
Reno-M-30	Instillation solution	14%	30% diatrizoate meglumine	Retrograde or ascending pyelography
Reno-M-60	Injection	28%	60% diatrizoate meglumine	Arthrography Cerebral angiography Cholangiography Discography Excretory urography Peripheral arteriography Pyelography Splenoportography Venography
Reno-M-Dip	Injection	14%	30% diatrizoate meglumine	Computed tomography (CT) Drip-infusion pyelography
Renovist	Injection	37%	34.3% diatrizoate meglumine and 35% diatrizoate sodium	Angiocardiography Aortography Excretory urography Peripheral arteriography and venography Venocavography
Renovist II	Injection	31%	28.5% diatrizoate meglumine and 29.1% diatrizoate sodium	See Renovist, above
Renovue-65	Injection	30%	65% iodamide meglumine	Excretory urography
Renovue-Dip	Injection	11.1%	24% iodamide meglumine	Excretory urography
Sinografin	Injection	38%	52.7% diatrizoate meglumine and 26.8% iodipamide meglumine	Hysterosalpingography
Telepaque	Tablets	66.7%	500 mg iopanoic acid	Cholecystography
Urovist Cysto	Instillation solution	14.1%	30% diatrizoate meglumine	Cystourethrography Retrograde pyelography
Urovist Meglumine DIU/CT	Injection	14.1%	30% diatrizoate meglumine	Drip-infusion pyelography Computed tomography (CT) Venography
Urovist Sodium 300	Injection	30%	50% diatrizoate sodium	See Hypaque 50%, above
Vascoray	Injection	40%	52% iothalamate meglumine and 26% iothalamate sodium	Angiocardiography Aortography Arteriography (coronary and renal) Excretory urography

In addition to barium and the iodine-containing compounds, other substances used as radiolabeled agents for diagnostic purposes (with their uses in parentheses) include chromium (red cell volume), cobalt (B_{12} absorption), gadopentetate dimeglumine (magnetic resonance imaging [MRI] for intracranial or spinal visualization), mercury (kidney function), polyvinyl chloride (GI tract), and technetium and phosphorus (brain tumors).

Barium Sulfate

Barium sulfate is the most commonly used substance for visualization of the GI tract. It is a highly insoluble compound; thus, only minimal amounts are absorbed systemically, and toxicity is quite low. Barium sulfate can be administered orally as a thick paste for examination of the esophagus or as a more dilute suspension for visualization of the stomach and upper intestinal tract. Radiographic studies of the lower GI tract and colon may be performed after a cleansing enema and rectal instillation of barium sulfate suspension. Barium sulfate may be constipating, and complete expulsion of the suspension from the GI tract after the examination usually requires use of a laxative or an enema. The barium-containing diagnostic agents are listed in Table 80-4.

Iodinated Radiopaque Agents

A variety of iodine-containing organic compounds can be used either orally or parenterally to visualize a number of different body organs. The opacity of these agents depends on the percentage of iodine in the molecule and the amount of drug concentrated at a particular site. Patients should be questioned concerning iodine hypersensitivity before administration of one of these compounds. Severe, *sometimes fatal*, allergic reactions have occurred with use of these agents, and patients with a history of bronchial asthma or other allergies must be closely monitored during administration and for at least 1 hour afterward. Appropriate antidotal measures, including respiratory aids, epinephrine, and corticosteroids, should be available.

Adverse reactions are uncommon, but the possibility of their occurrence must not be overlooked. Among the untoward reactions reported with use of radiographic contrast media are urticaria, wheezing, dyspnea, angioneurotic edema, laryngeal spasm, anaphylaxis, hyperthermia, headache, chest tightness, and tremor. Reactions that are probably attributable to volume, speed, and site of injection are flushing, dizziness, nausea, generalized vasodilation, and hypotension. Pain and irritation at the injection site have been noted, as well as paresthesias, numbness, hematomas, ecchymoses, and thrombophlebitis.

The iodinated radiographic contrast agents are listed in Table 80-5. Their dosage forms, iodine content, composition, and diagnostic uses are given as well. Because their dosage and route of administration depend on their diagnostic intent, the information included with each drug must be consulted before administration.

An adjunctive drug that is sometimes used in lymphography to facilitate visualization of the lymphatic system is isosulfan blue (Lymphazurin 1%). After subcutaneous injection of 0.5 mL into three interdigital spaces of each extremity per study, isosulfan is selectively concentrated in the lymphatic vessels, which it colors a bright blue. Adverse reactions are relatively infrequent (1%–2%) and are largely of an allergic nature, ranging from itching and swelling of the hands to generalized edema and respiratory distress in rare instances.

Another adjunctive agent that is used in certain radiographic studies is potassium perchlorate (Perchloracap). This agent provides perchlorate ion (ClO_4), which suppresses accumulation of pertechnetate ion ($CTcO_4$) in the choroid plexus and salivary and thyroid glands of patients receiving radioactive sodium pertechnetate (^{99m}Tc) for brain imaging or placenta localization. Perchlorate competes for plasma protein-binding sites with TcO_4, with a resultant shift of a portion of TcO_4 from the plasma to the red blood cell. The drug is given orally as capsules in a dose of 200 to 400 mg 30 to 60 minutes before a dose of sodium pertechnetate.

Selected Bibliography

Chard T: Pregnancy tests: A review. Hum Reprod 7:701, 1992
Collins WP: Early pregnancy tests. Br J Obstet Gynaecol 97:204, 1990
Davidud J et al: Reliability and feasibility of pregnancy home-use tests: Laboratory validation and diagnostic evaluation by 638 volunteers. Clin Chem 39:53, 1993
Greegor DH: Screening for colorectal cancer: The accuracy of fecal occult blood. J Am Med Assoc 270:451, 1993
Kestel F: Using blood glucose meters: What you and your patient need to know. Nursing 23:34, 1993
Lance P: Fecal occult blood tests: What's new? Gastroenterology 104: 1852, 1993
Lopez M, Fleisher T, deShazo RD: Use and interpretation of diagnostic immunologic laboratory tests. J Am Med Assoc 268:2970, 1992
Tomky DM, Clarke DH: A comparison of user accuracy, techniques, and learning time of various systems for self blood glucose monitoring. Diabet Educ 16:483, 1990
Virella G: Diagnostic immunology. Immunol Series 58:251, 1993
Winawer SJ: Colorectal cancer screening comes of age. N Engl J Med 328:1416, 1993

Nursing Bibliography

Baxter A: Management of adverse reactions to iodinated contrast media. Applied Radiology (Suppl):9, 1993
Boutotte J: TB the second time around . . . and how you can help to control it. Nursing '93 23(5):42, 1993
Lavin J: Anergy testing—a vital weapon. RN 56(9):31–33, 1993
Use "two step" testing to take another look at negative skin test results. Hospital Employee Health 12(2):22, 1993
White D: Diagnostic imaging. PT—Magazine of Physical Therapy June: 62, 1993

81

Miscellaneous Drug Products

- Adenosine
- Alglucerase
- Alprostadil
- Antidotes
- Binding–Chelating Agents
- Botulinum Toxin Type A
- Bromocriptine
- Capsaicin
- Dimethyl Sulfoxide
- Disulfiram
- Enzyme Preparations
- Flavoxate
- Gallium Nitrate
- Hemin
- Mesalamine
- Octreotide
- Olsalazine
- Pegademase
- Perfluorochemical Emulsion
- Plasma Expanders
- Plasma Protein Fractions
- Sclerosing Agents
- Sumatriptan
- Tiopronin
- Yohimbine

Several pharmacologic agents do not fall into one of the previously discussed categories of drugs and thus are reviewed here under a miscellaneous heading.

• Adenosine Phosphate

Cobalasine, Kaysine

Adenosine phosphate injection (25 mg/mL) is used for symptomatic relief of varicose vein complications accompanying stasis dermatitis. It has also been used experimentally in treating herpes infections. In addition, adenosine, as Adenocard injection (6 mg/2 mL) has been used to convert sinus rhythm to normal in paroxysmal supraventricular tachycardia, and this indication is considered in Chapter 32.

In stasis dermatitis, the drug is administered IM at a dose of 25 to 50 mg once or twice daily until symptoms have abated. Maintenance doses are 25 mg two to three times a week. Side effects usually include flushing, dizziness, and palpitations, because the drug is a vasodilator. Adenosine is contraindicated in patients with a history of myocardial infarction.

• Alglucerase

Ceredase

Alglucerase is used in the treatment of Gaucher's disease, which is characterized by a deficiency of the enzyme beta-glucocerebrosidase, resulting in accumulation of lipid glucocerebroside in macrophages, which become enlarged and are termed Gaucher's cells. This can lead to enlargement of the liver and spleen, severe anemia, thrombocytopenia, and osteonecrosis with resultant fractures, a characteristic feature of Gaucher's disease.

Mechanism

A modified form of the enzyme beta-glucocerebrosidase, alglucerase catalyzes the hydrolysis of glucocerebroside to glucose, thus replacing the deficient endogenous enzymatic activity. The drug reduces the size of the enlarged liver and spleen, usually within 6 months, and improves the hematologic picture by increasing hemoglobin, hematocrit, and erythrocyte and platelet counts.

Uses

Provides enzyme replacement therapy for patients with type 1 Gaucher disease, who exhibit one or more of the following symptoms: severe anemia, thrombocytopenia, bone disease, or significant hepatomegaly or splenomegaly.

Dosage

60 U/kg by slow intravenous (IV) infusion over 1 to 2 hours, usually once every 2 weeks. Dosage may be adjusted downward at intervals of 3 to 6 months as patient response dictates.

Significant Adverse Reactions

Burning and swelling at injection site, fever, chills, nausea, abdominal discomfort.

Nursing Management

Pretherapy Assessment

Assess and record baseline data necessary for detection of adverse effects of alglucerase: General: vital signs (VS), body weight, skin color and temperature.

Review medical history and documents for existing or previous conditions that:

a. require cautious use of alglucerase: breast-feeding.
b. contraindicate use of alglucerase: allergy to alglucerase, **pregnancy (Category C)**.

Nursing Interventions

Medication Administration

Administer by slow infusion over 1 to 2 hours.

Medication should not be shaken, should be stored at 2° to 8°C, and visually inspected for particulate matter and discoloration.

Surveillance During Therapy

Monitor for adverse effects, toxicity, and interactions.

Monitor for signs of hypersensitivity, which may require discontinuation of drug.

Interpret results of diagnostic tests and contact practitioner as appropriate.

• Alprostadil

Prostin VR Pediatric

Alprostadil (prostaglandin E_1) is a solution for IV infusion that is used in neonates with congenital heart defects temporarily to maintain the patency of the ductus arteriosus until corrective surgery can be performed.

Mechanism

Relaxes smooth muscle of the ductus arteriosus, thereby providing for adequate blood oxygenation. Other actions of prostaglandin E_1 include vasodilation, increased tone of intestinal and uterine smooth muscle, and inhibition of platelet aggregation.

Uses

Palliative therapy of neonates with congenital heart defects (eg, pulmonary stenosis, tricuspid atresia, tetralogy of Fallot, aortic coarctation) to maintain patency until corrective surgery can be performed.

Dosage

Initially, 0.1 μg/kg/min until improvement is noted; reduce infusion rate to lowest dose that maintains the response (0.01–0.05 μg/kg/min); maximum dose, 0.4 μg/kg/min.

Fate

Rapidly metabolized on first-pass through the lungs; metabolites are excreted primarily by the kidneys; does not appear to be retained in body tissue.

Common Side Effects

Fever, apnea, flushing, bradycardia, hypotension.

Significant Adverse Reactions

CV: tachycardia, edema, second-degree heart block, hyperemia, shock, congestive heart failure, ventricular fibrillation, cardiac arrest
CNS: seizures, hyperirritability, lethargy, hypothermia, cerebral bleeding, hyperextension of the neck
Hematologic: disseminated intravascular coagulation, anemia, thrombocytopenia, bleeding
GI: diarrhea, regurgitation, hyperbilirubinemia
Respiratory: wheezing, hypercapnia, respiratory depression
Other: anuria, hematuria, sepsis, peritonitis, hypokalemia, hypoglycemia, cortical proliferation of long bones

Contraindications

Respiratory distress syndrome (hyaline membrane disease). *Cautious use* in neonates with bleeding tendencies, because drug inhibits platelet aggregation.

Nursing Management

Pretherapy Assessment

Assess and record baseline data necessary for detection of adverse effects of alprostadil: General: VS, body weight, skin color and temperature, cyanosis, skeletal development; CNS: reflexes, state of agitation; Cardiovascular system (CVS): arterial pressure, peripheral perfusion; Respiratory system: adventitious sounds; Laboratory: bleeding times, arterial blood gases, blood pH.

Review medical history and documents for existing or previous conditions that:

a. require cautious use of alprostadil: neonates with bleeding tendencies.
b. contraindicate use of alprostadil: allergy to alprostadil; respiratory distress syndrome (hyaline membrane disease).

Nursing Interventions

Medication Administration

Prepare fresh solutions for administration by pump delivery system with sodium chloride injection or dextrose injection every 24 hours.

Surveillance During Therapy

Always monitor the drug dose being administered.

Monitor respiratory status closely during infusion, and always have respiratory assistance immediately available because apnea occurs in 10% to 20% of neonates treated with alprostadil, most often in those weighing less than 2 kg at birth.

Assess for indications of overdosage (eg, bradycardia, apnea, flushing, pyrexia). Infusion should be discontinued if these occur, then cautiously reinitiated when they subside.

Expect drug to be infused at lowest dose and for shortest time that will produce desired effect.

Monitor arterial pressure during drug administration. Perfusion rate should be reduced if pressure falls significantly.

Monitor results of blood oxygenation determinations in infants with decreased pulmonary flow and systemic blood pressure, and results of blood pH determinations in infants with compromised systemic blood flow.

Monitor for signs of hypersensitivity, which may require discontinuation of drug.

Monitor diagnostic test results obtained over the course of therapy.

Interpret results of diagnostic tests and contact practitioner as appropriate.

Monitor for possible drug–laboratory test interactions.

Monitor for possible drug–drug and drug–nutrient interactions.

Patient Teaching

Instruct patient or significant others about expected actions and possible adverse effects of prescribed drug.

Antidotes

Most drugs used as specific antidotes (eg, acetylcysteine, digoxin immune FAB, leucovorin, naloxone, physostigmine, pralidoxime, protamine sulfate, vitamin K) have been considered previously in the individual chapters dealing with the pharmacologic agents that they specifically antagonize. Certain other drugs are also useful as antidotes for specific types of poisonings, and are reviewed in the following sections.

• *Activated Charcoal*

Actidose-Aqua, Actidose with Sorbitol, Charcoaid, Liqui-Char

(CAN) InstaChar, Charcodote

Activated charcoal is a carbon residue that has a very large surface area owing to its fine, network-like structure, thus providing great adsorptive capacity per unit of weight. The amount of drug or other substance that can be adsorbed by activated charcoal is approximately 100 to 1000 mg/g of charcoal. The drug is used as a powder or liquid suspension for the emergency treatment of poisoning by most drugs and chemicals *except* cyanide, alkalis, and mineral acids. It is also largely ineffective against poisoning with ethanol, methanol, and iron salts.

The initial dosage is 1 g/kg or approximately 5 to 10 times the amount of poison ingested. The charcoal powder is given as a suspension in 6 to 8 oz of water, as soon as possible after the poisoning. Although the black solution does not appear palatable, it is odorless and tasteless. Either constipation or diarrhea may occur, and the stools will be blackened. The preparation may be mixed with sweet syrup to enhance palatability. Emesis should be induced if possible before administration of charcoal except in cases of poisoning with strong acids or alkalis, petroleum distillates, or other caustic substances. Concurrent use of syrup of ipecac or laxatives with charcoal should be avoided because charcoal can adsorb and inactivate these agents as well.

• *Sodium Thiosulfate*

Sodium thiosulfate, as an injection containing either 1 or 2.5 g/10 mL may be used either alone or in combination with sodium nitrite in treating cyanide toxicity. Sodium thiosulfate supplies an exogenous source of sulfur, which accelerates the activity of the rhodanase enzyme system responsible for the conversion of cyanide to the nontoxic thiocyanate ion. After administration of 300 mg sodium nitrite IV, 12.5 g of sodium thiosulfate is given by slow IV injection over 10 minutes. Both drugs may be repeated at one-half the dose if necessary. The half-life of sodium thiosulfate is approximately 30 minutes, and it is excreted unchanged in the urine.

• *Heavy Metal Antagonists*

Deferoxamine mesylate
Dimercaprol
Edetate calcium disodium

Several drugs have the ability to complex with various heavy metals (such as iron, lead, gold, mercury) and are used to treat poisoning with these substances. Such poisoning can occur either from drug overdosage—for example, with use of gold salts for rheumatoid arthritis or iron for severe anemias—or from accidental ingestion of substances such as lead-containing paints, insecticides, or pesticides. Heavy metal intoxication often impairs enzymatic function, and, if severe, impairment can lead to cellular anoxia and possibly death.

Table 81-1 lists the heavy metal antagonists, together with their indications, dosages, and nursing considerations.

Binding–Chelating Agents

Drugs capable of binding or chelating other substances, such as metals, are useful in treating certain diseases characterized by excessive body levels of these substances. One such drug, penicillamine, is an effective copper chelating agent useful in treating Wilson's disease and also in the symptomatic management of rheumatoid arthritis. It is reviewed in detail with other antiinflammatory drugs in Chapter 21. Three other binding–chelating drugs, trientine (which binds copper), succimer (which binds lead), and cellulose sodium phosphate (which binds calcium) are considered here.

• *Trientine*

Syprine

Mechanism

Removes excess copper from the body by chemically complexing with the metal.

Uses

Treatment of patients with Wilson's disease who are intolerant of penicillamine, which is normally the drug of choice.

CAUTION

Unlike penicillamine, trientine is *not* recommended for use in cystinuria, rheumatoid arthritis, or biliary cirrhosis.

Dosage

Adults: 750 to 1250 mg orally in 2 to 4 divided doses (maximum dose is 2 g/day)
Children: 500 to 750 mg orally in 2 to 4 divided doses (maximum dose is 1500 mg/day)

Average duration of therapy is 4 years.

Significant Adverse Reactions

Iron deficiency, dermatitis, heartburn, epigastric distress, malaise, anorexia, cramps, muscle pain or weakness, and systemic lupus-like symptoms.

Contraindications

Cystinuria, rheumatoid arthritis, or biliary cirrhosis. *Cautious use* in people with iron deficiency or systemic lupus erythematosus, and in pregnant or nursing women.

Interactions

Concurrent administration of mineral supplements and trientine may retard the absorption of each.

Nursing Management

Pretherapy Assessment

Assess and record baseline data necessary for detection of adverse effects of trientine: General: VS, body weight, skin color and temperature; Respiratory system: adventitious sounds; Laboratory: complete blood count (CBC), hemoglobin, antinuclear antibody titer, serum and 24-hour urine copper levels.

Table 81-1. **Heavy Metal Antidotes**

Drug	*Indications*	*Usual Dosage Range*	*Nursing Considerations*
Deferoxamine Mesylate *Desferal*	Acute iron intoxication Chronic iron overload (eg, multiple transfusions) Management of aluminum accumulation in bone in renal failure (investigational use)	*Acute intoxication* 1 g IM, followed by 0.5 g every 4 h for 2 doses, then every 4–12 h as needed IV infusion: same as IM dose at rate of 15 mg/kg/h *Chronic overload* IM: 0.5–1 g/day IV: 2 g at a rate of 15 mg/kg/h SC: 1–2 g/day over 8 to 24 h with a mini-infusion pump *Children*: 50 mg/kg IM *or* IV every 6 h or up to 15 mg/kg/h by IV infusion	Chelates iron in the ferric state, forming a stable, water-soluble, readily excretable complex; no effect on electrolyte or trace metal excretion; *contraindicated* in severe renal disease; should be used in conjunction with other appropriate antidotal measures (emesis, lavage, correction of acidosis, control of shock, respiratory assistance); pain on injection, allergic reactions, blurred vision, diarrhea, abdominal pain, tachycardias, and fever have been reported; urine may be colored red; use an infusion pump to control drip rate and monitor blood pressure every 5 min until stable; too-rapid infusion can cause hypotension, urticaria, erythema, and shock
Dimercaprol-BAL *Bal in Oil*	Arsenic, gold and mercury poisoning Acute lead poisoning (in combination with calcium EDTA)	*IM only* Arsenic/gold poisoning: 2.5–3 mg/kg 4 to 6 times a day for 2 d, then 2 to 4 times a day on the third day, then 1 to 2 times a day for 10 d Mercury poisoning: 5 mg/kg initially, then 2.5 mg/kg 1 to 2 times a day for 10 d Lead poisoning: 4 mg/kg at 4-h intervals in combination with calcium sodium EDTA at a different site	Complexes with a number of heavy metals forming stable, water-soluble chelates that are readily excreted by the kidney; sulfhydryl enzymes are thus protected from the toxic action of the metals; do *not* use in iron, cadmium, or selenium poisoning because resultant complexes are more toxic than the metals; most effective when given as soon as possible after metal ingestion; urine should be kept alkaline to minimize kidney damage as chelate is being excreted; local pain is frequent at site of injection; *contraindicated* in hepatic insufficiency; large doses may increase blood pressure and heart rate; other adverse effects include fever in children (30% frequency), nausea, vomiting, headache, burning in the mouth and throat, chest constriction, lacrimation, salivation, and paresthesias; other supportive measures are necessary (fluids, electrolytes, respiratory assistance)
Edetate Calcium Disodium–Calcium EDTA *Calcium Disodium Versenate*	Acute and chronic lead poisoning and lead encephalopathy	IV: 1 g diluted to 250–500 mL and infused over 1 h; administer twice a day for up to 5 d, stop 2 d, then resume for another 5 d if necessary IM (preferred in children): 50–75 mg/kg/d in 2 equally divided doses for 3 to 5 d	Calcium in the compound is displaced by a heavy metal (eg, lead), resulting in formation of a stable metal-drug complex that is removed by the kidneys—potentially a very toxic compound; recommended dosage levels should not be exceeded; do *not* infuse rapidly in patients with lead encephalopathy; increased intracranial pressure can be fatal; IM is the preferred route of administration; procaine should be added to the solution to reduce pain on injection; closely monitor renal function; do *not* give to patients with impaired kidney function; refer to package instructions for mixing and administering directions; *Edetate disodium* injection (Disotate, Endrate) is also available and is indicated for emergency treatment of hypercalcemia and control of ventricular arrhythmias associated with digoxin toxicity

EDTA, ethylenediaminetetraacetic acid.

Review medical history and documents for existing or previous conditions that:

a. require cautious use of trientine: pregnancy, breastfeeding; iron deficiency; systemic lupus erythematosus.
b. contraindicate use of trientine: allergy to trientine; cystinuria, rheumatoid arthritis, or biliary cirrhosis; **pregnancy (Category C)**.

Nursing Interventions

Medication Administration

Administer on an empty stomach 1 hour before or 2 hours after meals.

Ensure that patient swallows capsule whole with water.

Carefully wash any area that comes into contact with capsules because of risk of contact dermatitis.

Surveillance During Therapy

Monitor for toxicity and interactions.

Monitor results of serum copper levels, CBC with differentials, and urinalyses, which should be performed before initiating therapy and regularly thereafter. Changes in copper level indicate drug effectiveness. Decrease in hemoglobin or hematocrit may indicate iron deficiency anemia, in which case iron supplements may be required. Appearance of urinary protein or casts may indicate early drug-induced renal changes.

Monitor for signs of hypersensitivity, which may require discontinuation of drug.

Interpret results of diagnostic tests and contact practitioner as appropriate.

Patient Teaching

Instruct patient to take drug at least 1 hour before or after taking any other drugs or food. If epigastric distress occurs, as it often does, instruct patient to consult drug prescriber.

Teach patient how to recognize and immediately report systemic lupus-like symptoms (eg, malaise, anorexia, arthralgia, fever, decreased urinary output) because drug may need to be discontinued.

Encourage patient to eat iron-rich foods, including red meats, dark green vegetables, egg yolks, whole grains, legumes, raisins, prunes, brewer's yeast, and nuts. Collaborate with dietitian or refer patient for assistance as indicated.

• Succimer

Chemet

Mechanism

Forms water-soluble chelates with lead, increasing its urinary excretion; zinc excretion is also increased; no significant effect on urinary elimination of iron, calcium, or magnesium.

Uses

Treatment of lead poisoning in children with blood level greater than 45 μg/dL.

Treatment of poisonings with mercury and arsenic (investigational use only)

Dosage

Initially, 10 mg/kg orally every 8 hours for 5 days; reduce to 10 mg/kg every 12 hours for an additional 2 weeks. Repeated courses of therapy may be needed; allow at least 2 weeks between courses of therapy.

Fate

Oral absorption is rapid; peak plasma levels occur between 1 and 2 hours. Approximately half the dose is excreted, largely in the feces; the elimination half-life is 2 days.

Common Side Effects

GI distress, loose stools, anorexia, metallic taste, chills, rash, flu-like symptoms, headache, drowsiness, elevated serum aminotransferases.

Significant Adverse Reactions

Increased serum cholesterol, dizziness, paresthesias, backache, monilial infections, cloudy vision.

Contraindications

Cautious use in patients with liver or kidney disease, and a history of allergic reactions.

Interactions

Succimer may interfere with serum and urinary laboratory tests.

• Cellulose Sodium Phosphate

Calcibind

Mechanism

Binds calcium by an ion-exchange mechanism; the complex of calcium and cellulose phosphate is then excreted in the feces; also binds dietary magnesium and may increase urinary phosphorus and oxalate; no apparent alteration in serum levels of copper, zinc, or iron.

Uses

Treatment of absorptive hypercalciuria type 1 with recurrent calcium oxalate or calcium phosphate nephrolithiasis.

Dosage

Initially, 5 g orally with each meal. When urinary calcium declines to less than 150 mg/day, reduce dosage to 10 g/day in three divided doses.

Significant Adverse Reactions

Diarrhea, dyspepsia, loose bowels, bad taste in mouth.

Contraindications

Primary or secondary hyperparathyroidism, hypocalcemia, hypomagnesemia, osteomalacia, osteoporosis. *Cautious use* in patients with congestive heart failure or ascites (sodium content of drug is high), and in pregnant women and in children.

Nursing Management

Pretherapy Assessment

Assess and record baseline data necessary for detection of adverse effects of cellulose sodium phosphate: General: VS, body weight, skin color and temperature; GI: bowel sounds, output.

Review medical history and documents for existing or previous conditions that:

a. require cautious use of cellulose sodium phosphate: congestive heart failure or ascites (sodium content of drug is high); in pregnant women and in children.
b. contraindicate use of cellulose sodium phosphate: primary or secondary hyperparathyroidism, hypocalcemia, hypomagnesemia, osteomalacia, osteoporosis.

Nursing Interventions

Medication Administration

Administer oral form of drug with meals.

Ensure adequate fluid intake.

Surveillance During Therapy

Monitor for adverse effects and toxicity.

Monitor intake and output, and encourage fluid intake to maintain urinary output of at least 2000 mL/day.

Monitor results of periodic determinations of serum magnesium and parathyroid hormone, serum and urinary calcium and oxalate, and CBC to detect drug effects. Urinary calcium and oxalate levels reflect responsiveness to therapy.

Collaborate with dietitian, drug prescriber, and patient to develop acceptable dietary plan as adjunct to drug

therapy. Restriction of sodium, calcium, oxalate, and ascorbic acid increases drug's effectiveness.
Interpret results of diagnostic tests and contact practitioner as appropriate.
Monitor for possible drug–laboratory test interactions.
Monitor for possible drug–drug and drug–nutrient interactions.

Patient Teaching

Instruct patient that the prescribed drug is to be taken for the condition for which it is prescribed and not to be be used to treat any other infections.
Explain that powder may be mixed with full glass of water, fruit juice, or soft drink. It is not very palatable.
Ensure that patient understands need to take drug with meals or at least within 30 minutes of a meal. Otherwise, it is ineffective.
Explain that oral magnesium supplementation, which should be administered to prevent hypomagnesemia, can be taken any time so long as it is at least 1 hour before or after cellulose sodium phosphate administration to avoid binding magnesium.
Verify that patient understands dietary plan. Refer patient for additional instruction as necessary.

• Botulinum Toxin Type A

Botox

Botulinum toxin type A is a sterile, lyophilized form of purified botulinum toxin that is intended for injection into the extraocular muscles of the eye for the treatment of strabismus and blepharospasm associated with dystonia or nerve disorders in patients older than 12 years of age. Botulinum toxin blocks neuromuscular conduction by binding to receptor sites on nerve terminals, inhibiting release of acetylcholine. This effect is useful in reducing the excessive contractions associated with blepharospasm. The drug has been used experimentally for other dystonias as well as head and neck spasms. The most common side effects are ptosis, drying of the eye, photophobia, and altered vision. Dosing requirements must be followed closely and the drug administered by personnel skilled in the treatment of ocular diseases. Cautious use of botulinum toxin must be undertaken in patients receiving aminoglycosides or other drugs that exert a neuromuscular blocking action (see Chapter 17).

• Bromocriptine

Parlodel

An ergot derivative exhibiting dopamine agonist activity, bromocriptine markedly reduces secretion of prolactin with minimal effects on other pituitary hormones. It is used for treating amenorrhea and galactorrhea resulting from hyperprolactinemia and as adjunctive therapy in treating Parkinson's disease (see Chapter 28).

Mechanism

Activates postsynaptic dopamine receptors in the tuberoinfundibular dopaminergic neuronal system, resulting in secretion of prolactin inhibitory factor from the hypothalamus; prolactin inhibitory factor blocks liberation of prolactin from the anterior pituitary in patients with hyperprolactinemia; also stimulates dopamine receptors in the corpus striatum, thus relieving some of the symptoms of parkinsonism.

Uses

Short-term treatment of amenorrhea–galactorrhea associated with hyperprolactinemia, except where a demonstrable pituitary tumor is present (not indicated in patients with normal prolactin levels)
Treatment of female infertility associated with hyperprolactinemia
Adjunctive treatment of parkinsonism (see Chapter 28)
Treatment of acromegaly, either alone or in conjunction with pituitary irradiation or surgery
Investigational uses include treatment of pituitary adenomas (to reduce elevated prolactin levels), neuroleptic malignant syndrome, and cocaine addiction

Dosage

Amenorrhea–galactorrhea: 1.25 to 2.5 mg daily; increase by 2.5 mg every 3 to 7 days; usual dosage range 5 to 7.5 mg/day
Treatment of infertility: initially 2.5 mg once daily; increase to two to three times a day within the first week
Parkinsonism: initially 1.25 mg twice daily; increase every 2 to 4 weeks by 2.5 mg/day as necessary
Acromegaly: initially, 1.25 to 2.5 mg daily; increase gradually every 3 to 7 days until optimal response; usual dosage range is 20 to 30 mg daily

See Chapter 28 for additional information and Nursing Management.

• Capsaicin

Zostrix

Capsaicin is a plant extract that is believed to render skin insensitive to pain on topical application. Its precise mechanism of action is not completely understood, but the drug appears to deplete substance P in peripheral sensory nerve endings. Substance P is believed to be a neurotransmitter in afferent spinal cord sensory pathways that mediate pain. Capsaicin cream is available in two strengths (0.025%, 0.075%) and is indicated for temporary alleviation of pain associated with arthritis and neuralgias, such as shingles or diabetic neuropathy. It is also being investigated for use in intractable pruritus, postamputation pain ("phantom limb syndrome"), and reflex sympathetic dystrophy. The cream is applied three to four times a day, and optimal response is usually achieved within 14 to 28 days. Topical application can elicit a warm or burning sensation, which may be intensified by bathing. This burning sensation occurs more often when the drug is applied less than three or four times a day and diminishes with repeated use. Contact with the eyes or broken or irritated skin should be avoided.

• Dimethyl Sulfoxide

Rimso-50

(CAN) Kemsol

Dimethyl sulfoxide (DMSO) is a clear, colorless solvent possessing a wide range of pharmacologic actions; however, because the compound has not been adequately tested and its potential toxicity is rather high, its clinical applications are limited. DMSO is approved for use as a bladder irrigant for the treatment of interstitial cystitis, but has been used experimentally by topical application for treatment of musculoskeletal disorders and collagen diseases. The drug can also serve as a vehicle to enhance percutaneous absorption of other drugs, and has been reported to possess diuretic, local anesthetic, vasodilatory, muscle-relaxant, and bacteriostatic activity, although data to support these latter claims are insufficient. Principal adverse effects are a garlic-like odor on the breath and skin, topical irritation, and allergic reactions due to histamine release. Ocular disturbances have been noted in experimental animals. The following discussion is limited to the use of DMSO as a bladder irrigant. Its topical application should be discouraged until the efficacy and safety of the drug have been conclusively established.

Mechanism

Not established; appears to exert antiinflammatory, local anesthetic, diuretic, muscle-relaxing, vasodilatory, and bacteriostatic activity.

Uses

Symptomatic treatment of interstitial cystitis

Investigational uses include topical treatment of a variety of musculoskeletal disorders and enhancement of the percutaneous absorption of other drugs

Dosage

Instill 50 mL into the bladder and allow to remain at least 15 minutes; repeat every 2 weeks or more as needed.

Common Side Effects

Garlic-like taste and odor, discomfort on bladder instillation.

Significant Adverse Reactions

Hypersensitivity reactions (nasal congestion, dyspnea, angioedema, pruritus, urticaria).

Contraindications

No absolute contraindications. *Cautious use* in pregnant or nursing women, in children, and in patients with liver or kidney disease.

• Disulfiram

Antabuse

Disulfiram is an antioxidant that blocks the oxidative metabolism of alcohol at the acetaldehyde stage. Thus, ingestion of even small amounts of alcohol in the presence of disulfiram results in a 5- to 10-fold increase in blood acetaldehyde levels, which elicits a range of unpleasant symptoms known as the disulfiram reaction or *mal rouge*. Thus, disulfiram is used for the management of properly motivated chronic alcoholics who *desire* to be placed in a situation of enforced sobriety. The threat of illness on consumption of alcohol is the prime deterrent with this drug. The drug is slowly absorbed and excreted, and the effects persist for up to 2 weeks after the last dose has been taken. Users must be made aware of the consequences of ingesting even small amounts of alcohol in any form whatsoever (eg, cough syrups, mouthwashes, cold preparations, food sauces, vinegars). Also, application of alcohol-containing liniments or lotions (rubbing alcohol, colognes, toilet waters, aftershaves) should be avoided, because the alcohol may be absorbed systemically. The disulfiram–alcohol reaction consists of flushing, nausea, sweating, thirst, throbbing in the head, dyspnea, palpitations, chest pain, tachycardia, hypotension, weakness, vertigo, blurred vision, confusion, and syncope. With large amounts of alcohol, serious adverse reactions can occur, including arrhythmias, congestive heart failure, respiratory depression, convulsions, and even death. The intensity of the reaction depends on the amounts of disulfiram and alcohol ingested. Symptoms are usually fully developed at a blood alcohol level of 50 mg/dL, and unconsciousness occurs at 125 to 150 mg/dL.

Mechanism

Blocks conversion of acetaldehyde to acetate during alcohol metabolism by inhibiting the enzyme aldehyde dehydrogenase, thereby elevating plasma levels of acetaldehyde, a toxic intermediate.

Uses

Adjunctive treatment of chronic alcoholism, in conjunction with supportive therapy and proper motivation.

Dosage

Initially 500 mg/day in a single dose for 1 to 2 weeks; maintenance doses range from 125 to 500 mg once daily until patient is fully recovered.

Fate

Rapidly and completely absorbed orally; optimal effects occur within 8 to 12 hours; highly lipid soluble and localized initially in fatty tissue; slowly metabolized by the liver and excreted in the urine; effects persist for up to 2 weeks after withdrawal of medication.

Common Side Effects

Drowsiness.

Significant Adverse Reactions

Impotence, headache, restlessness, fatigability, skin eruptions, metallic taste, optic or peripheral neuritis, polyneuritis, tremor, psychotic reactions, and arthropathy.

See introductory section for disulfiram–alcohol reaction syndrome.

Contraindications

Severe myocardial disease, coronary occlusion, psychoses, pregnancy, and in patients who have recently received alcohol or alcohol-containing products, metronidazole, or paraldehyde. *Cautious use* in patients with epilepsy, diabetes, cerebral damage, hypothyroidism, hepatic cirrhosis, or nephritis.

Interactions

Disulfiram may potentiate the effects of diazepam, chlordiazepoxide, oral anticoagulants, and phenytoin.
Disulfiram plus isoniazid can result in coordination difficulties and behavioral changes.
Paraldehyde is partially metabolized to acetaldehyde and can produce toxic reactions in the presence of disulfiram.
Metronidazole given together with disulfiram can elicit psychotic reactions.

Nursing Management

Pretherapy Assessment

Assess and record baseline data necessary for detection of adverse effects of disulfiram: General: VS, body weight, skin color and temperature; GI: liver evaluation; CNS: orientation, affect, reflexes; Respiratory system: adventitious sounds; Endocrinologic system: thyroid palpation; Laboratory: renal and liver function tests, CBC, SMA-12.
Review medical history and documents for existing or previous conditions that:
a. require cautious use of disulfiram: epilepsy, diabetes, cerebral damage, hypothyroidism, hepatic cirrhosis, or nephritis.
b. contraindicate use of disulfiram: severe myocardial disease, coronary occlusion, psychoses; and in patients who have recently received alcohol or alcohol-containing products, metronidazole, or paraldehyde; **pregnancy (Category C)**.

Nursing Interventions

Medication Administration

Do not administer until patient has abstained from alcohol for at least 12 hours.
Administer orally; tablet may be crushed and mixed with nonalcoholic beverages.
Arrange for treatment with antihistamines if skin reaction occurs.
Ensure that patient and family are *fully* informed of rationale for therapy and consequences of ingesting or absorbing alcohol in any form (see introductory paragraph) before treatment with disulfiram is undertaken. Never administer to an intoxicated patient.
Assist with institution of appropriate measures (eg, oxygen, IV ascorbic acid, ephedrine, antihistamines) if severe disulfiram reactions occur.

Surveillance During Therapy

Interpret results of diagnostic tests and contact practitioner as appropriate.
Monitor for possible drug–laboratory test interactions.
Monitor for possible drug–drug and drug–nutrient interactions.
Provide for patient safety needs if CNS side effects occur.

Patient Teaching

Ensure that patient understands that disulfiram is not a cure for alcoholism but is merely an adjunct to other forms of therapy in managing chronic alcoholism in the person who *desires* to abstain.
Inform patient that tolerance does not develop with prolonged use. Instead, sensitivity to alcohol increases the longer the drug is used.
Instruct patient to abstain from alcohol for at least 12 hours before initiating disulfiram use.
Suggest that drug be taken in the morning unless sedation becomes a problem. Tablet may be crushed and mixed with a liquid if necessary.
Reassure patient that the side effects that may occur during the first 2 weeks of therapy (metallic taste, drowsiness, headache, weakness, skin eruptions) usually disappear with continued treatment.
Caution patient to exercise care in driving and performing other hazardous activities because drowsiness can occur.
Encourage patient always to carry identification indicating drug being taken, prescriber's name and phone number, and other pertinent information in case of an unexpected reaction. Inform patient that blood studies (CBC, SMA-12) and liver function tests are advised at regular intervals during treatment.
Warn patient that *mal rouge* reactions can occur up to 2 weeks after disulfiram has been discontinued if alcohol is ingested during that time.

Enzyme Preparations

Chymopapain
Chymotrypsin
Collagenase
Fibrinolysin and deoxyribonuclease
Hyaluronidase
Papain
Sutilains
Trypsin

A number of enzymes are available for either topical, intravertebral, or systemic use. Most are used topically to assist removal of excess fluids, tissue exudates, or clotted blood from ulcerated, inflamed, infected, or otherwise injured areas. Topical enzyme preparations may also be used for debriding surface ulcers, surgical or other types of wounds, and second- and third-degree burns. Systemically administered preparations may be useful in aiding the dispersion of other injected drugs or diagnostic agents, and possibly in relieving symptoms of healing surgical lesions. Finally, chymopapain is injected into herniated lumbar intervertebral disks to assist in reducing intradiscal pressure.

Because the enzyme preparations differ with regard to route of administration, indications, and precautions to be observed with their use, they are considered individually in Table 81-2.

• Flavoxate

Urispas

Mechanism

Exerts a direct relaxant effect on smooth muscle of the urinary tract; also possesses anticholinergic, local anesthetic, and possibly analgesic properties.

Table 81-2. Enzyme Preparations

Drug	*Indications*	*Administration and Dosage*	*Nursing Considerations*
TOPICAL ONLY			
Collagenase *Santyl*	Debridement of dermal ulcers and severe burns	Apply once daily	Digests collagen and promotes formation of granulation tissue and epithelization of ulcers and burns; optimal pH range for enzymatic activity is 6 to 8; clean lesion before application and cover wound with sterile gauze after using ointment; remove excess ointment each time dressing is changed; a suitable antibacterial ointment is used when infection is present; *avoid* soaks or washing with solutions containing metal ions or acidic substances, because they reduce enzymatic activity
Fibrinolysin and Desoxyribonuclease *Elase*	Topically: debridement of inflamed or infected lesions Intravaginal: adjunctive treatment of vaginitis and cervicitis	Topically: apply as ointment or solution prepared from powder in the form of a spray or wet dressing Change dressing 2 or 3 times a day, removing debris and exudates each time Vaginally: instill 5 g of ointment or 10 mL of solution (1 vial/10 mL) deep into vagina at bedtime for 5 days	Combination of two enzymes that attack both DNA and fibrin, thus breaking down necrotic tissue and fibrinous exudates; do *not* use parenterally, because bovine fibrinolysin may be antigenic; solutions from dry powder must be used within 24 h; after instillation of solution into vagina, wait 1 to 2 min, then insert a tampon for 12 to 24 h; affected area must be cleaned and dense, dry, escharotic tissue removed before application of drug, because enzymes must be in contact with the tissue to be removed to be effective; also available as ointment with 10 mg/g chloramphenicol as Elase-Chloromycetin
Papain *Panafil*	Debridement of surface lesions	Apply directly to lesion 1 to 2 times a day	Enzyme derived from *Carica papaya*; cover with gauze and remove accumulated necrotic tissue at each redressing; hydrogen peroxide may inactivate papain; itching or stinging can occur with topical application
Sutilains *Travase*	Debridement of burned areas, decubitus ulcers, incisional or traumatic wounds, and surface ulcers resulting from peripheral vascular diseases	Apply in a thin layer to moistened wound area 3 or 4 times a day	Proteolytic enzyme that digests necrotic tissue, thus facilitating formation of granulation tissue; avoid contact of ointment with eyes; a moist environment is essential for optimal enzymatic activity; action of enzyme is reduced by iodine, thimerosal, hexachlorophene, benzalkonium chloride, and nitrofurazone; side effects include mild pain, paresthesias, dermatitis, and possibly bleeding
Trypsin *Dermuspray, Granulderm, Granulex, GranuMed*	Treatment of decubitus and varicose ulcers, wounds, and severe sunburn	Spray twice daily	Used as a spray for debriding necrotic areas; spray contains balsam of Peru and castor oil
SYSTEMIC ONLY			
Hyaluronidase *Wydase* *(CAN) Hyalase*	Aid to increasing absorption and dispersion of other injected drugs and diagnostic agents Adjunct in subcutaneous urography Aid in hypodermoclysis	*Absorption of other drugs*: 150 U added to injected drug solution *Hypodermoclysis*: 150 U injected SC before injection of solution or into rubber tubing during procedure *Urography*: 75 U SC injected over each scapula	Mucolytic enzyme that hydrolyzes hyaluronic acid, thus aiding diffusion of fluids through tissues; extent of diffusion depends on amount of enzyme present and volume of solution; do *not* inject into acutely inflamed, infected, or cancerous areas; use *caution* when adding to solution to be injected to prevent overhydration because enzyme can facilitate excess water absorption; monitor infusion rate carefully; preliminary skin test (0.02 mL intradermally) is often used to detect sensitive individuals; whealing and itching are positive signs of hypersensitivity; may be antigenic with repeated use
OPHTHALMIC ONLY			
Chymotrypsin *Alpha Chymar, Catarase, Zolyse* *(CAN) Alpha Chymolean, Zonulyn*	Aid in intracapsular lens extraction to facilitate enzymatic zonulysis	0.25–2.0 mL to irrigate the posterior chamber; repeat every 2–4 min until extraction	Proteolytic enzyme that lyses peptide bonds of amino acids in zonular fibers that support the lens of the eye; complete lysis occurs within 30 min; inactivated by serum, blood, alkalies, acids, antiseptics, detergents, epinephrine, chloramphenicol, and isofluorophate; may increase intraocular pressure transiently; does not lyse adhesions between lens and other ocular structures

(*continued*)

Table 81-2. Enzyme Preparations (Continued)

Drug	Indications	Administration and Dosage	Nursing Considerations
INTRAVERTEBRAL ONLY			
Chymopapain *Chymodiactin (CAN) Discase*	Treatment of documented herniated lumbar intervertebral disks whose symptoms have not responded to more conservative therapy	2–4 U per disk as a single injection (maximum is 8 U in patients with multiple disk involvement)	Proteolytic enzyme that hydrolyzes the polypeptides and proteins that maintain the mucoprotein internal discal structure; compressive symptoms are thus lessened; used *only* in a hospital setting by trained personnel; paraplegia, CNS bleeding, and anaphylaxis have occurred; *avoid* intrathecal injection because drug is highly toxic by this route; risk increases with multiple injections

Uses

Symptomatic relief of dysuria, urgency, nocturia, suprapubic pain, and incontinence resulting from cystitis, urethritis, prostatitis, and other genitourinary conditions.

Dosage

100 to 200 mg orally three to four times a day.

Significant Adverse Reactions

Drowsiness, dizziness, blurred vision, dry mouth, headache, nervousness, increased intraocular tension, confusion, urticaria, dermatoses, tachycardia, palpitation, hyperpyrexia, eosinophilia, and leukopenia.

Contraindications

Pyloric or duodenal obstruction, obstructive intestinal lesions, achalasia, and GI hemorrhage. *Cautious use* in patients with glaucoma and in pregnant women.

Nursing Management

Pretherapy Assessment

Assess and record baseline data necessary for detection of adverse effects of flavoxate: General: VS, body weight, skin color and temperature; GI: liver evaluation, oral mucous membranes; CNS: orientation, affect, reflexes, ophthalmic examination, ocular pressure; Laboratory: CBC, stool guaiac.

Review medical history and documents for existing or previous conditions that:

a. require cautious use of flavoxate: glaucoma.
b. contraindicate use of flavoxate: pyloric or duodenal obstruction, obstructive intestinal lesions, achalasia, and GI hemorrhage; **pregnancy (Category C)**.

Nursing Interventions

Medication Administration

Provide small, frequent meals if GI upset occurs.

Arrange for definitive treatment of urinary tract infections causing symptoms being managed by flavoxate.

Surveillance During Therapy

Interpret results of diagnostic tests and contact practitioner as appropriate.

Monitor for possible drug–laboratory test interactions.

Monitor for possible drug–drug and drug–nutrient interactions.

Provide for patient safety needs if CNS side effects occur.

Patient Teaching

Urge patient to exercise caution in driving or performing tasks requiring alertness because drowsiness, dizziness, and blurred vision may occur.

Teach patient interventions to alleviate dry mouth.

• Gallium Nitrate

Ganite

Gallium nitrate inhibits calcium resorption from bone and is used in treating symptomatic cancer-related hypercalcemia that is unresponsive to sufficient hydration. It is administered in a dose of 200 mg/m^2 by IV infusion over 24 hours daily for 5 consecutive days. If serum calcium levels are lowered into the normal range in less than 5 days, treatment may be discontinued. The patient should be adequately hydrated before drug administration to increase the renal excretion of calcium.

Gallium is contraindicated when the serum creatinine is greater than 2.5 mg/dL. Renal function and serum calcium must be closely monitored during gallium therapy. Concurrent use of gallium with other nephrotoxic drugs (eg, aminoglycosides, amphotericin B, vancomycin) may increase the risk of renal insufficiency. Adverse effects may include hypotension, tachycardia, visual impairment, decreased hearing, tinnitus, dyspnea, GI distress, paresthesias, skin rash, fever, lethargy and hypothermia.

• Hemin

Panhematin

Mechanism

Iron-containing metalloporphyrin that decreases the hepatic or marrow synthesis of porphyrin, probably by inhibiting an enzyme necessary for porphyrin–heme synthesis.

Uses

Symptomatic management of recurrent attacks of acute intermittent porphyria.

Dosage

1 to 4 mg/kg/day by IV infusion over 10 to 15 minutes for 3 to 14 days. Maximum dose is 6 mg/kg/24 hours.

Significant Adverse Reactions

Phlebitis, pyrexia, leukocytosis, decreased hematocrit.

Contraindications

Porphyria cutanea tarda. *Cautious use* in patients with renal dysfunction, altered coagulability, thrombophlebitis; in pregnant or nursing women.

Interactions

Hemin may enhance the anticoagulant effects of oral anticoagulants and heparin.

The effects of hemin may be reduced by barbiturates, estrogens, and steroids, because these agents increase the activity of an enzyme that is inhibited by hemin.

Nursing Management

Pretherapy Assessment

Assess and record baseline data necessary for detection of adverse effects of hemin: General: VS, body weight, skin color and temperature; Laboratory: CBC, hematocrit (Hct).

Review medical history and documents for existing or previous conditions that:

a. require cautious use of hemin: renal dysfunction, altered coagulability, thrombophlebitis; in pregnant or nursing women.
b. contraindicate use of hemin: allergy to hemin or components of the product, porphyria cutanea tarda; **pregnancy (Category C)**.

Nursing Interventions

Medication Administration

Ensure that the presence of acute porphyria is established before hemin therapy is undertaken.

Freeze and store powder until time of use.

Reconstitute immediately before use (contains no preservatives). Discard unused portions.

Administer through large arm vein or central venous catheter to reduce risk of phlebitis.

Use terminal filtration through a 0.45-μm or smaller filter, as recommended, to ensure that no undissolved particles are injected.

Surveillance During Therapy

Monitor intake and output, particularly in patient receiving high doses. Promptly report onset of oliguria or anuria.

Monitor for toxicity.

Interpret results of diagnostic tests and contact practitioner as appropriate.

Monitor for possible drug–laboratory test interactions.

Monitor for possible drug–drug and drug–nutrient interactions.

• Mesalamine (5-aminosalicylic acid)

Asacol, Rowasa

(CAN) Salofalk

Mechanism

Exerts an antiinflammatory action in the colon, presumably by inhibiting production of prostaglandins and possibly leukotrienes; possesses a topical action to reduce pain and discomfort associated with chronic inflammatory bowel conditions

Uses

Treatment of distal ulcerative colitis, proctitis, or other inflammatory bowel syndromes.

Dosage

Oral: 800 mg 3 times a day for 6 weeks

Suppository: 1 suppository (500 mg) twice daily for 3 to 6 weeks. Retain suppository in the rectum for 1 to 3 hours if possible

Rectal suspension: 4 g (60 mL) once daily, usually at bedtime; should be retained for 8 hours; duration of treatment is 3 to 6 weeks

Fate

Poorly absorbed rectally; approximately 15% to 25% of a dose appears in the urine in 24 hours; primarily eliminated in the feces; approximately one fourth of an oral dose is absorbed, the remainder exerts a local action in the ileum and beyond and is excreted in the feces.

Common Side Effects

Oral: Abdominal pain and cramping, belching, nausea, headache, pharyngitis

Rectal: Flatulence, cramping, nausea, headache

Significant Adverse Reactions

Flu-like syndrome (weakness, malaise, fever), rhinitis, diarrhea, dizziness, rectal pain, skin rash, bloating, back or leg pain, hemorrhoids, peripheral edema, and urinary infections.

Contraindications

No absolute contraindications. *Cautious use* in patients with renal dysfunction or sulfa allergies; in pregnant or nursing women; and in children.

Nursing Management

Pretherapy Assessment

Assess and record baseline data necessary for detection of adverse effects of mesalamine: General: VS, body weight, skin color and temperature; CNS: reflexes, affect; GI: abdominal, rectal examination; Genitourinary: output, renal function; Laboratory: renal function tests.

Review medical history and documents for existing or previous conditions that:

a. require cautious use of mesalamine: renal dysfunction, sulfa allergies; in pregnant or nursing women; and in children.
b. contraindicate use of mesalamine: allergy to mesalamine, sulfites, or components of the product; **pregnancy (Category B)**.

Nursing Interventions

Medication Administration

Shake bottle well to ensure a homogenous suspension to administer; apply as a retention enema; patient must retain medication for approximately 8 hours.
Arrange for appropriate measures to deal with GI discomfort, CNS effects, headache, fever, and flu-like symptoms.

Surveillance During Therapy

Monitor for adverse effects and toxicity.
Interpret results of diagnostic tests and contact practitioner as appropriate.
Monitor for possible drug–laboratory test interactions.
Monitor for possible drug–drug and drug–nutrient interactions.

Patient Teaching

Teach patient proper administration and use of retention enema.
Inform patient that potential changes in renal function may be monitored by periodic urinalyses and blood urea nitrogen and serum creatinine determinations.
Teach patient how to recognize the acute intolerance syndrome associated with mesalamine use (eg, cramping, bloody diarrhea, acute abdominal pain, and, sometimes, fever, headache, and rash) and to report occurrence to prescriber, because the drug should be stopped promptly.
Warn patient hypersensitive to sulfites that the drug contains potassium metabisulfite, which may trigger the allergy.

• Octreotide

Sandostatin

Octreotide is a long-acting peptide whose actions resemble those of somatostatin; therefore, it decreases secretion of many endogenous peptides, such as gastrin, vasoactive intestinal peptide, insulin, glucagon, secretin, and pancreatic polypeptide, as well as serotonin. It is used subcutaneously for the symptomatic treatment of patients with metastatic carcinoid tumors to alleviate severe diarrhea and flushing. Octreotide may also be given to reduce the profuse, watery diarrhea resulting from vasoactive intestinal peptide tumors (VIPomas). Initial dosage is 50 μg subcutaneously (SC) once or twice daily; dosage may be increased thereafter depending on the response and tolerance by the patient. Octreotide has been used in a wide range of patients, from infants to the elderly. Most frequently occurring side effects are nausea, diarrhea, abdominal pain, and pain at the injection site. A wide range of other adverse reactions have been associated with octreotide, although the incidence is quite low. Like somatostatin, however, octreotide can lead to cholelithiasis, and patients must be closely monitored for gallbladder disease. Altered pancreatic and thyroid function can also occur during octreotide therapy.

• Olsalazine

Dipentum

Olsalazine is a sodium salt of a salicylate that is biotransformed into 5-aminosalicylic acid (see Mesalamine), and exhibits a similar pharmacologic profile. It is indicated for the maintenance treatment of ulcerative colitis in patients intolerant of sulfasalazine (see Chapter 59). The recommended oral dose is 2 capsules (500 mg) twice a day. Common side effects include diarrhea, abdominal pain or cramping, nausea, and headache. Refer to the previous monograph on mesalamine for additional information pertaining to olsalazine.

• Pegademase Bovine

Adagen

Pegademase is a modified enzyme used for replacement therapy in the treatment of severe combined immunodeficiency disease associated with decreased levels of adenosine deaminase (ADA), a rare, inherited and frequently fatal disease. In the absence of ADA, accumulation of adenosine and 2′-deoxyadenosine results in toxic effects on lymphocytes. The disease is curable by bone marrow transplantation, but in cases in which a donor is unavailable, pegademase administration can replace the deficient ADA, thereby eliminating the accumulation of the toxic metabolites.

The drug is given as an IM injection every 7 days. The initial dose is 10 U/kg, the second dose is 15 U/kg, and the third and succeeding doses are 20 U/kg. The optimal dosage and scheduling are based on close monitoring of the plasma ADA levels, and only personnel thoroughly familiar with the prescribing and monitoring information for pegademase should administer the drug.

• Perfluorochemical Emulsion, Intravascular

Fluosol

A stable emulsion of oxygen-carrying perfluorochemicals in Water for Injection, perfluorochemical emulsion, when oxygenated and injected transluminally through a coronary artery angioplasty balloon catheter, delivers oxygen to the myocardium. It is used to prevent or decrease myocardial ischemia during percutaneous transluminal coronary angioplasty in patients at high risk (eg, recent infarction, unstable angina, low baseline ejection fraction). The preparation is injected at a rate of 60 to 90 mL/min at approximately 37°C during the period of balloon inflation. Infusion of solution *at room temperature* has been associated with ventricular fibrillation. It should not be administered more than once every 6 months. Only personnel familiar with the product and the procedures for its administration should be involved in its use.

Plasma Expanders

Dextran, low molecular weight (Dextran 40)
Dextran, high molecular weight (Dextran 70, 75)
Hetastarch

Dextran, a synthetic polysaccharide of varying molecular weights, and hetastarch, a chemically modified corn starch, are used to expand reduced plasma volume, which can occur in hypovolemic shock resulting from hemorrhage, extensive burns, surgery, sepsis, or other forms of trauma. Their principal advantages over whole blood or plasma for volume replacement are their relatively low cost, wide availability, and lack of incompatibility problems, as well as the fact that they are not associated with the danger of transmitting diseases such as viral hepatitis or acquired immunodeficiency syndrome. These synthetic polysaccharides, however, can produce allergic reactions, occasionally severe, and may also interfere with platelet function, resulting in increased bleeding tendencies. Prior IV injection of dextran-1 (Promit), a monovalent hapten, may be used to prevent severe anaphylactic reactions to dextran infusion. Plasma expanders should *not* be viewed as substitutes for whole blood or plasma proteins when such are available.

The agents used as plasma expanders are considered as a group in the following, and are listed individually in Table 81-3.

Mechanism

Elevate the osmotic pressure of the blood, thus drawing water from extravascular spaces into the bloodstream. Plasma volume expands slightly in excess of the volume of drug solution infused. The drugs also decrease blood viscosity and reduce erythrocyte aggregation and rouleau formation, thus improving microcirculation. They reduce platelet adhesiveness and can alter the structure of fibrin clots, thus reducing the likelihood of thrombus formation. Secondary cardiovascular effects include increases in blood pressure, venous return, cardiac output, and urine flow, and decreased heart rate and peripheral resistance

Uses

Adjunctive treatment of shock due to hemorrhage, burns, surgery, sepsis, or other trauma (*not* to be viewed as a substitute for blood or plasma)

Priming fluid in pump oxygenators during extracorporeal circulation (dextran *40* only)

Prophylaxis against venous thrombosis and pulmonary embolism in patients undergoing high-risk procedures, for example, hip surgery (dextran *40* only)

Adjunctive use in leukapheresis to increase granulocyte yield (hetastarch only)

Dosage

See Table 81-3.

Fate

Onset of volume-expanding action varies from several minutes (dextran 40) to about 1 hour (dextran 75); hemodynamic status is improved for at least 12 hours (dextran 40) to over 24 hours (dextran 75, hetastarch) with a single infusion; molecules of molecular weight less than 50,000 daltons are eliminated by the kidneys, 40% to 75% within 24 hours; larger–molecular-weight molecules are slowly metabolized to smaller sugars and either excreted in the urine or eliminated as breakdown products (eg, carbon dioxide and water); small amounts of drugs are excreted in the feces.

Significant Adverse Reactions

Allergic reactions (nasal congestion, urticaria, wheezing, dyspnea, hypotension), anaphylactic reactions (rare), nausea,

Table 81-3. **Plasma Expanders**

Drug	Usual Dosage Range	Nursing Considerations
Dextran 40—low molecular weight *Gentran 40, 10%* *LMD, Rheomacrodex* *(CAN) Hyskon*	*Shock*: 20 mL/kg/24 h by IV infusion the first day; thereafter, 10 mL/kg/d for a maximum of 5 d *Extracorporeal circulation*: 10–20 mL/kg added to perfusion circuit *Prophylaxis of venous thromboses*: 10 mL/kg on day of surgery, then 500 mL/d for 2 to 3 d, then 500 mL every 2 to 3 d for 2 wk	Low–molecular-weight dextran is effective in reducing erythrocyte clumping and sludging and is reported to be able to disrupt thrombi; bleeding time can be prolonged and platelet function may be depressed by large doses; monitor coagulation time closely during therapy and observe for early signs of bleeding (epistaxis, petechiae)
Dextran 70, 75—high molecular weight *Gentran 75, Macrodex*	*Shock* Adults: 10–20 mL/kg/24 h by IV infusion; usually, 500 mL is given at a rate of 20–40 mL/min for emergency treatment Children: Maximum dose 20 mL/kg	High–molecular-weight dextran is slower in onset but more prolonged acting than low–molecular-weight dextran; be alert for allergic reactions, which most often develop in first few minutes of infusion; may adversely affect capillary flow by increasing blood viscosity; can interfere with platelet aggregation and transiently prolong bleeding time
Hetastarch *Hespan*	*Volume expansion*: 500–1000 mL/d (maximum 1500 mL/d); in acute situations, infusion rate is 20 mL/kg/h *Leukapheresis*: 250–700 mL infused at a fixed ratio (eg, 1:8) to venous whole blood	Synthetic polymer prepared from amylopectin; similar to dextran in action and can also increase erythrocyte sedimentation rate; thus is used to improve efficiency of granulocyte collection by centrifugation; may elevate bilirubin levels; use with *caution* in patients with liver disease; during leukapheresis, hemoglobin and platelet counts may be temporarily reduced owing to volume-expanding effects of hetastarch; blood counts, hemoglobin determinations, and prothrombin times should be performed during therapy

vomiting, headache, fever, joint pain, infection at injection site, phlebitis, hypervolemia, pulmonary edema, osmotic nephrosis, renal failure (rare), prolongation of bleeding time; *also with hetastarch*—submaxillary and parotid gland enlargement, flu-like symptoms, and edema of the lower extremities.

Contraindications

Severe cardiac decompensation, renal failure, and marked hemostatic defects (hyperfibrinogenemia, thrombocytopenia). *Cautious use* in patients with active hemorrhaging, liver or kidney impairment, severe dehydration, or history of allergic reactions, and in pregnant women.

Interactions

Dextran may cause false elevations in blood glucose, urinary proteins, bilirubin, and total protein assays, and its use can lead to unreliable readings in blood typing and cross-matching procedures.

Abnormally prolonged bleeding times can occur if plasma expanders are used together with anticoagulants or antiplatelet drugs.

Nursing Management

Pretherapy Assessment

Assess and record baseline data necessary for detection of adverse effects of plasma expanders: General: VS, body weight, skin color and temperature; GI: submaxillary and parotid gland evaluation, liver evaluation; CVS: adventitious sounds, peripheral and periorbital edema; Laboratory: renal and liver function tests, clotting times, prothrombin time, partial thromboplastin time, hemoglobin, Hct.

Review medical history and documents for existing or previous conditions that:

a. require cautious use of plasma expanders: active hemorrhaging, liver or kidney impairment, severe dehydration, history of allergic reactions, and in pregnant women.
b. contraindicate use of plasma expanders: severe cardiac decompensation, renal failure, and marked hemostatic defects (hyperfibrinogenemia, thrombocytopenia); **pregnancy (Category C)**.

Nursing Interventions

Medication Administration

Administer by IV infusion only.

Observe patient closely during infusion and discontinue drug at first sign of allergic reaction. Have resuscitative measures available (eg, epinephrine, antihistamines, corticosteroids).

Monitor central venous pressure during drug administration, and assess patient for signs of circulatory overload (dyspnea, wheezing, coughing, increased pulse and respiratory rate). Discontinue drug and inform prescriber if signs appear.

Question administration of solution containing sodium chloride to a patient with congestive heart failure or renal insufficiency or to one receiving corticosteroids.

Discard partially used containers because solution contains no bacteriostatic agent. Store at room temperature to prevent crystallization. Do not use if solution is not clear or under vacuum.

Surveillance During Therapy

Determine urine output and specific gravity at regular intervals. Oliguria, anuria, or altered specific gravity should be reported immediately. Marked elevations in specific gravity may indicate reduced urine flow. Recommended dosage and flow rate should not be exceeded because excessive doses can precipitate renal failure.

Check results of Hct determinations, which should be obtained after administration. Advise prescriber if value falls below 30 mg/dL.

Distinguish low–molecular-weight dextran (40) from high–molecular-weight dextran (70, 75). High–molecular-weight dextran is reportedly associated with fewer adverse reactions (except allergenic) but it is slower in onset, is not cleared as rapidly, is more viscous, and exhibits much less of an effect in retarding rouleau formation and erythrocyte clumping.

Interpret results of the following laboratory tests cautiously because dextran may cause false elevations: blood glucose, urinary proteins, bilirubin, and total protein assays. Readings in blood typing and cross-matching procedures may also be unreliable.

Interpret results of diagnostic tests and contact practitioner as appropriate.

Monitor for possible drug–laboratory test interactions.

Monitor for possible drug–drug and drug–nutrient interactions.

Plasma Protein Fractions

Albumin, human
Plasma protein fraction

The plasma protein fractions, which are obtained by fractionating human plasma, include normal serum albumin and plasma protein fraction. These products are primarily used to expand plasma volume, because they raise the osmotic pressure of the blood. Because they both are heat treated to destroy hepatitis B virus, they are considered somewhat safer than whole blood or plasma as volume expanders.

Normal serum albumin is available in two concentrations, a 5% solution, which is approximately osmotically and isotonically equivalent to human plasma, and a 25% solution, osmotically equivalent to five times the volume of plasma. Plasma protein fraction is a 5% solution of human plasma proteins (83%–90% albumin with small amounts of alpha- and beta-globulins) that is osmotically equivalent to human plasma. These albumin preparations do not appear to interfere with normal coagulation mechanisms and do not require cross-matching. The absence of cellular elements, moreover, greatly reduces the risk of sensitization with repeated administration.

The plasma protein fractions are discussed together in the following, and listed individually in Table 81-4.

Table 81-4. **Plasma Protein Fractions**

Drug	Usual Dosage Range	Nursing Considerations
Albumin, human *Albuminar, Albutein, Buminate, Plasbumin*	Variable, depending on diagnosis, severity of condition, patient's age, and concentration of solution; usually, the equivalent of 25–100 g albumin per day is given by slow IV infusion (1–4 mL/min depending on concentration); maximum recommended dose is 250 g/48 h	Available in two strengths, 5% and 25%, both containing 130–160 mEq/L; the 25% solution allows administration of large amounts of albumin quickly, and 100 mL provides as much plasma protein as 500 mL plasma or 2 pints whole blood; concentrated solution usually requires supplemental fluids in dehydrated patients, thus 5% solution may be preferred for routine use because maximum osmotic effect is attained without additional fluids; preparations may cause an elevation of alkaline phosphatase levels; the 25% solution is preferred in most patients requiring sodium restriction
Plasma Protein Fraction *Plasmanate, Plasma-Plex, Plasmatein, Protenate*	*Hypovolemic shock* Adults: 250–500 mL by IV infusion Children: 20–30 mL/kg *Hypoproteinemia*: 1000–1500 mL/d	Rate of infusion is determined by condition and patient's age and body weight; maximum infusion rate is 10 mL/min in shock and 5–8 mL/min in hypoproteinemia; do *not* give more than 250 g in 48 h; monitor patients carefully for signs of volume overload; slow infusion if blood pressure declines; use *cautiously* in sodium-restricted patients—solution contains 130–160 mEq/L; if edema is present or if large amounts of protein are lost, use 25% albumin solution

Mechanism

Increase intravascular osmotic pressure, thereby drawing extracellular fluid into the bloodstream, expanding plasma volume; bind bilirubin in the plasma.

Uses

Adjunctive emergency treatment of hypovolemic shock
Temporary replacement of blood loss to prevent hemoconcentration following severe burns
Treatment of hypoproteinemia due to nephrotic syndrome, hepatic cirrhosis, toxemia of pregnancy, and tuberculosis, and in postoperative patients and premature infants
Adjunctive therapy during exchange transfusions in hyperbilirubinemia and erythroblastosis fetalis
Adjunctive treatment of acute liver failure, adult respiratory distress syndrome, acute peritonitis, pancreatitis, or mediastinitis, and during cardiopulmonary bypass or renal dialysis

Dosage

See Table 81-4.

Significant Adverse Reactions

Hypotension, allergic reactions (fever, chills, flushing, urticaria, rash), headache, nausea, vomiting, tachycardia, salivation, back pain, and respiratory irregularities.

Vascular overload and pulmonary edema can occur with too-rapid infusion.

Contraindications

Cardiac failure, severe anemia, and normal or increased intravascular volume. In addition, plasma protein fraction is contraindicated in patients on cardiopulmonary bypass. *Cautious use* in patients with mild anemia, low cardiac reserve, hepatic or renal failure, or congestive heart failure.

Nursing Management

Pretherapy Assessment

Assess and record baseline data necessary for detection of adverse effects of albumin: General: VS, body weight, skin color and temperature; CVS: peripheral perfusion; Respiratory system: adventitious sounds; Laboratory: renal and liver function tests, electrolytes, Hct.

Review medical history and documents for existing or previous conditions that:

a. require cautious use of albumin: mild anemia, low cardiac reserve, hepatic or renal failure, or congestive heart failure.
b. contraindicate use of albumin: cardiac failure, severe anemia, and normal or increased intravascular volume. In addition, plasma protein fraction is contraindicated in patients on cardiopulmonary bypass, and in **pregnancy (Category C)**.

Nursing Interventions

Medication Administration

Administer by IV infusion only.

Monitor central venous pressure during drug administration, and assess patient for signs of circulatory overload (dyspnea, wheezing, coughing, increased pulse and respiratory rate). Discontinue drug and inform prescriber if signs appear.

Question administration of solution containing sodium chloride to a patient with congestive heart failure or renal insufficiency or to one receiving corticosteroids.

Maintain a slow infusion rate (see Table 81-4) because rapid infusion may produce vascular overload and hypotension. Observe patient for signs of vascular overload (coughing, dyspnea, tachycardia, distended neck veins).

Monitor blood pressure, pulse, and respiratory pattern during infusion.

Be prepared to administer supplemental whole blood or plasma to satisfy large volume requirements. Albumin preparations are not a substitute for whole blood.

Expect to administer additional fluids to patient with severe dehydration to minimize excessive depletion of tissue fluid.

Assess patient for signs of external bleeding because blood pressure may be elevated following too-rapid administration. If bleeding is noted, be prepared to deal with new hemorrhaging or possibly shock.

Use *only* solutions that do not appear turbid and show no evidence of sedimentation.

Use promptly after opening (ie, within 4 hours), and discard unused portions because solution contains no preservatives or bacteriostatic substances.

Do *not* infuse together with solutions containing alcohol or protein hydrolysates because albumin may precipitate, although drug solution can be added to usual IV infusion solutions.

Surveillance During Therapy

Monitor for adverse effects and toxicity.

Interpret results of diagnostic tests and contact practitioner as appropriate.

Monitor for possible drug–laboratory test interactions.

Monitor for possible drug–drug and drug–nutrient interactions.

Patient Teaching

Instruct the patient to report any of the following: headache; nausea, vomiting; difficulty breathing; back pain.

Sclerosing Agents

Ethanolamine oleate
Morrhuate sodium
Sodium tetradecyl sulfate

Sclerosing agents are injected IV and act by irritating the intimal endothelium of veins, producing a sterile inflammatory response. Ethanolamine is used to treat bleeding esophageal varices, whereas the other two agents are usually used to treat uncomplicated varicose veins of the lower extremities. The drugs are reviewed as a group in the following, and listed individually in Table 81-5.

Mechanism

Directly irritate the venous intimal endothelium after IV injection, resulting in development of a blood clot that occludes the vein and leads to formation of fibrous tissue and obliteration of the vein

Uses

Treatment of small, uncomplicated varicose veins of the lower extremities (morrhuate sodium, sodium tetradecyl sulfate)

Supplement to venous ligation to obliterate residual varicose veins or to reduce risk of surgery (morrhuate sodium, sodium tetradecyl sulfate)

Treatment of internal hemorrhoids (morrhuate sodium—effectiveness has not been conclusively established)

Treatment of esophageal varices that have recently bled

Dosage

See Table 81-5.

Common Side Effects

Burning and cramping at injection site.

Significant Adverse Reactions

Urticaria, tissue sloughing and necrosis; rarely, drowsiness, headache, hypersensitivity reactions (dizziness, weakness, respiratory difficulty, GI upset, vascular collapse, anaphylaxis).

In addition, ethanolamine has caused esophageal ulcer, pyrexia, retrosternal pain, pneumonia, pleural effusion, bacteremia, and acute renal failure.

Contraindications

Acute thrombophlebitis, uncontrolled diabetes, sepsis, blood dyscrasia, thyrotoxicosis, tuberculosis, neoplasms, asthma, acute respiratory or skin disease, varicosities due to abdominal or pelvic tumors; in bedridden patients; and persistent occlusion of deep veins. *Cautious use* in patients with local or systemic infections and in pregnant or nursing women.

Nursing Management

Pretherapy Assessment

Assess and record baseline data necessary for detection of adverse effects of sclerosing agents: General: VS, body weight, skin color and temperature; GI: liver evaluation; Laboratory: liver function tests.

Review medical history and documents for existing or previous conditions that:

a. require cautious use of sclerosing agents: local or systemic infections and in pregnant or nursing women.
b. contraindicate use of sclerosing agents: acute thrombophlebitis, uncontrolled diabetes, sepsis, blood dyscrasia, thyrotoxicosis, tuberculosis, neoplasms, asthma, acute respiratory or skin disease, varicosities due to abdominal or pelvic tumors; in bedridden patients; and persistent occlusion of deep veins; **pregnancy (Category C)**.

Nursing Interventions

Medication Administration

Store at room temperature; protect from light.

Have emergency measures (eg, antihistamines, epinephrine, corticosteroids) readily available for treatment of possible allergic reactions.

Be prepared to assist with injection procedure. Agents should not be used unless deep vein patency has been established. A preinjection evaluation for valvular competence should be performed, and a small amount (2 mL) of drug solution should be slowly injected into the varicosity. Only clear solutions should be used. Severe ischemia may result from intraarterial injection.

Table 81-5. **Sclerosing Agents**

Drug	*Usual Dosage Range*	*Nursing Considerations*
Ethanolamine *Ethamolin*	1.5–5 mL injected into bleeding vein; repeat after 1 wk, 6 wk, 3 mo, and 6 mo	Mild sclerosing agent used to obliterate bleeding esophageal varices; local inflammatory reaction produces fibrosis and occlusion of the vein; *not* recommended for varicosities of the leg; rare reports of anaphylaxis and acute renal failure have been noted; severe necrosis can occur with improper injection
Morrhuate Sodium *Scleromate*	50–250 mg IV (1–5 mL) depending on size of vein, given as multiple injections at the same time, *or* as a single dose; repeat at 5- to 7-d intervals as needed	To determine patient sensitivity, 0.25–1 mL is given into a varicosity 24 h before administration of a large dose; vial should be warmed before injecting; use a large-bore needle to fill syringe because solution froths easily; however, a small-bore needle is used for injection; pulmonary embolism has occurred
Sodium Tetradecyl Sulfate *Sotradecol (CAN) Trombovar*	0.5–2 mL of either strength solution depending on size of varicosity	Initially 0.5 mL of 1% solution should be given to determine patient sensitivity; observe for several hours before giving a larger amount; may *permanently* discolor vein at injection site; do *not* use for injecting veins for cosmetic purposes; *caution* in patients taking oral anticoagulants

Surveillance During Therapy

Monitor for adverse effects and toxicity.
Monitor liver function; injection does not alleviate underlying portal hypertension.
Interpret results of diagnostic tests and contact practitioner as appropriate.
Monitor for possible drug–laboratory test interactions.
Monitor for possible drug–drug and drug–nutrient interactions.

Patient Teaching

Warn patient that, after injection, the vein will become hard and swollen and will be tender to touch. Aching and a feeling of stiffness usually occur and may persist for 48 hours.

• Sumatriptan

Imitrex

Sumatriptan is a selective serotonin receptor agonist that is able to relieve the pain of migraine headache after injection. It is *not* intended for use as a migraine prophylactic agent.

Mechanism

Selectively binds to and activates vascular 5-hydroxytryptamine (serotonin) receptor subtype 5-HT_{1D} to cause vasoconstriction; this receptor subtype is present on cranial arteries, the basilar artery, and the vasculature of the dura mater; constriction of these vessels relieves the pain of migraine.

Uses

Acute treatment of migraine attacks
Investigational use for treatment of cluster headache.

Dosage

6 mg, injected SC; may repeat once within 24 hours, at least 1 hour after first injection.

Fate

Peak serum levels occur within 10 to 20 minutes after injection; half-life is approximately 2 hours; protein binding is minimal; excreted in the urine as both unchanged drug (25%) and metabolites.

Common Side Effects

Sensation of warmth, tingling or burning sensation, dizziness, vertigo, pain or redness at injection site.

Significant Adverse Reactions

CV: hypertension, tachycardia, flushing, palpitations, transient electrocardiographic changes, ventricular premature beats, syncope, angina-like pain, arrhythmias
GI: diarrhea, GI reflux, liver function abnormalities
Neurologic: confusion, anxiety, agitation, paresthesias, chills, lightheadedness, drowsiness, tremor, shivering, taste alterations, facial or neck pain, lacrimation
Other: dyspnea, erythema, pruritus, rash, skin eruptions, dysuria, urinary frequency, dysmenorrhea, thirst, joint pain and stiffness, muscular weakness, chest discomfort,

Contraindications

Ischemic heart disease, history of myocardial infarction, in controlled hypertension, concurrent use with ergotamine preparations (see Interactions). *Cautious use* in patients with renal or hepatic disease, history of cardiac arrhythmias, and asthma; and in pregnant or nursing mothers.

Interactions

Increased vasospasm can occur if sumatriptan is given concurrently with ergot-containing drugs, such as ergotamine.

Nursing Management

Pretherapy Assessment

Assess and record baseline data necessary for detection of adverse effects of sumatriptan: General: VS, body weight, skin color and temperature; CVS: electrocardiogram, peripheral perfusion; GI: liver evaluation, output; CNS: orientation, reflexes, bilateral grip strength; Laboratory: liver and renal function tests, electrolytes.

Review medical history and documents for existing or previous conditions that:

a. require cautious use of sumatriptan: renal or hepatic disease, history of cardiac arrhythmias, asthma, pregnancy, and breast-feeding.

b. contraindicate use of sumatriptan: ischemic heart disease, history of myocardial infarction, uncontrolled hypertension, concurrent use with ergotamine preparations (see Interactions); **pregnancy (Category C)**.

Nursing Interventions

Medication Administration

The maximum recommended adult dose is 6 mg SC; an autoinjection device is available for use by the patient for self-administration.

Ensure ready access to bathroom facilities if diarrhea occurs.

Surveillance During Therapy

Monitor injection site(s) for reaction to the drug because more than 50% of the patients using this agent report injection site reactions.

Interpret results of diagnostic tests and contact practitioner as appropriate.

Monitor for possible drug–laboratory test interactions.

Monitor for possible drug–drug and drug–nutrient interactions.

Provide for patient safety needs if CNS or cardiovascular side effects occur.

Patient Teaching

Teach the patient the proper use of the autoinjection device available for use with this drug.

Inform the patient to inspect the drug dosage form for particulates and discoloration; store the medication away from heat and light.

• Tiopronin

Thiola

Mechanism

Exchanges with cystine to form a mixed disulfide of tiopronin–cysteine, thus reducing the amount of sparingly soluble cystine.

Uses

Prevention of cystine kidney stone formation in patients with severe cystinuria who are resistant to more conservative treatment (eg, high fluid intake, diet modification).

Dosage

Average adult dose: 800 to 1000 mg daily in 3 divided doses, given orally; adjust dosage based on urinary cystine value

Children: average dose is 15 mg/kg/day

Fate

Cystine excretion falls on the first day of therapy; effects cease as soon as drug is stopped; up to 50% of a dose appears in the urine within the first 4 hours and up to 78% within 72 hours.

Significant Adverse Reactions

Drug fever, generalized rash, wrinkling and friability of skin, systemic lupus-like reaction, blood dyscrasias.

Contraindications

History of agranulocytosis, thrombocytopenia, or aplastic anemia on this medication. *Cautious use* in patients with myasthenia gravis, and in pregnant or nursing women; *not* recommended in children younger than 9 years of age.

Nursing Management

Pretherapy Assessment

Assess and record baseline data necessary for detection of adverse effects of tiopronin: General: VS, body weight, skin color and temperature; Genitourinary: output; Laboratory: liver and renal function tests, electrolytes, urinalysis, urinary cysteine, 24-hour urinary protein, CBC with differential, Hct.

Review medical history and documents for existing or previous conditions that:

a. require cautious use of tiopronin: myasthenia gravis, and in pregnant or nursing women; *not* recommended in children younger than 9 years of age.

b. contraindicate use of tiopronin: allergy to tiopronin, history of agranulocytosis, thrombocytopenia, or aplastic anemia on this medication; history of severe reaction to penicillamine; **pregnancy (Category C)**.

Nursing Interventions

Medication Administration

Administer in divided doses, three times a day, at least 1 hour before or 2 hours after meals.

Assure ready access to bathroom facilities if diarrhea occurs.

Assure that fluid intake and output are maintained to achieve a minimum urinary output of 2 L/day in a pH range of 6.5 to 7.

Arrange to initiate therapy at a lower than normal dose if the patient has a history of severe reaction to penicillamine.

Surveillance During Therapy

Monitor results of CBC with differentials, which should be performed periodically, because blood dyscrasias may occur.

Monitor results of urinary cystine determinations. Dosage adjustments are based on these values.

Monitor patient for any abnormal urinary findings.

Interpret results of diagnostic tests and contact practitioner as appropriate.

Monitor for possible drug–laboratory test interactions.

Monitor for possible drug–drug and drug–nutrient interactions.

Patient Teaching

Assist patient to develop plan to maintain high fluid intake to help deter stone formation.
Teach patient how to recognize symptoms of possible blood dyscrasias, which necessitate drug discontinuation, and to report them.

• *Yohimbine*

Aphrodyne, Yocon, Yohimex

Yohimbine is an alkaloid that chemically resembles reserpine. The drug is primarily an $alpha_2$-adrenergic blocker and can enhance the release of norepinephrine from presynaptic neuronal sites. In addition, it also appears to block peripheral serotonin receptors and readily enters the CNS, where it causes central excitation (irritability, tremor), increased blood pressure and heart rate, and increased release of antidiuretic hormone.

Yohimbine has no FDA-sanctioned uses, but has been used with some success in overcoming male erectile impotence because it can dilate penile vessels. The recommended dose is 5.4 mg three times a day. Yohimbine may also have activity as an aphrodisiac.

The adverse effects are largely caused by the CNS actions of the drug, and include elevated blood pressure and heart rate, irritability, increased motor activity, dizziness, flushing, sweating, nausea, and vomiting. The drug should not be used in people with renal disease or in pregnant women.

Selected Bibliography

Allgayer H: Sulfasalazine and 5-ASA compounds. Gastroenterol Clin North Am 21:643, 1992
Alter BP, Schofield JM, He LY, Weinberg RS: Effects of hemin on erythropoiesis. Adv Exp Med Biol 271:95, 1989
Angle CR: Childhood lead poisoning and its treatment. Annu Rev Pharmacol Toxicol 33:409, 1993
Deal CL, Schnitzer TJ, et al: Treatment of arthritis with topical capsaicin: A double-blind trial. Clin Ther 13:383, 1991
Ferraccioli GF, Salaffi F, et al: Long-term outcome with gold thiosulphate and tiopronin in 200 rheumatoid patients. Clin Exp Rheumatol 7: 577, 1989
Gait JE, Simerl NA: Comparisons of olsalazine and mesalazine in prevention of relapse in ulcerative colitis. Lancet 340:486, 1992
Goldberg DM: Enzymes as agents for the treatment of disease. Clin Chim Acta 206:45, 1992
Hollander E, McCarley A: Yohimbine treatment of sexual side effects induced by serotonin reuptake blockers. J Clin Psychiatry 53: 207, 1992
Kosnett MJ:. Unanswered questions in metal chelation. J Toxicol Clin Toxicol 30:529, 1992
Maggi CA: Therapeutic potential of capsaicin-like molecules: Studies in animals and humans. Life Sci 51:1777, 1992
McNichol RW, Sowell JM, et al: Disulfiram: A guide to clinical use in alcoholism treatment. Am Fam Physician 44:481, 1991
Pathak MA, Fitzpatrick TB: The evolution of photochemotherapy with psoralens and UVA (PUVA): 2000 BC to 1992 AD. J Photochem Photobiol 14:3, 1992
Sinoff SE, Hart MB: Topical capsaicin and burning pain. Clin J Pain 9: 70, 1993
Tsuji A, Wang J, Stenzel KH, Novogrodsky A: Immune stimulatory and anti-tumor properties of haemin. Clin Exp Immunol 93:308, 1993

Nursing Bibliography

Ross A: Nursing interventions for persons receiving immunosuppressive therapies for demyelinating pathology. Nursing Clinics of North America 28(4):829,1993
Roth S: Nursing care of the patient undergoing combined kidney-pancreas transplantation. Critical Care Nursing Quarterly 14(3):30, 1991

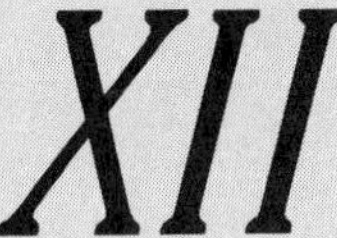

XII

Drug Dependence and Addiction

82 Drug Abuse

CNS Depressants
- Alcohol
- Barbiturates
- Nonbarbiturate Sedatives
- Antianxiety Agents
- Narcotics

Inhalants
- Acetone
- Benzene
- Toluene
- Trichloroethylene
- Others

Marijuana

CNS Stimulants
- Amphetamines
- Anorectics
- Cocaine

Psychotomimetics
- DMT
- DOM
- LSD
- Mescaline
- Psilocybin
- STP

Phencyclidine (PCP)

Nicotine

Despite recent major increases in educational and punitive (ie, jail) approaches, drug abuse remains a significant problem in the United States. Unfortunately, improper use of psychoactive substances—either prescribed legally or obtained illegally—appears resistant to currently available efforts.

A general definition of "drug abuse" is "the use of any psychoactive substance (eg, benzodiazepines, alcohol, volatile solvents) in a manner that deviates from the accepted sociologic norm." A more precise interpretation of this definition—*and* standards determining acceptable patterns of behavior for persons who use drugs—varies among cultures, and what is perceived as abuse of a substance in one culture may been deemed acceptable in another.

Drug abuse has many causes and perpetuating factors. Precipitating circumstances include indiscriminate prescribing of psychoactive drugs by physicians, inadequate monitoring of psychoactive drug use by physicians, pharmacists, and nurses, emotional instability, peer pressure, and a family or neighborhood environment that permits—and even encourages—illegal drug use. A very important indicator of the potential to become a substance abuser is a person's self-image. It is generally concluded by many drug counselors that those teenagers with a negative self-concept are more likely to demonstrate antisocial behavior—which includes the abuse of psychoactive substances—than children who think positively about themselves. Crucial in the development of a positive self-image is the ability of the family to provide love, respect, and discipline. The compulsion to continue to abuse drugs is reinforced by many factors, including availability, parental behavior patterns, stressful demands of everyday life, and a desire for social acceptance. Drug abuse, therefore, is an extremely complex phenomenon involving environmental, sociological, and psychological aspects.

Drug testing is another complex issue. Detection of a psychoactive substance or its metabolites in urine means *only* that use has occurred at some point in the immediate past. There are, however, several problems with even this interpretation. First, a nonuser may passively inhale enough marijuana smoke of others to give a positive urine test (this is *not* likely, but it can happen). Second, because some drugs and their respective metabolites have extremely long half-lives (eg, delta-9-THC, the major psychoactive component of marijuana, has a half-life ranging from approximately 25 to 60 hours), they will appear in the urine from 1 to 6 days *after* use. Third, depending on both the laboratory and the test kit being used, an error can occur; that is, some persons tested may show up as *false* positive (this problem is almost completely eliminated by confirming any result with mass spectrometer/gas chromatograph methodology). Fourth, substances other than those being looked for can give a false reading of an abused substance (eg, decongestants in over-the-counter cold medications can show up as amphetamine in some tests). Fifth, and most important, is the simple fact that the degree of impairment can be accurately correlated only to *blood* levels (or, in the case of alcohol, also to breath levels); it is scientifically invalid to measure the amount of drug in the urine and then attempt to determine the extent to which the person is impaired.

The discussion that follows focuses primarily on the pharmacology of the drugs of abuse and reviews methods for proper recognition and treatment of the drug-intoxicated state. An extensive listing of street names of abused drugs is provided at the end of this chapter to acquaint the reader with some of the terminology used by many drug abusers.

In discussing the drugs of abuse, frequent reference is made to the schedules in which controlled drugs are categorized. These schedules reflect the different regulations governing the prescribing and dispensing of each agent and the penalties for illegal possession. Descriptions of the schedules for controlled substances and a listing of drugs in each schedule are found in Chapter 10.

Before reviewing the pharmacology of abused drugs, it is necessary to describe briefly a few generally accepted terms that appear throughout the discussion (see Chapter 4 for additional information):

Psychological dependence (*Addiction*): A compulsive need to experience a pleasurable drug reaction, ranging from a mild desire to an overwhelming need to use the drug at any cost; **NOTE**: it is *NOT* necessary to develop "tolerance" *or* "physical dependence" for addiction to occur; all "addictions" (eg, "gambling," "sex") have the same psychological characteristics.

Tolerance: The initial adaptive response in which the repeated use of a drug leads to a reduction of its pharmacologic effects; when this decrease in effectiveness includes similar drugs in the same category, it is known as *cross-tolerance*; mechanisms include receptor upregulation or downregulation (eg, receptors that are continually activated by a drug decrease in number or affinity to counteract the excessive stimulation).

Physical dependence: A continuation of the altered physiologic state resulting from prolonged use of a drug; daily drug usage is now *necessary* to avoid experiencing withdrawal reactions, which can be severe and life-threatening (eg, convulsive seizures that can occur during withdrawal from alcohol); severity of withdrawal reactions increases as both the amount of substance abused per day *and* the length of time of abuse increase (for example, the person who had 4 drinks daily for 6 months will have withdrawal reactions less severe than someone who took 10 drinks daily for 5 years).

Long-term treatment of drug addiction is the same as treatment for all other addictions: psychological counseling (single or group) to identify—and try to correct—abnormal self-destructive behaviors.

Central Nervous System Depressants

Alcohol

Alcohol abuse is the major drug problem in the United States in terms of accidents, damaged health, family strife, business interruptions, and socially unacceptable behavior. The actions produced by *acute* alcohol intoxication depend largely on the blood level; in the *non*tolerant drinker effects range from euphoria and altered judgment (50 mg/dL) to reduction in night vision (80 mg/dL) to *noticeable* impairment of motor coordination, concentration, and memory (100–150 mg/dL) to severe depression of respiration and cardiovascular activity and coma (300–400 mg/dL) to death (>400 mg/dL). *Chronic* alcohol abuse produces many toxic—and potentially fatal—effects; they include gastrointestinal (GI) ulceration, liver damage (eg, hepatitis; cirrhosis), pancreatitis, peripheral nerve damage, cardiac impairment, malnutrition, psychotic disturbances (eg, Wernicke's encephalopathy and Korsakoff's psychosis), and cancer (esophageal, liver, pancreatic, rectal). In addition, alcohol when taken with other central nervous system (CNS) depressants (eg, benzodiazepines, such as Valium) is a a frequently observed drug-related hospital emergency and is responsible for more fatalities than any other drug or combination of drugs.

Chronic alcohol ingestion also results in development of tolerance and physical dependence similar to that which occurs with barbiturates. Abrupt and complete cessation of alcohol use after several weeks of steady consumption may result in tremors, GI disturbances, anxiety, confusion, weakness, insomnia, and possibly delusions. Longer periods of alcohol abuse can, on abrupt complete termination, cause delirium tremens (fever, tachycardia, tremors, profuse sweating), agitation, disorientation, intense hallucinations, and convulsions.

Treatment of *acute* alcohol withdrawal is largely symptomatic and usually involves use of sedatives or anticonvulsants (eg, benzodiazepines, barbiturates, phenytoin) along with necessary medical supportive therapy. The most effective management of *chronic* alcoholism involves a combination of supportive social interaction (eg, Alcoholics Anonymous) and psychological counseling. Pharmacotherapy should be avoided because use of antianxiety agents interferes with the need of an alcoholic to adjust to living as a drug-free person, and use of disulfiram (Antabuse; see Chapter 81) can be dangerous and is potentially fatal.

Barbiturates

Barbiturates have declined in therapeutic use because of the availability of drugs that are safer and equally—or more—efficacious (eg, benzodiazepines); they are still employed as anticonvulsants in treatment of epilepsy and, to some degree, as agents for induction of general anesthesia. Members of the drug abuse culture, however, use barbiturates for their significant sedative (ie, anxiety-reducing) effects alone or to minimize central excitatory activity resulting from abuse of CNS stimulants. Barbiturates are classified into either schedule II, III, or IV, depending on their potency, duration of action, and tendency to produce dependence. The shorter-acting drugs (amobarbital, pentobarbital, secobarbital—and combinations thereof) are sought most by abusers because they produce a degree of euphoria after ingestion; they are all schedule II drugs.

Daily barbiturate use for more than 1 week reduces the amount of time spent in rapid eye movement (REM) sleep, which causes irritability and possibly personality and behavioral changes. Because quality sleep is decreased, the user begins to increase the dose to obtain the original depth of sleep (ie, that which occurred during the first few days of barbiturate use).

Symptoms of acute barbiturate intoxication closely resemble those of alcohol intoxication and are related the blood level of the drug; in the drug addict who has developed physical dependence, higher blood levels are required to produce such effects compared with the nontolerant user. Slurred speech, disorientation, impaired motor coordination, poor judgment, confusion, and emotional instability are frequent occurrences with excessive barbiturate usage. Serious overdosage can produce significant depression of respiration, rapid and weak pulse, cyanosis, mydriasis, coma, and ultimately death (of respiratory failure). The CNS effects of barbiturates are additive to those of other CNS depressants, and combinations with alcohol or narcotics often prove fatal.

Withdrawal reactions occur on abrupt termination of excessive barbiturate use; they range from anxiety, weakness, confusion, anorexia, insomnia (due to rebound REM sleep) and mild tremors to delirium, disorientation, hallucinations, and convulsions. Symptoms are generally more severe with the shorter-acting derivatives. Management of the withdrawal state is symptomatic. Treatment of chronic barbiturate dependence may be accomplished by substituting phenobarbital for the barbiturate being abused at a dose that initially provides a similar effect, then gradually reducing the phenobarbital dose over a period of weeks (see also Chapter 22).

Nonbarbiturate Sedatives

Chronic use of a number of other sedative-hypnotics can also result in development of both psychological and physical dependence; a withdrawal syndrome resembling that of the barbiturates also occurs. Glutethimide, methyprylon, and ethchlorvynol are among the hypnotic drugs employed as barbiturate alternatives but offer no significant advantages. Glutethimide in particular is an undesirable agent, inasmuch as convulsions and toxic psychoses have occurred during its continued administration, and its long duration of action makes reversal of acute overdosage extremely difficult (see also Chapter 23).

Although methaqualone (also known as "Ludes") has been withdrawn from the market, it is still manufactured in illegal laboratories and therefore is available for abuse by drug addicts. Methaqualone is used orally and produces effects resembling those of the barbiturates; in addition, paresthesias are experienced by many persons before the onset of the hypnotic effect. Acute toxicity can produce respiratory and cardiovascular depression, convulsions, rigidity, and coma; prolonged use invariably leads to dependence. Withdrawal symptoms noted after cessation of methaqualone use include nausea, headache, cramping, insomnia, and occasionally toxic psychoses and severe convulsions. A combination of methaqualone and the antihistamine diphenhydramine is marketed in Great Britain as Mandrax; it is a more dangerous preparation than methaqualone alone because the antihistamine can produce excitation, ataxia, and psychotic behavior in large doses.

Meprobamate is occasionally used for relief of anxiety, tension, and accompanying muscle spasms. It is somewhat less potent than the barbiturates and correspondingly less toxic, although tolerance occurs rather easily and physical dependence has been reported with as little as 3 g/day for several weeks. Meprobamate withdrawal is usually characterized by insomnia, anxiety, and tremors but can include hallucinations, convulsions, and coma. Fatalities have occurred with meprobamate overdosage.

Antianxiety Agents

The benzodiazepines are the most widely used antianxiety drugs, primarily because their margin of safety is greater than with other sedatives or hypnotics. In addition to being used as "street drugs," benzodiazepines frequently are misused by patients being treated for anxiety neuroses or other psychosomatic disorders. Diazepam (eg, Valium), alprazolam (eg, Xanax) and lorazepam (eg, Ativan) are among the more frequently prescribed benzodiazepines; as with alcohol, they are involved in many emergency room cases. A principal hazard with these drugs is the possibility of serious intoxication when they are combined with other depressants, most notably alcohol; deaths have resulted from this combination. Prolonged use of benzodiazepines has resulted in both psychological and physical dependence; abrupt discontinuation after several months of treatment has resulted in the appearance of cramping, sweating, agitation, disorientation, confusion, tremors, depression, auditory and visual hallucinations, and paranoia. Some patients exhibit these effects after withdrawing from even lower doses (see Chapter 25 for further discussion).

Flurazepam, temazepam, estazolam, quazepam, and triazolam are benzodiazepine analogues used for short-term treatment of insomnia and are claimed to have several advantages over the barbiturates (no hangover, less depression of REM sleep, greater safety margin). Because there is the potential for psychological dependence, these derivatives should be accorded the same respect as other hypnotic agents (eg, barbiturates).

Narcotics (Opioids)

Narcotic drugs include the natural alkaloids morphine and codeine (from the opium plant) and many semisynthetic and synthetic derivatives (see Chapter 20); they are widely used for their antitussive, antidiarrheal, and powerful analgesic actions. The reduction of pain induced by opioids frequently results in a temporary state of euphoria; relief from the accompanying anxiety can be a very pleasurable sensation, especially in patients with long-term pain (eg, cancer). Whereas legitimate patients *rarely* develop psychological dependence, nonpatient drug abusers can rapidly become addicted.

Heroin (schedule I) and Dilaudid (schedule II) are widely abused street drugs. Pure heroin is usually not available; most illicit heroin usually contains only 1% to 10% active drug, the remainder consisting of fillers such as sugars, starches, or quinine. This variable composition is a major cause of overdosage (ie, when the percentage of opiate is significantly larger than expected). Most other narcotics are qualitatively if not quantitatively similar in their effects and are variously classified as schedule II, III, IV, or V. Other frequently abused narcotics are *oxycodone* (alone or in combination with aspirin [eg, Percodan] or acetaminophen [eg, Percocet or Tylox]), *hydrocodone* (usually in combination with acetaminophen [Lortab, Vicodin] or in cough syrups [Hycodan, Tussionex]) and *codeine* (usually codeine-containing cough syrups [eg, Bromanyl, Ambenyl, Tussi-Organidin] or in combination with acetaminophen [eg, Tylenol w/Codeine]).

Intravenous injection of heroin and other powerful narcotics results in a sensation similar to a sexual orgasm (eg, the "rush") and a feeling of extreme contentment. Oral use of narcotics does not produce the "rush" but usually leads to relaxation, euphoria, and a feeling of detachment or indifference to anxiety or pain. Other effects of narcotic drugs unrelated to their abuse potential are miosis, drowsiness, constipation, nausea, vomiting, and depression of vital functions.

Repeated use of narcotics produces tolerance to their pleasurable effects, which consequently causes the need to continually increase the dosage. Eventually, physical dependence develops and the abuser soon requires the drug—not to provide the euphoric effect but to prevent the emergence of withdrawal symptoms. In the physically dependent abuser, doses are pushed to extreme limits to continue to experience the "rush"; overdosage can occur, leading to respiratory failure, which is the most common cause of narcotic-induced death. Other related hazards of narcotic addictions are malnutrition, infections—including acquired immunodeficiency syndrome (AIDS)—attributable to unsterile injection equipment and poor hygiene, toxic reactions to contaminants injected along with the narcotic, hepatitis, vasculitis, and thromboembolic complications.

Acute opioid overdosage is marked by stupor, slow and shallow respiration, pinpoint pupils (**NOTE**: patients may present with *dilated* pupils because of activation of the sympathoadrenal system in cases of extreme overdosage), cold and clammy skin, hypotension, bradycardia, and possibly coma. Treatment involves a narcotic antagonist (naloxone) along with necessary supportive treatment (respiratory assistance, vasopressors). Dosage of the narcotic antagonist must be carefully controlled to avoid precipitation of acute withdrawal symptoms.

When narcotics are unavailable to a physically dependent individual, withdrawal symptoms usually begin within 8 to 12 hours, reach a maximum intensity in 36 to 72 hours, and can persist for up to 7 to 10 days. The persistence and severity of these symptoms depends on the drug involved, the degree of dependence (a function of the length of time the drugs have been used), and the average amount administered. Initial signs of withdrawal include yawning, perspiration, lacrimation, sneezing, and restlessness. Progressively severe symptoms encompass anorexia, irritability, insomnia, anxiety, vomiting, generalized body aches, stomach cramping, diarrhea, fever, chills, tremors, jerking movements, muscle spasms, tachycardia, and elevated blood pressure. Although frightening to the patient, symptoms experienced during narcotic withdrawal are not usually life threatening, in contrast to those associated with barbiturate withdrawal, which have resulted in fatalities.

Withdrawal symptoms can be suppressed by administration of another narcotic, frequently oral methadone; the initial stabilizing dose of methadone depends on the amount of narcotic abused per day. Methadone's long duration of action (up to 24 hours) permits use of one dose per day. This procedure is designed to stabilize a narcotic addict on a regular oral dose of methadone to develop *cross-tolerance* to the abused opioid (eg, heroin). Thus, the addict no longer experiences the narcotic-induced "rush" when it is injected (or taken orally). After stabilization, an eventual—and gradual—reduction of the dose should begin. Of course, the addict should also receive psychotherapy because use of methadone alone will *not* result in elimination of the narcotic abuse problem. It should be understood that because methadone is also a powerful narcotic, its abuse has now become a significant problem as well. Withdrawal from methadone is more prolonged than withdrawal from opiates, but symptoms are often less severe. A newer chemically related compound, levomethadyl (ORLAAM), has an even longer duration of action (48–72 hours) and is also being employed for management of narcotic addiction in a similar manner to utilization of methadone.

Naltrexone (Trexan) is a long-acting *antagonist* that is also available for treatment of narcotic addiction; effects of even intravenous heroin can be blocked for up to 3 days, depending on the naltrexone dose. The patient must be narcotic free for at least 7 days and have normal liver function before receiving naltrexone.

Detoxification programs work best in conjunction with psychiatric and social counseling. Because the addict's daily behavior is usually structured completely around obtaining and using narcotic drugs, withdrawal alone will not be successful in overcoming narcotic dependence.

Inhalants

Volatile hydrocarbons such as acetone, benzene, carbon tetrachloride, trichloroethane, trichloroethylene, and toluene are present in many household products, including glue, paint, lighter fluid, nail polish remover, and varnish thinner, and are frequently abused by young persons. These volatile liquids are commonly placed on a rag or handkerchief or in a bag, and inhaled. The initial effects are CNS excitation, characterized by a sense of exhilaration, dizziness, and occasionally auditory or visual hallucinations, accompanied by tinnitus, blurred vision, slurred speech, and a staggering gait. These effects generally last 30 to 60 minutes. Larger amounts of inhaled vapors can lead to drowsiness, hypotension, delirium, stupor, unconsciousness, and possibly coma. Amnesia frequently follows recovery. Fatalities have resulted, either from drug-induced respiratory failure or from suffocation from the plastic bags placed over the face. Cardiac arrest also has been reported.

Recent reports indicate that several deaths among teenagers resulted from inhalation of correction fluid (eg, Liquid Paper, White-Out); the halogenated hydrocarbons in these products appear to induce ventricular fibrillation. Also, several teenagers have died after inhalation of *butane gas* (used to refill cigarette lighters); some of these victims died of burns to their lungs when the butane caught fire and traveled along the vapor trail directly into their bodies.

Although psychological dependence can develop, physical dependence is rare (primarily because the duration of action is short). *Chronic* direct inhalation of volatile hydrocarbons can result in significant organ damage, especially to the liver, kidneys, heart, and CNS (eg, cerebellar ataxia, equilibrium disorders, optic neuropathy, hearing loss, impaired memory, and a decreased ability to concentrate); such damage also can occur when inhaled indirectly from the workplace. These dangerous aspects of volatile inhalant abuse are overlooked by youthful users.

Treatment of acute intoxication resembles that of barbiturate overdosage and employs oxygen and respiratory assistance along with other supportive care as needed. Injections of vasopressors (such as epinephrine) should be avoided, however, because there is danger that myocardial sensitization by volatile halogenated hydrocarbons may precipitate arrhythmias in the presence of adrenergic amines.

Marijuana

Marijuana is obtained from the hemp plant, *Cannabis sativa*, and constitutes a mixture of dried leaves, flowering tops, and other parts of the plant. The biologically active constituents of marijuana are termed *cannabinoids;* among the more than 60 known compounds, delta-9-tetrahydrocannabinol (THC) appears to be the major psychoactive chemical. Marijuana can be taken orally but is more powerful when rolled into cigarettes (joints) and smoked. Depending on the potency, peak psychopharmacologic effects occur within 10 to 20 minutes of inhalation and persist for 1 to 4 hours. The average joint contains between 2% and 4% THC (approximately 10–20 mg), of which approximately one-half is usually absorbed. More powerful varieties are grown in countries located in warmer climates; the THC content may be 10% or higher.

The resinous secretions from the flowering tops of the cannabis plant are also available as hashish. These secretions are usually dried and then either smoked or compressed into a variety of other dosage forms, such as cookies, cakes, or candies. Although hashish ranges in potency depending on the source, it is generally between 5 and 10 times more potent than marijuana itself. Hashish oil, a concentrated liquid extract of cannabis plant materials, contains a high percentage of THC (10%–50%), and several drops are equivalent to a single joint of marijuana. Hashish oil has also been administered IV, but this procedure is associated with a significant mortality.

The psychological effects of marijuana vary widely among individuals and depend on the mental status, mood, previous experience, and expectations of the users, as well as the environment and circumstances surrounding its use. Typical reactions include a sense of relaxation and wellbeing (possibly even euphoria), impaired time and space orientation, altered sensory perception (especially sound and color), and spontaneous—often uncontrolled—laughter. Short-term memory may be affected, psychomotor performance may be somewhat impaired, and attention span can be reduced. Driving ability may be compromised because marijuana can *decrease* both reaction time and psychomotor performance; such impairment has reduced these critical skills needed to safely operate a vehicle, and car accidents have occurred in which the drivers were found to have measurable levels of THC in their blood!

Physiologic changes accompanying marijuana usage can include elevated pulse rate and conjunctival congestion, which occur routinely, and erythema, enhanced appetite, disturbed equilibrium, xerostomia, oropharyngeal irritation, tinnitus, and paresthesias.

Adverse reactions may appear to be minimal with occasional use in emotionally stable persons. Reported untoward reactions to marijuana comprise mild depression, anxiety, agitation, and a panic state, most frequently observed in first-time users. Acute intoxication from high doses may produce a *toxic psychosis* manifested by paranoia, image distortion, depersonalization, disorganized thought and speech, fantasies, and, rarely, hallucinations. Acute psychoses can also develop in patients with schizophrenia (known or undiagnosed), even in those currently being treated with antipsychotic medications. This condition usually resolves within 24 hours. Even though there is no significant clinical evidence of marijuana-induced teratogenicity, marijuana has caused birth defects in animals; therefore, it should *not* be used during pregnancy. THC can disrupt pituitary production of gonadotropic hormones and is excreted in breast milk; women who are breast-feeding should not use marijuana.

Although acute overdosage with marijuana is rare, episodes can be managed by appropriate support of respiration, blood pressure, and other vital functions as required. A quiet environment and reassuring attitude are helpful during the acute psychotic phase; extreme agitation is best treated with benzodiazepines (eg, diazepam).

Psychological dependence may occur, but physical dependence is rare. A phenomenon of reverse tolerance has been reported in some marijuana users, whereby smaller amounts of the drug are able to elicit the desired psychic effects with repeated administration. This may be caused in part by cumulation effects of the drug with frequent use.

Chronic use of marijuana has been implicated in pulmonary toxicity (precancerous cellular changes); this is not surprising because many of the cancer-causing chemicals that are in cigarette tobacco are also found in marijuana. In male users, there may be a decrease in both sperm production and sperm motility and an increased number of abnormal forms of sperm; women may experience menstrual irregularities. Animal studies in primates indicate some abnormal changes in brain cells (eg, increased width of synapses) after prolonged exposure to marijuana smoke; although there is no such clinical evidence, some chronic marijuana users have reported reductions in their short-term memory that still exist years after stopping their marijuana use.

Regarding clinical applications, delta-9-THC, as dronabinol (Marinol), is now available in the United States for anorexia (and weight loss) in AIDS patients and for reducing nausea and vomiting caused by cancer chemotherapy.

Another area of potential therapeutic use of cannabinoids, especially THC, is reduction of elevated intraocular pressure in glaucoma. Other pharmacologic actions of THC currently being studied for possible clinical use include its possible analgesic, anti-inflammatory, tranquilizing, bronchodilatory, and anticonvulsant effects.

CNS Stimulants

Amphetamines

The three amphetamines (DL-amphetamine, dextroamphetamine, methamphetamine), as well as the structural analogues phenmetrazine and methylphenidate, are schedule II drugs. Their approved clinical indications are limited, including only treatment of the attention deficit disorder syndrome in children, short-term treatment of obesity, and symptomatic control of narcolepsy. Amphetamines are, however, a widely abused group of drugs and, together with the anorectics (see next discussion), are misused for their CNS-stimulating effects. Students, truck drivers, housewives, executives, athletes, and health professionals (eg, doctors, nurses, pharmacists) have used amphetamines to suppress fatigue, increase alertness, enhance psychomotor performance, and produce euphoria. Although potentially hazardous, and in some instances illegal, this type of amphetamine administration is usually not labeled "abusive." Amphetamine abuse refers to the parenteral or oral administration of large doses of the drugs to attain the intense "rush" or "high" characteristic of these agents. Methamphetamine (eg, "Speed") is a favorite among drug abusers because an IV injection elicits immediate euphoria (orgasmic-like reaction). However, tolerance to this effect develops rapidly so that in a short time increasingly larger doses must be administered to experience the same sensation. Whereas normal therapeutic doses are in the 5-mg to 15-mg/day range, "speed freaks" have been known to use as much as 5,000 mg/day. Obviously such large-dose administration cannot continue for long, and after a period of several days to weeks, the person becomes exhausted to the point of lapsing into long periods of sleep and depression—the so-called "crash."

Symptoms of mild amphetamine intoxication include insomnia, increased blood pressure and pulse rate, excitation, hyperactive reflexes, mydriasis, anorexia, and palpitations. More severe overdosage is reflected by extreme agitation, hostility, impulsiveness, hallucinations, confusion, bizarre behavior, aggressiveness, paranoid ideation, convulsions, and possibly death. The social implications of amphetamine abuse are obvious. Methamphetamine abuse, moreover, can result in cerebral vascular spasm, systemic necrotizing angiitis, cerebral hemorrhaging (cerebrovascular accident; CVA), arrhythmias, and severe abdominal pain. Effects of acute amphetamine intoxication have been treated with haloperidol, a dopamine antagonist with minimal anticholinergic effects. Acidification of the urine markedly increases the excretion of amphetamines and can be employed to facilitate renal elimination.

Prolonged use of amphetamines can produce physical dependence; abrupt withdrawal results in an increased appetite, fatigue, lethargy, and depression. Withdrawal should be accomplished by allowing the patient to remain in a quiet environment and providing support of vital functions where necessary.

Although the legal production of amphetamines has been sharply curtailed by the federal government, illegal laboratories currently provide these drugs—especially methamphetamine—for the street market. Amphetamine abuse remains a serious sociological and medical problem.

Phenmetrazine, an anorectic (see below), and methylphenidate, a drug principally used in attention deficit disorder (see Chapter 29), are two structurally related compounds classified as schedule II drugs that possess pharmacologic and toxicologic actions similar to those of the amphetamines. Although administered orally for their clinical indications, the tablets are frequently dissolved in water by abusers and injected IV. A major danger associated with parenteral use of these drugs is the presence of insoluble talc particles in the injection solution, which can result in circulatory impairment and talc deposits in the lungs and eye.

Anorectics

A number of other amphetamine-related drugs termed "anorectics" are employed as adjuncts in the treatment of obesity and are discussed in Chapter 29. Their pharmacology in most cases is similar to that of the amphetamines but they are less potent CNS stimulants and generally not as desirable as street drugs. They are, however, frequently misused as appetite suppressants, and chronic ingestion of these agents produces many of the symptoms of prolonged amphetamine use, namely insomnia, elevated blood pressure, tachycardia, and anxiety. Severe overdosage can result in a syndrome resembling amphetamine intoxication; these drugs should never be used continuously for longer than several weeks at a time. Most of these drugs are found in schedule III, whereas phentermine and fenfluramine are listed in schedule IV.

Cocaine

Cocaine, a natural product extracted from leaves of the coca plant, has been employed clinically as a local anesthetic (especially for the nose and oral cavity). Currently a very popular drug of abuse, cocaine has systemic effects very similar to those of amphetamine but more powerful and of much shorter duration. The powdered drug is most commonly administered by inhalation or snorting through the nasal passages; IV injection is also a favored route. "Crack," a hardened form of cocaine, is heated in a glass pipe and smoked; it rapidly (almost equal to IV administration) produces an intense euphoria. Irrespective of its route of administration, cocaine quickly elicits a pleasurable "high" accompanied by tachycardia, elevated blood pressure, restlessness, and mydriasis. Repeated use can lead to a strong psychological—and physical—dependence; the cocaine addict is extremely involved in obtaining—and using—it on a daily (sometimes hourly) basis. Cocaine powder is often adulterated with various sugars and local anesthetics at every level of distribution; clinical studies have shown that cocaine users are unable to distinguish between lidocaine and cocaine.

Chronic use of cocaine is associated with the following effects:

Cardiovascular
- Arrhythmias
- Acute myocardial infarction
- Rupture of the ascending aorta
- Cerebrovascular accident (CVA; stroke)

Respiratory
- Pulmonary edema
- Pneumomediastinum
- Rhinorrhea
- Rhinitis
- Ulceration and perforation of the nasal septum

Gastrointestinal
- Intestinal ischemia (may cause gangrene, requiring resection)
- Weight loss
- Nausea

Central nervous system
- Anxiety
- Irritability
- Tactile hallucinations (imaginary skin insects, or "cocaine bugs")
- Visual disturbances (flashing lights, or "snow effect")
- Paranoia
- Insomnia
- Assertive behavior

Genitourinary
- Difficulty in maintaining erection
- Delay in orgasm for both men and women

Overdosage with cocaine can lead to arrhythmias, tremors, convulsions, respiratory failure, and death. Treatment of acute intoxication involves many considerations but primary attention to cardiovascular (hypertension; arrhythmias) and CNS (eg, seizures) events is extremely important.

Use of cocaine during pregnancy is associated with spontaneous abortion. Infants born to such women show deficits in both sensory and motor functions, which persist to at least 2 years of age.

Withdrawal from cocaine results in excessive fatigue, hypersomnia, depression (with possible suicidal tendencies), and extreme craving for the drug. Bromocriptine (Parlodel), a dopamine agonist, is of benefit in reducing the latter effect.

Psychotomimetics

Psychotomimetic drugs, often termed hallucinogens, include both naturally occurring (eg, psilocybin; mescaline) and synthetic (eg, lysergic acid diethylamide [LSD]; 2,5 dimethoxy-4-methyl amphetamine [DOM]) compounds, which produce significant distortions of reality. Psychotomimetics are schedule I drugs that can cause serious psychological harm to the occasional—as well as the frequent—user. They have the capacity to distort mental function (often producing confusion, delirium and amnesia) and senses of direction, time, and distance. With large doses, delusions and hallucinations are common [Note: because users usually know that the distortions they are seeing are *not* real, the more accurate term is "*pseudo*hallucination;" however, in this chapter, the more commonly used term—hallucination—is employed]. Seriously impaired judgment and severe depression have frequently resulted from ingestion of these drugs. Although hallucinations are usually employed to experience pleasant psychic alterations (eg, euphoria, elation, vivid color imagery, synesthesias ["hearing" colors; "seeing" sounds]), the actual experience depends on both the "*set*" (psychological state of user, eg, depressed, anxious) and "*setting*" (immediate environment [eg, inside a room; outside in a park]). Some users experience anxiety, dysphoria, panic, severe depression, and despair; this is known as a "bad trip." These latter effects tend to occur in inexperienced, nontolerant persons, especially those with preexisting psychological problems;

they can occur in anyone after large doses. Treatment of "bad" trips involves placing the patient in a nonthreatening, supportive environment and maintaining reassuring verbal contact (the "talk-down"). Reassure patients that the "bad trip" will end, the frightening visions are due to the drug, and they are not "going crazy." The "talk-down" should also include *reality-defining* (gently urge patients to talk about what they are now experiencing and have them repeat simple, concrete statements, eg, "this is a table [book; chair]," etc.); it also can be reassuring to repeatedly tell patients their names. If unsuccessful in calming the patient and pharmacotherapy is indicated, benzodiazepines are recommended. Phenothiazines should be avoided because they have anticholinergic effects; if the person on a "bad trip" actually has ingested high doses of an over-the-counter (OTC) sleeping pill such as Nytol or Sominex (both contain diphenhydramine, which also has anticholinergic activity) and is given a phenothiazine, an "anticholinergic crisis" can develop, which then has to be reversed with cholinergic drugs (eg, physostigmine [Antilirium]).

Most "bad trips" end within 24 to 48 hours but do not discuss it immediately after it ends because patients are still recovering psychologically. Even with optimal treatment, some "bad trips" push the patient into a prolonged psychotic episode that can be indistinguishable from a schizophrenic reaction. A reliable sign of recovery from "bad trip" is a good night of sleep; it ends the state of tension and helps to restore psychological equilibrium.

Recurrences of the perceptual distortions are experienced by a large number of psychotomimetic drug users, especially with LSD, and can occur up to 5 years after initial usage. These flashbacks vary in duration from seconds to minutes and, although occasionally spontaneous, are most frequently triggered by periods of stress or anxiety or by use of other psychotropic drugs, such as marijuana. These flashback episodes may be potentially harmful to the person, depending on their severity and place of occurrence.

A degree of tolerance to the behavioral and psychological effects of LSD develops within a short period, but marked psychological dependence is rare, and physical dependence does not occur. There are no characteristic symptoms after abrupt discontinuation of drug usage.

Chronic episodes of psychotic behavior are not uncommon after use of psychotomimetic drugs. Most occur in persons who exhibit underlying emotional instability. The extent to which use of hallucinogens contributes to the protracted disturbed behavior of these people is difficult to assess accurately. Unfortunately, it is just such unstable persons who frequently become involved with use of psychotomimetic agents.

Many commonly used hallucinogens are *tryptaminergic*, that is, they have molecular similarity to serotonin and apparent specific affinity for postsynaptic 5-HT_2 receptors. Psychoactive drugs of this category include:

LSD: synthetic drug; most potent hallucinogen currently available; effects usually last 8 to 12 hours; tolerance develops quickly and effects usually cannot be duplicated for several days; sold as tablets, thin squares of gelatin (window panes), or impregnated paper (blotter acid); average effective oral dose is 25 to 50 μg.

Mescaline: active ingredient of flowering heads of the peyote cactus; oral doses of 250 to 500 mg produce hallucinations lasting 6 to 12 hours

DOM ("STP" [Serenity, Tranquility, Peace]): synthetic drug (2,5-dimethoxy-4-methylamphetamine); similar to mescaline; powerful psychotomimetic drug producing intense, prolonged psychic alterations that can last for several days after a single oral dose; frequently sold on the illicit market as mescaline

DMT: naturally occurring hallucinogen; *N, N*-dimethyltryptamine is not effective orally; must be inhaled or smoked; produces a rapid, brief alteration in perception and mood

Psilocybin ("Magic mushrooms"; "Shrooms"): a natural product (mushrooms of the "Psilocybe" variety); biotransformed to **psilocin** (active metabolite); chemically related to LSD but less potent and shorter acting; usually administered orally

Other substances used for their hallucinogenic effects include:

Anticholinergics: large doses of either natural products, eg, plants (eg, jimson weed) which contain Belladonna alkaloids (eg, atropine and scopolamine) or various drugs with anticholinergic activity (eg, diphenhydramine found in OTC products for treatment of insomnia [eg, Nytol; Sominex]), can produce hallucinogenic activity.

Adrenergics: drugs with a molecular structure related to amphetamine; includes **MDMA** (3,4,-*M*ethylene*D*ioxy*M*eth*A*mphetamine; "Ecstasy"; "Adam") and **MDEA** (3,4-*M*ethylene*D*ioxy*E*thyl*A*mphetamine; "Eve"); pharmacologic and toxicologic effects are very similar to those of the amphetamines except hallucinations are more likely to develop; death has occurred in a number of users; chances of a fatality increase in users who have ingested "smart" drinks containing amino acids (especially tryptophan) *and/or* are very active physically (eg, "rave dancing") and dehydrated (because of sweating and/or reduced fluid intake); toxic reactions should be attended to *immediately*, including treatment of hypertension, tachycardia, and hyperthermia (agitation and seizures also have occurred); early deaths (within 24 hours) are related to cardiac arrhythmias and seizures; late deaths (24–48 hours) are usually caused by development of the "Neuroleptic Malignant Syndrome."

Phencyclidine

Related to ketamine, phencyclidine (PCP; "Angel Dust") had been used as a veterinary anesthetic. However, this potent psychotomimetic, one of the most dangerous drugs of abuse, is no longer manufactured legally in the United States; it is, however, still produced by illegal laboratories. The PCP available on the street, often highly contaminated, is frequently misrepresented as LSD, THC, cocaine, or mescaline. Although occasionally administered orally or IV, it is most often used by smoking or nasal inhalation (snorting).

Effects of PCP depend on the dose and route of administration. Small amounts elicit euphoria, numbness of the extremities, and a sense of detachment. Larger amounts can result in analgesia, impaired speech, loss of coordination, agitation, muscle rigidity, tachycardia, elevated blood pressure (which may cause death by a CVA), exaggerated gait, auditory hallucinations, acute anxiety, self-destructive behavior, and severe mood disorders, including paranoia, violent hostility, and feelings of depersonalization or doom. A psychotic state indistinguishable from paranoid schizophrenia is often a result of prolonged use of the drug but has occurred after only one dose. Delayed psychological reactions have been observed for up to several weeks after administration.

"Bad trips" can readily occur with PCP; these behavioral disturbances are often severe and prolonged. A very effective method of treating the "bad trip" includes placing the user in a room with *minimal* sensory stimuli; the room should be **quiet** and **dark**. *In contrast* to treatment of LSD-induced "bad trips," verbal contact should be **avoided** during the acute recovery stage from the adverse PCP reaction. Involuntary movements, facial grimacing, torticollis, and catatonic-like posturing are frequently present. If needed, benzodiazepines can be used to control agitation. It must be understood that the PCP user who becomes agitated will be *extremely difficult to control*, even when three or four staff members combine to intervene; because PCP has powerful analgesic properties, use of physical force (even in self-defense) will not be felt—and may only further enrage—the out-of-control user. Because recovery can take several days, patients should be kept under close observation during this time. Urinary acidifiers increase the renal excretion of PCP.

Nicotine

Cigarettes kill approximately 420,000 American smokers every year; the *yearly* healthcare cost for treating such patients is approximately $72 *billion*!

In addition, nonsmokers—including children—who passively inhale cigarette smoke in the workplace or home also experience increased sickness and death.

Nicotine is an alkaloid found in tobacco (concentration usually between 1% and 2%). When a cigarette is smoked, nicotine

Table 82-1
Glossary of Street Names for Drugs of Abuse

Street Name	***Drug***	***Street Name***	***Drug***
Acapulco gold	Marijuana	Dexies	Dextroamphetamine
Acid	LSD	Dillies	Dilaudid
Angel dust	Phencyclidine	Dollies	Methadone
Aurora	Phencyclidine	Double cross	Amphetamines
Bennies	Amphetamines	Downers	Barbiturates
Big H	Heroin	Estuffa	Heroin
Black beauties	Amphetamines	First line	Morphine
Black mollies	Amphetamines	Flake	Cocaine
Blockbusters	Barbiturates	Footballs	Amphetamines
Blotter acid	LSD	Ganga	Marijuana
Blow	Cocaine	Giri	Cocaine
Bluebirds	Barbiturates	Glass	Methamphetamine
Blue devils	Barbiturates	Goma	Morphine
Blue velvet	Paregoric *plus* Amphetamine	Grass	Marijuana
Blues	Barbiturates	Green dragons	Barbiturates
Boy	Heroin	Griffa	Marijuana
Brown	Heroin	Guerilla	Phencyclidine
Brownies	Amphetamines	H	Heroin
Brown sugar	Heroin	Hash	Hashish
Buttons	Peyote	Haze	LSD
C	Cocaine	Hazel	Heroin
Caballo	Heroin	Hearts	Dextroamphetamine
Cactus	Peyote	Heaven dust	Cocaine
California sunshine	LSD	Hemp	Marijuana
Cannabis	Marijuana	Herb	Marijuana
Charley	Cocaine	Hero	Heroin
Christmas tree	Barbiturates	Hog	Phencyclidine, chloral hydrate
Chiva	Heroin	Hombre	Heroin
Coca	Cocaine	Horse	Heroin
Coke	Cocaine	Ice	Methamphetamine
Colombian	Marijuana	J	Marijuana
Copilots	Amphetamines	Jay	Marijuana
Crack	Cocaine	Jet	Phencyclidine
Crank	Methamphetamines	Joint	Marijuana
Crap	Heroin	Junk	Heroin
Crossroads	Amphetamines	Lady	Cocaine
Crystal	Methamphetamine, phencyclidine	Log	Marijuana
Cube	Morphine, LSD	Ludes	Methaqualone
Cubes	LSD	Mary Jane	Marijuana
Cyclone	Phencyclidine		

(continued)

is rapidly absorbed by the lungs and produces many effects, including:

CV: peripheral vasoconstriction, tachycardia, increased blood pressure
GI: reduced appetite, diarrhea, constipation, nausea and vomiting (novice users)
CNS: insomnia, headache, dizziness, paresthesia
GU: dysmenorrhea

Because of the strong psychological and physical dependence, it is very difficult for many cigarette users to stop smoking even though most agree that it is a harmful—even life-threatening—addiction! Another factor that decreases the chance for a smoker to successfully terminate such use is that cigarettes still are available legally for sale in the United States (cigarettes remain a significant source of tax revenue for the federal and many state governments).

Disorders caused by cigarette smoking include periodontal disease, cancer of the oral cavity, emphysema and lung cancer; in **female** smokers, the death rate from lung cancer has increased greatly during the past 10 years and now causes more deaths than breast cancer. Cardiovascular disorders include peripheral vascular disease, coronary artery disease (eg, myocardial infarction) and cerebral infarction. Damage to the gastrointestinal tract includes gastritis and ulceration. Smokers also have more cataracts and bladder cancer than nonsmokers. These toxicities are caused not only by the nicotine content but also from constant exposure to the many carcinogenic products found in cigarette tobacco.

Women who smoke during their pregnancy have higher rates of miscarriage, spontaneous abortion, prenatal mortality, and premature births than nonsmokers.

The newborn of female smokers are underweight and shorter than normal.

Switching to smokeless (chewing) tobacco is not safe either; many users of these products develop gum shrinkage (gingival recession) and leukoplakic lesions in the mouth; *oral cancer* is a definite threat with use of chewing tobacco and has already caused the death of users, including teenagers!

Recent data indicate that *non*smokers also suffer when

Table 82-1
Glossary of Street Names for Drugs of Abuse (Continued)

Street Name	*Drug*	*Street Name*	*Drug*
Mesc	Peyote, mescaline	Reefer	Marijuana
Mescal	Peyote	Roach	Marijuana
Meth	Methamphetamine	Rock	Cocaine
Mexican mud	Heroin	Rocket fuel	Phencyclidine
Mexican reds	Barbiturates, secobarbital	Roses	Amphetamines
Microdots	LSD, Morphine	Sativa	Marijuana
Minibennies	Amphetamines	Scag	Heroin
Mist	Phencyclidine	Shermans	Phencyclidine
Morf	Morphine	Sleeping pills	Barbiturates
Morpho	Morphine	Smack	Heroin
Morphy	Morphine	Smoke	Marijuana
Mota	Marijuana	Snow	Cocaine
Mud	Morphine	Soapers	Methaqualone
Mujer	Cocaine	Soles	Hashish
Mutah	Marijuana	Sparklers	Amphetamines
Nebbies	Barbiturates, pentobarbital	Speed	Methamphetamine
Nimbies	Barbiturates, pentobarbital	Speedball	Heroin *plus* Cocaine
Nose candy	Cocaine	Stick	Marijuana
Oranges	Amphetamines	Stumblers	Barbiturates
Owsleys	LSD	Stuff	Heroin
Panama red	Marijuana	Sunshine	LSD
Paper acid	LSD	Supergrass	Phencyclidine
Paradise	Cocaine	T's and blues	Pentazocine and tripelennamine
PCP	Phencyclidine	Tar	Opium
Peace pill	Phencyclidine	Tea	Marijuana
Pep pills	Amphetamines	THC	Tetrahydrocannabinol
Perico	Cocaine	Thing	Heroin
Pink ladies	Barbiturates	Thrusters	Amphetamines
Pinks	Barbiturates, secobarbital	Tic tac	Phencyclidine
Pinks and Grays	Propoxyphene	Truck drivers	Amphetamines
Polvo	Heroin	Uppers	Amphetamines
Polvo blanco	Cocaine	Wake-ups	Amphetamines
Pot	Marijuana	Wedges	LSD
Purple haze	LSD	Weed	Marijuana
Quacks	Methaqualone	Whack	Phencyclidine
Quads	Methaqualone	Whites	Amphetamines
Rainbows	Barbiturates, Tuinal	Window panes	LSD
Reds and blues	Barbiturates, Tuinal	Yellow jackets	Barbiturates, pentobarbital
Redbirds	Barbiturates, secobarbital	Yellows	Barbiturates, pentobarbital
Red devils	Barbiturates, secobarbital		

exposed to cigarette smoke; reported diseases increased by passive inhalation include bronchitis and lung cancer. Children who live with one or smokers exhibit higher rates of respiratory disease and otitis media with effusion; in addition, they also appear to present with higher rates of cancers such as acute lymphocytic leukemia, lymphomas, and brain cancer.

Psychotherapeutic intervention and continued support are the most effective methods by which a person can permanently stop smoking. Because physical dependence to nicotine does occur, withdrawal can result in nausea, diarrhea, headache, insomnia, irritability, and poor concentration. Weight gain often occurs because of both an increased appetite and the substitution of food for oral gratification. Utilization of nicotine replacement therapy (eg, nicotine patches; see Chapter 12) can be a useful adjunct in programs designed to help a person give up cigarette smoking.

Selected Bibliography

Abraham HD, Aldridge AM: Adverse consequences of lysergic acid diethylamide. Addiction 8:1327, 1993

Anderson P, Cremona A, Paton A, Turner C, Wallace P: The risk of alcohol. Addiction 88:1493, 1993

Cone EJ, Huestis MA: Relating blood concentrations of tetrahydrocannabinol and metabolites to pharmacologic effects and time of marijuana usage. Ther Drug Monitor 15:527, 1993

Conway T, Balson A: Concomitant abuse of clonidine and heroin. J Southern Med Assoc 86(8):954, 1993

Des Jarlais DC, Friedman SR: AIDS and the use of injected drugs. Sci Am 270(2):82, 1994

Drugs of Abuse. Trends Pharmacol Sci 13:169, 1992

Hunt WA, Nixon SJ (eds): Alcohol-induced brain damage. Research Monograph #22, National Institute on Alcohol Abuse and Alcoholism, 1993

Kain ZN, Rimar S, Barash PG: Cocaine abuse in the parturient and effects on the fetus and neonate. Anesth Analg 77:835, 1993

Kupari M, Koskinen P: Comparison of the cardiotoxicity of ethanol in women versus men. Am J Cardiol 70:645, 1992

Loiselle JM, Baker MD, Templeton JM, Schwartz G, Drott H: Substance abuse in adolescent trauma. Ann Emerg Med 22(10):1530, 1993

Paraf F, Lewis J, Jothy S: Acute fatty liver of pregnancy after exposure to toluene. J Clin Gastroenterol 17(2):163, 1993

Watters JK, Estilo MJ, Clark GL, Lorvick J: Syringe and needle exchange as HIV/AIDS prevention for injection drug users. JAMA 271(2):115, 1994

Wood JH, Katz JL, Winger G: Benzodiazepines: Use, abuse and consequences. Pharmacol Rev 44:151, 1992

Nursing Bibliography

Belcaster A: Caring for the alcohol abuser. Nursing '94 24(2):56, 1992

Lindblom L, et al: Chemical abuse: An intervention program for the elderly. J Gerontol Nurs 18(4):6, 1992

Solari-Twadell P: Recreational drugs: Societal and professional issues. Nurs Clin North Am 26(2):499, 1991

Appendices

A
Common Abbreviations

aa	of each (equal parts)
abd.	abdomen
ac	before meals
AD	right ear
ad	up to
ad lib	as much as needed
Adm.	admission, admitted
alb.	albumin
alk.	alkaline
ALT	alanine aminotransferase
AM	morning
amp.	ampule
amt.	amount
appt.	appointment
aq. (dest.)	water (distilled)
AS	left ear
AST	aspartate aminotransferase
AU	each (both) ear(s)
aur.	ear
AV	atrioventricular
bid	twice daily
bm	bowel movement
BP	blood pressure
BPH	benign prostatic hypertrophy
c̄	with
Ca	calcium
CAD	coronary artery disease
Cal.	calories
caps	capsule
CBC	complete blood count
cc	cubic centimeter
CHF	congestive heart failure
Cl	chloride
CNS	central nervous system
c/o	complained of
col. ct.	colony count
comp.	compound
conc.	concentrated
COP	cardiac output
COPD	chronic obstructive pulmonary disease
CP	cerebral palsy
CPR	cardiopulmonary resuscitation
cv	cardiovascular
cxr	chest x-ray
d/c	discontinue
diarr.	diarrhea
dil.	dilute
disch.	discharge
disp.	dispense
dist.	distilled
dL, dl	deciliter
DOA	date of admission
DOB	date of birth
DPT, DTP	diphtheria, pertussis, tetanus immunization
dr.	dram
dsg./dssg.	dressing
dtd	dispense such doses
DTR	deep tendon reflexes
Dx.	diagnosis
ECG (EKG)	electrocardiogram
ECR	emergency chemical restraint
ED	emergency department
EEG	electroencephalogram
eg	for example
elix.	elixir
EMG	electromyogram
ENT	ear, nose, throat
EOM	extraocular movements
ER	emergency room
etc.	et cetera
eval	evaluation
ex.	example
extrem.	extremity
FBS	fasting blood sugar
Fe	iron
fl.	fluid
ft	foot; feet
FUO	fever of unknown origin
g, gm	gram
G-6-PD	glucose-6-phosphate dehydrogenase
gal	gallon
GFR	glomerular filtration rate
GC	gonorrhea, gonococcus
GI	gastrointestinal
gr	grain
gt (gtt)	drop(s)
GU	genitourinary
gyn	gynecology
h, hr	hour
Hct	hematocrit
HDL	high-density lipoprotein
Hgb	hemoglobin
HEENT	head, eyes, ears, nose, and throat
HIV	human immunodeficiency virus
Hosp.	hospital
H-S	hepato-spleno
h.s.	hour of sleep, bedtime
hx.	history
IA	intraarterial
ICP	intracranial pressure
ie	that is
IM	intramuscular

I&O, I/O	intake and output
IPPB	intermittent positive pressure breathing
IPV	inactivated polio vaccine
IV	intravenous
K	potassium
L, l	liter
Ⓛ	left
Lab.	laboratory
Lat.	lateral
lb	pound(s)
LDH	lactate dehydrogenase
LDL	low-density lipoprotein
LE	lower extremities
liq.	liquid; a solution
LLQ	left, lower quadrant
LMP	last menstrual period
ltd.	limited
LUQ	left, upper quadrant
mcg, μg	microgram
MDI	metered dose inhaler
Med.	medical
mEq	milliequivalent
mg	milligram
MI	myocardial infarction
MIC	minimum inhibitory concentration
min	minute
mixt	mixture
mL, ml	milliliter
mo	month
MRI	magnetic resonance imaging
Mx. (m)	minim
n/c/o	no complaint of
neg.	negative
Neuro.	neurology
NG	nasogastric
noct.	night
non rep., NR	do not repeat
NPO	nothing by mouth
Nsg.	nursing
NSR	normal sinus rhythm
NSS	normal saline solution
N&V (N/V)	nausea and vomiting
OCP	oral contraceptive pills
OD	right eye
o.d. (q.d.)	daily
oint.	ointment
OPV	oral polio vaccine immunization
os	mouth
OS	left eye
OT	occupational therapy
OTC	over-the-counter
OU	each eye
oz	ounce
pc	after meals
PCA	patient-controlled analgesia
PCP	*Pneumocystis carinii* pneumonia
per	through *or* by
PERLA	pupils equal and reactive to light and accommodation
PERRLA	pupils equal, round, and reactive to light and accommodation
plt.	platelet
PM	afternoon, evening
PMH	past medical history
PO, p.o.	by mouth
PPD	purified protein derivative
ppm	parts per million
prn	when necessary
PT	physical therapy (or prothrombin time)
PTT	partial thromboplastin time
pulv.	a powder
q	every
q4h	every 4 hours
qd	every day
qh	every hour
qid	four times a day
qod	every other day
qs	quantity sufficient (up to a specified amount)
Ⓡ	right
RBC	red blood cell
RDA	recommended dietary allowance
re	that is; regarding; in reference to
REM	rapid eye movement
rep.	repeat; may refill
RLQ	right, lower quadrant
R/O	rule out
ROM	range of motion
RUQ	right, upper quadrant
℞	prescription
s, sec	second
$\bar{s}$	without
s&s	signs and symptoms
SC (SQ)	subcutaneously
sens.	sensitive
SG	specific gravity
SGOT	serum glutamic oxaloacetic transaminase
SGPT	serum glutamic pyruvic transaminase
sig.	give directions; label
sl, SL	under tongue; sublingual
sol.	solution
span.	spansule
$\overline{ss}$	half (one half)
STAT	immediate
STS	serologic test for syphilis
sub.q., SC	subcutaneous
suppos.	suppository
sx.	symptoms
syr.	syrup
t, tsp	teaspoon
T, tbsp	tablespoon
tab.	tablet
TB	tuberculosis
tet-tox.	tetanus toxoid
tid	three times daily
TM	tympanic membrane
TNTC	too numerous to count
TPN	total parenteral nutrition
TPR	temperature, pulse, respirations
tinc.	tincture
(Tr)	tincture
Tx.	treatment
u	unit
UA	urinalysis
UE	upper extremities

ung. ointment
ut dict, UD as directed
UTI urinary tract infection
URI upper respiratory infection
vag. vaginal
VD venereal disease
VLDL very–low-density lipoprotein
V.O. verbal order
V/S vital signs
WBC white blood cell
wk week
WNL within normal limits
w/o without
wt weight

B

Normal Laboratory Values and Pulmonary Function Tests

Representative Laboratory Values

The following table lists laboratory values according to traditional units and, whenever possible, according to the International System of Units. Readers are advised to determine the system used in their institution's laboratory before comparing values to those given in this chart. The values are often dependent on the method used and "normal values" may differ between laboratories.

Laboratory Test	*Traditional Units*	*International (SI*) Units*
ACTH, 8 AM, plasma	<80 pg/mL	<3.8 pmol per liter
Albumin, serum	3.5 g–5.5 g/100 mL	35 g–55 g per liter
Aldosterone, 8 AM (patient supine, 100 mEq Na and 60–100 mEq K intake)	1 ng–5 ng/dL	0.03 nmol–0.15 nmol per liter
Ammonia, urine	30 mEq–50 mEq in 24 h	30 mmol–50 mmol per day
Ammonia, whole blood venous	80 μg–110 μg/dL	47 μmol–65 μmol per liter
Amylase, serum	60–180 Somogyi units/dL 0.8 U–3.2 U/Liter	13 nmol–53 nmol per second per liter
Amylase, urine	35–260 Somogyi units per hour	
Arterial blood gases (sea level)		
Bicarbonate (HCO_3^-)	21 mEq–28 mEq per liter	21 mmol–28 mmol per liter
Carbon Dioxide (pCO_2)	35–45 mmHg	4.7 kPa–6.0 kPa
pH (arterial blood)	7.38–7.44	
Oxygen (pO_2)	80–100 mmHg	11 kPa–13 kPa
Oxygen saturation (S_aO_2)	95%–99%	
Base excess (BE)	0 ± 2 mEq/L	
Ascorbic acid, serum	0.4 mg–1.0 mg/dL	23 μmol–57 μmol
Ascorbic acid, leukocytes	25 mg–40 mg/dL	1420 μmol–2270 μmol per liter
Base, total, serum	145 mEq–155 mEq/L	145 mmol–155 mmol per liter
β (beta)-Hydroxybutyrate, plasma	<0.5 mmol/L	
Bilirubin, total, serum	0.3 mg–1.0 mg/dL	5.1 μmol–17 μmol per liter
Direct serum	0.1 mg–0.3 mg/dL	1.7 μmol–5.1 μmol per liter
Indirect serum	0.2 mg–0.7 mg/dL	3.4 μmol–12 μmol per liter
Bleeding time, (Ivy) 5-mm wound	1 min–9 min	
Bromides, serum toxic levels	>17 mEq/L	17 mmol per liter
Calcitonin, plasma	0–28 pg/mL	0–8.2 pmol per liter
Calcium, ionized	2.3 mEq–2.8 mEq/L 8.5 mg–10.5 mg/dL	2.2 mmol–2.7 mmol per liter
Calcium, urine	<7.5 mEq/24 h *or* <150 mg/24 h	<3.8 mmol per day
Carbon dioxide content, plasma (at sea level)	21 mEq–30 mEq/L *or* 50–70 volume %	21 mmol–30 mmol per liter
Carcinoembryonic antigen (CEA)	0 ng–2.5 ng/mL (healthy nonsmokers)	0 μg–2.5 μg per liter
Carotenoids, serum	50 μg–300 μg/dL	0.9 μmol–5.6 μmol per liter
Catecholamines, urinary excretion		
Free catecholamines	<100 μg per day	<590 nmol per day
Epinephrine	<50 μg per day	<295 nmol per day
Metanephrine	<1.3 mg per day	<6.2 μmol per day
Vanillylmandelic acid (VMA)	<8 mg per day	<40 μmol per day
Chloride, serum (Cl^-)	98 mEq–106 mEq/L	98 mmol–106 mmol per liter
Copper, serum	80 μg–140 μg/dL	12 μmol–24 μmol per liter

Laboratory Test	*Traditional Units*	*International (SI*) Units*
Cortisol		
8 AM	5 μg–24 μg/dL	140 nmol–662 nmol per liter
4 PM	3 μg–12 μg/dL	82 nmol–331 nmol per liter
Creatine phosphokinase, serum (CPK)	10 U–70 U/mL (women)	0.17 mmol–1.18 mmol per second per liter
	25 U–90 U/mL (men)	0.42 mmol–1.51 mmol per second per liter
Isoenzymes serum	Fraction 2 (MB) <5% total	
Creatinine, serum	0.6 mg–1.5 mg/dL	53 μmol–133 μmol per liter
Creatinine clearance, urine	91 mL–130 mL/min	1.5 mL–2.2 mL per second
Digoxin, serum		
Therapeutic level	1.2 ± 0.4 ng/mL	1.54 ± 0.5 nmol per liter
Toxic level	>2.4 ng/mL	>3.2 nmol per liter
Dilantin, plasma		
Therapeutic level	10 μg–20 μg/mL	40 μmol–79 μmol per liter
Toxic level	>30 μg/mL	>119 μmol per liter
Estradiol, plasma		
Women (higher at ovulation)	20 pg–60 pg/mL	0.07 nmol–0.22 nmol per liter
Men	<50 pg/mL	<0.18 nmol per liter
Ethanol, blood		
Mild to moderate intoxication	80 mg–200 mg/dL	17 mmol–43 mmol per liter
Marked intoxication	250 mg–400 mg/dL	54 mmol–87 mmol per liter
Severe intoxication	>400 mg/dL	>87 mmol per liter
Fatty acids, free (nonesterified), plasma	<0.7 mmol/L	
Ferritin, serum	15 ng–200 ng/mL	15 μg–200 μg per liter
Fibrinogen, plasma	160 mg–415 mg/dL	0.5 μmol–1.4 μmol per liter
Fibrinogen split products	titer 1:4 or less	
Folic acid, serum	6 ng–15 ng/mL	14 nmol–34 nmol per liter
Folic acid, red blood cell	150 ng–450 ng/mL of cells	340 nmol–1020 nmol per liter cells
Gastrin, serum	40 pg–200 pg/mL	40 ng–150 ng per liter
Globulins, serum	2.0 g–3.0 g/dL	20 g–30 g per liter
Glucagon, plasma	50 pg–200 pg/mL	14 pmol–56 pmol per liter
Glucose (fasting) plasma		
Normal	75 mg–105 mg/dL	4.2 mmol–5.8 mmol per liter
Diabetes mellitus	>140 mg/dL (on more than one occasion)	>7.8 mmol per liter
Glucose, 2-h postprandial, plasma		
Normal	<140 mg/dL	<7.8 mmol per liter
Impaired glucose tolerance	140 mg–200 mg/dL	7.8 mmol–11.1 mmol per liter
Diabetes mellitus	>200 mg/dL (on more than one occasion)	>11.1 per liter
Glucose, true, urine	50 mg–300 mg/24 h	0.3 mmol–1.7 mmol per day
Gonadotropins, plasma		
Women, mature, premenopausal (except during ovulation)		
FSH	5 mU–30 mU/mL	5 units–30 units per liter
LH	5 mU–25 mU/mL	5 units–25 units per liter
Women, ovulatory surge		
FSH	5 mU–20 mU/mL	5 units–20 units per liter
LH	15 mU–40 mU/mL	15 units–40 units per liter
Women, postmenopausal		
FSH	>40 mU/mL	>40 units per liter
LH	>40 mU/mL	>40 units per liter
Men, mature		
FSH	5 mU–20 mU/mL	5 units–20 units per liter
LH	5 mU–20 mU/mL	5 units–20 units per liter
Children, both sexes, prepubertal		
FSH	<5 mU/mL	<5 units per liter
LH	<5 mU/mL	<5 units per liter
Growth hormone (after 100 g glucose by mouth)	<5 ng/dL	<230 pmol per liter
Haptoglobin, serum	103 mg–153 mg/dL	1.3 ± 0.2 g per liter
Hemoglobin, blood		
Adult men	14 g–18 g/dL	8.7 mmol–11.2 mmol per liter
Adult women	12 g–16 g/dL	7.4 mmol–9.9 mmol per liter

Laboratory Test	*Traditional Units*	*International (SI*) Units*
Infant: Days 1–13	14.5 g–24.5 g/dL	
Days 14–60	11.3 g–17.3 g/dL	
Child: 3 months–10 years	9.9 g–14.5 g/dL	
11 years–15 years	13.4 g/dL	
Hemoglobin A	up to 6% of total hemoglobin	
Immunoglobulins, serum		
IgA	90 mg–325 mg/dL	0.9 g–3.2 g per liter
IgE	<0.025 mg/dL	<0.00025 g per liter
IgG	800 mg–1500 mg/dL	8.0 g–15 g per liter
IgM	45 mg–150 mg/dL	0.45 g–1.5 g per liter
Insulin, serum or plasma, fasting	6 μU–26 μU/mL	43 pmol–186 pmol per liter
Iron, serum (mean ± 1 SD)	105 ± 35 μg/dL	19 ± 6 μmol per liter
Iron binding capacity, serum (mean ± 1 SD)	305 ± 32 μg/dL	55 ± 6 μmol per liter
saturation	20%–45%	
Ketones, total, plasma	0.5 mg–1.5 mg/dL	5.0 mg–15.0 mg per liter
Ketones, total, urine	19.8 mg–81.2 mg/24 h	
Lactate dehydrogenase, serum	200 units–450 units/mL (Wrobleski) 60 units–100 units/mL (Wacker) 25 units–100 units/L	0.4 μmol–1.7 μmol per second per liter
Lactic acid, blood	<1.2 mmol/L	
Lead, serum	<20 μg/dL	<1.0 μmol per liter
Leukocytes, total	4,300–10,000 per mm³ (avg. 7,000)	
Neutrophils, juvenile and band	100–2,100 per mm³ (avg. 520)	
Neutrophils, segmented	1,100–6,050 per mm³ (avg. 3,000)	
Eosinophils	0–700 per mm³ (avg. 150)	
Basophils	0–150 per mm³ (avg. 30)	
Lymphocytes	1,500–4,000 per mm³ (avg. 2,500)	
Monocytes	200–950 per mm³ (avg. 430)	
Lipase, serum	1.5 units (Cherry Crandall)	
Lipids, total	400 mg–1000 mg/dL	
Total plasma cholesterol	150 mg–250 mg/dL	
Triglycerides	40 mg–150 mg/dL	
Phospholipids	150 mg–250 mg/dL	48 mmol–81 mmol per liter
Lithium, serum		
Therapeutic level	0.6 mEq–1.5 mEq/L	0.5 mmol–1.5 mmol per liter
Toxic level	>2.0 mEq/L	>2 mmol per liter
Magnesium, serum	1.5 mEq–2.5 mEq per liter 2 mg–3 mg/dL	0.8 mmol–1.3 mmol per liter
Nitrogen, nonprotein, serum	15 mg–35 mg/dL	0.15 g–0.35 g per liter
Oxygen content: (see also arterial blood gases)		
Arterial blood (sea level)	17–21 volume %	
Venous blood, arm (sea level)	10–16 volume %	
Oxytocin, plasma		
Men, preovulatory women	0.5 μU–2 μU/mL	0.5 mU–2 mU per liter
Ovulating women	2 μU–4 μU/mL	2 mU–4 mU per liter
Lactating women	5 μU–10 μU/mL	5 mU–10 mU per liter
Partial thromboplastin time (PTT)	(Standard) 68–82 seconds (Activated) 32–46 seconds	
Phosphatase, alkaline, serum	21–91 IU per liter at 37°C	0.4 μmol–1.5 μmol per second per liter
Phosphorus, inorganic, serum	3 mg–4.5 mg/dL	1.0 mmol–1.4 mmol per liter
Platelets (Brecher-Cronkite method)	150,000–440,000 per cubic mL	2.9 × 10¹¹ per liter
Potassium, serum	3.5 mEq–5.0 mEq/L	3.5 mmol–5.0 mmol per liter
Potassium, urine	25 mEq–100 mEq/24 h	25 mmol–100 mmol per day
Progesterone		
Men, prepubertal girls, postmenopausal women	<2 ng/mL	6 nmol per liter
Women, luteal, peak	>5 ng/mL	>16 nmol per liter
Prolactin, serum	2 ng–15 ng/mL	0.08 nmol–6.0 nmol/L
Protein, total, serum	5.5 g–8.0 g/dL	55 g–80 g per liter
Protein, urine	<150 mg/24 hr	<0.05 g per day

Laboratory Test	*Traditional Units*	*International (SI*) Units*
Protein fractions, serum (see albumin, globulin)		
Prothrombin time	11 seconds–15 seconds	
Quinidine, serum		
Therapeutic level	1.5 μg–3 μg/mL	4.6 μmol–9.2 μmol per liter
Toxic level	5 μg–6 μg/mL	15.4 μmol–18.5 μmol per liter
Reticulocytes	0.5%–2.0% of red blood cells	
Salicylate, plasma		
Therapeutic level	20 mg–25 mg/dL	1.4 mmol–1.8 mmol per liter
Toxic level	>30 mg/dL	>2.2 mmol per liter
Sedimentation rate (Westergren)		
Men	≤15 mm/h	
Women	≤20 mm/h	
Children	≤10 mm/h	
Sodium, serum	136 mEq–145 mEq/L	136 mmol–145 mmol per liter
Sodium, urine	100 mEq–260 mEq/24 h	100 mmol–260 mmol per day
Specific gravity, urine		
After 12-h fluid restriction	1.025 or more	
After 12-h deliberate water intake	1.003 or less	
Testosterone		
Women	<100 ng/dL	<3.5 nmol per liter
Men	300 ng–1000 ng/dL	105 nmol–350 nmol per liter
Prepubertal boys and girls	5 ng–20 ng/dL	0.175 nmol–0.702 nmol per liter
Thyroid function tests		
Radioactive iodine uptake 24 hr.	5%–30% (range varies in different areas of the thyroid owing to variable uptake)	
Reverse triiodothyronine (rT_3), serum	10 ng–40 ng/dL	0.128 nmol–0.512 nmol per liter
Thyroxine (T_4), serum radioimmunoassay	4 μg–12 μg/dL	50 nmol–154 nmol per liter
Triiodothyronine (T_3), serum radioimmunoassay	80 ng–100 ng/dL	1.2 nmol–1.5 nmol per liter
Thyroid-stimulating hormone (TSH)	<5 μU/mL	<5 mU per liter
Transaminase, serum glutamic oxaloacetic (AST)	10 to 40 Karmen units/mL 6 units–18 units/L	0.10 μmol–0.30 μmol per second per liter
Transaminase, serum glutamic pyruvic (ALT)	10 to 40 Karmen units/mL 3 units–26 units/L	0.05 μmol–0.43 μmol per second per liter
Urea nitrogen, whole blood (BUN)	10 mg–20 mg/dL	3.6 mmol–7.1 mmol per liter
Uric acid, serum		
Men	2.5 mg–8.0 mg/dL	0.15 mmol–0.48 mmol per liter
Women	1.5 mg–6.0 mg/dL	0.09 mmol–0.36 mmol per liter
Vitamin A, serum	20 μg–100 μg/dL	0.7 μmol–3.5 μmol per liter
Vitamin B_{12}, serum	200 pg–600 pg/mL	148 pmol–443 pmol per liter
White blood cells (see leukocytes)		
Zinc, serum	100 μg–140 μg/dL	15 μmol–21 μmol per liter

* From the French name, Système International d'Unités.

Pulmonary Function Tests

The following table lists values for pulmonary function tests. Normal values are listed for men and women.

	Normal Values	
Test Name (symbol)	*Men*	*Women*
Spirometry		
Forced vital capacity (FVC)	≥4.0 L	≥3.0 L
Forced expiratory volume in 1 second (FEV)	>3.0 L	>2.0 L
FEV/FVC (FEV, %)	>60%	>70%
Lung volumes		
Total lung capacity (TLC)	6 L–7 L	5 L–6 L
Functional residual capacity (FRC)	2 L–3 L	2 L–3 L
Residual volume (RV)	1 L–2 L	1 L–2 L
Inspiratory capacity (IC)	2 L–4 L	2 L–4 L
Expiratory reserve volume (ERV)	1 L–2 L	1 L–2 L
Vital capacity (VC)	4 L–5 L	3 L–4 L

C
FDA Pregnancy Categories

Category	***Description***
A	No demonstrated fetal risk in humans during any stage of pregnancy
B	No demonstrated fetal risk in animal studies but no adequate studies in pregnant women *or* Animal studies have shown an adverse effect but studies in pregnant women have not demonstrated a risk during any stage of pregnancy
C	Animal studies have shown an adverse effect on the fetus but there are no adequate studies in humans *or* No animal or human studies are available (use of the drug *may be acceptable* despite the risks)
D	Evidence of human fetal risk *but* the benefits from use of the drug *may be acceptable* despite the risks
X	Animal or human studies have demonstrated fetal abnormalities or adverse reaction reports give evidence of fetal risk (risk to a pregnant woman clearly outweighs the possible benefit)

D
Drug Compatibility Guide

The following table presents a compilation of drug compatibility information obtained from several sources. It is intended to be used as a general guide to drug compatibilities rather than as a definitive information source, inasmuch as the compatibility of two or more drugs in solution depends on a number of variables, such as the solution itself, the concentration of drugs present, and the method of mixing (bottle, syringe, or Y-site).

Drugs reported to be compatible in solution are indicated by Y in the table, and drugs documented to be incompatible as reflected by the development of cloudiness, turbidity, or precipitation within the solution are indicated by an N. Where no information was found on the compatibility of two drugs, the corresponding space was left blank.

For some drug combinations, conflicting information was obtained about compatibility, especially where different parameters were used in obtaining the data. In such cases, a conservative approach was followed, and the combination was indicated as not compatible in the table, although compatibility may depend on solution strength, vehicle, time after mixing before used, or any number of other factors.

Before mixing any drugs, it is imperative that healthcare personnel ascertain if a potential incompatibility problem exists by referring to an appropriate information source or by contacting the pharmacist. The accompanying table is intended solely to provide a handy guide from which one can quickly obtain a general idea of drug solution compatibility.

	aminophylline	amphotericin B	ampicillin	atropine	calcium gluconate	carbenicillin	cefazolin	cimetidine	clindamycin	diazepam	dopamine	epinephrine	erythromycin	fentanyl	furosemide	gentamicin	glycopyrrolate	heparin sodium	hydrocortisone	hydroxyzine	levarterenol	lidocaine	meperidine	morphine	nitroglycerin	pentobarbital	potassium chloride	sodium bicarbonate	tetracycline	vancomycin	verapamil	vitamin B & C complex
aminophylline	•		Y		Y	N	N		N	Y	Y	N	N					Y	Y	N	N	Y	N	N	Y	Y	Y	Y	N	N	Y	N
amphotericin B		•	N		N	N		N			N					N		Y	Y			N					N	Y	N		N	
ampicillin	Y	N	•	N	N	Y	Y		N		N		N			N		Y	N			Y					Y		N		Y	Y
atropine			N	•				Y		N		N		Y			Y	N		Y	N		Y	Y		N	Y	N			Y	Y
calcium gluconate	Y	N	N		•		N		N		Y	N	Y					Y	Y		Y	Y					Y	N	N	Y	Y	Y
carbenicillin	N	N	Y			•		Y	Y		Y	N	N			N			Y		N	Y					Y		N		Y	N
cefazolin	N		Y		N		•	N		Y			N			N			Y		N	N				N	Y		N		Y	Y
cimetidine		N		Y		Y	N	•	Y			Y	Y		Y	Y		Y			Y	Y				N	Y		Y	Y	Y	Y
clindamycin	N		N		N	Y		Y	•							Y		Y	Y							N	Y	Y			Y	Y
diazepam	Y			N			Y			•		N			N		N	N		N	N	N	N	N		N	N	N			Y	N
dopamine	Y	N	N		Y	Y					•					N		Y	Y			Y			Y		Y		Y		Y	Y
epinephrine	N			N	N	N		Y		N		•	N		N			Y			N	N	Y				N	N			Y	Y
erythromycin	N		N		Y	N	N	Y				N	•					N	Y			Y				N	Y	Y	N	Y	Y	N
fentanyl				Y										•						Y			Y	Y		N						
furosemide								Y		N		N			•	N		Y			N				Y		Y		N		Y	Y
gentamicin		N	N			N	N		Y		Y				N	•		N													Y	Y
glycopyrrolate				Y						N							•			Y		Y	Y	Y		N		N				
heparin sodium	Y	Y	Y	N	Y			Y	Y	N	Y	Y	N		Y	N		•	N	N	Y	Y	N	N			Y	Y	N	N	Y	Y
hydrocortisone	Y	Y	N		Y	Y	Y		Y		Y		Y					N	•		Y	Y				N	Y	Y	N	Y	Y	Y
hydroxyzine	N			Y						N				Y			Y	N		•		Y	Y	Y		N						N
levarterenol	N			N	Y	N	N	Y		N		N			N			Y	Y		•					N	Y		Y		Y	Y
lidocaine	Y	N	Y		Y	Y	N	Y		N	Y	N	Y				Y	Y	Y	Y		•			Y	Y	Y	Y	Y		Y	Y
meperidine	N			Y						N		Y		Y			Y	N		Y			•	N		N		N			Y	
morphine	N			Y						N				Y			Y	N		Y			N	•		N	Y	N			Y	Y
nitroglycerin	Y										Y				Y							Y			•						Y	
pentobarbital	Y			N			N	N	N	N			N	N			N		N	N	N	Y	N	N		•		N	N	N	Y	
potassium chloride	Y	N	Y	Y	Y	Y	Y	Y	Y	N	Y	N	Y		Y			Y	Y		Y	Y		Y			Y	Y	Y	Y	Y	
sodium bicarbonate	Y	Y		N	N				Y	N		N	Y				N	Y	Y			Y	N	N		N	Y	•	N	N	Y	N
tetracycline	N	N	N		N	N	N	Y			Y		N		N			N	N		Y	Y				N	Y	N	•			Y
vancomycin	N				Y			Y					Y					N	Y							N	Y	N		•	Y	Y
verapamil	Y	N	Y	Y	Y	Y	Y	Y	Y	Y	Y	Y	Y		Y	Y		Y	Y		Y	Y	Y	Y	Y	Y	Y	Y		Y	•	Y
vitamin B & C complex	N		Y	Y	Y	N	Y	Y	Y	N	Y	Y	N		Y	Y		Y	Y	N	Y	Y		Y				N	Y	Y	Y	•

E

General Bibliography

Pharmacology and Nursing

American Drug Index (yearly). Philadelphia, JB Lippincott, 1995

Annual Review of Pharmacology and Toxicology. Palo Alto, CA, Annual Reviews (yearly)

Cooper JR, Bloom FE: The Biochemical Basis of Neuropharmacology, 6th ed. New York, Oxford University press, 1991

Craig CR, Stitzel RE (eds): Modern Pharmacology, 4th ed. Boston, Little, Brown & Co, 1994

Drug Information for the Health Care Professional, 15th ed. Rockville, Md, United States Pharmacopeial Convention, 1995

Facts and Comparisons—Drug Information. Philadelphia, JB Lippincott (updated monthly)

Gilman AG, Goodman LS, Rall TW, Murad F (eds): The Pharmacological Basis of Therapeutics, 9th ed. New York, Macmillan, 1995

Handbook of Nonprescription Drugs, 10th ed. Washington, DC, American Pharmaceutical Association, 1993

Katzung BC (ed): Basic and Clinical Pharmacology, 5th ed. Los Altos, CA, Appleton & Lange, 1992

The Medical Letter on Drugs and Therapeutics. New Rochelle, NY, Medical Letter (biweekly)

Physiology

Fox SI: Human Physiology, 4th ed. Dubuque, IA, WC Brown, 1993

Ganong WF: Review of Medical Physiology, 16th ed., Norwalk, CT, Appleton & Lange, 1993

Guyton AC: Human Physiology and Mechanisms of Disease, 5th ed. Philadelphia, WB Saunders, 1992

Rhoades R, Pflanzer R: Human Physiology, 2nd ed. Philadelphia, WB Saunders, 1992

Roitt I: Essential Immunology, 8th ed. Oxford, Blackwell Scientific Publications, 1994

Sherwood L: Human Physiology: From Cells to Systems, 2nd ed. St. Paul, MN, West Publishing Co., 1993

Tortora GS, Grabowski SR: Principles of Anatomy and Physiology, 7th ed. New York, HarperCollins, 1993

Index

Note: Page numbers followed by f indicate figures; page numbers followed by t indicate tables.

B

C

D

E

G

H

I

J

K

L

M

N

O

P

Q

R

T

U

V

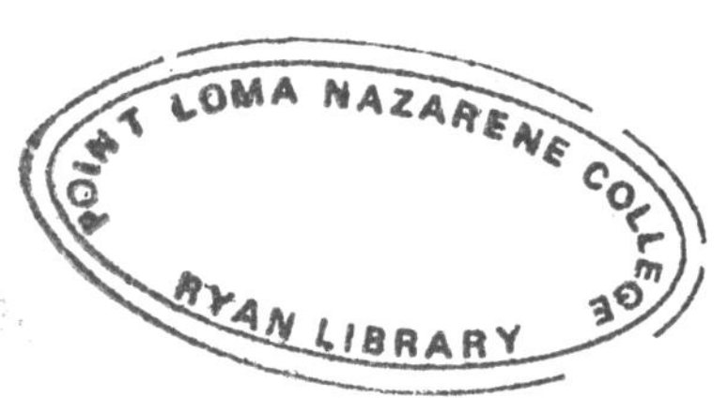

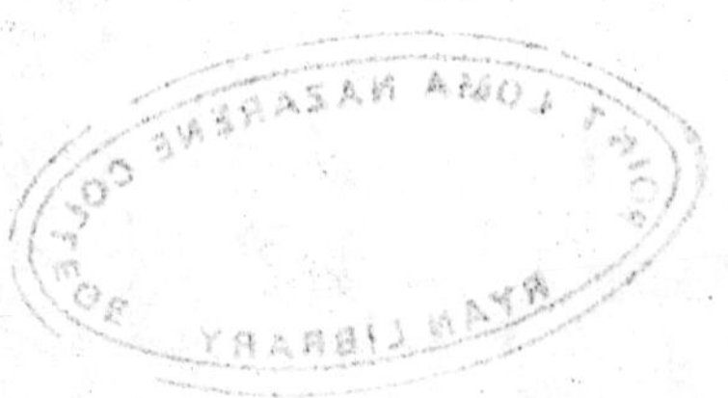